MOSBY'S
Comprehensive Review of
DENTAL
HYGIENE

MOSBY'S
Comprehensive Review of
DENTAL
HYGIENE

SEVENTH edition

MICHELE LEONARDI DARBY, BSDH, MS

Eminent Scholar, University Professor, Chair
Gene W. Hirschfeld School of Dental Hygiene
Old Dominion University
Norfolk, Virginia

3251 Riverport Lane
St. Louis, Missouri 63043

Notices

Knowledge and best practice in this field are constantly changing. As new research and experience broaden our understanding, changes in research methods, professional practices, or medical treatment may become necessary.

Practitioners and researchers must always rely on their own experience and knowledge in evaluating and using any information, methods, compounds, or experiments described herein. In using such information or methods they should be mindful of their own safety and the safety of others, including parties for whom they have a professional responsibility.

With respect to any drug or pharmaceutical products identified, readers are advised to check the most current information provided (i) on procedures featured or (ii) by the manufacturer of each product to be administered, to verify the recommended dose or formula, the method and duration of administration, and contraindications. It is the responsibility of practitioners, relying on their own experience and knowledge of their patients, to make diagnoses, to determine dosages and the best treatment for each individual patient, and to take all appropriate safety precautions.

To the fullest extent of the law, neither the Publisher nor the authors, contributors, or editors, assume any liability for any injury and/or damage to persons or property as a matter of products liability, negligence or otherwise, or from any use or operation of any methods, products, instructions, or ideas contained in the material herein.

Library of Congress Cataloging-in-Publication Data or Control Number
Mosby's comprehensive review of dental hygiene / [edited by] Michele Darby.—7th ed.
    p. ; cm.
  Comprehensive review of dental hygiene
  Includes bibliographical references and index.
  ISBN 978-0-323-07963-1 (pbk. : alk. paper)
  1. Dental hygiene.   2. Dental hygiene—Examinations, questions, etc.   I. Darby, Michele Leonardi,
1949–   II. Title: Comprehensive review of dental hygiene.
  [DNLM: 1. Dental Prophylaxis—Examination Questions.   2. Dental Prophylaxis—Outlines.
WU 18.2]
  RK60.7.M67 2012
  617.6'01076—dc22
                                                              2011014560

Publisher: Linda Duncan
Acquisitions Editor: Kristin Hebberd
Developmental Editor: Joslyn Dumas
Publishing Services Manager: Catherine Jackson
Project Manager: Sara Alsup
Design Direction: Teresa McBryan

Printed in the United States of America

Last digit is the print number: 9 8 7 6 5 4 3

To my husband, Dennis,
and our children, Devan and Blake,
for the joy and peace they bring me.

M.L.D.

CONTRIBUTORS

Stephen C. Bayne, MS, PhD, FADM
Professor and Chair
Cariology, Restorative Sciences, and Endodontics
University of Michigan
School of Dentistry
Ann Arbor, Michigan

Christine French Beatty, PhD
Professor
Department of Dental Hygiene
Texas Woman's University
P.O. Box 425796
Denton, Texas

Christine M Blue, RDH, MS
Director and Assistant Professor
Primary Dental Care
School Of Dentistry
University of Minnesota
Minneapolis, Minnesota

Denise M. Bowen, RDH, BS, MS
Professor Emeritus
Department of Dental Hygiene
Idaho State University
Pocatello, Idaho

Kristin Hamman Calley, BSDH, MS
Associate Professor
Department of Dental Hygiene
Division of Graduate Studies
Idaho State University
Pocatello, Idaho

Irene Connolly, BSDH, MS
Adjunct Assistant Professor
Gene W. Hirschfeld School of Dental Hygiene
Old Dominion University
Norfolk, Virginia

Barbara Leatherman Dixon, RDH, BS, MEd
Vice President (2004–2010)
WREB, A National Dental and Dental Hygiene
    Testing Agency
Phoenix, Arizona
Commissioner (2006–2010)
Joint Commission National Dental Examination
Chicago, IL

JoAnn R. Gurenlian, RDH, PhD
President and CEO
Gurenlian & Associates
Haddonfield, New Jersey

Lisa F. Harper Mallonee, BSDH, MPH, RD, LD
Associate Professor
Department of Dental Hygiene
Texas A&M Health Science Center
Baylor College of Dentistry
Dallas, Texas

Elena Bablenis Haveles, BS, Pharm.D.
Adjunct Associate Professor of Pharmacology
Gene W. Hirschfeld School of Dental Hygiene
College of Health Sciences
Old Dominion University
Norfolk, Virginia

Gwen L. Hlava, RDH, MS
Professor and Chair
Department of Dental Hygiene
University of Nebraska Medical Center
College of Dentistry
Lincoln, Nebraska

Olga A. C. Ibsen, RDH, BS, MS
Adjunct Professor
Department of Oral and Maxillofacial Pathology,
    Radiology, and Medicine
New York University
College of Dentistry
New York, New York
Adjunct Professor
Department of Dental Hygiene
University of Bridgeport
Bridgeport, Connecticut

Todd N. Junge, RDH, BS
Assistant Professor
Department of Dental Hygiene
University of Nebraska Medical Center
College of Dentistry
Lincoln, Nebraska

Jill S. Nield-Gehrig, RDH,MA
Dean Emeritus
Division of Allied Health & Public Service Education
Asheville-Buncombe Technical Community College
Asheville, North Carolina

Darnyl Palmer, RDH, BA, MS
Clinical Instructor
Department of Dental Hygiene
Georgia Perimeter College
Dunwoody, Georgia

Jessica C. Peek, BSDH, MS
Department of Dental Ecology
School of Dentistry
University of North Carolina at Chapel Hill
Chapel Hill, North Carolina

John M. Powers, PhD
Professor of Oral Biomaterials
Department of Restorative Dentistry and Biomaterials
University of Texas Dental Branch at Houston
Houtson, Texas
Senior Vice President
Dental Consultants
Ann Arbor, Michigan

Maureen Savner, RDH, MS
Associate Professor, Clinical Coordinator
Department of Dental Health
Luzerne County Community College
Nanticoke, Pennsylvania

Heidi Schlei, BSDH, MS, EMT
Instructor
Department of Allied Health
Waukesha County Technical College
Pewaukee, Wisconsin

M. Anjum Shah, BSDH, RDH, MS
Assistant Professor
Division of Dental Hygiene
Virginia Commonwealth University
School of Dentistry
Richmond, Virginia

Rebecca Sroda, CDA, RDH, MA
Associate Dean of Allied Health
Director of Dental Education
Southern Florida Community College
Avon Park, Florida

Edward J. Swift, Jr., DMD, MS
Professor and Chair
Department of Operative Dentistry
University of North Carolina
Chapel Hill, North Carolina

Evelyn M. Thomson, BSDH, MS
Adjunct Assistant Professor
Gene W. Hirschfield School of Dental Hygiene
Old Dominion Univerisity
Norfolk, Virginia

Jeffrey Y. Thompson, PhD
Professor
Department of Prosthodontics
College of Dental Medicine
Nova Southeastern University
Ft. Lauderdale, Florida

Lynn Tolle, BSDH, MS
Professor and Director of Clinics
Gene W. Hirschfeld of Dental Hygiene
Old Dominion University
Norfolk, Virginia

Pamela Zarkowski, JD, MPH
Vice President for Academic Affairs and Professor
University of Detroit Mercy
Detroit, Michigan

Meg Zayan, RDH, MPH, EdD
Dean and Associate Professor
Fones School of Dental Hygiene
Division of Health Sciences
University of Bridgeport
Bridgeport, Connecticut

PREFACE

The success of earlier editions of *Mosby's Comprehensive Review of Dental Hygiene*, the plethora of new knowledge from rigorous research, and the need for evidence-based education and practice serve as the prime forces guiding the development of the seventh edition. Publishing a book that comprehensively reviews the foundation for dental hygiene competencies is a challenge. Demographic, societal, and educational trends, issues surrounding access to care for all citizens, and new healthcare delivery and finance systems require successful dental hygienists to possess competence in the biological, social, behavioral, and dental hygiene sciences, and in general education. The book and the accompanying Evolve website offer a complete learning package to:

- assist individuals in reviewing the theory, skills, and judgments required on national, regional, and state dental hygiene board examinations;
- prepare dental hygienists for reentry into professional dental hygiene roles—clinician, educator, advocate, researcher, and administrator/manager;
- provide educators with salient information used for course and curriculum development and outcomes assessment.

"CLIENT" VS. "PATIENT"

Throughout the book, "client" (instead of "patient") is used predominantly because the term is congruent with the profession's disease prevention, health promotion, and wellness focus. Most important, the term "client" conveys dental hygiene's partnership with consumers and communities inclusive of individuals, families, and target groups who are fast becoming the focus of community-based dental hygiene practice. Both the American Dental Hygienists' Association and the Canadian Dental Hygienists' Association have embraced the term "client" in their policies and actions. When the client is debilitated by disease or disability, the term "patient" is used.

A special effort was made to design testlets for the community oral health content and case-based questions that include client health; dental, pharmacologic, and cultural history; and dental charts, radiographs, and photographs. Other multiple-choice test items mimic the various types used on the actual National Board Dental Hygiene Examination.

ORGANIZATION

The seventh edition of *Mosby's Comprehensive Review of Dental Hygiene* is divided into 22 independent, interrelated chapters. Chapter 1 provides guidance and confidence-boosting recommendations for anyone preparing for a board examination. Emphasis is on understanding board examinations, test-taking strategies, and trends in standardized board examinations. Given the global economy, basic information on licensure/practice requirements for dental hygienists interested in international employment is also included. Chapters 2 to 22 cover subject areas found on the National Board Dental Hygiene Examination and contain theoretical and applied information in an outline format. End-of-chapter review questions, with rationales on Evolve, explain why the correct answer is appropriate and why each incorrect choice is wrong. The rationales for the correct and incorrect answers provide an additional strategy for efficient board preparation. This information enables the reviewer to assess both decision making and judgment in integrating professional knowledge, and facilitates mastery of each chapter's content, further increasing the likelihood of success on examination day.

Internet links and a comprehensive index that enables users to locate information quickly and easily are included. Illustrations and the appendices minimize the need to search alternative sources; however, reference lists and website resources are provided for those who desire more in-depth study or enrichment.

SIMULATED NATIONAL BOARD DENTAL HYGIENE EXAMINATIONS/ ELECTRONIC RESOURCES

Resources for Students

This edition includes four Simulated National Board Dental Hygiene Examinations with rationales for correct and incorrect answers. One examination is at the end of the book and three more interactive examinations are found on the text's Evolve website. Answers for all four examinations are provided on the Evolve site. Paralleling the National Board Dental Hygiene Examination in content, length, and question format, these tests permit the student to experience the reality of a board examination in four separate practice opportunities in hard copy and computerized format. We have even included a clock on the Evolve site so students can take the examination with real-time guidelines.

The examinations will improve students' test-taking abilities, identify areas of weakness, and explain, via the rationales, gaps in each individual's knowledge base. By first identifying specific areas for study and then systematically reviewing the comprehensive information provided in the logical outline, the student will feel confidently prepared for the board examination.

Resources for Faculty

Providing four Simulated National Board Dental Hygiene Examinations in different formats will thoroughly test your students at all levels. The examination at the back of the book is also on the Evolve site. There, you have the ability to scramble the questions or quiz students using excerpts of the full examination. The Evolve site also allows faculty to publish class syllabi and lecture notes, set up virtual office hours and email communication, and encourage student responsibility through chat rooms and discussion boards. This service is available for WebCT, Blackboard, and Angel systems with qualified adoptions.

Both students and faculty have access to additional resources on Evolve; see the inside front cover for a complete listing.

ACKNOWLEDGMENTS

I would like to express my sincere appreciation to those who helped make this edition of *Mosby's Comprehensive Review of Dental Hygiene* a reality. Detailed outlines, board questions, answers, and rationales were developed by renowned experts identified in the table of contents. Comments and suggestions from students, faculty, and returning dental hygienists who have used the book are embodied in this edition. The exemplary work of these contributors has made *Mosby's Comprehensive Review of Dental Hygiene* a board-preparation experience that is second to none.

My special thanks go to John Dolan, Executive Editor; Kristin Hebberd, Managing Editor; Joslyn Dumas, Developmental Editor, and Sara Alsup, Project Manager, who facilitated the many steps of the publication process at Elsevier.

Also acknowledged are the authors, corporations, and publishers who granted permission to use quotes, concepts, photographs, figures, and tables.

Since the work of those who contributed to the earlier editions remains central to this revision, I want to gratefully acknowledge their efforts, particularly the work of Dr. Eleanor Bushee and Linda E. DeVore, whose competence and good humor as oral health professionals, teachers, administrators, colleagues, and friends will forever be missed, and Marilyn Beck, Dr. Marcia Brand, Patricia Regener Campbell, Karen Caspers, Marie A. Collins, Patricia Damon-Johnson, Judith A. Davidson, Dr. Catherine C. Davis, Mary-Catherine Dean, Susann Duncan, Diane M. Frazier, Jacquelyn L. Fried, Barbara Heckman, Jan Shaner Greenlee, Charlotte Hangorsky, Kara Hansen, Beverly Entwistle Isman, Dr. Donald E. Isselhard, Sandra Kramer, Mary M. Lee, Shirley Kuhn, Kathy Macciocca, Sally Mauriello, Susan Schwartz Miller, Cara Miyasaki, Lynn Ray, Dr. Marlene Moss-Klyvert, Dr. Peggy Reep, Dr. Lindsay Rettie, Danielle Leigh Ryan, Michelle Sensat, Dr. Lynn Utecht, Venkat Varkala, Nancy Webb, K. Cy Whaley, and Susan Zimmer. Without the earlier contributions of these talented people, the current edition of *Mosby's Comprehensive Review of Dental Hygiene* would not be possible.

— **Michele Leonardi Darby**

TABLE OF CONTENTS

Preparing for National, Regional, and State Dental Hygiene Board Examinations

Barbara Leatherman Dixon

Preparing for board examinations requires deliberate planning, study and review, time management, organization of information and schedules for applications, and a positive "can-do" attitude. Conscientious dental hygienists will organize a plan for success well in advance and be prepared to satisfy board requirements with confidence in their professional knowledge and skills. This book is a guide through the evidence-based knowledge on which dental hygiene practice is based. Systematic use of this book enables one to reinforce professional education, integrate concepts and ideas from many dental hygiene educators, and identify subject areas where additional study is warranted.

The introductory chapter is a primer in navigating the licensure system—whether a new graduate, a practicing dental hygienist who is moving to another licensing jurisdiction, or a dental hygienist returning to practice after a lapse of activity—to prepare for both didactic and clinical board examinations. A dental hygienist must master all subject matter and skills necessary for practice; therefore, each chapter focuses on different aspects of such knowledge and skills. However, success on board examinations also relies on being psychologically, emotionally, and physically prepared to demonstrate competence. It is essential to become thoroughly familiar with the format, logistics, and requirements of any preparatory examination for licensure.

This chapter discusses licensure structure and explains how it functions with the interaction of numerous agencies and organizations. Information on the National Board Dental Hygiene Examination (NBDHE) as well as a discourse on clinical board examinations is provided. The chapter concludes with an overview of this review book, including its purpose and organization, as well as instructions on how to use the text effectively.

DENTAL HYGIENE LICENSURE

In the United States, licensure is under the authority of an individual state or jurisdiction. Licensure of dental hygienists is a means of regulation to protect the public from unqualified individuals and unsafe practice of the profession. Each state has a *state practice act* that defines the practice of dental hygiene, establishes educational and testing requirements for licensure, sets parameters for enforcement of the law within that jurisdiction, and creates a state board of dentistry or dental hygiene to serve in accordance with the statute. A certificate for successful completion of an examination is *not* authorization to practice. Beginning practice without a license is illegal. Dental hygiene licensure requirements vary from state to state, but nearly every state has three requirements:

- Graduation from a dental hygiene program accredited by the Commission on Dental Accreditation (CODA) or, based on reciprocity, by the Commission on Dental Accreditation of Canada (CDAC)
- Successful completion of the NBDHE
- Successful completion of a regional or state clinical board examination

It should be noted that recognition of an accrediting agency is a governmental function. In health care fields with a domain of specialized education, accreditation is conducted by a dedicated agency within the profession. In dentistry, the U.S. Department of Education (USDE) has recognized the CODA of the American Dental Association (ADA) as the official accrediting body for schools of dentistry, dental hygiene, dental assisting, and dental laboratory technology. The CODA is also listed in the publications of accreditation agencies by the Council for Higher Education Accreditation (CHEA). A diploma, certificate, associate's degree, or baccalaureate degree in dental hygiene indicating graduation from an accredited program is an essential

---

BOX 1-1 Membership in the Five Regional Testing Agencies in the United States

CITA
Alabama
Louisiana
Mississippi
North Carolina
West Virginia
Puerto Rico

CRDTS
Colorado
Georgia
Hawaii
Illinois
Iowa
Kansas
Minnesota
Missouri
Nebraska
North Dakota
South Carolina
South Dakota
Washington
West Virginia
Wisconsin
Wyoming

NERB
Connecticut
District of Columbia
Illinois
Indiana
Maine
Maryland
Massachusetts
Michigan

New Hampshire
New Jersey
New York
Ohio
Oregon
Pennsylvania
Rhode Island
Vermont
West Virginia
Wisconsin

SRTA
Arkansas
Kentucky
South Carolina
Tennessee
Virginia
West Virginia

WREB
Alaska
Arizona
California
Idaho
Kansas
Missouri
Montana
New Mexico
North Dakota
Oklahoma
Oregon
Texas
Utah
Washington
Wyoming

CITA, *Council of Interstate Testing Agencies;* CRDTS, *Central Regional Dental Testing Service, Inc.;* NERB, *Northeast Regional Board of Dental Examiners, Inc.;* SRTA, *Southern Regional Testing Agency, Inc.;* WREB, *WREB: A National Dental and Dental Hygiene Testing Agency.*

---

component for licensure that is based on the accreditation system carried out under the auspices of the CODA. States that provide for licensure of a dentist or dental hygienist from a nonaccredited school generally require evidence of an educational program that is equivalent to an accredited program. The NBDHE is developed and administered by the Joint Commission on National Dental Examinations (JCNDE). Client-based clinical examinations are conducted by five regional testing agencies (Boxes 1-1 and 1-2). The licensure boards of California, Delaware, Florida, and the Virgin Islands of the United States administer independent examinations. Nevada, administers the American Dental Hygiene Licensing Examination (ADHLEX). Clinical examinations accepted for initial licensure are shown in Figure 1-1.

A license is applicable only within the geographic boundaries of the issuing state. However, most states have some provision for granting dental hygiene licensure by credentials or endorsement. Requirements generally include an active license in good standing, recent practice experience, successful completion of the NBDHE, successful completion of a clinical examination, and graduation from an accredited program. Specifics differ from state to state and are subject to change. For example, some states accept NBDHE scores only if earned within the last 5 to 10 years, or limit recognition of clinical board examination results to those from particular testing agencies.

Applicants for dental hygiene licensure must contact the state licensing board for current requirements and procedures (Box 1-3).

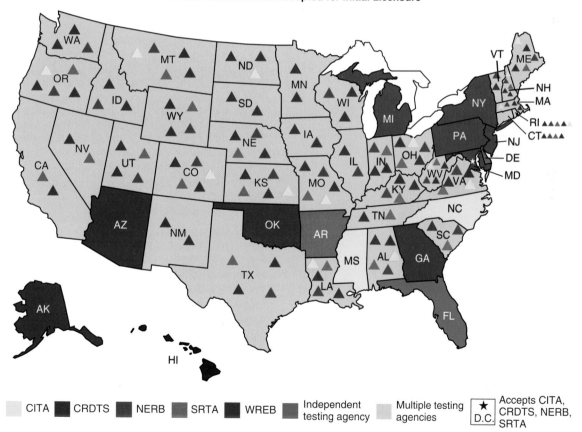

Clinical Examinationa Accepted for Initial Licensure

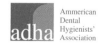

Please note that recognizing jurisdictions and licensing requirements are subject to change. While this document is updated yearly, candidates are encouraged to contact the State Board where they wish to seek licensure to confirm information.

Information is based upon individual calls to the respective State Boards of Dentistry.

ADHA defines Initial Licensure as state licensure sought immediately following graduation from an accredited dental hygiene program.

FIGURE 1-1 Clinical examinations accepted for licensure. (*From the American Dental Hygienists' Association.*)

BOX 1-3 State Boards, Regional Testing Agency Membership,* and Contact Information†

Alabama (CITA)*
State Board of Dental Examiners of Alabama
5346 Stadium Trace Parkway, Suite 112
Hoover, AL 35244
Phone: 205-955-7267
Fax: 205-985-0674
www.dentalboard.org

Alaska (WREB)
Alaska State Board of Dental Examiners
Division of Occupational Licensing
P.O. Box 110806
Juneau, AK 99811-0806
Phone: 907-465-2542
Fax: 907-465-2974
www.dced.state.ak.us/occ/

Arizona (WREB)
Arizona State Board of Dental Examiners
5060 N. 19th Avenue, #406
Phoenix, AZ 85015
Phone: 602-242-1492
Fax: 602-242-1445
www.azdentalboard.org

Arkansas (SRTA)
Arkansas State Board of Dental Examiners
101 East Capitol, Suite 111
Little Rock, AR 72201
Phone: 501-682-2085
Fax: 501-682-3543
www.asbde.org

California (WREB)
Dental Hygiene Committee of California
2005 Evergreen Street, Suite 1050
Sacramento, CA 95815
Phone: 916-263-1978
Fax: 916-263-2688
www.dhcc.ca.gov/index.shtml

Colorado (CRDTS)
Colorado State Board of Dental Examiners
1560 Broadway, Suite 1350
Denver, CO 80202
Phone: 303-894-7800
Fax: 303-894-7764
www.dora.state.co.us/dental

Connecticut (NERB)
Connecticut State Dental Commission
Department of Public Health
410 Capitol Avenue
Hartford, CT 06134-0308
Phone: 860-509-7553
Fax: 860-509-8457
www.state.ct.us/dph

Delaware
Delaware State Board of Dental Examiners
861 Silver Lake Boulevard
Cannon Building, Suite 203
Dover, DE 19903

Phone: 302-744-4533
Fax: 302-739-2711
http://dpr.delaware.gov/boards/dental/index.shtml

District of Columbia (NERB)
District of Columbia Board of Dentistry
Department of Health
717 14th Street NW, Suite 600
Washington, DC 20002
Phone: 202-724-8745
Fax: 202-727-8471
http://dchealth.dc.gov/prof_license/services/boards_main_action.asp?strappid=5

Florida
Florida Board of Dentistry
4052 Bald Cypress Way
Bin C08
Tallahassee, FL 32399-3258
Phone: 850-245-4474
Fax: 850-921-5389
www.doh.state.fl.us/mqa

Georgia (CRDTS)
Georgia Board of Dentistry
237 Coliseum Drive
Macon, GA 31217-3858
Phone: 478-207-2440
Fax: 866-888-1308
www.sos.state.ga.us/plb/dentistry

Hawaii (CRDTS)
Hawaii State Board of Dental Examiners
Department of Commerce and Consumer Affairs
P.O. Box 3469
Honolulu, HI 96801
Phone: 808-586-2702
Fax: 808-586-2689
http://hawaii.gov/dcca/areas/pvl/

Idaho (WREB)
Idaho State Board of Dentistry
P.O. Box 83720
Boise, ID 83720-0021
Phone: 208-334-2369
Fax: 208-334-3247
www.idaho.gov/isbd

Illinois (NERB, CRDTS)
Illinois State Board of Dentistry
Department of Professional Regulation and Education
320 W. Washington, 3rd Floor
Springfield, IL 62786
Phone: 217-785-0800
Fax: 217-782-7645
www.idfpr.com/dpr/WHO/dent.asp

Indiana (NERB)
Indiana State Board of Dental Examiners
Indiana Professional Licensing Agency
402 W. Washington, Room W 072
Indianapolis, IN 46204

BOX 1-3 State Boards, Regional Testing Agency Membership,* and Contact Information†—cont'd

Phone: 317-234-2054
Fax: 317-233-4236
www.in.gov/pla/dental.htm

Iowa (CRDTS)
Iowa Dental Board
400 S.W. 8th Street, Suite D
Des Moines, IA 50309-4687
Phone: 515-281-5157
Fax: 515-281-7969
www.dentalboard.iowa.gov

Kansas (CRDTS, WREB)
Kansas Dental Board
900 SW Jackson Street, Suite 564-S
Topeka, KS 66612-1230
Phone: 785-296-6400
Fax: 785-296-3116
www.accesskansas.org/kdb

Kentucky (SRTA)
Kentucky Board of Dentistry
312 Whittington Parkway, Suite 101
Louisville, KY 40222
Phone: 502-429-7280
Fax: 502-429-7282
http://dentistry.ky.gov

Louisiana (CITA)
Louisiana State Board of Dentistry
365 Canal Street, Suite 2680
New Orleans, LA 70130
Phone: 504-568-8574
Fax: 504-568-8598
www.lsbd.org

Maine (NERB)
Maine Board of Dental Examiners
143 State House Station
Augusta, ME 04333
Phone: 207-287-3333
Fax: 207-287-8140
www.mainedental.org

Maryland (NERB)
Maryland State Board of Dental Examiners
Spring Grove Hospital Center
The Benjamin Rush Building
55 Wade Avenue
Baltimore, MD 21228
Phone: 410-402-8501
Fax: 410-402-8505
www.dhmh.state.md.us/dental/

Massachusetts (NERB)
Massachusetts Board of Registration in Dentistry
239 Causeway Street, 5th Floor
Boston, MA 02114
Phone: 617-973-0973
Fax: 617-973-0982
www.mass.gov/dph/boards/dn

Michigan (NERB)
Michigan Board of Dentistry
Department of Commerce/Industry Services
P.O. Box 30670
Lansing, MI 48909-8170
Phone: 517-335-0918
Fax: 517-373-2179
www.michigan.gov/healthlicense

Minnesota (CRDTS)
Minnesota Board of Dentistry
2829 University Avenue SE, Suite 450
Minneapolis, MN 55414
Phone: 612-617-2250
Fax: 612-617-2260
www.dentalboard.state.mn.us

Mississippi (CITA)
Mississippi State Board of Dental Examiners
600 E. Amite Street, Suite 100
Jackson, MS 39201-2801
Phone: 601-944-9622
Fax: 601-944-9624
www.dentalboard.ms.gov

Missouri (CRDTS, WREB)
Missouri Dental Board
P.O. Box 1367
Jefferson City, MO 65102-1367
Phone: 573-751-0042
Fax: 573-751-8216
http://pr.mo.gov/dental.asp

Montana (WREB)
Montana Board of Dentistry
301 South Park
P.O. Box 200513
Helena, MT 59620-0513
Phone: 406-841-2390
Fax: 406-841-2305
http://www.dentistry.mt.gov

Nebraska (CRDTS)
Nebraska Board of Dentistry
Credentialing Division
P.O. Box 94986
Lincoln, NE 68509-4986
Phone: 402-471-2115
Fax: 402-471-3577
www.dhhs.ne.gov/crl/medical/dent/Dentist/Dentist.htm#Board

Nevada‡
Nevada State Board of Dental Examiners
6010 S. Rainbow Boulevard, Suite A-1
Las Vegas, NV 89118
Phone: 702-486-7044
Fax: 702-486-7046
www.nvdentalboard.nv.gov

Continued

BOX 1-3 State Boards, Regional Testing Agency Membership,* and Contact Information†—cont'd

New Hampshire (NERB)
New Hampshire Board of Dental Examiners
2 Industrial Park Drive
Concord, NH 03301-8520
Phone: 603-271-4561
Fax: 603-271-6702
www.state.nh.us/dental

New Jersey (NERB)
New Jersey State Board of Dentistry
124 Halsey Street
P.O. Box 45005
Newark, NJ 07102
Phone: 973-504-6405
Fax: 973-273-8035
www.njconsumeraffairs.gov/dentistry

New Mexico (WREB)
New Mexico Board of Dental Health Care
2550 Cerrillos
Santa Fe, NM 87505-5101
Phone: 505-476-4680
Fax: 505-476-4545
http://www.rld.state.nm.us/

New York (NERB)
New York State Board of Dentistry
89 Washington Avenue, 2nd Floor—West Wing
Albany, NY 12234-1000
Phone: 518-474-3817, ext. 550
Fax: 518-473-6995
www.op.nysed.gov/proflist.htm

North Carolina (CITA)
North Carolina State Board of Dental Examiners
507 Airport Boulevard, Suite 105
Morrisville, NC 27560-8200
Phone: 919-678-8223
Fax: 919-678-8472
www.ncdentalboard.org

North Dakota (CRDTS, WREB)
North Dakota Board of Dentistry
P.O. Box 7246
Bismarck, ND 58507-7246
Phone: 701-258-8600
Fax: 701-244-9824
www.nddentalboard.org

Ohio (NERB)
Ohio State Dental Board
77 S. High Street, 17th Floor
Columbus, OH 43215-6135
Phone: 614-466-2580
Fax: 614-752-8995
www.dental.ohio.gov

Oklahoma (WREB)
Oklahoma Board of Dentistry
201 N.E. 38th Terrace, #2
Oklahoma City, OK 73105
Phone: 405-524-9037

Fax: 405-524-2223
www.dentist.state.ok.us

Oregon (WREB, NERB)
Oregon Board of Dentistry
1600 SW 4th Avenue, Suite 770
Portland, OR 97201
Phone: 971-673-3200
Fax: 971-673-3202
http://oregon.gov/dentistry

Pennsylvania (NERB)
Pennsylvania State Board of Dentistry
P.O. Box 2649
Harrisburg, PA 17105
Phone: 717-783-7162
Fax: 717-787-7769
www.dos.state.pa.us/dent

Puerto Rico (CITA)
Puerto Rico Board of Dental Examiners
Department of Health
P.O. Box 70184
San Juan, PR 00936-8184
Phone: 787-765-2929
Fax: 787-725-7903

Rhode Island (NERB)
Rhode Island State Board of Examiners in Dentistry
3 Capitol Hill
Providence, RI 02908
Phone: 401-222-5960
Fax: 401-222-6548
www.health.ri.gov/hsr/professions/dental.php

South Carolina (CRDTS, SRTA)
South Carolina State Board of Dentistry
P.O. Box 11329
Columbia, SC 29211-1329
Phone: 803-896-4665
Fax: 803-896-4719
www.llr.state.sc.us/pol/dentistry

South Dakota (CRDTS)
South Dakota State Board of Dentistry
P.O. Box 1079
105 S. Euclid Avenue, Suite C
Pierre, SD 57501
Phone: 605-224-1282
Fax: 888-425-3032
www.sdboardofdentistry.com

Tennessee (SRTA)
Tennessee Board of Dentistry
227 French Landing, Suite 300
Heritage Place Metro Center
Nashville, TN 37243
Phone: 800-278-4123
Fax: 615-770-7444
http://health.state.tn.us/Boards/Dentistry/

BOX 1-3 State Boards, Regional Testing Agency Membership,* and Contact Information†—cont'd

Texas (WREB)
Texas State Board of Dental Examiners
333 Guadalupe Street, Suite 3-800
Austin, TX 78701
Phone: 512-463-6400
Fax: 512-463-7452
www.tsbde.state.tx.us

Utah (WREB)
Utah Board of Dentists and Dental Hygienists
Division of Occupational and Professional Licensing
P.O. Box 146741
Salt Lake City, UT 84114-6741
Phone: 801-530-6621
Fax: 801-530-6511
http://www.dopl.utah.gov/licensing/dentistry.html

Vermont (NERB)
Vermont Board of Dental Examiners
Office of the Secretary of State
North FL 2 National Life Building
Montpelier, VT 05620-3402
Phone: 802-828-2390
Fax: 802-828-2465
www.vtprofessionals.org

Virgin Islands
Virgin Islands Board of Dental Examiners
Department of Health
48 Sugar Estate
St. Thomas, VI 00802
Phone: 340-774-0117
Fax: 340-777-4001

Virginia (SRTA)
Virginia Board of Dentistry
9960 Maryland Drive, Suite 300
Richmond, VA 23233-1463
Phone: 804-367-4538
Fax: 804-527-4428
http://www.dhp.virginia.gov/dentistry/default.htm

Washington (CRDTS, WREB,)
Dental Health Care Quality Assurance
Washington State Department of Health
Dental Hygiene Examining Committee
Quality Assurance Commission
310 Israel Road SE
Tumwater, WA 98501
Phone: 360-236-4700
Fax: 360-236-4818
http://www.doh.wa.gov/hsqa/Professions/Dental_Hygiene/default.htm

West Virginia (CRDTS, NERB, SRTA,)
West Virginia Board of Dental Examiners
P. O. Box 1447
Crab Orchard, WV 25827-1447
Phone: 304-252-8266
Fax: 304-253-9454
E-mail: wvbde@charterinternet.com
www.wvdentalboard.org

Wisconsin (CRDTS, NERB)
Wisconsin Dentistry Examining Board
P.O. Box 8935
1400 E. Washington Avenue
Madison, WI 53708
Phone: 608-266-2812
Fax: 608-261-7083
http://www.drl.state.wi.us/board_detail.asp?boardid=13&locid=0

Wyoming (CRDTS, WREB)
Wyoming Board of Dental Examiners
1800 Carey Avenue, 4th Floor
Cheyenne, WY 82002
Phone: 307-777-6529
Fax: 307-777-3508
http://plboards.state.wy.us/dental/index.asp

*The letters in parentheses ( ) after a state indicate membership in that regional clinical testing examination agency. Jurisdictions without a regional board affiliation conduct boards independently. CITA, Council of Interstate Testing Agencies; CRDTS, Central Regional Dental Testing Service, Inc.; NERB, Northeast Regional Board of Dental Examiners, Inc.; SRTA, Southern Regional Testing Agency, Inc.; WREB, WREB: A National Dental and Dental Hygiene Testing Agency.
†State board information can also be found on the Web site of the American Association of Dental Boards (AADB), www.dentalboards.org.
‡Nevada administers examinations developed by ADEX with examiners from any of the ADEX member states.

STATE BOARDS OF DENTISTRY/ DENTAL HYGIENE AND PROFESSIONAL ASSOCIATIONS

State boards of dentistry or dental hygiene are governmental agencies that control and manage dental hygiene licensure in accordance with laws adopted by the legislature of the states. In general, boards have the power or influence to grant, deny, and revoke licenses. Board members are charged with the following duties:

- Enforcing the state practice act and its rules and regulations
- Conducting or recognizing examinations for competence
- Reviewing and investigating complaints concerning unlawful or unprofessional conduct by licensees

Significant variations exist from jurisdiction to jurisdiction in the way regulatory boards are organized, in the power or authority they have, and even in their titles. For the purpose of clarity in this text, the term *state board* or *state board of dentistry* is used to refer to the *regulatory body* in a respective legal jurisdiction that is empowered to determine prerequisites for licensure and issue licenses to practice dental hygiene (see Box 1-3).

Frequently, licensure candidates and even licensed practitioners confuse the state board with the state dental association. Although strong ties may exist between a state board and the state dental association, distinct legal differences exist between these two bodies. The state board of dentistry is a *governmental agency*, established by law, which functions as an arm of the state legislature to regulate the practice of dentistry and dental hygiene. Its sole purpose is to protect the public from incompetent or unethical practitioners. In contrast, a state dental or dental hygiene association is a *voluntary organization* of practitioners, who join together to promote the oral health of the public and to advance the profession.

Practitioners need to understand both this distinction and the interplay between state boards and professional associations. Professional associations *do not* determine requirements for licensure or regulate practice; this is founded by law and implemented through state boards. Professional associations do, however, initiate programs and research projects and propose legislative changes that may ultimately be incorporated into the legal requirements for practice. In most states, state board members are appointed by the governor. Alabama, Nebraska, North Carolina, Oklahoma, and the District of Columbia are the exceptions, with designation being done through election by members of the profession or through appointment by another governmental body. Typically, professional associations nominate and influence these appointments.

All states have some form of dental hygiene representation on the board. Recent years have seen a trend toward self-regulation, with the establishment of separate dental hygiene state boards and advisory committees. Currently, about 17 states have varying degrees of self-regulation for dental hygienists (Arizona, California, Connecticut, Delaware, Florida, Iowa, Maine, Maryland, Michigan, Missouri, Montana, Nevada, New Mexico, Oklahoma, Oregon, Texas, and Washington). In Canada, over 90% of dental hygienists are self-regulated (in the provinces of Alberta, British Columbia, Manitoba, New Brunswick, Nova Scotia, Ontario, Quebec, and Saskatchewan).

The legislative and political arenas in dentistry are constantly changing, as are technologic advancements in health. As a result, revision to state practice acts—including the definitions of *dental hygiene* and the scope of practice—is ongoing. Likewise, as the standards of competence in dental hygiene are redefined in terms of requisite professional skills and knowledge, examinations undergo continual updating. Although this places demands on the individual practitioner, the educational system, and the agencies responsible for evaluating competence, it is the means by which the profession advances its standards of care. State practice acts charge the state board with conducting or sanctioning both didactic and practical examinations to determine competence to practice. Some state laws even define the content of such examinations and specify the passing score. The majority of practice acts authorize the state board to recognize multiple examinations (see Figure 1-1). Although other agencies are part of the licensure process, the fundamental authorization to recognize qualifications for licensure lies with the state regulatory board.

JOINT COMMISSION ON NATIONAL DENTAL EXAMINATIONS

The JCNDE is the agency responsible for the development and administration of the NBDHE. It comprises a 15-member panel of representatives, as follows:
- American Dental Association, ADA (3)
- American Dental Education Association, ADEA (3)
- American Association of Dental Boards, AADB (6)
- American Dental Hygienists Association, ADHA (1)
- Public Member (1)
- American Student Dental Association, ASDA (1)

A standing committee of the JCNDE, the Committee on Dental Hygiene (CDH), consists of five dental hygienists (including the ADHA Commissioner)—two educators and two practitioners and a dental hygiene student representative appointed by the ADHA—plus one Commissioner from the ADA, the ADEA, and the AADB. The CDH's responsibilities relate primarily to the NBDHE, including the following:
- Examination content and specifications
- Test construction procedures, including nomination of test constructors
- Information to publicize or explain the testing program
- Examination regulations that affect dental hygiene candidates
- Matters pertaining to finances, the ADA and the Joint Commission Bylaws, and the Joint Commission Standing Rules that affect the NBDHE

The Commission has final authority to act on committee recommendations, but historically, the CDH has been the guiding force of the dental hygiene examination program.

NATIONAL BOARD DENTAL HYGIENE EXAMINATION

Examination Format

The NBDHE is designed to "assess the ability of a candidate to understand important information from biomedical, dental, and dental hygiene sciences, and to apply such information in a problem-solving context."[1] The examination is computer-based and includes approximately 350 multiple-choice items in independent, case-based, and testlet formats. The NBDHE is a comprehensive examination with two components. Component A presents 200 discipline-based items in three major areas:

- Scientific basis for dental hygiene practice
- Provision of clinical dental hygiene services
- Community health/research principles

Component B presents 150 case-based items, which relate to no more than 15 dental hygiene patient cases. Case material includes dental and health histories, dental charting, radiographs, and clinical photographs. Every examination includes one or more of the following patient types: geriatric, adult with periodontitis, pediatric, special needs, and medically compromised. The case-based items address knowledge, skills, and judgments necessary for the following:

- Assessing client characteristics
- Obtaining and interpreting radiographs
- Planning and managing dental hygiene care
- Performing periodontal procedures
- Using preventive agents
- Providing supportive treatment services
- Professional responsibility

The NBDHE tests the candidate's ability to apply the essential knowledge and skills as a beginning safe practitioner to solve oral health care problems and answer questions related to dental hygiene care. The examination is based on 56 competencies underlying entry-level dental hygiene practice as promulgated by the ADEA and the *Accreditation Standards* published by the CODA. As part of its validity analyses to verify that the examination content supports these competencies, the JCNDE conducts a nationwide practice survey every 5 years. For more information, read the *NBDHE Technical Report* available at http://www.ada.org/prof/ed/testing/nbdhe/index.asp. The *NBDHE Test Specifications* document, accessible in the *National Board Dental Hygiene Examination Guide*, is the blueprint for test development. The outline lists the specific categories of subject matter included in the examination, with an itemization of the number of items devoted to each area. It should be referenced as a guide for study and review.

Examination items are written and selected in accordance with the Dental Hygiene Test Specifications by test construction committees. The committees comprise test constructors, who represent locations across the country and are selected on the basis of their expertise in eight areas: (1) basic sciences, (2) oral medicine/oral diagnosis, (3) radiology, (4) periodontics, (5) dental hygiene curriculum, (6) clinical dental hygiene, (7) special needs, and (8) community dental health. Test construction committees author new examination items and develop new cases, revise and clone test items, create multiple versions of the examination, and review examination drafts before publishing. Committees strive toward higher cognitive levels—understanding, application, and reasoning—in test development.

Item Format

The multiple-choice items on the NBDHE consist of a stem, which poses a problem, and a set of four to five possible responses. The stem is usually either a question or an incomplete statement. Key words in the stem such as *best, most, first, not, except,* or *least* are usually highlighted or italicized. Only one response is correct or clearly the best choice by universally agreed-on standards of care.

A variety of item formats are used in the NBDHE. Descriptions of formats as well as sample items from the *NBDHE Candidate's Guide* are provided below.

Completion

As indicated by the name, *completion* items necessitate the correct completion of a theory or idea. For example

---

The sensation of touch, pain, pressure, or temperature is determined by the:
a. Specific nerve fiber stimulated
b. Method of stimulation of a nerve fiber
c. Degree of myelinization of a nerve fiber
d. Strength of the stimulation to a nerve fiber
e. Frequency of the stimulation to a nerve fiber

Question

A *question* item asks a question. Response choices could include only one best answer. For example:

Which of the following is innervated by the phrenic nerve?
a. Diaphragm
b. Abdominal muscles
c. Sternocleidomastoid muscle
d. Internal intercostal muscles
e. External intercostal muscles

Negative

A *negative* item is characterized with words such as *except*, *least*, or *not* in the stem. These key words are emphasized by capitalization, italics, or both. For example:

Each of the following is affected by saliva **EXCEPT** one. Which one is the **EXCEPTION?**
a. Swallowing
b. Dental caries
c. Oral microflora
d. Protein digestion
e. Carbohydrate breakdown

Paired True-False

In a *paired–true-false* item, the stem consists of two sentences on the same topic. The candidate is asked to determine whether the statements are true or false. For example:

Protection from excessive exposure to radiation is aided by use of aluminum filters and a lead diaphragm. The filters reduce the amount of soft radiation reaching the patient's face and the diaphragm controls the area exposed.
a. Both statements are TRUE.
b. Both statements are FALSE.
c. The first statement is TRUE, the second is FALSE.
d. The first statement is FALSE, the second is TRUE.

Cause and Effect

In *cause-and-effect* items, the stem includes a statement and a reason joined by the word "because." This item requires the candidate to judge both the accuracy and the relationship of the two statements. First, the candidate should determine whether each statement is correct or incorrect and then how the statements are related. For example:

A traumatic injury can cause the pulp space to calcify BECAUSE the accident can trigger odontoclasts into accelerated activity.
a. Both the statement and reason are correct and related.
b. Both the statement and reason are correct but NOT related.
c. The statement is correct, but the reason is NOT.
d. The statement is NOT correct, but the reason is correct.
e. NEITHER the statement NOR the reason is correct.

Testlet

Testlet items are used for testing knowledge and application of community health and research principles; they are also used in the case-based section of the examination. A short scenario describing a situation, event, or problem is followed by a set of associated multiple-choice items. For example:

A dental hygienist employed at a school for mentally challenged teens received a grant to improve the oral health status of enrolled students. Before receiving the grant, the dental hygienist collected data on all of the students using the Gingival Index (GI), the Plaque Index (PI), the Tooth Surface Index of Fluorosis (TSIF), and the Community Periodontal Index of Treatment Needs (CPITN). The teachers and school nurse also were queried on the health curriculum and the healthy behaviors taught and practiced in the classroom, as well as their perceptions of the students' oral health needs.

1. The dental hygienist determined the oral health status of the mentally challenged teens. What was used to determine their oral health status?
   A. The teens' school records
   B. The dentist's records
   C. The teachers and the school nurse
   D. Dental indices, including GI, PI, TSIF, and CPITN
2. The mean TSIF for the students was 5.7 on a scale of 0 to 7, with 0 indicating no evidence of fluorosis. The *best* action for the dental hygienist to take is to:
   A. Plan additional fluoride therapy for the teens
   B. Conduct a decayed-missing-filled (DMF) survey
   C. Talk with the school administrators about defluoridating the school's water supply
   D. Investigate why these students have fluorosis so that fluorosis can be prevented from occurring in future cohorts of students
3. The severely mentally challenged teens had CPITN scores (codes) of 2,3,3,4,4,4,4,4. Which of the following represents the mean CPITN score of this subsample of teens?
   A. 2.5
   B. 3.5
   C. 4
   D. Answer not given
4. In analyzing the dental indices data, the dental hygienist found that the correlation between the diminished I.Q. level and the oral disease status was $r = +0.95$. Which of the following represents the relationship between the degree of mental incapacity and the oral disease status?
   A. No correlation
   B. Weak positive correlation
   C. Moderate positive correlation
   D. Strong positive correlation
5. In a correlation coefficient, the number represents the direction of the correlation. The sign (+ or −) represents the strength of the correlation.
   A. Both statements are TRUE.
   B. Both statements are FALSE.

C. The first statement is TRUE, and the second statement is FALSE.

D. The first statement is FALSE, and the second statement is TRUE.

6. From querying the teachers and the school nurse, the dental hygienist discovered that oral hygiene was neither taught nor practiced at this school. Which of the following should be done *first* to institute oral hygiene as a component of the health and daily living skills curriculum?

A. Educate teens about plaque removal

B. Provide teachers, the school nurse, and teens with toothbrushes

C. Provide an in-service education program on "Oral Health in the Curriculum"

D. Send a note home to the teens' parents or guardians to remind them about the importance of oral health

Case-Based

The *case-based* portion of the examination presents the candidate with medical and dental histories along with pharmacologic and social histories, a chief complaint, dental and periodontal charting, a full mouth radiographic survey and panographic survey, and clinical photographs. Ten to 15 items based on observations and judgments about the client's clinical conditions and needs follow. These items may be presented in any of the test formats previously described.

Examples of cases and other items are provided in the NBDHE samples at the end of this book and on the Evolve Web site. *Sample Examination Items* can also be accessed from the JCNDE Web site.

Proposed NBDHE Item Formats

The Joint Commission on National Dental Examinations has proposed the addition of new question formats for the NBDHE. Although test takers may see these questions on the 2012 examinations, the new items will only be included for field testing purposes. Candidates' performance on these new items will not influence their scores until a later date when these proposed formats have been deemed to be valid and reliable measures. Given that these items are still under development at the time of publication, and that the Joint Commission on National Dental Examinations will continue to evaluate their inclusion, examination candidates should be advised to check the Joint Commission's website for the latest information: www.ada.org/JCNDE.aspx. If the Joint Commission decides to adopt these new item formats on the NBDHE, sample questions will be posted on this book's EVOLVE site. To ensure that candidates and faculty are familiar with these three proposed item formats, examples follow:

Multiple Correct Responses

A multiple correct item uses a multiple choice format and includes several correct answers that must be identified from a long list of options. To get credit and earn a score of one point, all correct options must be identified and selected by the test taker.

From the following list, select the four client-related factors that MOST influence the dental hygiene diagnosis and care plan.

a. Smoking behavior

b. History of heart transplant with valvulopathy

c. A1c score of 8

d. Occupation

e. Stage 2 hypertension

f. Marital status

g. Height

Extended Match

Extended match items consist of lettered options and a list of numbered terms, problems or questions. The one lettered option that most closely answers the question or relates to the term or condition must be selected. Lettered options can be used once, more than once, or not at all. This format is used to evaluate knowledge of relationships between factors. For example:

Select the corresponding gingival change associated with each of the medications listed below:

Drug	Gingival Condition
1. ___ Methotrexate	a. Masked gingival inflammation
2. ___ Hydrochlorothiazide	b. Gingival enlargement
3. ___ Warfarin	c. Gingival sensitivity
4. ___ Nifedipine	d. Lichenoid reaction
5. ___ Prednisone	e. Gingival bleeding
	f. Gingival hyperplasia
	g. Gingival pigmentation

Ordering

Sequence-of-ordering items are designed to test aspects of clinical judgment used to carry out the proper sequence of actions in a protocol or procedure, or to demonstrate knowledge of the steps in a cycle. For example:

Order the initial five steps of emergency response as BEST performed for a collapsed or unconscious person. Arrange five letters in proper succession.

1. ____   a. Open the airway
2. ____   b. Establish unresponsiveness
3. ____   c. Check for pulse
4. ____   d. Check breathing
5. ____   e. Activate the EMS (emergency medical system)
         f. Start compressions
         g. Initiate defibrillation

National Board Dental Hygiene Examination Eligibility and Application

Eligibility for the NBDHE requires qualification via one of the following stipulations:

- A student in an accredited dental hygiene program is eligible when certified by the program director to be prepared for the examination.
- A graduate of an accredited dental hygiene program is eligible following the JCNDE's receipt of evidence of graduation.
- A graduate of a nonaccredited program is eligible only if the program was equivalent to an accredited program (i.e., length of study, curriculum content, hours of clinical instruction, etc.).
- A dental student from an accredited dental school is eligible if the dean of that school certifies that the student has completed the equivalent of a dental hygiene program.
- A dentist is eligible if the National Board Dental Examination (NBDE) eligibility requirements have been met.

Applications may be submitted either electronically or on paper to the Joint Commission. The steps involved in the application process include the following:

- Read the *NBDHE Guide* before applying. During the application process, candidates will be asked to confirm and agree to the rules and regulations.
- Obtain a Dental Personal Identifier Number (DENTPIN) from the ADA. The DENTPIN is a unique number to identify students and test candidates for the secure reporting, transmission of test scores, and tracking of academic data in the educational system of the United States.
- Apply for the examination. Include requests for score reporting to state boards where licensure is sought, and, if applicable, submit appropriate documentation to support a request for testing accommodation for reasons of a disability.
- After processing the application, the Joint Commission will send the notification of eligibility.
- Schedule an appointment to take the examination at a Pearson VUE Testing Center. The computer-delivered NBDHE is scheduled and administered on an individual basis year round.

Examination Day

Candidates for the NBDHE must present two original, current forms of identification to the testing center.

- One government issued ID with a photograph and signature
- One ID with a signature
  No personal items (e.g., cell phones, study materials, backpacks or purses, watches, "good luck charms," food or water bottles, etc.) are allowed in the secure

testing area. The two testing sessions have an optional 1-hour break between the sessions. Three and a half hours are allowed for the first session, Component A (200 discipline-based items). Four hours are allowed for the second session, Component B (150 client case-based items). National board candidates receive a *Notice of Completion* on finishing the examination, before leaving the testing center.

Examination Results

A candidate's examination score is dependent on two factors: (1) The first is the number of correct responses that were selected (the raw score). On the NBDHE, no penalty is levied for selecting an incorrect response; however, if two or more responses are marked for a single test item, no credit is awarded. (2) The second factor in score determination is the score scale conversion for the examination. The NBDHE is criterion referenced, that is, candidates are graded against a predetermined standard. The raw score necessary to achieve a particular standard score is based on the judgment of experts and by other methods, including equating, to ensure that scores accurately and fairly reflect the candidate's ability to solve oral health care problems and to answer items relating to dental hygiene practice on the examination. Detailed specifics on the scoring system are outlined in the Technical Report on the Joint Commission's Web site. The NBDHE is a comprehensive examination; for that reason, one score is reported. This total score is a standard score, not the percentage of correct answers. The raw score is converted to a scaled score and reported in standard scores ranging from 49 to 99. Each standard score represents a range of raw scores. The minimum passing score on the NBDHE is a standard score of 75. A candidate whose standard score is at 74 likely missed the passing score by more than one item. The performance of those who pass and those who fail tends to be distinctly different. All examination results are audited for decision accuracy of the pass/fail point before being reported.

Effective from January 1, 2012, the Joint Commission will transition from the reporting of numerical scores to just "pass" or "fail" for both the NBDHE and the NBDE; however, the raw scores in each of the subject areas on the examination will be provided to failing candidates. The pass/fail reporting system provides the information needed by state boards to determine the qualifications of dental hygienists or dentists who seek licensure to practice dental hygiene or dentistry.

Official score reports for the computer-based examination are mailed approximately 3 to 4 weeks after the examination. The candidate receives an individual score report, the dental hygiene program director receives an NBDHE school report once a month for the previous month of testing, and scores are sent to those state boards specified on candidates' applications.

Candidates who have passed the NBDHE may not retake the examination unless required by a state board or licensing jurisdiction. An unsuccessful candidate may reapply after 90 days from the date of the previous examination attempt. After three failures, the candidate must wait 12 months before re-applying.

Ethical and Legal Issues

The Joint Commission maintains a program to identify any irregularities or cheating on the examination. As professionals, applicants for the NBDHE are obliged to uphold ethical standards of behavior. All candidates are expected to pass the examination on individual merit, without assistance or prior knowledge of examination items. The National Board's *Rules of Conduct* are regulations that prohibit retaining or sharing test items so that no candidate has an unfair advantage. Maintaining the confidentiality of the examination protects the integrity of the examination process and ensures valid outcomes in determining satisfactory achievement to practice safely and responsibly. Violating the Confidentiality Agreement by distributing or seeking unreleased examination items is an infraction of the law and carries stiff penalties, including voiding of examination results and civil liability or criminal penalties or both. In some cases, misconduct may be reported to school or licensing authorities. Unethical conduct carries the risk of delay, denial, or loss of licensure. When the Joint Commission discovers, or is informed, that a breach of examination regulations has occurred, the candidate's results are withheld or invalidated. In some cases, the candidate must wait up to 2 years to be considered eligible for re-testing.

In addition to unauthorized access, or the written or oral distribution of confidential exam content, other irregularities include the following:

- Falsifying information on the application
- Attempting to take the exam for someone else
- Bringing prohibited items (e.g., pens, cell phones, candy/gum, medicines, religious items, etc.) to the test center or the testing area
- Creating a disturbance of any kind
- Taking unscheduled breaks during the examination

Study the rules of conduct in the *Candidate's Guide*, and follow all examination regulations.

The JCNDE's systematic security control procedures to identify and investigate irregularities preserve the examination's legitimacy.

Preparing for the National Board Dental Hygiene Examination

1. Organize a study plan 4 to 6 months in advance to allow an orderly, progressive review without undue pressure.

2. Obtain the *NBDHE Candidates Guide* and application materials provided by the JCNDE. Study the information thoroughly to gain a clear understanding of the format and design of the examination and the protocol for its administration.

3. Obtain a copy of the most recently released NBDHE from the Joint Commission. Released examinations, protected by copyright and available for a fee, are valuable as examples. Retired examinations may contain out-of-date subject material and should not be relied on as the sole study activity. Simulated board examinations, such as the ones in this text and on the Evolve Web site, may also prove beneficial during review.

4. Outline the areas of weakness. Be guided by school experience as indicated by grades or difficulty in certain subjects and by the items from the released or simulated examinations missed or marked as questionable. Dental hygienists who have been out of school or practice for some period should focus on basic science material and any developments in dental technology or services that may have expanded or changed the evidence base for practice since graduation.

5. Gather a personal resource library for ready reference throughout the review process. Properly used, this book should be the mainstay study guide; directions for its use are included at the end of this chapter. This book is designed to direct a comprehensive review of dental hygiene, provide questions to assess mastery of the subject material, and offer documentation for correct and incorrect responses. This review book may be supplemented with textbooks, class notes, or pertinent journal articles, and Web sites for further study in particular areas. Dental hygienists whose textbooks and reference material are outdated should obtain current resources. The JCNDE does not approve or recommend any particular texts or review courses. Programs or conferences that profess to be "National Board Review Courses" are not affiliated in any way to the JCNDE.

6. If considering a study club, recruit three to five colleagues whose study habits, personal habits, and self-discipline complement the group's efforts for collaboration. Otherwise, study alone. Never rely exclusively on someone else for your preparation for the examination.

7. If a study group is formed, organize a schedule and procedures for operation. Content areas can be assigned to individuals for specific study and research, and then members of the group can pool information and notes. Discussion of items or content areas can contribute to the review process.

8. Create an orderly system to guide the review, and establish target dates to complete each area. It would be logical to set deadlines for the review of

BOX 1-4 Tips for Managing Examination Anxiety

- Be well prepared. Nothing boosts confidence like good advance preparation.
- Schedule studying over several weeks. Do not rely on last minute cramming.
- Maintain a positive attitude when preparing for the examination.
- Become familiar with the contents and requirements listed in the *Candidate's Guide.*
- Get physical exercise for a few days prior to the test—it will help reduce stress.
- Eat healthy meals, and get plenty of rest in the days leading up to the examination.
- Avoid negative thoughts and messages. Anxiety is contagious.
- Plan a relaxing activity the evening before the examination.
- *On the Day of the Examination:*
  Allow plenty of time for traffic, parking difficulties, and bad weather.
  Dress comfortably, and layer clothing in case the room temperature is too hot or too cold.
  Bring your admission card and identification to the examination site.
  Leave study materials and cell phones at home or outside the examination center.
  Stay relaxed. If nervous, take a few deep breaths, and keep focused.
  Read the directions slowly and carefully. Follow all instructions.

each chapter in this book. Alternatively, organize your review around the NBDHE test specifications. Another option is to assess and prioritize perceived needs. The point is to plan a system of review with goals and deadlines to monitor progress.

9. Get going, and stick with the plan. If progress slows, assess the obstacles and make modifications to continue with a comprehensive review. Aim to complete the study at least 3 to 5 days before the examination date.

10. Take positive steps to manage examination anxiety (Box 1-4).

Fundamental Guidelines for Taking Multiple-Choice Tests

Using a system for reading and responding to test items will facilitate performance. Here are some general strategies in dealing with any multiple-choice examination items:

1. Read the stem of the item carefully and completely before looking at the responses.

A. Determine what the item is asking; identify key words; and try to formulate the answer before looking at the responses.

B. Consider each response carefully, and determine whether the response is appropriate and complete.

C. Immediately eliminate responses that are obviously incorrect, and attempt to narrow the choices to just two.

D. For combination items, narrow the choices by eliminating any response that is incorrect and consider only those choices confidently known to be correct.

E. When the choices have been narrowed as much as possible and the correct answer is still not clear, make an educated guess. No penalty is levied for wrong guessing on the NBDHE.

2. Exercise caution in selecting any response that contains words such as *always, never, none, all,* or *every.* Unconditional responses are frequently incorrect.

3. Look for the answer that *best* applies to the conditions presented in the item.

A. Avoid selecting responses that are based on isolated rules, are applicable only to certain locales or regions, or refer to procedures and techniques that are not universally practiced.

B. If the item asks for an immediate action, such as the *first* thing one would do, all of the options may be correct. The *best* answer would be based on identified priorities and conditions stipulated in the item.

4. The approach to case-based items includes a slightly different strategy.

A. Case-based items require time to read and assimilate pertinent information; good time management is of critical importance. Before beginning a case-based section, estimate the reasonable amount of time that you can dedicate to each case and still complete the entire examination (divide the total time allowed by the number of cases in the section). If a case requires extra time, answer as many items as possible with confidence, then flag the remaining items and return to them when the other cases have been finished.

B. When beginning a case, review *all* of the case material—client history; health, dental, and pharmacologic histories; chief complaint; clinical charts; radiographs; and photographs. Make a mental note of significant findings, and begin formulating a concept of specific problems or concerns about the case before attempting to answer the test items. Answering items *before* reviewing all of the case material will result in overlooking important aspects of the case and incorrect responses.

C. A well-constructed case will *require* referencing the case material to make clinical decisions and respond to the items. Before marking a response, consider what information is needed to answer an item correctly and where that information is documented in the case. For example, an item on an artifact in a radiograph may require looking only at a specific radiograph to determine the nature of the artifact. In contrast, an item on clinical attachment loss may necessitate review of periodontal probing depths, radiographs, and perhaps clinical photographs or client history. Items that ask for disease classification or appropriate care plans are more likely to require consideration of *all* available information before responding.

5. Watch for grammatical clues. A well-edited item will offer responses that are grammatically consistent with the stem. If the item indicates a plural response, all the options should be in plural form. Any response that is incompatible with the flow of the question may be an indication of an incorrect response.

6. Take heed of the words *not, least,* or *except* in the item's stem. Read the stem carefully.

7. Carefully review questions that include "all of the above" or "none of the above." These responses impose broadly inclusive and exclusive conditions.

8. The pattern of letters for correct responses is likely to be fairly random. Do not be overly concerned if the same-lettered response is selected repeatedly; it is not advisable to base response selections on a pattern of letters.

Future Trends in the National Board Testing Program

In its mission to develop and conduct reliable, state-of-the-art cognitive examinations that assist regulatory boards in making valid decisions regarding licensure of dental hygienists and dentists, the JCNDE periodically incorporates modifications to its policies for the fair and secure administration of its examinations. Development of a secure Web site through which scores and pass/fail status could be released to candidates, dental hygiene schools, and state boards is progressing. In addition to expanding item pools, increasing the number of test versions, and ongoing forensic analyses to audit quality control and monitor trends in candidate performance, several actions to enhance examination security are under investigation. Alternatives being considered include using computer-adaptive testing or linear-on-the-fly testing (LOFT) as delivery methods to reduce item exposure and moving to a more restricted testing window format to reduce stress on the item pool.

▌CLINICAL TESTING STRUCTURE

The emphasis of the examinations conducted by state and regional boards is on evaluating entry-level clinical competence. The methodology for assessing clinical ability involves hands-on clinical treatment of clients. In addition, some testing agencies include a didactic test or some type of clinical simulation exercise. Testing agencies are obliged to adhere to published psychometric guidelines such as those from the AADB, the American Psychological Association (APA), the National Council on Measurement in Education (NCME), the American Educational Research Association (AERA), and others in the development and administration of their examinations. Committees of examiners and educators collaborate to determine the appropriate criteria, standards, and technical aspects of clinical testing. Examination content and format are similar among state board and regional examinations. A candidate's performance on the examination is reported to the regulatory board (or in the case of regional boards, any of the boards of the jurisdictions accepting that particular examination, which the candidate has requested). (See Figure 1-1 and Box 1-1.) A particular state's practice act delineates all provisions for licensure, including the authority for approval of performance on an examination as meeting its requirements for licensure to practice. A license *must* be obtained before beginning practice.

Regional examining boards are nonprofit agencies that comprise individual state boards of dentistry, dental hygiene, or both. Regional agencies have no authority over state boards and cannot implement policy that supersedes the statutory powers of its member state boards. The state board makes the determination to accept the results of the regional board as satisfaction of its requirements for licensure. A regional agency consists of states that have opted to standardize clinical testing requirements and to pool resources to develop and administer reliable clinical examinations. Regional examinations are developed with the consensus of the member states (see Boxes 1-1 and 1-2).

The membership of regional agencies fluctuates as states join or withdraw. Some states belong to more than one regional board, while other states belong to a regional board but accept the results of one or more other regional examining boards (see Box 1-3 and Figure 1-1). The five existing regional testing agencies are similar in their organization and structure. Each maintains an office and employs staff separate from any of its member state board headquarters (see Box 1-2). A board of directors, steering committee, or general membership is responsible for determining agency policies and managing finances. A second key component of the organization is an examination review committee; typically each member state board is represented. The examination review committee may also include a dental hygiene program director or faculty member representing the region's educational institutions. The examination review committee is charged with analyzing the examination, and developing the examination through modification and revision. The American Board of Dental Examiners (ADEX) is a test development organization serving its member state boards. Member state boards are identified on the ADEX Web site, www.adex.org. The ADEX dental and dental hygiene examinations are currently administered by NERB and Nevada.

For jurisdictions conducting an independent examination, the state board is the testing agency.

EXAMINER SELECTION AND TRAINING

Typically, dental hygienists and dentists who are state board members are eligible to serve as examiners. The pool of examiners for regional testing agencies comes primarily from its member state boards. In addition, many state boards have the authority to designate other examiners; these appointed examiners are usually active licensed practitioners from the state. The number of examiners assigned to the examination is based on the examination agency's administrative protocols. Testing dates and sites are arranged in advance by the examining agency. Training programs for examiners vary but typically emphasize standardization and grading exercises to calibrate examiners in the application of examination criteria. Examiners do not use their personal criteria during evaluations. Most testing agencies have some type of *examiner performance review system* to monitor scoring and ensure compliance with the agency's standards. The result is a thorough and uniform assessment of clinical competence.

CLINICAL EXAMINATION ADMINISTRATION

Most clinical board examinations are administered anonymously or in a double-blind manner. Candidates are identified only by a number, and examiners are segregated from the candidates. Clients are brought to the examiners' clinics; candidates are not present when the examiners conduct their evaluations. The purpose of this practice is to eliminate any potential for examiner bias based on a candidate's personality, race, gender, religion, or personal background. Evaluations are focused solely on clinical performance. Predictably, candidates may be curious and seek information from their clients for any perceived clues about the grading assessments. Examiners are typically prohibited from sharing any information on scoring, so

making assumptions on the basis of reports of clients, who generally understand little about the examination process, will only lead to misinformation and erroneous conclusions.

CLINICAL FACILITIES

Most testing agencies use school clinical facilities to administer board examinations. Schools release their facilities for several days for the examination. Accommodating examination requirements necessitates scheduling adjustments, substantial loss of income from the clinic, and increased demands on faculty and staff. Most schools charge a "school use fee" for services and supplies. This cost is added to the examination fee.

If testing will take place in a facility unfamiliar to you, visit the site before the testing date, if possible. Most testing agencies schedule a candidate's orientation session and clinic tour before the day of examination. The clinical facility is *not* under the management and control of the board examiners, and the school may have its own institutional requirements or record keeping for which the candidate is responsible. Renting of equipment or instruments is handled through the testing site. After an examination application has been processed, most testing agencies will mail examination-related documents as well as an information package from the school that includes a description of the clinic facilities, a list of supplies provided, emergency and infection control protocols, compatibility of hand pieces, instrument rental policies, and so on. Many schools have maintenance personnel on call to handle school equipment breakdown during the examination.

Any concerns must be directed to the appropriate source. The testing site, or school, deals with questions about the facilities, the testing agency addresses questions about the examination itself, and the state board attends to jurisprudence and licensure applications.

INSTRUMENT REQUIREMENTS

Because examiners are calibrated with select instruments, testing agencies are likely to require certain instruments for the examination. Although such requirements may impose some inconvenience, they help the examination process to be better standardized. Typically, instrument requirements pertain only to the examining instruments (e.g., the mirror, explorer, and periodontal probe). Hand piece and instrument selection for performing treatment is left to the candidate's discretion. Most clinical examinations allow the use of power scaling devices.

If you are unfamiliar with the required instruments, obtain them and practice with them in advance.

Reference the instrument's task analysis, seek guidance in correct adaptation and usage, or do both.

Instruments should be in excellent condition and *sharp*. Examiners may stipulate replacements if instruments are incorrect or defective. Have extra sets of sterile instruments in case a client is not accepted or an instrument is dropped.

EXAMINATION FORMS

Forms are an important consideration in charting, record keeping, or documentation necessary during the examination. Innumerable systems for charting and for taking client histories exist. Obtain examination forms (or facsimiles) in advance, and study them carefully. Practice using them. If these forms are not available before the examination, take the time to read and review them at the examination site to understand how to use the forms *before* beginning any charting procedures. When charting procedures are part of the examination, their function is to measure a candidate's ability to recognize and record oral conditions, *not* to be a copying exercise. Familiarity with examination forms will help avoid confusion and facilitate recording of data on clinical judgments in the appropriate places. Follow exactly instructions on *how* and *when* to complete the forms.

CLASSIFICATION OF ORAL CONDITIONS OF CLIENTS

The selection of a board client is the single most important factor in preparing for and successfully completing a clinical examination. Testing agencies detail specific oral conditions as criteria for client acceptability, including the number of teeth and surfaces that must have subgingival calculus and acceptable ranges of sulcular probing depths. Most examinations require a client with "moderate" to "heavy" subgingival calculus deposits. Clients exhibiting only plaque biofilm or light deposits are probably inadequate to present a valid test of the candidate's skills. A person with grossly heavy, tenacious calculus or severe periodontal disease is most likely too difficult for the purposes of a clinical examination.

Testing agencies develop and maintain highly defined and precise criteria in an effort to equalize difficulty in the examination.

CLIENT RECRUITMENT

Testing agencies do not provide clients for candidates. This responsibility belongs to the candidate. Some schools assist their students in client recruitment and

may allow candidates who are not students to screen clients before a board examination. Ultimately, however, *it is the responsibility of the candidate to present an appropriate client*. Examiners make the final decision regarding acceptability. Dental hygiene educators and other licensed practitioners are not calibrated to testing agency standards. Client selection is integral to the examination; it is part of the test. Success or failure on the examination often hinges on submitting a client who meets the criteria—this crucial decision must not be delegated to an instructor or other licensed dental professionals. It is risky to present a marginally qualifying client or to *design* the treatment selection by prescaling in hopes of an "easier" examination. Having a client rejected results in enormous stress on the candidate, grading penalties or failure of the examination, the loss of operating time, or all of these consequences.

Historically, candidates have exhibited incredible resourcefulness in recruiting clients. Family and friends are primary sources. The college campus or one's personal dentist or dental hygienist also serves as a potential client source. Students and staff at hospitals are frequently recruited. Many candidates have contacted local police and fire stations. Sometimes, graduating classes organize a collective effort to recruit clients as well as backup clients for the entire class. Candidates have been known to advertise in local newspapers or post notices on community center bulletin boards to obtain clients. Some candidates have resorted to literally "beating the streets." Stories of bizarre and unprofessional methods of client recruitment are directly proportional to the desperation of the candidates. Stress can be avoided by beginning a search for clients well in advance of the examination. Maintain professionalism in all contacts with potential clients. The pressures of a high-stakes board examination do not supersede ethical considerations. A client's personal, oral, and systemic health needs extend beyond the day of the examination and therefore must be given due consideration. Most testing agencies require some type of "continuing care" form to advise the client of additional treatment that may be necessary but not provided during the examination.

Client selection is dictated by the testing agency's defined criteria. Criteria may stipulate requirements for age; systemic health status; minimum number of teeth; combination of molars, premolars, and incisors; calculus deposits; periodontal conditions; radiographs; and more. The requirements also include informed consent from the client for treatment, confidentiality, and adherence to universal precautions for infection control. Carefully review *all* prerequisites before recruiting clients.

In addition to published criteria, take into consideration the attitude and cooperativeness of the client. Ascertain the client's pain threshold or tolerance to treatment procedures. Advise the client of the time commitment. Clinical examinations usually require long treatment sessions, possible waiting periods, and evaluation and instrumentation by multiple examiners. If clients are not adequately prepared for the demands of the examination, difficult situations can develop. Refusing to cooperate, threatening to leave, and actually leaving the examination are potential scenarios that must be circumvented. Advise the client of the purposes of the examination, its importance to your future career, the treatment that will be provided, the examiners' role, the examination schedule, and delays that may arise. When the clients understand the purpose and format of the board examination, most are supportive of the profession's efforts to ensure the competence of practitioners and appreciative of the dental hygiene care to be received.

Finding the "perfect" client who satisfies all criteria is challenging. It is prudent to recruit more than one client to ensure that you have a backup. Inform these clients that they may not be needed for the examination but if they are willing, they may be able to sit for another candidate. Stay in contact with any clients who have been recruited. Confirm the time and date, transportation or parking arrangements, and exact meeting locations.

CONTENT AND DESIGN OF CLINICAL EXAMINATIONS

Clinical examinations provide a reliable third-party assessment of candidates' client-focused skills and judgments. Each testing program has unique examination protocols, procedures, requirements, and forms. Candidates preparing to take a clinical examination *must contact the testing agency responsible for administering the examination* to obtain its test specifications (see Box 1-2). This chapter provides only a general overview.

Four basic categories of clinical competencies are typically included in regional and state clinical examinations: (1) appropriate client and treatment selection, (2) calculus detection and removal, (3) periodontal assessment, and (4) tissue management. Components within these areas may include dental and periodontal charting, extraoral and intraoral evaluation, charting the location of subgingival deposits, and removal of extrinsic stain, plaque, and supragingival calculus. Root debridement and removal of subgingival calculus are universal requirements. As previously noted, specific requirements for case difficulty vary among examinations. Some agencies mandate a treatment submission of 6 to 10 teeth; others require one quadrant, with a limited number of additional teeth. Client acceptability criteria also include a specific number of "qualifying" subgingival deposits. Typically, the number of anterior teeth that may be included in the treatment submission is limited, and a certain number of posterior teeth in proximal contact must be included. Examiners evaluate the treatment selection. If the client does not meet the criteria, at a minimum, points are deducted; at a maximum, client rejection results in failure of the examination.

Some examination requirements, while they potentially affect the examination outcome, are not actually scored. Acceptable client age and health criteria are prime examples of "nongraded" requirements. Acceptable probing depths are another such requirement. Diagnostic quality radiographs must be submitted with the client, although the radiographs may not be a graded feature. Some agencies require a full-mouth series (exposed within 2 to 3 years), including bitewings (exposed within 6 to 12 months). Others require only periapicals and bitewings (within 1 year) of the teeth in the treatment submission. Radiographs of "nondiagnostic quality" will result in point deductions, negative impact on client acceptance and the ability to continue the examination, or both.

Allotted clinic time is another variable factor. Most board examinations place specific time limits for the completion of assignments. If a candidate has one or more treatment selections rejected, it is likely that a point deduction, loss of treatment time, failure of the exam, or all of these consequences will be incurred.

Pain management for the client is addressed by various means. Some examinations allow the use of topical anesthetic only. Others permit administration of local anesthetic agents by the candidate in compliance with the host school's state practice act. Testing agency protocols range from confirmation of formal education in administration of local anesthesia to successful completion of an examination on local anesthesia delivery. Some agencies also have provisions for "qualified" licensed practitioners to administer the local anesthesia. Verify the authorization for the delivery of local anesthetics with the testing agency, the regulatory board, or both *before* the examination.

In addition to client-based testing in the clinic, some regional testing agencies require assessment on computer-simulated clients at testing centers or at school testing sites. The knowledge, skills, and judgments necessary to provide competent entry-level dental hygiene care are evaluated in a standardized examination. Both the physical client-based section and the simulation section must be passed for successful completion of the examination.

EXAMINATION SCORING

No uniform scoring system for regional or state board clinical examinations exists. Scoring is linked to the composition and structure of each examination. In general, clinical board examinations use a system of "weighting" to emphasize the importance or recognize the complexity of certain skills sets and treatment procedures. For example, dental hygiene practice surveys show that competency in root debridement is more critical than that in stain removal. Consequently, in examination development, when both components are measured, root debridement is weighted with more point value than is stain removal. A candidate should strive to demonstrate competence in all skills that are evaluated in an examination but may choose to concentrate time and effort on each area in proportion to the weighted significance built into the examination.

Because professional conduct and ethical behavior are central to the practice of dental hygiene, all testing agencies have stipulations for penalties such as point deduction or immediate failure of the examination for infractions. Examples of improper conduct include, but are not limited to, the following:

- Violating standards as defined in the *Candidate's Guide*
- Evidence of dishonesty or misrepresentation during the application or course of the examination
- Treatment of teeth other than those approved or assigned by examiners
- Receiving assistance from another practitioner or using unauthorized aids
- Improper record keeping or failure to properly document anesthetic use
- Breach of infection control standards
- Causing excessive tissue trauma
- Rude or abusive behavior
- Continuing to work after the established cut-off time
- Disregard for patient welfare or comfort
- Use of cellular telephones, cameras, or electronic devices

The testing agency must be contacted for all performance criteria and the definition of the cut-off point separating acceptable performance from unacceptable performance (see Box 1-2).

Preparing for State or Regional Clinical Board Examinations

Contact the state board office of the state in which licensure is desired. Obtain a licensure application, noting all requirements, including which board examinations are accepted and any related conditions or restrictions. Consult the current state dental practice act as well as the rules and regulations for these specifics. Some jurisdictions require successful completion of local anesthesia administration, nitrous oxide-oxygen administration, and restorative therapy examinations in addition to the dental hygiene examination.

Prepare a scheduled time line of all pertinent dates for completing examinations (and receiving results) for licensure requirements.

1. Obtain the testing agency's examination schedule, application forms, *Candidate's Guide* and any information pertaining to the examination that is published or available online. Read the information carefully at least twice. Do this several months before the examination.

2. Review all of the application material, and highlight or list all the requirements for the examination, including forms or documentation that must be provided, client requirements, instruments, supplies, and so on. The application procedures of many testing agencies are available online. Make a note of the desired examination's application deadline.

3. Gather the credentials necessary to sit for the examination. These credentials may include items such as school transcripts, the NBDHE score, a copy of the diploma, current cardiopulmonary resuscitation (CPR) certification, evidence of malpractice or liability insurance, and a passport-quality photograph. Retain photocopies of everything.

4. Check the testing agency's Web site for *Frequently Asked Questions* or *Advice to Candidates*. These sections provide insights and coping strategies to enhance confident preparation. Advice from candidates who have taken the examination offers a candid link to others' experiences and perceptions and may help combat examination anxiety.

5. Begin searching for suitable clients. Present a prospective client, with a clear and professional explanation of the client's role as well as yours in the examination.

6. For candidates still in school, many programs conduct "mock boards" as a trial practice run. But make an effort to gain additional experience with clients whose difficulty level is commensurate with board requirements.

7. Practicing dental hygienists should set up clinical simulations of board requirements, for example, client difficulty level, time constraints, and so on. Evaluate your clinical skills through critical self-assessment.

8. For dental hygienists who have been out of practice for some period, a number of dental and dental hygiene schools offer continuing education programs. Review courses should be investigated and pursued well before the examination date.

9. Obtain the specific instruments required for the examination, and practice using them.

10. Obtain examination forms before the test, and become familiar with them. If unavailable, study the Forms section of the *Candidate's Guide*.

11. Be cognizant of the numbering system used in the examination—it must be applied accurately. Not complying with the prescribed system can cause charting errors or result in not correctly identifying which teeth are assigned by examiners.

12. A few days before the examination, get clinic attire ready, and organize the instruments and supplies. Confirm the arrangements with the client(s) regarding time, date, location, and relevant directions. Check in with the client again the night before the examination.

13. If taking the examination at an unfamiliar testing site, tour the clinical facilities before the examination.

14. Plan to arrive at the testing site on time taking into consideration mishaps, traffic, and parking problems that may be encountered and the time required for locating the operatory, setting up, and orienting to the clinic. Avoid starting the day feeling rushed and distracted.

15. At the examination, listen closely to instructions, and read thoroughly all of the material provided. Failure to read and follow instructions is a common denominator in problems experienced by candidates.

16. *Relax*, and concentrate on the high-quality dental hygiene care that you are able to provide because of your professional education and experience. Test-taking strategies are provided in Box 1-4 and on the Web sites presented in the Web Site Information and Resources table at the end of this chapter.

Future Trends in Clinical Examinations and Licensure

Given the highly mobile nature of today's society, the commitment to increased access to professional oral care, and the frustration and expense for candidates of repeated clinical examinations, demand for greater portability of credentials in dental hygiene and dentistry has grown. This has increased broader implementation of *licensure by credentials* for active practitioners and has spawned debates on the need for a uniform national clinical examination that would be recognized by most, if not all, states. Another disputed topic is the appropriateness of using humans in clinical examinations. Several organizations advocate discontinuation of the use of clients in testing, for both ethical and practical reasons. Others believe that a patient-based examination is essential for the evaluation of clinical skills. While consensus on these issues is difficult to achieve, it

is generally agreed that any clinical examination developed would have to be equal to or better in terms of fidelity and reliability than what is currently available in the examination system. A dental hygiene examination that is constructed, directed, and administered by dental hygienists, with input and consideration from other constituencies of dentistry, would best serve the dental hygiene community and the public.

Many testing agencies are implementing electronic scoring systems to augment efficiency in compiling examination data. The resulting shorter time to release examination results facilitates obtaining licensure in a timely manner.

International Requirements

In our global culture, interest in working outside the United States is becoming increasingly appealing. International licensure requirements vary significantly. A dental hygienist contemplating employment in another country should contact the ADHA, the International Federation of Dental Hygienists (IFDH), and the ADA for pertinent information and potential links. (Contact ADHA at www.adha.org, the IFDH at www.ifdh.org, and the ADA at www.ada.org). Individual resources or personal contacts within the country of destination should also be pursued.

As a starting point, documentation for all credentials—passports or visas, school transcripts, licenses, diplomas, employment history, and so on—must be gathered. Some countries require language proficiency before certification is granted; others require employment *before* issuing a work permit. Most countries require proof of graduation from an accredited school and successful completion of cognitive and clinical board or case-based examinations; other counties request merely "reporting to employer" (Table 1-1).[2]

Special citation is warranted of the National Dental Hygiene Certification Board of Canada (NDHCB), which was established in 1994 in response to a priority concern of Canadian dental hygienists for portability of licensure. The NDHCB examination is a multiple-choice examination (225–250 items) to assess a candidate's readiness for entry into practice and is accepted for licensure by all provinces, except Quebec and the Northwest Territories. Clinical practice evaluations are conducted by most Canadian dental hygiene regulatory authorities only for graduates of nonaccredited dental hygiene programs.

The NDHCB operates and delivers its examinations in both English and French, the official languages of Canada. Examination information can be obtained

TABLE 1-1 International Dental Hygiene: Educational and Legal Requirements to Practice in Various Countries

	ENTRY LEVEL EDUCATION Type & Length		TYPE OF REGULATION Self-Regulation	Dental Board	Govt. Agency	IMMIGRANT REQUIREMENTS Proof of Graduation	Written Exam	Clinical Exam	Case Review
Australia	Diploma 2 yrs	Degree 3 yrs		X		X	X	X	
Austria*				Not regulated			To employer		
Canada^	Diploma 2–3 yrs	Degree 3 yrs	X	X	X	X	X	X	X
Denmark	Diploma 2.5 yrs	Degree 1 yr		X		X			X
Finland		Degree 3 yrs	X		X	X			
Germany*				Not regulated					
Ireland*	Diploma 2 yrs		X	X		X	X	X	X
Isreal	Diploma 2 yrs				X	X	X	X	
Italy		Degree 3 yrs + 2 yrs**	X		X				
Japan	Diploma 3 yrs	Degree 4 yrs			X		Not specified		
Korea	Diploma 3 yrs	Degree 4 yrs	X		X	X	X	X	X
Latvia	Diploma 2 yrs DN + 1 yr DH					X	X	X	X
Netherlands		Degree 4 yrs	X		X	X			X^^
New Zealand	Diploma 2 yrs			X		X	X	X	X
Norway	Diploma 2 yrs	Degree 3 yrs	X		X	X			X
Slovakia		Degree 3 yrs		Not regulated			To employer		
South Africa	Diploma 2 yrs	Degree 3 yrs	X			X			X
Sweden	Diploma 2–3 yrs	Degree 3 yrs			X	X			X
Switzerland	Diploma 3 yrs		X		X	X			X
United Kingdom	Diploma 3 yrs	Degree 3 yrs**			X	X	X	X	X
United States	Diploma 2 yrs	Degree 4 yrs	X	X		X	X	X	

Note: Countries also known to have formal dental hygiene education programs and dental hygiene practice include New South Wales, Queensland, Kuwait, Jordan, Bahrain, Saudi Arabia, Iceland, Spain, Portugal, Czech Republic, Lithuania, Poland, Russia, Slovakia, Hong Kong, Jamaica, Puerto Rico, and Nigeria. A program is planned for Nicaragua.
*Austria, Germany, and Ireland also require a work permit.
^Canadian regulation varies by province and territory.
**Italy and the United Kingdom require successful completion of an additional prescribed course of study.
^^Netherlands requires unsuccessful applicants to complete further dental hygiene schooling.
(From Johnson P: International profiles of dental hygiene, 2007: A 21-nation comparison, Int Dent J *59(2):63–77, 2009.)*

directly from the NDHCB using the following contact information:

> National Dental Hygiene Certification Board
> 1929 Russell Road, Suite 322
> Ottawa, Ontario K1G 4G3
> Canada
> Phone: 613-260-8156
> Fax: 613-260-8511
> General inquiries: exam@ndhcb.ca; http://www.ndhcb.ca/en/about.php

The rigors of a country's requirements appear to be strongly correlated with the number of dental hygienists in the country, how long dental hygiene has been established, and the size and strength of its educational system. The information displayed in Table 1-1 summarizes data on licensure requirements available through the IFDH and the *International Dental Journal.*

CONTENT AND ORGANIZATION OF THIS REVIEW BOOK

This book presents a review, in outline form, of basic, dental, dental hygiene, and clinical sciences. Each review outline is followed by related questions that test the reader's knowledge of concepts, principles, and theories underlying the practice of dental hygiene.

Each chapter contains a section on Evolve entitled "Answers and Rationales," which provides justification for the correct answer and every response in the review questions covering the subject matter. The rationale supporting the correct answer is specified, as well as explanations for incorrect responses. By reviewing these rationales, the reader will be able to confirm facts and reinforce knowledge. An example is provided below.

CHAPTER 1 REVIEW QUESTION

Answers and Rationales to Chapter Review Questions are available on this text's accompanying Evolve site. See inside front cover for details.

*e*volve

1. An isolated radiopaque area in the periodontal ligament space is observed on a client's radiographs. This radiopaque structure might be a/an:
   a. Denticle
   b. Cementicle
   c. Epithelial rest
   d. Cementum spur
   e. Exostosis of alveolar bone

CHAPTER 1 ANSWER AND RATIONALE

b. **Calcified bodies, or cementicles, are sometimes found and seen radiographically in the periodontal space and appear as radiopaque structures.**

a. A denticle is a calcified body but is related to dentin formation and is found in the pulp of the tooth, not in the periodontal space.

c. An epithelial rest would not appear on a radiograph as a radiopaque structure but as a radiolucent structure because it is a soft tissue.

d. A cementum spur does not float free but is attached to the cementum.

e. An exostosis of bone would be attached to the wall of the alveolar bone proper.

How to Use This Book in Studying

1. Review one section of the content at a time. Study the material outlined in the section. Refer to other textbooks, Web sites, and references to research additional details if any area is unclear.

2. After reviewing the content, answer the review questions that immediately follow. As each question is answered, write a few words about why that response is correct; justify the response selected. If your response is a guess, make a special mark to identify it as such. This will enable ready identification of areas that need further review and clarification. Remember that analyzing a question, narrowing the choices, and then making an educated guess, if necessary, can improve performance. On board examinations, guessing is preferable to not answering at all.

3. Score yourself using the answers provided on the Evolve Web site. If the item was answered correctly, compare the reason noted for selecting that answer with the listed rationales. For each item answered

incorrectly, review the correct answer and its rationale. Go back to the chapter pertaining to that subject, and research information in your reference material. Carefully review all the questions and rationales for the items identified as guesses to ensure mastery of the material.

4. After an interval of several days or weeks, review the chapters and answer the questions again. If the same items are missed, further study of that content material is necessary.

Completion of the Review Process

Board examinations can be completed with confidence and success after completing the comprehensive review presented in this book; assessing areas of strength and weaknesses with the aid of the chapter review questions; reinforcing concentrated study of particular material pinpointed by the review; becoming familiar with the board examination process, protocol, and purpose; and following instructions for preparation. Preparation for board examinations actually begins with the first class in the accredited entry-level dental hygiene program and continues throughout the educational process. This book is designed to present a cohesive, comprehensive review of that professional educational base, to reinforce existing knowledge, and to provide guidance for areas requiring more concentrated study.

REFERENCE

1. American Dental Association: *Candidate's guide*, Chicago, 2011, American Dental Association, Commission on National Board Dental Examinations.
2. Johnson PM: International profiles of dental hygiene 2007: a 21-nation comparison, *Int Dent J* 59(2):63–77, 2009.

@ WEB SITE INFORMATION AND RESOURCES

SOURCE	WEB SITE ADDRESS	DESCRIPTION
State University of New York at Buffalo	http://ub-counseling.buffalo.edu/stresstestanxiety.shtml	Causes of examination anxiety, physical signs of examination anxiety, effects of examination anxiety, and how to reduce examination anxiety. Includes an anxiety checklist and goal setting strategies
University of Illinois at Chicago, Academic Center for Excellence	http://www.uic.edu/depts/ace/strategies.shtml	"College Study Strategies & Study Tips" section. Includes extensive information on time management, studying, lectures and reading, taking examinations, and controlling stress
University of Texas at Austin, Learning Center	http://www.utexas.edu/student/utlc/learning_resources/	Advice on time management, anxiety and stress management, concentration, note-taking, and test taking
Pennsylvania State University	http://www.uic.edu/depts/ace/strategies.shtml	Tips for examination preparation, examination taking do's and don'ts, and how to beat examination anxiety
Massachusetts Institute of Technology	http://web.mit.edu/uaap/learning/teach/tests/index.html	"Learning to Learn" section. Includes assessing personal skills and needs, studying efficiently, time management, tackling tests, and maintaining academic integrity

Barbara Leatherman Dixon and the publisher acknowledge the past contributions of Lynn Ray to this chapter.

CHAPTER 2

Histology and Embryology

Maureen Dotzel Savner

During the process of care, the dental hygienist must distinguish normal structures, variants of normal structures, and developmental abnormalities from pathology. A clear sense of developmental processes and tissue histology provides the background for competent assessment and evaluation.

Knowledge of tissue components and embryologic tissue origin supports an understanding of the physiologic changes that take place during the course of disease progression. This knowledge also provides insight into how tissue is capable of responding to a pathologic condition. This chapter contains basic general histologic information, with a focus on oral tissue components and oral and facial development. A clinician uses this knowledge to formulate a feasible dental hygiene care plan, evaluate the success of care, and make appropriate referrals to dentists and physicians when necessary.

GENERAL HISTOLOGY

Cells

A. Smallest structures and functionally self-contained units in the body; they vary in size, shape, and surface, depending on functional specialization (Figure 2-1)
B. Cells possess similar common physiologic properties that permit:
  1. Excitability
    a. Change in the environment stimulates the cell to bring about a response to adapt to the change
    b. Example—nerve cells conduct impulses
  2. Synthesis
    a. Cells must have the ability to form substances that produce products to aid in the body's function

  b. Example—glands synthesize and secrete products to aid bodily functions
  3. Membrane transport
    a. Fluids, chemical elements, and compounds must have the ability to move both in and out of cells
    b. Example—nutrients are transported across the epithelial lining of the gastrointestinal tract
  4. Reproduction
    a. Cells must have the ability to preserve the species by giving rise to offspring
    b. Example—union of a sperm and ovum can lead to the formation of an offspring
C. The building blocks of tissues in the body are attached to each other and to noncellular surfaces by cell junctions; the structures of various types of cell junctions depend on location and function; the types of junctions are:
  1. Desmosomes—cell-to-cell attachments; this type of attachment is found between ameloblasts (enamel-forming cells) and cells of the stratified squamous epithelium that lines the oral cavity
  2. Tight junctions—cells attach to each other by fusion of their cell membranes; adjacent odontoblasts (dentin-forming cells) form tight junctions that prevent substances in the pulp from passing into the dentin
  3. Gap junctions—contain a channel that runs between cells for communication of cell electrical impulses and passage of molecules; this type of junction is present among some odontoblasts, allowing them to coordinate their activity
  4. Hemidesmosome—the attachment of a cell to a noncellular surface; the basal layer cells of stratified squamous epithelium attach to the basement membrane by hemidesmosomes; this attachment mechanism is present in the epithelial

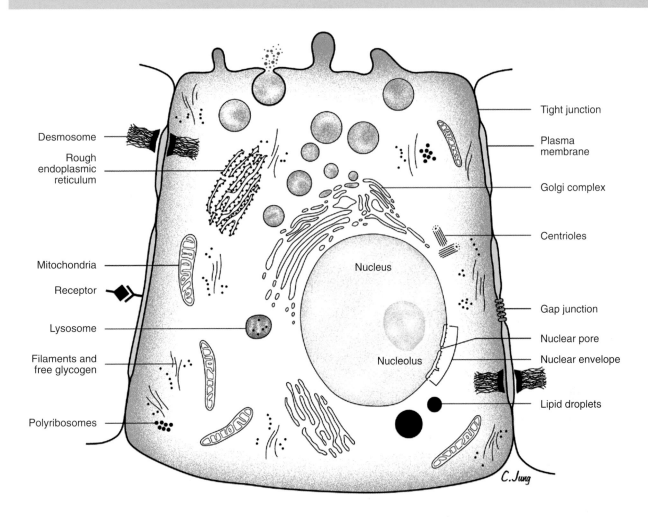

Desmosome

Rough
endoplasmic
reticulum

Mitochondria

Receptor

Lysosome

Filaments and
free glycogen

Polyribosomes

Tight junction

Plasma
membrane

Golgi complex

Centrioles

Nucleus

Gap junction

Nuclear pore

Nucleolus

Nuclear envelope

Lipid droplets

C. Jung

FIGURE 2-1 Typical cell. *(From Avery JK, Chiego DJ:* Essentials of oral histology and embryology: A clinical approach, *ed 3, St Louis, 2006, Mosby.)*

attachment to the tooth; the epithelial attachment refers to the basal lamina and hemidesmosomes that connect the junctional epithelium of the soft tissue to the tooth surface

D. Cells are surrounded by a cell membrane that separates them from the extracellular environment; cell membrane encloses all components of the cell:

1. Cytoplasm

2. Organelles

3. Inclusions

4. Nucleus

Specialization

A. Differentiation

1. Cells that recognize one another will group together.

2. Cancer cells do not recognize each other.

B. Organization of chemicals

1. Chemicals appear early in the development of the embryo

2. Endocrine substances are produced by one type of cell and can affect other types of cells

C. Cells → tissues → organs → organ systems

Cell Membrane

A. Referred to as plasma membrane or plasmalemma; usually too thin to be seen with a light microscope; average width is approximately 7 nanometers (nm); considered selectively permeable because it controls passage of materials in and out of the cell

1. It surrounds the cell and is semi-permeable, allowing some substances to pass through it and others to be excluded

2. Its permeability may vary selectively by porous openings

3. Selective permeability characteristics:

a. Protecting cell from external environment

b. Permitting entrance and exit of selected substrates

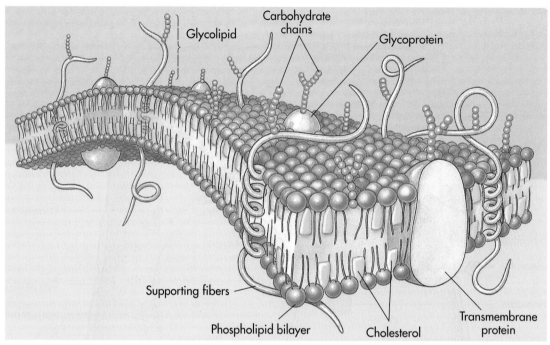

FIGURE 2-2 Fluid mosaic model. Schematic, three-dimensional view of the fluid mosaic model of membrane structure. The lipid bilayer provides the basic structure and serves as a relatively impermeable barrier to most water-soluble molecules. *(Modified from Thibodeau GA, Patton KT: Structure and function of the human body, ed 13, St Louis, 2008, Mosby.)*

c. Using active transport, passive transport, or facilitated diffusion
4. Its composition is a 3:2 ratio of proteins to lipids; lipids and proteins are the major components
5. Its structure is trilaminar, with a bipolar membrane and a central core of lipids between two layers of protein
6. The 0.8 nm pores in the surface allow diffusion of small lipid-insoluble substances
B. Trilaminar structure composed of two facing layers of lipid molecules, into which large globular proteins are inserted (Figure 2-2)
1. Lipid bilayers consist mainly of phospholipid molecules; they are oriented such that the hydrophilic ends face the outer and inner surfaces of the cell; the hydrophobic ends attract and face each other
2. Globular proteins are of two types:
a. Integral proteins that extend through the full width of the cell membrane and protrude; these may have carbohydrate units attached to them
b. Peripheral proteins that are linked or attached to the cell-membrane surface

Cytoplasm

A. Translucent, aqueous, homogeneous gel enclosed in the cell by the cell membrane; organelles and inclusions are suspended in the cytoplasmic gel

B. All metabolic activities of the cell occur in the cytoplasm, including:
1. Assimilation (digestion)
2. Synthesis of substances such as proteins, proteoglycans, and glycoproteins
3. A transport medium in which all nutrients and metabolites are carried from one organelle to another
4. Presence of enzymes and electrolytes, in which specific metabolic reactions take place (e.g., glycolysis)

Nucleus

A. Controls the two major functions of the cell
1. Chemical reactions—synthesizing activities; determines nutrient needs
2. Stores genetic information of the cell
B. Genetic information stored in chromosomes for cell duplication; chromosomal deoxyribonucleic acid (DNA); the human nucleus contains 46 chromosomes
C. Chromosomes are visible only during cell division, when they become long, coiled strands; at other times, chromosomal material is dispersed in granular clumps of material called *chromatin*
D. Each nucleus contains one or more round, dense structures referred to as the *nucleolus* (plural, *nucleoli*); these produce ribosomal ribonucleic acid (RNA)—protein plus RNA; the nucleus also is

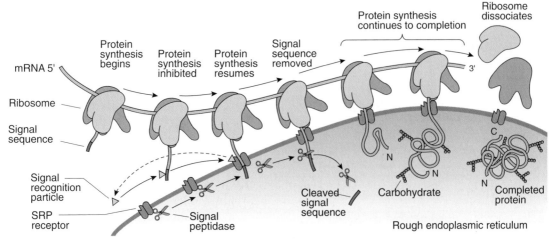

FIGURE 2-3 Ribosomes showing protein synthesis on rough endoplasmic reticulum. Messenger RNA is being passed through ribosomes on endoplasmic reticulum where transfer RNA becomes incorporated in protein (being formed) that is assembled in the ribosome. *(From Gartner LP, Hiatt JL: Color textbook of histology, ed 3, St. Louis, 2007, Saunders.)*

surrounded by a nuclear membrane and contains nuclear matrix with chromosomes

Synthesis Activities

A. Three types of RNA are necessary for protein synthesis
  1. Messenger RNA (mRNA)—copies of short segments of deoxyribonucleic acid (DNA), the genetic code
    a. mRNA can be compared with a tape that contains all the genetic information of proteins, but it must pass through the ribosomes attached to the endoplasmic reticulum (ER)
    b. As the tape passes through the ribosomes, transfer RNA (tRNA) adds the exact amino acid to the newly forming proteins (Figure 2-3)
  2. tRNA—carrier of specific amino acids (building blocks of proteins)
  3. Ribosomal RNA—found floating freely in the cytoplasm (polyribosomes) or attached to the ER
B. Protein synthesis also can occur on polyribosomes floating freely in the cytoplasm; proteins synthesized on the free polyribosomes are used in cellular metabolic processes; proteins synthesized on the ribosomes attached to the ER are transported out of the cell

Inclusions

A. Transitory, nonliving metabolic byproducts found in the cytoplasm of the cell
B. May appear as lipid droplets, carbohydrate accumulations (such as mucopolysaccharides), or engulfed foreign substances

Lysosomes

A. Membrane-bound organelles responsible for the breakdown of foreign substances that are engulfed by the cell by the process of phagocytosis or pinocytosis
B. Produced by a budding process from the Golgi complex, lysosomes form spherical vesicles containing powerful degradative or hydrolytic enzymes; enzymes are first produced by the ER and then transported to the Golgi complex
C. During phagocytosis, lysosomes fuse with engulfed substances to form a secondary vesicle; the vesicle with digestive materials may remain in the cell as a residual body or be discharged outside of the cell
D. Vitamins A and E and zinc are important stabilizers for the lysosome's membrane

Golgi Complex

A. The structure consists of stacks of closely spaced membranous sacs, in which newly formed proteins are concentrated and prepared for export out of the cell (Figure 2-4)
  1. Small membrane-bound vesicles pinch off from the Golgi complex and form secretory granules (newly formed proteins)
  2. Secretory granules attach to the inside of the cell membrane and are then discharged outside of the cell
B. Responsible for secreting to the external environment a variety of proteins synthesized on the ER
C. Major site of membrane formation and recycling
D. Storage site for newly synthesized proteins
E. Site for packaging and transporting many cell products (e.g., polysaccharides, proteins, and lipids)
F. Synthesis site for lysosomes

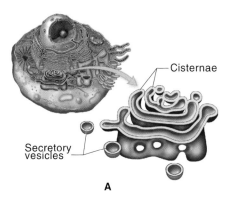

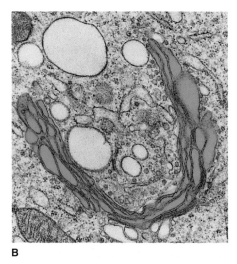

FIGURE 2-4 Golgi complex. **A,** Schematic representation of the Golgi complex showing a stack of flattened sacs, or cisternae, and numerous small membranous bubbles, or secretory vesicles. **B,** Transmission electron micrograph showing the Golgi complex high-lighted with color. *(From Patton KT, Thibodeau GA: Anatomy and physiology, ed 7, St Louis, 2010, Mosby.)*

G. Also involved in the production of large carbohydrate molecules and lysosomes

Mitochondria

A. Membranous structure bounded by inner and outer cell membranes; the membranes contain enzyme complexes in a particular array (e.g., tricarboxylic acid cycle enzymes); the inner part is formed into folds (cristae) that extend, like shelves, inside the mitochondria to provide an additional work surface area for the organelle; usually more than one mitochondria are present in a cell; the number depends on the amount of energy required by the cell

B. Provides the chief source of energy for the cell ("powerhouse of the cell" by oxidation of nutrients) by enzymatic breakdown of fats, amino acids, and carbohydrates; transforms the chemical energy bond of nutrients into the high-energy phosphate bonds of adenosine triphosphate (ATP)

C. A single cell may contain 50 to 2500 mitochondria, depending on the cell's energy needs (Figure 2-5)

Endoplasmic Reticulum

A. Extensive membranous system found throughout the cytoplasm of the cell; composed of lipoprotein membranes existing in the form of connecting tubules and broad, flattened sacs (cisternae); the outer membrane may or may not be covered with ribosomes. The two types are:
  1. Granular or rough-surfaced endoplasmic reticulum (RER)
    a. Contains ribosomes that are attached to the cytoplasmic side of the membrane
    b. Site of protein synthesis
  2. Agranular or smooth-surfaced endoplasmic reticulum (SER)
    a. No ribosomes are present
    b. Site of steroid synthesis
  3. The membrane system functions to synthesize, circulate, and package intracellular and extracellular materials

B. Proteins are synthesized on ribosomes attached to the ER and are transported to the Golgi complex for packaging

C. The system contains enzymes involved in a variety of metabolic activities (e.g., lipogenesis and glycogenesis)

D. SER has a number of diverse roles and is found in a variety of cell types

Filaments and Tubules

A. Thread-like structures approximately 7 to 10 nm thick; thicker filaments are the same as those seen in muscle (protein myosin strands) and have been associated with contractility in cells

B. Microfilaments act as a support system for the cell cytoskeleton

C. Bundles of microfilaments form tonofibrils and become part of the attachment apparatus (desmosomes) between cells (see Figure 2-21, *B*).

Microtubules

A. Delicate tubes, 20 to 27 nm wide, found in cells that are undergoing mitosis and alterations in cell shape (cell morphology)

B. They have an internal support function, particularly in long cellular processes such as neurites or odontoblastic processes

C. They have the capacity to direct intracellular transport through the cytoplasm

Centrioles

A. Cylindrical structures composed of microtubule-like components

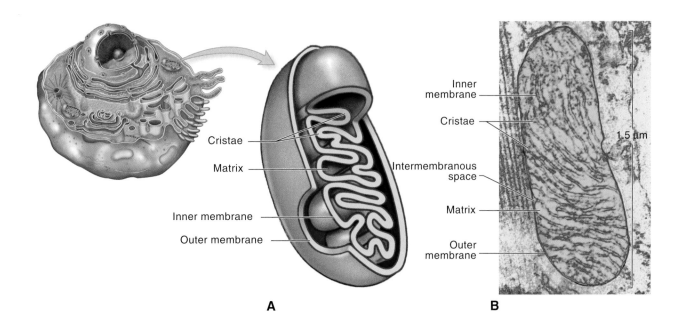

FIGURE 2-5 Mitochondrion. **A,** Cutaway sketch showing outer and inner membranes. Note the many folds (cristae) of the inner membrane. **B,** Transmission electron micrograph of a mitochondrion. Although some mitochondria have the capsule shape shown here, many are round or oval. *(From Patton KT, Thibodeau GA:* Anatomy and physiology, *ed 7, St Louis, 2010, Mosby.)*

B. Centrioles function in cell replication and the formation of cellular extensions

Internal Environment and Homeostasis

A. Extracellular fluid
   1. Fluid mass that circulates outside and between cells
   2. Fluid composition must be regulated exactly

$$[Na^+] = 142 \, mEq/L$$
$$[K^+] = 5 \, mEq/L$$
$$[Cl^-] = 103 \, mEq/L$$
$$[Ca^{+2}] = 5 \, mEq/L$$
$$pH = 7.4$$

B. Intracellular fluid
   1. Fluid located inside the cells of the body
   2. Intracellular composition must be regulated exactly

$$[Na^+] = 10 \, mEq/L$$
$$[K^+] = 141 \, mEq/L$$
$$[Cl^-] = 4 \, mEq/L$$
$$[Ca^{+2}] = <1 \, mEq/L$$
$$pH = 7.0$$

C. Homeostasis—the delicate balance maintained between the two fluid compositions

Transport Through the Cell Membrane

A. Diffusion
   1. Definition—continuous movement of molecules among one another in liquids or gases
   2. Molecules may move across a membrane
   3. Direction of diffusion of a substance is from a region of high concentration to a region of low concentration, which is the diffusion gradient
   4. If equal amounts of a substance are placed at either end of a chamber such as a cell, they diffuse toward each other, and the net rate of diffusion equals zero
   5. Factors that affect the diffusion rate are as follows:
      a. The greater the concentration difference, the greater is the diffusion rate
      b. The greater the cross-sectional area of the chamber, the greater is the diffusion rate
      c. The higher the temperature, the greater is the reaction rate
      d. The lesser the square root of the molecular weight, the greater is the reaction rate
      e. The shorter the distance traveled through the cell membrane, the greater is the reaction rate
   6. How rapidly a substance can diffuse through the lipid matrix of the cell membrane is determined by the substance's solubility in lipids

a. Oxygen, carbon dioxide, and alcohol can diffuse rapidly through the cell membrane because they are lipid soluble

b. Water is not lipid soluble and therefore must depend on another mechanism to diffuse through the cell membrane

7. Facilitated diffusion involves the use of a carrier substance to transport a non–lipid-soluble substance across the cell membrane

a. Once the substance reaches the opposite side of the membrane, it breaks away from the carrier

b. This system does not involve the use of energy

8. Diffusion through pores

a. Substances must be less than 0.8 nm in diameter to move through the pore

b. Calcium ions line the pores; therefore, positive elements such as potassium are repelled

c. Antidiuretic hormone (ADH) from the hypothalamus can cause the pores in kidney tubule cells to decrease in diameter

B. Osmosis

1. Definition—process of net diffusion of water through a semi-permeable membrane caused by a concentration difference

2. Osmotic pressure—pressure that develops in a solution as a result of the net osmosis into that solution; pressure is affected by the number of dissolved particles per unit volume of fluid

3. Isotonic solution—when placed on the outside of a cell, will not cause osmosis (e.g., 0.9% sodium chloride)

4. Hypertonic solution—when placed on the outside of a cell, will cause osmosis out of the cell (e.g., greater than 0.9% sodium chloride) and lead to crenation (shrinking) of the cell

5. Hypotonic solution—when placed on the outside of a cell, will cause osmosis into the cell (e.g., less than 0.9% sodium chloride) and lead to cell lysis

C. Active transport

1. Process used by a cell when large quantities of a substance are needed inside of the cell and only a small amount of the substance is present in the extracellular fluid

2. Involves pumping the substance against its concentration gradient

3. Uses a carrier system and energy (ATP)

4. Keeps sodium extracellularly (sodium pump) and potassium intracellularly; important for the transmission of nerve impulses

5. Almost all monosaccharides are actively transported into the body

D. Phagocytosis—movement of a solid particle into the cell

1. Cell wall invaginates around the particle

2. Pinches off from the rest of the membrane and floats inward

E. Pinocytosis—movement of fluid into a cell; similar to phagocytosis, except that the cell invaginates around fluid

Cell Replication

A. Mitosis—process of cell replication (Figure 2-6)

1. Interphase

a. The genetic material of each chromosome replicates

b. Chromosomes are dispersed as chromatin material in the nucleus

2. Prophase

a. Chromosomes coil and contract; each chromosome consists of a pair of strands called *chromatids*, which are held together by a centromere

b. The nuclear envelope disappears

c. The centriole divides, and the two centrioles move to opposite poles of the cell

d. Spindle fibers develop

3. Metaphase

a. Chromatids line up at the center

b. Spindle fibers attach at the centromere

c. The centromere replicates, allowing the separation of chromatids

4. Anaphase

a. Spindle fibers pull the new chromosomes to opposite poles of the cell

5. Telophase

a. A nuclear membrane forms around each set of chromosomes

b. Centrioles replicate in each cell

Concepts Relating to Dental Tissues

A. All calcified dental tissues are produced by secretory cells that require a great amount of energy in producing their organic matrices, which become calcified; organelles such as mitochondria play an important role in providing energy

B. Mitochondria have been associated with the calcification (mineralization) process that occurs in dental tissues

C. Cell organelles help maintain tissues after the initial formation by the cell; fibroblasts (i.e., connective tissue cells that are present in all tooth tissues except enamel) contain increased numbers of cell organelles; these additional organelles aid fibroblasts in their synthesizing and secretory functions

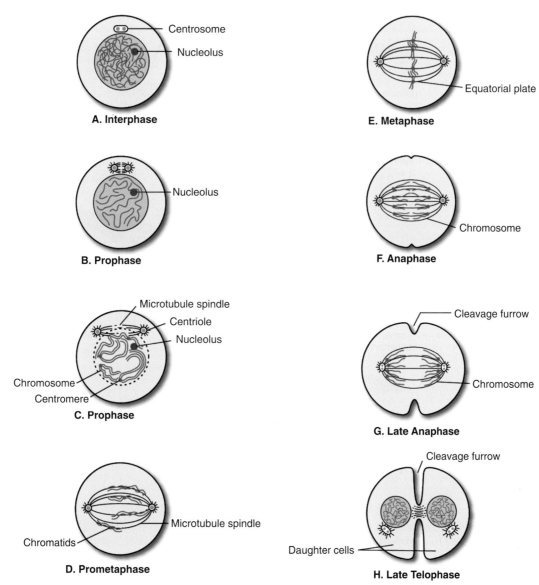

FIGURE 2-6 Phases of mitosis. *(From Avery JK, Chiego DJ: Essentials of oral histology and embryology: A clinical approach, ed 3, St Louis, 2006, Mosby.)*

Basic Tissues

A. At the beginning of human development, individual cells multiply and differentiate to perform specialized functions; groups of cells with similar morphologic characteristics and functions come together and form tissues

B. Tissue components
   1. Cells
   2. Intercellular substance—a product of living cells; a medium for the passage of nutrients and waste within the tissue; the amount of substance varies with different tissues
   3. Tissue fluid—blood plasma that diffuses through capillary walls; the fluid carries nutrients to the intercellular substance and waste materials to capillaries

C. Tissues in the human body can be classified into four types:
   1. Epithelial tissue
   2. Connective tissue
   3. Nerve tissue
   4. Muscle tissue

D. Each of the four basic tissues may be further subdivided into several variations

Epithelial Tissue

A. Main categories
   1. Surface epithelia
   2. Glandular tissue

CELL SHAPES   SIMPLE   STRATIFIED

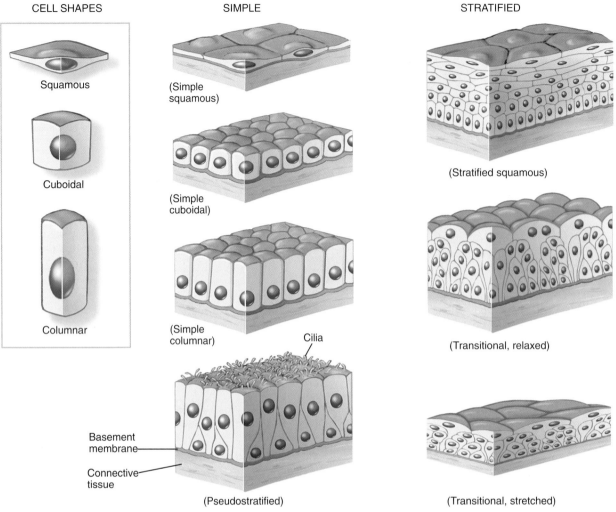

Squamous

(Simple squamous)

(Stratified squamous)

Cuboidal

(Simple cuboidal)

Columnar

(Simple columnar)

Cilia

(Transitional, relaxed)

Basement membrane

Connective tissue

(Pseudostratified)

(Transitional, stretched)

FIGURE 2-7 Classification of epithelia according to morphologic shape and number of cell layers. *(From Patton KT, Thibodeau GA:* Anatomy and physiology, *ed 7, St Louis, 2010, Mosby.)*

B. The epithelium consists exclusively of cells held together by specialized cell junctions (little intercellular material is present between cells); cells rest on an underlying connective tissue, the basement membrane

C. Epithelial cells (keratinocytes) form continuous sheets (tissues) and perform the following functions:
  1. Protection—covering all outer surfaces of the body (e.g., skin)
  2. Absorption—forming the lining of all inner surfaces of the body (e.g., digestive tract)
  3. Secretion—forming glands (glandular tissue)

D. Epithelial tissue varies, depending on function—it may have surface specializations on its free surfaces
  1. Microvilli—for absorption
  2. Cilia—for surface transportation

E. Replicates through mitosis

Surface Epithelia

A. The epithelium is classified according to:
  1. The shape of the most superficial cells:
    a. Squamous (flat)
    b. Cuboidal (cubical)
    c. Columnar (tall, narrow—cylindrical or prismatic)
  2. Number of cell layers present:
    a. One cell layer—simple; found in areas of little or no friction (e.g., lining of blood vessels)
    b. Several cell layers—stratified; capable of withstanding more functional use (e.g., mucous membranes)

B. Combined characteristics allow for six different types of epithelia (Figure 2-7) and locations:
  1. Simple squamous—found in the walls of vessels
  2. Simple cuboidal—lines the ovaries
  3. Simple columnar—lines the intestines and the cervix of the uterus

4. Stratified squamous—lines the oral cavity
5. Stratified cuboidal and stratified columnar—line the large ducts of the major salivary glands

C. Other intermediate forms of epithelium:
   1. Pseudo-stratified columnar (e.g., trachea)—appears stratified but is, in fact, only one layer
   2. Transitional (e.g., urinary tract)—resembles both stratified squamous and stratified cuboidal epithelia

D. Other cell types found in the epithelium:
   1. Melanocytes—produce melanin (pigmentation); intensity of brown skin color is not caused by the difference in the number of melanocytes present but by the difference in the rate of melanin production, the size of pigment granules, and the length of time of their preservation
   2. Inflammatory cells—transient cells usually associated with inflammation
   3. Langerhans' cells—antigen-presenting cells
   4. Merkel cells—mechano-receptors

E. The epithelium lining the oral cavity (oral mucosa) and the skin (dermis) is an example of stratified squamous epithelium

Glandular Tissue

A. Most glands develop from the epithelium; the epithelial basal cell grows downward into the underlying connective tissue

B. Types:
   1. Exocrine:
      a. Serous; mucous or seromucous secretions
      b. Ducts carry secretions
         (1) Simple—nonbranching duct
         (2) Compound—branching duct
   2. Endocrine:
      a. Hormone secretions directly into the bloodstream
      b. The bloodstream carries secretions; no ducts

Connective Tissue

Connective Tissue Proper

A. All connective tissue proper develops from the embryonic mesenchyme; contains large amounts and various types of intercellular material and few cells; highly vascular; has two main functions:
   1. Provides mechanical and biologic support (supports organs and other structures)
   2. Provides pathways for metabolic substances and thus aids in the distribution of nutrients

B. Types of connective tissue:
   1. Bone—hard and calcified; serves supportive and protective functions
   2. Cartilage—firm but flexible; serves a supportive function
   3. Reticular—network of branching fibers; acts as a filter; loose and elastic; provides a connection between structures
   4. Bone marrow—site where blood cells are manufactured
   5. Lymphoid tissue (tonsils and lymph nodes)
   6. Fat or adipose (special type of connective tissue composed of fat cells)—located under the skin; provides insulation
   7. Dental tissues:
      a. Pulp
      b. Dentin
      c. Cementum

C. Types of connective tissues—differ in composition of cell products and proportions of products present:
   1. Dense connective tissue—consists predominantly of heavy, tightly packed collagen fibers; main function is to resist tension; this dense collagenous connective tissue is present in the gingiva
   2. Loose connective tissue—collagen and reticulin fibers extending in all directions; the main function is to provide biologic support and fill the spaces between organs and tissues

Connective Tissue Components

A. Cells
   1. Types of cells normally present:
      a. Fibroblasts—produce the fibrous matrix and ground substance of connective tissue
      b. Macrophages—capable of digestive activity
      c. Mast cells—contain vesicles filled with heparin and histamine
      d. Mesenchymal cells—primitive cells with the capability of differentiating into various connective tissue cells; they play a key role in the replacement of connective tissue lost as a result of injury or disease
   2. Cells that are normally in the bloodstream but move in and out of the blood vessels into surrounding connective tissue when needed (wandering cells):
      a. Monocytes
      b. Polymorphonuclear leukocytes
      c. Lymphocytes
      d. Plasma cells

B. Fibrous matrix
   1. Matrix of connective tissue composed of some or all of the following fibers:
      a. Collagen fibers—consist of three long polypeptide chains coiled in a left-handed helix to form a tropocollagen unit, which is assembled in a "quarter-stagger" model outside of the cell; fibers are highly resistant to tension and are part of the anchoring mechanism by which the connective tissue attaches the basement membrane (see Figure 2-20, *B*); the most abundant fibers found in connective tissue

b. Reticulin fibers—comparable with collagen fibers in their protein composition; usually found in the border areas between connective tissue and other tissues

c. Elastic fibers—consist of long fibrous proteins that differ in composition from collagen; are the branching fibers responsible for recoiling tissues when they are stretched

d. Oxytalan fibers—resemble elastic fibers in morphology and chemical composition; are believed to be immature elastic fibers

C. Ground substance

1. Amorphous substance that consists of many large, highly organized carbohydrate chains attached to long protein cores (e.g., proteoglycans)

2. Molecular structure and composition are responsible for the ground substance's resistance to compression, or compressive loading, from any direction

Types (Cartilage and Bone)

Cartilage

A. Cartilage and bone are sister tissues, both highly specialized forms of connective tissue, whose intercellular substances have assumed particular properties that allow them to perform support functions

1. Very "bouncy," resilient tissue that is specialized to resist compression; has a gel-like matrix in which the ground substance predominates over the intercellular matrix

2. Relatively avascular tissue

3. In humans, most of the embryonic skeleton is preformed as hyaline cartilage that is eventually replaced by bone (during endochondral ossification); depending on the location and loading pattern imposed on the cartilage, it may specialize to form fibrous or elastic cartilage

4. All mature cartilage is surrounded by the perichondrium, a fibrous connective tissue, which serves a biomechanical function; it acts as an attachment site for muscles and tendons

B. Cartilage, like all types of connective tissue, has three components:

1. Cells—chondroblasts and chondrocytes

2. Fibrous matrix—type II collagen fibers and, in some cases, elastic fibers

3. Ground substance—proteoglycans, which have a protein core with side chains of chondroitin sulfate and keratan sulfate (glycosaminoglycans); because of the chemical nature and organization of proteoglycans, the ground substance can readily bind and hold water, which allows the tissue to assume a gelatinous nature that can resist compression and also permit some degree of diffusion through the matrix

C. Types

1. Hyaline cartilage

a. Found in the adult human

(1) Covering articular surfaces of movable long bones

(2) Forms the skeletal support parts of:

(a) Trachea

(b) Larynx

(c) External ear

(d) Nasal septum

(e) Ends of ribs

b. Most abundant type of cartilage; forms the embryonic skeleton in humans; is best suited to resist compression; appears as a homogeneous, translucent tissue because its intercellular matrix dominates its collagenous fibers; the major type of fiber in collagen

2. Fibrous cartilage (fibrocartilage)

a. Has a very sparse amount of intercellular substance dominated by collagen fibers, which are in such proportion that they are visible through a light microscope and are seen running between the chondrocytic cells in the cartilage

b. Resembles tendons except for the presence of the chondrocytes enclosed in lacunae

c. Usually found in areas that are subjected to both compression and tension, as in:

(1) Intervertebral disc

(2) Temporomandibular joint of older adults

(3) Pubic symphysis

3. Elastic cartilage

a. In areas that are in need of elastic recoil, hyaline cartilage becomes highly specialized, and elastic fibers are added to its intercellular matrix, as in:

(1) External ear

(2) Epiglottis

b. Elastic fibers are highly branched and form a delicate fibrous matrix, often obscuring the intercellular substance; fibers can be seen only through a light microscope when stained with a specific elastic stain

Bone

A. A specialized vascular connective tissue composed of a mineralized organic matrix; the inorganic component of bone is hydroxyapatite:

$$Ca_{10}(PO_4)_6(OH)_2$$

B. Two main functions:

1. Provides skeletal support and protection of soft tissues

2. Acts as a reservoir for calcium and phosphorus ions; when these two ions drop below a critical level in the blood (100 mg of calcium per

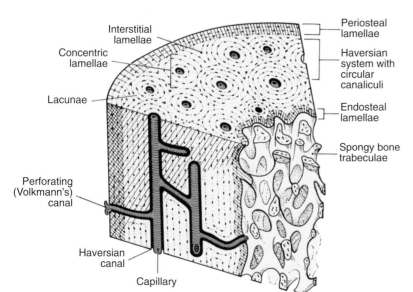

FIGURE 2-8 Microscopic morphology of bone tissue. Haversian system bone is composed of lamellae arranged in concentric circles around a canal. Interstitial bone fills the space between the concentric circles. Circumferential lamellar bone is found on the outer aspects of compact bone; endosteal lamellar bone covers the inner aspect of compact bone. Spongy bone is composed of trabeculae and marrow cavity. *(From Avery JK, Chiego DJ: Essentials of oral histology and embryology: A clinical approach, ed 3, St Louis, 2006, Mosby.)*

100 mL of blood, and 600 mg of phosphorus per/100 mL of blood), they can be withdrawn from the bone

C. Characteristic of all bones
   1. Compact bone—dense bone that appears as a continuous solid mass
   2. Trabecular (cancellous or spongy) bone—composed of a central medullary cavity filled with either red or yellow marrow and with intervening spicules of bone (trabeculae); these trabeculae act to reinforce bone by increasing in number with increased function

D. Bone morphology
   1. Bone-forming cells (osteoblasts) are produced from undifferentiated mesenchymal cells of the periosteum, the endosteum, and the periodontal ligament
      a. The periosteum is the connective tissue that covers the outer aspects of bone
      b. The endosteum is a more delicate connective tissue lining the inner aspects of bone, the trabeculae, and Volkmann's canals (canals of the bone containing blood vessels)
      c. The periodontal ligament is specialized periosteum because it covers the outer aspects of the alveolar bone; it is also capable of forming bone and of forming cells that produce cementum (cementoblasts)
   2. Osteoblasts become incorporated into bone during their formation; they occupy a space called *lacuna* (plural, *lacunae*)
   3. Lacunae are connected to each other by means of a system of canals named *canaliculi*; these canals house the cytoplasmic extension of the osteocytes and provide a means for the transport of vascular components

4. Both compact and trabecular mature bones are formed in layers, or *lamellae*. Lamellae are found in three distinct types of arrangements present in all mature human bones (Figure 2-8):
   a. Concentric, or haversian system, bone makes up the bulk of compact bone; it consists of lamellae arranged in concentric circles around a blood vessel (haversian canal) to form an osteon. An osteon, which consists of this concentrically arranged bone and haversian canal, is the basic metabolic unit of bone
   b. Interstitial lamellae fill the space between the concentric circles of the haversian system bone
   c. Lamellar bone is not arranged in concentric circles and is found on the surfaces of most bones. This bone is further defined by its location. When found on the outer aspects or the circumference of the bone underneath the periosteum, it is referred to as *circumferential*, or *(sub)periosteal, bone*; when found on the surfaces of trabeculae or the inner aspect of compact bone, it is referred to as *(sub)endosteal bone*

E. Bone tissue
   1. Bone, like all connective tissues, has three main components:
      a. Cells
         (1) Osteoblasts—bone-forming cells
         (2) Osteoclasts—bone-resorbing cells
         (3) Osteocytes—osteoblasts that are embedded in the lacunae of bone matrix and that maintain bone tissue
      b. Fibrous matrix—collagen fibers (type I), which are the dominant component of bone matrix

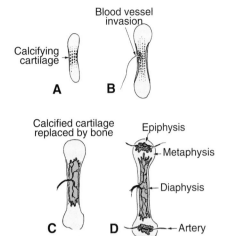

FIGURE 2-9 Stages of endochondral bone formation in long bone growth. **A,** Original hyaline cartilage is calcified in the center of the diaphysis. **B,** A blood vessel invades the center of the shaft. **C,** The marrow space appears in the center of the shaft, and bone forms around the diaphysis. **D,** Bone formation continues in the shaft, and secondary ossification sites appear in the heads (*epiphyses*) of the bones. A disc of cartilage remains between bone forming in the head and the shaft (epiphyseal line). *(From Avery JK, Chiego DJ: Essentials of oral histology and embryology: A clinical approach, ed 3, St Louis, 2006, Mosby.)*

   c. Ground substance—proteoglycans containing chondroitin sulfates and seeded with the mineral salt hydroxyapatite

  2. Bone is formed by osteoblasts developed in one of two ways:

   a. Intramembranous ossification—mesenchymal cells move closer together (condensation), differentiate into osteoblasts, and begin to deposit bone matrix; this is how the maxilla and the mandible are formed

   b. Endochondral ossification—future bone is preformed in a cartilage model that is eventually resorbed and replaced by new bone formed by osteoblasts (Figure 2-9)

    (1) Cartilage must undergo two important changes before being resorbed and replaced by new bone:

     (a) Chondrocytic hypertrophy

     (b) Calcification of the cartilage model

    (2) Endochondral ossification is the process by which all long bones in the human body are formed

     (a) Bone growth in length—occurs in the cartilaginous epiphyseal growth plate

     (b) Bone growth in diameter—occurs in the cellular layer of the fibrous covering of connective tissue periosteum, which produces a periosteal bone collar on the outer bone surface

F. Structure of long bones (macroscopic)

  1. The typical long bone is composed of:

   a. Diaphysis (shaft)—thick compact bone forming a hollow cylinder with a central marrow cavity; this is the primary center of ossification in a long bone

   b. Epiphyses (ends)—spongy bone covered by a thin layer of compact bone; these are the secondary growth centers

   c. Metaphysis—transitional region between the epiphyses and the diaphysis, where the cartilage growth plate is located

   d. All articular surfaces of long bones are covered by articular cartilage

  2. While active, the epiphyseal growth plate usually has four zones, proceeding from first to last:

   a. Primary spongiosa with resorption

   b. Hypertrophy and provisional calcification

   c. Proliferation

   d. Resting zone (see Figure 2-9)

Blood and Lymph

A. Vascular system

  1. Develops embryonically from mesenchymal cells that come together and form delicate tubular structures composed of endothelial cells

  2. Consists of the heart, blood vessels, and lymphatics

   a. Is a closed system that runs from the heart to the organs of the body and back to the heart

   b. Between the heart and the organs, the blood vessels branch progressively into finer and finer vessels and finally enter the organs

    (1) Here a delicate network of capillaries forms, called the *capillary bed*—the most essential part of the vascular system

    (2) Exchanges of gases and substances occur in this capillary bed

   c. Blood is then carried back to the heart via larger vessels, the veins

  3. Functions

   a. Carries nutrients, oxygen, and hormones to all parts of the body

   b. Carries metabolic waste products to the kidneys

   c. Transports inflammatory cells and antibodies

   d. Maintains a constant body temperature

B. Lymph vessels empty into filtering organs (nodes) and generally flow toward larger lymph vessels, the thoracic duct, and the right lymphatic duct; lymph enters the venous branches of the circulatory system

Blood Vessels

A. Arteries—the largest of the blood vessels; walls are composed of:

  1. A thick layer of smooth muscle cells

2. Elastic tissue—the largest amount is found in the large arteries close to the heart

B. Veins—usually accompany arteries but carry blood in the opposite direction

1. Walls are composed of:

a. A layer of endothelial cells

b. A connective tissue layer

c. Occasionally a few smooth muscle cells

2. Veins contain about 70% of total blood volume of the body at any given time

C. Capillaries—the simplest of the blood vessels in the structure

1. Walls consist of a simple layer of endothelial cells and a basal lamina

2. Usually, the diameter of a capillary lumen is so small that only one blood cell at a time can pass through it

3. Capillaries form a barrier between blood and tissues

4. Transport of substances occurs at the capillary level through:

a. Pores in the endothelial wall of the capillary

b. Openings between adjacent endothelial cells

c. Pinocytotic vesicles formed by the wall of the capillary

Microvasculature

A. Composed of the smallest arteries and veins located in the capillary bed

1. At the end of the arterioles is a preferential channel that has several side branches entering the capillary bed

2. Blood passes through the capillary bed from the arterial side to the venous side

B. Selective openings and closings of the capillary bed occur in the microvasculature to ensure regulation of the amount of blood throughout the body at any given time

Blood Components

A. Cells

1. Red blood cells—erythrocytes; most numerous

2. White blood cells—leukocytes (granular and nongranular)

3. Platelets—cell fragments of a specific cell type found in red bone marrow; have no nuclei

B. Plasma—liquid portion of blood

Functions of Blood Cells

A. Red blood cells (erythrocytes) contain hemoglobin, which carries oxygen from lungs to tissues

B. White blood cells (leukocytes) function chiefly to fight infection, to scavenge foreign invaders, and to repair injured tissue

1. Granular leukocytes

a. Polymorphonuclear neutrophils (PMNs)—first line of defense against bacterial invasion

b. Eosinophils—involvement in allergic reactions

c. Basophils—antigen involvement

2. Nongranular leukocytes

a. Monocytes—can become macrophages in connective tissue

b. Lymphocytes—produce antibodies

C. Platelets—promote blood clotting

Lymphatic System

A. Made up of a series of vessels that carry excess tissue fluid from the capillaries to filtering organs such as lymph nodes on the return to the bloodstream

B. Lymph nodes are found along the lymphatic pathway

1. Consist of masses of lymph tissue that serve as a filtering system for the body

2. The tonsils and the spleen are both filtering organs for the body

3. Swollen and palpable lymph nodes may indicate that an infection is present somewhere in the body

C. The function of lymph is to protect and maintain the internal fluid environment of the body

Nerve Tissue

A. Main functions of the nervous system

1. Directs and maintains the complex internal environment of the body

2. Integrates and interprets incoming stimuli and directs appropriate responses at a conscious or unconscious level

B. The nervous system can be classified as follows:

1. Central nervous system (CNS)

2. Peripheral nervous system (PNS)

3. Autonomic nervous system (ANS)

C. Afferent nerves transmit impulses (sensations) from the periphery to the CNS (sensory input); efferent nerves transmit impulses (commands) from the CNS to muscles and other organs (motor output) (Figure 2-10)

D. Divisions of the nervous system

1. Central nervous system

a. Includes the brain and the spinal cord

b. Main functions:

(1) Receives incoming information at a conscious or unconscious level (sensory)

(2) Integrates outgoing responses (motor) that are transmitted to various parts of the brain and the spinal cord

2. Peripheral nervous system

a. Composed of 31 pairs of spinal nerves and 12 pairs of cranial nerves

b. All nerves transmit information to and from the CNS

c. Contains both sensory and motor nerves (neurons)

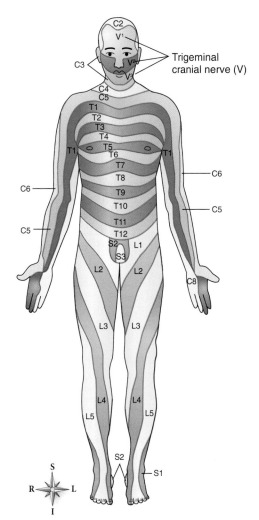

FIGURE 2-10 Cross-section of a spinal cord showing pathways used to transmit nerve impulses from the periphery to the central nervous system. *(From Patton KT, Thibodeau GA: Anatomy and physiology, ed 7, St Louis, 2010, Mosby.)*

3. Autonomic nervous system (Figure 2-11)
   a. Controls, regulates, and coordinates visceral activities (digestion, body temperature, blood pressure, and glandular secretions) at an unconscious level
   b. Is further subdivided into:
      (1) Sympathetic division—acts to regulate and mobilize activities during emergency or stress (flight activities); activities that require high outputs of energy produce an accelerated heart rate and increase in blood pressure
      (2) Parasympathetic division—works in the opposite manner of the sympathetic division; stimulates activities that restore or conserve energy (e.g., decreased heart rate, constricted pupils, contraction of ciliary muscle)

      (3) These two divisions are seen as acting reciprocally rather than antagonistically

Structural Components
A. Neurons (Figure 2-12)
   1. Structural components of nerve tissue
   2. Receive and transmit information
   3. Highly specialized cells consisting of:
      a. Cell body—contains the nucleus and organelles; located in the ganglia in the CNS and the PNS
      b. One or more cytoplasmic extensions:
         (1) Dendrites—conduct impulses toward the cell body
         (2) Axons—conduct impulses away from the cell body
   4. Classified according to the number of cell processes (Figure 2-13):
      a. Multi-polar neurons—located in the CNS and autonomic ganglia; usually, one process is the axon and the other processes are the dendrites
      b. Unipolar neurons—have a short cell process that leaves the cell body and divides into two long branches; one branch goes to the CNS, and the other goes to the PNS (sensory neurons)
   5. Interneurons—lie within the CNS; receive and link sensory and motor impulses to bring about appropriate responses in the body
B. Glial cells—provide structural support and nourishment for the neurons; Schwann cells in the PNS and satellite cells in the ganglia

Definitions
A. *Synapse*—an area that occurs between two neurons or between a neuron and its effector (muscle or gland); found between the cell surfaces are:
   1. Synaptic cleft—intercellular space separating a presynaptic and postsynaptic membrane
   2. Presynaptic membrane—situated before the synapse
   3. Postsynaptic membrane—situated after the synapse
B. *Neurotransmitters*—chemicals released from the neuron as electrical impulses travel along the axon and reach the terminal end
   1. Neurotransmitters increase the permeability of the cell membranes; impulses are relayed to the effector; impulses can be excitatory or inhibitory
   2. Two-membrane junctions
   3. Types of neurotransmitters:
      a. Acetylcholine—secreted by cholinergic fibers
      b. Norepinephrine—secreted by adrenergic fibers
C. *Myelin sheath*—fatty layer surrounding the axon of the nerve

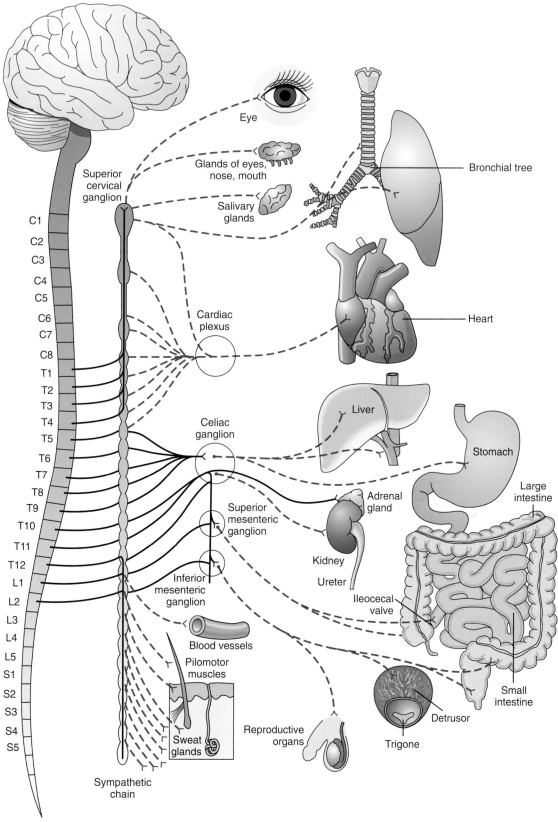

FIGURE 2-11 Distribution of sympathetic nerves. *(From Copstead-Kirkhorn LC, Banasik JL: Pathophysiology, ed 4, St Louis, 2010, Saunders.)*

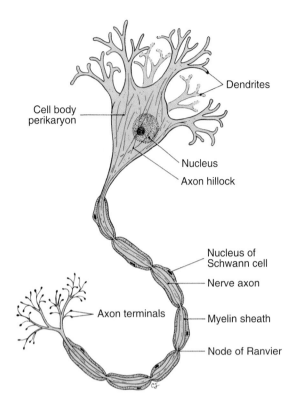

FIGURE 2-12 Neuron with its cell body, axon, dendrites, and synaptic relationships with the muscle tissue and another neuron. *(From Avery JK, Chiego DJ: Essentials of oral histology and embryology: A clinical approach, ed 3, St Louis, 2006, Mosby.)*

1. Myelinated—contains a fatty sheath
2. Unmyelinated—contains no fatty sheath

D. *Neurilemma*—continuous sheath that encloses the segmented myelin sheath of some nerves

E. *Neuroglia*—extremely soft tissue that supports the nervous tissue of the brain and the spinal cord

F. *Free nerve endings*—end portions of afferent (sensory) axons no longer covered by a supportive Schwann cell; found in:
1. Dental pulp
2. Oral epithelium

G. *Encapsulated nerve endings*—composed of several portions of afferent axons surrounded by a capsule of several Schwann cells without a myelin sheath and some connective tissue; they are associated with:
1. Touch perception (Meissner's corpuscles) found in the lamina propria of the oral mucosa
2. Periodontal ligament

Cranial Nerves See the sections titled "Nervous System" in Chapters 3 and 4.

A. Twelve pairs of cranial nerves originate from the brain
1. Cranial nerves transmit information to the brain from the special sensory receptors and regulate the functions of:

a. Smell
b. Sight
c. Hearing
d. Taste

2. Cranial nerves bring impulses from the CNS to the voluntary muscles of:
a. Eyes
b. Mouth (masticatory muscles)
c. Face (facial expression)
d. Tongue (swallowing and speech)
e. Larynx

B. In oral health care, a local anesthetic agent is injected into a sensory peripheral nerve; it diffuses through the nerve fibers and blocks the transmission of impulses to the brain in an area of several teeth or in a localized area of soft tissue (see the section titled "Characteristics and Physiology of Pain" in Chapter 18).

Muscle Tissue

A. Composed mainly of cells called *muscle fibers,* which have differentiated from the embryonic mesenchyme and have become highly specialized in contracting (shortening)

B. Contracting ability of muscle fibers is a result of large amounts of actin and myosin, which are intracellular, contractile protein filaments

C. The three muscle tissue types are:
1. Skeletal (striated) muscle
   a. Under conscious control; referred to as voluntary muscle
   b. Has rapid, short, strong contractions; requires a great deal of energy
   c. Innervated by motor nerves
   d. Skeletal muscles of the head region:
      (1) Muscles of mastication
      (2) Muscles of facial expression
   e. Muscle attachments are possible because of the connective tissues surrounding the muscle, bone, or cartilage; connecting tissues of the muscle run directly into the periosteum, cover the bone or perichondrium, cover the cartilage or perimysium, or cover the muscle. The exact nature of the attachment depends on the site and function of the muscle. The intermediate structures may be:
      (1) Tendons
      (2) Ligaments
      (3) Aponeuroses
   f. Muscles that change the shape of the tongue by their contractions are attached on both sides to the lamina propria of the oral mucosa of the tongue
2. Smooth muscle
   a. Under the control of the ANS and not under conscious control

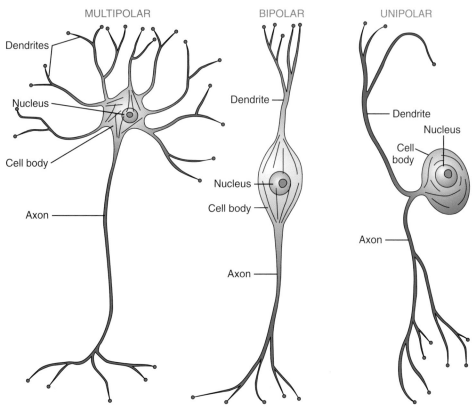

MULTIPOLAR   BIPOLAR   UNIPOLAR

Dendrites

Nucleus

Cell body

Axon

Dendrite

Nucleus

Cell body

Axon

Dendrite

Nucleus

Cell body

Axon

FIGURE 2-13 Classification of neurons based on the location of the cell body and the relative length and number of dendrites and axons. *(From Copstead-Kirkhorn LC, Banasik JL: Pathophysiology, ed 4, St Louis, 2010, Saunders.)*

b. Contractions are slow and can be maintained over a long period without the use of much energy

3. Cardiac muscle

a. Has some of both skeletal (striated) and smooth muscle characteristics

b. Is involuntary; has fast, powerful contractions

c. Purkinje fibers—specialized cells present in heart muscle that act like nerves to conduct messages through the heart

d. Bundle of His—a band of specialized cardiac muscle fibers

Muscle Contraction

A. Muscle can be stimulated to contract by one nerve or by many nerves

B. Each striated muscle contains bundles of highly organized contractile proteins called *myofibrils*; each myofibril consists of regularly arranged protein filaments: actin and myosin (Figure 2-14)

C. Protein filaments are attached to a *Z* band; the section of a myofibril between two *Z* bands is called a *sarcomere*, which is the contractile unit

D. As a muscle unit contracts, actin and myosin filaments slide past each other, shorten the length of

the individual sarcomere (sliding mechanism), and cause total shortening of the muscle fiber

GENERAL EMBRYOLOGY

A. All human development begins by fertilization, the union of a female germ cell (ovum) and a male germ cell (sperm)

B. Each germ cell contains 23 chromosomes (haploid number); during the process of fertilization, the number of chromosomes is restored to 46 (diploid number)

C. The developing organism, called the *zygote*, goes through a series of mitotic divisions:

1. Morula—16 to 32 cells, appearance resembles that of a mulberry

2. Blastocele—a central cavity with an embryonic pole

3. Blastocyst—thin-walled hollow ball of cells that attaches to and embeds in the uterine wall

a. Two distinct layers become visible:

(1) Epiblast (ectoderm) layer

(2) Hypoblast (endoderm) layer

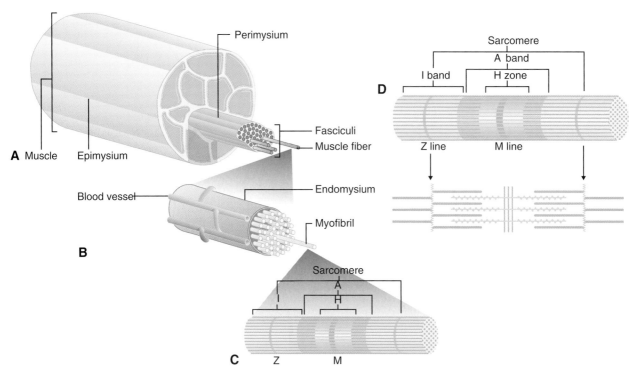

FIGURE 2-14 Muscle fiber. **A,** The epimysium runs continuously with the endomysium and the perimysium. **B,** The arrangement of fasciculi varies among muscles. **C,** The banding pattern apparent on microscopic inspection of a muscle cell results from the organized structure of the proteins (myofibrils) of the contractile apparatus. **D,** Thick and thin filaments are organized into contractile units called *sarcomeres. (From Copstead-Kirkhorn LC, Banasik JL:* Pathophysiology, *ed 4, St Louis, 2010, Saunders.)*

b. These two layers constitute the embryonic disc, which will give rise to the future embryo

D. Three distinct periods in human development:
1. Period of the ovum (first week)—fertilized ovum develops an embryonic disc
2. Embryonic period (second week to eighth week)—most of the organs and organ systems develop
   a. A period of differentiation
   b. At the end of this period, a recognizable individual has developed
   c. Most congenital malformations occur during this time
3. Fetal period (third month to ninth month)—growth of existing structures takes place

E. Development of some facial and oral structures is dependent on a group of cells (neural crest cells) derived from the ectoderm as the neural tube is forming; these cells migrate cephalad and interact with the cephalic ectoderm and mesoderm to result in the development of:
1. Facial skeleton—Meckel's cartilage
2. Neck skeleton—hyoid bone

3. Connective tissue components
4. Tooth development

F. Neural crest cells migrate into each of the branchial arches and surround the existing mesoderm; in each arch, the following components develop:
1. Cartilage rod (skeleton of each arch)—first branchial arch, Meckel's cartilage
2. Muscular component—second branchial arch, facial musculature
3. Vasculature component
4. Nerve component—first branchial arch, trigeminal nerve

G. On the internal aspect of the branchial arches are corresponding pharyngeal pouches that give rise to:
1. External auditory meatus
2. Pharyngotympanic tube
3. Palatine tonsils
4. Parathyroid glands

Facial Development

A. Initiation of the development of the oral cavity occurs in the third prenatal week (embryonic period) and is complete in the twelfth week

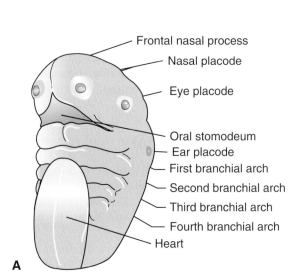

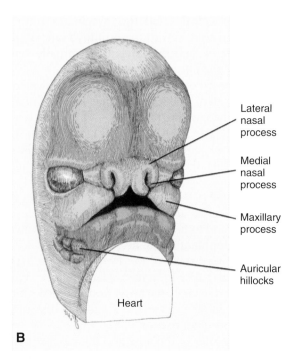

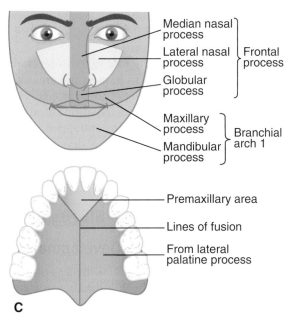

FIGURE 2-15 Facial development. **A** and **B,** Facial development begins with the outgrowth of branchial arches. Note the relationship of the oral stomodeum to the heart and the developing face. Nasal pits develop from the frontal nasal process and grow to become nostrils. The nasal pits separate the frontal nasal process into the medial nasal process and the right and left lateral nasal processes. **C,** Note the developmental processes and the lines of fusion on the adult face illustration. (**B,** From Avery JK, Chiego DJ: Essentials of oral histology and embryology: A clinical approach, ed 3, St Louis, 2006, Mosby.)

B. The future facial region is located among the bulging forebrain, the frontal nasal process, and the developing heart

C. At the beginning of the fourth week, five facial swellings, called *branchial arches,* appear on the embryo

1. Located between the first branchial arch and the frontal process (forebrain) is the oral stomodeum (primitive oral cavity) (Figure 2-15); the stomodeum is the first sign of facial development

2. The stomodeal ectoderm invaginates until it comes in contact with the primitive foregut; the stomodeum and the foregut are initially separated by the buccopharyngeal membrane, which is composed of the ectoderm and the endoderm. It is located in the region that will eventually house the palatine tonsils
3. Rathke's pouch—a small invagination in the roof of the stomodeum; deepens into the brain and forms the anterior lobe of the pituitary gland
4. The maxilla and the mandible develop from the first branchial arch
5. The second to fifth branchial arches are involved in development of the neck

D. On the lower aspect of the frontal process, nasal pits (nostrils) arise from nasal placodes (see Figure 2-15, B) and separate the lower frontal process into:
1. Medial nasal process (area between the nasal pits); this gives rise to:
   a. The center of the nose and the nasal septum
   b. The globular process that develops into:
      (1) the center of the upper lip (philtrum)
      (2) the primary palate (premaxilla): the anterior portion of the palate
2. Lateral nasal processes (area to the right and left of the nasal pits) that form the sides of the nose

E. Maxillary processes arise from the superolateral border of the first branchial arch; they grow:
1. Downward to merge with the mandibular processes and form the closure at the corner of the mouth
2. Medially to form the sides of the upper lip, which unite with the globular process (forms the center of the lip)
3. Inward to form the lateral palatine processes that fuse together with the primary palate (premaxilla) to form the palate

F. The lower face is formed by the bilateral swellings (mandibular processes) of the mandibular arch

G. Several facial or oral processes merge or fuse together during development; incomplete merging or fusing can result in cleft formation—cleft lip or cleft palate

Palatal Development

A. The globular process develops as medial nasal processes grow downward and gives rise to:
1. The philtrum of the upper lip
2. The primary palate (premaxillary process), which carries the incisor tooth buds

B. During the sixth week of embryonic life, two lateral palatine processes (palatal "shelves") develop from each side of the maxilla and lie vertically on each side of the tongue (these palatal shelves form the secondary palate)

C. During the seventh week of embryonic life, the developing tongue drops down, and the vertical lateral palatine processes flip up, assume a horizontal position, and fuse with the primary palate

D. Where the two palatal processes (shelves) fuse in the midline, trapped epithelium between the two processes may result in epithelial remnants, which may produce cysts

Tongue Development

During the fourth week of embryonic life, the tongue develops from several swellings arising on the internal aspect of branchial arches 1 to 4 (pouches); these swellings eventually merge and form the body and root of the tongue.

A. Branchial arch 1—two lateral swellings and one medial swelling (tuberculum impar) merge to form the body of the tongue

B. Branchial arches 2, 3, and part of 4—copula merge to form the base of the tongue

C. Branchial arch 4—site where the epiglottis is formed

D. Thyroid gland—develops from an invagination of ectoderm in the area of the foramen cecum of the tongue; the thyroid gland eventually migrates down to its position in the neck; thyroid tissue that remains entrapped in the tissue of the tongue may result in a developmental abnormality known as *lingual thyroid nodule*

| ORAL HISTOLOGY

Tooth Development

A. Begins in the seventh week of embryonic life with the 20 primary teeth; continues until the late teens with sequential exfoliation of the primary dentition and development and eruption of the secondary dentition—the 32 permanent teeth

B. Tissues of the tooth
1. Each tooth consists of four tissues (Figure 2-16):
   a. Enamel—calcified
   b. Cementum—calcified
   c. Dentin—calcified
   d. Pulp—uncalcified
2. All tissues of the tooth are specialized forms of connective tissue, except enamel
3. Each tooth is the product of two tissues that interact during tooth development:
   a. Mesenchyme (ectomesenchyme)—derived from neural crest cells

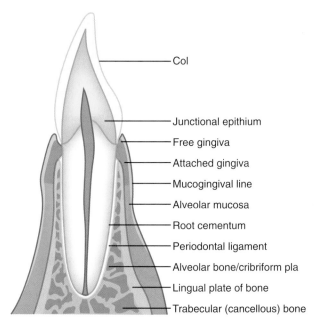

FIGURE 2-16 Four tissues of the tooth: enamel, cementum, dentin, and pulp. The periodontal ligament and alveolar bone are supporting tissues; junctional epithelium is the area where the enamel or cementum of the tooth and the epithelium of the gingival tissue form an attachment.

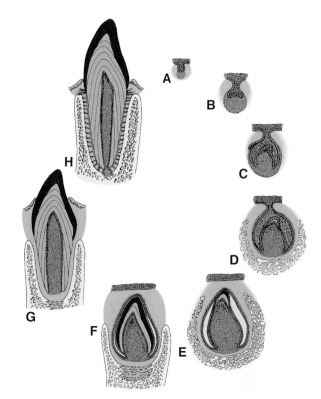

FIGURE 2-17 Sequential stages of tooth development. **A,** Bud stage. **B,** Cap stage. **C,** Bell stage. **D,** Dentinogenesis. **E,** Amelogenesis. **F,** Appositional dentin and enamel. **G,** Eruption and root development. **H,** Functional stage. *(From Avery JK, Chiego DJ: Essentials of oral histology and embryology: A clinical approach, ed 3, St Louis, 2006, Mosby.)*

b. Epithelium—oral epithelium derived from the ectoderm
C. Involves two major events:
  1. Morphodifferentiation—shaping of the tooth
  2. Cytodifferentiation—cells differentiating into specific tissue-forming cells:
    a. Ameloblasts—enamel-forming cells
    b. Cementoblasts—cementum-forming cells
    c. Odontoblasts—dentin-forming cells
    d. Fibroblasts—pulp-forming cells (also capable of differentiating into a chondroblast, collagenoblast, or osteoblast)

Morphodifferentiation

A. Oral epithelium and underlying ectomesenchyme are responsible for shaping the tooth
  1. Both primary and permanent tooth germs go through the same stages of development
  2. The oral epithelium grows down into the underlying ectomesenchyme; small areas of condensed mesenchyme form future tooth germs
B. Stages (Figure 2-17)
  1. Bud stage—condensed areas of ectomesenchymal cells that are continuous with the oral epithelium; connection between the two is referred to as the *dental lamina*
  2. Cap stage—future shape of the tooth becomes evident; cells specialize to form the enamel organ

  3. Bell stage—final stage of morphodifferentiation; in the latter part of this stage, cytodifferentiation begins in the enamel organ
  4. Dentinogenesis—origin or initial stages of dentin formation
  5. Amelogenesis—differentiated cells begin initial enamel formation
  6. Apposition stage—formation of dental tissue matrix; this matrix will then undergo maturation or calcification
  7. Eruption and root development
  8. Functional stage—the tooth is fully erupted in the mouth

Cytodifferentiation

A. Stages of cytodifferentiation and morphodifferentiation overlap; both the epithelial and mesenchymal components of the tooth germ become organized
  1. Epithelial components become the enamel organ, which is organized into four distinct cell layers (Figure 2-18):
    a. Outer enamel epithelium (OEE)—outlines the shape of the future developing enamel

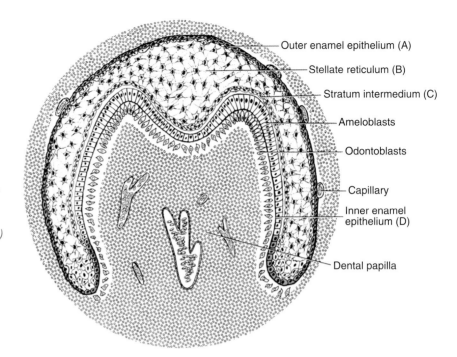

FIGURE 2-18 The four distinct layers of the enamel organ. **A,** Outer enamel epithelium. **B,** Stellate reticulum. **C,** Stratum intermedium. **D,** Inner enamel epithelium. *(Modified from Avery JK, Chiego DJ: Essentials of oral histology and embryology: A clinical approach, ed 3, St Louis, 2006, Mosby.)*

organ on the outer surface; composed of small cuboidal cells, one cell layer thick

  b. Inner enamel epithelium (IEE)—innermost layer of the enamel organ on the concave side of the developing tooth germ; this will become the future enamel-producing cells, the ameloblasts; composed of cuboidal-type cells, one cell layer thick

  c. Stratum intermedium (STI)—flat, supporting squamous-type cells; two to three cell layers thick, lying on top of the inner enamel epithelial cells

  d. Stellate reticulum (STR)—mechanically and nutritionally supporting cells that fill the bulk of the developing enamel organ; are star-shaped with large amounts of intercellular space between them

 2. Mesenchymal components—become subdivided into:

  a. Dental sac (follicle)—surrounds the developing tooth germ and provides cells that will form the periodontal ligament, which, in turn, will produce the cementum and the alveolar bone proper

  b. Dental papilla—condensed ectomesenchyme located on the concave side of the enamel organ; peripheral cells facing the IEE will differentiate into odontoblasts, dentin-forming cells

  c. The center of the dental papilla will become the dental pulp

B. Tooth development is dependent on a series of sequential cellular interactions between the epithelial and mesenchymal components of the tooth germ

 1. First interaction—between the oral epithelium and the mesenchyme; the ectomesenchyme instructs the epithelium to grow down into the ectomesenchyme and shape the tooth

 2. Second interaction—signal given by cells of the inner enamel epithelium (preameloblasts) to the mesenchymal cells on the periphery of the dental papilla to differentiate into odontoblasts and begin the deposition of dentin

 3. Third interaction—as soon as odontoblasts begin to deposit dentin, preameloblasts become true secreting ameloblasts and begin the deposition of enamel

 4. Fourth interaction—occurs with the development of root dentin and cementum

Dentin and Enamel Formation

A. Both enamel-forming and dentin-forming cells are polarized, tall, columnar, secreting cells; just before ameloblasts and odontoblasts begin to deposit enamel and dentin, organelles, especially the mitochondria, increase in number; organelles move to the basal nonsecretory end of the cell; both cells require tremendous amounts of energy for the production of their calcified tissues

B. All dentin and enamel formation begins at the dento-enamel junction (DEJ) of the cup or the

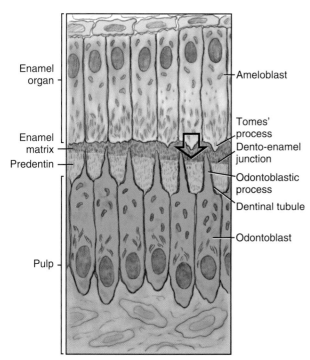

FIGURE 2-19 Odontoblasts and ameloblasts with their cell extensions. Tall, secretory odontoblast with its cell extension (odontoblastic extension). Tall, secretory ameloblast with its cell extension (Tomes' process). *(From Bath-Balogh M, Fehrenbach MJ: Illustrated dental embryology, histology, and anatomy, ed 3, St Louis, 2011, Saunders.)*

incisal edge of the tooth and continues in an apical direction

C. The permanent tooth germ grows off the primary (deciduous) tooth germ by an epithelial attachment similar to dental lamina, called *successional lamina*; this applies to all the developing permanent teeth except the first, second, and third molars; these develop from the dental lamina, which continues to grow back in oral arches

D. Dentin formation
1. Odontoblasts produce collagen fibers that unravel to produce a fibrous connective tissue matrix (fibrillar matrix) of predominantly collagen fibers with a rich proteoglycan ground substance; dentinal tissue is calcified by the deposition of the crystals of the calcium salt hydroxyapatite into the matrix
2. Each odontoblast has a long cell extension, the odontoblastic process, left behind in the calcified dentin and enclosed in a dentinal tubule (Figure 2-19)
3. Dentin remains a vital tissue throughout the life of the tooth; cells continue to produce dentin when needed

E. Enamel formation
1. Ameloblasts produce an enamel matrix with protein components called *amelogenins* and *enamelins*; the matrix is calcified immediately by the deposition of the crystals of the calcium salt hydroxyapatite
2. Ameloblasts deposit enamel; each ameloblast has a secretory process called *Tomes' process*; Tomes' process has a six-sided pyramidal shape and is responsible for prism-shaped microscopic patterns of enamel rods; unlike the odontoblastic process, Tomes' process is not left behind embedded in the calcified tissue (see Figure 2-19)
3. When the tooth emerges into the oral cavity, the enamel has no vital cells associated with the tissue; enamel is not a true tissue like other dental tissues and is incapable of tissue growth or repair; once formed, the mineral substance cannot be physiologically withdrawn from the tooth
4. A final product of the ameloblasts is the primary enamel cuticle, a calcified coating on the enamel surface
5. Secondary cuticle—a noncalcified coating; product of the reduced enamel organ

F. Dento-gingival junction formation
1. After the enamel formation is complete, remains of the enamel organ (OEE, IEE, STI, and STR) come together to form the reduced enamel epithelium
2. Reduced enamel epithelium—plays an important role in the formation of the dento-gingival junction as the tooth emerges into the oral cavity

G. Cementum formation
1. Formation of root dentin and cementum follows after the formation of the crown of the tooth is complete
2. Hertwig's root sheath is formed by the joining of the outer enamel epithelium and the inner enamel epithelium; the sheath continues to grow down, shapes the root of the tooth and the formation of root dentin, and is followed by differentiation of cells from the dental sac; these cells produce:
   a. Cementum
   b. Periodontal ligament
   c. Alveolar bone proper

Soft Tissue of the Oral Cavity

Oral Mucosa
A. Oral epithelium (Figure 2-20)
1. Covered by a layer of the stratified squamous epithelium that:
   a. Acts as a mechanical barrier
   b. Protects the underlying tissues

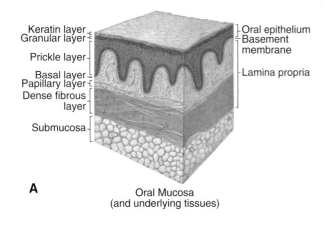

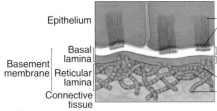

FIGURE 2-20 Basic structure of the oral epithelium. **A,** Two basic tissues comprise the oral mucosa: the oral epithelium and connective tissue. Connective tissue is composed of a papillary layer and a reticular layer. A submucosal layer may or may not be present, depending on the location of the oral mucosa. Note the arrangement of rete ridges (or pegs) and connective tissue papillae. **B,** Basal lamina interface between oral epithelium and connective tissue. Note the hemidesmosomes with attachment plaque between epithelial cells and the basal lamina. *(From Bath-Balogh M, Fehrenbach MJ: Illustrated dental embryology, histology, and anatomy, ed 3, St Louis, 2011, Saunders.)*

2. Three types of stratified squamous epithelia are found in the oral cavity:
   a. Orthokeratinized
      (1) Effective as a mechanical protector and barrier against fluids
      (2) Least common of the three types
      (3) Layers:
          (a) Basal cell layer—deepest layer
          (b) Prickle cell layer
          (c) Granular layer—contains the keratohyaline granules, the precursor to keratin
          (d) Keratinized layer—contains degenerative cells with no nuclei or organelles; cells are filled with keratin, become hard (cornified), and are eventually lost from the surface epithelium
   b. Nonkeratinized
      (1) Functions as a selective barrier; acts as a cushion and as protection against mechanical stress and wear

   (2) Layers:
       (a) Basal cell layer
       (b) Prickle cell layer
       (c) Outer surface of nonkeratinized cells (squamae); no distinctly recognizable layer above the prickle cell layer; superficial cells in the outermost layer undergo a gradual increase in size; look empty but are filled with fluid sacs; cells act as a cushion and are firmly attached to each other
   c. Parakeratinized
      (1) Intermediate form of the epithelium located between the orthokeratinized and nonkeratinized oral mucosa
      (2) Layers:
          (a) Basal cell layer
          (b) Prickle cell layer
          (c) Keratinized layer—no distinct granular layer present; gradually becomes filled with keratin; nuclei and other cell organelles remain until the cell becomes cornified, and then they are eventually lost
3. The stratified squamous epithelium is constantly renewed by mitosis at the basal cell layer; turnover time ranges from 5 to 16 days
4. Other cell types in the oral epithelium—nonepithelial cells; these cells are normally found in the oral epithelium and perpetuate themselves:
   a. Melanocytes—usually found in the basal cell layer; responsible for the production of pigment (melanin)
   b. Langerhans' cells—located in the more superficial cell layers; they are antigen-presenting cells—part of the body's immune system
   c. Merkel cells—usually found in the basal cell layer; are associated with nerve terminals (endings)
   d. Inflammatory cells—transient cells associated with inflammation: lymphocytes, monocytes, neutrophils
B. Connective tissue—referred to as *lamina propria*
   1. Subdivided into two layers:
      a. Papillary layer—directly under the epithelial layer
      b. Reticular layer—dense fibrous layer located under the papillary layer
   2. Forms a mechanical support system and carries:
      a. Blood vessels
      b. Nerves
C. Submucosa
   1. Layer of loosely organized connective tissue
   2. Present only in areas that require a high degree of compressibility and flexibility (e.g., cheeks, soft palate)

3. When present, it is located between the lamina propria and areas of muscle tissue
D. Interface
   1. Area of interdigitation between the oral epithelium and connective tissue
   2. Epithelial extensions into connective tissue (lamina propria) are called *ridges* or *rete pegs* (see Figure 2-20, *A*)
   3. Connective tissue extensions into overlying epithelium are called *connective tissue papillae*
   4. Corrugated arrangement
      a. Increases the surface area between the two tissues
      b. Increases the strength of the junction between the two tissues
      c. Decreases the distance between the blood supply and the epithelium, which does not have its own blood supply; blood vessels are carried to the epithelium in connective tissue through connective tissue papillae
      d. This rete peg arrangement is found in healthy attached gingiva. The stippling of healthy attached gingiva is caused by this arrangement. The healthy sulcular epithelium does not have rete pegs
E. Basement membrane (see Figure 2-20, *B*)
   1. Located between oral epithelium and connective tissue
   2. Noncellular
   3. Produced partly by epithelial cells and connective tissue cells
   4. Composed of two layers (laminae):
      a. Basal lamina (densa)—20 to 70 nm thick, seen as a thin, dark line; produced by epithelial cells
      b. Reticular lamina (lucida)—much thicker than the basal lamina; produced by connective tissue cells
   5. Epithelial cells form hemidesmosome attachments to the basal lamina (see Figure 2-20)
F. Clinical changes in the oral mucosa
   1. Inflammation, friction, heat, and chronic irritation produce changes in the degree of keratinization
      a. Inflammation causes a reduction in keratinization
      b. Friction, heat, and chronic irritation cause an increase in keratinization
      c. Increased keratinization causes tissue appearance to be lighter or whitish; in areas of the mouth that have minor salivary glands, such as the soft palate, increased keratin may obstruct the gland openings, producing the appearance of red dots on hyperkeratinized tissue (nicotine stomatitis)
   2. The appearance of the oral mucosa changes in response to pathologic, dermatologic, systemic, allergic, and localized factors

Classifications of Mucosa

A. Masticatory—gingiva, hard palate (orthokeratinized epithelial covering)
   1. Histologic structure
      a. Keratinized stratified squamous epithelium; rete pegs—projections into the underlying connective tissue
      b. No submucosa; no salivary glands
      c. Fibrous connective tissue; gingival fibers
   2. Clinical appearance
      a. Coral pink; influenced by vascularity, the thickness and degree of keratinization of the epithelium, and the presence of pigment cells
      b. Texture—stippled; the result of the rete peg arrangement
      c. Consistency—firm; owing to the fibrous content (mostly collagen) of the underlying connective tissue
B. Lining—lips, cheeks, floor of mouth, ventral surface (underside) of tongue, soft palate, alveolar mucosa (nonkeratinized epithelial covering)
   1. The floor of the mouth is the thinnest of the nonkeratinized squamous epithelial lining mucosa (100 μm)
   2. Connective tissue of the lining mucosa has more elastic fiber than that of the masticatory mucosa; fluid disperses readily in this area, making it an ideal site for local anesthetic injections

Specialized Mucosa of the Tongue

A. Specialized covering found only on the top of the tongue; covered with lingual papillae
B. Epithelial layer—stratified squamous epithelium that varies in thickness and degree of keratinization
C. Taste buds are epithelial organs of special sense (taste); most taste buds are found on lingual papillae; isolated ones may be found on the soft palate and on the walls of the pharynx
D. Connective tissue papillae form specialized lingual papillae
   1. Fungiform papillae—located on the dorsal aspect of the tongue; mushroom-shaped; a single taste bud may be present on the top surface
   2. Filiform papillae—most abundant of papillae; found covering the entire top surface of the tongue; have no taste buds; elongated in cases of "hairy" tongue
   3. Circumvallate papillae—large papillae located in a V-shaped groove at the base of the tongue; encircled by a deep groove; mushroom shaped; taste buds are located on their sides; small salivary glands (Ebner's glands) empty into surrounding grooves of taste buds

4. Foliate papillae—located along the sides of the tongue, near the base; taste buds may be located on only one of the sides
E. No submucosa is present

Tissues of the Tooth

Dentin

A. Mature dentin composition
  1. Chemical composition
    a. Organic matter, 18%
    b. Inorganic matter, 70%
    c. Water, 12%
  2. Tissue composition
    a. Cells—odontoblasts
    b. Fibrous material—collagen fibers (type I)
    c. Ground substance—proteoglycans and glycoproteins
  3. Calcification—deposition of crystals of the calcium salt hydroxyapatite in the dentin, fibrous matrix, and ground substance
B. Process of dentogenesis
  1. Dentin begins to form in the late bell stage of the developing tooth germ (see Figure 2-17)
  2. Newly differentiated odontoblasts deposit the dentin matrix; odontoblastic processes become surrounded by predentin (a newly deposited, uncalcified dentin matrix); predentin becomes calcified as cells deposit more dentin; predentin is adjacent to the pulp in young teeth
  3. Each cell process in mature calcified dentin is enclosed in a dentinal tubule (Figure 2-21)
    a. Dentinal tubules can run from the DEJ to the periphery of the dental pulp, where cell bodies of odontoblasts are located
    b. Tubules follow a primary S-shaped curve (pathway) and secondary S-shaped curves along the length of the tubules
      (1) Primary S-shaped curves are caused by the movement of odontoblasts from a wider area to a narrower area, which produces crowding of the odontoblasts; because of the S-shaped curved movement, odontoblasts adjust to the new crowding while moving back toward the dental pulp
      (2) Secondary S-shaped curves are seen along the length of the dentinal tubule as small waves in the tubules, about 4 μm apart; may possibly be reflecting changes in the movement of the odontoblasts during night and day
    c. Tubules tend to have more branching at their terminal ends in the crown of the tooth than in root dentin; root dentin has more lateral branching, with fewer primary S-shaped curves

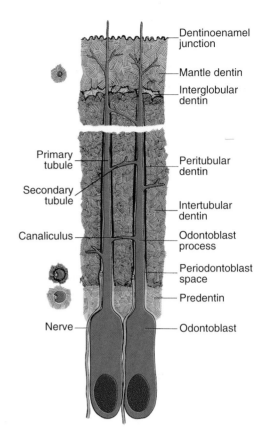

FIGURE 2-21 Odontoblastic process with its cell process enclosed in dentinal tubule. *(From Avery JK, Chiego DJ: Essentials of oral histology and embryology: A clinical approach, ed 3, St Louis, 2006, Mosby.)*

    d. Higher tubular density in peripheral dentin makes teeth particularly sensitive when exposed, almost as sensitive as the dentin near the pulp
    e. The diameter of tubules changes during the process of dentin formation; the widest dentinal tubules are found in children and are about 4 μm wide
  4. The first layer of dentin immediately adjacent to the DEJ is called *mantle dentin*; the remainder of the deposited dentin is called *circumpulpal dentin* (around the pulp)
    a. Mantle dentin
      (1) The layer of dentin that is about 10 to 30 μm thick
      (2) Differs from circumpulpal dentin because in addition to collagen fibers normally found in dentin, it contains a second group of thicker and heavier collagen fibers
        (a) These fibers are deposited perpendicular to the DEJ
        (b) These heavier collagen fibers are referred to as *Korff's fibers*

(3) Mantle dentin is less calcified than is circumpulpal dentin

   b. Circumpulpal dentin

     (1) Contains finer collagen fibers than does mantle dentin

     (2) Fibers are deposited parallel to the DEJ

5. Dentin that forms immediately around the odontoblastic process is called *peritubular dentin*

   a. Forms a sheath around each odontoblastic process about 1 μm thick

   b. Consists of a matrix of delicate collagen fibers

   c. Is highly calcified

   d. Is the first dentin to be decalcified by bacterial enzymes when exposed to caries

6. The remainder of dentin is called *intertubular dentin*

   a. Consists of large, coarse collagen fibers

   b. The matrix is less calcified than that of peritubular dentin

   c. Produced first by the odontoblast; then the odontoblast produces its peritubular dentin

7. Once dentin is deposited, it does not undergo any remodeling

C. Types

  1. Primary dentin—refers to dentin deposited before completion of the apical foramen

  2. Secondary dentin—refers to dentin formed after completion of the apical foramen; tends to be more calcified than primary dentin; forms at a slower rate

  3. Reactive (reparative) dentin—forms rapidly in localized areas where dental tubules have been exposed to external traumas such as:

   a. Dental caries

   b. Attrition or bruxism (enamel has been mechanically worn away)

   c. Thermal extremes

  4. Sclerotic dentin—forms when the dentinal fibers have degenerated and the tubules become filled with calcium salts

  5. Dead tracts—dentinal tubules that remain unfilled after dentinal fiber degeneration

  6. Interglobular dentin—small areas of unmineralized dentin near the DEJ

  7. Tomes' granular layer—small unmineralized areas of dentin beneath the cementum (may play a role in root sensitivity)

D. Sensory conduction

  1. Nerves associated with dentin are located in the dental pulp, but it is believed that they monitor the changes in the environment of odontoblasts, which allows for the perception of pain

  2. When dentinal tubules become exposed to the outside environment, a direct contact is made with the dental pulp; fluid in open, exposed tubules begins to evaporate, and the movement of fluid caused by evaporation may stimulate the nerves closest to odontoblasts to produce pain (dentinal hypersensitivity) (see the section titled "Control of Dentinal Hypersensitivity" in Chapter 16)

Pulp Tissue

A. Structure

  1. Most centrally located tissue in the tooth

  2. Loose connective tissue

  3. Cells

   a. Fibroblasts—undifferentiated mesenchymal cells

   b. Histiocytes—found along blood vessels; sometimes referred to as *macrophages* when filled with ingested materials

   c. Lymphocytes—when present, tend to be near the odontoblastic layer

   d. Cells present in diseased pulp include monocytes, polymorphonuclear leukocytes, eosinophils, and plasma cells

   e. No fat cells are present

  4. Structural arrangement

   a. The outer periphery of the pulp gives rise to the odontoblastic cell layer

   b. The layer subjacent to the odontoblastic layer is called the *cell-free zone*, or the *zone of Weil*

   c. Next to the cell-free zone is a relatively cell-rich zone

   d. The core of the pulp is centrally located

B. Functions

  1. Nutritive functions—very rich blood supply that forms a capillary plexus surrounding odontoblasts

  2. Formative function—peripheral layer of pulp cells gives rise to odontoblasts

  3. Sensory function—naked nerve fibers travel as free nerve endings and make contact with odontoblasts

  4. Protective function—the pulp can respond to stimuli that occur outside the tooth; response may trigger the formation of reactive dentin

C. Blood supply and nerves

  1. Blood vessels enter the pulp through the apical foramen; one or more small arterioles form a rich capillary plexus under the odontoblastic layer; exchange of nutrients occurs across the capillary wall

  2. Two types of nerve fibers enter the pulp:

   a. Autonomic nerve fibers—only the sympathetic autonomic nerve fibers are present; they regulate blood flow in the vessels

   b. Afferent nerve fibers—come from the second and third branches of the trigeminal nerve; they lose their myelin sheath and terminate as free nerve endings in close association with odontoblasts. It is thought that the presence of free nerve endings is responsible for the perception of pain by the dental pulp

D. Pulp changes
  1. Changes resulting from aging
    a. As the tooth ages, the amount of collagen fibers increases and the number of reticulin fibers decreases; in addition, the ground substance loses considerable water
    b. The pulp becomes less cellular and more fibrous
    c. The size of the pulp decreases because of the continued deposition of dentin
  2. Small calcified bodies, called *denticles*, may be present
    a. The three types of denticles are:
      (1) True denticles—form during tooth development in the root; have dentinal tubules in their structure; odontoblasts are present on the periphery
      (2) False denticles—form when the components of the pulp start to degenerate; calcify and grow into irregular calcified bodies; dentinal tubules are not usually present
      (3) Diffuse calcifications—occur in diseased pulp in many locations; are likely to grow and cause problems
    b. Both true and false denticles may be loose in the dental pulp, attached to the dentin wall, or embedded in the dentin tissue
    c. Calcified structures in the pulp appear radiopaque on radiographs

Comparison of Pulp and Dentin

A. Dentin and the dental pulp are closely related functionally and developmentally; both are products of the dental papilla (derived from neural crest cells)
B. Two major differences exist between these tissues:
  1. The pulp is a loose, noncalcified connective tissue; dentin is a highly specialized calcified connective tissue
  2. The pulp is a very vascular tissue; dentin is avascular
C. Dentin and the pulp form the bulk of the fully developed tooth
D. During tooth development, the peripheral cells of the dental papilla differentiate into odontoblasts and form dentin, while the core of the dental papilla becomes the pulp

Enamel

A. Composition
  1. Most highly calcified of all the dental tissues

  2. Composed mainly of inorganic calcium salt and hydroxyapatite, with a small amount of protein material and water in the matrix
    a. Inorganic component, 95%
    b. Organic component, 1%
    c. Water, 4%
B. Process of amelogenesis
  1. Enamel formation, like dentin formation, begins in the late bell stage of tooth development
  2. Shortly after the deposition of dentin, the inner enamel epithelial cells of the enamel organ become secretory ameloblasts
    a. Ameloblasts begin to deposit the enamel matrix, which is mineralized almost immediately
    b. Ameloblasts have tall columnar cell bodies that appear hexagonal in cross-section
    c. The secretory process of the ameloblast is shovel shaped and is called *Tomes' process*; the shape of the process is closely related to the form of the structural units that make up the fully developed enamel tissue
  3. Ameloblasts pass through two main stages while depositing enamel:
    a. Secretory stage—ameloblasts deposit the enamel matrix, which contains both organic and inorganic components
    b. Resorbing stage—ameloblasts remove most of the water and organic components from the matrix
  4. Enamel maturation begins before the completion of enamel formation
    a. First, very thin and needle-like hydroxyapatite crystals are deposited in the matrix
    b. During the process of enamel maturation, the crystals increase in all dimensions, which is made possible by the continual removal of water and organic components from the matrix
    c. The hydroxyapatite crystals in enamel are four times larger than those in bone, dentin, and cementum
C. Enamel rods—structural units of enamel
  1. Enamel is composed of tightly packed masses of hydroxyapatite crystals called *enamel rods*, or *prisms*
  2. Rod formation is related to the shape of the Tomes' process and the orientation of crystals as they are deposited by ameloblasts
  3. The prisms are rod-shaped structures that run from the DEJ to the outer edge of the enamel surface
  4. They are stacked in interlocking rows, one on top of the other; the stacking arrangement causes the rods to appear as keyhole-shaped prisms when viewed in cross-section, with the top of the

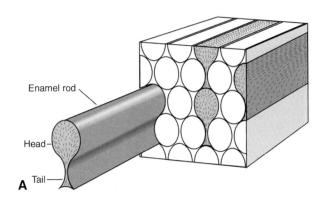

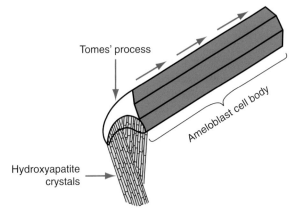

FIGURE 2-23 Ameloblast depositing hydroxyapatite crystals from the Tomes' process; note the angular change in the orientation of crystals being deposited, which accounts for the rod sheath around the head of the rod. *(Modified from Dr. Marlene Klyvert, Columbia University, School of Dental and Oral Surgery, New York.)*

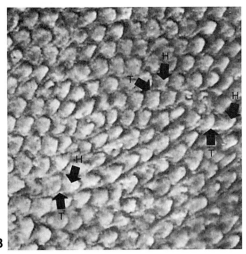

FIGURE 2-22 Enamel rod, the basic unit of enamel. **A,** Relationship of the rod to enamel. **B,** Scanning electron micrograph of enamel showing head (*H*) and tail (*T*). (*B, From Bath-Balogh MB, Fehrenbach MJ: Illustrated dental embryology, histology, and anatomy, ed 3, St Louis, 2011, Saunders.*)

keyhole facing the occlusal or incisal edge of the tooth and the tail facing the cervical portion; four ameloblasts contribute to form one keyhole (Figure 2-22)
5. The average width of an enamel rod is approximately 4 μm; the rods are narrower near the DEJ and wider near the outer surface of the enamel
6. The crystals in the head region of the rod are oriented with their long axis parallel to the long axis of the rod; in the tail region, crystals are perpendicular to the long axis of the rod
7. Adjacent rods are separated from each other by rod sheaths approximately 0.1 to 2.0 μm wide; they can be observed in the head region of the rods but are not as clearly defined in the tail region; and they are produced by an abrupt change in the angulation (orientation) of the crystals as they are deposited by the moving ameloblast (Figure 2-23)
8. Rodless enamel may be found near the DEJ and the outer surface of the enamel

9. The rods are perpendicular to the outer surface of the enamel; near the cervix of the tooth, they tend to be oriented apically; toward the inner third of the enamel, groups of rods curve but then straighten out to form right angles with the enamel surface
D. Microscopic structures
1. Bands of Hunter–Schreger—alternating light and dark bands; perpendicular to the DEJ; manifest as a result of enamel rod curvature
2. Stripes of Retzius—narrow brown lines that extend diagonally from enamel rods; on the tooth surface, they end in shallow furrows known as *perikymata*
3. Enamel lamellae—cracks that occur during enamel crystallization
4. Enamel tufts—hypomineralized inner ends of some enamel rods; located in the DEJ area
5. Enamel spindles—terminal portions of dentinal fibers that extend across the DEJ into the enamel
E. Clinical importance
1. Dental procedures performed on enamel
a. Application of fluoride—because enamel is semi-permeable, fluoride ions are attracted to the hydroxyapatite crystals; fluoride also changes hydroxyapatite into fluorapatite; the tooth becomes more resistant to acids produced by bacteria
b. Acid etching of enamel—the structure of enamel (rods and rod sheaths) allows acid to penetrate it for a limited distance (30 μm), and the acid attacks the mineral at the periphery of the sheaths; the acid thus creates a rough enamel surface, which helps bonding materials adhere more readily; the acid may

attack the rod core and produce the same effect

c. Cavity preparations—all rods are supported by dentin; margins will fail if enamel is left unsupported

2. Tetracycline stains

a. Appear clinically as dark bands through enamel, especially near the cervix of the tooth where enamel is thin

b. Caused by the administration of tetracycline (antibiotic) during the formation of teeth

c. Tetracycline binds chemically to organic and inorganic components of bone and dentin

d. The resulting darkened area shows through enamel, making the fully developed tooth appear unattractive

e. Stains are difficult to bleach out; affected teeth may need crowns or veneers, but only for aesthetic purposes

3. Pits and fissures in enamel

a. Are often present in less calcified areas

b. Form where ameloblasts become crowded between adjacent areas (cusps), resulting in incomplete maturation of enamel

c. Place teeth at increased risk for dental caries

d. Require the application of dental sealants to prevent caries and arrest incipient caries

Cementum

A. General properties and functions

1. Calcified connective tissue that covers the roots of teeth; in conjunction with the alveolar bone proper and the periodontal ligament, forms the attachment apparatus of the teeth, allowing the teeth to become suspended in the jaw

2. Derived from the dental sac (dental follicle)

3. Resembles bone in structure and composition; major differences are:

a. Bone is a vascularized tissue

b. Cementum is avascular

4. Least mineralized of the calcified tissues of the tooth

B. Mature cementum composition

1. Chemical composition

a. Organic components, 23%

b. Inorganic components, 65%

c. Water, 12%

2. Tissue composition

a. Cells—cementoblasts, cementocytes

b. Fibrous matrix—collagen fibers (type I); dominant component of the tissue, 90%

c. Ground substance—proteoglycans

C. Process of cementogenesis (Figure 2-24)

1. After crown formation is complete, the epithelial root sheath (*Hertwig's root sheath*) begins to grow down

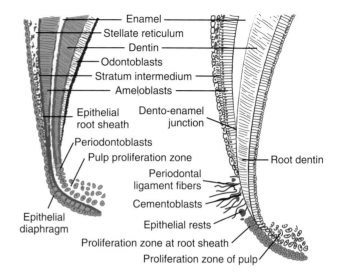

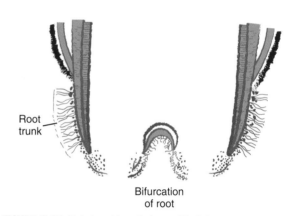

FIGURE 2-24 Relationship of the epithelial root sheath to the forming root and the formation of cementum.

a. Shapes the root of the tooth

b. Induces the formation of root dentin

2. After the first root dentin is deposited, the root sheath breaks down; cells from the dental sac migrate onto the newly deposited dentin and differentiate into cementoblasts

D. Mature cementum (fibrous matrix)

1. Very little cementum is deposited on the developing root until the tooth reaches functional occlusion (only approximately two thirds of the root has been formed when the tooth erupts)

2. Two groups of fibers are found in cementum:

a. Group I

(1) Collagen fibers produced by cementoblasts

(2) Fibers that form in the fibrous component of cementum

(3) Run parallel to the long axis of the root (internal fibers)

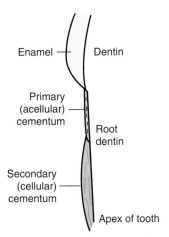

FIGURE 2-25 Relationship of the primary acellular cementum to the secondary (cellular) cementum, or root of tooth; note the thickness of the cellular cementum near the tooth apex.

   b. Group II
      (1) Fibers produced by cells from the dental sac
      (2) Fibers of the periodontal ligament (external fibers)
      (3) Insert into cementum at right angles to the DEJ or at right angles to the internal fibers of cementum
      (4) Coarser than internal fibers; cores of fibers remain uncalcified in the calcified cementum; referred to as *Sharpey's fibers*
E. Cellular and acellular cementum (Figure 2-25)
   1. Acellular cementum (primary cementum)
      a. Cervical half of the tooth is covered with a thin layer of cementum, approximately 10 μm thick
      b. Does not contain any embedded cementocytes (cementoblasts) in lacunae
      c. Forms at a slower rate than does cellular cementum
      d. Does not increase during the life of the tooth
      e. Appears to be involved more in maintenance than in the production of the tissue
      f. Contains less inorganic matrix than does cellular cementum
      g. Better calcified than cellular cementum
   2. Cellular cementum (secondary cementum)
      a. Apical portion of the tooth is covered with cellular cementum, reaching a thickness of 100 to 150 μm
      b. Contains cementocytes trapped in the lacunae of the tissue
      c. Deposited throughout the life of the tooth
      d. Deposited at intervals (pauses), producing arrest lines—highly calcified lines similar to those seen in bone tissue

F. Abnormalities
   1. Reversal lines
      a. May be present in cementum as in bone tissue
      b. Reflect resorption of tissue (remodeling)
      c. Resorption of cementum does not occur as frequently as in bone tissue; when it does occur, it is usually associated with:
         (1) Extreme orthodontic movement of the teeth
         (2) Trauma to teeth
   2. Cementicles
      a. Small, abnormal calcified bodies occasionally found in the periodontal ligament
      b. Result of cellular debris (i.e., degenerating remnants of the epithelial root sheath)
      c. May be found:
         (1) Attached to the cementum surface
         (2) Free in the periodontal ligament
         (3) Embedded in the cementum of the root
   3. Hypercementosis
      a. Local abnormal thickening of parts of the cementum
      b. Usually found in the apical region, occurring on one or all of the teeth
      c. May be seen in cases of:
         (1) Chronic inflammation of the tooth
         (2) Loss of an antagonist tooth (no opposing tooth in the jaw)
         (3) Additional eruption; compensatory cementosis takes place
         (4) Tooth becoming fused with the surrounding alveolar bone proper

Cemento-Enamel Junction
A. Three types of cemento-enamel relationships can occur during the development of the tooth
   1. Cementum meets enamel edge-to-edge—occurs in approximately 76% of all teeth
   2. Cementum overlaps a small part of enamel—occurs in approximately 14% of all teeth
   3. Cementum is ditched with no exposed dentin—occurs in approximately 10% of all teeth
B. Cemento-enamel relationships occur when root–cementum development begins; this is related to the timing of the disruption (breakdown) of the epithelial root sheath and allows the cells from the dental sac to differentiate and begin depositing cementum
C. Differentiation of root dental papillae into odontoblasts is mediated by a cell-to-matrix type of inductive interaction (between the basal lamina of Hertwig's root sheath and the undifferentiated root dental papilla)
D. Differentiation of dental sac cells into cementoblasts is mediated by a cell-substrate type of inductive interaction between sac cells and newly deposited dentin

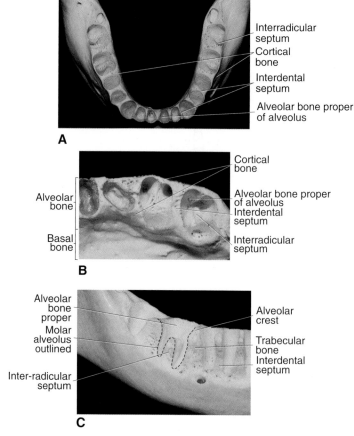

FIGURE 2-26 Components of alveolar bone.
A, Mandibular arch of the skull with teeth removed.
B, Portion of the maxilla of a skull with teeth removed.
C, Cross-section of mandible with teeth removed.
(From Bath-Balogh MB, Fehrenbach MJ: Illustrated dental embryology, histology, and anatomy, ed 3, St Louis, 2011, Saunders.)

E. Practicing dental hygienists should use caution during instrumentation in areas where cementum is thin or absent; conservation of tooth structure is recommended

F. Recession of gingiva and loss of clinical attachment may also leave exposed cementum or dentin, creating root sensitivity and increased risk of root caries

Supporting Tissues

Alveolar Bone

A. The part of the bony maxilla and mandible, the alveolar process, in which teeth are suspended in alveoli (bony sockets)

B. Existence or presence of alveolar bone is totally dependent on the presence of dental roots; when teeth do not develop and erupt, alveolar bone does not develop; when teeth are extracted, alveolar bone is resorbed

C. Formed during the development and eruption of teeth; developing teeth, primary or permanent, are located in bony crypts in the bone of the maxilla or of the mandible

D. Has the same biophysical and chemical properties as other bone tissue in the body; has the same basic components as other connective tissue

1. Cells—osteoblasts, osteocytes, osteoclasts
2. Fibrous matrix—collagen fibers are the dominant component; calcified by deposition of the calcium salt hydroxyapatite into the matrix
3. Ground substance—proteoglycans

E. Gross anatomy of a mature bone socket (Figure 2-26)
   1. Each tooth is suspended in its own alveolus (socket), with each alveolus having the same structure and anatomy
      a. Outer cortical (compact lamellar) plate of bone—faces the cheek and lips (buccal)
      b. Inner cortical (compact lamellar) plate of bone—faces the tongue and palate (lingual)
      c. Spongiosa—cancellous bone sandwiched between the cortical plates of bone
   2. Alveolar bone proper—the part of the alveolus directly facing the root of the tooth; follows the general outline of the root; sometimes referred to as the *cribriform plate*, or *lamina dura*
      a. Cribriform plate
         (1) Contains numerous small openings; allows blood vessels and nerves in the periodontal ligament and bone to communicate

(2) Consists of two layers of bone:
    (a) Compact lamellar bone
    (b) Layer of bundle bone into which the periodontal fibers insert themselves; the cores of the fibers remain uncalcified in the calcified tissues of bone or cementum—called *Sharpey's fibers*

  b. *Lamina dura* is purely a radiographic term based on the fact that this area appears more radiopaque on radiographs; it is not more calcified than the rest of the bone socket; rather, the opacity is caused by the two-dimensional view of the compact bone in the area

  c. Alveolar bone proper that forms sockets around multiple-rooted teeth consists of the cribriform plates of both roots and some spongy bone, called *inter-radicular alveolar bone*

  d. The alveolar bone proper between teeth consists of the cribriform plates of both teeth and some spongy bone, called *interdental alveolar bone*

  e. Spongiosa is composed of small trabeculae of bone with large narrow spaces between the trabeculae

3. The alveolar bone proper (cribriform plate) is the only essential part of the bone socket; spongiosa and outer and inner cortical plates of bone are not always present; spongiosa may be absent, and outer and inner cortical plates may be fused together

4. Trabeculae of the spongiosa reflect functional forces or loading patterns imposed on teeth; the pattern changes when the forces are altered; two principal directions of the trabeculae are parallel and perpendicular to the direction of the imposed forces; trabecular bone orientation can be observed on radiographs; the number of trabeculae increases with increased function

5. Orthodontic movement of teeth always causes remodeling of the alveolar bone proper to accommodate movement of teeth; it affects the insertion of periodontal ligament fibers in the bundle bone but is a localized type of resorption; when the bundle bone is redeposited, fibers become firmly attached again; with pressure, bone is resorbed; when tension is applied, bone formation occurs

6. Radiographs of teeth may be used to show the height, slope, or both, of the interdental bone septum, which may reflect periodontal disease or other disease; the crest of the alveolar bone is usually between 0.75 mm and 1.49 mm from the cemento-enamel junction

7. The periosteum is a dense connective tissue layer on the outer portion of bone and is active in bone formation. The endosteum lines the inner aspects (medullary cavity) of bone

F. Alveolar bone is constantly remodeled by means of resorption and formation; this makes it the least stable of periodontal tissues
  1. Alveolar bone is affected by function, age-related and disease-related changes, hormones, and other systemic and host factors
  2. Remodeling affects the height, contour, and density of alveolar bone

Periodontal Ligament

A. A specialized form of connective tissue derived from the dental sac, which contributes to the attachment of teeth

B. Made up of groups of fiber bundles called *gingival fibers* and principal fiber bundles; areas of loose connective tissue, blood vessels, and nerves are present between principal fiber bundles; areas of loose connective tissue are called *interstitial spaces*

C. Tissue components
  1. Fibroblasts of the periodontal ligament (PDL) are responsible for the production of the fibrous matrix and the ground substance; they are continually engaged in synthetic activities, rebuilding and producing new fibers to be incorporated into existing fibers, which are constantly being remodeled; PDL has a very fast turnover rate
  2. Ground substance—proteoglycans
  3. The fibrous matrix is the dominant component of the PDL
    a. The fibers are collagen and oxytalan, with a few elastic fibers associated with blood vessels
    b. The fibers are arranged in dense bundles inserted into the alveolar bone proper and cementum
    c. The fibers are arranged into two groups:
      (1) Gingival fiber groups (Figure 2-27, *B*; see also Chapter 14, Figure 14-2):
        (a) Dento-gingival fibers—extend from the cervical cementum to the free gingiva and from the cervical cementum to the lamina propria of the gingiva, over the alveolar crest
        (b) Dento-periosteal fibers—extend from cervical cementum over the alveolar crest to the periosteum of the cortical plates of bone
        (c) Trans-septal fibers—extend from the cementum of the tooth to the adjacent tooth, over the alveolar crest
        (d) Circular fibers—extend horizontally around the most cervical part of the root and insert themselves into the

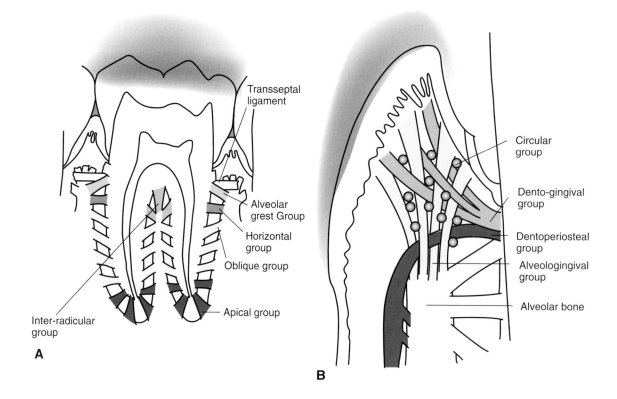

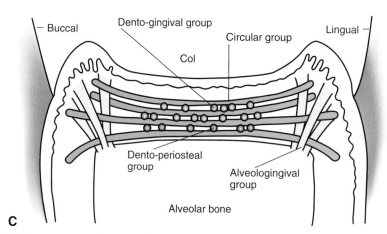

FIGURE 2-27 Connective tissue fibers. **A,** Principal fiber groups of the periodontal ligament. **B,** Gingival fiber groups. **C,** Gingival ligament fibers in the col area. *(Modified from Ten Cate AR: Oral histology: development, structure, and function, ed 6, St Louis, 2003, Mosby.)*

cementum and lamina propria of the gingiva and the alveolar crest

(2) Principal fiber groups (see Figure 2-27, *A;* see also Chapter 14, Figure 14-4):
   (a) Alveolar crest fibers—extend from cervical cementum and insert themselves into the alveolar crest
   (b) Horizontal fibers—extend at right angles to the long axis of the root of the tooth in a horizontal plane from

alveolar bone to cementum; found in the cervical third of the root

(c) Oblique fibers—slant occlusally from cementum to alveolar bone; most abundant of the fiber bundles; start at the apical two thirds of the root
(d) Apical fibers—radiate from apical cementum into alveolar bone
(e) Inter-radicular fibers (seen only in multiple-rooted teeth)—extend from

the cementum in the furcation area of the tooth to the inter-radicular alveolar bone

    d. Sharpey's fibers—the terminal portion of a PDL fiber that is embedded in bone and cementum

    e. Fiber groups are oriented to give the tooth optimal resistance to all kinds of functional loading patterns

      (1) Circular fibers resist rotational movements of the tooth (see Figure 2-27, C)

      (2) Alveolar crest and apical fibers resist pull of the tooth from its socket

      (3) Trans-septal fibers connect all teeth and maintain the integrity of the dental arches

    f. Elastic fibers in the PDL do not contribute to the support of the tooth; the role of the oxytalan fibers is not clear

D. Blood vessels

    1. The blood supply of the PDL is very rich and highly developed, more than in any other connective tissue; blood vessels are found in the interstitial spaces of the ligament

    2. Each tooth, with its PDL and alveolar bone, has a common blood supply; a small artery branches off the main artery that supplies the jaw and enters the following:

      a. Apical foramen of the tooth—which supplies the pulp of the tooth

      b. Periodontal ligament—which supplies the areas all around the tooth

      c. Alveolar bone of the tooth

    3. Once blood vessels enter the pulp chambers, they are isolated from surrounding tissues, but vessels supplying the PDL and alveolar bone are richly interconnected via openings in the cribriform plate

E. Nerves

    1. The PDL contains two types of nerves:

      a. Autonomic—sympathetic fibers that travel with blood vessels; these regulate blood flow to the tissues

      b. Afferent sensory fibers—mostly myelinated nerves from the branches of the second and third divisions of the trigeminal nerve (fifth cranial nerve)

    2. Two types of nerve endings are found in the PDL:

      a. Free, unmyelinated nerve endings—responsible for pain sensation

      b. Encapsulated nerve endings—responsible for registering pressure changes

F. The width of the PDL varies with the functional forces placed on the tooth and at different levels of the root (apex and cervix)

    1. The width is greater in young adults (0.21 mm) than in older adults (0.15 mm)

    2. The width is greater near the cervical and apical areas than in the middle of the root

    3. Minimal movement (rotations) of any tooth occurs around the axis in the middle of the root; greatest movement occurs near the apex and the cervix, accounting for the difference in the width of the PDL along the root

    4. The width is related to the amount of function and cellularity; an actively functioning tooth has a slightly wider PDL and more cellularity than does a nonfunctioning tooth

G. Abnormalities

    1. Cementicles

    2. Epithelial rests (cell rests of Malassez)

      a. Remnants of the epithelium from the root sheath that did not disintegrate; formed from a cluster of epithelial cells surrounded by a basement membrane

      b. In most cases, these rests are harmless, but they have the potential to become cystic

    3. Untreated periodontal disease can result in damage to the supporting apparatus of the tooth and eventual loss of the tooth

Dento-Gingival Junction

A. The area on the tooth where enamel and the epithelium form a junction; with aging, the junction is displaced more apically between cementum and the epithelium

B. First established as the tooth emerges into the oral cavity (Figure 2-28)

    1. Developing tooth is covered with reduced enamel epithelium (REE), consisting of:

      a. A layer of outer enamel epithelial cells

      b. Remnants of the stratum intermedium cell layers

      c. Stellate reticulum

      d. Postsecretory ameloblasts

    2. Basal cells of oral epithelium covering the emerging tooth and outer layer of cells of the REE begin to proliferate. They soon grow together to form one continuous unit. As the tooth emerges through the combined epithelia, it forms the initial dento-gingival junction on the enamel of the tooth

C. Dento-junctional epithelium

    1. Gingival epithelium that faces the tooth

    2. Composed of nonkeratinized stratified squamous epithelium without rete pegs and divided into:

      a. Sulcular epithelium

        (1) Found occlusally at the same height as the free gingiva

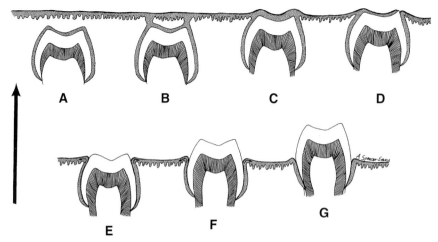

FIGURE 2-28 Tooth emerging into the oral cavity. Note that the reduced enamel epithelium covering the tooth joins the oral epithelium. The reduced enamel epithelium will form the initial junctional epithelium. **A,** Crown penetrating bone and connective tissue. **B,** Contact of crown with oral epithelium. **C,** Fusion of epithelia. **D,** Thinning of the epithelium. **E,** Rupture of the epithelium. **F,** Crown emergence. **G,** Occlusal contact. *(From Avery JK, Chiego DJ: Essentials of oral histology and embryology: A clinical approach, ed 3, St Louis, 2006, Mosby.)*

(2) The sulcus forms a shallow pocket around the tooth, about 0.5 mm deep

(3) In the disease state, the sulcus deepens and exhibits rete pegs and ulcerations

b. Junctional epithelium (see Figures 2-28 and 2-29)

(1) Begins at the base of the sulcus

(2) Firmly attached to the tooth, enamel, cementum, or all by hemidesmosomes

(3) Located between two basal laminae:

(a) One basal lamina faces the enamel surface

(b) The second basal lamina faces the connective tissue of the gingiva

(c) Basal laminae are continuous at the base of the junctional epithelium (see Figure 2-29)

3. A membrane called the *primary cuticle* intervenes between the basal lamina of the junctional epithelium and the tooth surface

a. The primary cuticle is formed during the late stages of eruption of the tooth

b. The composition of the cuticle is not known, but the cuticle thickens with aging

4. The newly erupted tooth is covered with a thin, delicate membrane called *Nasmyth's membrane*

a. Will float off of the tooth surface if placed in a 10% solution of hydrochloric acid

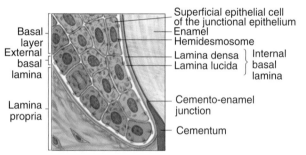

FIGURE 2-29 The epithelial attachment is the part of the junctional epithelium that attaches the junctional epithelium to the tooth surface. Note that the outer external basal lamina is continuous with the inner basal lamina, and between them are the cells of the junctional epithelium. *(From Bath-Balogh M, Fehrenbach MJ: Illustrated dental embryology, histology, and anatomy, ed 3, St Louis, 2011, Saunders.)*

b. Contains some cells of the REE and the dental cuticle

5. In the area of the dento-gingival junction, the junctional epithelium has the capacity to repair itself

6. The site of the dento-gingival junction is easily invaded by microorganisms and is the area where periodontal disease often begins

7. For a review of the histology, see the table below.

WEB SITE INFORMATION AND RESOURCES

SOURCE	WEB SITE ADDRESS	DESCRIPTION
University of Pennsylvania and Temple University 1999	http://www.dental.pitt.edu/informatics/periohistology/en/guin01m.htm	Histology slides of periodontal tissues and quiz questions
Leeds University	http://www.dentistry.leeds.ac.uk/oroface/virtlab/histolab/histintr.html	Pictures of ground sections and slides
University of North Carolina at Chapel Hill	http://www.med.unc.edu/embryo_images/	Images and text on normal and abnormal human embryology

SUGGESTED READINGS

Avery JK, Chiego DJ: *Essentials of oral histology and embryology*, ed 3, St Louis, 2006, Mosby.

Bath-Balogh M, Fehrenbach MJ: *Dental embryology, histology and anatomy*, ed 3, St Louis, 2011, Saunders.

Galilis KA: Anatomy and histology quizzes, University of Western Ontario Department of Anatomy and Cell Biology: http://www.drgalil.ca: Accessed April 18, 2010.

Ibsen OAC, Phelan JA: *Oral pathology for the dental hygienist*, ed 5, St Louis, 2009, Saunders.

University of Oklahoma College of Dentistry: Oral histology slides: http://dentistry.ouhsc.edu/oral-histology: Accessed April 18, 2010.

CHAPTER 2 REVIEW QUESTIONS

Answers and rationales to chapter review questions are available on this text's accompanying Evolve site. See inside front cover for details.
Use Case A to answer questions 1 to 8.
Use Case B to answer questions 9 to 23.
Use Case C to answer questions 24 to 36.

evolve

CASE A

A 28-year-old client has a mandibular labial oral piercing. On oral assessment, she exhibits a palpable nodule in the area of the piercing. She states that she noticed the "little lump" about a year after she received the piercing. She received the mandibular labial and tongue piercings approximately 2 years ago. She does not remember biting her lip. She has come to the dental office because she chipped the enamel of her mandibular central incisor and she is experiencing dentinal hypersensitivity.

1. **The nodule in the area of the labial piercing is diagnosed as a cyst. A cyst is all of the following EXCEPT:**
   a. An abnormal pathologic sac
   b. A cavity lined by epithelial tissue
   c. Enclosed by connective tissue
   d. Diagnosed on the basis of histologic appearance and location
   e. Composed entirely of connective tissue

2. **The client habitually removed the labial piercing during the first year after she received the piercing. The layer of stratified squamous epithelium that constantly undergoes mitosis was pushed down into the underlying connective tissue. These epithelial cells served as the source of cyst formation. In which layer of the epidermis are cells undergoing mitosis most likely to be seen?**
   a. Stratum basal
   b. Stratum luciderm
   c. Stratum corneum
   d. Stratum spinosum
   e. Stratum granulosum

3. **The sensitivity of the client's mandibular incisors is MOST likely related to:**
   a. Fluid entering the sulcular epithelium
   b. Fluid entering the rodless enamel
   c. Fluid entering the dentinal tubules
   d. Fluid entering the lacuna of the cementum

4. **Of the following tissues, which one or more have nerve innervations?**
   a. Dentin and enamel
   b. Enamel and cementum
   c. Pulp and periodontal ligament
   d. Dentin, pulp and periodontal ligament
   e. Enamel, dentin, pulp and periodontal ligament

5. **Because of the proximity of odontoblastic cell bodies to nerve terminal endings in the tooth, clinical exposure of dentin may result in sensitivity. What is the location of the odontoblastic bodies?**
   a. Dentin
   b. Pulp
   c. Enamel
   d. Cementum
   e. Periodontal ligament

6. **Some loss of enamel is evident on the lingual aspects of the client's maxillary central incisors because of their contact with the lingual piercing. The tooth structure loss that occurs from pathologic wear of teeth by foreign substance is called:**
   a. Attrition
   b. Erosion
   c. Abfraction
   d. Abrasion
   e. Dental caries

7. **Bone loss is noted on the periapical radiograph of the mandibular incisors. The crest of the alveolar bone is usually apical to the cemento-enamel junction (CEJ) by:**
   a. The CEJ
   b. 0.75 to 1.49 mm
   c. 3 mm to 4 mm
   d. 4 mm to 5 mm
   e. 0.5 mm

8. **When a cyst shows up radiographically, it has a well-defined border; this cyst of the mandibular labial tissue will show up radiographically.**
   a. Both statements are true
   b. Both statements are false
   c. The first statement is true; the second is false
   d. The first statement is false; the second is true

CASE B

A 48-year-old woman is being treated by the dental hygienist for the first time. She states that she is in very good health. Clinical examination reveals generalized bleeding of the gingiva with generalized rolled margins, bulbous interdental papillae, and no signs of inflammation of the attached gingiva. A 1-mm zone of attached gingiva on the facials of the mandibular central incisors and a class

l furcation on the facial of tooth #30 are noted. She has a 7-mm clinical attachment loss reading on the facial of #30. Radiographs do not reveal the furcation, but a radiopacity that is continuous with the coronal enamel and extends into the furcation is noted. No other attachment loss or bone loss is noted throughout the mouth. Occlusal evaluation reveals no premature contacts or signs of tooth wear.

9. **The tissue lining of an unhealthy gingival sulcus consists of:**
   a. Keratinized epithelium with rete pegs
   b. Keratinized epithelium without rete pegs
   c. Nonkeratinized epithelium with rete pegs
   d. Nonkeratinized epithelium without rete pegs
   e. Parakeratinized epithelium with rete pegs

10. **The bottom of the gingival sulcus is marked by the:**
    a. Marginal gingiva
    b. Junctional epithelium
    c. Alveolar crest
    d. Sulcular epithelium
    e. Periodontal ligament

11. **Which of the following tissues have little or no keratinization?**
    a. Attached gingiva
    b. Interdental papilla
    c. Lingual papilla
    d. Hard palate
    e. Sulcular epithelium

12. **What does bleeding caused by probing indicate?**
    a. Loss of crestal bone
    b. An increase in gingival vasculature
    c. Fibrosis in the connective tissue
    d. Ulceration of crevicular epithelium
    e. Apical migration of junctional epithelium

13. **Which of the following tissue changes result in erythematous gingiva?**
    a. Increased keratinization
    b. Presence of inflammatory cells
    c. Increased vascularization
    d. Increased production of collagen
    e. Necrosis of epithelium

14. **What type of connective tissue underlies the epithelium of the gingival?**
    a. Reticular
    b. Elastic
    c. Fibrous
    d. Submucosa
    e. Oxytalan

15. **In gingivitis, poor tissue tone is caused by:**
    a. Bleeding
    b. Dilation of blood vessels
    c. Destruction of collagen fibers
    d. Large numbers of inflammatory cells

16. **The MOST likely periodontal diagnosis for this client would be:**
    a. Generalized severe chronic periodontitis
    b. Generalized severe chronic gingivitis
    c. Generalized moderate chronic gingivitis with localized area of severe chronic periodontitis
    d. Generalized moderate chronic periodontitis with localized severe chronic periodontitis
    e. Generalized mild chronic periodontitis

17. **The possible cause of the furcation involvement on the facial area of #30 is:**
    a. Enamel projection onto the root surface
    b. Palato-gingival groove
    c. Occlusal trauma
    d. Frena pull
    e. None of the above; no furcation involvement is noted radiographically

18. **Definitive diagnosis of furcation involvement is made by:**
    a. Clinical probing
    b. Reviewing the client's history
    c. Checking the mobility of the tooth
    d. Inspecting the radiographs of the area

19. **Enamel projections on the root surface are attributed to the differentiation of:**
    a. Cementoblasts
    b. Enamel spindles
    c. Primary enamel cuticle
    d. Enamel tufts
    e. Hertwig's epithelial root sheath

20. **Hertwig's epithelial root sheath is derived from the:**
    a. Inner enamel epithelium
    b. Reduced enamel epithelium
    c. Primary enamel cuticle
    d. Rests of Malassez
    e. Periodontal ligament

21. **Hertwig's epithelial root sheath is entirely composed of:**
    a. All layers of the enamel organ
    b. Enamel organ and dental papilla
    c. Inner and outer cells of the dental papilla
    d. Inner and outer enamel epithelium
    e. Dental papilla and dental sac

22. **When is root formation completed?**
    a. On tooth eruption
    b. 2 to 3 months after eruption
    c. 6 to 8 months after eruption
    d. 1 to 4 years after eruption
    e. Never

23. **Remnants of Hertwig's epithelial root sheath found in the periodontal ligament of a functioning tooth are called:**
    a. Enamel pearls
    b. Denticles
    c. Rests of Malassez
    d. Cementicles
    e. Intermediate plexus

CASE C

A 12-year-old client with orthodontics has generalized healthy gingiva that is coral pink and stippled. The orthodontist has stated that the tooth movement is on schedule. Some recession is noted on the maxillary left canine and the first premolar. The first premolar demonstrates some mobility. Orthodontic tooth movement involves the function of the periodontal ligament, cementum, and alveolar bone.

24. **The stippled texture of the gingiva may be attributed to:**
    a. Keratinization
    b. Connective tissue projections
    c. Presence of submucosa
    d. Optimal blood supply
    e. Pigmentation

25. **The color of the gingiva may be attributed to all of the following EXCEPT one. Which one is the EXCEPTION?**
    a. Keratinization
    b. Connective tissue projections
    c. Thickness of the epithelium
    d. Blood supply
    e. Pigmentation

26. **During orthodontic treatment, pressure applied to the periodontal ligament is intended to produce bone formation. Pressure on the periodontal ligament stimulates bone formation.**
    a. Both statements are TRUE
    b. Both statements are FALSE
    c. The first statement is TRUE; the second statement is FALSE
    d. The first statement is FALSE; the second statement is TRUE

27. **A specialized periosteum which forms and resorbs bone and cementum is called:**
    a. Circumferential bone
    b. Endosteum
    c. Cortical bone
    d. Lamina dura
    e. Periodontal ligament

28. **Cementum resorbs less readily than does bone. Cementoid, the outer, less calcified layer of cemental tissue, results in cementum resorbing less readily than bone.**
    a. Both statements are TRUE
    b. Both statements are FALSE
    c. The first statement is TRUE; the second statement is FALSE
    d. The first statement is FALSE; the second statement is TRUE

29. **Cementum is a product of:**
    a. Periodontal ligament
    b. Dentin
    c. Pulp
    d. Hertwig's root sheath
    e. Alveolar bone

30. **The outer, less calcified layer of cementum is called:**
    a. Cellular cementum
    b. Acellular cementum
    c. Cementoid
    d. Cementicles
    e. Sharpey's fibers

31. **Which of the following cells does the periodontal ligament contain?**
    a. Fibroblasts and osteocytes
    b. Osteoclasts and cementoblasts
    c. Cementocytes and fibroblasts
    d. Osteocytes and cementocytes
    e. Osteoblasts and osteocytes

32. The maxillary right canine and the first premolar were orthodontically moved labially outside of the outer cortical plate. A cleft-like absence of the alveolar cortical plate resulting in a denuded root surface is called:
    a. Lability
    b. Physiologic migration
    c. Dehiscence
    d. Fenestration

33. Which of the following are characteristics of bundle bone (the alveolar bone proper)?
    a. Covered by endosteum and adjacent to periodontal ligament
    b. Adjacent to periodontal ligament and adjacent to fatty marrow
    c. Adjacent to fatty marrow and containing Sharpey's fibers
    d. Adjacent to the periodontal ligament and containing Sharpey's fibers

34. Which of the following tissues of the normal periodontium is the alveolar bone directly adjacent to?
    a. Periodontal ligament and gingival epithelium
    b. Cementum, epithelial attachment, and gingival epithelium
    c. Periodontal ligament and gingival connective tissue
    d. Periodontal ligament and epithelial attachment
    e. Periodontal ligament and cementum

35. Alveolar bone is the most stable of all periodontal tissues. Pressures used in orthodontic therapy encourage the bone to be stable.
    a. Both statements are TRUE
    b. Both statements are FALSE
    c. The first statement is TRUE; the second statement is FALSE
    d. The first statement is FALSE; the second statement is TRUE

36. Through tooth movement, the periodontal ligament fibers must be reoriented. The cells that are important in the formation of the principal fibers of the periodontal ligament are:
    a. Cementoblasts
    b. Cementoclasts
    c. Osteoblasts
    d. Osteoclasts
    e. Fibroblasts

37. The types of epithelia found lining the oral cavity include:
    a. Simple and stratified squamous
    b. Stratified, cuboidal, and squamous
    c. Keratinized, simple, and stratified squamous
    d. Keratinized and nonkeratinized stratified squamous

38. Epithelial tissues are characterized by:
    a. Much intercellular substance and few cells
    b. No intercellular substance
    c. Little intercellular substance and many cells
    d. Intercellular substance in surface layer only

39. Embryonically, the mandible is derived from the:
    a. Stomodeum
    b. First branchial arch
    c. Frontal process
    d. Second branchial arch
    e. Third branchial arch

40. The anterior portion, or body, of the tongue develops from the:
    a. Second branchial arch
    b. Maxillary process
    c. Mandibular process
    d. Globular process
    e. Rathke's pouch

41. A cleft lip occurs when the maxillary process fails to fuse with the:
    a. Palatine process
    b. Globular process
    c. Lateral nasal process
    d. Mandibular process
    e. Opposing maxillary process

42. One of the first structures of the face to develop in the primitive embryo is the:
    a. Mandible
    b. Nose
    c. Stomodeum
    d. Maxilla
    e. First branchial arch

43. The lateral palatine processes initially grow downward toward the future floor of the mouth. This is caused by the presence of the:
    a. Tongue
    b. Nasal septum
    c. Maxillary process
    d. Premaxilla
    e. Mandibular process

44. When a cleft of the alveolar process is present, it occurs between the:
    a. First and second premolars
    b. Central incisors
    c. Lateral incisor and canine
    d. Canine and first premolar
    e. Central and lateral incisor

45. The cementum is derived from the:
    a. Reduced enamel epithelium
    b. Dental papilla
    c. Outer enamel epithelium
    d. Dental sac
    e. Alveolar bone

46. During embryonic development, neural crest cells migrate to the branchial arches and surround the:
   a. Ectoderm
   b. Mesoderm
   c. Endoderm
   d. Ectoderm, mesoderm, *and* endoderm

47. All of the following tooth tissues are derived from the mesoderm EXCEPT one. Which one is the EXCEPTION?
   a. Enamel
   b. Dentin
   c. Cementum
   d. Periodontal ligament
   e. Alveolar bone

48. Which of the following is NOT part of the enamel organ?
   a. Outer enamel epithelium
   b. Dental papilla
   c. Stratum intermedium
   d. Inner enamel epithelium
   e. Stellate reticulum

49. The periodontal ligament is derived from the:
   a. Dental sac
   b. Dental papilla
   c. Dental lamina
   d. Cementum
   e. Alveolar bone

50. Dentin is a product of the:
   a. Dental lamina
   b. Dental organ
   c. Dental papilla
   d. Dental cuticle
   e. Dental sac

Anatomy and Physiology

Christine Blue

Anatomy and physiology are subjects that focus on the organization, structure, and function of the human body. Dental hygienists use knowledge of anatomy and physiology most often during client assessment, treatment, and evaluation; during oral radiographic and pathologic examinations; and for the administration of local anesthetic agents. This knowledge also allows the dental hygienist to determine whether clients are functioning within normal limits, deviating from the normal, or presenting with structures that are ectopic. Moreover, this knowledge enables dental hygienists to link systemic and oral health and disease. This chapter covers basic concepts; definitions of terms, cell structure, and function; and body systems, including the skeletal, muscular, nervous, circulatory, lymphatic, digestive, endocrine, urinary, and reproductive systems.

BASIC CONCEPTS

Anatomy

A. Study of the structure of an organism and the relationships of its parts; derived from the Greek word meaning "the act of cutting up." Dissection is the principal technique used to isolate and study the structural components of the body
B. Branches of anatomy
   1. Gross anatomy—study of structures that can be identified with the naked eye (see Chapter 4)
   2. Microscopic anatomy—study of cells (cytology) and tissues (histology) (see Chapter 2)
   3. Developmental anatomy (embryology)—study of human growth and development (see Chapter 2)

Physiology

A. Study of body functions—how the body parts work

Levels of Organization

See Figure 3-1.
A. Chemical level—organization of chemical structure separates living and nonliving material; atoms, molecules, and macromolecules result in living matter
B. Organelle level—organelles are structures made of molecules and organized to perform specific functions; allow the cell to perform vital functions; types include:
   1. Mitochondria
   2. Golgi apparatus
   3. Endoplasmic reticulum
C. Cellular level—cells comprise the basic structural and functional units of an organism; the smallest living units in the human body
   1. Nucleus surrounded by cytoplasm within a limiting membrane
   2. Differentiate to perform unique functions
D. Tissue level—groups of cells and materials surrounding them that work together to perform a particular function
   1. Four major tissue types:
      a. Epithelial tissue
      b. Connective tissue
      c. Muscle tissue
      d. Nervous tissue
E. Organ level—different types of tissues joined together to form body structures
   1. Each organ has a unique size, shape, appearance, and placement in the body (e.g., stomach, heart, liver, lungs, brain)
F. System level—related organs that have a common function (e.g., digestive system breaks down and absorbs molecules in food; organs include the mouth, salivary glands, pharynx, esophagus, stomach, liver, gallbladder, pancreas, small intestine, and large intestine)

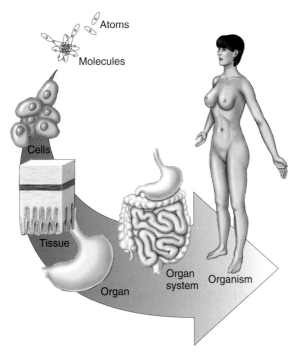

FIGURE 3-1 Levels of organization, from simple to complex; from atom to human organism. *(From Herlihy B: The human body in health and illness, ed 4, St Louis, 2011, Saunders.)*

G. Organism level—all the systems of the body combine to make up an organism

Anatomic Nomenclature

(See the section on "Anatomic Nomenclature" in Chapter 4.)

A. Anatomic position—erect body position with arms at the sides and palms upward (Figure 3-2)

B. Plane or section—imaginary flat surfaces that pass through the body (Figure 3-3)

  1. Sagittal plane—vertical plane dividing the body into right and left sides; midsagittal plane bisects the body at the exact midline

  2. Coronal or frontal plane—divides the body or organ into anterior and posterior portions

  3. Transverse plane—divides the body or organ into superior and inferior portions (may also be called *cross-sectional* or *horizontal plane*)

Body Cavities

See Figure 3-4.

A. Dorsal cavity

  1. Cranial cavity—formed by the cranial bones of the skull; contains the brain

  2. Vertebral cavity—formed by the vertebrae; contains the spinal cord

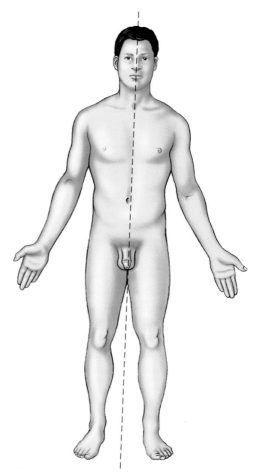

FIGURE 3-2 Anatomic position and bilateral symmetry. *(Modified from Herlihy B: The human body in health and illness, ed 4, St Louis, 2011, Saunders.)*

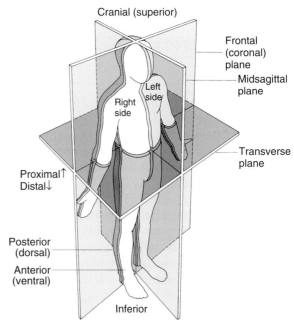

FIGURE 3-3 Directions and planes of the body. *(Modified from Solomon EP: Introduction to human anatomy and physiology, ed 2, St Louis, 2008, Saunders.)*

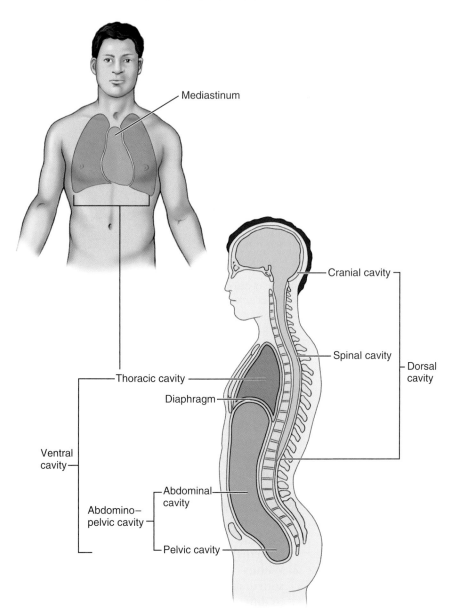

FIGURE 3-4 Major body cavities. *(From Herlihy B: The human body in health and illness, ed 4, St Louis, 2011, Saunders.)*

B. Ventral cavity
   1. Thoracic (chest) cavity comprises the upper portion
      a. Pericardial cavity—contains the heart
      b. Pleural cavities—contain the lungs
      c. Mediastinum—mass of tissue between pleural cavities; contains all thoracic viscera except the lungs; includes the heart, esophagus, trachea, and several large blood vessels
   2. Abdomino-pelvic cavity
      a. Upper (abdominal) cavity contains the stomach, spleen, liver, gallbladder, small intestine, and most of the large intestine
      b. Lower (pelvic) cavity contains the bladder, rectum, sigmoid, and reproductive organs

CELLS

(See the section on "General Histology" in Chapter 2.)

Cellular Structure

See Figure 3-5.
A. Plasma or cell membrane
   1. Surrounds and contains the cytoplasm of a cell; composed of proteins and lipids
   2. Selective permeability characteristics
      a. Protects cell from external environment
      b. Permits the entrance and exit of selected substrates

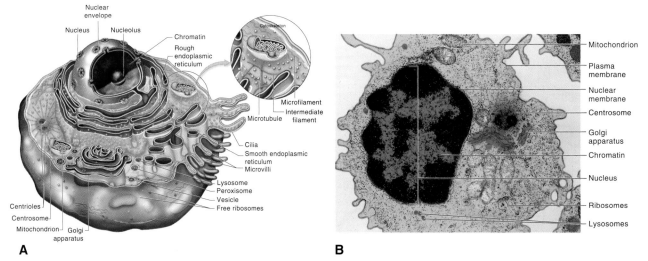

FIGURE 3-5 Typical, or composite, cell. **A,** Artist's interpretation of cell structure. **B,** Color-enhanced electron micrograph of a cell. Both show the many mitochondria, known as the "power plants of the cell." Note, too, the innumerable dots bordering the endoplasmic reticulum. These are ribosomes, the cell's "protein factories." *(From Patton KT, Thibodeau GA: Anthony's textbook of anatomy and physiology, ed 19, St Louis, 2010, Mosby.)*

  c. Membrane proteins have several functions—channels and transporters are integral proteins that help specific solutes across the membrane; receptors serve as cellular recognition sites; some membrane proteins are enzymes

 3. Basic framework—lipid bilayer; two layers of phospholipids, cholesterol, and glycolipids

B. Cytoplasm—all cellular contents between the plasma membrane and the nucleus; includes:

 1. Cytosol—fluid portion of cytoplasm; site of many chemical reactions for the cell's existence

 2. Cytoskeleton—network of several kinds of protein filaments that extend throughout the cytoplasm; structural framework for the cell; generates movement

 3. Organelles—specialized cellular structures with characteristic shapes and specific functions

C. Ribosomes

 1. Free ribosomes—not attached to other organelles; synthesize proteins used inside the cell

 2. Bound ribosomes—attached to the endoplasmic reticulum (ER); form rough ER; synthesize proteins destined for use in the plasma membrane or for export from cell

D. Endoplasmic reticulum—network of membranes that form flattened sacs called *cisterns*; arranged in parallel rows within the cytoplasm of a cell; contains enzymes involved in a variety of metabolic activities

 1. Rough (granular)
  a. Contains ribosomes
  b. Site of protein synthesis

 2. Smooth (agranular)
  a. No ribosomes present
  b. Synthesizes certain lipids and carbohydrates
  c. Contains enzymes that release glucose into the bloodstream and inactivate or detoxify a variety of drugs and potentially harmful substances, including alcohol, pesticides, and carcinogens

E. Golgi complex

 1. Stack of 3 to 20 flattened membranous sacs (cisterns)

 2. Within the cisterns, proteins are modified, sorted, and packaged into vesicles for transport to different destinations

F. Lysosomes

 1. Membrane-enclosed vesicles that form in the Golgi complex

 2. Contain digestive enzymes

 3. Function in the digestion of worn-out organelles (autophagy) and self (autolysis)

G. Mitochondria

 1. Ellipsoid bodies that consist of two membranes that contain enzyme complexes in a particular array (e.g., tricarboxylic acid cycle enzymes)

 2. Function as the powerhouse of the cell by transforming the chemical energy bond of nutrients into the high-energy phosphate bonds of adenosine triphosphate (ATP)

 3. A single cell may contain 50 to 2500 of these organelles, depending on the cell's energy needs

H. Nucleus

 1. Consists of a double nuclear membrane, nuclear pores (control the movement of substances into and out of nucleus), nucleoli (produce ribosomes), and deoxyribonucleic acid (DNA)

Movement of Substances Through Cell Membranes

See Table 3-1.

A. Passive transport processes—do not require energy expenditure of the cell membrane

1. Diffusion—a passive process

a. Molecules spread through the membranes

b. Molecules move from an area of high concentration to an area of low concentration (down a concentration gradient)

c. Eventually a state of equilibrium is reached

d. Membrane channels—pores in cell membranes through which specific ions or small water-soluble molecules can pass

2. Simple diffusion—substances diffuse across a membrane in one of two ways: lipid-soluble substances diffuse through the lipid bilayer, and ions diffuse through pores

3. Osmosis

a. Diffusion of water through a selectively permeable membrane (limits diffusion of at least some solute particles); results in gain of volume on one side of the membrane and loss of volume on the other side of the membrane

b. A solution containing solute particles that cannot pass through a membrane exerts osmotic pressure on the membrane

c. Potential osmotic pressure—maximum pressure that could develop in a solution when it is separated from pure water by a selectively permeable membrane; knowledge of potential osmotic pressure allows the prediction of the direction of osmosis and resulting change of pressure

(1) Isotonic—when two fluids have the same potential osmotic pressure

(2) Hypertonic (higher pressure)—cells placed in solutions that are hypertonic to intracellular fluid shrivel as water flows out of cells by osmosis faster than it enters

(3) Hypotonic (lower pressure)—a solution that has a lower concentration of solutes than the cytosol inside the cell; water molecules enter the cells by osmosis faster than they leave

4. Facilitated diffusion (carrier-mediated passive transport)

a. Movement of molecules made more efficient by the action of specific transport mechanisms in the plasma membrane; facilitated by channel proteins or carrier proteins

b. Transports substances down a concentration gradient

c. Substances moved by facilitated diffusion include glucose, fructose, galactose, urea, and some vitamins

5. Filtration

a. Passage of water and permeable solutes through a membrane by the force of hydrostatic pressure; occurs most often in capillaries

b. Small molecules travel down a hydrostatic pressure gradient and through a sheet of cells; results in the separation of large and small particles

B. Active transport processes—require the expenditure of metabolic energy by the cell

1. Active transport

a. Process that moves substances against a concentration gradient (from an area of low concentration to an area of high concentration)

b. Opposite of diffusion

c. Substances moved by "pumps," for example, calcium pumps and sodium–potassium pumps

2. Endocytosis and exocytosis—allow substances to enter or leave the interior of a cell without actually moving through its plasma membrane

a. Endocytosis—process by which the plasma membrane "traps" some extracellular material and brings it into the cell in a vesicle; the two basic types are:

(1) Phagocytosis (cell eating)—large particles are engulfed by the plasma membrane and enter the cell in vesicles; vesicles fuse with lysosomes, where particles are digested

(2) Pinocytosis (cell drinking)—the plasma membrane folds inward, forming a pinocytic vesicle containing a droplet of extracellular fluid; the vesicle detaches from the plasma membrane and enters the cytosol

b. Exocytosis—process by which large molecules, notably proteins, can leave the cell, even though they are too large to move through the plasma membrane; large molecules are enclosed in membranous vesicles and then pulled to the plasma membrane by the cytoskeleton, where the contents are released

(1) Provides a way for new material to be added to the plasma membrane

TABLE 3-1 Some Important Transport Processes

Process	Type	Description		Examples
Simple diffusion	Passive	Movement of particles through the phospholipid bilayer or through channels from an area of high concentration to an area of low concentration—that is, down the concentration gradient		Movement of carbon dioxide out of all cells; movement of sodium ions into nerve cells as they conduct an impulse
Channel-mediated passive transport (facilitated diffusion)	Passive	Diffusion of particles through a membrane by means of channel structures in the membrane (particles move down their concentration gradient)		Diffusion of sodium ions into nerve cells during a nerve impulse
Osmosis	Passive	Diffusion of water through a selectively permeable membrane in the presence of at least one impermanent solute		Diffusion of water molecules into and out of cells to correct imbalances in water concentration
Facilitated diffusion	Passive	Diffusion of particles through a membrane by means of carrier molecules; also called *carrier-mediated passive transport*		Movement of glucose molecules into most cells
Pumping	Active	Movement of solute particles from an area of low concentration to an area of high concentration (up the concentration gradient) by means of an energy-consuming pump structure in the membrane		In muscle cells, pumping of nearly all calcium ions to special compartments—or out of a cell
Phagocytosis	Active	Movement of cells or other large particles into a cell by trapping it in a section of plasma membrane that pinches off to form an intracellular vesicle; type of endocytosis		Trapping of bacterial cells by phagocytic white blood cells
Pinocytosis	Active	Movement of fluid and dissolved molecules into a cell by trapping them in a section of plasma membrane that pinches off to form an intracellular vesicle; type of endocytosis		Trapping of large protein molecules by some body cells
Exocytosis	Active	Movement of proteins or other cell products out of a cell by fusing a secretory vesicle with a plasma membrane		Secretion of the hormone prolactin by pituitary cells

(Art from Patton KT, Thibodeau GA: Anthony's textbook of anatomy and physiology, ed 19, St Louis, 2010, Mosby.)

Cell Metabolism

A. Metabolism—chemical reactions in a cell
  1. Catabolism—breaking of large molecules into smaller ones; usually releases energy
  2. Anabolism—building of large molecules from smaller ones; usually consumes energy
B. Role of enzymes
  1. Enzymes—chemical catalysts, reducing activation energy needed for a reaction
  2. Regulate cell metabolism
  3. Chemical structure of enzymes
    a. Proteins of a complex shape
    b. Active site—where the enzyme molecule fits the substrate molecule; lock-and-key model
  4. Enzyme nomenclature
    a. Enzymes usually have an "-ase" suffix; the first part of the word often signifies the substrate or the type of reaction catalyzed
    b. Oxidation-reduction enzymes—known as *oxidases, hydrogenases,* and *dehydrogenases;* energy release depends on these enzymes
    c. Hydrolyzing enzymes—hydrolases, for example, digestive enzymes
    d. Phosphorylating enzymes—phosphorylases or phosphatases; add or remove phosphate groups
    e. Carboxylases and decarboxylases—add or remove carbon dioxide
    f. Mutases or isomerases—rearrange atoms within a molecule
    g. Hydrases—add water to a molecule without splitting it
  5. Functions of enzymes
    a. Regulate cell functions by regulating metabolic pathways; specific in their actions
    b. Chemical and physical agents called *allosteric effectors* alter enzyme action by changing the shape of the enzyme molecule, for example:
      (1) Temperature
      (2) Hydrogen ion (H^+) concentration (pH)
      (3) Ionizing radiation
      (4) Cofactors
      (5) End products of certain metabolic pathways
    c. Most catalyze chemical reactions in both directions
    d. Continually being destroyed and replaced
    e. Many are first synthesized as inactive proenzymes
C. Catabolism
  1. Cellular respiration—pathway in which glucose is broken down to yield its stored energy; an important example of cell catabolism; has three chemically linked pathways:

  a. Glycolysis
    (1) Pathway in which glucose is broken apart into two pyruvic acid molecules to yield a small amount of energy (which is transferred to ATP and nicotinamide adenine dinucleotide [NADH])
    (2) Includes many chemical steps (reactions that follow one another), each regulated by specific enzymes
    (3) Is anaerobic (requires no oxygen)
    (4) Occurs within the cytosol (outside the mitochondria)
  b. Citric acid cycle (Krebs cycle)
    (1) Pyruvic acid (from glycolysis) is converted into acetyl coenzyme A (CoA) and enters the citric acid cycle after losing carbon dioxide (CO_2) and transferring some energy to NADH
    (2) A cyclic sequence of reactions that occurs inside the inner chamber of a mitochondrion. The acetyl splits from the CoA and is broken down, yielding CO_2 and energy (in the form of energized electrons), which is transferred to ATP, NADH, and flavin adenine dinucleotide (FADH2)
  c. The electron transport system (ETS)
    (1) Energized electrons are carried by NADH and FADH2 from glycolysis and the citric acid cycle to electron acceptors embedded in the cristae of the mitochondrion
    (2) As electrons are shuttled along a chain of electron-accepting molecules in the cristae, their energy is used to pump accompanying protons (H^+) into the space between mitochondrial membranes
    (3) Protons flow back into the inner chamber through carrier molecules in the cristae; their energy of movement is transferred to ATP
    (4) Low-energy electrons coming off the ETS bind to oxygen and rejoin their protons, forming water (H_2O)
D. Anabolism
  1. Protein synthesis is a central anabolic pathway in cells
  2. DNA (see the section on "Genetics" in Chapter 7)
    a. A double-helix polymer (composed of nucleotides); functions to transfer the information encoded in genes, which directs protein synthesis
    b. Gene—a segment of a DNA molecule that consists of approximately 1000 pairs of nucleotides; contains the code for synthesizing one polypeptide

3. Transcription
   a. Messenger ribonucleic acid (mRNA) forms along a segment of one strand of DNA
   b. Noncoding introns are removed, and the remaining exons are spliced together to form the final edited version of the mRNA copy of the DNA segment
4. Translation
   a. After leaving the nucleus and being processed, mRNA associates with a ribosome in the cytoplasm
   b. Transfer ribonucleic acid (tRNA) molecules bring specific amino acids to the mRNA at the ribosome; the type of amino acid is determined by the fit of a specific tRNA's anticodon with an mRNA's codon
   c. As amino acids are brought into place, peptide bonds join them, eventually producing an entire polypeptide chain
5. Processing—enzymes in the ER and Golgi apparatus link polypeptides into whole protein molecules or process them in other ways

Cell Growth and Reproduction

A. Cell growth and reproduction of cells are the most fundamental of all functions in a living being; together they constitute the life cycle of the cell
   1. Cell growth—depends on the use of the genetic information in DNA to make structural and functional proteins for cell survival
   2. Cell reproduction—ensures that genetic information is passed from one generation to the next
B. Cell growth
   1. Production of cytoplasm—more cell material is made, including growth and replication of organelles and plasma membrane; a largely anabolic process
   2. DNA replication
      a. Replication of the genome prepares the cell for reproduction; mechanics similar to RNA synthesis
      b. DNA replication
         (1) DNA strand uncoils, and strands come apart
         (2) Along each separate strand, a complementary strand forms
         (3) The two new strands are called *chromatids* (attached pairs); their point of attachment is called a *centromere*
   3. Growth phase of the cell's life cycle—subdivided into the first phase (G1), the DNA synthesis phase (S), and the second growth phase (G2)

C. Cell reproduction
   1. Mitosis—process of organizing and distributing nuclear DNA during cell division; cells reproduce by splitting themselves into two smaller daughter cells (see the section on "Cell Replication" and Figure 2-6 in Chapter 2)
   2. Meiosis—germ cell division; produces gametes (sperm and oocytes), the cells needed to form the next generation of sexually reproducing organisms
D. Regulating the cell's life cycle
   1. Cyclin-dependent kinases (CDKs)—activating enzymes that drive the cell through the phases of its life cycle
   2. Cyclins—regulatory proteins that control the CDKs and "shift" them to start the next phase; important in cancer pathways

TISSUES

(See the sections on "Concepts Relating to Dental Tissues," "Basic Tissues," "Epithelial Tissue," "Connective Tissue," "Blood and Lymph," "Nerve Tissue," and "Muscle Tissue" in Chapter 2.)

Body Membranes

A. Thin tissue layers that cover surfaces, line cavities, and divide spaces or organs
B. Epithelial membranes are the most common
   1. Cutaneous membranes (skin)
      a. Primary organ of the integumentary system
      b. One of the most important organs
      c. Comprises approximately 16% of body weight
   2. Serous membranes
      a. Parietal membranes—line closed body cavities
      b. Visceral membranes—cover visceral organs
      c. Pleura—surround the lung and line the thoracic cavity
      d. Peritoneum—covers the abdominal viscera and lines the abdominal cavity
   3. Mucous membranes (see the section on "Soft Tissue of the Oral Cavity" and Figure 2-21 in Chapter 2)
      a. Line and protect orifices that open to the exterior of the body, for example, anus, vagina, and oral cavity
      b. Line ducts and passageways of respiratory and digestive tracts
C. Connective tissue membranes
   1. Have smooth and slick synovial membranes to reduce friction between opposing surfaces in a movable joint; contain no epithelial components

2. Synovial membranes—line bursae and the spaces between the bones in joints; secrete synovial fluid

SYSTEMS OF THE BODY AND THEIR COMPONENTS

The Integumentary System

A. Functions—regulation of body temperature, protection, sensation, excretion, immunity, synthesis of vitamin D

B. Parts
   1. Epidermis—thin outer portion composed of keratinized stratified squamous epithelium
      a. Components include keratin, melanin, Langerhans' cells, Merkel cells
      b. Four layers:
         (1) Stratum basale
         (2) Stratum spinosum
         (3) Stratum lucidum
         (4) Stratum corneum
   2. Dermis—deeper, thicker, connective tissue
      a. Components include collagen and elastic fibers that give skin its extensivity and elasticity; dermal papillae that produce fingerprints and facilitate gripping objects; corpuscles of touch (Meissner's corpuscles); and nerve endings that are sensitive to touch
      b. One layer

C. Skin color—from melanin, carotene, and hemoglobin pigments

D. Accessory structures—hair, skin glands, and nails
   1. Hair—threads of fused, dead keratinized cells that function in protection
      a. Consist of a shaft above the surface, a root that penetrates the dermis and subcutaneous layer, and a hair follicle
   2. Sebaceous glands—usually connected to hair follicles; absent in palms and soles of feet; produce sebum, which moistens hair and waterproofs skin
   3. Sudoriferous glands—produce perspiration; carry waste to the skin's surface; assist in maintaining body temperature
   4. Nails—hard keratinized epidermal cells covering terminal portions of fingers and toes; the principal parts are body, free edge, root, lunula, cuticle, and matrix

Tissues and Membranes of the Body

A. Epithelial tissues
   1. Form membranes that contain and protect the internal fluid environment
   2. Absorb nutrients
   3. Secrete products that regulate functions involved in homeostasis

B. Connective tissues
   1. Hold organs and systems together
   2. Form structures that support the body and permit movement

C. Muscle tissues—work with connective tissues to permit movement

D. Nervous tissues—work with glandular epithelial tissue to regulate body function

The Skeletal System

(See Figure 3-6 and the section on "Connective Tissue" in Chapter 2.)

A. Functions
   1. Provides rigid support system
   2. Provides protection, for example, cranial bones protect the brain
   3. Serves as a source and a sink for calcium; involved in the formation of blood cells (hemopoiesis)
   4. Basis of attachment of muscles; allows movement

B. Types of bones
   1. Classified by shape
      a. Long bones
      b. Short bones
      c. Flat bones
      d. Irregular bones
   2. Sutural bones—found between the sutures of certain cranial bones

C. Parts of a long bone
   1. Diaphysis—shaft
   2. Epiphyses—ends
   3. Articular cartilage—layer of hyaline cartilage that covers the articular surfaces of epiphyses; cushions jolts and blows to bone
   4. Periosteum—white fibrous membrane that covers bone; contains cells that form and destroy bone, blood vessels; point of attachment for ligaments and tendons
   5. Medullary (marrow) cavity
      a. Tube-like hollow space in the diaphysis
      b. Filled with narrow marrow in adult
   6. Endosteum—epithelial membrane that lines the medullary cavity

D. Bone tissue
   1. Most distinctive form of connective tissue
   2. Extracellular components are hard and calcified
   3. Rigidity allows its supportive and protective functions
   4. Tensile strength nearly equal to cast iron at less than one third the weight
   5. Bone matrix composition
      a. Inorganic salts

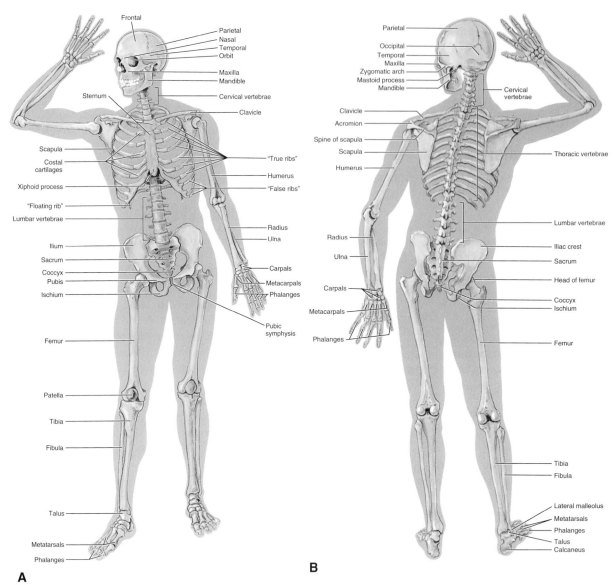

FIGURE 3-6 Skeleton. **A,** Anterior view. **B,** Posterior view. *(From Solomon EP:* Introduction to human anatomy and physiology, *ed 2, St Louis, 2008, Saunders.)*

(1) Hydroxyapatite—highly specialized chemical crystals of calcium and phosphate contribute to the hardness of bone

(2) Slender needle-like crystals oriented to resist stress and mechanical deformation

(3) Magnesium and sodium are also present

b. Organic matrix

(1) Ground substance—composite of collagenous fibers and an amorphous mixture of protein and polysaccharides; secreted by connective tissue cells

(2) Adds to the overall strength and resilience of bone

Microscopic Structure of Bone

(See the section on "Bone" and Figure 2-9 in Chapter 2.)

A. Compact bones' microstructures

1. Osteons, or haversian systems—cylinder-shaped structural units (living bone cells are located in these units); constitute the structural framework of compact bone; surround canals that run lengthwise through bone and are connected by transverse Volkmann's canals; permit the delivery of nutrients and removal of waste products

2. Four types of structures make up each osteon:

a. Lamella—concentric, cylinder-shaped layers of calcified matrix

b. Lacunae—small spaces containing tissue fluid; bone cells are located between the hard layers of the lamella

c. Canaliculi—ultra-small canals radiating in all directions from the lacunae and connecting them to each other and to the haversian canal

d. Haversian canal—extends lengthwise through the center of each osteon; contains blood vessels and lymphatic vessels

B. Cancellous (spongy) bone

  1. No osteons in cancellous bone; instead, it has trabeculae

  2. Nutrients are delivered and waste products are removed by diffusion through tiny canaliculi

  3. Bony spicules are arranged along the lines of stress, enhancing the bone's strength

C. Blood supply

  1. Bone cells are metabolically active and need a blood supply, which comes from the bone marrow in the internal medullary cavity of cancellous bone

  2. Blood vessels, lymphatic vessels, and nerves from the periosteum penetrate bone by way of Volkmann's canals; connect with vessels in the haversian canals

D. Types of bone cells

  1. Osteoblasts—bone-forming cells found in all bone surfaces; synthesize and secrete osteoid, an important component of ground substance; collagen fibrils line up in the osteoid and serve as a framework for the deposition of calcium and phosphate

  2. Osteoclasts—giant multi-nucleate cells that contain powerful lysosomal enzymes that destroy bone matrix (resorption); contain large numbers of mitochondria and lysosomes

  3. Osteocytes—mature bone cells; maintain metabolism such as exchange of nutrients and wastes with the blood

Bone Marrow

A. Myeloid tissue—specialized type of soft, diffuse connective tissue found in the medullary cavities of long bones and in the spaces of spongy bone; site for the production of blood cells

B. Two types of marrow occur during a person's lifetime:

  1. Red marrow

    a. Found in virtually all bones in an infant or child's body; in an adult, red marrow found in ribs, bodies of the vertebrae, humerus, pelvis, and femur

    b. Produces red blood cells

  2. Yellow marrow

    a. As an individual ages, red marrow is replaced by yellow marrow

    b. Marrow cells become saturated with fat and are no longer active in blood cell production

    c. Yellow marrow can revert to red marrow during times of decreased blood supply, for example, anemia, exposure to radiation, and certain diseases

Regulation of Blood Calcium Levels

A. The skeletal system serves as a reservoir for approximately 98% of body calcium reserves

  1. Helps maintain the constancy of blood calcium

    a. Calcium is mobilized in and out of blood during bone remodeling

    b. During bone formation, osteoblasts remove calcium from blood and lower circulating levels

    c. During breakdown of bone, osteoclasts release calcium into blood and increase circulating levels

  2. Homeostasis of calcium ion concentration essential for:

    a. Bone formation, remodeling, and repair

    b. Blood clotting

    c. Transmission of nerve impulses

    d. Maintenance of skeletal and cardiac muscle contraction

Divisions of the Skeleton

A. Axial skeleton—made up of 80 bones of the head, neck, and torso

B. Appendicular skeleton—made up of 126 bones that form the appendages to the axial skeleton; the upper and lower extremities

Axial Skeleton

A. Skull (see Chapter 4)

B. Vertebral column (Figure 3-7)

  1. Consists of 24 vertebrae plus the sacrum and the coccyx

  2. Segments of the vertebral column

    a. Cervical vertebrae (7)

    b. Thoracic vertebrae (12), T1 to T12 are stronger than cervical vertebrae; have facets for articulating with the ribs

    c. Lumbar vertebrae (5), L1 to L5 are the largest and strongest; well adapted for the attachment of large back muscles

    d. Sacrum (5 fused vertebrae)—provides strong foundation for pelvic girdle

    e. Coccyx (4 or 5 fused vertebrae)—articulates with the sacrum

  3. Characteristics of vertebrae

    a. All vertebrae, except the first, have a flat, rounded body anteriorly and centrally, a spinous process posteriorly, and two transverse processes laterally

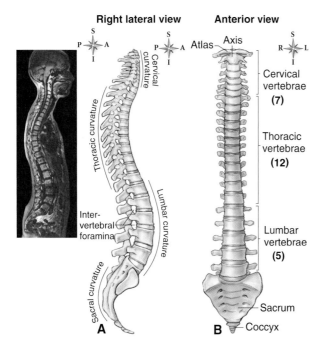

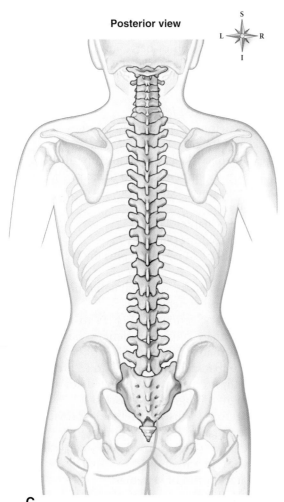

FIGURE 3-7 The vertebral column. *(From Patton KT, Thibodeau GA: Anthony's textbook of anatomy and physiology, ed 19, St Louis, 2010, Mosby.)*

b. All but the sacrum and the coccyx have a vertebral foramen
c. The first cervical vertebra, the atlas, supports the head
d. The second cervical vertebra, the axis, has an upward projection (dens) to allow the rotation of the head
4. The vertebral column as a whole articulates with the head, ribs, and iliac bones
5. Individual vertebrae articulate with each other in joints between their bodies and between their articular processes

C. Sternum
1. Dagger-shaped bone in the middle of the anterior chest wall made up of three parts:
   a. Manubrium—upper handle part
   b. Body—middle blade part
   c. Xiphoid process—blunt cartilaginous lower tip; ossifies during adult life
2. The manubrium articulates with the clavicle and the first and second ribs
3. Ribs join the body of the sternum, either directly or indirectly, by means of costal cartilages

D. Ribs
1. Twelve pairs of ribs form the sides of the thoracic cavity
2. Each rib articulates with the body and the transverse process of its corresponding thoracic vertebra
3. From its vertebral attachment, each rib curves outward and then forward and downward
4. Rib attachment to the sternum:
   a. Ribs 1 to 8 join a costal cartilage that attaches it to the sternum
   b. The costal cartilage of ribs 8 to 10 indirectly joins the cartilage of the rib above to the sternum (false ribs)
   c. Ribs 11 and 12 are floating ribs, since they are not attached to the sternum

Appendicular Skeleton
A. Upper extremity (Figure 3-8)
1. Consists of the bones of the shoulder girdle, upper arm, lower arm, wrist, and hand
2. Shoulder girdle
   a. Made up of the scapula and the clavicle
   b. The clavicle forms the only bony joint with the trunk (sternoclavicular joint)
   c. At its distal end, the clavicle articulates with the acromion process of the scapula
3. Humerus (Figure 3-9)
   a. Longest bone of the upper arm
   b. Articulates proximally with the glenoid fossa of the scapula and distally with the radius and the ulna
4. Ulna (Figure 3-10)

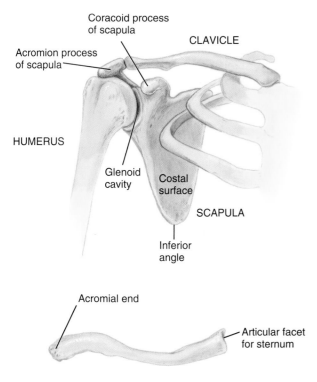

CLAVICLE (right, superior view)

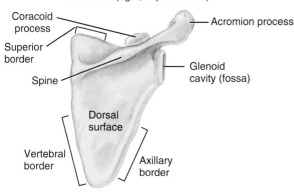

SCAPULA (right, posterior view)

FIGURE 3-8 Right scapula and clavicle. *(From Applegate E: The anatomy and physiology learning system, ed 2, St Louis, 2011, Saunders.)*

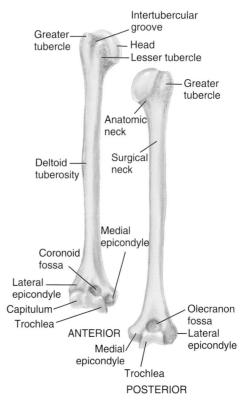

FIGURE 3-9 Humerus (upper arm). *(Modified from Applegate E: The anatomy and physiology learning system, ed 4, St Louis, 2011, Saunders.)*

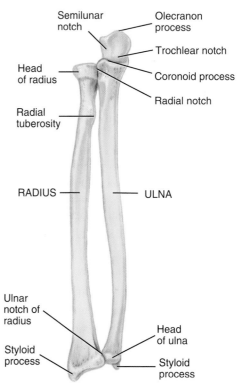

FIGURE 3-10 Radius and ulna (lower arm). *(Modified from Applegate E: The anatomy and physiology learning system, ed 4, St Louis, 2011, Saunders.)*

   a. Long bone found on the little finger side of the forearm
   b. Articulates proximally with the humerus and the radius and distally with the fibrocartilaginous disc
5. Radius (see Figure 3-10)
   a. Long bone found on the thumb side of the forearm
   b. Articulates proximally with the capitulum of the humerus and the radial notch of the ulna; articulates distally with the scaphoid and lunate carpals of the wrist

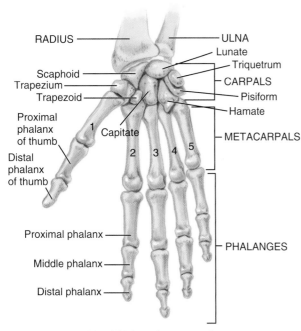

RADIUS — ULNA
— Lunate
— Triquetrum
Scaphoid — CARPALS
Trapezium — Pisiform
Trapezoid — Hamate
Proximal phalanx of thumb
1 Capitate
METACARPALS
Distal phalanx of thumb
2 3 4 5
Proximal phalanx —
— PHALANGES
Middle phalanx —
Distal phalanx —

Hand (right, palmar aspect)

FIGURE 3-11 Bones of the hand and wrist. *(Modified from Applegate E: The anatomy and physiology learning system, ed 4, St Louis, 2011, Saunders.)*

6. Carpal bones (Figure 3-11)
   a. Eight small bones that form the wrist; bound closely and firmly by ligaments; arranged in two transverse rows:
      (1) Top row made up of the pisiform, the triquetrum, the lunate, and the scaphoid
      (2) Bottom row made up of the hamate, the capitate, the trapezoid, and the trapezium
   b. Joints between the radius and carpals allow wrist and hand movements
   c. Carpal tunnel—concavity formed by the pisiform and the hamate (on the ulnar side) and the scaphoid and the trapezium (on the radial side), through which the median nerve passes; narrowing of the carpal tunnel gives rise to carpal tunnel syndrome
7. Metacarpal bones
   a. Form the framework of the hand
   b. The thumb metacarpal forms the most freely movable joint with the carpals
   c. The heads of the metacarpals (knuckles) articulate with the phalanges
8. Phalanges—bones of the fingers
B. Lower extremity
1. Consists of the bones of the hip, thigh, lower leg, ankle, and foot

2. The pelvic girdle is made up of the sacrum and the two coxal (hip) bones bound tightly by strong ligaments
   a. A stable circular base that supports the trunk and attaches the lower extremities to the axial skeleton
   b. Each coxal bone is made up of three fused bones:
      (1) Ilium—largest and uppermost part
      (2) Ischium—strongest and lowermost part
      (3) Pubis—anterior and inferior part
3. Femur—longest and heaviest bone in the body (Figure 3-12)
4. Patella—kneecap; small triangular bone in front of the joint between the femur and the tibia
5. Tibia
   a. Larger bone of the leg; bears the weight of the body
   b. Articulates proximally with the femur to form the knee joint
   c. Articulates distally with the fibula and the talus of the ankle
6. Fibula
   a. Smaller, more laterally and deeply placed of the two shin bones
   b. Articulates with the tibia
7. Foot (Figures 3-13 and 3-14)
   a. The structure is similar to that of the hand, with adaptations for supporting weight
   b. Foot bones are held together to form spring arches
      (1) Tarsus (ankle)—contains seven bones: calcaneus (heel bone), talus (ankle bone), cuneiforms, cuboid, and navicular

Joints
A. Classification of joints
1. Structural—based on the presence or absence of synovial cavity and type of connecting tissue; classified as fibrous, cartilaginous, or synovial
2. Functional—based on the degree of movement permitted; joints may be synarthroses (immovable), amphiarthroses (slightly movable), or diarthroses (freely movable)
B. Fibrous joints (Figure 3-15)
1. Bones held together closely by fibrous connective tissue
   a. Syndesmoses—joints in which ligaments connect two bones
   b. Sutures—found only in the skull; tooth-like projections from adjacent bones interlock with each other
   c. Gomphoses—found between the root of the tooth and the alveolar process of the mandible or the maxilla

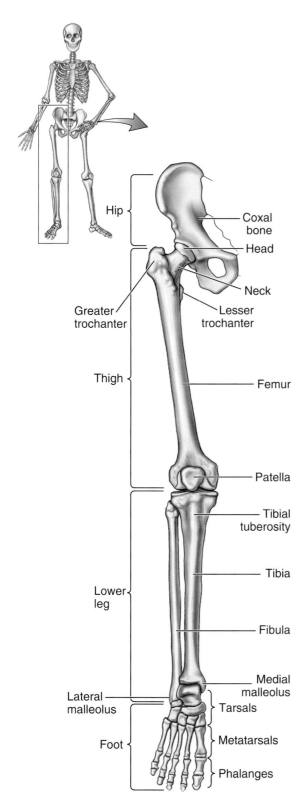

FIGURE 3-12 Bones of the thigh and leg. *(Modified from Herlihy B: The human body in health and illness, ed 3, St Louis, 2011, Saunders.)*

Labels in figure: Hip, Coxal bone, Head, Neck, Greater trochanter, Lesser trochanter, Thigh, Femur, Patella, Tibial tuberosity, Tibia, Fibula, Lower leg, Lateral malleolus, Medial malleolus, Tarsals, Foot, Metatarsals, Phalanges

C. Cartilaginous joints (Figure 3-16)
   1. Bones held together by hyaline cartilage or fibrocartilage; allow little motion
      a. Synchondroses—hyaline cartilage present between articulating bones
      b. Symphysis—joints in which a pad or disc of fibrocartilage connects two bones
D. Synovial joints
   1. Structures of synovial joints (Figure 3-17)
      a. Joint capsule—sleeve-like casing around the ends of bones, which binds them together
      b. Synovial membrane—membrane lining the joint capsule; secretes synovial fluid
      c. Articular cartilage—hyaline cartilage covering the articular surfaces of the joint cavity
      d. Menisci (articular discs)—pads of fibrocartilage located between articulating bones
      e. Bursae—sac-like body cavities; reduce friction in joints
      f. Ligaments—strong cords of dense white fibrous tissue; hold the bones of a synovial joint more firmly together (the temperomandibular joint [TMJ] has three ligaments)
   2. Types of synovial joints
      a. Uniaxial joints—permit movement around only one axis and in only one plane
         (1) Hinge joints—the articulating ends of bones form a hinge-shaped unity that allows only flexion and extension
         (2) Pivot joints—a projection of one bone articulates with a ring or notch of another bone
      b. Biaxial joints—permit movements around two perpendicular axes in two perpendicular planes
      c. Saddle joints—the articulating ends of bones that resemble reciprocally shaped miniature saddles, for example, thumbs
      d. Condyloid (ellipsoidal) joints—a bony projection that fits into an elliptical socket
      e. Multi-axial joints—permit movements around three or more axes in three or more planes
         (1) Ball-and-socket (spheroid) joints—most movable joints; the ball-shaped head of one bone fits into a concave depression, for example, shoulder
         (2) Gliding joints—relatively flat articulating surfaces that allow limited gliding movements along various axes, for example, neck

Anatomy of the Muscular System

See Figure 3-18.
A. Muscle tissue has five key functions:
   1. Producing body movements
   2. Stabilizing body positions

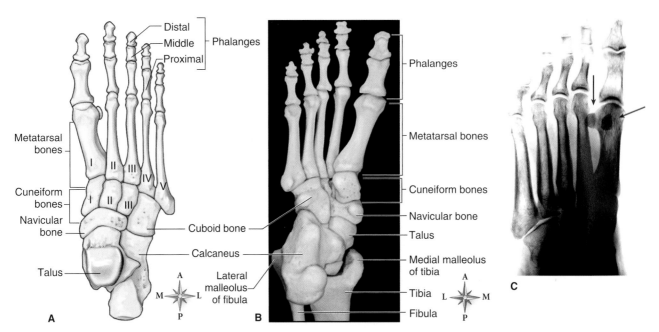

FIGURE 3-13 The foot. **A,** Bones on the right foot viewed from above. Tarsal bones consist of cuneiforms, navicular, talus, cuboid, and calcaneus. **B,** Posterior aspect of the right ankle skeleton and inferior aspect of the right foot skeleton. **C,** X-ray film of the left foot showing prominent sesamoid bones near the distal end (head) of the first metatarsal bone of the great toe. *(From Patton KT, Thibodeau GA: Anthony's textbook of anatomy and physiology, ed 19, St Louis, 2010, Mosby.)*

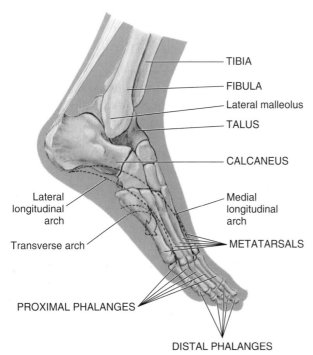

FIGURE 3-14 Arches of the foot. *(From Solomon EP: Introduction to human anatomy and physiology, ed 2, St Louis, 2008, Saunders.)*

3. Regulating organ volume
4. Moving substances within the body
5. Producing heat

B. Characteristics
1. Excitability—property of receiving and responding to stimuli by producing electrical signals; ability of muscle fibers (and neurons) to respond to a stimulus and convert it into an action potential
2. Contractibility—ability to contract (shorten and thicken)
3. Extensibility—ability to be stretched
4. Elasticity—ability to return to original shape after contraction or extension

C. Types
1. Skeletal muscle—mostly attached to bones; striated and voluntary
2. Cardiac muscle—forms most of the walls of the heart; striated and involuntary
3. Smooth muscle—located in viscera; participates in internal processes

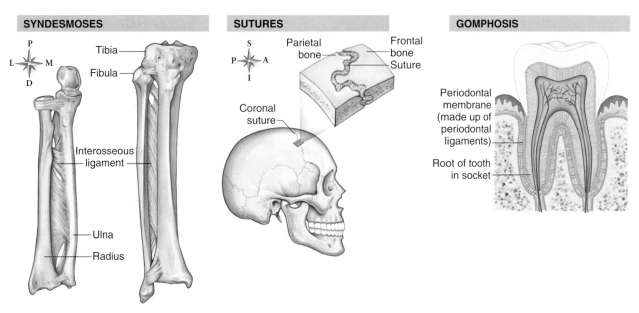

| SYNDESMOSES | SUTURES | GOMPHOSIS |

FIGURE 3-15 Fibrous joints. *(From Patton KT, Thibodeau GA:* Anthony's textbook of anatomy and physiology, *ed 19, St Louis, 2010, Mosby.)*

Skeletal Muscle Structure

See Figure 3-19.
A. Connective tissue components (may become a tendon or an aponeurosis)
   1. Endomysium—delicate connective tissue membrane that covers specialized skeletal muscle fibers
   2. Perimysium—tough connective tissue binding fascicles together
   3. Epimysium—coarse sheath covering the muscle as a whole
B. Size, shape, and fiber arrangement
   1. Size—ranging from extremely small to large masses
   2. Shape—variety of shapes such as broad, narrow, long, tapering, short, blunt, triangular, quadrilateral, or irregular and as flat sheets, or bulky masses
   3. Arrangement—variety of arrangements; the direction of fibers is significant because of its relationship to function
C. Attachment of muscle
   1. Origin—point of attachment that does not move when the muscle contracts
   2. Insertion—point of attachment that moves when the muscle contracts
D. Muscle actions
   1. Most movements produced by the coordinated actions of several muscles; some muscles in the group contract while others relax
      a. Prime mover (agonist)—muscles that directly perform a specific movement
      b. Antagonist—when contracting, directly oppose prime movers; relax while the agonist is contracting to produce movement; provide precision and control during contraction of prime movers
      c. Synergists—contract at the same time as prime movers do; facilitate prime mover actions to produce a more efficient movement
      d. Fixator muscles—stabilize joints
E. Lever systems—bones serve as levers, and joints serve as fulcrums; the muscle applies a pulling force on a bone lever at the point of the muscle's attachment to the bone, causing the insertion bone to move about its joint fulcrum

Head and Neck Muscles (See the section on "The Muscular System of the Head and Neck" and Figure 4-4 in Chapter 4.)
A. Muscles of facial expression—unique in that at least one point of attachment is to the deep layers of the skin over the face or neck
B. Muscles of mastication—responsible for chewing movements
C. Muscles that move the head—paired muscles on either side of the neck that are responsible for head movements

Trunk Muscles
A. Muscles of the thorax—critical in respiration
B. Muscles of the abdominal wall—arranged in three layers, with fibers in each layer running in different directions to increase strength
C. Muscles of the pelvic floor—support structures in the pelvic cavity

SYNCHONDROSES

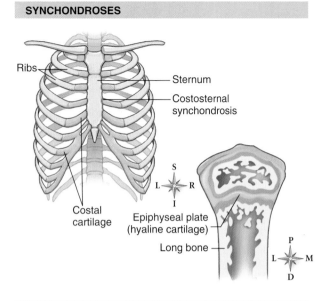

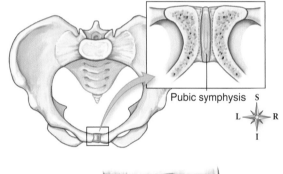

SYMPHYSES

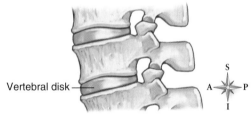

FIGURE 3-16 Cartilaginous joints. *(From Patton KT and Thibodeau GA: Anthony's textbook of anatomy and physiology, ed 19, St Louis, 2010, Mosby.)*

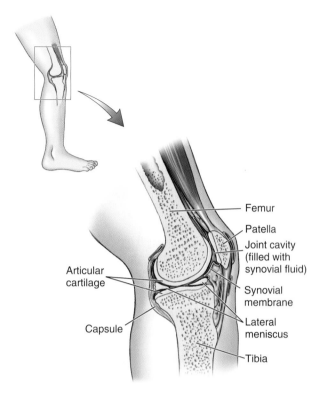

FIGURE 3-17 Structure of synovial joints. *(From Herlihy B: The human body in health and illness, ed 3, St Louis, 2011, Saunders.)*

D. Muscles that move the wrist, hand, and fingers—located on the anterior or posterior surfaces of the forearm

Lower Limb Muscles

A. The pelvic girdle and the lower extremity function in locomotion and maintenance of stability
B. Muscles that move the thigh and the lower leg
C. Muscles that move the ankle and the foot
    1. Extrinsic foot muscles—located in the leg; exert their actions by pulling on tendons that insert on bones in the ankle and foot; responsible for dorsiflexion, plantar flexion, inversion, and eversion
    2. Intrinsic foot muscles—located within the foot; responsible for flexion, extension, abduction, and adduction of the toes

Posture

A. Maintaining body posture is an important function of muscles
B. Good posture—body alignment that favors function and requires the least muscular work to maintain, keeping the body's center of gravity over its base
C. How posture is maintained:
    1. Muscles exert a continual pull on bones in the opposite direction from gravity

Upper Limb Muscles

A. Muscles acting on the shoulder girdle—muscles that attach the upper extremity to the torso; located anteriorly (chest) or posteriorly (back and neck); allow extensive movement
B. Muscles that move the upper arm—the shoulder is a synovial joint allowing extensive movement in every plane of motion
C. Muscles that move the forearm—found proximal to the elbow and attached to the ulna and radius

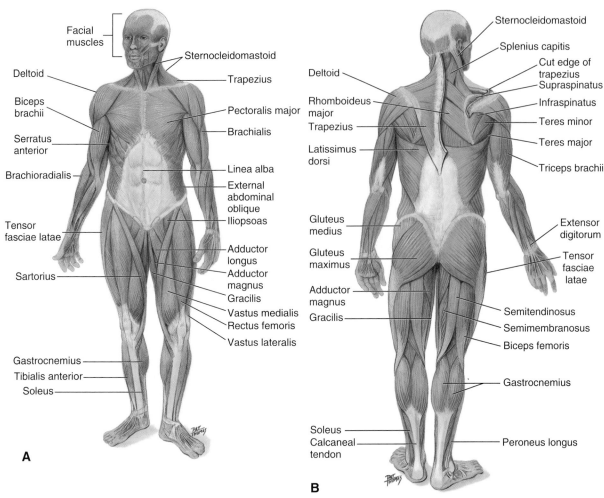

FIGURE 3-18 General overview of the body musculature. **A,** Anterior view. **B,** Posterior view. *(Modified from Applegate E: The anatomy and physiology learning system, ed 4, St Louis, 2011, Saunders.)*

2. Structures other than muscle and bone have a role in maintaining posture

  a. The nervous system—responsible for the existence of muscle tone and for the regulation and coordination of the amount of pull exerted by individual muscles

  b. Respiratory, digestive, excretory, and endocrine systems all contribute to maintain posture

Function of Skeletal Muscle

A. Overview of muscle cells

  1. Muscle cells are called *fibers* because of their thread-like shape

  2. Sarcolemma—plasma membrane of muscle fibers

  3. Sarcoplasmic reticulum

    a. A network of tubules and sacs found within muscle fibers

  b. The membrane of the sarcoplasmic reticulum continually pumps calcium ions from the sarcoplasm and stores the ions within sacs

4. Muscle fibers contain many mitochondria and several nuclei

5. Myofibrils—numerous fine fibers packed close together in the sarcoplasm

6. Sarcomere

  a. The segment of myofibril between two successive Z lines

  b. Each myofibril consists of many sarcomeres

  c. The contractile unit of muscle fibers

7. Striated muscle

  a. Dark stripes are called *A bands*; the light H zone runs across the midsection of each dark A band

  b. Light stripes are called *I bands*; the dark Z line extends across the center of each light I band

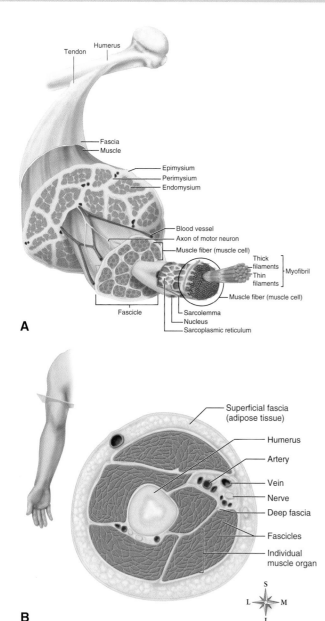

A

B

FIGURE 3-19 Structure of a muscle organ. *(From Patton KT, Thibodeau GA: Anthony's textbook of anatomy and physiology, ed 19, St Louis, 2010, Mosby.)*

8. T tubules
   a. Transverse tubules that extend across the sarcoplasm at right angles to the long axis of the muscle fiber
   b. Formed by the inward extension of the sarcolemma
   c. The membrane has ion pumps that continually transport calcium ions inward from the sarcoplasm
   d. Allow electrical impulses traveling along the sarcolemma to move deeper into the cell

9. Triad
   a. Triplet of tubules; a T tubule is sandwiched between two sacs of the sarcoplasmic reticulum; allows an electrical impulse traveling along a T tubule to stimulate the membranes of adjacent sacs of the sarcoplasmic reticulum

B. Myofilaments
   1. Each myofibril contains thousands of thick and thin myofilaments
   2. Four different kinds of protein molecules make up myofilaments
      a. Myosin
         (1) Makes up almost all of the thick filament
         (2) Myosin "heads" are chemically attracted to actin molecules; known as *cross-bridges* when attached to actin
      b. Actin—globular protein that forms two fibrous strands twisted around each other to form the bulk of the thin filament
      c. Tropomyosin—protein that blocks the active sites on actin molecules
      d. Troponin—protein that holds tropomyosin molecules in place
   3. Thin filaments attached to both Z lines of a sarcomere and extend partway toward the center
   4. Thick myosin filaments are not attached to Z lines

C. Mechanism of contraction
   1. Excitation and contraction
      a. A skeletal muscle fiber remains at rest until stimulated by a motor neuron
      b. Neuromuscular junction—motor neurons connect to the sarcolemma at the motor endplate
      c. Neuromuscular junction—synapse where neurotransmitter molecules transmit signals
      d. Acetylcholine—neurotransmitter released into the synaptic cleft, which diffuses across the gap, stimulates receptors, and initiates an impulse in the sarcolemma
      e. A nerve impulse travels over the sarcolemma and inward along T tubules to trigger the release of calcium ions
      f. Calcium binds to troponin, causing the tropomyosin to shift and expose the active sites on actin
      g. Sliding filament theory
         (1) When active sites on actin are exposed, myosin heads bind to them
         (2) Myosin heads bend, pulling the thin filaments past them
         (3) Each head releases itself, binds to the next active site, and pulls again
         (4) The entire myofibril becomes shortened

2. Relaxation
  a. Immediately after calcium ions are released, the sarcoplasmic reticulum begins actively pumping them back into sacs
  b. Calcium ions are removed from troponin molecules, ending the contraction
3. Energy sources for muscle contraction
  a. Hydrolysis of ATP yields the energy required for muscular contraction
  b. ATP binds to the myosin head to perform the work of pulling the thin filament during contraction
  c. Muscle fibers continually synthesize ATP from the breakdown of creatine phosphate
  d. Catabolism by muscle fibers requires glucose and oxygen
  e. At rest, excess oxygen (O_2) in the sarcoplasm is stored by myoglobin
    (1) Red fibers—muscle fibers with high levels of myoglobin
    (2) White fibers—muscle fibers with little myoglobin
  f. Aerobic respiration occurs when adequate O_2 is available
  g. Anaerobic respiration occurs when low levels of O_2 are available and results in the formation of lactic acid
  h. Skeletal muscle contraction produces excess heat that can be used to maintain body temperature

Function of Skeletal Muscle Organs
A. Motor unit
  1. Motor unit—comprises the motor neuron and the muscle fibers to which it is attached
  2. Some motor units can consist of only a few or numerous muscle fibers
  3. Generally, with a smaller number of fibers in a motor unit, more precise movements are possible; the larger the number of fibers in a motor unit, the more powerful is the contraction
B. Twitch contraction
  1. A quick jerk of a muscle that is produced as a result of a single, brief threshold stimulus (generally occurs only in experimental situations)
  2. Three phases:
    a. Latent phase—the nerve impulse travels to the sarcoplasmic reticulum to trigger the release of calcium
    b. Contraction phase—calcium binds to troponin, and the sliding of filaments occurs
    c. Relaxation phase—the sliding of filaments ceases
C. Treppe—the "staircase phenomenon"
  1. Gradual, step-like increase in the strength of a contraction; observed in a series of twitch contractions that occur 1 second apart

2. Eventually, the muscle responds with less forceful contractions, and the relaxation phase becomes shorter
3. If the relaxation phase disappears completely, a contracture (abnormal shortening of muscle tissue that can cause disability) occurs
D. Tetanus—smooth, sustained contractions
  1. Multiple wave summation—multiple twitch waves are added together to sustain muscle tension for a longer time
  2. Incomplete tetanus—very short periods of relaxation occur between peaks of tension
  3. Complete tetanus—twitch waves fuse into a single sustained peak
E. Muscle tone
  1. Tonic contraction—continual, partial contraction of a muscle
  2. At any one time, a small number of muscle fibers within a muscle contract, producing tightness of muscle tone
  3. Muscles with less tone than normal are flaccid
  4. Muscles with more tone than normal are spastic
  5. Muscle tone is maintained by negative feedback mechanisms
F. Principle of graded strength
  1. Skeletal muscles contract with varying degrees of strength at different times
  2. Factors that contribute to the phenomenon of graded strength:
    a. The metabolic condition of individual fibers
    b. The number of muscle fibers contracting simultaneously; the greater the number of fibers contracting, the stronger is the contraction
    c. The number of motor units recruited
    d. The intensity and frequency of stimulation
  3. Length–tension relationship
    a. The maximal strength that a muscle can develop bears a direct relationship to the initial length of its fibers
    b. A shortened muscle's sarcomeres are compressed; therefore, the muscle cannot develop much tension
    c. An overstretched muscle cannot develop much tension because the thick myofilaments are too far from the thin myofilaments
    d. The strongest maximal contraction is possible only when the skeletal muscle has been stretched to its optimal length
  4. Stretch reflex
    a. The load imposed on a muscle influences the strength of a skeletal contraction
    b. The body tries to maintain a consistency of muscle length in response to increased load

c. Maintains a relatively constant length as the load is increased up to a maximum sustainable level

G. Isotonic and isometric contractions

1. Isotonic contraction
   a. Contraction in which the tone or tension within a muscle remains the same as the length of the muscle changes
      (1) Concentric—the muscle shortens as it contracts
      (2) Eccentric—the muscle lengthens as it contracts
   b. Isotonic means "same tension"
   c. All of the energy of contraction is used to pull on the thin myofilaments and thereby change the length of a fiber's sarcomeres
2. Isometric contraction
   a. Contraction in which muscle length remains the same while muscle tension increases
   b. Isometric means "same length"
3. Body movements occur as a result of both types of contractions

Function of Cardiac and Smooth Muscle Tissue

A. Cardiac muscle (also known as *striated involuntary muscle*)

1. Found only in the heart; forms bulk of the walls of each chamber
2. Contracts rhythmically and continuously to maintain a constant blood flow
3. Resembles skeletal muscle but has specialized features related to its role in continuous pumping of blood
   a. Each cardiac muscle contains parallel myofibrils
   b. Cardiac muscle fibers form strong, electrically coupled junctions (intercalated discs) with other fibers; individual cells also exhibit branching
   c. Syncytium—continuous, electrically coupled mass; important for coordinating muscle contractions
   d. Cardiac muscle fibers form around the heart chambers a continuous, contractile band that conducts a single impulse across a virtually continuous sarcolemma
   e. T tubules are larger, and form diads with a rather sparse sarcoplasmic reticulum
   f. Cardiac muscle sustains each impulse longer than does skeletal muscle; therefore, impulses cannot come rapidly enough to produce tetanus
   g. Cardiac muscle does not run low on ATP and does not experience fatigue
   h. Cardiac muscle is self-stimulating

B. Smooth muscle

1. Smooth muscle is composed of small, tapered cells with single nuclei
2. T tubules are absent; only a loosely organized sarcoplasmic reticulum is present
3. Calcium comes from outside the cell and binds to calmodulin instead of troponin to trigger a contraction
4. No striations are present because both the thick and thin myofilaments have an arrangement different from that in skeletal or cardiac muscle fibers; myofilaments are not organized into sarcomeres
5. Two types of smooth muscle tissue:
   a. Visceral muscle (single unit)
      (1) Gap junctions join smooth muscle fibers into large, continuous sheets
      (2) Most common type; forms a muscular layer in the walls of hollow structures such as the digestive, urinary, and reproductive tracts
      (3) Exhibits autorhythmicity, which produces peristalsis
   b. Multi-unit
      (1) Does not act as a single unit; is composed of many independent cell units
      (2) Each fiber responds only to input from nerves

The Nervous System

(See the section on "Nerve Tissue" in Chapter 2.)

A. Two main subsystems (Figure 3-20):

1. The central nervous system (CNS)—consists of the brain and the spinal cord
2. The peripheral nervous system (PNS)—includes all nervous tissue outside the CNS; contains the nerves to and from the body wall

B. Functions

1. Sensory—detection of different types of stimuli both inside and outside the body
   a. Afferent or sensory neurons—carry information from the PNS to the CNS
2. Integrative—processing of sensory information by analyzing and storing some of it and by making decisions regarding appropriate responses; interneurons carry out this function
3. Motor—responses to integrative decisions
   a. Efferent or motor neurons carry information from the CNS to the PNS

C. The central nervous system

1. Brain—housed within the skull; contains about 100 billion neurons
2. Spinal cord—contains about 100 million neurons; is connected directly to the brain and is protected by the vertebral column

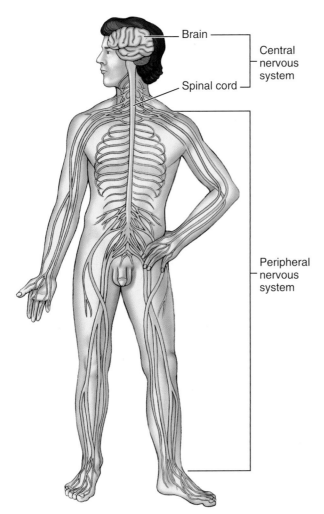

Brain
Central
nervous
system
Spinal cord

Peripheral
nervous
system

FIGURE 3-20 The nervous system. *(From Herlihy B: The human body in health and illness, ed 3, St Louis, 2011, Saunders.)*

from the receptors for the special senses of vision, hearing, taste, and smell
   (2) Motor neurons—conduct impulses from the CNS to skeletal muscles only; motor responses are voluntary
b. The autonomic nervous system (ANS)
   (1) Divisions
c. Sympathetic division (thoracolumbar) involves motor (afferent) nerves from the ANS
d. Parasympathetic division (craniosacral)
e. The enteric nervous system
   (1) "Brain of the GI system"; enteric motor neurons govern the contraction of GI tract smooth muscle, secretions of the GI tract organs such as acid secretions by the stomach, and activity of GI tract endocrine cells

Cellular Organization

Nervous system structure (Figure 3-21; see also the section on "Nerve Tissue" and Figures 2-13 and 2-14 in Chapter 2.)
A. Each neuron (nerve cell) consists of a cell body containing a nucleus
B. Dendrite—sends impulses toward the cell body or to a muscle or gland
C. Axon—conducts nerve impulses away from the cell body
D. Neuroglia—specialized tissue cells that support neurons, attach neurons to blood vessels, produce the myelin sheath around the axons of the CNS, and carry out phagocytosis
E. Myelin—fatty substance around axons; provides insulation and increases the speed of nerve conduction; deposited by Schwann cells in layers in the PNS
   1. Neurilemma—outermost layer of the Schwann cell
   2. Nodes of Ranvier—located between myelin segments; unmyelinated
   3. Oligodendrocytes myelinate CNS axons
F. White matter consists of aggregations of myelinated processes from many neurons
G. Gray matter contains the neurons, dendrites, and axon terminals of unmyelinated axons and neuroglia; forms an H-shaped inner core in the spinal cord that is surrounded by white matter; a superficial shell of gray matter covers the cerebrum and the cerebellum
H. The nervous system exhibits plasticity—the capability to change on the basis of experiences; limited ability to regenerate
I. Axons and dendrites that are associated with a neurilemma in the PNS may undergo repair if the cell body is intact, Schwann cells are functional, and scar tissue does not form too rapidly

3. Source of thoughts, emotions, memories; source of most nerve impulses that stimulate muscles to contract and glands to secrete
4. Communication to and from CNS accomplished by:
   a. Cranial nerves
   b. Spinal nerves
   c. Ganglia—small clusters of neuronal cell bodies that relay signals traveling along cranial and spinal nerves
   d. Enteric plexuses—in the walls of the organs of the gastrointestinal (GI) tract; help regulate the digestive system
D. The peripheral nervous system
   1. Subdivisions
      a. The somatic nervous system
         (1) Sensory neurons—convey information to the CNS from the somatic receptors in the head, body wall, and limbs and also

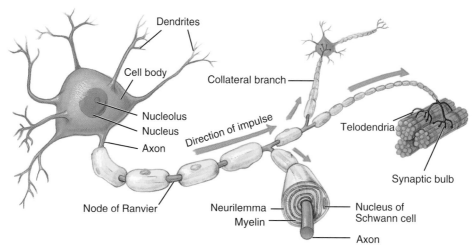

FIGURE 3-21 Structure of a typical neuron. *(From Applegate E: The anatomy and physiology learning system, ed 4, St Louis, 2011, Saunders.)*

Action Potentials (See the section on "Characteristics and Physiology of Pain" in Chapter 18.)

A. Neurons communicate by means of nerve action potentials (impulses)

B. Generation of action is dependent on:

1. The presence of special types of ion channels and the existence of a resting membrane potential

2. Membrane potential—a difference in electrical charge across the plasma membrane; a cell that has a membrane potential is said to be *polarized*

3. A nerve impulse results from the concentration of two ions on the inside and outside of the nerve

4. Resting membrane potential—the outside surface of plasma membrane has a positive charge; the inside surface has a negative charge; the resting membrane in neurons is ≈70 millivolts (mV)

5. During an action potential, voltage-gated sodium (Na⁺) and potassium (K⁺) channels open in sequence. Opening of voltage-gated Na⁺ channels results in depolarization, followed by the loss and then reversal of membrane polarization (from −70 mV to +30 mV). Then, the opening of voltage-gated K⁺ channels allows repolarization, the recovery of the resting membrane potential

6. According to the "all-or-none" principle, if a stimulus is strong enough to generate an action potential, the impulse generated is of a constant size. A stronger stimulus does not generate a larger impulse

7. During the absolute refractory period, another impulse cannot be generated; during the relative refractory period, an impulse can be triggered only by a supra-threshold stimulus

8. Nerve impulse conduction that occurs as a step-by-step process along an unmyelinated axon is called *continuous conduction*. In *salutatory conduction*, a nerve impulse "leaps" from one node of Ranvier to the next along a myelinated axon

9. Axons with larger diameters conduct impulses faster than those with smaller diameters; myelinated axons conduct impulses faster than unmyelinated axons

Synaptic Transmission

A. Neurons communicate with each other and with effectors at synapses in a series of events known as *synaptic transmission.*

B. Two types of synapses:

1. Electrical synapses—gap junctions allow ions to flow from one cell to another

2. Chemical synapses—neurotransmitter is released from a presynaptic neuron into the synaptic cleft and then binds to receptors on the postsynaptic plasma membrane

C. Types of neurotransmitters

1. Excitatory neurotransmitter—depolarizes the membrane of the postsynaptic neuron to bring the membrane potential closer to threshold

2. Inhibitory neurotransmitter—hyperpolarizes the membrane of the postsynaptic neuron

D. The postsynaptic neuron integrates excitatory and inhibitory signals in a process called *summation* and then responds accordingly

E. The neurotransmitter is removed from the synaptic cleft in three ways: diffusion, enzymatic degradation, and reuptake by neurons or neuroglial cells

F. Important neurotransmitters include acetylcholine, glutamatic aminobutyric acid (GABA), glycine, norepinephrine, epinephrine, dopamine, serotonin, neuropeptides, and nitric oxide

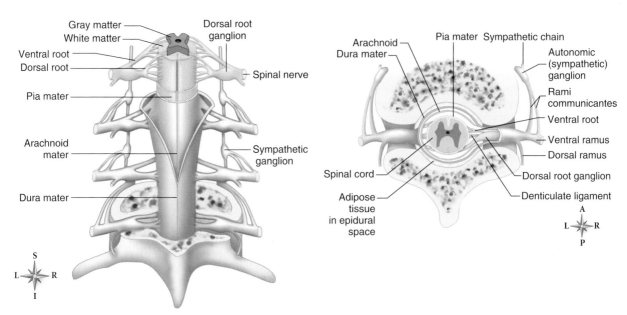

FIGURE 3-22 Coverings of the spinal cord. *(From Patton KT, Thibodeau GA:* Anthony's textbook of anatomy and physiology, *ed 19, St Louis, 2010, Mosby.)*

Spinal Cord

See Figure 3-22; see also Figure 2-11.
A. Location—in the vertebral canal; extends from the foramen magnum of the occipital bone of the skull to the superior border of the second lumbar vertebrae in the vertebral column; approximately 42 to 45 cm (16 to 18 inches)
B. Meninges—three layers of connective tissue coverings that extend around the spinal cord and the brain
  1. Dura mater—outermost of three layers
  2. Arachnoid—middle layer composed of collagen and elastic fibers
  3. Pia mater—inner layer composed of collagen and elastic fibers that adhere to the surface of the spinal cord and brain; contains numerous blood vessels
C. Spinal cord does not run the entire length of the vertebral column; nerves called *cauda equina* arise from the lowest portion of a cord and angle down the vertebral canal
D. Functions
  1. White matter tracts in the spinal cord are pathways for nerve impulse conduction; sensory impulses flow from the periphery to the brain, and motor impulses flow from the brain to the periphery
  2. Gray matter receives and integrates incoming and outgoing information
  3. Spinal reflexes—fast automatic responses to sensory impulses that enter the spinal cord via spinal nerves

  4. Reflex arc—pathway followed by nerve impulses that produce a reflex
    a. Somatic reflex—reflex involving involuntary contraction of skeletal muscles (e.g., knee-jerk reflex)
    b. Withdrawal reflex—causes immediate withdrawal of a limb from a source of injury before awareness of pain
    c. Autonomic reflex—reflexes involving smooth muscle, cardiac muscle, and glands (e.g., swallowing, urinating)
E. Spinal nerves
  1. Thirty-one pairs of spinal nerves; each has a dorsal (afferent) root and a ventral (efferent) root
  2. Named and numbered according to the region and level of the vertebral column from which they emerge
  3. Emerge from the spinal cord to form plexuses along the spinal cord except in the thoracic region
    a. The cervical plexus (C1 to C4) innervates muscles, skin, posterior head, neck, upper shoulders, and diaphragm
    b. Brachial plexus (C5 to T1) nerves supply upper limbs, neck, and muscles
      (1) Radial—lateral side of the arm
      (2) Medial—middle portion of the arm
      (3) Ulnar—medial side of the arm
    c. T2 to T12 comprise the intercostal nerves; do not form a plexus
    d. Lumbosacral plexus—includes L1 to S4

(1) Lumbar portion—first four lumbar nerves contribute to the femoral nerve; supplies abdominal wall, external genitals, and part of lower limbs

(2) Sacral portion—sacral nerves, the last lumbar nerve, and the coccygeal nerve supply the pelvis and legs; contribute to the sciatic nerve (longest nerve in the body)

Brain See Figure 3-23.

A. Principal parts—brain stem (consists of the medulla oblongata, pons, and midbrain), diencephalon (consists of the thalamus and hypothalamus), cerebrum, and cerebellum

B. Supplied with oxygen and nutrients by the cerebral arterial circle, or circle of Willis; any interruption of the oxygen supply may permanently damage or kill brain cells; glucose deficiency may produce dizziness, convulsions, and unconsciousness.

C. The blood–brain barrier (BBB) limits the passage of certain materials from the blood into the brain.

D. The brain is protected by cranial bones, meninges, and the cerebrospinal fluid
  1. Cranial meninges are continuous with the spinal meninges (dura mater, arachnoid, and pia mater)
  2. Cerebrospinal fluid—formed in the choroid plexuses; circulates continually through the subarachnoid space, ventricles, and central canal; protects the brain and spinal cord by serving as a shock absorber; delivers nutritive substances from the blood and removes wastes

E. Medulla oblongata (also called *medulla*)—is continuous with the upper part of the spinal cord;

contains regions for regulating heart rate, diameter of blood vessels, respiratory rate, swallowing, coughing, vomiting, sneezing, and hiccupping; the vestibulocochlear, accessory, vagus, and hypoglossal nerves originate at the medulla

F. Pons—connects the spinal cord to the brain; links parts of the brain to one another; relays impulses related to voluntary skeletal movements from the cerebral cortex to the cerebellum; contains two regions that control respiration. The trigeminal, abducens, facial, and vestibular branches of the vestibulocochlear nerves originate at the pons.

G. Midbrain—conveys motor impulses from the cerebrum to the cerebellum and the spinal cord, and sensory impulses from the spinal cord to the thalamus

H. Reticular formation—net-like arrangement of gray and white matter extending throughout the brain stem; alerts the cerebral cortex to incoming sensory signals; helps regulate muscle tone

I. Diencephalon—consists of the thalamus and the hypothalamus
  1. Thalamus—contains nuclei that serve as relay stations for sensory impulses to the cerebral cortex; provides crude recognition of pain, temperature, touch, pressure, and vibration
  2. Hypothalamus—located below the thalamus; controls and integrates the ANS and pituitary gland; functions in rage and aggression; controls body temperature; regulates food and fluid intake; maintains consciousness and sleep patterns

J. The reticular activating system—functions in arousal (awakening from deep sleep) and consciousness (wakefulness)

K. Cerebrum—largest part of the brain; the cortex contains convolutions, fissures, and sulci
  1. Cerebral lobes—frontal, parietal, temporal, and occipital
  2. White matter under the cerebral cortex consists of myelinated axons extending in three principal directions
  3. Sensory areas receive and interpret sensory impulses; motor areas govern muscular movement
  4. Contains tissues associated with emotional and intellectual processes
  5. Generates brain waves measurable by electroencephalogram (EEG), which may be used to diagnose epilepsy, infections, and tumors

L. Basal ganglia—paired masses of gray matter in the cerebral hemispheres that control muscular movements

M. The limbic system—found in cerebral hemispheres and the diencephalon; functions in the emotional aspects of behavior and memory

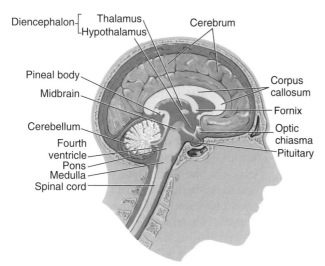

FIGURE 3-23 Divisions of the brain. *(From Solomon EP: Introduction to human anatomy and physiology, ed 2, St Louis, 2008, Saunders.)*

N. Hemispheres of the brain
1. Left hemisphere—receives sensory signals from and controls the right side of the body; more important for language, numerical and scientific skills, and reasoning
2. Right hemisphere—receives sensory signals from and controls the left side of the body; more important for musical and other artistic awareness, spatial and pattern perception, recognition of faces, emotional content of language, and generating mental images of sight, sound, touch, taste, and smell

O. Cerebellum—occupies the inferior and posterior aspects of the cranial cavity. It consists of two hemispheres with a cerebellar cortex of gray matter and an interior of white matter tracts; attaches to the brain stem by three pairs of cerebellar peduncles; coordinates skeletal muscles and maintains normal muscle tone and body equilibrium

Cranial Nerves (See the section on "The Nervous System" in Chapter 4.)

A. Twelve pairs of cranial nerves originate from the brain

B. Like spinal nerves, cranial nerves are part of the PNS

The Autonomic Nervous System

A. Regulates smooth muscle, cardiac muscle, and certain glands; usually operates without conscious control by the centers in the brain, in particular by the hypothalamus

B. Two principal divisions—sympathetic and parasympathetic; most organs have dual innervation; in general, nerve impulses from one division stimulate excitation, and impulses from the other division cause inhibition
1. Sympathetic (thoracolumbar division)—sympathetic ganglia are classified as sympathetic trunk ganglia (lateral to the vertebral column) and prevertebral ganglia (anterior to the vertebral column)
2. Parasympathetic—parasympathetic ganglia are called *terminal ganglia*; located near or within visceral effectors
3. Neurons of preganglionic autonomic neurons are myelinated; those of postganglionic autonomic neurons are unmyelinated

C. Functions
1. Cholinergic neurons release acetylcholine (Ach); adrenergic neurons release norepinephrine (NE)
2. Activation of the sympathetic division causes widespread responses; the "fight-or-flight" response
3. Activation of the parasympathetic division produces more restricted responses that typically are concerned with "rest-and-digest" activities

Special Senses

A. Sensation—conscious or subconscious awareness of external and internal conditions of the body; for a sensation to occur, three conditions must be satisfied:
1. A stimulus, or change in environment, capable of activating certain sensory neurons must occur
2. A sensory receptor must convert the stimulus to nerve impulses
3. The nerve impulses must be conducted along a neural pathway from the sensory receptor to the brain

B. Components of the eye (Figure 3-24)
1. Conjunctiva—thin mucous membrane that covers the front of the eye and lines the eyelid
2. Lacrimal glands—located bilaterally on the outer borders of the orbital cavity; secrete about 1 milliliter (mL) of fluid per day; contain lysozyme to destroy bacteria
3. Nasolacrimal duct—carries fluid away from the gland
4. Iris—the colored part of the eye that is a circular diaphragm; regulates the amount of light that enters the eye
5. Pupil—where light enters the eye; black in color
6. Lens—biconvex disc without blood
7. Sclera—white covering on the anterior aspect of the eye
8. Vitreous body—colloid inside of the eyeball; maintains the shape
9. Optic disc—located on the posterior surface of the eyeball; contains no rods or cones, only optic nerves
10. Retina—contains cones in its center (fovea) and rods on the outer periphery; process of forming an image on the retina is much like that of a camera to produce a picture
    a. Light rays are bent as they enter the eye
    b. The lens adjusts to the amount of light

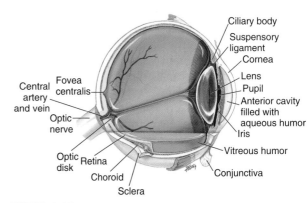

FIGURE 3-24 Horizontal cross section of the eye. *(From Applegate E: The anatomy and physiology learning system, ed 4, St Louis, 2011, Saunders.)*

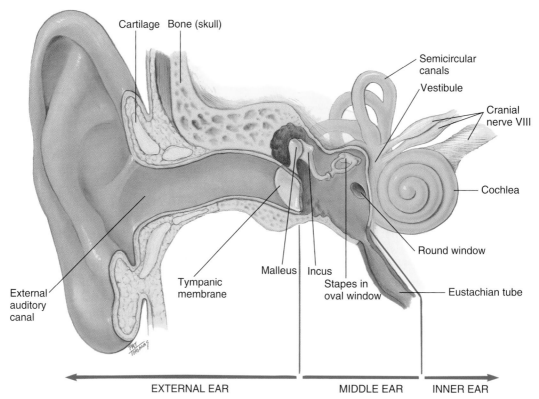

FIGURE 3-25 The ear. *(From Jarvis C: Physical examination and health assessment, ed 5, St Louis, 2007, Saunders.)*

c. Light rays are converged on the fovea

d. Rays cause changes in the chemistry of rods and cones

e. Optic nerve sends impulses to the occipital lobes of the brain

C. Hearing and equilibrium (Figure 3-25)

1. The external ear consists of an ear flap

2. The middle ear is separated by the tympanic membrane (eardrum); contains the ossicles (malleus, incus, and stapes) and the eustachian tube (to equalize pressure)

3. The inner ear contains the vestibule, the cochlea, and semicircular canals

a. Cranial nerve VIII innervates this structure

b. Small hairs detect various frequencies and pitches; impulses are sent to the temporal lobes of the brain

c. Semi-circular canals maintain equilibrium

D. Tongue

1. Cranial nerve VII provides sensory fibers to the anterior two thirds of the tongue, including fungiform and foliate papillae; sensations of sweet, sour, and salty tastes are detected

2. Cranial nerve IX provides sensations of taste to the posterior one third of the tongue's circumvallate papillae; the bitter taste is detected there

3. Food must be in solution in the mouth before taste buds can transfer the information to the brain

4. Most taste sensations are made up of various combinations of the four basic tastes

E. Olfactory sense

1. Stimulates hairs (cilia) that are sensitive to slight odors

2. On each side of the nose, bundles of slender, unmyelinated axons of olfactory receptors extend through holes in the cribriform plate of the ethmoid bone

3. These bundles of axons form cranial nerve I, the olfactory nerve; they terminate in the brain in olfactory bulbs, which are located inferior to the frontal lobes of the cerebrum

4. Within the olfactory bulbs, the axon terminals of olfactory receptors synapse with the dendrites and cell bodies of the next neurons in the olfactory pathway

5. The axons of the neurons extending from the olfactory bulb form the olfactory tract

6. The olfactory tract projects into the primary olfactory area in the temporal lobe, where the conscious awareness of smell begins

F. Tactile sensation (Table 3-2)

1. Meissner's corpuscles—receptors that control the sensation of touch

2. Pacinian corpuscles—receptors that control the sensation of pressure

3. Ruffini's corpuscles—receptors that control the sensation of heat

4. Krause's end bulbs—receptors that control the sensation of cold

5. Nociceptors—sensory receptors for pain; during tissue irritation or injury, release of chemicals such as prostaglandins (PGs) stimulates nociceptors

G. Proprioceptive sensations—inform consciously and subconsciously; sense the degree of muscle contraction, amount of tension present in tendons, position of joints, and orientation of head and equilibrium

The Endocrine System

A. Communication, integration, and control of body processes; secreting cells send hormone molecules via the blood to specific target cells contained in target tissues or target organs

1. Works in conjunction with the nervous system to achieve and maintain homeostasis

2. The neuroendocrine system—interaction of the endocrine and nervous systems to perform similar functions

B. Endocrine glands—"ductless glands"; many are made of glandular epithelium whose cells manufacture and secrete hormones; a few endocrine glands are made of neurosecretory tissue; widely scattered throughout the body

Hormones

A. Function of hormones—regulate most cells to stimulate a physiologic activity; work more slowly and last longer than neurotransmitters; carried to almost every point in the body

B. Classification of hormones

1. Classification by general function

a. Tropic hormones—target other endocrine glands and stimulate their growth and secretion

b. Sex hormones—target reproductive tissues

TABLE 3-2 Classification of Somatic Sensory Receptors

By Structure	By Location and Type	By Activation Stimulus	By Sensation or Function
Free Nerve Endings Nociceptors	Both exteroceptors and visceroceptors—most body tissues	Almost any noxious stimulus; temperature change; mechanical	Pain; temperature; itch; tickle; stretching
Merkel discs	Exteroceptors	Light pressure; mechanical	Discriminative touch
Root hair plexuses	Exteroceptors	Hair movement; mechanical	Sense of "deflection" hair movement
Nociceptors	Merkel discs		Root hair plexuses
Encapsulated Nerve Endings *Touch and Pressure Receptors* Meissner's corpuscle	Exteroceptors; epidermis, hairless skin	Light pressure, mechanical	Discriminative touch; low-frequency vibration
Krause's corpuscle	Mucous membranes	Mechanical; thermal?	Touch; low-frequency vibration
Ruffini's corpuscle	Dermis of skin, exteroceptors	Mechanical; thermal?	Crude and persistent touch
Pacinian corpuscle	Dermis of skin, joint capsules	Deep pressure, mechanical	Deep pressure; high-frequency vibration; stretch

Continued

TABLE 3-2 Classification of Somatic Sensory Receptors—cont'd

By Structure	By Location and Type	By Activation Stimulus	By Sensation or Function
Stretch Receptors Muscle spindles	Skeletal muscle	Stretch, mechanical	Sense of muscle length
Golgi tendon receptors	Musculotendinous junction	Force of contraction and tendon stretch, mechanical	Sense of muscle tension
Meissner's corpuscle			Ruffini's corpuscle
Krause's end bulb			Intrafusal fibers Muscle spindles
Pacinian corpuscle			Golgi tendon receptors

(Modified from Patton KT, Thibodeau GA: Anthony's textbook of anatomy and physiology, ed 19, St Louis, 2010, Mosby.).

c. Anabolic hormones—stimulate anabolism in target cells
2. Classification by chemical structure
   a. Steroid hormones
      (1) Synthesized from cholesterol
      (2) Lipid-soluble; can easily pass through plasma membrane of target cells
      (3) Examples include cortisol, aldosterone, estrogen, progesterone, and testosterone
   b. Nonsteroid hormones—synthesized primarily from amino acids
   c. Protein hormones—long, folded chains of amino acids, for example, insulin and parathyroid hormone
   d. Glycoprotein hormones—protein hormones with carbohydrate groups attached to the amino acid chain
   e. Peptide hormones—smaller than protein hormones; short chain of amino acids, for example, oxytocin, antidiuretic hormone (ADH)
   f. Amino acid derivative hormones—each is derived from a single amino acid molecule
      (1) Amine hormones—synthesized by modifying a single molecule of tyrosine; produced by neurosecretory cells and by neurons, for example, epinephrine, norepinephrine
      (2) Amino acid derivatives produced by the thyroid gland; synthesized by adding iodine to tyrosine
C. Mechanism of action
   1. General principles
      a. Hormones signal a cell by binding to the specific receptors of a target cell in a "lock-and-key" fashion
      b. Different hormone-receptor interactions produce different regulatory changes within the target cell through chemical reactions
      c. Combined hormone actions
         (1) Synergism—combinations of hormones acting together have a greater effect on a

target cell than the sum of the effects that each would have if acting alone

    (2) Permissiveness—when a small amount of one hormone allows a second one to have its full effects on a target cell

    (3) Antagonism—one hormone produces the opposite effects of another hormone; used to "fine tune" the activity of target cells with great accuracy

  d. Endocrine glands produce more hormone molecules than needed; unused hormones are quickly excreted by the kidneys or broken down by metabolic processes

2. Mechanism of steroid hormone action

  a. Steroid hormones are lipid soluble, and their receptors are normally found within the target cell

  b. After a steroid hormone molecule has diffused into the target cell, it binds to a receptor molecule to form a hormone-receptor complex

  c. Mobile receptor hypothesis—the hormone passes into the nucleus, where it binds to a mobile receptor and activates a certain gene sequence to begin transcription of mRNA; newly formed mRNA molecules move into the cytosol, associate with ribosomes, and begin synthesizing protein molecules that produce the effects of the hormone

  d. The amount of steroid hormone present determines the magnitude of the target cell's response

  e. Because transcription and protein synthesis take time, responses to steroid hormones are often slow

3. Mechanisms of nonsteroid hormone action

  a. Second messenger mechanism—also known as the *fixed-membrane-receptor hypothesis*

    (1) A nonsteroid hormone molecule acts as a "first messenger" and delivers its chemical message to receptors that are fixed in the plasma membrane of the target cell

    (2) The message is then passed by way of a G-protein into the cell where a "second messenger" triggers the appropriate cellular response

    (3) The second messenger mechanism produces target cell effects that differ from steroid hormone effects in several important ways:

      (a) The effects of the hormone are amplified by a cascade of reactions

      (b) The second messenger mechanisms, for example, inositol trisphosphate (IP3), guanosine monophosphate (GMP), calcium calmodulin mechanisms

      (c) The second messenger mechanism operates much more quickly than the steroid mechanism does

  b. Nuclear receptor mechanism—small iodinated amino acids (T4 and T3) enter the target cell and bind to receptors associated with a DNA molecule in the nucleus; this binding triggers transcription of mRNA and synthesis of new enzymes

D. Regulation of hormone secretion

  1. Usually part of a negative feedback loop called an *endocrine reflex*; the simplest regulatory mechanism is when an endocrine gland is sensitive to the physiologic changes produced by its target cells

  2. Regulated by a hormone produced by another gland

  3. May be influenced by the input of the nervous system; this fact emphasizes the close functional relationship between the two systems

Prostaglandins

A. Unique group of lipid molecules (20-carbon fatty acid with 5-carbon ring); serve important, widespread integrative functions, but do not meet the usual definition of a hormone; tend to integrate activities of neighboring cells

B. Called *tissue hormones* because the secretion is produced in a tissue and diffuses only a short distance to other cells within the same tissue

C. Structural classes of prostaglandins

  1. Prostaglandin A (PGA)—intra-arterial infusion resulting in an immediate drop in blood pressure accompanied by an increase in regional blood flow to several areas

  2. Prostaglandin E (PGE)—regulation of red blood cell deformability and platelet aggregation; regulation of hydrochloric acid secretion in the GI tract

  3. Prostaglandin F (PGF)—causes uterine contractions; affects intestinal motility; required for normal peristalsis

Pituitary Gland

A. Structure of the pituitary gland

  1. Also known as *hypophysis*; the "master gland"

  2. Size: 1.2 to 1.5 cm

  3. Located on the ventral surface of the brain within the skull

  4. Infundibulum—stem-like stalk that connects the pituitary to the hypothalamus

  5. Composed of two separate glands, the adenohypophysis (anterior pituitary gland) and the neurohypophysis (posterior pituitary gland)

B. Adenohypophysis (anterior pituitary)
1. Divided into two parts:
   a. Pars anterior—forms the major portion of the adenohypophysis
   b. Pars intermedia
2. Tissue is composed of irregular clumps of secretory cells supported by fine connective tissue fibers and surrounded by a rich vascular network
3. Three types of cells can be identified by their stain affinity:
   a. Chromophobes—do not stain
   b. Acidophils—stain with acidic stains
   c. Basophils—stain with basic stains
4. Five functional types of secretory cells:
   a. Somatotrophs—secrete growth hormone (GH)
   b. Corticotrophs—secrete ACTH
   c. Thyrotrophs—secrete TSH
   d. Lactotrophs—secrete prolactin
   e. Gonadotrophs—secrete LH and FSH
C. Hormones secreted by the adenohypophysis
1. Growth hormone; also known as *somatotropin* (*STH*)
   a. Promotes growth of bone, muscle, and other tissues by accelerating amino acid transport into the cells
   b. Stimulates fat metabolism by mobilizing lipids from storage in adipose cells and speeding up the catabolism of lipids after they have entered another cell
   c. Shifts cell chemistry away from glucose catabolism and toward lipid catabolism as an energy source; this leads to increased blood glucose levels
   d. Functions as an insulin antagonist; vital to maintaining the homeostasis of blood glucose levels
2. Prolactin (PRL); also known as *lactogenic hormone*
   a. Produced by acidophils in the pars anterior
   b. Promotes breast development during pregnancy in anticipation of milk secretion; stimulates lactation after delivery
3. Tropic hormones—have a stimulating effect on other endocrine glands; four principal tropic hormones are produced and secreted by the basophils of the pars anterior
   a. Thyroid-stimulating hormone (TSH), or thyrotropin—promotes and maintains the growth and development of the thyroid; causes the thyroid to secrete its hormones
   b. Adrenocorticotropic hormone (ACTH), or adrenocorticotropin—promotes and maintains normal growth and development of the cortex of the adrenal gland; stimulates the adrenal cortex to secrete some of its hormones

c. Follicle-stimulating hormone (FSH)—stimulates primary graafian follicles to grow toward maturity in females; also stimulates follicle cells to secrete estrogens; in males, stimulates the development of the seminiferous tubules of the testes and maintains spermatogenesis
d. Luteinizing hormone (LH)—stimulates the formation and activity of the corpus luteum of the ovary in females; the corpus luteum secretes progesterone and estrogens when stimulated by LH; LH also supports FSH in stimulating the maturation of follicles; in males, LH stimulates the interstitial cells in the testes to develop and secrete testosterone; FSH and LH are called *gonadotropins* because they stimulate the growth and maintenance of the gonads
4. Control of secretion in the adenohypophysis
   a. The hypothalamus secretes releasing hormones into the blood, which are then carried to the hypophyseal portal system; through negative feedback, the hypothalamus adjusts the secretions of the adenohypophysis, which then adjusts the secretions of the target glands, which, in turn, adjust the activity of their target tissues
   b. The hypophyseal portal system carries blood from the hypothalamus directly to the adenohypophysis, where the target cells of the releasing hormones are located; releasing hormones influence the secretion of hormones by acidophils and basophils
   c. Under stress, hypothalamus translates nerve impulses into hormone secretions by endocrine glands, creating a neuroendocrine link
D. Neurohypophysis (posterior pituitary)
1. Serves as storage and release site for ADH and oxytocin (OT), which are synthesized in the hypothalamus
2. ADH and OT are released into blood; controlled by nervous stimulation
3. Antidiuretic hormone
   a. Prevents the formation of a large volume of urine, thereby helping the body conserve water
   b. Causes the tubules in the kidney to resorb water from urine
   c. Dehydration triggers the release of ADH
4. Oxytocin—has two actions:
   a. Causes the release of milk from the lactating breast; regulated by the positive feedback mechanism; PRL cooperates with OT
   b. Stimulates the contractions of uterine muscles during childbirth; regulated by positive feedback mechanism

Pineal Gland

A. Tiny, pinecone-shaped structure located on the dorsal aspect of the brain's diencephalon

B. A member of the nervous system because it receives visual stimuli; also a member of the endocrine system because it secretes hormones

C. Supports the body's biologic clock

D. Principal pineal secretion is melatonin

Thyroid Gland

(See the section on "Glands of the Head and Neck Region" and Figure 4-8 in Chapter 4.)

A. Structure of the thyroid gland

1. Two large lateral lobes and a narrow connecting isthmus; located in the neck, on the anterior and lateral surfaces of the trachea, just below the larynx

2. A thin worm-like projection of thyroid tissue often extends upward from the isthmus

3. The weight of the thyroid in an adult is approximately 30 g

4. Composed of follicles
   a. Small hollow spheres
   b. Filled with thyroid colloid that contains thyroglobulins

B. Thyroid hormone

1. Two different hormones:
   a. Triiodothyronine (T3)—contains three iodine atoms; considered to be the principal thyroid hormone; T3 binds efficiently to the nuclear receptors in target cells
   b. Tetraiodothyronine (T4), or thyroxine—contains four iodine atoms; approximately 20 times more abundant than T3; its major importance is its role as a precursor to T3

2. The thyroid gland stores considerable amounts of a preliminary form of its hormones prior to secreting them

3. Before being stored in the colloid of follicles, T3 and T4 are attached to globulin molecules to form thyroglobin complexes

4. On release, T3 and T4 detach from globulin and enter the bloodstream

5. Once in the blood, T3 and T4 attach to plasma globulins and travel as a hormone–globulin complex

6. T3 detaches from plasma globulin as it nears the target cells; T4 also detaches, but to a lesser extent

7. Thyroid hormone—helps regulate the metabolic rate of all cells, cell growth, and tissue differentiation; it is said to have a "general" target

C. Calcitonin

1. Produced by the thyroid gland in the parafollicular cells

2. Influences the processing of calcium by bone cells by decreasing blood calcium levels and promoting the conservation of the hard bone matrix

3. Parathyroid hormone acts as antagonist to calcitonin to maintain calcium homeostasis

Parathyroid Glands

A. Structure of the parathyroid glands

1. Four or five parathyroid glands are embedded in the posterior surface of the thyroid's lateral lobes

2. Tiny, rounded bodies within thyroid tissue formed by compact, irregular rows of cells

B. Parathyroid hormone (PTH)

1. An antagonist to calcitonin; acts to maintain calcium homeostasis

2. Acts on bone and the kidneys
   a. Causes more bone to be dissolved, yielding calcium and phosphate, which enter the bloodstream
   b. Causes phosphate to be secreted by the kidney cells into urine to be excreted
   c. Increases the intestinal absorption of calcium by stimulating the kidney to produce active vitamin D

Adrenal Glands

A. Structure of the adrenal glands

1. Located on top of the kidneys like caps

2. Made up of two portions:
   a. Adrenal cortex—composed of endocrine tissue
   b. Adrenal medulla—composed of neurosecretory tissue

B. Adrenal cortex

1. All cortical hormones are steroids; known as *corticosteroids*

2. Composed of three distinct layers of secreting cells:
   a. Zona glomerulosa—outermost layer, directly under the outer connective tissue capsule of the adrenal gland; secretes mineralocorticoids
   b. Zona fasciculata—middle layer; secretes glucocorticoids
   c. Zona reticularis—inner layer; secretes small amounts of glucocorticoids and gonadocorticoids

3. Mineralocorticoids—important role in regulating sodium levels
   a. Aldosterone
      (1) The only physiologically important mineralocorticoid; the primary function is maintenance of sodium homeostasis in blood by increasing sodium resorption in the kidneys
      (2) Increases water retention; promotes the loss of potassium and hydrogen ions

(3) Secretion is controlled by the renin–angiotensin mechanism and by blood potassium concentration

4. Glucocorticoids
   a. Secreted by the zona fasciculata
   b. Examples include cortisol, cortisone, and corticosterone
   c. Affect every body cell
   d. Are protein mobilizing, gluconeogenic, and hyperglycemia inducing
   e. Tend to cause a shift from carbohydrate catabolism to lipid catabolism
   f. Essential for maintaining normal blood pressure by helping norepinephrine and epinephrine to have their full effect; cause vasoconstriction
   g. High blood concentration causes eosinopenia and marked atrophy of lymphatic tissues
   h. Act with epinephrine to bring about normal recovery from injury produced by inflammatory agents
   i. Secretion increases in response to stress
   j. Except during stress response, secretion is mainly controlled by a negative feedback mechanism involving ACTH from the adenohypophysis
5. Gonadocorticoids—sex hormones (androgens) released from the adrenal cortex
C. Adrenal medulla
   1. Neurosecretory tissue—composed of neurons specialized to secrete their products into blood
   2. Secretes epinephrine and norepinephrine, part of the class of nonsteroid hormones called *catecholamines*; both hormones bind to the receptors of sympathetic effectors to prolong and enhance the effects of sympathetic stimulation by the ANS

Pancreatic Islets

A. Structure of the pancreatic islets
   1. Elongated gland; its head lies in the duodenum; extends horizontally behind the stomach and touches the spleen
   2. Composed of endocrine and exocrine tissues
      a. Islets of Langerhans—endocrine portion; each islet contains four primary types of endocrine glands joined by gap junctions:
         (1) Alpha cells (α-cells)—secrete glucagon
         (2) Beta cells (β-cells)—secrete insulin; account for up to 75% of all pancreatic islet cells
         (3) Delta cells (δ-cells)—secrete somatostatin
         (4) Pancreatic polypeptide cells (F- or PP-cells)—secrete pancreatic polypeptides

   b. Acini—exocrine portion; secretes a serous fluid containing digestive enzymes into the ducts draining into the small intestine
B. Pancreatic hormones—work as a team to maintain the homeostasis of food molecules
   1. Glucagon—produced by α-cells; tends to increase blood glucose levels; stimulates gluconeogenesis in liver cells
   2. Insulin—produced by β-cells; lowers the blood concentration of glucose and fatty acids; promotes their metabolism by tissue cells
   3. Somatostatin—produced by δ-cells; primary role is regulating the other endocrine cells of pancreatic islets
   4. Pancreatic polypeptide—produced by F- (PP-) cells; influences the digestion and distribution of food molecules to some degree

Gonads

A. Testes
   1. Paired organs within the scrotum in the male
   2. Composed of seminiferous tubules and a scattering of interstitial cells
   3. Testosterone—produced by interstitial cells; responsible for the growth and maintenance of male sexual characteristics; secretion is mainly regulated by gonadotropin levels in blood
B. Ovaries
   1. Primary sex organs in the female
   2. Set of paired glands in the pelvis that produce several types of sex hormones
      a. Estrogens—steroid hormones secreted by ovarian follicles; promote development and maintenance of female sexual characteristics
      b. Progesterone—secreted by the corpus luteum; maintains the lining of the uterus necessary for successful pregnancy
      c. Ovarian hormone secretion depends on the changing levels of FSH and LH from the adenohypophysis

Placenta

A. Tissues that form on the lining of the uterus as a connection between the circulatory systems of the mother and the developing fetus
B. Serves as a temporary endocrine gland; produces human chorionic gonadotropin, estrogens, and progesterone

Thymus Gland

A. Located in the mediastinum just beneath the sternum
B. Large in children, begins to atrophy at puberty, and is a vestige of fat and fibrous tissue by old age
C. Considered to be primarily a lymphatic organ

D. Thymosin—isolated from thymus tissue; stimulates development of T cells

Gastric and Intestinal Mucosa
A. The mucous lining of the GI tract contains cells that produce both endocrine and exocrine secretions
B. GI hormones such as gastrin, secretin, and cholecystokinin–pancreozymin (CCK) play regulatory roles in coordinating the secretory and motor activities involved in the digestive process
C. Ghrelin—a hormone secreted by endocrine cells in the gastric mucosa; stimulates the hypothalamus to boost appetite; slows metabolism and fat burning; may be a contributor to obesity

Heart
A. Has a secondary endocrine role; hormone-producing cells produce atrial natriuretic hormone (ANH)
B. ANH opposes increases in blood volume or blood pressure; also an antagonist to ADH and aldosterone

The Cardiovascular System

The cardiovascular system consists of three interrelated components: blood, the heart, and blood vessels.
A. Blood
  1. A vital liquid that has three general functions: transportation, regulation, and protection
    a. Transportation—transports oxygen from the lungs to the cells throughout the body and carbon dioxide from the cells to the lungs; carries nutrients from the GI tract to body cells, heat and waste products away from cells, and hormones from endocrine glands to other body cells
    b. Regulation—helps regulate the pH of body fluids; helps adjust body temperature; blood osmotic pressure also influences the water content of cells.
    c. Protection—blood clots in response to injury to protect against excessive blood loss; white blood cells protect against disease by carrying out phagocytosis and by producing antibodies; contains interferons that also help protect against disease
B. Characteristics
  1. Viscosity greater than that of water; temperature of 38°C (100.4°F); pH ranges between 7.35 and 7.45
  2. Blood constitutes about 8% of body weight in an adult
C. Components (Figure 3-26)
  1. Consists of 55% plasma; 45% formed elements that include red blood cells (erythrocytes), white blood cells (leukocytes), and platelets
  2. Hematocrit—the percentage of red blood cells in whole blood

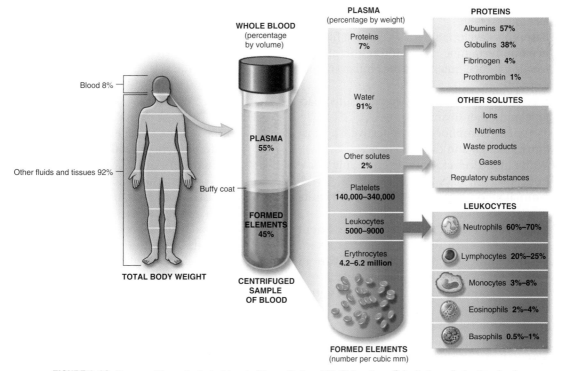

FIGURE 3-26 Composition of whole blood. (*From Patton KT, Thibodeau GA:* Anthony's textbook of anatomy and physiology, *ed 19, St Louis, 2010, Mosby.*)

3. Plasma contains 91% water, 7% proteins, and 2% solutes
4. Principal solutes include proteins (albumins, globulins, fibrinogen), nutrients, hormones, respiratory gases, electrolytes, and waste products
5. Hemopoiesis—the formation of blood cells from pluripotent stem cells, occurs in red bone marrow
6. Red blood cells—biconcave discs without a nucleus that contain hemoglobin
   a. Hemoglobin transports oxygen
   b. Red blood cells live for about 120 days; in terms of a normal blood count, a healthy male has about 4.7 to 6.1 million/mm³ red blood cells; a healthy female has about 4.2 to 5.4 million/mm³ red blood cells
   c. After phagocytosis of aged red blood cells by macrophages, hemoglobin is recycled
   d. Erythropoiesis—red blood cell formation occurring in adult red bone marrow; stimulated by hypoxia, which stimulates the release of erythropoietin by the kidneys
7. White blood cells—nucleated cells with two principal groups:
   a. Granular leukocytes (neutrophils, eosinophils, basophils)
   b. Agranular leukocytes (lymphocytes and monocytes)
   c. Function—to combat inflammation and infection. Neutrophils and monocytes do so by phagocytosis
   d. Eosinophils combat the effects of histamine in allergic reactions, and increase with allergies and parasites
   e. Basophils develop into mast cells that liberate heparin, histamine, and serotonin in allergic reactions that intensify the inflammatory response
   f. B cells (lymphocytes)—effective against bacteria and other toxins
   g. T cells (lymphocytes)—effective against viruses, fungi, and cancer cells
   h. White blood cells usually live for only a few hours or a few days
   i. Normal blood contains 5,000 to 10,000 white blood cells /mm³
8. Platelets—disc-shaped cell fragments without nuclei
   a. Formed from megakaryocytes; take part in hemostasis by forming a platelet plug
   b. Normal blood contains 150,000 to 450,000 platelets /mm³
D. Hemostasis—stoppage of bleeding
   1. Three mechanisms:
      a. Vascular spasm—when a blood vessel is damaged, the smooth muscle in its walls contracts immediately

      b. Platelet plug—when platelets come into contact with parts of a damaged blood vessel, their characteristics change drastically, and they come together to form a plug that helps fill the gap in the injured vessel
      c. Blood clotting—a series of reactions
         (1) Prothrombinase is formed
         (2) Conversion of prothrombin into thrombin
         (3) Conversion of soluble fibrinogen into insoluble fibrin
   2. Clot—a network of insoluble protein fibers (fibrin), in which formed elements of blood are trapped
   3. Normal coagulation requires vitamin K and also involves clot retraction and fibrinolysis
   4. Anticoagulants prevent clotting
   5. Thrombosis—clotting in an unbroken blood vessel; a thrombus that moves from its site of origin is called an *embolus*
E. Blood groups
   1. Surfaces of red blood cells contain a genetically determined assortment of glycolipids and glycoproteins called *isoantigens*. Based on the presence or absence of various isoantigens, blood is categorized into different blood groups. Within a blood group, two or more different blood types may be present:
   2. ABO blood group system—based on isoantigens A and B
      a. Type A—red blood cells display only antigen A
      b. Type B—red blood cells display only antigen B
      c. Type AB—red blood cells display both antigens A and B
      d. Type O—red blood cells display neither antigen A nor B
F. Heart
   1. Located in the space between the lungs, behind the sternum, in the thoracic cavity known as the *mediastinum*; size of a human fist; apex of the heart points down and to the left
   2. Consists of four chambers: two atria and two ventricles (Figure 3-27)
      a. Blood from superior and inferior venae cavae fills the right atrium and passes into the right ventricle through the tricuspid valve (three flaps)
      b. From the right ventricle, the unoxygenated blood is sent to the lungs by passing through the semi-lunar valve and the pulmonary artery
      c. Oxygenated blood is sent from the lungs to the left atrium through the pulmonary veins; the left semi-lunar valve separates the left atrium from the pulmonary veins

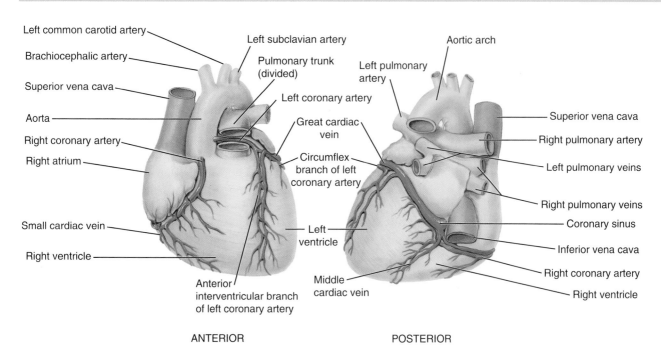

Left common carotid artery

Brachiocephalic artery

Superior vena cava

Aorta

Right coronary artery

Right atrium

Small cardiac vein

Right ventricle

Left subclavian artery

Pulmonary trunk (divided)

Left coronary artery

Great cardiac vein

Circumflex branch of left coronary artery

Left ventricle

Anterior interventricular branch of left coronary artery

Middle cardiac vein

Aortic arch

Left pulmonary artery

Superior vena cava

Right pulmonary artery

Left pulmonary veins

Right pulmonary veins

Coronary sinus

Inferior vena cava

Right coronary artery

Right ventricle

ANTERIOR   POSTERIOR

FIGURE 3-27 The heart and great vessels. *(From Applegate E: The anatomy and physiology learning system, ed 4, St Louis, 2011, Saunders.)*

d. From the left atrium, blood flows through the mitral valve (two flaps) into the left ventricle

e. Blood enters the circulation by passing through the left semilunar valve into the aorta

3. The heart walls consist of three layers:
    a. Visceral pericardium or epicardium
    b. Myocardium—heaviest covering
    c. Endocardium—smooth continuous covering
    d. All valves and chambers are lined by the endothelium

4. The valves of the heart are unique
    a. Atrioventricular (AV) valves—tough, fibrous tissue; open except when ventricles contract; hang into the ventricle like a leaf; held in place by chordae tendineae at the edge of the valves
        (1) Tricuspid AV valve—formed by three flaps
        (2) Bicuspid AV valve (mitral valve)— formed by two parts
    b. Semi-lunar (SL) valves—pressure opens them, and reverse pressure closes them; remain closed until ventricles contract
        (1) Pulmonary SL valve—located at the right
        (2) Aortic SL valve—located at the left

5. Heart rate averages 70 to 72 beats per minute; the heart cannot contract without nerve impulses; nerves regulate heart rate
    a. Sinoatrial (SA) node—located in the walls of the right atrium near the superior vena cava; the heart beat begins there
        (1) From there, the action current spreads out and passes down to the fibrous layer and stops
        (2) The current goes through the AV node at the upper end of the interventricular septum
        (3) Modified cardiac muscle divides into right and left branches
        (4) Along the AV bundle, fibers pass out into the cardiac muscle (Purkinje fibers)
    b. The action current consists of the impulse starting at the SA node, spreads to the atria, passes to the AV node, is picked up and sent down through all the cardiac fibers from Purkinje fibers, and ends by spreading up over the ventricles; muscle contracts after the impulse spreads over the heart
        (1) Purkinje fibers provide for uniform contraction
        (2) If the AV node is blocked, ventricles will set up their own rhythm

6. Cardiac cycle—includes all the events associated with one heart beat (Figure 3-28)
    a. In a normal cardiac cycle, the two atria contract while the two ventricles relax; then, while the two ventricles contract, the two atria relax
        (1) Systole—phase of contraction
        (2) Diastole—phase of relaxation
    b. Three phases of cardiac cycle (each cycle lasts about 0.8 second):

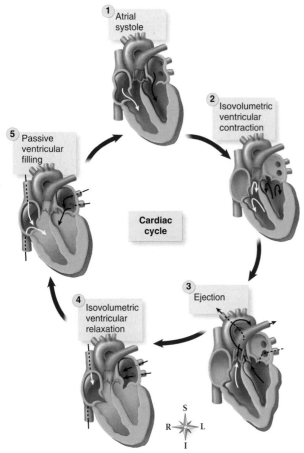

FIGURE 3-28 The cardiac cycle. *(From Patton KT, Thibodeau GA: Anthony's textbook of anatomy and physiology, ed 19, St Louis, 2010, Mosby.)*

(1) Relaxation period—begins at the end of a cardiac cycle; ventricles start to relax, and all four chambers are in diastole; repolarization of ventricular muscle fibers initiates relaxation; as ventricles relax, pressure within them drops; when ventricular pressure drops below atrial pressure, AV valves open, and ventricular filling begins

(2) Contraction (atrial systole)—an action potential from the SA node causes atrial depolarization; atria contract and force the last 25% of blood into ventricles; AV valves are still open, and semi-lunar valves are closed

(3) Contraction (ventricular systole)—ventricular contraction pushes blood against AV valves, forcing them to shut; pressure inside chambers rises when left ventricular pressure surpasses aortic pressure; right ventricular pressure rises above the pressure in the pulmonary trunk; both semi-lunar valves open, and ejection of

blood from the heart begins; ejection continues until ventricles start to relax; ventricular pressure drops, semi-lunar valves close, and another relaxation period begins

c. Heart sounds
   (1) First sound—AV valves close
   (2) Second sound—SL valves close

d. Cardiac output—volume of blood ejected per minute from the left ventricle into the aorta; determined by:
   (1) Stroke volume (SV)—amount of blood ejected by the left ventricle during each contraction or beat; in a resting adult, stroke volume averages 70 mL, and heart rate is about 75 beats per minute
   (2) Number of heart beats per minute
   (3) Regulation of stroke volume depends on three factors:
      (a) Starling's law—the more the heart is stretched as it fills during diastole, the greater is the force of contraction during systole.
      (b) The forcefulness of the contraction of individual ventricular muscle fibers
      (c) The pressure required to eject blood from the ventricles
   (4) Regulation of heart rate—adjustments of heart rate are important in the short-term control of cardiac output and blood pressure, for example, during exercise, cardiac output rises to supply working tissues with increased amounts of oxygen and nutrients
      (a) The most important factors are the autonomic nervous system and the hormones epinephrine and norepinephrine released by adrenal glands
      (b) The regulation of the nervous system originates in the cardiovascular center in the medulla oblongata
      (c) Sympathetic impulses increase heart rate and force of contraction; parasympathetic impulses decrease heart rate
      (d) Sensory receptors help adjust heart rate, for example, baroreceptors (neurons sensitive to blood pressure) are strategically located in the arch of the aorta and carotid arteries. If an increase in blood pressure occurs, baroreceptors send nerve impulses along the sensory neurons that are part of the glossopharyngeal and vagus nerves (X) to the cardiovascular center. The cardiovascular center

responds, and the result is a decrease in heart rate that lowers cardiac output, thus lowering blood pressure

    (5) Chemical regulation of heart rate
        (a) Epinephrine and norepinephrine enhance the heart's pumping effectiveness by increasing both heart rate and contraction force
        (b) Thyroid hormones also increase heart rate; a sign of hyperthyroidism is tachycardia
        (c) Ions—elevated blood levels of K^+ or Na^+ decrease heart rate and contraction force

The Circulatory System

The circulatory system contributes to the homeostasis of other body systems by transporting and distributing blood throughout the body to deliver oxygen, nutrients, hormones and so on and to carry away wastes.

A. Types of blood vessels
  1. Arteries—carry blood away from the heart to body tissues; walls have three layers of tissue surrounding a hollow space called the *lumen*
    a. Inner layer composed of endothelium
    b. Middle layer composed of smooth muscle and elastic tissue
    c. Outer layer composed mainly of elastic and collagen fibers
    d. Vasoconstriction—increase in sympathetic stimulation stimulates smooth muscle to contract, squeezing the vessel wall and narrowing the lumen
    e. Vasodilation—sympathetic stimulation decreases; smooth muscle fibers relax
  2. Arteriole—very small artery that delivers blood to capillaries
  3. Capillaries—microscopic vessels that connect arterioles to venules; present near almost every body cell; permit the exchange of nutrients and wastes between the body's cells and blood; the number of capillaries varies with the metabolic activity they serve
    a. Because capillaries are so numerous, blood flows more slowly through them than through larger blood vessels
    b. Slow flow aids the prime mission of the entire cardiovascular system—to keep blood flowing through capillaries so that capillary exchange (movement of substances into and out of capillaries) can occur
    c. Methods of capillary exchange
        (1) Diffusion
        (2) Bulk flow (filtration and resorption)—capillary blood pressure "pushes" fluid out of capillaries into interstitial fluid (filtration); blood colloid osmotic pressure "pulls" fluid into capillaries from interstitial fluid (resorption)

  4. Venules—small vessels that emerge from capillaries and merge to form veins; they receive blood from capillaries and empty blood into veins, which return blood to the heart
  5. Venous return—volume of blood flowing back to the heart occurs because of the pumping action of the heart, aided by skeletal muscle contractions (skeletal muscle pump) and breathing (respiratory pump).
  6. Hormonal regulation of blood pressure—several hormones regulate blood pressure and blood flow by altering cardiac output, changing vascular resistance, or adjusting the total blood volume
    a. Renin–angiotensin–aldosterone (RAA)—when blood volume or blood flow to the kidneys decreases, certain cells in the kidneys secrete renin into the bloodstream.
        (1) Renin and angiotensin together produce the hormone angiotensin II, which raises blood pressure by causing vasoconstriction
        (2) Angiotensin II also stimulates the secretion of aldosterone, which increases resorption of sodium ions (Na^+) and water by the kidneys; water resorption increases the total blood volume, which, in turn, increases blood pressure
    b. Epinephrine and norepinephrine—in response to sympathetic stimulation, the adrenal medulla releases these hormones, which, in turn, increase cardiac output by increasing the rate and force of heart contractions; they also cause vasoconstriction of arterioles

B. Blood pressure—pressure exerted by blood on the walls of a blood vessel; generated by the contraction of ventricles (see the sections on "Health History Evaluation" in Chapter 15 and "Vital Signs" in Chapter 21)
  1. Blood pressure is highest in the aorta and in the large systemic arteries; it drops progressively as distance from the left ventricle increases
  2. An increase in blood volume increases blood pressure; a decrease in blood volume decreases blood pressure
  3. Vascular resistance—the opposition to blood flow because of friction between blood and the walls of blood vessels; depends on the size of the blood vessel lumen, blood viscosity, and total length of the blood vessel
  4. Neural regulation—the nervous system regulates blood pressure via negative feedback loops that

occur as two types of reflexes: baroreceptor and chemoreceptor reflexes

    a. Baroreceptors—neurons sensitive to pressure; send impulses to the cardiovascular center to regulate blood pressure

    b. Chemoreceptors—neurons sensitive to concentrations of O_2, CO_2, and hydrogen ions (H^+); chemoreceptors detect changes in the blood levels of O_2, CO_2, and H^+ and in the veins in skin and abdominal organs

    c. Antidiuretic hormone—produced by the hypothalamus and released from the pituitary gland in response to dehydration or decreased blood volume; also causes vasoconstriction

    d. Atrial natriuretic peptide—released by cells in the atria of the heart; lowers blood pressure by causing vasodilation and by promoting loss of salt and water in urine, which reduces blood volume

  5. Autoregulation refers to local adjustments of blood flow in response to physical and chemical changes in a tissue

C. Assessing circulation via pulse and blood pressure (see the section on "Health History Evaluation" and Table 15-5 in Chapter 15, and the section on "Pulse, Blood Pressure, and Shock" and Figures 21-1 and 21-2 in Chapter 21)

  1. Pulse—alternative expansion and elastic recoil of an artery with each heart beat

  2. Blood pressure—pressure exerted by blood on the walls of an artery when the left ventricle undergoes systole and then diastole

  3. Shock—failure of the cardiovascular system to adequately circulate blood or deliver adequate amounts of oxygen and nutrients to meet the metabolic needs of cells

D. Circulatory route

  1. Systemic circulation—takes oxygenated blood from the left ventricle through the aorta to all parts of the body and returns deoxygenated blood to the right atrium

    a. Parts of the aorta include the ascending aorta, the arch of the aorta, and the descending aorta; each part gives off arteries that branch to supply the whole body

    b. Blood leaving the aorta and traveling through systemic arteries is of a bright red color; as it moves through the capillaries, it loses some of its O_2 and takes on CO_2 so that the blood in systemic veins is of a dark red color

  2. Pulmonary circulation—takes deoxygenated blood from the right ventricle to the air sacs of the lungs and returns oxygenated blood from the air sacs to the left atrium; allows blood to be oxygenated for systemic circulation; deoxygenated blood is returned to the heart through

systemic veins; all veins of systemic circulation flow into either the superior vena cava, the inferior vena cava, or the coronary sinus, which empty into the right atrium

  3. Hepatic portal circulation—collects deoxygenated blood from the veins of the GI tract and spleen and directs it into the hepatic portal vein of the liver; allows the liver to extract, modify, and detoxify harmful substances in blood; the liver also receives oxygenated blood from the hepatic artery

The Lymphatic and Immune System

A. Components (Figure 3-29)

  1. Lymph

  2. Lymphatic vessels

  3. Structures and organs that contain lymphatic tissue (specialized reticular tissue containing large numbers of lymphocytes)

  4. Red bone marrow

B. Function

  1. Drains tissue spaces of excess interstitial fluid

  2. Transports dietary lipids (triglycerides, cholesterol, and lipid-soluble vitamins A, D, E, K) from the GI tract to blood

  3. With the help of macrophages, protects the body from foreign invasion by microbes and cancer cells

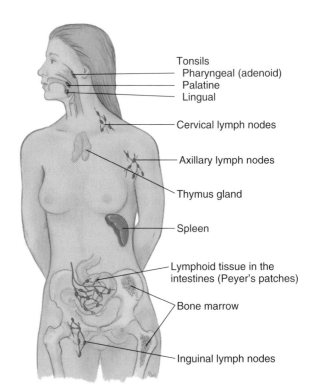

FIGURE 3-29 Components of the lymphatic system. *(From Jarvis C: Physical examination and health assessment, ed 5, St Louis, 2007, Saunders.)*

4. The major difference between the interstitial fluid and lymph is location; when fluid bathes tissue cells, it is called *interstitial fluid*, or *intercellular fluid*; when it flows through lymphatic vessels, it is called *lymph*

C. Lymphatic vessels and lymph circulation
   1. Lymphatic vessels—begin as lymphatic capillaries in tissue spaces between cells; have thinner walls and more valves than veins
   2. Lymphatic capillaries—merge to form larger vessels, called *lymphatic vessels*, which ultimately converge into the thoracic duct or the right lymphatic duct
   3. Lymph flows from the interstitial fluid, to lymphatic capillaries, to lymphatic vessels, to lymph trunks, to the thoracic duct or right lymphatic duct, to the subclavian veins as a result of skeletal muscle contractions, respiratory movements, and the valves in the lymphatic vessels
      a. The milking action of skeletal muscle contractions compresses lymphatic vessels and forces lymph toward subclavian veins (skeletal muscle pump)
      b. Lymphatic vessels contain valves that ensure the one-way movement of lymph; lymph flow is also maintained by pressure changes that occur during inhalation (respiratory pump); lymph flows from the abdominal region, where the pressure is higher, toward the thoracic region, where it is lower; when the pressures reverse during exhalation, valves prevent the backflow of lymph
      c. Edema—accumulation of the interstitial fluid in tissue spaces caused by an obstruction such as an infected lymph node, blockage of lymphatic vessels, injury, or inflammation (see the section on "Inflammation" in Chapter 7).

D. Lymphatic organs and tissues (see Chapter 9, Table 9-9, and Figures 9-1 and 9-2)
   1. Primary lymphatic organs (red bone marrow)—sites where stem cells divide and mature into B cells and T-cells
   2. Secondary lymphatic organs and tissues—lymph nodes, spleen, and lymphatic nodules; sites where most immune responses occur
   3. Thymus—a two-lobed organ located posterior to the sternum and medial to the lungs
      a. Site of T cell maturation
      b. Produces hormones
      c. Large in infants; after puberty, much of thymic tissue is replaced by fat and connective tissue; the gland continues to function throughout life
   4. Lymph nodes—approximately 600 bean-shaped organs located along lymphatic vessels; scattered throughout the body, both in superficial and deep locations; usually occur in groups (see the section on "Blood and Lymph" in Chapter 2; the section on "The Lymphatic System" and Figure 4-7 in Chapter 4; and the section on "Extraoral and Intraoral Assessment" and Figure 15-6 in Chapter 15)
      a. Contain B cells that develop into plasma cells, which secrete antibodies, T cells, and macrophages
      b. Function as filters of lymphatic fluid

The Immune System

Comprises a wide variety of body reactions or responses to fight the invasion of pathogens (Figure 3-30; see the section on "Disease Barriers," Tables 9-8 and 9-9, and Figures 9-1 and 9-2 in Chapter 9).

A. Two major categories:
   1. Nonspecific immunity—mechanisms that provide general defense by acting against anything recognized as "not self" or foreign
   2. Specific immunity—mechanisms that recognize specific threatening agents

Nonspecific Immunity

A. Species resistance—genetic characteristics of an organism or species that defend against pathogens
B. First line of defense—mechanical and chemical barriers, for example, skin, mucous membranes, sebum, mucus, enzymes, and hydrochloric acid in the stomach

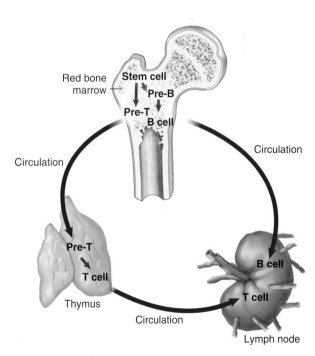

FIGURE 3-30 Lines of defense. *(From Patton KT, Thibodeau GA: Anthony's textbook of anatomy and physiology, ed 19, St Louis, 2010, Mosby.)*

C. Second line of defense—inflammation (see Figure 3-30; see the sections on "Inflammation," "Acute Inflammation," and "Chronic Inflammation" in Chapter 7)
   1. Inflammatory response—tissue damage elicits responses to counteract injury and promote normalcy
   2. Phagocytosis—ingestion and destruction of microorganisms or other small particles by phagocytes, for example, neutrophils, macrophages, histiocytes in connective tissue, microglia in the nervous system, and Kupffer cells in the liver
D. Third line of defense—natural killer cells (lymphocytes that kill tumor cells and cells infected by viruses); method of killing cells—lysing cells by damaging plasma membranes
   1. Interferon—protein synthesized and released into the circulation by certain cells if invaded by viruses
   2. Complement—group of enzymes lyse cells when activated by either specific or nonspecific mechanisms

Specific Immunity
A. Specific immunity—part of the third line of defense consisting of lymphocytes; lymphocytes are densest where they develop in bone marrow, thymus gland, lymph nodes, and spleen; lymphocytes flow through the bloodstream, become distributed in tissues, and return to the bloodstream in a continuous recirculation; lymphocytes are named by the CD protein surface markers that the cells carry, for example, CD4 and CD cells (called the CD system)
B. Two classes of lymphocytes—B lymphocytes (B cells) and T lymphocytes (T cells)
   1. B cells—produce antibodies that attack pathogens (antibody-mediated immunity)
   2. T cells—attack pathogens more directly (cell-mediated immunity)

B Cells and Antibody-Mediated Immunity (See the section on "Disease Barriers" and Figure 9-1 in Chapter 9.)
A. B cells develop in two stages:
   1. Pre–B cells develop by a few months of age
   2. The second stage occurs in lymph nodes and the spleen—activation of B cell when it binds to a specific antigen
   3. B cells serve as ancestors to antibody-secreting plasma cells
B. Antibodies—proteins (immunoglobulins) secreted by activated B cell; resist disease first by recognizing foreign abnormal substances
C. Antibody molecule—consists of two heavy and two light polypeptide chains; each molecule has two antigen-binding sites and two complement-binding sites; produces antibody-mediated immunity (humoral immunity) within plasma
D. Classes of immunoglobulins (Ig) (see Table 9-9 in Chapter 9)
   1. IgM—inactive B cells synthesize and insert themselves into their own plasma membranes; predominant class produced after initial contact with an antigen
   2. IgG—makes up 75% of antibodies in blood; predominant antibody of the secondary antibody response
   3. IgA—major class of antibody in external secretions of the mucous membranes, saliva, and tears
   4. IgE—role in immediate hypersensitivity reactions and parasitic infections
   5. IgD—small amount in blood; precise function unknown; thought to activate B cells
E. Complement—component of blood plasma consisting of several protein compounds; serves to kill foreign cells by cytolysis; causes vasodilation and enhances phagocytosis and other functions; complement protein 3 activated without antigen stimulation; produces full complement effect by binding to bacteria or viruses in presence of properdin
F. Clonal selection theory
   1. The human body contains many diverse clones of cells, each committed by its genes to synthesize a different antibody
   2. When an antigen enters the body, it selects the clone whose cells are synthesizing its antibody and stimulates them to proliferate and create more antibodies
   3. The clones selected by antigens consist of lymphocytes and are selected by the shape of antigen receptors on the lymphocyte's plasma membrane

T Cells and Cell-Mediated Immunity (See the section on "Disease Barriers" and Figure 9-1 in Chapter 9.)
A. T cells—lymphocytes that go through the thymus gland before migrating to the lymph nodes and spleen; function to produce cell-mediated immunity and regulate specific immunity in general
   1. Pre–T cells develop into thymocytes while in the thymus
   2. Thymocytes stream into blood and are carried to the T-dependent zones in the spleen and lymph nodes
B. T cells display antigen receptors on their surface membranes; the T cell is activated when an antigen (presented by a macrophage) binds to its receptors, causing it to divide repeatedly to form a clone of identical sensitized T cells

1. Sensitized T cells go to the site where the antigen entered, bind to antigens, and release cytokines (lymphokines)

C. Killer T cells—release lymphotoxin to kill cells

D. Helper T cells—regulate the function of B cells

E. Suppressor T cells—suppress B cell differentiation into plasma cells

The Respiratory System

A. The respiratory system functions as an air distributor and gas exchanger that supplies O_2 and removes CO_2 from cells, and warms, filters, and humidifies air (Figure 3-31)

 1. Alveoli serve as gas exchangers; all other parts of the respiratory system serve as air distributors

 2. Respiratory organs influence speech, homeostasis of body pH, and olfaction

B. Divided into two parts:

 1. Upper respiratory tract—organs located outside of the thorax and consist of the nose, nasopharynx, oropharynx, laryngopharynx, and larynx

 2. Lower respiratory tract—organs located within the thorax and consist of the trachea, bronchial tree, and lungs

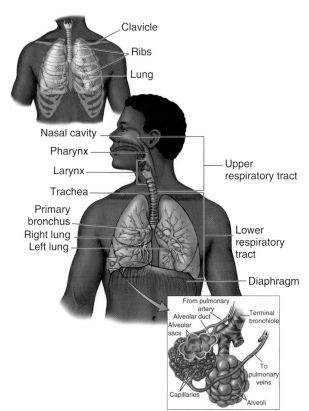

FIGURE 3-31 Structural plan of the respiratory system. *(From Herlihy B: The human body in health and illness, ed 3, St Louis, 2011, Saunders.)*

C. Accessory structures—oral cavity, rib cage, and diaphragm

Upper Respiratory Tract

(See the section on "Osteology of the Head and Neck" in Chapter 4.)

A. Nose—passageway for air traveling to and from the lungs; filters air, aids speech, and makes the sense of smell possible

 1. The external portion of the nose consists of a bony and cartilaginous frame covered by skin containing sebaceous glands; two nasal bones meet and are surrounded by frontal bone to form the roof; the floor of the nose is bound by the maxilla

 2. The internal nose (nasal cavity) lies over the roof of the mouth, separated by the palatine bones

  a. Cribriform plate—separates the roof of the nose from the cranial cavity

  b. Septum—separates the nasal cavity into right and left cavities; consists of four structures: the perpendicular plate of the ethmoid bone, the vomer bone, the vomeronasal cartilages, and the septal nasal cartilage

 3. Each nasal cavity is divided into three passageways: superior, middle, and inferior meati

 4. Anterior nares—external openings to nasal cavities, open into the vestibule

 5. Nasal mucosa—a mucous membrane over which air passes; contains a rich blood supply

  a. Olfactory epithelium—specialized membrane containing many olfactory nerve cells and a rich lymphatic plexus

 6. Paranasal sinuses (see the section on "Paranasal Sinuses" in Chapter 4)

B. Pharynx (throat) (see the section on "Clinical Oral Structures" and Figures 5-1 and Table 5-1 in Chapter 5)

C. Larynx

 1. Located between the root of the tongue and the upper end of the trachea; functions as part of the airway to the lungs and produces the voice

 2. Consists of cartilages attached to each other by muscle; lined by a ciliated mucous membrane that forms two pairs of folds:

  a. Vestibular (false) vocal folds

  b. True vocal cords

 3. The framework of the larynx is formed by nine cartilages:

  a. Single laryngeal cartilages—the three largest cartilages: the thyroid cartilage, the epiglottis, and the cricoid cartilages

  b. Paired laryngeal cartilages—three pairs of smaller cartilages: the arytenoid, the corniculate, and the cuneiform cartilages

4. Muscles of the larynx
  a. Intrinsic muscles both insert and originate within the larynx
  b. Extrinsic muscles insert in the larynx but originate on another structure

Lower Respiratory Tract

A. Trachea (windpipe)—extends from the larynx to the primary bronchi; furnishes part of the open airway to the lungs; obstruction causes death
B. Bronchi and alveoli
  1. The lower end of the trachea divides into two primary bronchi (one at the right and one at the left), continue into each lung, and then divide into secondary bronchi that branch into bronchioles, which then divide into alveolar ducts
  2. Alveoli—the primary gas exchange structures
    a. Respiratory membrane—the barrier between which gases are exchanged by alveolar air and blood; consists of the alveolar epithelium, the capillary endothelium, and their joined basement membranes
    b. Surfactant—a component of the fluid coating the respiratory membrane that reduces surface tension
  3. Bronchi and alveoli distribute air to the lung's interior
C. Lungs
  1. Cone-shaped organs extending from the diaphragm to above the clavicles; function in air distribution and gas exchange
    a. Hilum—slit on lung's medial surface, where primary bronchi and pulmonary blood vessels enter
    b. Base—the inferior surface of the lung; rests on the diaphragm
    c. Costal surface—lies against the ribs
    d. Left lung—divided into two lobes (superior and inferior)
    e. Right lung—divided into three lobes (superior, middle, and inferior)
    f. Lobes—further divided into functional units called *bronchopulmonary segments*
      (1) Ten segments in the right lung
      (2) Eight segments in the left lung
D. Thorax
  1. Part of the body between the neck and the abdomen; partially encased by the ribs and containing the heart and lungs; functions to bring about inspiration and expiration

Respiratory Physiology

The respiratory system includes pulmonary ventilation, gas exchange in the lungs and tissues, transport of gases by blood, and regulation of respiration.

A. Pulmonary ventilation (breathing)
  1. Mechanism
    a. Establishes two gas pressure gradients: one in which the pressure within the alveoli of the lungs is lower than atmospheric pressure to produce inspiration; the other in which the pressure in the alveoli of the lungs is higher than atmospheric pressure to produce expiration
    b. Pressure gradients—established by changes in the size of the thoracic cavity via the contraction and relaxation of muscles
    c. Boyle's law—the volume of gas varies inversely with pressure at a constant temperature (expansion of the thorax results in decreased intrapleural pressure, leading to a decreased alveolar pressure causing air to move into the lungs)
  2. Two components of respiration:
    a. Inspiration—contraction of the diaphragm produces inspiration; as the diaphragm contracts, the thoracic cavity enlarges; the ability of pulmonary tissues to stretch, which makes inspiration possible, is termed *compliance*
    b. Expiration—a passive process that begins when the inspiratory muscles are relaxed, decreasing the size of the thorax and increasing intrapleural pressure from about −6 mm Hg to a preinspiration level of −4 mm Hg
      (1) The pressure between the parietal and visceral pleura is always less than atmospheric pressure
      (2) Elastic recoil—tendency of pulmonary tissues to return to a smaller size after having been stretched passively during expiration
  3. Pulmonary volumes—amount of air moved in and out and remaining; important in order for a normal exchange of O_2 and CO_2 to take place
    a. Spirometer—instrument used to measure the volume of air
    b. Tidal volume (TV)—amount of air exhaled after normal inspiration
    c. Expiratory reserve volume (ERV)—largest volume of additional air that can be forcibly exhaled (normal ERV is 1.0 and 1.2 liters [L])
    d. Inspiratory reserve volume (IRV)—amount of air that can be forcibly inhaled after normal inspiration (normal IRV is 3.3 L)
    e. Residual volume—amount of air that cannot be forcibly exhaled (1.2 L)
    f. Pulmonary capacity—the sum of two or more pulmonary volumes

g. Vital capacity—the sum of IRV TV + ERV; depends on many factors, including the size of the thoracic cavity and posture

h. Minimal volume—amount of air remaining after RV

i. Functional residual capacity—amount of air at the end of a normal respiration

j. Total lung capacity—sum of all four lung volumes; the total amount of air a lung can hold

k. Anatomic dead space—air in passageways that does not participate in gas exchange

l. Physiologic dead space—anatomic dead space plus the volume of any nonfunctioning alveoli (as in pulmonary disease)

m. Alveolar ventilation—volume of inspired air that reaches the alveoli; alveoli must be properly ventilated for adequate gas exchange

B. Pulmonary gas exchange

1. Partial pressure of gases—pressure exerted by a gas in a mixture of gases or a liquid

a. Law of partial pressures (Dalton's law)—the partial pressure of a gas in a mixture of gases is directly related to the concentration of that gas in the mixture and to the total pressure of the mixture

b. Arterial blood partial pressure of O_2 (PO_2) and partial pressure of CO_2 (PCO_2) equals alveolar PO_2 and PCO_2

2. Gas exchange in the lungs takes place between alveolar air and blood flowing through lung capillaries

a. Four factors determine the amount of oxygen that diffuses into blood:

(1) Oxygen pressure gradient between alveolar air and blood

(2) Total functional surface area of the respiratory membrane

(3) Respiratory minute volume

(4) Alveolar ventilation

b. Structural facts that facilitate O_2 diffusion from alveolar air to blood

(1) The walls of alveoli and capillaries form only a very thin barrier for gases to cross

(2) Alveolar and capillary surfaces are large

(3) Blood is distributed through capillaries in a thin layer so that each red blood cell comes close to alveolar air

C. How blood transports gases

1. O_2 and CO_2 are transported as solutes and as parts of the molecules of certain chemical compounds

2. Transport of O_2

a. Hemoglobin—made up of four polypeptide chains (two α-chains, two β-chains), each

with an iron-containing heme group; CO_2 can bind to amino acids in the chains, and O_2 can bind to iron in the heme groups

b. Oxygenated blood contains about 0.3 mL of dissolved O_2 per 100 mL of blood

c. Hemoglobin increases the O_2-carrying capacity of blood

d. O_2 travels in two forms: as dissolved O_2 in plasma (PO_2) and associated with hemoglobin (oxyhemoglobin)

(1) Increasing blood PO_2 accelerates the association of hemoglobin with O_2

(2) Oxyhemoglobin carries the majority of the total O_2 transported by blood

3. Transport of CO_2

a. A small amount of CO_2 dissolves in plasma and is transported as a solute (10%)

b. Less than one fourth of blood CO_2 combines with NH_2 (amine) groups of hemoglobin and other proteins to form carbaminohemoglobin (20%)

c. The association of CO_2 with hemoglobin is accelerated by an increase in blood PO_2

d. More than two thirds of the CO_2 in plasma is bicarbonate ions (70%)

D. Systemic gas exchange

1. Gas exchange in tissues takes place between arterial blood flowing through tissue capillaries and cells

a. O_2 diffuses out of arterial blood because the O_2 pressure gradient favors its outward diffusion

b. As dissolved O_2 diffuses out of arterial blood, blood PO_2 decreases, which accelerates oxyhemoglobin dissociation to release more O_2 to plasma for diffusion to cells

2. CO_2 exchange between tissues and blood takes place in the opposite direction from O_2 exchange

a. Bohr effect—increased PO_2 decreases the affinity between O_2 and hemoglobin

b. Haldane effect—increased CO_2 loading is caused by a decrease in PO_2

E. Regulation of respiration

1. Respiratory control centers—main integrators that are located in the brain stem and control the nerves that affect inspiratory and expiratory muscles

a. Medullary rhythmicity center—generates the basic rhythm of the respiratory cycle

(1) Consists of two interconnected control centers:

(a) Inspiratory center, which stimulates inspiration

(b) Expiratory center, which stimulates expiration

b. The basic breathing rhythm can be altered by different inputs to the medullary rhythmicity center

   (1) Input from the apneustic center in the pons stimulates the inspiratory center to increase the length and depth of inspiration

   (2) Pneumotaxic center in the pons—inhibits the apneustic center and the inspiratory center to prevent overinflation of the lungs

2. Factors that influence breathing—sensors from the nervous system provide feedback to the medullary rhythmicity center

   a. Changes in the PO_2, PCO_2, and pH of arterial blood influence the medullary rhythmicity area

   (1) PCO_2 acts on the chemoreceptors in the medulla; an increase in PCO_2 results in faster breathing; a decrease results in slower breathing

   (2) A decrease in blood pH stimulates the chemoreceptors in the carotid and aortic bodies

   (3) Arterial blood PO_2 presumably has little influence if it stays above a certain level

   b. Arterial blood pressure controls breathing through the respiratory pressoreflex mechanism

   c. Hering-Breuer reflexes control respirations by regulating the depth of respirations and the volume of tidal air

   d. The cerebral cortex influences breathing by increasing or decreasing the rate and strength of respirations

The Digestive System

See Figure 3-32.

A. System of organs that breaks down food into molecules small enough for cells to use; the two groups are:

1. Gastrointestinal tract—continuous tube that extends from the mouth to the anus; organs include the mouth, pharynx, esophagus, stomach, and small and large intestines

2. Accessory digestive organs—teeth, tongue, salivary glands, liver, gallbladder, and pancreas; teeth and tongue only accessory organs that come into direct contact with food

B. Functions

1. Ingestion—taking foods and liquids into mouth

2. Secretion—cells within the walls of the GI tract and accessory organs secrete a total of about 7 L of water, acid, buffers, and enzymes into the lumen of the tract

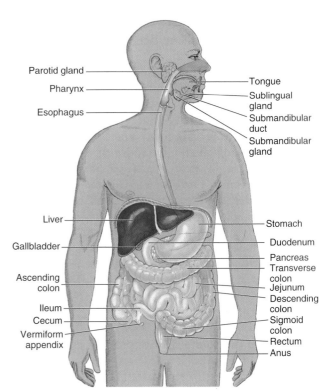

FIGURE 3-32 Location of digestive organs. *(Modified from Solomon EP: Introduction to human anatomy and physiology, ed 2, St Louis, 2008, Saunders.)*

3. Mixing and propulsion—alternating contraction and relaxation of smooth muscle in the walls of the GI tract mix food and secretions and propel them toward the anus; motility is the ability of the GI tract to mix and move material along its length

4. Digestion—mechanical and chemical processes break down ingested food into small molecules

5. Absorption—entrance of ingested and secreted fluids, ions, and small molecules that are products of digestion into the epithelial cells lining the lumen of the GI tract; absorbed substances pass into blood or lymph and circulate to cells throughout the body

6. Defecation—wastes, indigestible substances, microorganisms, and digested materials that were not absorbed leave the body through the anus; the eliminated material is called *feces*

C. Organs

1. Mouth

   a. Formed by cheeks, palates, lips, and tongue, which aid mechanical digestion

   b. Fauces—opening from the mouth to the throat

   c. Tongue—composed of skeletal muscle covered with mucous membrane and forms the floor of the oral cavity; superior and lateral surfaces covered with papillae, some of which contain taste buds

  d. Salivary glands empty via ducts into the oral cavity; three pairs of parotid, submandibular, and sublingual; secrete saliva that lubricates food and starts the chemical digestion of carbohydrates (salivary amylase begins the digestion of starches in the mouth); salivation is entirely under the control of the nervous system

  e. Teeth—see the sections on "Dental Terminology" and "Dental Anatomy" in Chapter 5.

  f. Mastication—food is chewed, mixed with saliva, and shaped into a bolus

2. Pharynx

  a. Food that is swallowed passes from the mouth into the oropharynx

  b. From the oropharynx, food passes into the laryngopharynx

3. Esophagus

  a. Muscular tube that connects the pharynx to the stomach

  b. Swallowing—moves the bolus from the mouth to the esophagus, which passes the food bolus into the stomach by peristalsis; consists of a voluntary stage, a pharyngeal stage (involuntary), and an esophageal stage (involuntary)

4. Stomach

  a. Is attached to the esophagus and ends at the pyloric sphincter

  b. Anatomic subdivisions: cardia, fundus, body, and pylorus

  c. Adaptations for digestion include rugae; glands that produce mucus, hydrochloric acid, a protein-digesting enzyme (pepsin), intrinsic factor, and gastrin; and a three-layered muscularis for efficient mechanical movement

  d. Mechanical digestion consists of mixing waves; chemical digestion consists of conversion of proteins into peptides by pepsin; mixing waves and gastric secretions reduce food to chyme

  e. Gastric secretion and motility are regulated by neural and hormonal mechanisms; parasympathetic impulses and gastrin cause the secretion of gastric juices; food in the small intestine, secretin, and cholecystokinin inhibit gastric secretion

  f. Gastric emptying

   (1) Stimulated in response to stretching; gastrin released in response to the presence of certain foods

   (2) Inhibited by reflex action and hormones (secretin and cholecystokinin)

  g. Impermeable to most substances; the stomach can absorb water, certain ions, drugs, and alcohol

5. Pancreas

  a. Connected to the duodenum by the pancreatic duct

  b. Pancreatic islets (islets of Langerhans)—secrete hormones; endocrine portion of the pancreas

  c. Acinar cells—secrete pancreatic juice; exocrine portion of the pancreas

  d. Pancreatic juice—contains enzymes that digest starch, glycogen, and dextrins (pancreatic amylase); proteins (trypsin, chymotrypsin, and carboxypeptidase); triglycerides (pancreatic lipase); and nucleic acids (nucleases)

6. Liver and gallbladder

  a. Liver—has left and right lobes; produces bile

  b. Gallbladder—a sac located in a depression under the liver; stores and concentrates bile

D. Layers of the GI tract

1. Basic arrangement from deep to superficial: mucosa, submucosa, muscularis, and serosa (visceral peritoneum)

2. The mucosa contains extensive patches of lymphatic tissue

The Urinary System

A. Kidneys—principal organs of the urinary system; accessory organs are ureters, urinary bladder, and urethra

B. Regulates content of blood plasma to maintain the "dynamic constancy," or homeostasis, of the internal fluid environment within normal limits

C. Anatomy of the urinary system

1. Structure

  a. Kidneys (Figure 3-33)

   (1) Shape, size, and location

    (a) Roughly oval, with a medial indentation; each kidney approximately $11 \times 7 \times 3$ cm

    (b) The left kidney is often larger than the right; the right kidney is located a little lower

    (c) The kidneys are located in the retroperitoneal position; lie on either side of the vertebral column between T12 and L3

    (d) Superior poles of both kidneys extend above the level of the twelfth rib and the lower edge of the thoracic parietal pleura

(e) The renal fascia anchors the kidneys to surrounding structures; heavy cushion of fat surrounds each kidney
(2) Internal structures of the kidney
  (a) Cortex and medulla
  (b) Renal pyramids: comprise much of the medullary tissue

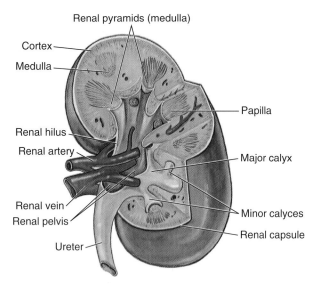

FIGURE 3-33 Internal structure of the kidney. *(From Solomon EP: Introduction to human anatomy and physiology, ed 2, St Louis, 2008, Saunders.)*

(c) Renal columns: where cortical tissue dips into the medulla between the pyramids
(d) Calyx: cup-like structure at each renal papilla that collects urine; the structures join together to form the renal pelvis
(e) Renal pelvis: narrows as it exits the kidney to become the ureter
(3) Kidneys are highly vascular
b. Renal artery: a large branch of the abdominal aorta; brings blood into each kidney (Figure 3-34)
c. Interlobular arteries—the renal artery branches between the pyramids of the medulla; interlobular arteries extend toward the cortex, arch over the bases of the pyramids, and form arcuate arteries; from arcuate arteries, interlobular arteries penetrate the cortex
d. Juxtaglomerular apparatus—located where the afferent arteriole brushes past the distal tubule; important for the maintenance of blood flow homeostasis by reflexively secreting renin when blood pressure in the afferent arteriole drops
e. Ureter—tube running from each kidney to the urinary bladder; composed of three layers:

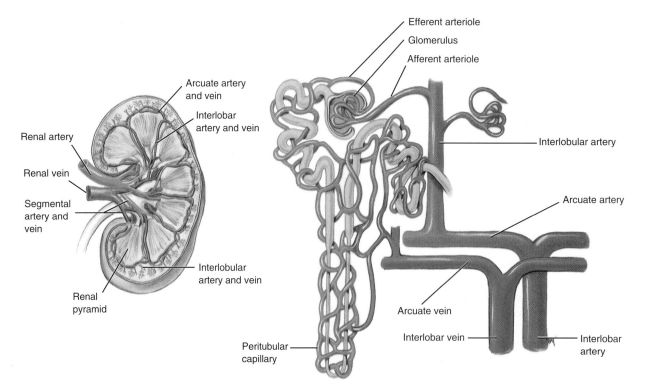

FIGURE 3-34 Circulation of blood through the kidney. *(Modified from Applegate E: The anatomy and physiology learning system, ed 4, St Louis, 2011, Saunders.)*

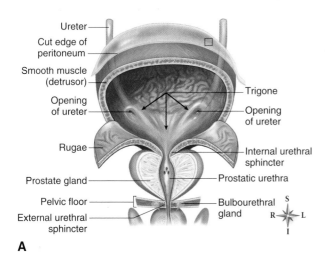

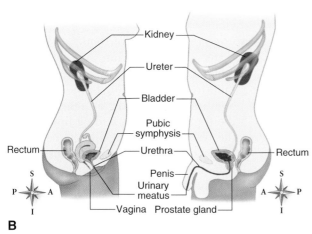

FIGURE 3-35 Structure and location of the urinary bladder. **A,** Frontal view of a dissected urinary bladder (male) in a fully distended position. **B,** Sagittal view of the female urinary system (*left*) and male urinary system (*right*), each showing a partially distended bladder. *(From Patton KT, Thibodeau GA:* Anthony's textbook of anatomy and physiology, *ed 19, St Louis, 2010, Mosby.)*

mucous lining, muscular middle layer, and fibrous outer layer

  f. Urinary bladder (Figure 3-35)
    (1) Collapsible, bag-like structure located behind the symphysis pubis; made mostly of smooth muscle tissue; linim forms rugae; can distend considerably
    (2) Functions
      (a) Reservoir for urine before it is voided
      (b) Expels urine from the body with the aid of the urethra
    (3) Mechanism for voiding
      (a) Voluntary relaxation of external sphincter muscle
      (b) Reflexive contraction of regions of the detrusor muscle

      (c) Urine forced out of bladder via the urethra
  g. Urethra
    (1) Small mucous membrane–lined tube; extends from the trigone to the exterior of the body
    (2) In the female, lies posterior to the symphysis pubis and anterior to the vagina; approximately 3 cm long
    (3) In the male, after leaving the bladder, passes through the prostate gland, where it is joined by two ejaculatory ducts; from the prostate, it extends to the base of the penis and then through the center of the penis and ends as the urinary meatus; approximately 20 cm long; the male urethra is part of the urinary system as well as the reproductive system

D. Microscopic structure of the nephron
  1. Nephrons—microscopic functional units; make up the bulk of the kidney; those located in the renal cortex are called *cortical nephrons*; those near the junction of the cortical and medullary layers are called *juxtamedullary nephrons*; each nephron is made up of various structures
    a. Renal corpuscle
    b. Bowman's capsule—cup-shaped mouth of the nephron
      (1) Formed by parietal and visceral walls, with a space between them
      (2) Pedicels in the visceral layer are packed closely together to form filtration slits; slit diaphragm prevents filtration slits from enlarging under pressure
      (3) Glomerulus—network of fine capillaries in Bowman's capsule; together called *renal corpuscle*; located in the cortex of the kidney
      (4) The basement membrane lies between the glomerulus and Bowman's capsule
      (5) Glomerular–capsular membrane— formed by the glomerular endothelium, the basement membrane, and the visceral layer of Bowman's capsule; function is filtration
    c. Proximal tubule—first part of the renal tubule nearest to Bowman's capsule; follows a winding, convoluted course; also known as *proximal convoluted tubule*
    d. Loop of Henle
      (1) Renal tubule segment just beyond proximal tubule
      (2) Consists of a thin descending limb, a sharp turn, and a thick ascending limb

(3) Juxtamedullary nephron—a nephron with a loop of Henle that dips far into the medulla

(4) Cortical nephron—a nephron with a loop of Henle that does not dip into the medulla but remains almost entirely within the cortex; constitutes about 85% of the total number of nephrons

e. Distal tubule—convoluted tubule beyond the loop of Henle; also known as *distal convoluted tubule*

f. Collecting duct

(1) Straight tubule joined by the distal tubules of several nephrons

(2) Joins larger ducts; larger collecting ducts of one renal pyramid converge to form one tube that opens at a renal papilla into a calyx

E. Physiology of the urinary system

1. Overview of kidney function

a. Processes blood and forms urine

b. Nephron—basic functional unit; forms urine through:

(1) Filtration—movement of water and protein-free solutes from the plasma in the glomerulus into the capsular space of Bowman's capsule

(2) Tubular resorption—movement of molecules out of the tubule and into peritubular blood

(3) Tubular secretion—movement of molecules out of peritubular blood and into the tubule for excretion

2. Filtration—first step in blood processing that occurs in the renal corpuscles

a. From the blood in glomerular capillaries, about 180 L of water and solutes filter into Bowman's capsule each day; takes place through the glomerular–capsular membrane

b. Occurs as a result of the existence of a pressure gradient

c. Occurs rapidly because of the increased number of fenestrations

d. Glomerular hydrostatic pressure and filtration are related to systemic blood pressure

3. Resorption—second step in urine formation; occurs as a result of passive and active transport mechanisms from all parts of the renal tubules; major portion of resorption occurs in proximal tubules

a. Resorption in the proximal tubule—most water and solutes are recovered by blood, leaving only a small volume of tubule fluid to move on to the loop of Henle

(1) Sodium—actively transported out of the tubule fluid and into blood

(2) Glucose and amino acids—passively transported out of the tubule fluid by means of the sodium co-transport mechanism

(3) Chloride, phosphate, and bicarbonate ions passively move into blood because of an imbalance of electrical charge

(4) Water—movement of sodium and chloride into blood causes an osmotic imbalance, moving water passively into blood

(5) Urea—approximately one half of urea passively moves out of the tubule; the remaining urea moves on to the loop of Henle

b. Resorption in the loop of Henle

(1) Water is resorbed from the tubule fluid, and urea is picked up from the interstitial fluid in the descending limb

(2) Sodium and chloride are resorbed from the filtrate in the ascending limb, where the resorption of salt dilutes the tubule fluid and creates and maintains a high osmotic pressure of the medulla's interstitial fluid

4. Resorption in the distal tubules and collecting ducts

a. The distal tubule resorbs sodium by active transport but in smaller amounts than in the proximal tubule

b. ADH—secreted by the posterior pituitary gland; targets the cells of distal tubules and collecting ducts to make them more permeable to water

c. With the resorption of water in the collecting duct, urea concentration of the tubule fluid increases, causing urea to diffuse out of the collecting duct into the medullary interstitial fluid

d. Urea participates in a countercurrent multiplier mechanism that, along with countercurrent mechanisms of the loop of Henle and the vasa recta, maintains the high osmotic pressure needed to form concentrated urine and to avoid dehydration

5. Tubular secretion

a. Tubular secretion—movement of substances out of blood and into the tubular fluid

b. The descending limb of the loop of Henle secretes urea via diffusion

c. Distal and collecting tubules secrete potassium, hydrogen, and ammonium ions

d. Aldosterone—hormone that targets the cells of distal and collecting tubules; causes increased activity of sodium–potassium pumps

e. Secretion of hydrogen ions increases with increased concentration of hydrogen ions in blood

6. Regulation of urine volume
   a. ADH influences water resorption; as water is resorbed, the total volume of urine is reduced by the amount of water removed by the tubules; ADH reduces water loss
   b. Aldosterone—secreted by the adrenal cortex; increases the absorption of sodium by the distal tubule, raising the sodium concentration of blood and thus promoting the resorption of water
   c. Atrial natriuretic hormone—secreted by specialized atrial muscle fibers; promotes the loss of sodium via urine; opposes aldosterone, causing the kidneys to resorb less water and thereby produce more urine
   d. Tubuloglomerular feedback mechanism—maintains constant glomerular filtration rate (GFR) by regulating resistance in afferent arterioles; protects kidney GFR function from rapid blood pressure variations; dependent on macula densa cells and the juxtaglomerular apparatus; may influence the renin–angiotensin mechanism
   e. Myogenic mechanism—rapid and effective regulation of GFR via changes in the contraction and relaxation of afferent arteriole smooth muscle
   f. Related to the total amount of solutes other than sodium excreted in urine; generally, the more solutes present, the higher is the volume of urine

7. Urine composition—approximately 95% water with several substances dissolved in it, for example:
   a. Nitrogenous wastes—result of protein metabolism; for example, urea, uric acid, ammonia, and creatinine
   b. Electrolytes—mainly the following ions: sodium, potassium, ammonium, chloride, bicarbonate, phosphate, and sulfate; amounts and kinds of minerals vary with diet and other factors
   c. Toxins—during disease, bacterial poisons leave the body in urine
   d. Pigments—especially urochromes
   e. Hormones—high hormone levels may spill into the filtrate
   f. Abnormal constituents such as blood, glucose, albumin, casts, or calculi

The Reproductive System

Male

A. Testes
   1. Two ovoid bodies that lie in the scrotum and are suspended in the inguinal region by the spermatic cord
   2. Sperm—formed and stored in the seminiferous tubules of the testes
   3. Testosterone—produced in the testes
   4. The epididymis is adjacent to the testes in the scrotum
      a. Acts as a storage reservoir for sperm along with the seminiferous tubules
      b. Sperm may live for as long as a month in both the epididymis and the seminiferous tubules
   5. If the testes fail to descend during infancy, the condition is referred to as *cryptorchidism*

B. Vas deferens
   1. Conducts sperm from the epididymis to the urethra
   2. Acts as a storage site for sperm

C. Urethra
   1. Passageway for semen from the vas deferens through the penis
   2. Passage for urine from the bladder through the penis
   3. Ends at the urinary meatus, which is the opening in the glans penis through which urine and semen are excreted

D. Seminal vesicles
   1. Membranous pouches located posterior to the bladder
   2. Produce a secretion that contains fructose, amino acids, and mucus
   3. Secrete mucoid material into the upper end of the vas deferens

E. Prostate gland
   1. Located inferior to the bladder
   2. Secretes an alkaline fluid to activate sperm
   3. Secretes its milky fluid into the vas deferens

F. Bulbo-urethral glands (Cowper's glands)
   1. Located inferior to the prostate gland
   2. Secrete a mucous secretion into the urethra before ejaculation to aid in lubrication

G. Penis
   1. Organ of copulation; divided into the shaft and the glans penis
      a. Glans penis—most sensitive portion of the penis
      b. The foreskin covers the glans penis (removed by circumcision)
   2. Erectile tissue (corpus cavernosum) surrounds the penile urethra; causes erection when engorged with blood

H. Sperm
  1. Spermatozoa formed in the testes
  2. Contains head, neck, body, and tail
    a. The head contains the genetic material of the male
    b. The tail provides motility through flagellar movement
    c. Sperm move through the female genital tract to seek the ovum at a velocity of approximately 1 to 4 mm per minute
  3. Spermatogenesis
    a. After a spermatogonium has been divided by mitosis for the last time, it increases in size and forms a primary spermatocyte
    b. The primary spermatocyte is divided by meiosis to form the secondary spermatocyte, with a haploid number of chromosomes
    c. Division of the secondary spermatocytes results in the formation of spermatoids
    d. Spermatoids are transformed into motile cells called *spermatozoa*
I. Physiology of ejaculation
  1. Erection—stiffening of a flaccid penis
  2. Rhythmic peristalsis in the genital ducts during orgasm causes semen to be propelled through the epididymis, vas deferens, seminal ducts, and urethra
  3. Semen—a thick, whitish fluid of high viscosity
    a. Between 2.5 and 5 mL are secreted at ejaculation
    b. Each milliliter contains 10 to 150 million sperm
    c. Sperm usually move at about 3 mm per minute
J. Hormonal influences
  1. Hormones are essential to the mechanism of reproduction and to the development and maintenance of secondary sex characteristics
  2. The anterior pituitary gland secretes FSH and LH, which cause the growth and function of testes at puberty
  3. Secondary sex characteristics in the male (appear during adolescence)
    a. Deepening of voice; widening of the musculature of the chest and shoulders
    b. Growth of facial and body hair

Female

A. Pelvis
  1. Wider and shallower than the male's pelvis
  2. Shaped like a funnel with a wide mouth
  3. Divided into true and false pelvis by the inlet, or brim; the sacral promontory and ileopectineal lines are dividing points between true and false pelvis
  4. Forms part of the birth canal
  5. The perineum, vagina, muscles, and ligaments form the soft structures of the pelvis
    a. Retain pelvic organs in place
    b. During labor, the direct presenting part of the infant is forward
B. Ovaries
  1. Flat, oval-shaped bodies about 2.5 cm long
  2. Supported in the pelvis by the broad ligament and suspensory ligament
  3. Three types of follicles in the ovaries:
    a. Primordial follicles contain a primary oocyte
      (1) Present at birth
      (2) Follicles complete their first maturation under the influence of FSH
    b. Growing follicles—contain a mature ovum and spaces that contain fluid
    c. Mature follicles—bulge from the surface of the ovary
C. Fallopian tubes (oviducts)
  1. Lie in the folds of the broad ligaments
  2. Fimbriae (finger-like projections) located at the ovarian ends; the isthmus portion is connected to the uterus
  3. Important events occurring in the fallopian tube are fertilization of the ovum by a spermatozoon, segmentation, and formation of the blastocyst
D. Uterus
  1. Hollow, pear-shaped organ with thick muscular walls; located behind the bladder and in front of the rectum
  2. Divided into three parts:
    a. Fundus—rounded upper part
    b. Body—narrows from the fundus
    c. Cervix—tapering projection
  3. Muscular layers
    a. Endometrium—one layer of ciliated columnar cells except for the lower one third of the cervical canal where it changes to stratified squamous epithelium; contains glands and a good blood supply
    b. Myometrium—contains smooth muscle and large blood vessels
    c. Exometrium—contains the pelvic peritoneum
  4. Serves as the womb for a developing fetus
E. External genitalia
  1. Vagina—female organ of copulation
    a. Passageway for menstrual flow
    b. Connects the uterus to the external surface (vaginal orifice)
    c. Serves as the birth canal
  2. Mons pubis—rounded eminence in front of the pubic symphysis
  3. Labia majora—two longitudinal folds; protect the inner vulva
  4. Labia minora—two smaller inner folds; protect the clitoris

5. Clitoris
   a. Homologue of the penis in the male
   b. Increases in size with sexual stimulation
F. The perineum contains the structures found between the pubic symphysis and the coccyx
G. Mammary glands
   1. Composed of compound alveolar glands
   2. Secrete milk to the nipples under the influence of lactogenic hormone from the pituitary gland
   3. Pigmented circular region (areolae surround the nipple)
   4. Active glandular growth occurs during pregnancy to prepare mammary glands to produce milk (lactation)
H. Hormonal cycle
   1. Begins at puberty and ends at menopause
   2. FSH—secreted by the anterior pituitary gland; activates the primary graafian follicle; maturing follicle produces estrogen; causes the endometrium to become engorged with blood and prepares it to receive the fertilized ovum
   3. Both hormones (FSH and estrogen) allow the ovum to mature
   4. The mature ovum is released into the fallopian tube by a ruptured graafian follicle; LH assists ovulation; the follicle forms the corpus luteum and secretes progesterone
   5. Increased progestogen levels reduce FSH and increase LH; cause the corpus luteum to secret progesterone
      a. Stimulate the uterus to store glycogen and increase the uterine blood supply
      b. The corpus luteum begins to involute as a result of lowered FSH levels
   6. Menstrual cycle lasts 21 to 35 days
      a. Menstruation begins if the ovum is not fertilized
      b. If fertilization occurs, the placenta will secrete chorionic gonadotropin to maintain the corpus luteum; estrogens and progesterone continue to be secreted to maintain the rich vascular supply in the endometrium for the developing embryo
I. Secondary sex characteristics (appear during puberty)
   1. Widening of hips
   2. Breast and genital enlargement
   3. Growth of axillary and pubic hair

SUGGESTED READINGS

Janson CB: *Memmler's the human body in health and disease*, ed 11, Philadelphia, 2009, Lippincott Williams & Wilkins.

Patton KT, Thibodeau GA: *Anatomy and physiology*, ed 7, St Louis, 2010, Mosby.

Snell RS: *Clinical anatomy*, ed 7, Philadelphia, 2004, Lippincott Williams & Wilkins.

Tortora GJ, Derrickson BH: *Introduction to the human body*, ed 8, New York, 2010, John Wiley & Sons.

CHAPTER 3 REVIEW QUESTIONS

Answers and Rationales to Chapter Review Questions are available on this text's accompanying Evolve site. See inside front cover for details.

evolve

1. In what phase is a cell highly active and growing?
   a. Anaphase
   b. Prophase
   c. Metaphase
   d. Telophase
   e. Interphase

2. Which one of the following statements best describes mucous membranes?
   a. Composed of two layers
   b. Found in body cavities that open to the body's exterior
   c. Located at the ends of bones
   d. Found lining the thoracic cavity
   e. Capable of producing synovial fluid

3. Which of the following is NOT a type of connective tissue?
   a. Blood
   b. Adipose tissue
   c. Reticular tissue
   d. Cuboidal tissue
   e. Cartilage

4. Where is smooth muscle tissue found in the body?
   a. In the heart
   b. Attached to the bones
   c. Between skin and underlying tissues and organs
   d. In the discs between the vertebrae
   e. In the walls of hollow organs

5. Which connective tissue cells secrete antibodies?
   a. Mast cells
   b. Adipocytes
   c. Macrophages
   d. Plasma cells
   e. Chondrocytes

6. In which of the following would articular cartilage and bursae most likely be found?
   a. Gomphosis
   b. A suture
   c. The symphysis pubis
   d. The knee
   e. A synchondrosis

7. Moving the femur forward when walking is an example of:
   a. Abduction
   b. Circumduction
   c. Flexion
   d. Gliding
   e. Inversion

8. The portion of the nervous system that regulates the gastrointestinal (GI) tract is the:
   a. Somatic nervous system
   b. Sympathetic division
   c. Integrative division
   d. Central nervous system
   e. Enteric nervous system

9. The depolarizing phase of a nerve impulse is caused by a:
   a. Rush of sodium ions (Na^+) into the neuron
   b. Rush of Na^+ out of the neuron
   c. Rush of potassium ions (K^+) into the neuron
   d. Rush of K^+ out of the neuron
   e. Pumping of K^+ into the neuron

10. The speed of nerve impulse conduction is increase by:
    a. The cold
    b. A very strong stimulus
    c. The small diameter of an axon
    d. Myelination
    e. Astrocytes

11. What part of the brain contains the centers that control heart rate and breathing rhythm?
    a. Medulla
    b. Midbrain
    c. Cerebellum
    d. Thalamus
    e. Pons

12. What part of the brain serves as a link between the nervous and endocrine systems?
    a. Reticular formation
    b. Hypothalamus
    c. Pons
    d. Brain stem
    e. Cerebellum

13. What part(s) of the brain is/are concerned with memory, reasoning, judgment, and intelligence?
    a. Sensory areas
    b. Limbic system
    c. Motor areas
    d. Cerebellum
    e. Association areas

14. Which of the following cranial nerves is NOT involved in controlling the movement of the eyeball?
    a. Oculomotor
    b. Trochlear
    c. Facial
    d. Abducens

15. **Which of the following pairs is mismatched?**
    a. Acetylcholine, parasympathetic nervous system
    b. Fight-or-flight, sympathetic nervous system
    c. Conserves body energy, parasympathetic nervous system
    d. Cholinergic, acetylcholine
    e. Norepinephrine, parasympathetic nervous system

16. **Which part of the central nervous system contains centers that regulate the autonomic nervous system?**
    a. Hypothalamus
    b. Cerebellum
    c. Spinal cord
    d. Basal ganglia
    e. Thalamus

17. **Which nerve carries most of the parasympathetic output from the brain?**
    a. Spinal
    b. Vagus
    c. Oculomotor
    d. Facial
    e. Glossopharyngeal

18. **Which of the following would NOT be affected by the autonomic nervous system?**
    a. Heart
    b. Intestines
    c. Urinary system
    d. Skeletal system
    e. Reproductive organs

19. **Which of the following pairs is NOT correctly matched?**
    a. Exteroceptors, monitor external environment
    b. Proprioceptors, monitor body position
    c. Nociceptors, detect pain
    d. Mechanoreceptors, detect pressure
    e. Interoceptors, located in the ear

20. **All of the following are characteristics of taste EXCEPT one. Which one is the EXCEPTION?**
    a. Olfaction can affect taste
    b. Three cranial nerves conduct the impulses for taste to the brain
    c. Taste adaptation occurs quickly
    d. Humans can recognize about 10 primary tastes
    e. Taste receptors are located in taste buds on the tongue and roof of the mouth

21. **All of the following are true of nociceptors *except* one. Which one is the EXCEPTION?**
    a. They respond to stimuli that may cause tissue damage
    b. They consist of free nerve endings
    c. They can be activated by excessive stimuli from other sensations
    d. They are found in virtually every body tissue except the brain
    e. They adapt very rapidly

22. **All of the following are functions of tears EXCEPT one. Which one is the EXCEPTION?**
    a. Moisten the eye
    b. Wash away eye irritants
    c. Destroy certain bacteria
    d. Lubricate the eye
    e. Provide nutrients to the cornea

23. **Transmission of vibration (sound waves) from the tympanic membrane to the oval window is accomplished by:**
    a. Nerve fibers
    b. Tectorial membrane
    c. The auditory ossicles
    d. The endolymph
    e. The auditory (eustachian) tube

24. **Which of the following structures refracts light rays entering the eye?**
    a. Cornea
    b. Sclera
    c. Pupil
    d. Retina
    e. Conjunctiva

25. **All of the following statements concerning the actions are true EXCEPT one. Which one is the EXCEPTION?**
    a. Hormones bring about changes in the metabolic activities of cells
    b. Target cells must have receptors for a hormone
    c. Lipid-soluble hormones may directly enter target cells and activate genes
    d. A hormone that attaches to a membrane receptor is termed the *first messenger*
    e. Adenosine triphosphate (ATP) is a common second messenger in target cells

26. **A female who is sluggish, gaining weight, and has a low body temperature may be having problems with her:**
    a. Pancreas
    b. Parathyroid gland
    c. Adrenal medulla
    d. Ovaries
    e. Thyroid gland

27. **A patient exhibiting liver failure would tend to have a(an):**
    a. Higher than normal blood levels of circulating hormones
    b. Higher than normal blood levels of local hormones
    c. Lower than normal blood levels of circulating hormones
    d. Lower than normal blood levels of local hormones
    e. Excessive production of releasing hormones

28. All of the following are symptoms of Cushing's syndrome EXCEPT one. Which one is the EXCEPTION?
    a. "Moonface"
    b. Breakdown of muscle proteins
    c. "Buffalo hump" on back
    d. Twitches, spasms of skeletal muscles
    e. Spindly arms and legs

29. What is the purpose of a hematocrit?
    a. Determines the five types of white blood cells
    b. Determines blood type
    c. Determines the percentage of red blood cells in whole blood
    d. Determines the platelet count
    e. Determines blood clotting

30. A primary function of erythrocytes is to:
    a. Maintain blood volume
    b. Help blood clot
    c. Provide immunity against some disease
    d. Clean up debris following infection
    e. Deliver oxygen to the cells of the body

31. In a person with blood type A, the isoantibody(ies) that would normally be present in the plasma is (are):
    a. Anti-A antibody
    b. Anti-B antibody
    c. Both anti-A and anti-B antibodies
    d. Neither anti-A nor anti-B antibody
    e. Anti-O antibodies

32. Which statement about an individual with vitamin K deficiency is TRUE?
    a. Blood vessels undergo vascular spasms
    b. Thrombosis is stimulated
    c. Clotting is inhibited
    d. Hemoglobin cannot be produced
    e. Nutritional anemia develops

33. A thrombus that is being transported by the bloodstream is called:
    a. A plasma protein
    b. A platelet
    c. An embolus
    d. A wandering macrophage
    e. A reticulocyte

34. The blood vessels that allow the exchange of nutrients, wastes, oxygen, and carbon dioxide between the blood and tissues are the:
    a. Capillaries
    b. Arteries
    c. Venules
    d. Arterioles
    e. Veins

35. Which of the following represents pulmonary circulation as the blood flows from the right ventricle?
    a. Pulmonary trunk→pulmonary veins→pulmonary capillaries→pulmonary arteries
    b. Pulmonary arteries→pulmonary capillaries→pulmonary trunk→pulmonary veins
    c. Pulmonary capillaries→pulmonary trunk→pulmonary arteries→pulmonary veins
    d. Pulmonary trunk→pulmonary arteries→pulmonary capillaries→pulmonary veins
    e. Pulmonary veins→pulmonary capillaries→pulmonary arteries→pulmonary trunk

36. The characteristic of arteries that allows them to stretch is:
    a. Contractility
    b. Vasoconstriction
    c. Excitability
    d. Vascular resistance
    e. Elasticity

37. All of the following statements about blood vessels are false EXCEPT one. Which one is the EXCEPTION?
    a. Capillaries contain valves
    b. The walls of arteries are generally thicker and contain more elastic tissue than the walls of veins
    c. Veins carry blood away from the heart
    d. Blood flows most rapidly through veins
    e. The blood pressure in arteries is always lower than that in veins

38. Which of the following is a function of lymph nodes?
    a. To filter lymph
    b. To substitute for tonsils
    c. To produce lymph
    d. To serve as a primary storage site for blood
    e. To produce a protective mucus

39. The cells that attack and destroy foreign agents such as fungi, parasites, cancer cells, and foreign tissues are:
    a. T cells
    b. Plasma cells
    c. B cells
    d. Natural killer cells
    e. Memory cells

40. The ability of the body's immune system to recognize its own tissue is known as:
    a. Immunologic escape
    b. Autoimmunity
    c. Nonspecific resistance
    d. Hypersensitivity
    e. Immunologic tolerance

41. Most chemical digestion occurs in the:
  a. Liver
  b. Stomach
  c. Duodenum
  d. Colon
  e. Pancreas

42. The smell of your favorite food makes "your mouth water"; this reaction is caused by:
  a. Sympathetic stimulation of the salivary glands
  b. Mastication
  c. Parasympathetic stimulation of the salivary glands
  d. Increased mucus secretion by the pharynx
  e. The enteric nervous system

43. Which of the following is a function of bile?
  a. Breaks down sugar in the gallbladder
  b. Breaks down carbohydrates
  c. Emulsifies triglycerides
  d. Is required for the absorption of amino acids
  e. Enters the small intestine through the right hepatic duct

44. The purpose of villi in the small intestine is to:
  a. Aid in the movement of food through the small intestines
  b. Phagocytose microbes
  c. Produce digestive enzymes
  d. Increase the surface area for the absorption of digested nutrients
  e. Produce gastric juice

CASE A

Your patient has end-stage renal disease and is on dialysis. She is scheduled for a kidney transplantation, and her nephrologist has requested that she receive needed dental treatment prior to the organ transplantation surgery. Use Case A to answer questions 45 to 50.

45. What is the functional component of the kidney?
  a. Neuron
  b. Nephron
  c. Islet cells
  d. Plasma

46. All of the following are systemic complications associated with renal failure EXCEPT one. Which one is the EXCEPTION?
  a. Cardiovascular
  b. Neuromuscular
  c. Hematologic
  d. Diabetes

47. Your patient exhibits extreme pallor of the oral mucosa. This is most likely caused by:
  a. Decreased production of erythropoietin
  b. Uremic stomatitis
  c. Lichenoid disease
  d. Secondary hyperparathyroidism

48. What would uremic stomatitis most likely correspond to in the patient in question 47?
  a. A rise in blood pressure
  b. Hemodialysis
  c. A rise in blood urea nitrogen
  d. Sodium and potassium retention

49. All of the following are functions of the kidney EXCEPT one. Which one is the EXCEPTION?
  a. Eliminate waste from blood
  b. Release hormones
  c. Regulate potassium and sodium levels
  d. Regulate digestion

50. Anemia may occur in patients with chronic renal failure. This is because the kidneys cannot produce enough erythropoietin to activate red blood cell production.
  a. Both the statement and the reason are correct and related
  b. Both the statement and the reason are correct but NOT related
  c. The statement is correct, but the reason is NOT
  d. The statement is NOT correct, but the reason is correct
  e. NEITHER the statement *nor* the reason is correct

4 Head and Neck Anatomy and Physiology

Irene Mary Connolly

For the dental hygienist, knowledge of the skeletal, muscular, nervous, and circulatory systems of the head and neck region is essential for client assessment and evaluation; radiography and reading radiographs; and client referral for abnormal conditions. An understanding of the circulatory and lymphatic systems enables the dental hygienist to locate sources of oral infection, trace the spread of disease in the head and neck, and identify nerves and anatomic landmarks for safe and effective delivery of local anesthetic agents.

ANATOMIC NOMENCLATURE

A. Location of an anatomic structure is based on the body in the anatomic position; the term *anatomic position* denotes a body standing erect, head facing directly forward, with arms at the sides and palms facing forward (Figure 4-1)
B. Planes—the sections of the body are divided into imaginary flat surfaces called *planes*; a plane is a flat surface determined by the location of these three points in space:
　1. Median plane or midsagittal section—passes through the midline, vertically dividing the head and body into right and left sides
　　a. Sagittal plane or sagittal section—any plane parallel to the median or midsagittal plane
　2. Frontal or coronal plane—passes through the head and body, vertically dividing it into anterior and posterior sections
　3. Horizontal or transverse plane—divides the head and body into upper (superior) and lower (inferior) portions
C. Relative positions
　1. Anterior or ventral—structures nearest the front side of the body or head
　2. Posterior or dorsal—structures nearest the back side of the body or head

3. Tongue surfaces—an exception to the previous anatomic positions is the surfaces of the human tongue, which still has the anatomic orientation of a four-footed animal; the dorsal surface of the tongue is the top surface, and the ventral surface of the tongue is the bottom surface
4. Medial—structures closest to the median plane of the body and head
5. Lateral—structures farthest from the median plane of the body and head (for example, ears are lateral to the nose or eyes)
6. Superficial—structures located toward the surface of the body
7. Deep—structures located internally the surface of the body
8. Proximal—near the source of attachment
9. Apex—the tip or pointed end of a structure
10. Contralateral—structures on the opposite side of the body
11. Cranial or superior—toward the head
12. Caudal or inferior—toward the tail

OSTEOLOGY

A. Definition—the study of bones
B. Classification—bone and cartilage are classified as rigid and firm connective tissues; they contain large amounts and various types of intercellular material (or matrix; plural, matrices) and few cells; with the exception of cartilage, connective tissue is highly vascular
C. Function—bone supports organs and structures; provides attachments for muscles and ligaments; is involved in movement, body defense, and repair mechanism; protects the soft tissues and organs of the body
D. Histology of bone (see the section on "Connective Tissue" in Chapter 2)

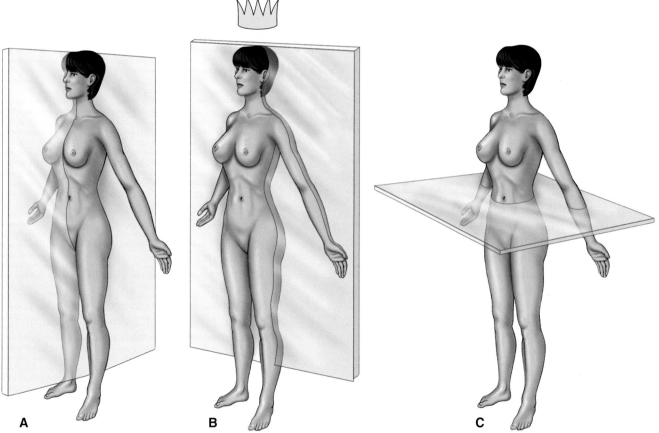

FIGURE 4-1 Anatomic directions and planes of section. **A,** Sagittal. **B,** Frontal. **C,** Transverse. *(From Herlihy B:* The human body in health and illness, *ed 4, St Louis, 2011, Saunders.)*

1. Intramembranous ossification—osteoblasts are formed from a network of mesenchymal cells; osteoblasts secrete collagen and a matrix of mucoproteins that form osteoids; this matrix initially forms bone
   a. Osteoblasts—cells that form bone
   b. Osteoclasts—cells that resorb (remove) bone
   c. Osteocytes—mature osteoblasts that are entrapped in bone matrix
2. Endochondral ossification—hyaline cartilage "template" becomes mineralized and is replaced by bone; osteoids are formed within cartilage
3. Cartilage—noncalcified, avascular, pliable connective tissue; three types of cartilage:
   a. Hyaline cartilage—serves as a template for bones
   b. Fibrous cartilage—transitional cartilage found between hyaline cartilage and tendons and ligaments; usually present in joints or articulations
   c. Elastic cartilage—contains elastic fibers in its matrix and found in structures such as the external ear, auditory tube, epiglottis, and parts of the larynx

E. Descriptive terminology
   1. Bony prominences—a *process* is a general term used to describe any prominence on a bony surface
      a. Condyle—the large convex, rounded articular end of a bone, usually involved in joints
      b. Tuberosity—a large rough prominence that typically serves as an attachment area for muscles or tendons
      c. Tubercle or eminence—rounded (small) elevation on the bony surface (e.g., genial tubercles on the mandible)
      d. Arch—a length of bone with a bow-like outline; shaped like a bridge
      e. Cornu—a horn-like prominence
      f. Crest—a thin, wedge-shaped ridge (e.g., crista galli of ethmoid bone)
      g. Spine—sharp prominences that serve as attachments for muscles
   2. Bony depressions
      a. Notch—an indentation at the edge of a bone
      b. Groove—a furrow

c. Fossa—a deep depression in a bone; usually is round in shape; can be an area for muscle attachment (plural, fossae)

d. Sulcus—a shallow depression or groove that usually marks the course of an artery or nerve (plural, sulci)

e. Sinus—a cavity within a bone

3. Bony openings

a. Foramen—a short tube-like opening in a bone (e.g., incisive foramen)

b. Canal—a long, tube-like opening in a bone (e.g., mandibular canal)

c. Meatus—an opening or canal in a bone (e.g., internal acoustic meatus)

d. Fissure—a narrow cleft-like opening; may be a line of fusion between two bones (e.g., superior orbital fissure of the orbit)

4. Skeletal articulations—areas where bones are joined; articulations can be movable or immovable

a. Sutures—line of union of generally immovable articulation; appears as jagged lines (e.g., bones of the skull)

b. Joints—movable articulation (e.g., jaw, shoulder, hip)

Axial Skeleton

Bones of the head are grouped into two categories:

A. Neurocranium, or cranial bones (eight bones)—bones that surround the brain

1. Frontal bone (single bone) (Figure 4-2)

a. Forms the forehead at the top and front of the skull

b. Contains the frontal sinuses

c. Supraorbital ridge forms the roof of the orbits of the eyes

d. Articulates with the parietal bones to form the coronal suture

e. Articulates with many of the cranial and facial bones

f. Landmarks are the supraorbital notch, the zygomatic process of the frontal bone, and the lacrimal fossa, which contains the tear-producing lacrimal gland

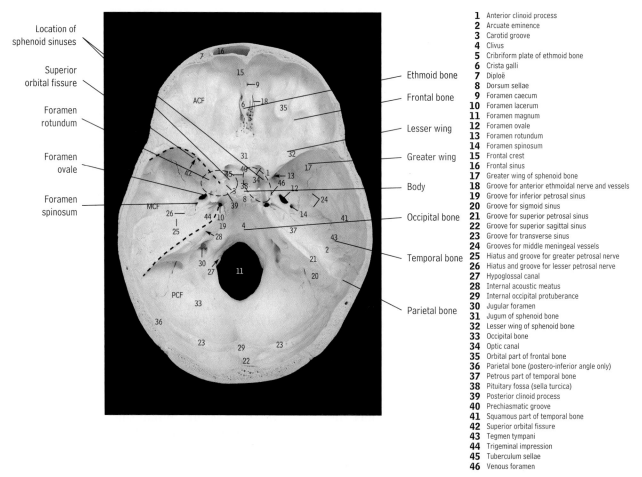

1 Anterior clinoid process
2 Arcuate eminence
3 Carotid groove
4 Clivus
5 Cribriform plate of ethmoid bone
6 Crista galli
7 Diploë
8 Dorsum sellae
9 Foramen caecum
10 Foramen lacerum
11 Foramen magnum
12 Foramen ovale
13 Foramen rotundum
14 Foramen spinosum
15 Frontal crest
16 Frontal sinus
17 Greater wing of sphenoid bone
18 Groove for anterior ethmoidal nerve and vessels
19 Groove for inferior petrosal sinus
20 Groove for sigmoid sinus
21 Groove for superior petrosal sinus
22 Groove for superior sagittal sinus
23 Groove for transverse sinus
24 Grooves for middle meningeal vessels
25 Hiatus and groove for greater petrosal nerve
26 Hiatus and groove for lesser petrosal nerve
27 Hypoglossal canal
28 Internal acoustic meatus
29 Internal occipital protuberance
30 Jugular foramen
31 Jugum of sphenoid bone
32 Lesser wing of sphenoid bone
33 Occipital bone
34 Optic canal
35 Orbital part of frontal bone
36 Parietal bone (postero-inferior angle only)
37 Petrous part of temporal bone
38 Pituitary fossa (sella turcica)
39 Posterior clinoid process
40 Prechiasmatic groove
41 Squamous part of temporal bone
42 Superior orbital fissure
43 Tegmen tympani
44 Trigeminal impression
45 Tuberculum sellae
46 Venous foramen

FIGURE 4-2 Superior view of the internal surface of the skull. *(From Abrahams PH, Marks SC Jr, Hutchings RT: McMinn's color atlas of human anatomy, ed 6, St Louis, 2008, Mosby.)*

2. Parietal bones (paired bones) (see Figure 4-2)
   a. Constitute a large part of the vault and sides of the cranium
   b. Articulates with its counterpart and various bones to form the coronal, sagittal, squamosal, and lambdoidal sutures of the skull

3. Temporal bones (paired bones)
   a. Form the lateral walls of the skull
   b. Articulate on each side of the skull with the zygomatic and parietal bones, and sphenoid and occipital bones
   c. Divided into three portions:
      (1) Squamous portion—forms the zygomatic process of the temporal bone, which is part of the zygomatic arch; this area provides the cranial portion of the temporomandibular joint (TMJ) containing the articular fossa, articular eminence, and postglenoid process
      (2) Tympanic portion—forms most of the external acoustic meatus; it is separated from the petrous portion by the petrotympanic fissure, through which the chorda tympanic nerve emerges
      (3) Petrous portion—contains the mastoid process that serves as an attachment for the sternocleidomastoid muscle; other landmarks include the styloid process, stylomastoid foramen, jugular notch, and internal acoustic meatus

4. Occipital bone (single bone) (see Figure 4-2)
   a. Forms the posterior portion of the skull
   b. Articulates with the parietal, temporal, and sphenoid bones
   c. Foramen magnum is formed completely by this bone
   d. Jugular notches on both the occipital and temporal bones form the jugular foramen
   e. Occipital condyles on each side form a movable articulation with the atlas
   f. Occipital bone has paired hypoglossal canals that are openings for cranial nerve XII

5. Sphenoid bone (single bone)
   a. Articulates with the ethmoid and frontal bones anteriorly and the temporal and occipital bones posteriorly
   b. Body of the sphenoid bone contains the sphenoid sinuses and the sella turcica, the seat of the pituitary gland, which supplies numerous hormones to the body
   c. Pterygoid processes project down from the body of the sphenoid bone in an inferior, backward direction; its landmarks include:
      (1) Medial and lateral pterygoid plates—attachment points for important muscles of mastication
      (2) Pterygoid fossa—located between the medial and lateral pterygoid plates
      (3) Hamulus—inferior termination of the medial pterygoid plate; also provides attachment for the muscles of the soft palate
   d. Greater sphenoid wings—lateral projections in the temporal area
      (1) Forms the outer wall and floor of the ocular orbits
      (2) Infra-temporal crest—divides the temporal and infra-temporal surfaces
      (3) Foramen rotundum—maxillary division of cranial nerve V
      (4) Foramen ovale—mandibular division of cranial nerve V
      (5) Foramen spinosum—opening in the greater wing of the sphenoid that gives passage to the middle meningeal artery
      (6) Foramen lacerum—contains the internal carotid artery
      (7) Superior orbital fissure—transmits cranial nerves III, IV, VI, and the ophthalmic division of cranial nerve V
   e. Lesser sphenoid wings—anterior process
      (1) Forms the posterior part (apex) of the orbit
      (2) Optic foramen—entrance point of cranial nerve II

6. Ethmoid bone (single bone) (see Figure 4-2)
   a. Single midline bone of the skull; forms the base of the cranium and orbits
   b. Articulates with the frontal, sphenoid, lacrimal, and maxillary bones; joins the vomer inferoposteriorly
   c. Contains ethmoid sinuses
   d. Cribriform plate—perforated to allow the passage of olfactory nerves
   e. Crista galli—an extension of the perpendicular plate that serves as an attachment for the meninges of the brain
   f. Perpendicular plate—along with the vomer and nasal septal cartilage, forms the nasal septum
   g. Superior nasal conchae and the middle nasal conchae are formed from the lateral portions of the ethmoid bone; their purpose along with the inferior nasal conchae is to increase the surface area of the respiratory epithelium

B. Viscerocranium, or facial bones (14 bones)—surround the face (Figure 4-3)
   1. Inferior nasal conchae (paired bones)
      a. Project from the maxilla to form part of the lateral walls of the nasal cavity
      b. Are separate from the ethmoid bone, but articulate with it

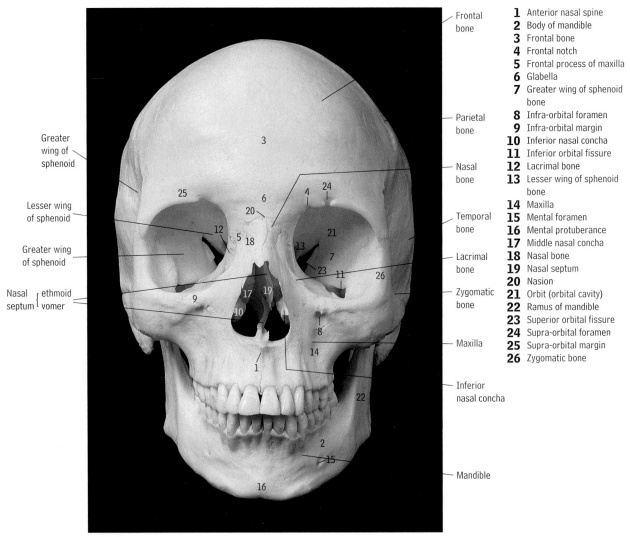

FIGURE 4-3 Anterior view of facial bones. *(From Abrahams PH, Marks SC Jr, Hutchings RT: McMinn's color atlas of human anatomy, ed 6, St Louis, 2008, Mosby.)*

1 Anterior nasal spine
2 Body of mandible
3 Frontal bone
4 Frontal notch
5 Frontal process of maxilla
6 Glabella
7 Greater wing of sphenoid bone
8 Infra-orbital foramen
9 Infra-orbital margin
10 Inferior nasal concha
11 Inferior orbital fissure
12 Lacrimal bone
13 Lesser wing of sphenoid bone
14 Maxilla
15 Mental foramen
16 Mental protuberance
17 Middle nasal concha
18 Nasal bone
19 Nasal septum
20 Nasion
21 Orbit (orbital cavity)
22 Ramus of mandible
23 Superior orbital fissure
24 Supra-orbital foramen
25 Supra-orbital margin
26 Zygomatic bone

2. Nasal bones (paired bones) (see Figure 4-3)
   a. Form the bridge of the nose, articulating with each other
   b. Articulate with the maxillae and frontal bone
3. Vomer (single bone)
   a. Forms the posterior portion of the nasal septum, articulating with the perpendicular plate of the ethmoid bone
4. Lacrimal bones (paired bones) (see Figure 4-3)
   a. Thin bones that form part of the anterior medial wall of the orbit of the eye
   b. The nasolacrimal duct is located at the junction of the lacrimal and maxillary bones
   c. Fluid (tears) from the lacrimal gland is drained through this duct into the inferior nasal meatus
5. Zygomatic bones (paired bones)—(see Figure 4-3)

   a. Zygomatic arch (cheekbone)—composed of the temporal process of the zygomatic bone and the zygomatic process of the temporal bone
   b. Three processes are named for the bones with which the zygomatic bones articulate: frontal process, maxillary process, and temporal process
6. Maxillae (paired bones)—have a body and four processes (see Figure 4-3)
   a. The body contains the maxillary sinus and forms the lower and medial rims of the orbits and the borders of the nasal cavity (piriform aperture); other landmarks are:
      (1) Infraorbital foramen—originates as the inferior orbital fissure and becomes the infraorbital canal that carries the infraorbital nerve, the inferior ophthalmic vein,

and the infraorbital artery; it is a landmark for the administration of local anesthesia to the maxillary premolars, canines, and incisors

    (2) Canine fossa—inferior to the infraorbital foramen and distal to the roots of the maxillary canines

  b. The frontal process articulates with the frontal bone, forming the medial orbital rim; it articulates with the lacrimal bone within the orbit

  c. The alveolar process (see the section on "Supporting Tissues" in Chapter 2)

    (1) Less dense bone containing the roots of the maxillary teeth

    (2) Sockets (alveoli) for maxillary teeth

    (3) Canine eminence—a protuberance over the root of the maxillary canine

    (4) Maxillary tuberosity—contains the posterosuperior alveolar fifth cranial nerve foramina, a soft tissue depression distal to the last maxillary molar; is a landmark for the posterosuperior alveolar injection to achieve anesthesia for the maxillary molar teeth

  d. Zygomatic process

    (1) Articulates with the zygomatic bone

    (2) Forms part of the infraorbital rim

  e. Palatine processes

    (1) Articulate with each other to form the anterior, major portion of the hard palate and the median palatine suture

    (2) Contains the incisive foramen, another landmark for the administration of local anesthesia to the nasopalatine nerve

7. Palatine bones (paired bones)

  a. The horizontal plates of the palatine bones articulate with each other to form the posterior portion of the hard palate, a continuation of the median palatine suture

  b. Articulate with the maxillary and sphenoid bones

  c. The vertical plates form part of the lateral walls of the nasal cavity and a small part of the orbital apex

  d. Contain the greater palatine foramen, a landmark for the administration of local anesthetic agent, and the lesser palatine foramen, where nerve and blood vessels pass through to the soft palate and tonsils

8. Mandible (single bone) (see Figure 4-3)

  a. Largest, strongest, and only movable facial bone; articulates with the temporal bones on both sides

  b. Body—horizontal portion runs from the anterior to the lateral aspects; landmarks include:

    (1) Mental protuberance—the chin

    (2) Symphysis—midline, nonmovable suture

    (3) Alveolar process of the mandible

    (4) Sockets (alveoli) for mandibular teeth

    (5) Mental foramen—located bilaterally on the external aspect, below and between the first and second premolars; the mental nerve transmits to the inferior alveolar nerve; the mental artery transmits to the inferior alveolar artery, the landmark for the administration of local anesthesia to premolars and anterior teeth

    (6) Genial tubercles—form the midline on the internal surface and provide points of muscle attachment

    (7) Retromolar triangle—distal to the third mandibular molar

    (8) Sublingual and submandibular fossae—on the internal aspect, these fossae contain their corresponding salivary glands

  c. Ramus—projects vertically and backward from the body of the mandible

    (1) External oblique line—located on the external surface; forms a crest where the ramus joins the body of the mandible

    (2) Mandibular foramen—located bilaterally on the internal surface; forms the opening of the mandibular canal and the exit for blood vessels and the inferior alveolar nerve

    (3) Lingual—a raised bony prominence; anterior to the mandibular foramen

    (4) Condyle—articulates with temporal bone, forming the movable part of the TMJ

    (5) Coronoid process—the superior margin, which forms the anterior border of the ramus and provides points of muscle attachment

    (6) Mandibular notch—concave area between the condyle and the coronoid process

C. Neck bones

  1. Hyoid bone—U-shaped bone suspended in the neck; located superior and anterior to the thyroid cartilage; landmarks are the greater and lesser horns for the attachment for many muscles and ligaments of the tongue and throat

  2. Atlas—first cervical vertebra; its lateral masses articulate superiorly with the occipital condyles of the skull and inferiorly with the axis

  3. Axis—second cervical vertebra; along with the atlas, the axis provides attachment points for many muscles responsible for the movement of the head

PARANASAL SINUSES

A. Air-filled, mucus-lined cavities or openings in the bones of the skull that function to lighten the weight of the skull and act as sound resonators; the four paired sinuses are:
1. Frontal sinuses—frontal bone above the orbit; drain into the middle nasal meatus
2. Sphenoid sinuses—body of sphenoid bone; drain into the superior nasal meatus
3. Ethmoid sinuses—consist of three small compartments: anterior and middle compartments, which drain into the middle meatus; posterior compartment, which drains into the superior meatus of the nasal cavity
4. Maxillary sinuses—triangle shaped, largest, and most complicated of the sinus cavities; drain into the middle meatus; infection of these sinuses can cause discomfort and complications of the maxillary posterior teeth

THE MUSCULAR SYSTEM

A. Descriptive terminology
1. Muscle tissue, one of the four classifications of body tissue, consists of specialized fibers for contraction; three types of muscle tissue are voluntary skeletal muscles, involuntary cardiac, and involuntary smooth muscles; muscles in the head and neck region are skeletal muscles
2. Movement—muscles are under neural control to shorten or contract; contraction is the action of the muscle fibers
3. Origin—attachment to a relatively immovable structure (e.g., sternocleidomastoid muscle originates on the clavicle and sternum)
4. Insertion—attachment to the more movable structure; insertion moves toward the origin (e.g., sternocleidomastoid muscle inserts on the mastoid process of the temporal bone and the muscles flex, moving the head downward)
B. Muscles of facial expression—most facial muscles are superficial, paired muscles originating in bone and inserting into skin; they are innervated by the seventh cranial or facial nerve and are responsible for functions related to speech, emotional expression, and mastication
1. Epicranial or occipitofrontalis muscle—scalp region; composed of two bellies (the fleshy, contractile part of a muscle), the frontal and occipital, which are connected by the epicranial aponeurosis; raise the eyebrows and scalp

2. Orbicularis oculi muscle—surrounds the eye; closes the eyelid
3. Corrugator supercilii muscle—superior to the orbicularis; wrinkles the forehead
4. Orbicularis oris muscle—encircles the mouth; closes lips
5. Buccinator muscle—anterior part of the cheek; originates on the maxilla, mandible, and pterygomandibular raphe and inserts into the angle of the mouth; functions to pull the mouth laterally, thereby shortening the cheek, and as an aid in keeping food on the chewing surfaces of the teeth
6. Risorius muscle—mouth region; acts in smiling and widening the mouth
7. Levator labii superioris muscle—upper lip; raises the upper lip
8. Levator labii superioris alaeque nasi muscle—upper lip; raises the upper lip and dilates the nose, as in sneering
9. Zygomaticus minor muscle—upper lip; raises the upper lip
10. Zygomaticus major muscle—angle of the mouth; pulls the angle of the mouth laterally, causing the appearance of a smile
11. Levator anguli oris muscle—angle of the mouth; elevates the corner of the mouth, as in smiling
12. Depressor labii inferioris muscle—lower lip; lowers the lower lip to expose lower teeth
13. Mentalis muscle—chin area; raises the chin, narrows the vestibule near mandibular incisors
14. Platysma muscle—neck region; originates in the clavicle fascia and inserts in the region of the mandible and facial muscles of the mouth; pulls down the corners of the mouth, raising the skin of the neck
C. Muscles of mastication—four paired muscles, all inserting on the mandible, innervated by the fifth cranial or trigeminal nerve; they are responsible for movement of the jaw
1. Masseter muscle—most superficial, largest, and strongest of the four muscles
   a. Originates on the zygomatic arch; originates from two heads, one superficial and one deep, and inserts on the lateral surface of the angle of the mandible
   b. Action—elevates the jaw
2. Temporalis muscle
   a. Originates from a fan-like attachment on the temporal fossa; inserts on the coronoid process of the mandible
   b. Action—when the entire muscle contracts, it elevates the mandible, raising the jaw; contraction of only the posterior portion causes retraction of the mandible

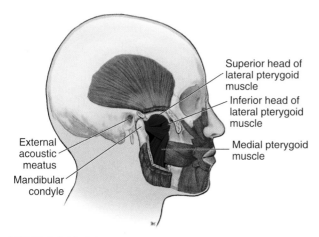

FIGURE 4-4 Medial pterygoid and lateral pterygoid muscles of mastication. The lower parts of the temporalis muscle, the zygomatic arch, and most of the mandible have been removed; some of the masseter muscle is present at the angle of the mandible. *(From Fehrenbach MJ, Herring SW: Illustrated anatomy of the head and neck, ed 3, St Louis, 2007, Saunders.)*

3. Medial (internal) pterygoid muscle (Figure 4-4)
  a. Originates from the pterygoid fossa; inserts on the medial surface of the angle of the mandible
  b. Action—elevates the mandible, thereby raising the jaw
4. Lateral pterygoid muscle; lies within the infratemporal fossa (see Figure 4-4)
  a. Originates from two heads: the superior head originates from the greater wing of the sphenoid, the inferior head originates from the lateral pterygoid plate of the sphenoid; both insert on the mandibular condyle
  b. Action—both heads working together depress (opens) and protrude the jaw; when only one side is contracted, the jaw shifts to the opposite side, causing lateral deviation of the mandible
D. Cervical muscles—paired superficial, large, easily palpated muscles, both innervated by cranial nerve XI (accessory nerve)
  1. Sternocleidomastoid muscle—well-defined, large muscle; important landmark for palpating lymph nodes
    a. Originates from the clavicle and sternum; inserts on the mastoid processes of the temporal bones on both sides of the head
    b. Action—contraction of one side makes the head bend to that side; contraction of both muscles makes the head bow
    c. Innervated by cranial nerve XI (accessory nerve)

2. Trapezius muscle—broad, paired, superficial muscles
  a. Originates from the occipital bone and the cervical and thoracic vertebrae, inserts on the clavicle and the scapula
  b. Action—functions in shrugging of shoulders
  c. Innervated by cranial nerve XI (accessory nerve) and third and fourth cervical nerves
E. Hyoid muscles—all are attached to the hyoid bone; usually grouped as suprahyoid or infrahyoid muscles, depending on their relationship to the hyoid; they aid in mastication and swallowing
  1. Suprahyoid muscle group—located superior to the hyoid; acts to raise the hyoid and the larynx
    a. Digastric muscle
      (1) Two separate bellies—anterior belly originates from the intermediate tendon on the hyoid bone and inserts near the symphysis of the mandible; posterior belly originates from the mastoid notch and inserts on the intermediate tendon of the hyoid
      (2) Action—pulls back the jaw; anteriorly innervated by the mylohyoid nerve; posteriorly by the posterior digastric nerve
    b. Mylohyoid muscle—forms the floor of the mouth
      (1) Originates from the inner surface of the mandible; unites medially with its counterpart and inserts on the body of the hyoid
      (2) Helps elevate the tongue and depress the mandible; innervated by the mylohyoid nerve, a division of cranial nerve V (trigeminal nerve)
    c. Stylohyoid muscle
      (1) Originates from the styloid process; inserts on the body of the hyoid; innervated by the seventh cranial, or facial, nerve
    d. Geniohyoid muscle—located on the floor of the mouth
      (1) Originates from the genial tubercles on the mandible; inserts into the body of the hyoid
      (2) Innervated by cranial nerve XII (hypoglossal nerve)
  2. Infrahyoid muscle group—acts to depress the hyoid bone; all muscles in the group innervated by the second and third cervical nerves
    a. Sternothyroid muscle
      (1) Originates on the sternum; inserts on the thyroid cartilage
      (2) Depresses the thyroid cartilage and the larynx (not the hyoid)

b. Sternohyoid muscle
  (1) Originates on the sternum; inserts on the body of the hyoid
  c. Omohyoid muscle
  (1) Two separate bellies—inferior belly originates from the scapula and attaches to the tendon of the superior belly, which is the origin of the superior belly that inserts on the body of the hyoid
  d. Thyrohyoid muscle
  (1) Originates on the thyroid cartilage; inserts on the body and greater cornu of the hyoid
F. Muscles of the tongue—all are innervated by cranial nerve XII (hypoglossal nerve); aid in speech, mastication, and swallowing; grouped into intrinsic and extrinsic muscles
  1. Intrinsic tongue muscles
    a. Located entirely within the tongue; include the superior longitudinal, transverse, vertical, and inferior longitudinal muscles; considered by some to be one muscle
  2. Extrinsic tongue muscles
    a. All insert inside the tongue but originate elsewhere; their names indicate their points of origin
      (1) Genioglossus muscle—acts in the protrusion of the tongue
      (2) Styloglossus muscle—acts in the retraction of the tongue
      (3) Hyoglossus muscle—depresses the tongue

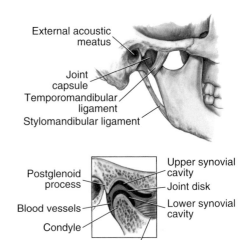

FIGURE 4-5 View of the temporomandibular joint depicting upper and lower synovial cavities and the joint disk. *(From Avery JK, Chiego DJ: Essentials of oral histology and embryology: A clinical approach, ed 3, St Louis, 2006, Mosby.)*

zygomatic arch to the posterior neck of the condyle; prevents posterior and inferior displacement of the mandible
  4. Sphenomandibular ligament—located medially; not part of the TMJ but assists in stabilizing the jaw; extends from the spine of the sphenoid to the lingula of the mandible
  5. Stylomandibular ligament—located medially; runs from the styloid process of the temporal bone to the angle of the mandible

TEMPOROMANDIBULAR JOINT

A. Description—bilaterally, the sites of articulation are between the immovable temporal bones of the skull and the movable mandible; innervated by the mandibular division of the fifth cranial, or trigeminal, nerve; blood supply comes from the external carotid artery
B. Type of joint—synovial joint; synovial fluid located in cavities above and below the joint disk lubricates the joint
C. Type of movement—gliding in the upper synovial cavities, rotating in the lower synovial cavities; the action allows for functions of speech and mastication
D. Structure of the joint (Figure 4-5)
  1. Joint disk—located between the temporal bone and the condyle of the mandible, between the upper and lower synovial cavities
  2. Joint capsule—fibrous capsule that completely surrounds the joint
  3. Temporomandibular joint ligament—located laterally on each joint, extending from the

THE CIRCULATORY SYSTEM

A. Classification and function
  1. Blood is classified as connective tissue that consists of freely moving cells
  2. Three functions of blood:
    a. Transportation—supplies oxygen (O_2) to all tissues of the body and nutrients to all cells of the body
    b. Regulation—sustains the pH of the body at 7.4; aids in the regulation of body temperature and maintains fluid balance
    c. Protection—defends the body against infections and blood loss
B. Basic components of blood (see the section on "Blood and Lymph" in Chapter 2)
  1. Plasma—clear liquid portion of blood; consists of 90% water, 10% proteins, and solids comprising more than half the total volume of blood
  2. Erythrocytes—red blood cells (RBCs); average 4.5–5 million/mm^3 of blood; they lack nuclei but contain the protein hemoglobin, which transports O_2 throughout the body

3. Leukocytes—white blood cells (WBCs); average 5000–10,000/mm^3 of blood; WBCs protect the body against infections

    a. Granulocytes—contain granules in their cytoplasm

        (1) Neutrophils average 54% to 62% of the volume of WBCs; they are the first to appear and fight infection by the process of phagocytosis

        (2) Eosinophils average 1% to 3% of the volume of WBCs, which increases during allergic reactions

        (3) Basophils average less than 1% of the volume of WBCs but increase during allergic and inflammatory reactions

    b. Agranulocytes—lack granules in their cytoplasm

        (1) Lymphocytes average 25% to 38% of WBCs; they provide an immune response

        (2) Monocytes average 3% to 7% of WBCs; they function during inflammatory and immune responses

4. Platelets—thrombocytes; cell fragments that participate in blood clotting

C. Vascular system—arteries carry blood from the heart to arterioles, capillaries, venules, and veins; the lymphatic system interacts with the circulatory system to maintain fluid pressure and to filter foreign particles

D. Descriptive terminology

    1. Anastomosis—connection between vessels

    2. Plexus—large network of blood vessels in a certain area

    3. Venous sinus—blood-filled space between two layers of tissue

E. Blood supply to the head and neck

    1. Pathways from the aorta to the head and neck differ on the right and left sides

    a. Right side—the brachiocephalic artery branches off from the aorta, giving rise to the right subclavian artery, which flows to the arm, and to the right common carotid artery, which flows to the head

    b. Left side—the left common artery and the left subclavian artery branch directly and separately from the aorta

    2. All arteries of the head and neck are symmetrically located on either side of the head, with the common carotid artery dividing into the internal carotid and external carotid arteries

    a. Internal carotid artery—enters the skull to the brain area

    b. External carotid artery—supplies the principal areas of the oral cavity and face

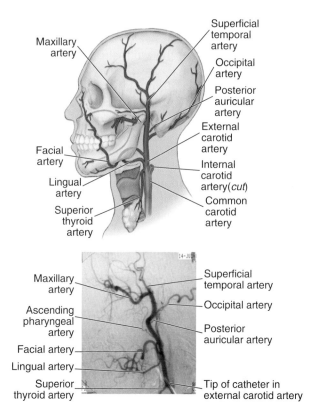

FIGURE 4-6 Carotid vasculature. Note the arteries branching from the external carotid artery. *(From Reynolds PA, Abrahams PH: McMinn's interactive clinical anatomy: Head and neck, ed 2, London, 2001, Mosby Ltd.)*

3. Anterior branches of the external carotid artery (Figure 4-6)

    a. Lingual artery—runs above the hyoid bone; supplies the floor of the mouth, the apex of the tongue, and the suprahyoid muscles; gives rise to the sublingual artery, which supplies the mylohyoid muscle, sublingual salivary gland, and mucous membranes of the floor of the mouth

    b. Facial artery—runs deep to the submandibular gland and crosses the lower border of the mandible laterally, supplies the muscles of the face to the nasal region; branches from the facial artery are:

        (1) Ascending palatine artery—supplies the soft palate, palatine muscles, and palatine tonsils

        (2) Submental artery—supplies the submandibular lymph nodes, the submandibular salivary gland, and mylohyoid and digastric muscles

        (3) Inferior labial artery—supplies lower lip tissue and some muscles of facial expression

(4) Superior labial artery—supplies the upper lip

4. Medial branch of the external carotid artery
   a. Ascending pharyngeal artery—supplies the pharyngeal walls; forms an anastomosis with the ascending palatine artery, which supplies the soft palate and meninges of the brain

5. Posterior branch of the external carotid artery
   a. Occipital artery—supplies the suprahyoid and sternocleidomastoid muscles, the scalp, and meningeal tissue
   b. Posterior auricular artery—supplies the inner ear and mastoid air cells

6. Terminal branches of the external carotid artery
   a. Superficial temporal artery—gives rise to arteries supplying the temporalis muscle and the transverse facial artery supplying the parotid salivary gland duct
   b. Maxillary artery—a large branch diverging from the external carotid artery near the neck of the condyle; runs between the mandible and the sphenomandibular ligament anteriorly and through the infratemporal fossa superiorly; after traversing the infratemporal fossa, it crosses the surface of the lateral pterygoid muscle and enters the pterygopalatine fossa behind and below the eye; within these fossae, the maxillary artery gives off many branches, generally supplying muscles of mastication, teeth, oral and nasal cavities, and the covering tissues of the brain
      (1) Inferior alveolar artery—enters the mandibular canal by way of the mandibular foramen, along with the inferior alveolar nerve; supplies the mandibular teeth and the floor of the mouth and diverges into many branches
      (2) Mylohyoid artery—arises from the inferior alveolar artery before it enters the mandibular canal; supplies the mylohyoid muscle and the floor of the mouth
      (3) Mental artery—exits the mandibular canal by the mental foramen; supplies the chin region; forms an anastomosis with the inferior labial artery
      (4) Incisive artery—remains in the mandibular canal, dividing into branches that supply the teeth, periodontium, and gingiva of the anterior mandibular region
      (5) Within the infratemporal fossa, branches of the maxillary artery supply the muscles of mastication; all these arteries accompany branches of the mandibular division of cranial nerve V (trigeminal nerve)
         (a) Deep temporal arteries—supply the temporalis muscle
         (b) Pterygoid arteries—supply the lateral and medial pterygoid muscles
         (c) Masseteric arteries—supply the masseter muscle
      (6) Posterosuperior alveolar artery—exits the infratemporal fossa and descends into the maxillary tuberosity; supplies the maxillary posterior teeth and maxillary sinus
      (7) Infraorbital artery—branches off the maxillary artery in the pterygopalatine fossa; travels through the inferior orbital fissure; enters the infraorbital canal, giving off branches to the orbit, and then branches off as the anterosuperior alveolar artery; it travels through the infraorbital foramen exiting on the face
      (8) Anterosuperior alveolar artery—travels down the maxillary sinus to supply the anterior maxillary teeth and the periodontium; forms an anastomosis with the posterosuperior alveolar artery
      (9) Greater palatine and lesser palatine arteries—travel to the palate through the pterygopalatine canal and the greater and lesser foramina, supplying the hard and soft palates

F. Venous drainage of the head and neck
   1. Generalizations—the venous system originates as small venules, which become larger veins in the neck region that carry blood back to the heart; veins anastomose freely with one another; as they lack one-way valves, which would prevent backflow, they are easily involved in the spread of infections
   2. Internal and external jugular veins
      a. Internal jugular vein—drains the brain and most of the facial area
      b. External jugular vein—drains the more superficial areas of the cranium
   3. Facial vein—drains into the internal jugular vein
      a. Drains the veins from the corner and orbit of the eye; communicates with the cavernous venous sinus
      b. Drains the veins of the lip and chin region
      c. Sometimes drains the lingual veins and sometimes drains directly into the internal jugular vein
   4. Retromandibular vein—formed by the superficial temporal and maxillary veins; divides and connects the internal and external veins

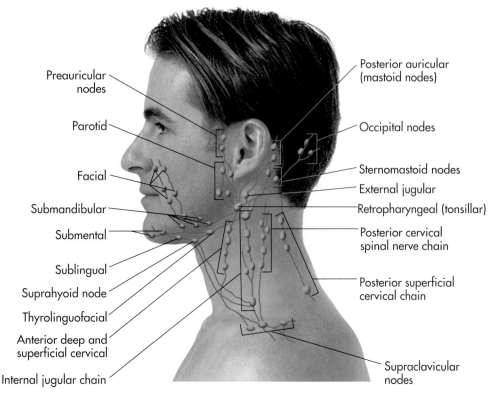

FIGURE 4-7 The lymphatic drainage system of the head and neck. If the group of nodes is often referred to by another name, the second name appears in parentheses. *(From Seidel HM, Ball JW, Dains JE, et al: Mosby's guide to physical examination, ed 6, St Louis, 2011, Mosby.)*

a. Posterior division—drains the temporal, maxillary, and posterior auricular areas and joins the external jugular vein

b. Anterior division—drains the facial vein and enters the internal jugular vein

5. Maxillary vein—located in the infratemporal fossa; drains the pterygoid plexus, which drains the veins from the area served by the maxillary artery, such as the middle meninges, oral cavity, nose, and palate

6. Pterygoid plexus of veins—collection of vessels that form anastomoses with the facial and retromandibular veins located in the infratemporal fossa

a. Drains portions of the face into the maxillary vein

b. Drains the meninges of the brain

c. Surrounds and protects the maxillary artery

d. Can be involved in the spread of dental infections

e. Can be pierced during the administration of a local anesthetic agent

7. External and internal jugular veins on both sides of the neck join their respective brachiocephalic veins, which then drain into the superior vena cava, directly to the heart

THE LYMPHATIC SYSTEM

A. Function—parallels the venous blood vessels; returns filtered fluids to the bloodstream from various body tissues; maintains fluid balance; plays a role in the immune system by the presence of lymphocytes that defend the body against disease; absorbs lipids from the intestine and transports them to the blood (Figure 4-7).

B. Descriptive terminology (see the section on "Blood and Lymph" in Chapter 2)

1. Lymph—tissue fluid that drains into the lymphatic vessels from the interstitial spaces of the body

2. Lymph nodes—clusters of bean-shaped interconnected lymphoid tissue located along the lymphatic vessels that contain lymphocytes

3. Lymphatic vessels—a system of tubules or vessels that drain a region, communicate with each other and have a one-way flow into the veins

C. Superficial cervical lymph nodes

1. Submental nodes

a. Located beneath the chin

b. Drain the mandibular incisors, apex of the tongue, tonsillar area, soft palate, and posterior nasal cavity

c. Empty into the submandibular nodes or deep cervical nodes

2. Submandibular nodes
   a. Located near the angle of the mandible
   b. Drain the maxillary teeth and maxillary sinus, mandibular canines, posterior teeth (except third molars), floor of the mouth, sublingual and submandibular salivary glands, tongue, cheek, hard palate, and anterior nasal cavity
   c. Empty into the superior deep cervical nodes

D. Superficial lymph nodes of the head
   1. Occipital nodes
      a. Drain the occipital region of the scalp
      b. Empty into the inferior deep cervical nodes
   2. Three nodes empty into the superior deep cervical nodes:
      a. Retroauricular nodes—located posterior to the ear and drain that region
      b. Anterior auricular nodes—located anterior to the ear and drain that region
      c. Superficial parotid nodes—located near the parotid gland and drain that region
   3. Facial lymph nodes
      a. Located along facial veins and drain the facial region
      b. Empty into submandibular nodes

E. Deep lymph nodes of the head—all located too medial for palpation
   1. Deep parotid lymph nodes
      a. Drain the middle ear, auditory tube, and parotid gland
      b. Empty into the superior deep cervical nodes
   2. Retropharyngeal lymph nodes
      a. Drain the palate, the paranasal sinuses, and the pharynx
      b. Empty into the superior deep cervical nodes

F. Deep cervical nodes
   1. Superior (upper) deep cervical nodes
      a. Located lateral to the internal jugular vein and beneath the sternocleidomastoid muscle, two inches below the ear
      b. Considered secondary nodes for most of the throat area, the third molar region, and the posterior nasal cavity region; often, these nodes provide the first indication of a throat infection
      c. Empty into the inferior deep cervical nodes or directly into the jugular trunk
   2. Inferior (lower) deep cervical lymph nodes
      a. Located lateral to the internal jugular vein and beneath the anterior border of the sternocleidomastoid muscle, two inches above the clavicle
      b. Considered secondary nodes for the regions at the base of the neck and some of the glands in the anterior neck
      c. Empty into the jugular trunk

G. Tonsils—part of the lymphatic system; drain into the superior deep cervical nodes
   1. Palatine tonsils—located between the anterior and posterior pillars
   2. Lingual tonsils—located on the base of the dorsal surface of the tongue
   3. Pharyngeal tonsils—located on the posterior wall of the nasopharynx
   4. Tubal tonsils—located posterior to the openings of the eustachian tube

GLANDS OF THE HEAD AND NECK REGION

A. General definition—a *gland* is a group of specialized cells that produce a substance used by other parts of the body; the two categories of glands are:
   1. Endocrine glands—have no ducts or tubes; functioning depends on the circulatory system; carry hormones internally to another organ (e.g., thyroid gland)
   2. Exocrine glands—have ducts or tubes; carry secretions externally to a body cavity or surface (e.g., salivary glands)

B. Function of salivary glands—produce saliva, which lubricates and cleanses the oral cavity

C. Role of saliva—remineralizes the tooth surface; supplies minerals for supragingival calculus formation; mixes with food as the initial part of the digestive system, producing a bolus that makes food easier to swallow, and begins to break down starches into digestible carbohydrates

D. Composition of saliva—consists of varying amounts of serous or mucous fluids, depending on the gland
   1. Serous fluid—a thin, watery, proteinaceous fluid containing enzymes
   2. Mucus—a thick, sticky fluid consisting mainly of carbohydrates

E. Exocrine glands of the head
   1. Major salivary glands
      a. Parotid salivary gland—located on the surface of the masseter muscle behind the ramus of the mandible, anterior and inferior to the ear; the largest salivary gland, but produces only 25% of the total salivary volume, mostly serous secretion; the associated duct is the parotid, or Stensen's; the duct pierces the buccinator muscle and opens opposite the second maxillary molar; innervated by the glossopharyngeal nerve and the branches of cranial nerve V (trigeminal nerve)
      b. Submandibular salivary gland—located medially underneath the angle of the mandible; the second largest salivary gland providing 60% to 65% of the total salivary

volume consisting of mixed serous and mucous secretion; the associated duct is the submandibular duct (Wharton's duct) on the floor of the mouth, which opens into the sublingual caruncle; innervated by the fibers of the chorda tympani and the submandibular ganglion of cranial nerve VII (facial nerve)

  c. Sublingual salivary gland—located in the sublingual fossa, in the anterior floor of the mouth; the smallest diffuse salivary gland providing 10% of the total salivary volume of mixed secretion, predominantly mucus; associated ducts are located along the sublingual fold; also shares the sublingual caruncle duct with the submandibular salivary gland; innervated by the fibers of the chorda tympani and the submandibular ganglion of cranial nerve VII (facial nerve)

2. Minor salivary glands—all innervated by cranial nerve VII (facial nerve)

  a. Numerous small glands—secrete mostly mucus; located on oral cavity tissues such as the soft palate; buccal, labial, and lingual mucosa; and the floor of the mouth

  b. Ebner's glands—secrete only serous saliva; located in the circumvallate lingual papillae of the tongue; cleanse the taste buds

3. Lacrimal glands—located in the lacrimal fossa of the frontal bone; secrete lacrimal fluid known as *tears*; the associated duct is formed by the union of the lacrimal and maxillary bones; drain into the inferior meatus of the nasal cavity; innervated by cranial nerve VII (facial nerve)

F. Endocrine glands of the neck region

  1. Thyroid gland—located in the neck area; consists of two lobes on either side of the larynx; largest of the endocrine glands; secretes the hormone thyroxine, which stabilizes the metabolism of the entire body (Figure 4-8)

  2. Parathyroid glands—located behind and embedded within the thyroid gland; secrete hormones regulating calcium metabolism and phosphorus uptake

  3. Thymus gland—located inferior to the thyroid in the upper part of the chest; secretes thymosin, which assists in the maturation of certain WBCs called T cell lymphocytes, which play a role in the immune system of the body; shrinks after puberty

THE NERVOUS SYSTEM

A. Classification and function—nerve tissue is a separate classification of body tissue; nerve tissue perceives information from one location and transmits

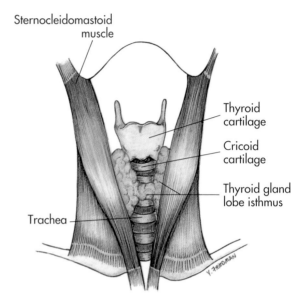

FIGURE 4-8 Anatomic position of the thyroid gland. *(From Potter PA, Perry AG:* Fundamentals of nursing, *ed 6, St Louis, 2009, Mosby.)*

it to another, responding to internal and external changes; the nervous system regulates body systems, causes muscles to contract and glands to secrete, allows for sensory perception, and performs many tasks without a person's conscious awareness

B. Descriptive terminology (see the section on "Nerve Tissue" in Chapter 2)

  1. Neuron—a nerve cell containing a nucleus; dendrites, which conduct impulses to the cell body; and axons, which conduct impulses away from the cell body

  2. Nerve—a bundle of neural processes outside the central nervous system (CNS) and within the peripheral nervous system (PNS)

  3. Myelin sheath—fatty tissue wrapped around the axons, which insulates and protects nerve fibers

  4. Nodes—small spaces between sheaths for speeding the conduction of an impulse

  5. Synapses—junction points where the transmission of nerve impulses occurs between two neurons or between a neuron and an effector organ

  6. Ganglion—a collection of nerve cells outside the CNS

  7. Afferent, or sensory, neurons transmit impulses toward the CNS; conduction transmits impulses *away* from a body structure

  8. Efferent, or motor, neurons transmit information from the brain to the periphery of the body; in this case, conduction is *toward* a body structure

C. The nervous system—coordinates the functions of the body; major divisions of the nervous system are:
1. The central nervous system—includes the brain and the spinal cord
2. The peripheral nervous system—includes all the nerves outside of the CNS, such as the cranial nerves carrying impulses to and from the brain and the spinal nerves carrying messages to and from the spinal cord
3. The autonomic nervous system—part of the PNS; operates without conscious control, and carries on automatically; both cranial and spinal nerves carry autonomic nervous system impulses; subdivisions of the autonomic nervous system are:
   a. The sympathetic nervous system—known as the "fight-or-flight" mechanism; responds to stressful situations (e.g., a decrease in salivary flow)
   b. The parasympathetic nervous system—the antagonist of the sympathetic nervous system; acts to return the body to its normal condition (e.g., salivary flow increases to its normal amount)
D. Cranial nerves (12 pairs)—part of the PNS; designated with Roman numerals, for example, cranial nerve V, VI, and VII; provide efferent, afferent, or mixed impulses
1. Cranial nerve I (olfactory nerve)—afferent type; carries odor impulses from the nasal cavity to the brain; enters the skull through the cribriform plate of the ethmoid bone
2. Cranial nerve II (optic nerve)—afferent type; carries visual impulses from the eye to the brain; enters the skull through the optic canal of the sphenoid bone
3. Cranial nerve III (oculomotor nerve)—efferent type; contraction of most eye muscles; exits the skull through the superior orbital fissure of the sphenoid bone
4. Cranial nerve IV (trochlear nerve)—efferent type; supplies one eyeball muscle; like the oculomotor nerve, exits the skull through the superior orbital fissure of the sphenoid bone
5. Cranial nerve V (trigeminal nerve)—both efferent and afferent types; largest cranial nerve; three branches transport sensory fibers from the eye, the maxilla, and the mandible; the third branch supplies motor fibers to the muscles of mastication and the mylohyoid muscle; knowledge of this nerve is critical for the successful administration of a local anesthetic agent (Tables 4-1 and 4-2; see Chapter 18, Management of Pain and Anxiety)

TABLE 4-1 Summary of Maxillary Injection Sites for Local Anesthetic Agent Administration

Landmark and Nerve	Injection	Teeth or Tissue
Maxillary tuberosity / posterosuperior alveolar nerve of the maxillary branch of the trigeminal nerve, V_2	Posterosuperior alveolar (PSA)	Maxillary first, second, and third molars and related tissues
Apex of the second premolar / middle superior alveolar nerve of the maxillary branch of the trigeminal nerve, V_2 (not present in all people)	Middle superior alveolar (MSA)	Maxillary first and second premolars, the mesiobuccal root of the maxillary first molar and related tissues
Apex of the maxillary canine / anterosuperior alveolar nerve of the maxillary branch of the trigeminal nerve, V_2	Anterosuperior alveolar (ASA)	Maxillary premolars, canines, and incisors and related tissues
Greater palatine foramen / greater palatine nerve off the maxillary branch of trigeminal nerve, V_2	Greater palatine (GP)	Palatal roots of the maxillary molars and premolars and related tissues
Incisive foramen / nasopalatine nerve of the maxillary branch of the trigeminal nerve, V_2	Nasopalatine (NP)	Anterior portion of palate or lingual aspects of anterior maxillary teeth
Infraorbital foramen / infraorbital nerve of the maxillary branch of the trigeminal nerve, V_2	Infraorbital (IO)	Facial aspects of the anterior maxillary teeth and buccal aspects of the premolars

6. Divisions or branches of the trigeminal nerve:
   a. Ophthalmic division, or V1—all afferent nerves; all branches enter the superior orbital fissure of the sphenoid bone
      (1) Frontal nerve—a merger of the supraorbital nerve (forehead and anterior scalp) and the supratrochlear nerve (bridge of

TABLE 4-2 Summary of Mandibular Injection Sites for Local Anesthetic Agent Administration

Landmark and nerve	Injection	Teeth or Tissue
Mandibular foramen / inferior alveolar nerve of the mandibular nerve of the trigeminal nerve, V_3	Inferior alveolar (IA)	Possibly all mandibular teeth on one side of the mouth
Mental foramen / inferior alveolar, incisive, mental nerves of the mandibular nerve of the trigeminal nerve, V_3	Mental block (MB) or incisive block (IB)	Mandibular premolars; anterior teeth, including lingual aspects on one side of the mouth
Buccal tissue distal and buccal to the most distal molar / buccal nerve of the mandibular nerve of the trigeminal nerve, V_3	Buccal block (LB)	Buccal periodontium and gingiva of the mandibular molars

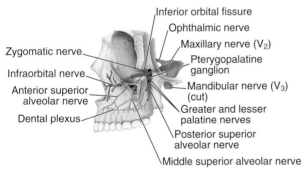

FIGURE 4-9 Branches of the maxillary division of the fifth cranial, or trigeminal, nerve. *(From Fehrenbach MJ, Herring SW: Illustrated anatomy of the head and neck, ed 3, St Louis, 2007, Saunders.)*

the nose and medial part of the upper eyelid and forehead)
(2) Lacrimal nerve—controls the upper eyelid, conjunctiva, and lacrimal gland
(3) Nasociliary nerve—several branches from the eyelids, sides of the nose, eyeball, nasal cavity, and paranasal sinuses
  b. Maxillary division, or V2—all afferent nerves; enter the skull through the foramen rotundum of the sphenoid bone and follow the same pathway as the arterial supply to the region (Figure 4-9)

(1) Zygomatic nerve—enters the orbit carrying sensations from the skin, cheek, and temple; carries postganglionic fibers from the pterygopalatine ganglion to provide parasympathetic innervation to the lacrimal gland
(2) Infraorbital nerve—enters through the infraorbital foramen and canal; carries sensations from the upper lip, medial portion of the cheek, lower eyelid, and side of the nose
(3) Anterosuperior alveolar (ASA) nerve—carries sensations from the dental branches in the pulp tissue of maxillary central incisors, lateral incisors, maxillary canines, and their associated tissues through the apical foramina; ascends the wall of the maxillary sinus, joining the infraorbital nerve in the infraorbital canal
(4) Middle superior alveolar (MSA) nerve—carries sensations from the dental branches in the pulp tissue of the maxillary premolar teeth and mesial buccal root of the maxillary first molar, the periodontium, and buccal gingiva through the apical foramina; ascends the wall of the maxillary sinus, joining the infraorbital nerve in the infraorbital canal (this nerve is not always present)
(5) Posterosuperior alveolar (PSA) nerve—carries sensations from the dental branches in the pulp tissue of the maxillary molars, periodontium, buccal gingiva, and part of the maxillary sinus through the apical foramina, exiting through the maxillary tuberosity; all branches of the PSA nerve exit from several PSA foramina on the maxillary tuberosity, and join the maxillary nerve in the pterygopalatine fossa
(6) Greater palatine nerve—carries sensations from the hard palate, and the lesser palatine nerve carries sensations from the soft palate and palatine tonsil; after entering the greater or lesser palatine foramina, both nerves enter the pterygopalatine canal to join the maxillary nerve in the pterygopalatine fossa
(7) Nasopalatine nerve—carries sensations from the anterior hard palate lingually to the anterior maxillary teeth; enters the incisive canal through the incisive foramen and travels along the nasal septum, thus causing numbness of the nose when a local anesthetic agent is

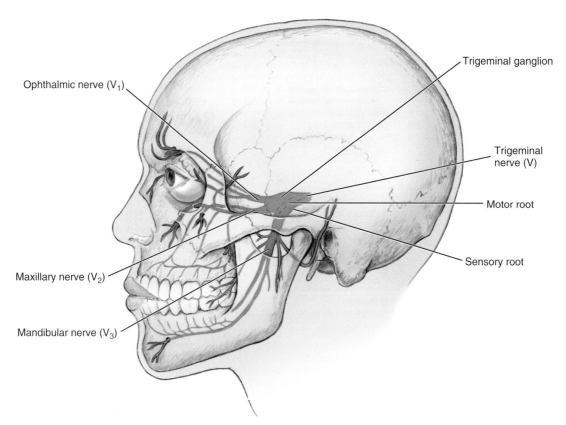

Ophthalmic nerve (V₁)

Trigeminal ganglion

Trigeminal nerve (V)

Motor root

Sensory root

Maxillary nerve (V₂)

Mandibular nerve (V₃)

FIGURE 4-10 Pathway of the mandibular division of the trigeminal nerve (V3, fifth cranial). *(From Fehrenbach MJ, Herring SW: Illustrated anatomy of the head and neck, ed 3, St Louis, 2007, Saunders.)*

administered in this area; communicates with the greater palatine nerve

c. Mandibular division, or V3—the only division containing both afferent and efferent types; largest of the trigeminal branches; enters the skull through the foramen ovale on the sphenoid bone (Figure 4-10)

(1) The buccal nerve carries sensations from the cheek, buccal mucosa, and buccal gingiva

(2) Muscular branches—efferent (motor) nerves supplying the four muscles of mastication, deep temporal nerves, masseteric nerve, and lateral pterygoid nerve

(3) Auriculo-temporal nerve—carries sensations from the ear and scalp; branches of this nerve innervate the parotid salivary gland through postganglionic parasympathetic fibers from the ninth cranial nerve (cranial nerve IX)

(4) Lingual nerve—carries sensations from the floor of the mouth, the lingual mandibular gingiva, and the anterior two thirds of the tongue through the chorda tympani; it communicates with cranial nerve VII (facial nerve)

supplying parasympathetic fibers to the submandibular and sublingual salivary glands and carries sensory fibers of taste perception from the anterior two thirds of the tongue; because of its location in the floor of the mouth, it is often inadvertently anesthetized when a mandibular block is administered

(5) Inferior alveolar (IA) nerve—carries sensations from mandibular teeth; it travels through the mandibular canal, along with the inferior alveolar artery and vein; it is a merger of the mental and incisive nerves

(a) Mental nerve—carries sensations from the chin, lower lip, and the anterior mandibular labial mucosa; enters the mental foramen between the premolars

(b) Incisive nerve—carries sensations from the dental branches of the pulp tissue of the anterior mandibular teeth through the apical foramina; merges with the mental nerve to form the inferior alveolar nerve and travels through the mandibular canal

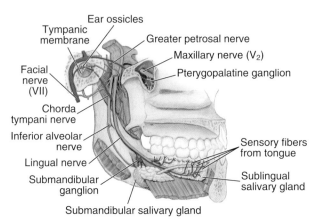

FIGURE 4-11 Two branches of the facial nerve: the greater petrosal nerve and the chorda tympani. *(From Fehrenbach MJ, Herring SW: Illustrated anatomy of the head and neck, ed 3, St Louis, 2007, Saunders.)*

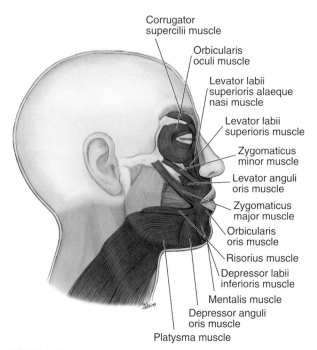

FIGURE 4-12 Branches of the facial nerve supplying the muscles of facial expression. *(Fehrenbach MJ, Herring SW: Illustrated anatomy of the head and neck, ed 3, St Louis, 2007, Saunders.)*

(6) Mylohyoid nerve—the other efferent (motor) nerve that supplies the mylohyoid muscle and the anterior belly of the digastric muscle; it joins the inferior alveolar nerve entering the foramen ovale

7. Cranial nerve VI (abducent)—efferent nerve; moves the lateral eyeball muscle; exits the skull through the superior orbital fissure of the sphenoid bone

8. Cranial nerve VII (facial)—efferent and afferent nerves, leaves the brain through the internal acoustic meatus in the petrous portion of the temporal bone and gives off two branches (Figure 4-11):
   a. Greater petrosal nerve—efferent nerve; fibers are carried through the pterygopalatine ganglion to the lacrimal gland, nasal cavity, and minor salivary glands of the hard and soft palate; the afferent nerve fibers carry taste sensations from the palate
   b. Chorda tympani nerve—parasympathetic efferent nerve supplying submandibular and sublingual salivary glands; has an afferent component, carrying taste sensations from the body of the tongue
   c. Facial nerve (cranial nerve VII)—continues anteriorly, passing through the parotid gland, and separates into efferent branches supplying the muscles of facial expression; temporal, zygomatic, buccal, mandibular, and cervical branches serve the muscles in their respective areas (Figure 4-12)
      (1) Although the facial nerve is embedded in the parotid gland, it does not innervate the gland
      (2) Damage or disease of the parotid gland can cause facial paralysis

9. Cranial nerve VIII (vestibulocochlear, or auditory nerve)—afferent nerve; carries sensory fibers for hearing and balance from the semicircular canals; enters the brain through the internal acoustic meatus of the temporal bone

10. Cranial nerve IX (glossopharyngeal nerve)—afferent and efferent nerve; carries sensory fibers from the back of the tongue and pharynx, providing taste sensation from the posterior third of the tongue; parasympathetic innervation of the parotid gland occurs through the lesser petrosal nerve; the efferent innervation controls the swallowing mechanism

11. Cranial nerve X (vagus nerve)—mixture of afferent and efferent nerves; the efferent component supplies the muscles of the soft palate, pharynx, larynx, and parasympathetic fibers to the organs in the thoracic and abdominal cavities; the afferent component carries sensations from the ear and epiglottis

12. Cranial nerve XI (accessory nerve)—efferent nerve; controls the trapezius and sternocleidomastoid muscles, soft palate, and pharynx

13. Cranial nerve XII (hypoglossal nerve)—efferent nerve; controls the muscles of the tongue; exits the skull through the hypoglossal canal of the occipital bone

Note: Cranial nerves IX, X, and XI are part of the pharyngeal plexus; all pass through the skull by way of the jugular foramen

@ WEBSITE INFORMATION AND RESOURCES

SOURCE	WEB ADDRESS	DESCRIPTION
DMOZ open directory project	http://dmoz.org/Health/Conditions_and_Diseases/	Links to universities, national institutions, and PubMed, with an array of tutorials and information about temporomandibular joint anatomy and disorders
Laboratory Dissections of the Head and Neck. Osteology of the Skull Laboratory	http://ect.downstate.edu/courseware/haonline/labs/headneck.htm	Laboratory dissections of the head and neck, along with quiz questions
Loyola University Medical Center, Chicago, Medical Education Network (images from the Visible Human Project)	http://www.meddean.luc.edu/lumen/meded/grossanatomy/	Cross-sectional, magnetic resonance imaging (MRI), computed tomography (CT), and cinematic images of human anatomy
Moorehouse School of Medicine, Human Morphology	http://www.msm.edu/human_morph/gross/head-neck.htm	Tutorials, slides, and CT and cinematic images of head and neck anatomy generated from several universities specializing in medicine

CHAPTER 4 REVIEW QUESTIONS

Answers and Rationales to the Review Questions are available on this text's accompanying Evolve site. See inside front cover for details.   ⊝volve

1. Several of the muscles of mastication are attached to the sphenoid bone. What is the name of the landmark on the sphenoid bone for these attachments?
   a. Greater wings
   b. Pterygoid process
   c. Pterygopalatine space
   d. Styloid process

2. The sphenoid bone is a complicated bone containing foramina, fissures, and landmarks for the passage or attachment of many important features of the head. An important nerve for dentistry that runs exclusively through this bone is the:
   a. Facial nerve
   b. Glossopharyngeal nerve
   c. Hypoglossal nerve
   d. Trigeminal nerve

3. Which of the following cells play a role in the resorption of bone?
   a. Osteoblasts
   b. Osteoclasts
   c. Osteocytes
   d. Chrondrocytes

4. Which of the following sentences best describes the alveolar process of the maxilla?
   a. This process contains the infraorbital foramen
   b. The genial tubercles are attached to this process
   c. The mental foramen is present on its lateral aspect
   d. This process is easily remodeled because of its lack of density

5. The perforated cribriform plate of the ethmoid bone allows for the passage of nerves affecting one of the senses. Identify the sense and the nerve.
   a. Sight/optic nerve
   b. Smell/olfactory nerve
   c. Sound/vestibulocochlear nerve
   d. Taste/facial nerve

6. The maxillary tuberosity is perforated by many foramina. It is the landmark for the administration of local anesthesia for the lingual aspect of the anterior maxillary teeth.
   a. Both statements are TRUE
   b. Both statements are FALSE
   c. The first statement is TRUE, and the second statement is FALSE
   d. The first statement is FALSE, and the second statement is TRUE

7. Which of the following features is located on the lateral or external surface of the mandible?
   a. Genial tubercles
   b. Lingula
   c. Mandibular foramen
   d. Mental foramen

8. The palate is formed by the palatine bones and _____.
   a. Ethmoid bone
   b. Nasal bones
   c. Maxillary bones
   d. Sphenoid bone

9. Paranasal sinuses:
   a. Hold fibers that perceive odors
   b. Drain through the nasal conchae
   c. Increase the surface area of the respiratory epithelium
   d. Increase the surface area of the olfactory epithelium

10. Tilting and rotating the head requires the action of the:
    a. Platysma muscle
    b. Sternocleidomastoid muscle
    c. Stylohyoid muscle
    d. Trapezius muscle

11. Which of the following muscles, when contracted, make the client's vestibule tight and shallow, thereby making it difficult to instrument the facial aspect of the anterior mandibular teeth?
    a. Levator anguli oris
    b. Depressor labii inferioris
    c. Mentalis
    d. Zygomaticus major

12. Which of the following is a muscle of mastication?
    a. Buccinator
    b. Zygomaticus major
    c. Temporalis
    d. Risorius

13. Which of the following muscles insert into the lateral surface of the angle of the mandible?
    a. Lateral pterygoid
    b. Masseter
    c. Medial pterygoid
    d. Temporalis

14. **Which of the following muscles causes the jaw to retract?**
    a. Temporalis
    b. Lateral pterygoid
    c. Masseter
    d. Medial pterygoid

15. **Which of the following statements concerning the masseter muscle is correct?**
    a. It is the most superficial muscle of facial expression
    b. It originates from the zygomatic arch
    c. It inserts on the medial surface of the mandible's angle
    d. It depresses the mandible during contraction

16. **Which of the following paired suprahyoid muscles unite medially to form the floor of the mouth?**
    a. Geniohyoid muscle
    b. Omohyoid muscle
    c. Digastric muscle
    d. Mylohyoid muscle

17. **The extrinsic muscles of the tongue are named for their:**
    a. Action
    b. Innervation
    c. Insertion
    d. Origin

18. **The muscles responsible for movement of the tongue are innervated by the:**
    a. Glossopharyngeal nerve
    b. Hypoglossal nerve
    c. Trigeminal nerve
    d. Vagus nerve

19. **The lateral pterygoid muscle is largely contained in the:**
    a. Greater wing of the sphenoid
    b. Infratemporal fossa
    c. Ptergyoid fossa
    d. Temporal fossa

20. **The masseter muscle is innervated by the:**
    a. Facial nerve
    b. Hypoglossal nerve
    c. Mandibular division of the trigeminal nerve
    d. Maxillary division of the trigeminal nerve

21. **Under which classification of basic tissues of the body does blood fall?**
    a. Connective
    b. Epithelial
    c. Muscle
    d. Nerve

22. **Concentrated study of which artery and its branches is important in the fields of dentistry and dental hygiene?**
    a. External carotid
    b. Internal carotid
    c. Subclavian
    d. Radial

23. **From which artery does the blood supply to mandibular teeth originate?**
    a. Facial
    b. Lingual
    c. Mandibular
    d. Maxillary

24. **Which of the following structures can be pierced during the administration of local anesthesia to maxillary molars?**
    a. Cavernous venous sinus
    b. Facial vein
    c. Pterygoid plexus of veins
    d. Retromolar vein

25. **Serious complications from facial or dental infections can occur because of the:**
    a. Limited anastomosis between the vessels in the head
    b. Inability of the vessels in the head and neck to clot
    c. Large size of the vessels in the head and neck
    d. Absence of valves in the veins of the head

26. **Which of the following is an example of an exocrine gland?**
    a. Parotid gland
    b. Thymus gland
    c. Cavernous venous sinus
    d. Deep lymph nodes

27. **The majority of the hard palate is directly vascularized by the:**
    a. Sphenopalatine artery
    b. Greater palatine artery
    c. Lesser palatine artery
    d. Ascending palatine artery

28. **The infratemporal fossa houses all of the following EXCEPT one. Which one is the EXCEPTION?**
    a. Lateral pterygoid muscles
    b. Maxillary artery
    c. Maxillary vein
    d. Temporalis muscle

29. **Which oral landmark marks the opening to the submandibular gland?**
    a. Lingual frenum
    b. Stensen's duct
    c. Sublingual fold
    d. Sublingual caruncle

30. **Dental and facial infections can spread through the:**
    a. Blood system
    b. Fascial spaces
    c. Lymphatic system
    d. All of the above

31. **If a nerve is an efferent nerve, it is a:**
    a. Motor nerve that travels to the brain
    b. Motor nerve that travels away from the brain
    c. Sensory nerve that travels to the brain
    d. Sensory nerve that travels away from the brain

32. **The central nervous system is composed of:**
    a. The autonomic nervous system
    b. Spinal nerves
    c. Cranial nerves
    d. The spinal cord

33. **Which of the following nerves are completely efferent?**
    a. Optic (cranial II)
    b. Vestibulocochlear (cranial VIII)
    c. Hypoglossal (cranial XII)
    d. Trigeminal (cranial V)

34. **Which of the following nerves exits the mandibular canal?**
    a. Inferior alveolar
    b. Lingual
    c. Mandibular
    d. Mylohyoid

35. **The chorda tympani is a branch of:**
    a. The fifth cranial nerve
    b. The seventh cranial nerve
    c. The ninth cranial nerve
    d. The twelfth cranial nerve

36. **Damaged to the _____ can result in Bell's palsy.**
    a. Facial nerve
    b. Glossopharyngeal nerve
    c. Vagus nerve
    d. Trigeminal nerve

37. **The three divisions of the trigeminal nerve enter the head through the following foramina:**
    a. Inferior orbital fissure, foramen rotundum, and foramen magnum
    b. Optic canal, foramen rotundum, and foramen ovale
    c. Superior orbital fissure, foramen rotundum, and foramen magnum
    d. Superior orbital fissure, foramen rotundum, and foramen ovale

38. **Where is the submandibular salivary gland located?**
    a. Anterior to the sublingual gland
    b. Inferior to the mylohyoid muscle
    c. Lateral to the angle of the mandible
    d. In the mandibular vestibule area

39. **The salivary gland that secretes a serous secretion is the:**
    a. Parotid gland
    b. Submandibular gland
    c. Sublingual gland
    d. Minor salivary glands

40. **Which of the following landmarks is present on the maxillary bone?**
    a. Foramen ovale
    b. Greater palatine foramen
    c. Infraorbital canal
    d. Superior orbital fissure

41. **Which of the following best describes the head of the condyle moving too far anteriorly on the articular eminence?**
    a. Subluxation
    b. Retraction
    c. Rotation
    d. Lateral deviation

42. **The spaces above and below the fibrous disk of the temporomandibular joint (TMJ) are termed:**
    a. Articulating cavities
    b. Joint cavities
    c. Mucosal cavities
    d. Synovial cavities

43. **After a clinician administers a local anesthetic agent near the infraorbital foramen landmark, the following structures will be anesthetized:**
    a. Mandibular molars
    b. Mandibular 1st and 2nd premolars
    c. Maxillary molars
    d. Maxillary canines and incisors

44. **Into which system does the lymphatic system drain?**
    a. Arterial
    b. Capillary
    c. Glandular
    d. Venous

45. **What structure or area would a clinician palpate to assess the condition of the retroauricular and anterior auricular lymph nodes?**
    a. The sternocleidomastoid muscle
    b. The angle of the mandible
    c. The region behind and in front of the ear
    d. The occipital region

46. **Which of the following cranial nerves and tissue pairs are correctly matched?**
    a. Abducens nerve, tongue muscles
    b. Facial nerve, sublingual and submandibular glands
    c. Trigeminal nerve, muscles of facial expression
    d. Vagus nerve, temporomandibular joint

47. **The paranasal sinuses drain through the:**
    a. Lacrimal ducts
    b. Nasal conchae
    c. Nasal meatuses
    d. Ethmoid air cells

48. **The floor of the maxillary sinuses is made up of the:**
    a. Zygomatic process
    b. Infratemporal crest
    c. Alveolar process of the maxilla
    d. Frontal process of the maxilla

49. **All of the following are branches of the mandibular division of the trigeminal nerve EXCEPT one. Which one is the EXCEPTION?**
    a. Buccal nerve
    b. Lingual nerve
    c. Mental nerve
    d. Nasopalatine nerve

50. **The reason that primary lymph nodes lying close to a cancerous lesion are often removed is to prevent the cancer from:**
    a. Metastasizing
    b. Spreading to the secondary nodes
    c. Entering the blood supply
    d. All of the above

Clinical Oral Structures, Dental Anatomy, and Root Morphology

Heidi A. Schlei

The practice of dental hygiene is based on oral anatomy, a fundamental dental science. A thorough knowledge of oral anatomy provides the basis for assessing, diagnosing, planning, implementing, and evaluating clients during the dental hygiene process of care. Oral structures reflect local and systemic health. Oral anatomy also provides the basis for client education, fluoride and pit-and-fissure sealant therapy, periodontal and tooth assessment, instrumentation, and non-surgical and periodontal maintenance care, all of which require imagery and tactile perception. The dental hygienist also uses oral anatomy to assess the relationship of teeth, both within and between the arches. These factors influence care plans, evidence-based decision making, professional recommendations, and referral to other health care practitioners.

CLINICAL ORAL STRUCTURES

Oral tissues are indicators of a client's oral and general health. Abnormal conditions can be recognized if the appearance of normal oral structures is known (Figures 5-1 to 5-8 and Table 5-1). Oral structures are identified according to their specific locations and functions. Generally, oral structures appear in shades of pink and may be pigmented in dark-complexioned individuals. In the oral cavity, the presence of melanin pigmentation is random, scattered, and unpredictable.

DENTAL TERMINOLOGY

A. Parts of a tooth (see the section on "Tissues of the Tooth" in Chapter 2)
   1. Crown
      a. Anatomic crown—part of the tooth covered by enamel

   b. Clinical crown—two definitions:
      (1) Portion of the tooth that is visible in the oral cavity; determined by the location of the gingival margin
      (2) Unattached portion of the tooth; determined by the junction of the epithelium to the tooth surface; includes the portion of the tooth that is bounded by the marginal gingiva
2. Root—part of the tooth covered by cementum
   a. Apex—rounded end of the root
   b. Periapex (periapical)—area around the apex of a tooth
   c. Foramen—opening at the apex through which blood vessels and nerves enter
   d. Furcation—area of a two-rooted or three-rooted tooth, where the root divides
      (1) Furcation entrance—area of opening into the furcation
      (2) Roof of the furcation—most coronal area of the furcation; the "ceiling" of a mandibular furcation; the base of a maxillary furcation
      (3) Interfurcal area—area between the roots of a two-rooted or three-rooted tooth
   e. Root trunk—area from the cemento-enamel junction (CEJ) to the furcation
   f. Root concavity—broad, shallow, vertical depression on the root; named by location: mesial, distal, and lingual; a concavity located on the furcation side of a root is called a *furcal concavity*
3. Enamel—hardest calcified tissue covering the dentin in the crown of the tooth; 96% mineralized
4. Cementum—bone-like calcified tissue covering the dentin in the root of the tooth; 50% mineralized

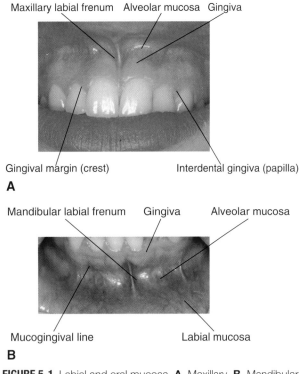

Maxillary labial frenum Alveolar mucosa Gingiva

Gingival margin (crest) Interdental gingiva (papilla)

A

Mandibular labial frenum Gingiva Alveolar mucosa

Mucogingival line Labial mucosa

B

FIGURE 5-1 Labial and oral mucosa. **A,** Maxillary. **B,** Mandibular.

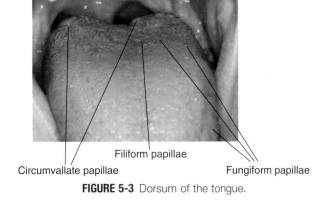

Circumvallate papillae Filiform papillae Fungiform papillae

FIGURE 5-3 Dorsum of the tongue.

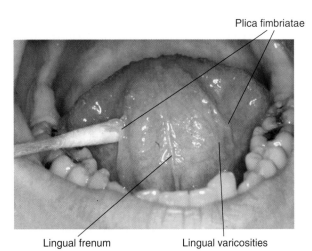

Plica fimbriatae

Lingual frenum Lingual varicosities

FIGURE 5-5 Ventral surface of the tongue.

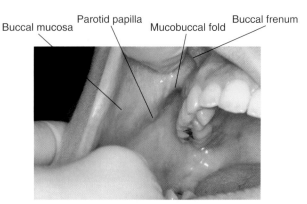

Buccal mucosa Parotid papilla Mucobuccal fold Buccal frenum

FIGURE 5-2 Buccal mucosa.

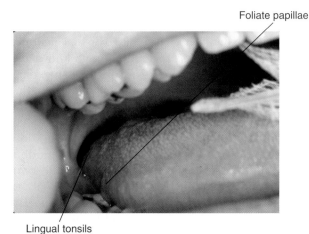

Foliate papillae

Lingual tonsils

FIGURE 5-4 Lateral surface of the tongue.

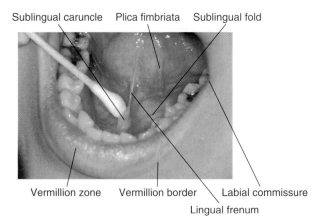

Sublingual caruncle Plica fimbriata Sublingual fold

Vermillion zone Vermillion border Labial commissure

Lingual frenum

FIGURE 5-6 Ventral surface of the tongue and the floor of the mouth.

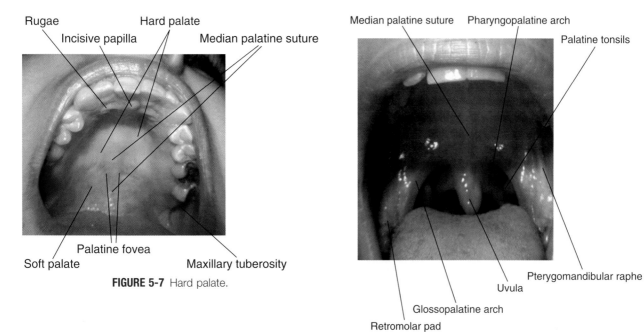

FIGURE 5-7 Hard palate.

FIGURE 5-8 Soft palate and oropharynx.

TABLE 5-1 Oral Structures

Structure	Clinical Description	Clinical Consideration
Lips, Cheeks, and Oral Mucosa (see Figure 5-1, *A*, and *B*, and Figure 5-2)		
Philtrum	Midline vertical depression of the skin between the nose and upper lip	Common location for cleft lip
Vermillion zone	Transitional area between the skin of the face and the oral mucosa of lips; medium pink in light-skinned individuals, and pigmented with melanin in dark-skinned individuals	The junction between the vermillion zone and the skin of the face is a frequent site of herpetic lesions; the lower lip is a frequent site of oral cancer; Fordyce's granules or spots (small white spots of ectopic sebaceous material) may be present
Labial commissure	Junction of upper and lower lips at the corner of the mouth	Frequent site of chafing, herpetic lesions, and cracking (angular cheilitis); avoid pulling with instrument handle
Vestibule	Space bounded by cheeks, lips, and facial surfaces of teeth and gingivae	Frequent site of aphthous ulcers
Labial mucosa	Mucosal lining of the inner lip; vascular; small elevations are external manifestation of numerous labial salivary glands	Frequent site of mucoceles, mucus-retention cysts, aphthous ulcers, and scars
Labial frenum (maxillary and mandibular)	Fold of tissue at the midline (maxillary and mandibular) between the inner surface of the lip and the alveolar mucosa	Maxillary fold is sometimes overdeveloped, which results in a space between the central incisors, called a *diastema*; frequently has an extra flap of tissue. If overextended onto the attached gingiva, mandibular fold may cause recession
Buccal mucosa	Mucous membrane lining of the inner cheek	Frequent site of linea alba, cheek bites, and Fordyce's granules
Parotid papilla	Flap of tissue on the cheek opposite the maxillary first molars; contains the opening of Stensen's duct, which carries saliva from the parotid gland	Large amounts of mainly serous saliva come from this duct; the opening can often be seen as a dark spot

Continued

TABLE 5-1 Oral Structures—cont'd

Structure	Clinical Description	Clinical Consideration
Buccal frena (muscle attachments)	Folds of epithelium between the cheek and attached gingivae (maxillary and mandibular) in the first premolar area	Overextension may cause gingival recession
Mucobuccal fold	Fold, or "gutter" area, between the alveolar and buccal or labial mucosa	The height of the mucobuccal fold above a maxillary tooth area to be anesthetized is the needle insertion area. The mental foramen of the mandible can be palpated in the mucobuccal fold area, facial to the mandibular premolars; this is the needle insertion site for a mental nerve block
Alveolar mucosa	Thin movable mucosal lining covering alveolar bone; between the attached gingiva and the mucobuccal fold on the facial aspect of maxillary and mandibular arches and between the attached gingiva and the floor of the mouth on the lingual aspect of the mandibular arch	Very thin and fragile epithelium. Frequent site of aphthous ulcers
Gingiva	Keratinized mucosa that surrounds teeth and alveolar bone	Ideally, except for a narrow band around the necks of teeth, it is firmly attached to teeth and bone
Mucogingival line or junction	A visible line where the pink keratinized gingiva meets the more vascular alveolar mucosa	Found on maxillary facial and mandibular facial and lingual areas
Gingival margin or crest	The most coronal edge of keratinized gingivae	The mandibular lingual lining is the site of tori (bony projections), which may interfere with exposing radiographs or taking impressions

Tongue (see Figures 5-3 to 5-6)
The tongue is a flat, muscular organ of speech and taste; the lateral border and undersurface are frequent sites of oral cancer.

Median sulcus	Midline depression on the dorsum of the tongue	Presence and depth vary. Additional deep depressions are called *fissures*; a fissured tongue
Fungiform papillae	Mushroom-shaped, red to dark-brown elevations scattered over the anterior third of the dorsum of the tongue	In dark-skinned individuals, they may contain melanin pigmentation. Function in taste sensations of sweet, sour, and salty
Filiform papillae	Fringe-like keratinized projections concentrated in the middle third of the dorsum of the tongue	Readily collect plaque and stain. Tongue with moving patches devoid of these papillae is called a *geographic tongue*
Circumvallate papillae	8–10 large papillae arranged in an inverted V-shaped row posterior to filiform papillae	Function in the taste sensation of bitter. Ducts of von Ebner's salivary glands open around them and secrete serous saliva
Foliate papillae	Vertical ridges on the lateral borders of the tongue	Function in the taste sensation of sour. May be a site of precancerous or cancerous findings (white or red areas, ulcers, masses, pigmentations)
Lingual tonsils	Mass of lymphoid tissue on the base of the tongue, posterior to circumvallate papillae	Difficult to observe; extend and move the tongue to the right and left to examine
Lingual frenum	Thin fold of epithelium attaching the undersurface of the tongue to the floor of the mouth	A short frenum limits movement (ankyloglossia, tongue-tied) and makes exposing radiographs and taking impressions difficult

TABLE 5-1 Oral Structures—cont'd

Structure	Clinical Description	Clinical Consideration
Sublingual folds	Two ridges of tissue on the floor of the mouth arranged in a V-shaped direction, from the lingual frenum to the base of the tongue	Contains Wharton's duct from the submandibular (also called *submaxillary*) salivary gland; Bartholin and Rivinis ducts; and the openings of the sublingual salivary glands. Limited amounts of mixed saliva secreted there
Sublingual caruncle	Round elevation of the floor of the mouth on either side of the lingual frenum. Contains the opening for Wharton's ducts	Wharton's duct carries large amounts of saliva from the submandibular (also called *submaxillary*) salivary gland
Lingual veins	Blue line on the undersurface of the tongue on either side of the lingual frenum	With age, these veins becomes more prominent in size and color; varicosities may be present
Plica fimbriatae	Fringe-like projections on the undersurface of the tongue, lateral to the lingual vein	May be dark colored, with more melanin pigmentation

Palate (see Figures 5-7 and 5-8)
The anterior two thirds of the roof of the mouth is the hard palate; the posterior third is the soft palate; a frequent site of oral cancer.

Incisive papilla	Midline pad of tissue lingual to the maxillary central incisors	Often burned or traumatized when eating. Protects the nasopalatine nerve, which enters through the underlying incisive foramen; the palatal mucosa immediately lateral to the papilla is the needle insertion site for nasopalatine nerve-block anesthesia
Rugae	Firm irregular ridges of masticatory mucosa on the anterior half of the hard palate	If prominent, rugae may be burned or traumatized more easily
Palatine fovea	Small dimple on either side of the midline at the junction of the hard and soft palates	Touching area posterior to this may initiate the gag reflex
Palatal salivary duct openings	Small, dark spots scattered on the hard and soft palates	Represent the duct openings of minor palatal salivary glands
Palatine raphe	Hard linear elevation along the midline of the hard palate; external manifestation of the palatine suture, which joins the right and left maxillary and palatine bones	Excess bone (tori) or a deep depression may be present there. Site of hyperkeratinization or associated nicotinic stomatitis
Maxillary tuberosity	Protuberance of alveolar bone distal to the last maxillary molar	Erupting third molar may be present there

Tonsillar Region (see Figure 5-8)

Retromolar area	Triangular area of bone and pad of tissue distal to the last mandibular molar	An erupting third molar may be present, and a flap of tissue (operculum) is often associated with infection in this area
Pterygomandibular raphe	Fold of tissue from the retromolar area to an area near the maxillary tuberosity; separates the soft palate from the cheek; lies medial to the posterior border of the ramus of the mandible	Covers a ligament from the mandible to sphenoid bone. Used as a guide to identify the posterior border of the ramus of the mandible when targeting the area for needle insertion for inferior alveolar-nerve anesthesia
Anterior or glossopalatine arch	Thin fold of epithelium extending laterally and inferiorly from both sides of the soft palate to the base of the tongue	Marks the entry into the pharynx; the anterior boundary of the tonsillar recess
Posterior or pharyngopalatine arch	Thin fold of epithelium that is more posterior and narrower than the anterior arch	Marks the posterior boundary of the palatine tonsillar recess
Tonsillar recess	Recessed area between the anterior and posterior arches	May or may not contain palatine tonsils

Continued

TABLE 5-1 Oral Structures—cont'd

Structure	Clinical Description	Clinical Consideration
Palatine tonsils	Globules of lymphoid tissue in the tonsillar recess	Vary greatly in size Not visible if removed or atrophied, or may be so large that the fauces is very narrow
Uvula	Fleshy tissue suspended from the midline of the posterior border of the soft palate	Closes the opening to the nasopharynx when swallowing. Varies in size and shape
Pharyngeal tonsils	Globules of lymphoid tissue on the oropharyngeal wall	Nontechnical term is *adenoids*. Appear as globules of reddish-orange tissue. Mucosal secretions from the sinuses may be seen here
Fauces or faucial isthmus	Isthmus (narrowing) of the space from the oral cavity into the pharynx	

5. Dentin—hard calcified tissue surrounding the pulp and underlying enamel and cementum; makes up the bulk of the tooth; 70% mineralized

6. Pulp—innermost noncalcified tissue containing blood vessels, lymphatics, and nerves

7. Pulp cavity—space containing the pulp
   a. Pulp canal—portion of the pulp cavity in the root of the tooth
   b. Pulp chamber—portion of the pulp cavity in the crown of the tooth
   c. Pulp horns—crown-ward extensions of the pulp chamber

B. Junction of parts
   1. CEJ (cervical line)—junction of cementum and enamel
   2. Dento-enamel junction (DEJ)—junction of dentin and enamel
   3. Cemento-dentin junction (CDJ)—junction of cementum and dentin

C. Tooth surfaces
   1. Facial—surface toward the face
      a. Labial (toward the lips)—facial surfaces of anterior teeth
      b. Buccal (toward the cheeks)—facial surfaces of posterior teeth
   2. Lingual—surface toward the tongue; may also be called *palatal* for maxillary teeth
   3. Proximal—surface toward the adjacent tooth
      a. Mesial—proximal surface toward the midline
      b. Distal—proximal surface farthest from the midline
   4. Contact area—area that touches the adjacent tooth in the same arch
   5. Incisal—surface of an incisor that is toward the opposite arch; the biting surface; newly erupted

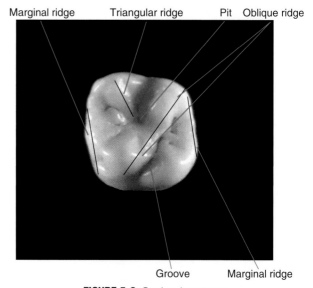

FIGURE 5-9 Occlusal anatomy.

permanent incisors have *mamelons* (projections of enamel) on this surface

6. Occlusal—surface of a posterior tooth that is toward the opposite arch; the chewing surface; this surface has elevations and depressions; the expression of these anatomic landmarks varies with the population from which they are derived (Figure 5-9)
   a. Cusp—large, rounded, elevated area of enamel
   b. Ridge—rounded, linear elevation of enamel
      (1) Marginal ridge—forms the mesial and distal borders of the lingual surface of anterior teeth and the occlusal surface of posterior teeth

(2) Triangular ridge—ridge from the tip of the cusp to the central developmental groove; formed by the junction of two cuspal inclines

(3) Oblique ridge—collective term referring to two triangular ridges meeting in an oblique line; a characteristic of maxillary molars

(4) Transverse ridge—collective term referring to two triangular ridges meeting in a faciolingual line

(5) Cingulum—large, rounded elevation of enamel on the linguocervical third of anterior teeth

c. Cuspal inclines—two surfaces of a cusp that slant or slope down and away from the crests of the triangular ridge toward developmental grooves

d. Groove—narrow linear depression

(1) Fissure—structural effect of enamel formation manifested as developmental lines or grooves on the external surface of a tooth; the area where the centers of calcification coalesce during tooth development

(2) Developmental groove—groove or line that indicates the primary anatomic divisions (cusps, lobes) of a crown

(3) Supplemental groove—a less distinct groove that branches from a developmental groove

e. Fossa—a shallow, broad depression

f. Pit—a sharp, pointed depression generally located at the junction of developmental grooves (fissures) or at their termination; the opening of a pit may be narrow or wide but is smaller than a toothbrush bristle; pits may be shallow or deep, and their apical descent may be steep or gradual; pits in primary teeth are not as deep as those in permanent teeth

D. Junction of surfaces—a tooth has curved surfaces; therefore, no "corner," where one surface begins and another ends, is present; the transition area is called the *line angle area* and is named for the surfaces that are involved (e.g., MB, mesiobuccal, DL, distolingual, MO, mesio-occlusal)

E. Embrasure—the interproximal space between teeth that begins at the contact area and widens in facial, lingual, occlusal–incisal, and cervical directions; functions as a spillway and escapement area by deflecting food and reducing the forces placed on the periodontium during chewing; also provides a self-cleaning area; the interproximal gingiva fills the cervical embrasure

DENTAL ANATOMY

A. Permanent dentition (Table 5-2)

1. Humans are diphyodonts, that is, they have two sets of teeth in a lifetime—a primary dentition and a permanent dentition—that span three dentition periods: primary, mixed, and permanent

2. The permanent dentition consists of:

a. Eight incisors, two in each quadrant, named central and lateral incisors, respectively. The four quadrants in a dentition are: maxillary right, maxillary left, mandibular right, and mandibular left

(1) Incisors are the only teeth with an incisal ridge; newly erupted incisors have mamelons—three rounded elevations on the incisal ridge—which are worn away shortly after eruption

(2) Incisal angles—formed by the proximal surfaces and the incisal ridge; central incisor angles are sharper than lateral incisor angles, and mesioincisal angles are sharper than distoincisal angles

(3) Maxillary lateral incisors vary the most in size and shape and may be congenitally missing

b. Four canines—one in each quadrant

(1) Only teeth with one cusp

(2) Considered the "cornerstone" of the dentition because of the long, large root, which is externally manifested by the canine eminence of maxillary alveolar bone

(3) Canines and incisors together are considered "anterior" teeth

c. Eight premolars, two in each quadrant, named first and second premolars

(1) Generally have two cusps, but the mandibular second premolar also has a three-cusped type, the tricuspidate, which is common

(2) Have one root, except maxillary first premolars, which have two roots 60% of the time

(3) Replace primary molars when they exfoliate

(4) In the past, first premolars were frequently extracted for orthodontic reasons

d. Twelve molars, three in each quadrant; named first, second, and third molars

(1) Largest teeth in the dentition

(2) Only teeth that do not replace primary teeth

TABLE 5-2 Characteristics of the Crowns and Roots of Permanent Teeth

Maxillary	Crown	Root(s)	Visual Characteristics
Central incisor	Largest of incisors. The mesiodistal width is greater than the faciolingual depth. The lingual anatomy is distinct: a broad cingulum with grooves, where it joins the lingual fossa; mesial and distal marginal ridges, linguoincisal ridge, and a lingual fossa. The lingual surface is smaller than the facial surface because of proximal surface convergence	One root, conical in shape. Proximal root concavities are uncommon. Prominent cemento-enamel junction (CEJ) incisal curvature on the proximal surface. The root is 1¼ times the length of the crown. Cervical cross-section is "rounded triangular" in shape with a flat mesial surface	Tooth #8
Lateral incisor	Similar to central but smaller. Cingulum is narrow, and a lingual pit is common	One root, conical in shape. The root is longer and more rounded than the central incisor. The root is 1⅓ times the length of the crown; may have a lingual or palatoradicular groove extending from the crown to the root	Tooth #7
Canine	Cusp ridges and tip are one third the length of the crown. The lingual anatomy is distinct, with a large cingulum, marginal ridges, and a vertical lingual ridge between two lingual fossae; rarely has pits	One long root, conical in shape. Generally has proximal root concavities. The distal crest of curvature in the middle third of the crown may hinder access to the mesial surface of the first premolar. Cervical cross-section is ovoid in shape. The root is 1½ times the length of the crown	Tooth #6
First premolar	Two cusps, facial longer than lingual. Long central developmental groove. Mesial and distal pits on occlusal surface. Prominent concavity in the cervical third of mesial surface	Two roots (40% have one root); one facial, one lingual. Bifurcated in the apical third to half; mesial and distal furcation entrances. Prominent mesial concavity begins on the crown cervical to the mesial contact and extends apically to the furcation	Tooth #4
Second premolar	Two cusps of more equal length. Occlusal outline is more rounded. Short central developmental groove. Many supplemental grooves. No mesial crown concavity or groove	One root. Proximal root concavities common; mesial root concavity not as pronounced as the first premolar. Elliptical in cross-section; broad proximally. The root is 1¾ times the length of the crown	Tooth #5

TABLE 5-2 Characteristics of the Crowns and Roots of Permanent Teeth—cont'd

Maxillary	Crown	Root(s)	Visual Characteristics
First molar	Largest tooth in the dentition. Rhomboidal occlusal view outline. Oblique ridge from mesiolingual to distobuccal cusp. Four cusps on the occlusal half and one minor cusp on the mesial half of the lingual surface, called the *cusp of Carabelli*. An occlusal lingual groove ends with a pit on the lingual surface. Pits on occlusal, in mesial, central, and distal fossae. Lingual surface wider than facial surface (exception)	Three roots: mesiofacial, distofacial, and lingual. Lingual root the longest; extends out beyond lingual surface of crown. Furcations on mesial, facial, and distal surfaces. Root concavities may be present on the palatal surface of the lingual root, the mesial surface of the mesiofacial root, and furcal surfaces (furcal concavities). Mesiofacial and distofacial roots may appear as a "pair," and their apices curve toward each other; resembles a pliers handle. Furcations begin gradually before the entrance, which is generally located near the junction of the cervical and middle third of the root; the mesial furcation is located more toward the lingual surface. Root is 1¾ times the length of the crown	Tooth #3
Second molar	Resembles the first molar, but is smaller. Four cusps; sometimes the distolingual cusp is not present. Pits on occlusal, in mesial, central, and distal fossae	Three roots: mesiofacial, distofacial, and lingual. Roots are closer together; more distally oriented; less inter-radicular bone. Longer root trunk The root is 1¾ times the length of the crown	Tooth #2
Third molar	Resembles the second molar, but varies frequently	May have three roots; varies frequently. Roots frequently fused	

Mandibular	Crown	Root(s)	Visual Characteristics
Central and lateral incisors	The central incisor is the smallest tooth; is symmetrical. The lateral incisor is only slightly larger; is asymmetrical. Incisal angles are sharp. Contact areas are near the incisal ridge. The lingual surface is concave, and the anatomy is not distinct. The lateral crown has a distal twist, and the cingulum is displaced toward the distal	One root, conical in shape. Proximal root concavities are likely. Cervical cross-section, elliptical in shape, narrow facial and lingual surfaces; broad proximally The root is 1½ times the length of the crown	Tooth #25 Tooth #26

TABLE 5-2 Characteristics of the Crowns and Roots of Permanent Teeth—cont'd

Mandibular	Crown	Root(s)	Visual Characteristics
Canine	Cusp ridges and tip occupy $\frac{1}{4}$ to $\frac{1}{5}$ of crown length The lingual anatomy is the same as that of the maxillary canine but not as prominent. The mesial surfaces of the crown and the root are in a straight line	One root, conical in shape. Proximal root concavities are present. In cervical cross-section, ovoid in shape, small lingual surface. Occasionally is bifurcated into a facial and lingual root in apical third. The root is $1\frac{1}{2}$ times the length of the crown	Tooth #27
First premolar	Two cusps, large facial and very small nonfunctional lingual. Triangular ridges form a prominent transverse ridge, two pits, and a mesiolingual groove. Crowns of all mandibular posterior teeth are inclined toward the tongue; may make instrument placement more difficult	One root, conical in shape. In cervical cross-section, may be ovoid or elliptical in shape. May have a deep proximal root concavity on the distal root surface. The root is $1\frac{2}{3}$ times the length of the crown	Tooth #28
Second premolar	Bicuspidate (2) or tricuspidate (3) forms. The bicuspidate form has an H-shaped groove pattern. The tricuspidate form has a Y-shaped groove pattern with a large facial cusp and smaller mesiolingual and distolingual cusps	One root, conical in shape. In cervical cross-section, may be ovoid or elliptical in shape. The root is $1\frac{2}{3}$ times the length of the crown	Tooth #29
First molar	Greater mesiodistal than faciolingual width. Five cusps: three facial, two lingual; Y-shaped occlusal groove pattern; extends onto facial surface and forms two facial grooves and pit. Occlusal pits in mesial, central, and distal fossae	Two roots, mesial and smaller distal. Furcations on facial and lingual surfaces; concavity before the furcation on facial surface begins just apical to the CEJ. Short root trunk; larger inter-radicular area. Proximal concavity and two root canals on the mesial root. Cervical enamel projections may occur. The root is $1\frac{3}{4}$ times the length of the crown	Tooth #30
Second molar	Similar to the first molar. Four cusps: two facial and two lingual "+"-shaped occlusal groove pattern; extends onto facial surface to form one groove and pit. Occlusal pits in mesial, central, and distal fossae	Two roots, mesial and distal. Roots are more likely to be closer together with a longer root trunk. Mesial root concavity is not as prominent. Roots are $1\frac{3}{4}$ times the length of the crown	Tooth #31

TABLE 5-2 Characteristics of the Crowns and Roots of Permanent Teeth—cont'd

Mandibular	Crown	Root(s)	Visual Characteristics
Third molar	Similar to the second molar. Varies greatly	Usually two roots. Roots are short, frequently fused, and angled to the distal	

Knowing the length of the crown of a tooth is helpful when assessing the length of its root and the amount of attachment. Maxillary central and lateral incisor crowns are the longest in the dentition, being approximately 9 to 10½ inches in length. Anterior crowns are 2 to 3 mm longer than posterior crowns. Roots range between 12 and 17 mm in length; incisor roots are the shortest, and canines are the longest. Proportionally, when comparing the length of roots with their crowns, molars have the "longest" roots overall because of their short crowns; maxillary incisors have the "shortest" roots

(3) Erupt distal to the second primary molars; the first mandibular molar is the first permanent tooth to erupt

(4) Multi-cusped, with each having a distinct cusp-and-groove pattern

(5) Maxillary molars have three roots; mandibular molars have two roots

(6) The presence, size, and shape of third molars vary greatly

(7) Premolars and molars together are considered "posterior" teeth

3. The Universal Numbering System (UNS) uses Arabic numerals 1 to 32 to specify permanent teeth, beginning with the maxillary right third molar and ending with the mandibular right third molar; the International Standards Organization (ISO) TC 106 designation system (also referred to as the *International Numbering System*) uses a two-digit code; the first digit—1 to 4—designates the quadrant in the dentition, clockwise from the upper-right quadrant. The second digit—1 to 8—designates the tooth, from the central incisor to the third molar. For example, tooth 11 is the permanent maxillary right central incisor

4. General characteristics of tooth form

a. All proximal surfaces converge toward the apex from the crests of curvature (height of contour) (Figure 5-10)

(1) This convergence provides spacing for the interproximal gingiva and bone

(2) In an ideal dentition, the proximal crest of curvature is also the contact area, which functions to stabilize adjacent teeth and protect the interproximal gingiva

(3) Proximal crests are located in the incisal or middle third of the crown

(4) As a general rule, the mesial crest is more incisal–occlusal than the distal crest, and mesial cusp ridges are shorter than distal cusp ridges; mesial outlines are straighter than distal outlines (Figure 5-11)

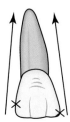

FIGURE 5-10 Apical convergence (*arrows*) of proximal surfaces.

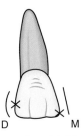

FIGURE 5-11 Comparison of mesial (*M*) and distal (*D*) outlines.

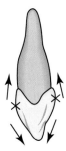

FIGURE 5-12 Apical and incisal occlusal convergence (*arrows*) of facial and lingual surfaces.

b. All facial and lingual surfaces converge toward the apex and toward the incisal–occlusal surface from the crests of curvature; this convergence facilitates mastication (Figure 5-12)

c. All facial surfaces of the crown are convex, and the crest of the curvature is located in the cervical third; the lingual surfaces of posterior teeth are convex, and the crest of curvature

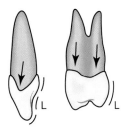

FIGURE 5-13 Facial and lingual contours (*arrows*) and the proximal curvature of the cemento-enamel junctions. *L*, lingual aspect.

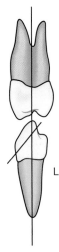

FIGURE 5-14 Lingual inclination of mandibular posterior crowns.

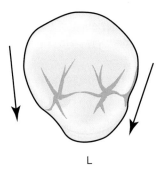

FIGURE 5-15 Lingual convergence (*arrows*) of proximal surfaces. *L*, lingual aspect.

is located in the middle third; the lingual surfaces of anterior teeth are concave in the middle third; these contours deflect food away from the gingiva and facilitate the function of teeth (Figure 5-13)

d. The CEJ on the proximal surface curves toward the incisal–occlusal surface and is more prominent on anterior teeth than on posterior teeth; the CEJ curves more on the mesial surface than on the distal surface (see Figure 5-13)

e. From a proximal view, the long axes of the crown and the root are in line except for the posterior mandibular teeth, which have the long axis of the crown tilting lingually to the long axis of the root; this lingual inclination enables the intercusping relationship of posterior teeth and the distribution of forces along their long axes (Figure 5-14)

f. Proximal surfaces converge toward the lingual; this is most prominent on maxillary incisors and canines (the two exceptions are the mandibular second premolar and the maxillary first molar) (see Table 5-2 and Figure 5-15)

5. General characteristics of roots
   a. Root anatomy is not as complex as crown anatomy, but variations in size, shape, and number frequently occur
   b. Teeth have one, two, or three roots
      (1) One root—incisors, canines, maxillary second premolars, mandibular premolars
      (2) Two roots—maxillary first premolars (buccal and lingual) and mandibular molars (mesial and distal)
      (3) Three roots—maxillary molars (mesiobuccal, distobuccal, and lingual)
   c. Teeth with two or three roots have a root trunk with depressions that deepen until the trunk divides at the furcation
      (1) The more cervical the furcation, the more stable is the tooth because of the divergence of roots with inter-radicular bone
      (2) Furcation involvement occurs when a loss of attachment exists apical to the furcation
      (3) Furcations that begin close to the CEJ are more likely to become involved in periodontal disease, but access is easier
      (4) Furcations are more cervical on the first molars, especially the mandibular first molar
   d. Some roots have longitudinal depressions called *root concavities*
   e. Individual roots are basically cone shaped, being widest at the CEJ and converging (tapering) to the apex; more root surface area is present in the cervical than apical third
   f. A cervical cross-section of a tooth with one root shows three basic shapes (Figure 5-16; see Table 5-2), which may be slightly altered by the presence of root concavities
      (1) Triangular—maxillary incisors
      (2) Ovoid (egg-shaped)—canines and some mandibular premolars

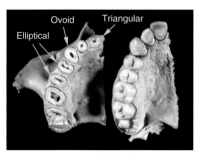

FIGURE 5-16 Root shapes as seen in cervical cross-section: elliptical, ovoid, and triangular.

(3) Elliptical—maxillary premolars, mandibular incisors, and some mandibular premolars
g. Roots that appear triangular or ovoid in cross-section have narrower lingual surfaces
h. A cervical cross-section of molars follows the form of the crown
i. From a facial or lingual view, roots have a distal inclination
j. Second-molar and third-molar roots are more likely to be closer together, fused, and distally inclined
k. The CEJs on posterior teeth have a much less pronounced curvature on all surfaces
l. Cementum is not as hard as enamel
m. Variations in root form
(1) Fused roots
(2) Supernumerary roots
(3) Dilaceration—unexpected root curvature
(4) Hypercementosis
(5) Enamel pearls
(6) Cervical enamel projections into a furcation
6. Clinical considerations of permanent tooth form
a. Clinical considerations of incisor form
(1) Maxillary lingual anatomy is more prominent than mandibular lingual anatomy; however, plaque, calculus, and stain readily collect on mandibular lingual surfaces
(2) The proximal surfaces of maxillary incisors are more accessible from the lingual approach because of the convergence of the proximal surfaces; the proximal surfaces of mandibular incisor roots are difficult to approach because of limited interproximal space and root concavities
(3) As people live longer and keep their teeth, repeated instrumentation on the roots of mandibular incisors places the crowns of these teeth in jeopardy; the very narrow facial and lingual root surfaces are

increasingly subject to loss of structure, resulting in unsupported cervical enamel
b. Clinical considerations of canine form
(1) Crown length and bulk make these teeth very stable
(2) The proximal surfaces are more accessible from the lingual approach than from the facial approach because of the convergence of the proximal surfaces
c. Clinical considerations of premolars
(1) Distinctive pit-and-groove patterns facilitate the identification of premolars
(2) Proximal root concavities, especially the mesial of the maxillary first premolar, make subgingival instrumentation difficult on the proximal surfaces
(3) Mandibular premolar crowns, with their small lingual surfaces and lingual inclinations, make instrumentation difficult
d. Clinical considerations of molars
(1) Complex pit-and-groove patterns make molars relatively susceptible to dental caries; they should be sealed shortly after eruption
(2) The lingual inclination of mandibular molar crowns makes the subgingival placement of instruments more difficult on the lingual surface
(3) Proximal furcation areas of maxillary molars should be approached from the lingual aspect because furcations are located closer to the lingual surface
(4) Roots with furcation involvement are especially difficult to manage; successful treatment may require surgery
B. Primary dentition
1. The primary (deciduous) dentition consists of 20 teeth: 8 incisors, 4 canines, and 8 molars
2. The UNS uses capital letters A through T for primary teeth, beginning with the maxillary right second primary molar and ending with the mandibular right second primary molar; the ISO TC 106 designation system uses a two-digit code. The first digit—5 to 8—designates the quadrant in the dentition, clockwise from the upper-right quadrant; the second digit—1 to 5—designates the tooth, from the central incisor to the second primary molar
3. The anatomy of primary teeth is similar to that of permanent teeth except (Figure 5-17):
a. Primary teeth are smaller in size than their permanent counterparts; primary molars are wider than the premolars that replace them but are smaller than permanent molars
b. Primary teeth are whiter than permanent teeth

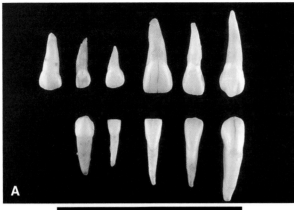

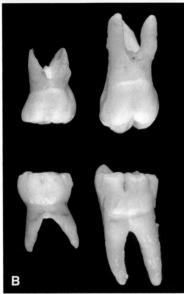

FIGURE 5-17 Comparison of dentitions. **A,** Comparison of primary and permanent anterior teeth. **B,** Comparison of primary second molars and permanent first molars.

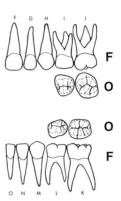

FIGURE 5-18 Primary teeth, designated according to the Universal Numbering System. *F,* facial; *O,* occlusal.

c. The crowns of primary teeth are shorter, with pronounced labial and lingual cervical ridges and a constricted cervical area

d. The occlusal tables of primary teeth are facio-lingually narrower, and the cuspal anatomy is not as pronounced as in permanent teeth

e. Enamel depth is more consistent and thinner (0.5 to 1 mm thick compared with that of permanent teeth, which is 2.5 mm)

f. Pulp chambers (relative to the size of the tooth) are larger, and pulp horns extend more occlusally than in permanent teeth; the amount of dentin is proportionately less

g. Roots are slender and longer than in permanent teeth, approximately twice the length of the crown

h. Root trunks are shorter, and roots are more divergent to accommodate the developing premolar crown

i. Primary teeth have fewer anomalies and variations in tooth form compared with permanent teeth

4. Anatomy of primary teeth (Figure 5-18)

a. Incisors—resemble the outline of their permanent counterparts except that they may have no mamelons on the incisal ridge and no pits on the lingual surface

b. Canines—resemble the outlines of their permanent counterparts; the maxillary canine has a sharp cusp and appears especially wide and short

c. Molars

(1) First primary molars

(a) Do not resemble any other teeth

(b) Have the same number and position of roots as that of permanent molars

(c) The CEJ on the mesial half of the buccal surface curves apically around a very prominent cervical ridge

(d) The maxillary first primary molar has an H-shaped groove pattern and usually has three cusps; the mesial cusps are the largest; a prominent cervical ridge present

(e) The mandibular first primary molar has four or five cusps; the mesial cusps are larger, and the mesiolingual cusp is long, pointed, and angled toward the occlusal surface

(2) The second primary molars are larger than the first primary molars and resemble the form of the first permanent molar

ERUPTION

A. General comments

1. *Eruption* frequently is defined as "the emergence of the tooth through the gingiva"

2. Also defined as the movements a tooth makes to attain and maintain a relationship with the teeth in the same and opposing arches; follows distinct stages:
   a. Beginning of hard tissue formation
   b. Enamel (crown) completion, after which actual tooth movement begins
   c. Eruption
   d. Root completion (approximately 50% of the root is formed when eruption begins)
3. Ages at which eruption occurs are given in classic eruption tables
5. Sequential patterns are reflected throughout the developmental stages, and knowledge of these patterns can be used to predict or approximate the age of one stage on the basis of another
6. As a generalization, the mandibular tooth of a type (incisor, canine, etc.) emerges before the maxillary tooth of the same type, and the first before the second (e.g., the central incisor emerges before the lateral incisor)
7. Clinically, eruption tables are helpful, but a better approach may be to correlate a given age with the teeth expected to be present
B. Primary dentition
   1. A guide for the emergence of teeth into the oral cavity is provided in Table 5-1.

	Mandibular	Maxillary
Central incisor	6 months	7½ months
Lateral incisor	7 months	9 months
Canine	16 months	18 months
First molar	12 months	14 months
Second molar	20 months	24 months

   2. The order of eruption for primary tooth development is: central incisor, lateral incisor, first molar, canine, and second molar
   3. Hard tissue formation begins in utero between 4 and 6 months
   4. Crowns are completed between 1½ and 10 months of age
   5. Roots are completed between 1½ and 3 years of age, 6 to 18 months after eruption
   6. By 3 years of age, all primary and permanent teeth (except the third molars) are in some stage of development
   7. Root resorption of a primary tooth is triggered by the pressure exerted by the developing permanent tooth; it is followed by primary tooth exfoliation in sequential patterns
   8. The primary dentition ends when the first permanent tooth erupts

C. Mixed dentition
   1. Transition dentition occurs between 6 and 12 years of age, with primary tooth exfoliation and permanent tooth eruption
   2. Physiologic and psychological effects on both parents and children may be noted
   3. Characteristic features have led to this stage being called the "ugly duckling" stage because of:
      a. Edentulated areas
      b. Disproportionately sized teeth
      c. Varying clinical crown heights
      d. Crowding
      e. Enlarged and edematous gingiva
      f. Different tooth colors
D. Permanent dentition
   1. Teeth that have primary predecessors are called *succedaneous teeth*: incisors, canines, and premolars
   2. Permanent tooth formation begins between birth and 3 years of age (except for the third molars)
   3. The crowns of permanent teeth are completed between 4 and 8 years of age, at approximately one half the age of eruption
   4. The order of eruption in permanent tooth development is provided in Table 5-2.

Mandibular	Maxillary
First molar	First molar
Central incisor	Central incisor
Lateral incisor	Lateral incisor
Canine	First premolar
First premolar	Second premolar
Second premolar	Canine
Second molar	Second molar
Third molar	Third molar

   5. A guide for the emergence of permanent teeth into the oral cavity is given table 5-2.

	Mandibular	Maxillary
Central incisor	6–7 years	7–8 years
Lateral incisor	7–8 years	8–9 years
Canine	9–10 years	11–12 years
First premolar	10–12 years	10–11 years
Second premolar	11–12 years	10–12 years
First molar*	6–7 years	6–7 years
Second molar	11–13 years	12–13 years
Third molar	17–21 years	17–21 years

First permanent tooth to erupt.

6. Roots of permanent teeth are completed between 10 and 16 years of age, 2 to 3 years after eruption.

E. Age changes in the dentition

1. After teeth have reached full occlusion, microscopic tooth movements occur to compensate for wear at contact areas (by mesial drift) and occlusal surfaces (by deposition of cementum at the root apex)

2. Attrition of incisal ridges and cusp tips may be so severe that dentin may become exposed and intrinsically stained

3. Noncarious cervical lesions (NCCL) related to loss of tooth structure
   a. Erosion—progressive uniform loss of structure by a chemical process
   b. Abrasion—abnormal loss of structure by external mechanical wear
   c. Abfraction—loss of weakened brittle enamel away from a point of biomechanical loading caused by tooth flexure and fatigue

4. Secondary dentin may be formed in response to dental caries, trauma, and aging; this results in a decrease in the size of the pulp cavity and tooth sensation

INTRA-ARCH AND INTERARCH RELATIONSHIPS

Each tooth has a relationship with adjacent teeth in the same and opposing arches. These relationships are influenced by a number of factors, including the size and shape of the maxilla, the mandible, and the teeth themselves, and a variety of external factors such as oral habits and dental disease.

A. Intra-arch relationship—the alignment of the teeth within an arch

1. Position of teeth in the jaw
   a. In an ideal alignment, teeth contact at their proximal crests of curvature; a continuous arch form is observed from an occlusal view
      (1) Some permanent dentitions have normal spacing with no contact
      (2) Primary dentitions often have developmental spacing in the anterior area; some primary dentitions have a pattern of spacing called *primate spaces* between the primary maxillary lateral incisor and the canine and between the primary mandibular canine and the first molar (Figure 5-19)
   b. Axial positioning—relationship of the long axis of individual teeth to an imaginary horizontal or median plane; ideally, each tooth

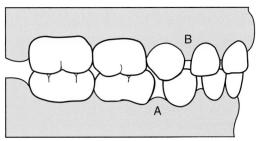

FIGURE 5-19 Primary teeth showing primate spaces. **A,** Mandibular primate space between the canine and the first molar. **B,** Maxillary primate space between the lateral incisor and the canine. *(Modified from Wilkins E: Clinical Practice of the Dental Hygienist, ed 10, Philadelphia, 2008, Lippincott, Williams, & Wilkins.)*

"sits" at an angle that best withstands the forces placed on it
      (1) Incisors are placed with their axes at approximately 60 degrees to the horizontal plane; the more posterior the tooth, the less acute is the angle (Figure 5-20)
      (2) The posterior mandibular teeth tip lingually toward the median plane; the long axes of the posterior maxillary teeth are more parallel to the median plane
   c. Curves of the occlusal plane (a line connecting the cusp tips of canines, premolars, and molars) are observed from the buccal and proximal views
      (1) Curve of Spee—when viewed from the buccal aspect in centric occlusion, the cusp tips of posterior teeth curve anteroposteriorly; for mandibular teeth, the curve is concave, and for maxillary teeth it is convex (Figure 5-21, A)
      (2) Curve of Wilson—medio-lateral curve connecting cusp tips of posterior mandibular teeth on opposite sides of the mouth; for mandibular teeth, the curve is concave due to their lingual tilt, and for maxillary molars it is convex. (see Figure 5-21, B)

2. Disturbances to the intra-arch alignment are described as:
   a. Open contacts—sites where an interproximal space exists because of normal alignment, missing teeth, oral habits, dental disease, or overdeveloped frena
   b. Versions—sites where a contact or position occurs at an unexpected area because of developmental disturbances, crowding, oral habits, dental caries, or periodontal disease; named for their misplaced positions: facio-version, linguo-version, mesio-version, disto-version, supra-version (super-erupted), infra-version (under-erupted), and torso-version (rotated)

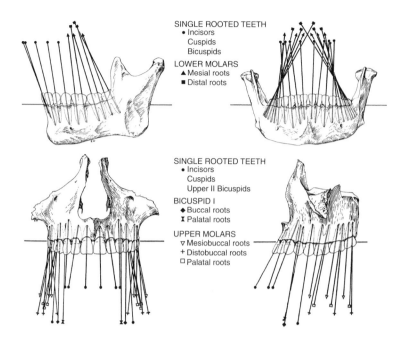

SINGLE ROOTED TEETH
- Incisors
  Cuspids
  Bicuspids

LOWER MOLARS
- ▲ Mesial roots
- ■ Distal roots

SINGLE ROOTED TEETH
- Incisors
  Cuspids
  Upper II Bicuspids

BICUSPID I
- ◆ Buccal roots
- ✗ Palatal roots

UPPER MOLARS
- ▽ Mesiobuccal roots
- + Distobuccal roots
- □ Palatal roots

FIGURE 5-20 Tooth positioning in relation to the horizontal plane. *(From Dempster WT, Adams WJ, Duddles RA: Arrangement in the Jaws of the Roots of the Teeth, J Am Dent Assoc 67:779, 1963.)*

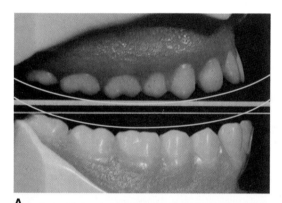

A

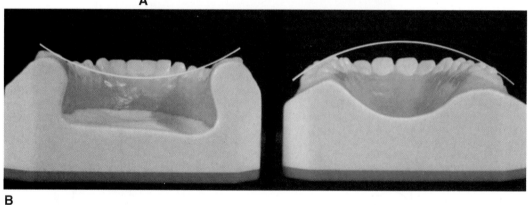

B

FIGURE 5-21 The curves of occlusion. **A,** Curve of Spee. **B,** Curve of Wilson. *(From Berkovitz BKB, Holland GR, Moxham BJ: Color atlas and textbook of oral anatomy, histology and embryology, ed 2, London, 1992, Mosby-Year Book, Inc.)*

B. Interarch relationships can be viewed from a stationary (fixed) perspective and a dynamic (movable) perspective
1. Stationary relationships
   a. Centric relationship—relationship of the condyle of the mandible to the articular fossa of temporal bone, as determined by the bones, ligaments, and muscles of the temporomandibular joint (TMJ); in an ideal dentition, the relationship is the same as in centric occlusion
   b. Centric occlusion—habitual occlusion where maximum intercuspation occurs (*Note*: A normal physiologic rest position of the mandible occurs during nonfunction when a freeway space with no interocclusal contact should occur); the characteristics of centric occlusion are:
      (1) Overjet—the characteristic of maxillary teeth to overlap mandibular teeth in a horizontal direction by 1 to 2 mm; the maxillary arch is slightly larger; it functions to protect the narrow edge of incisors and to provide for an intercusping relationship of posterior teeth (Figure 5-22)
      (2) Overbite—the characteristic of the anterior maxillary teeth to overlap the anterior mandibular teeth in a vertical direction by a third of the lower crown height; facilitates the scissors-like function of incisors (Figure 5-23)
      (3) Intercuspation—the characteristic of posterior teeth to intermesh in a faciolingual direction; mandibular facial cusps and maxillary lingual cusps are centric cusps that contact interocclusally in the opposing arch (Figure 5-24)
      (4) Interdigitation—the characteristic of each tooth to articulate with two opposing teeth (except for mandibular central incisors and maxillary last molars); a mandibular tooth occludes with its counterpart in the upper arch and the one mesial to it; a maxillary tooth occludes with its counterpart in the mandibular arch and the one distal to it (Figure 5-25)

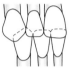

FIGURE 5-23 *Overbite*, the term used to describe the vertical overlap of the anterior maxillary teeth on the anterior mandibular teeth.

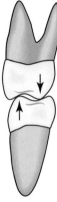

FIGURE 5-24 Intercuspation of posterior teeth. Centric cusps have interocclusal contact with opposing teeth.

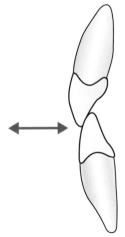

FIGURE 5-22 *Overjet*, the term used to describe the horizontal overlap of the anterior maxillary teeth on the anterior mandibular teeth.

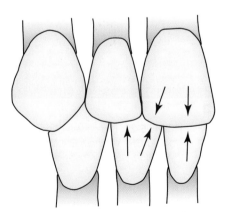

FIGURE 5-25 Interdigitation of teeth.

(a) Using the first permanent molars, Edward H. Angle classified these relationships as follows(Figure 5-26):

[1] Normal or neutral occlusion (ideal)—mesiobuccal groove of the mandibular first permanent molar aligns with the mesiobuccal cusp of the maxillary first permanent molar

[2] Class I malocclusion—normal molar relationships with alterations in other characteristics of the occlusion, such as versions, cross-bites, excessive overjets, or overbites

[3] Class II malocclusion—distal relationship of the mesiobuccal groove of the mandibular first permanent molar to the mesiobuccal cusp of the maxillary first permanent molar

[a] Division I—protruded anterior maxillary teeth

[b] Division II—one or more retruded anterior maxillary anterior teeth

[4] Class III malocclusion—a mesial relationship of the mesiobuccal groove of the mandibular first permanent molar to the mesiobuccal cusp of the maxillary first permanent molar

(b) Canines may also be used to confirm molar relationships or to classify an occlusion when a molar is missing; a class I canine relationship shows the cusp tip of the maxillary canine facial to and aligned with the interproximal space between the mandibular canine and the first premolar

(c) Occlusion in a primary dentition is assessed by the relationship of the distal terminus (surface) of second primary molars in centric occlusion; three relationships are possible: a flush terminal plane, a distal step, or a mesial step (Figure 5-27)

(d) Mixed dentition represents a transitional stage of occlusal development; the initial contact of permanent first molars usually begins at age 7, and by 12 years of age, the final occlusion of the first molars is established; distal-step primary dentitions always lead to a class II permanent molar

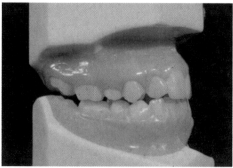

A

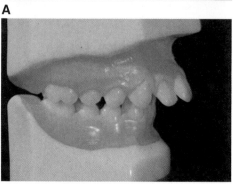

B

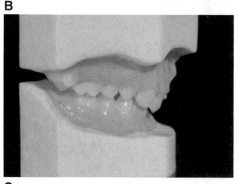

C

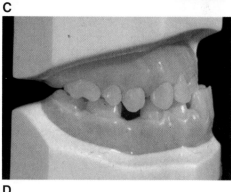

D

FIGURE 5-26 Malocclusion classified using Angle's system. **A,** Angle's class I malocclusion. **B,** Angle's class II malocclusion (division 1). **C,** Angle's class II malocclusion (division 2). **D,** Angle's class III malocclusion. *(Modified from Berkovitz BKB, Holland GR, Moxham BJ: Color atlas and textbook of oral anatomy, histology and embryology, ed 2, London, 1992, Mosby-Year Book, Inc.)*

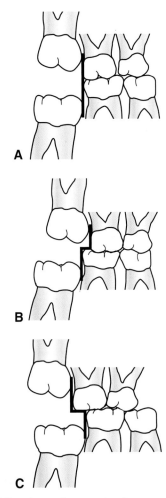

FIGURE 5-27 Terminus of second primary molars in centric occlusion. **A,** Flush terminal plane. **B,** Distal step. **C,** Mesial step.

occlusion; exaggerated mesial-step primary dentitions lead to a class III permanent molar occlusion; the development of occlusion from a flush terminus or a mild mesial-step primary dentition is variable but frequently leads to a class I first permanent molar relationship

2. Disturbances in interarch alignment are described as:
   a. Excessive overbite—the incisal edges of maxillary incisors extend to the cervical third of mandibular incisors
   b. Excessive overjet—maxillary teeth overjet mandibular teeth by more than 3 mm
   c. End-to-end relationships—edge-to-edge bite in which anterior teeth meet at their incisal edges with no overjet or overbite; cusp-to-cusp bite in which posterior teeth meet cusp to cusp with no intercuspation
   d. Open bite—no incisal or occlusal contact between maxillary and mandibular teeth; when teeth cannot be brought together, a space is created
   e. Cross-bites—the normal faciolingual relationship between maxillary teeth and mandibular teeth is altered; for anterior teeth, mandibular teeth are facial rather than lingual to maxillary teeth; for posterior teeth, normal intercuspation is not observed; numerous alterations are possible and result in maxillary or mandibular, buccal or lingual, or partial or total cross-bites

3. Dynamic interarch relationships are a result of functional mandibular movements that start and end with centric occlusion during mastication
   a. Mandibular movements are:
      (1) Depression (opening)
      (2) Elevation (closing)
      (3) Protrusion (thrusting forward)
      (4) Retrusion (bringing back)
      (5) Lateral movements right and left; one side is always the working, or chewing, side; the opposite side is the nonworking, or balancing, side. Ideally, these alternate during chewing
   b. Mandibular movements from a centric occlusion are guided by maxillary teeth
      (1) Protrusion is guided by incisors; called *incisal guidance*
      (2) Lateral movements are guided by the canines on the working side in young, unworn dentitions (canine-protected occlusion); lateral movements may be guided by incisors and posterior teeth in worn dentitions
   c. As mandibular movements commence from a centric occlusion, posterior teeth should disengage in protrusion; on the balancing side, posterior teeth should disengage in lateral movement
   d. If tooth contact occurs where teeth should be disengaged, occlusal interferences or premature contacts exist

ACKNOWLEDGMENT

Photographs in this chapter are provided courtesy of the former Program in Dental Hygiene, Marquette University, Milwaukee, Wisconsin; and Waukesha County Technical College, Pewaukee, Wisconsin.

@ WEB SITE INFORMATION AND RESOURCES

SOURCE	WEB SITE ADDRESS	DESCRIPTION
American Association of Orthodontists	http://www.aaortho.org	Information and links related to orthodontics. Includes a section for consumers with answers to frequently asked questions and media articles
National Institute of Dental and Craniofacial Research	http://www.nidcr.nih.gov	Information and links related to awareness of craniofacial development and disorders. Publications aimed at client/patient education are available.
Dental Hygiene Education Net	http://www.dhed.net/Main.htm	Links to both professional dental and dental hygiene organizations as well as numerous health care resource centers. Dental anatomy information for professionals and clients/patients is available, as well as resources such as journals and research sites for and by dental hygienists
Medscape from WebMD	http://emedicine.medscape.com	Numerous topics concerning oral health, including the oral examination, diseases of the oral cavity, and links to the Centers for Disease Control and Prevention (CDC) and other resources.
Medline Plus	http://www.nlm.nih.gov/medlineplu/	Current health information, including a medical encyclopedia; a service of the U.S. National Library of Medicine and the National Institutes of Health

SUGGESTED READINGS

Nelson S: *Wheeler's dental anatomy, physiology, and occlusion,* ed 9, Philadelphia, 2010, Saunders.

Bath-Balogh M, Fehrenbach MF: *Illustrated Dental Embryology, Histology, and Anatomy,* ed 3, St Louis, 2011, Saunders.

Beck M, Bryan, L: Root morphology and instrumentation implications. In Darby ML, Walsh MM, editors: *Dental hygiene theory and practice,* ed 3, Philadelphia, 2010, Saunders.

Norton N: *Netter's head and neck anatomy for dentistry,* Philadelphia, 2007, Saunders.

Wilkins E: *Clinical practice of the dental hygienist,* ed 10, Philadelphia, 2009, Lippincott Williams & Wilkins.

Woelfel JB, Scheid RC: *Dental anatomy: Its relevance to dentistry,* ed 7, Baltimore, 2007, Lippincott Williams & Wilkins.

Zwemer T, Thomas J, editors: *Mosby's dental dictionary,* St Louis, 2007, Mosby.

Heidi A. Schlei and the publisher acknowledge the past contributions of Marilyn Beck to this chapter.

CHAPTER 5 REVIEW QUESTIONS

Answers and Rationales to Review Questions are available on this text's accompanying Evolve site. See inside front cover for details.
Use Case A and Figure 5-28 to answer questions 1 to 12.

℮volve

CASE A Mixed Dentition

The mother of this young patient has expressed an interest in an orthodontic assessment for her child. The patient is cooperative and interested. Her oral hygiene is good. The hygienist notes several loose primary teeth. The gingiva surrounding the partially erupted teeth appears red and edematous. The mother has questions about when the partially erupted teeth will be fully formed and erupt into the oral cavity.

1. **Determine the age of this person by observing the teeth that are present. This patient is:**
   a. 8 to 9 years old
   b. 9 to 10 years old
   c. 10 to 11 years old
   d. 11 to 12 years old

2. **The cusp tips of which tooth are just erupting through the gingiva?**
   a. # 4
   b. # 5
   c. # 12
   d. # 13

3. **Choose the statement that BEST describes when root formation for the erupting tooth in question #2 will be complete.**
   a. The roots will be completely formed at the time of tooth eruption
   b. The roots will be completely formed within 6 months of tooth eruption
   c. The roots will be completely formed within 2 to 3 years after tooth eruption
   d. The roots will be completely formed no sooner than 3 to 5 years after tooth eruption

4. **Which primary tooth has an occlusal amalgam restoration?**
   a. Tooth A
   b. Tooth B
   c. Tooth I
   d. Tooth J

5. **To which anatomical structure is the arrow pointing?**
   a. Incisive papilla
   b. Median palatine suture
   c. Rugae
   d. Palatine fovea

6. **At what age would you expect all of the premolars to be at least partially erupted?**
   a. 9 years
   b. 10 years
   c. 11 years
   d. 12 years

7. **All of the following concerning tooth B are true *except* one. Which one is the *exception*?**
   a. The CEJ on the mesial half of the buccal curves apically
   b. Closely resembles the form of the first permanent molar
   c. Does not resemble any other tooth
   d. There is a prominent cervical ridge on the buccal

8. **Which tooth on the maxillary left appears to be in torso-version?**
   a. # 6
   b. # 7
   c. # 9
   d. # 10

9. **Which of the following is NOT a characteristic of the mixed dentition stage?**
   a. Clinical crowns appear to be consistently at the same height
   b. Crowding
   c. Different tooth colors
   d. Disproportionately sized teeth

10. **When this patient bites down, all maxillary teeth overlap mandibular teeth in a horizontal direction. This characteristic is referred to as:**
    a. Overbite
    b. Overjet
    c. Edge-to-edge bite
    d. Open bite

11. **Prior to the eruption of the first permanent molars, the relationship of the distal surfaces of the second primary molars was recorded as a "mild mesial step." Which Angle's Classification of Occlusion will most likely result when the permanent molars are fully erupted?**
    a. Class 0 malocclusion
    b. Class I malocclusion
    c. Class II malocclusion
    d. Class III malocclusion

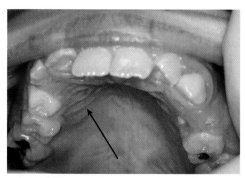

FIGURE 5-28 Facial view, mixed dentition.

12. **The root anatomy of the second primary molars is characterized by divergent roots and short root trunks. This anatomic feature is designed to accommodate the development of the first permanent premolar crowns.**
    a. Both the statement and the reason are correct and related
    b. Both the statement and the reason are correct but not related
    c. The statement is correct, but the reason is not correct
    d. Neither the statement nor the reason is correct

CASE B Permanent Dentition

An adult female client new to the dental practice expresses an interest in orthodontic treatment. The client has a moderate caries risk and a tongue thrust swallowing pattern. Three carious lesions on the proximal surfaces are recorded during the dental examination, and the client admits that she does not floss. She informs the hygienist that she has "a sore spot on the left side of her mouth" that hurts when she eats. Use Case B and Figures 5-29 and 5-30 to answer questions 13-20.

13. **Use canines to determine Angle's Classification of Malocclusion. Which of the following would be the best choice?**
    a. Class I malocclusion
    b. Class II division I malocclusion
    c. Class II division II malocclusion
    d. Class III malocclusion

14. **Which tooth appears to have a DO (disto–occlusal) amalgam restoration?**
    a. # 12
    b. # 13
    c. # 14
    d. # 21

15. **In a centric occlusion, the relationship of anterior teeth would be recorded in the client's dental chart as:**
    a. Edge-to-edge bite
    b. Excessive overbite
    c. Excessive overjet
    d. Open bite

16. **Which tooth is in linguo-version?**
    a. # 12
    b. # 13
    c. # 14
    d. # 21

17. **A round, reddened ulceration is observed near the mental foramen. This area is located within the:**
    a. Fauces
    b. Mucogingival junction
    c. Mucobuccal fold
    d. Sublingual fold

18. **The curve of Spee for this client can be described as:**
    a. Concave for maxillary teeth and convex for mandibular teeth
    b. Convex for maxillary teeth and concave for mandibular teeth
    c. Convex for both maxillary and mandibular teeth
    d. No curve of Spee is present

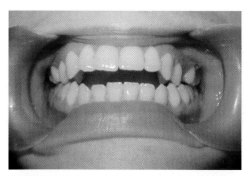

FIGURE 5-29 Lateral view, permanent dentition.

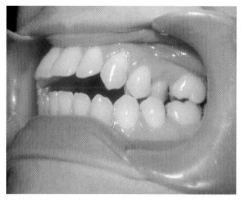

FIGURE 5-30 Facial view, permanent dentition.

19. **Protrusive movements in this client's dentition are not guided by incisors because incisors do not occlude with normal interdigitation and overbite in centric occlusion.**
    a. Both the statement and reason are correct
    b. The statement is correct, but the reason is not correct
    c. The statement is not correct, but the reason is correct
    d. Neither the statement nor reason is correct

20. **This client's posterior mandibular teeth exhibit normal axial positioning. This positioning is best described as:**
    a. More parallel to the median plane
    b. Tip buccally toward the median plane
    c. Tip lingually toward the median plane
    d. Tip lingually away from the median plane

21. **The lingual convergence of proximal surfaces facilitates instrumentation for all permanent teeth except:**
    a. Mandibular incisors and maxillary canines
    b. Mandibular second premolar and maxillary first molar
    c. Mandibular second premolar and maxillary second molar
    d. Mandibular first premolar and maxillary first molar

22. **When comparing mandibular molars, the mandibular first molar is more likely to have a concavity on the facial surface starting just apical to the cemento-enamel junction (CEJ). The mandibular second molar is more likely to have a prominent concavity and two root canals on the mesial surface of the mesial root.**
    a. Both statements are TRUE
    b. Both statements are FALSE
    c. The first statement is TRUE, and the second statement is FALSE
    d. The first statement is FALSE, and the second statement is TRUE

23. **Which one of the following statements concerning teeth with furcations is TRUE?**
    a. The more cervical a furcation, the more stable is the tooth due to more inter-radicular bone
    b. Furcation involvement occurs when the attachment level is coronal to the furcation roof
    c. Furcations are more cervical on second molars
    d. A concavity is found apical to the furcation on the lingual root of the maxillary first molar

24. **An inferior nerve block is indicated for periodontal debridement of the mandibular right quadrant. The target area for this injection is lateral to the:**
    a. Glossopalatine arch
    b. Retromolar area
    c. Pharyngopalatine arch
    d. Pterygomandibular raphe

25. **The mucogingival junction can be observed only in the vestibule on the maxillary arch because no alveolar mucosa is present on the palate.**
    a. Both the statement and reason are correct
    b. The statement is correct, but the reason is not correct
    c. The statement is not correct, but the reason is correct
    d. Neither the statement nor reason is correct

26. **All of the following are characteristics of primary teeth EXCEPT one. Which one is the EXCEPTION?**
    a. Primary teeth have pronounced buccocervical ridges that constrict at the CEJ
    b. Primary occlusal tables are narrower faciolingually than are permanent occlusal tables
    c. The primary enamel depth is thicker at cusp tips and thinner at the CEJ than permanent tooth enamel
    d. Pulp chambers are larger and pulp horns extend more occlusally than permanent tooth pulps

27. **Lateral movements are being assessed in a 14-year-old girl undergoing an orthodontic evaluation. The hygienist would expect these movements to be guided by:**
    a. Incisors
    b. Canines
    c. Premolars
    d. Molars

28. **Excessive retraction with the dental mirror or other instruments may cause cracking and irritation of this anatomic structure:**
    a. Mucobuccal fold
    b. Vermillion zone
    c. Labial mucosa
    d. Labial commissure

29. **A 17-year-old client complains of discomfort associated with the eruption of #17. An operculum is noted when examining the:**
    a. Maxillary tuberosity
    b. Buccal frenum
    c. Retromolar area
    d. Vestibule

30. **This salivary gland produces large amounts of saliva that is primarily serous in composition:**
    a. Parotid
    b. Palatal
    c. Sublingual
    d. Submandibular

31. **Which of the following statements about tooth form characteristics is true?**
    a. Distal cusp ridges are shorter than mesial cusp ridges
    b. The facial crest of curvature is located in the middle third on posterior teeth
    c. The proximal crests of curvature are located in the cervical third of all crowns
    d. Ideally, the proximal crest of curvature is also the contact area

32. **These permanent molars are susceptible to caries development in the occlusal pits found in mesial, central, and distal fossae:**
    a. All molars
    b. Maxillary molars
    c. Mandibular molars
    d. Maxillary and mandibular first molars only

33. **Which of the following characteristics facilitates the scissors-like action of incisors?**
    a. Overbite
    b. Overjet
    c. Protrusion
    d. Interdigitation

34. **When assessing an occlusion, the dental hygienist notes that tooth #30 is missing. Tooth #6 is facial to and mesial to tooth #27. All anterior teeth are slightly protruded. This occlusal relationship would be recorded as:**
    a. Class I
    b. Class II division I
    c. Class II division II
    d. Class III

35. **Which of the following characteristics of occlusion does the term INTERDIGITATION refer to?**
    a. Centric cuspation of maxillary lingual and mandibular buccal cusps
    b. Axial positioning of maxillary and mandibular teeth
    c. A tooth articulating with two teeth in the opposing arch
    d. Teeth contacting at their proximal crests of curvature

36. **During assessment, the dental hygienist observes wedge-shaped cervical defects on the maxillary left permanent canine and premolars. If the loss of cervical tooth structure is attributed to biomechanical loading, this would be recorded in the client's dental chart as:**
    a. Abrasion
    b. Abfraction
    c. Caries
    d. Erosion

37. **Which nonsuccedaneous teeth are present in the dentition of a 10-year-old child?**
    a. Permanent incisors
    b. Permanent premolars
    c. Permanent first molars
    d. Permanent second molars

38. **During an oral examination, which of the following structures appears to be the most posterior?**
    a. Circumvallate papillae
    b. Lingual frenum
    c. Lingual tonsils
    d. Pharyngeal tonsils

39. **This structure separates the soft palate from the cheek:**
    a. Glossopalatine arch
    b. Mucobuccal fold
    c. Pharyngopalatine arch
    d. Pterygomandibular raphe

40. **When assessing furcation involvement on the mesial aspect of tooth #14, the dental hygienist should check from the buccal aspect of the tooth because the mesial furcation is located more toward the buccal surface than toward the lingual surface.**
    a. Both the statement and reason are correct
    b. The statement is correct, but the reason is not correct
    c. The statement is not correct, but the reason is correct
    d. Neither the statement nor reason is correct

41. **During swallowing, movement of this structure helps seal the nasopharynx, decreasing the risk of food entering the nasal cavity.**
    a. Palatine fovea
    b. Palatine raphe
    c. Glossopalatine arch
    d. Uvula

42. **Which of the following statements concerning root anatomy is TRUE?**
    a. The proximal surfaces of maxillary incisors are more accessible from the facial approach
    b. Mandibular first premolars are oval or elliptical in cross-section and may have distal concavities
    c. Maxillary second premolars are broad proximally and oval in cross-section
    d. Mandibular canines have one root and are round in cross-section

43. **Which permanent tooth crown has a mesial surface that is in a straight line with the mesial surface of the root?**
    a. Maxillary central incisor
    b. Mandibular central incisor
    c. Mandibular lateral incisor
    d. Mandibular canine

44. **Of the following primary teeth, which one erupts first?**
    a. Maxillary canine
    b. Mandibular first molar
    c. Maxillary first molar
    d. Mandibular second molar

45. **Which permanent tooth does not have a transverse ridge?**
    a. Maxillary canine
    b. Maxillary first premolar
    c. Maxillary first molar
    d. Mandibular first premolar

46. **An H-shaped occlusal groove pattern is found on this primary tooth:**
    a. A
    b. I
    c. L
    d. T

47. **When comparing the maxillary first premolar and the maxillary second premolar, all of the following statements are true EXCEPT one. Which one is the EXCEPTION?**
    a. Both have a long central developmental groove
    b. Both have a transverse ridge
    c. The first premolar has a mesial crown concavity, but the second premolar does not
    d. The first premolar cusps are longer than lingual cusps, but the second premolar cusps are more equal in length

48. **When tooth M exfoliates, it will be replaced by this permanent tooth:**
    a. # 22
    b. # 23
    c. # 26
    d. # 27

49. **Which of the following permanent teeth erupts first?**
    a. # 20
    b. # 5
    c. # 22
    d. # 11

50. **During mastication, when a person chews on the right side, the right side is referred to as the BALANCING SIDE. The left side is referred to as the NON-WORKING SIDE.**
    a. Both statements are true
    b. Both statements are false
    c. The first statement is true, and the second statement is false
    d. The first statement is false, and the second statement is true

Oral and Maxillofacial Radiology

Evelyn M. Thomson

Although technology continues to create new diagnostic aids that advance the practice of dental hygiene, oral and maxillofacial radiographs remain an essential tool for comprehensive client care. Oral and maxillofacial radiographs play a key role in the assessment, care planning, and evaluation of oral health and disease. The goal of oral radiography is to obtain the highest quality radiographic image while maintaining the lowest possible radiation exposure risk to the patient.

Knowledge and skill in applying this information are critical for the safe use of ionizing radiation in the oral health care setting. This chapter emphasizes radiation physics, production, protection, and ethics; radiographic imaging techniques and receptor systems; radiographic film processing and quality assurance procedures; and radiographic anatomy and principles of interpretation.

GENERAL CONSIDERATIONS

Radiation Physics

A. Radiation is the emission or movement of energy through space in the form of particles or waves
B. Types of radiation
  1. Particulate radiation
    a. Particles have both mass and energy
    b. Some particles may have a positive, negative, or neutral charge
    c. Particles cannot reach the speed of light
    d. Examples—neutrons, protons, electrons, α-particles, and β-particles
  2. Electromagnetic radiation
    a. Nonparticulate radiations
    b. Energy charges and currents associated with electric and magnetic waves and frequencies
      (1) Wavelength—distance from one crest of a wave to the next; the shorter the wavelength, the greater are the energy and penetrating ability of the radiation; the shortest wavelengths are measured in nanometers (nm) (1×10^{-9} meters [m]), and the longer wavelengths are measured in meters
      (2) Frequency—number of wavelength crests passing a particular point per unit of time; measured in hertz (Hz); 1 Hz is equal to 1 cycle per second; the frequency of electromagnetic radiation ranges from $<3 \times 10^{9}$ to $>3 \times 10^{19}$ Hz
      (3) Photon and quantum—terms used to designate a single unit or bundle of energy
      (4) Energy—ability to do work; energy of electromagnetic radiation is measured in electron volts (eV); x-ray energy ranges from 100 to 100,000 eV (1 kiloelectron volt [keV] is equal to 1000 eV)
    c. Characteristics
      (1) Bundles of energy that have neither mass nor charge
      (2) Travels at a velocity of 186,000 miles per second (the speed of light)
      (3) Electromagnetic energies exist over a wide range of magnitudes; the range is termed the *electromagnetic spectrum*
      (4) The electromagnetic spectrum is measured according to frequency, energy, and wavelength
      (5) Interaction with biologic tissue causes changes in the tissue as a result of ionization
    d. Examples—radio waves, microwaves, infrared light, visible light, ultraviolet light, x-rays, gamma rays, and cosmic rays
  3. Ionizing radiation
    a. Definitions
      (1) Ion—charged particle; either positive or negative

(2) Ion pair—positive ion and negative ion

(3) Ionization—process by which radiant energy removes an orbital electron from an atom to yield an ion pair

(4) Ionizing radiation—particulate and electromagnetic radiation with sufficient energy to cause ionization of atoms; radiation must have energy greater than electron-binding energy

b. Biologic significance—damage of biologic systems results from the ionization process

c. Examples—α-particles, β-particles, x-rays, and gamma rays

C. Sources of radiation

1. Naturally occurring (or background) radiation constitutes 50% of the overall exposure to the United States population[1]

a. Radon gas, the result of naturally occurring radionuclides found in soil (a radionuclide is an unstable atom that decays by emitting particles and energy from the nucleus to become electrically stable) accounts for 37% of the natural background radiation (Figure 6-1)

b. Other terrestrial sources, cosmic radiation from outer space, and internal sources make up another 13% of natural exposure

2. Medical applications make up 48% the overall exposure to the United States population[1]

a. Computed tomography (CT) and nuclear medicine lead medical exposures by 24% and 12%, respectively

b. Other conventional radiographs, including oral and maxillofacial radiography, constitute 5% of medical exposures

3. Consumer products and industrial and occupational exposures account for the remaining 2% of total exposure to the United States population

D. Exposure—defined as the average annual effective dose equivalent of ionizing radiation

1. Average annual effective dose equivalent of ionizing radiation to a member of the U.S. population is 6.2 millisieverts (mSv) up from 3.6 (mSv) in the early 1980s[1] (Figure 6-2)

2. Significant increase largely arising from the increased use of large-dose medical imaging technologies[1]

Electricity

A. Definition—flow of electrons through a wire or other electrical conductor

B. Types

1. Direct current (DC)—electrons flow in one direction only along an electrical conductor

2. Alternating current (AC)—electrons flow in one direction and then reverse to flow in the opposite direction

a. Cycle—flow of electrons in one direction and then in the opposite direction

b. One cycle is equal to $\frac{1}{60}$ second

c. Designated as 60-Hz current in most of the Americas (including Canada) (European countries use 50-Hz current)

C. Units of measurement

1. Ampere (A)—the number of electrons flowing in an electrical circuit; one milliampere (mA) is equal to $\frac{1}{1000}$ ampere; modern dental machines commonly operate between 5 mA and 15 mA

2. Volt (V)—electrical potential or force that moves electrons along an electrical conductor; one kilovolt (kV) is equal to 1000 volts; kilovolt peak (kVp) refers to the peak voltage of an alternating current; dental units usually operate between 60 kVp and 100 kVp

D. Power supply to dental x-ray machines is primarily 110 -V, 60-Hz alternating current

X-Ray Machines

A. Types

1. Intraoral units—designed to provide sufficient radiation output for standard intraoral bitewing, periapical, and occlusal radiographs

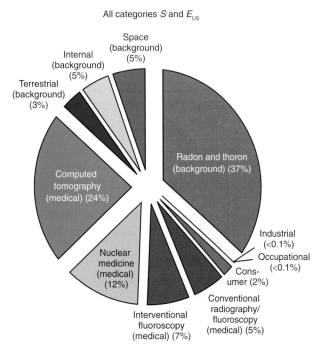

All categories S and E_{US}

Space (background) (5%)

Internal (background) (5%)

Terrestrial (background) (3%)

Computed tomography (medical) (24%)

Nuclear medicine (medical) (12%)

Radon and thoron (background) (37%)

Industrial (<0.1%)

Occupational (<0.1%)

Consumer (2%)

Interventional fluoroscopy (medical) (7%)

Conventional radiography/ fluoroscopy (medical) (5%)

FIGURE 6-1 Annual effective dose equivalent of ionizing radiations. This chart illustrates the approximate percentage of exposure of the U.S. population to background and artificial radiations. *(Reprinted with permission of the National Council on Radiation Protection and Measurements, http://NCRPonline.org)*

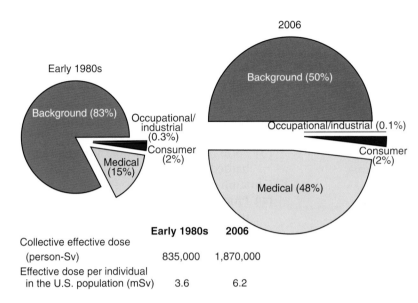

FIGURE 6-2 Comparison of effective dose equivalents. These charts illustrate the difference in approximate percentage of exposure of the U.S. population to background and artificial radiations in the early 1980s and 2006. *(Reprinted with permission of the National Council on Radiation Protection and Measurements,* http://NCRPonline.org)

	Early 1980s	**2006**
Collective effective dose (person-Sv)	835,000	1,870,000
Effective dose per individual in the U.S. population (mSv)	3.6	6.2

a. the x-ray beam is restricted to provide exposure of small anatomic sites
b. Kilovolt peak (kVp) and milliampere (mA) settings may be constant or variable, depending on the manufacturer

  2. Extraoral units—designed to provide greater radiation output as required by extraoral procedures; the x-ray beam is larger to accommodate larger anatomic areas under study

B. X-ray unit components
  1. Generator—device that supplies electrical power to the x-ray tube
    a. Transformer—device that changes the potential difference of incoming electrical energy to any desired level
    b. Types of transformers
      (1) Step-up transformer—increases the voltage sufficiently to propel electrons across the vacuum tube circuit to produce x-ray energy
      (2) Step-down transformer—decreases the voltage to generate the electrons needed at the filament circuit
      (3) Autotransformer—a special type of self-rectifying transformer designed to supply voltage of varying magnitude to several different circuits of the x-ray machine (e.g., filament circuit and high-voltage tube circuit)
    c. Rectification
      (1) Definition—process of changing an alternating current into a direct current
      (2) Rectifier—an electrical device that changes AC to DC
      (3) Dental x-ray units are considered to be self-rectified or half-wave rectified

    (a) In half-wave rectification, x-rays are generated during the first (positive) half of the electrical cycle; the filament is negative and the target is positive
    (b) X-rays are not generated during the second (negative) half of the electrical cycle
    (c) With a 60-cycle alternating current, 60 pulses of x-rays are generated per second, with each having a duration of $\frac{1}{120}$ second
      (4) In full-wave rectification, x-rays are generated during both phases of the alternating current cycle
    (a) Solid-state diodes (or vacuum-tube diodes) are used to redirect electrical current so that the filament remains negatively charged and the target remains positively charged for x-ray production
    (b) With a 60-cycle AC and full-wave rectification, 120 pulses of x-rays are generated per second
  2. X-ray tube (Figure 6-3)
    a. Protective housing
      (1) Lead-lined metal casing for the x-ray tube designed to prevent excessive radiation exposure and electrical shock
      (2) Limits amount of radiation leakage from unit
      (3) Provides mechanical support and protection for the x-ray tube
    b. Cooling system
      (1) Oil, gas, or air is sealed within protective housing and surrounds the x-ray tube

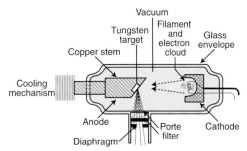

FIGURE 6-3 Component of the dental x-ray tube. *(From Frommer HH, Stabulas-Savage JJ: Radiology for the dental professional, ed 9, St Louis, 2011, Mosby.)*

(2) The system serves as both a thermal cushion and a lead-lined electrical insulator

c. Glass tube
   (1) Surrounds the electrodes of the x-ray tube to provide a vacuum
   (2) The aperture, or window, is a thin segment of the glass that allows maximum emission of x-rays and minimum absorption by the glass

d. Cathode
   (1) Electrically negative portion of the x-ray tube
   (2) Composed of:
      (a) Filament (tungsten wire)
      (b) Focusing cup
   (3) Milliamperage control regulates the:
      (a) Step-down transformer
      (b) Heating of the filament
      (c) Quantity of electrons are "boiled off" during thermionic emission (when electrical current is passed through a coil of tungsten wire, atoms of the wire absorb thermal energy, and some outer-shell electrons acquire enough energy to move a small distance away, forming an electron cloud)
   (4) Because like charges repel, the electron beam is directed to a small area on the anode

e. Anode
   (1) Electrically positive portion of an x-ray tube
   (2) Composed of the:
      (a) Tungsten target (tungsten is used as the target material because of its high atomic number, which yields higher efficiency in x-ray production plus higher-energy x-ray photons; conducts heat well; has high melting point [3380°C])

      (b) Copper stem—functions to conduct heat away from the target
   (3) Kilovoltage control regulates the:
      (a) Step-up transformer
      (b) Voltage between the cathode and the anode
      (c) Accelerating potential (speed) of electrons
   (4) Focal spot—portion of a target bombarded by electrons

f. Filtration
   (1) Process of selectively removing x-rays from the beam
   (2) Total filtration—the result of inherent and added filtration
      (a) Inherent filtration—filtering of a beam by a glass tube
      (b) Added filtration occurs by placing metal discs (usually aluminum) in the path of an x-ray beam
   (3) Low-energy, nonpenetrating x-rays are filtered from the beam
   (4) Federal regulations require 1.5 millimeters (mm) of aluminum-equivalent filtration for units operating below 70 kVp and 2.5 mm of aluminum-equivalent filtration for units capable of operating above 70 kVp

g. Collimation
   (1) Process of restricting the size and shape of the x-ray beam
   (2) Achieved by the use of a lead diaphragm disc with a circular or rectangular opening through which the beam is narrowed

3. Position-indicating device (PID)
   a. Definition—an open ended, circular or rectangular "cone" that extends from the tube head to direct the x-ray beam toward the image receptor
   b. Federal regulations limit the size of the intraoral x-ray beam to 7 cm (2.75 inches) in diameter
   c. Rectangular PIDs have an exit size of 3.5 × 4.4 cm (1.375 × 1.75 inches)
   d. Available lengths of PIDs are 20 cm (8 inches), 30 cm (12 inches), and 40 cm (16 inches)
   e. The longer PID produces an x-ray beam that is less divergent
      (1) Decreases radiation exposure to client
      (2) Provides better image resolution

4. Control panel
   a. Description—exposure factors (mA, kVp, and exposure time) are set, and electrical circuits are activated by using the controls located there

b. Function
  (1) Most intraoral machines available today have preset mA and kVp
  (2) Usually, settings of 5, 7, 10, or 15 mA are available; kVp settings range from 60 to 100
  (3) Depending on the machine type, the automatic timer is adjusted in impulses ($\frac{1}{60}$ of a second) or in fractions of a second
  (4) The exposure switch is depressed to initiate the emission of x-radiation
  (5) The emission of x-radiation from the machine is indicated by an audible "chirping" sound and the glow of an exposure indicator light
  (6) The control panel must be located in a protected area and still allow for observation of the client during exposure

Production of X-Radiation

A. X-ray machine preparation
  1. Initial process for x-radiation production is achieved by the activation of the on–off switch located on the unit control panel; this process completes the filament circuit, and the filament is heated
  2. Appropriate mA, kV, and exposure time are set by using the controls located on the unit console; if mA and kV are preset by the manufacturer, the control panel will be labeled with the preset values
    a. Milliamperage control, which is connected to the mA-filament circuit (step-down transformer), allows for warming of the cathode filament and determines the number of electrons available for x-ray production; the higher the mA, the hotter the filament becomes, resulting in a greater number of available electrons
    b. Kilovoltage control, which is connected to the high-voltage circuit (step-up transformer), establishes the high voltage needed for x-ray production; this control also provides the condition in which the anode is positively charged and the cathode is negatively charged for the attraction and high-speed acceleration of electrons from the cathode to the anode; the higher the kVp setting, the greater is the speed of acceleration of electrons from the cathode to the anode
    c. The exposure time establishes the time during which electrons are available for the bombardment of target material

B. Electronics of x-ray production
  1. X-rays are produced by the interactions that occur when high-speed electrons strike a target material
  2. The phenomenon of x-ray production occurs only when the exposure switch on the console is pressed, which completes the high-voltage circuit
    a. The heated filament provides electrons for x-ray production by thermionic emission
    b. Thermionic emission occurs when electrons absorb sufficient thermal energy (from the mA circuit) to allow for the electrons' short movement away from the filament; commonly referred to as a "boiling off" of electrons; an electron cloud surrounding the filament is formed
    c. The closure of the high-voltage circuit creates an electrical potential difference whereby electrons are attracted from the negative cathode to the positive anode
    d. The one-directional flow of electrons (from the negative cathode to the positive anode) is influenced by the focusing cup of the cathode; electrons are repelled away from the negatively charged focusing cup because like charges repel; this mechanism controls the size and shape of the electron stream

C. Electron–target interactions
  1. The electron stream is directed at a small portion of the target called the *focal spot*
  2. The actual production of x-radiation occurs by the interaction of accelerating electrons and target atoms
  3. Less than 1% of the kinetic energy leaving the cathode is converted into x-ray energy; just over 99% of the kinetic energy leaving the cathode is converted into heat energy
  4. Two types of interactions for x-ray production
    a. General (braking, or bremsstrahlung) radiation (Figure 6-4)

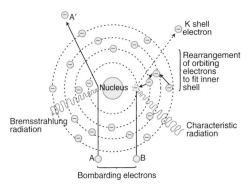

FIGURE 6-4 Illustration of the production of general and characteristic radiations. *(From Frommer HH, Stabulas-Savage JJ: Radiology for the dental professional, ed 9, St Louis, 2011, Mosby.)*

(1) 70% of x-ray photons produced by dental x-ray units in this manner[2]

(2) The accelerating electron passes near the nucleus of the target atom and is slowed down by the attraction of the nucleus

(3) The slowing-down process results in the transference of the electron's kinetic energy into x-ray energy plus a change in the traveling direction of the electron

(4) The energy of the photon produced depends on the amount of kinetic energy transferred

(5) The closer the accelerating electron passes by the nucleus, the greater is the nuclear attraction, which thereby yields greater energy transference and higher photon energy

  b. Characteristic radiation (see Figure 6-4)

(1) Can only occur at 70 kVp or higher with a tungsten target;[2] accounts for a small portion of x-rays produced by dental x-ray machines

(2) Occurs when an electron removes an orbital electron from the target atom

(3) During restabilization of the ionized atom, the hole created by the ejected orbital electron is filled by an outer-shell electron; the movement of the outer-shell electron results in the transference of electron-binding energy into x-ray energy

(4) The energy of the resulting characteristic x-ray photon occurs from the difference in binding energies of the orbital electrons involved

D. Characteristics of x-rays

  1. Represent a portion of the electromagnetic spectrum

  2. Exist as pure energy without mass or charge

  3. Travel at the speed of light (186,000 miles per second)

  4. Affect photographic emulsion

  5. Cause fluorescence of certain chemicals

  6. Can adversely affect biologic tissues

Interactions of X-Rays with Matter

A. Considerations

  1. When x-ray photons interact with matter, they may be either absorbed or scattered

    a. If an incident (initial) photon is absorbed, it ceases to exist

    b. If an incident photon is scattered, its direction of travel is altered; scattered photons do not aid in the formation of the radiographic image and only increase image density; scattered radiation causes fog (or "noise") that degrades image quality

  2. Attenuation (removal) of x-ray photons from the beam as they travel through matter (tissue) is determined by the intensity (energy) of the radiation and the density, atomic number, and electrons per gram of the matter

    a. As the energy of the radiation increases, the number of photons passing through the matter increases

    b. As the density, atomic number, or electrons per gram of the material increase, the number of photons passing through the matter decreases

  3. Definitions

    a. Primary radiation—photons coming directly from the target of the x-ray tube

    b. Secondary radiation—radiation resulting from the interaction of primary radiation and matter

    c. Scatter radiation—one form of secondary radiation in which the direction of travel has been altered

B. Types of interactions

  1. No interaction

    a. Refers to the passing of x-ray photons through a material without any alteration of the photon or the material; accounts for approximately 9% of interactions

    b. Photons proceed to strike the image receptor

  2. Photoelectric effect

    a. Results from an incident photon colliding with a tightly bound inner-shell electron

    b. The incident photon ceases to exist; the electron is ejected as a recoil electron (or photoelectron)

    c. Ionization of the atom occurs; the ejected electron leaves a vacancy in the shell that must be filled

    d. Low-energy characteristic radiation is produced by the shifting of an outer-shell electron to the inner vacancy

    e. In the energy range used for diagnostic applications, the photoelectric effect accounts for approximately 30% of interactions

  3. Compton scatter

    a. Results from an incident photon colliding with a loosely bound outer-shell electron

    b. Incident photon gives up part of its energy in the ejection of the orbiting electron

    c. Ionization of the atom occurs

    d. The direction of travel of the incident photon is changed; its energy is reduced

    e. The scattered photon and the ejected electron may have sufficient energy to undergo many more ionizing interactions before losing their entire energy

f. Compton-scattered x-radiations may exit the patient's tissues and cause image fogging

g. In the diagnostic energy range, Compton scattering accounts for approximately 60% of interactions

4. Coherent scatter

a. The interaction of an incident photon passing near an outer-shell electron and being scattered without losing energy

b. The incident photon ceases to exist, and a new photon of identical energy is released from the electron

c. In the diagnostic energy range, coherent scattering accounts for approximately 8% of total interactions

C. Image formation and differential attenuation

1. Radiographic image formation depends on the differential attenuation of x-ray photons from the primary beam by the client's tissues

2. If all photons exited the client's tissues (no absorption), the image receptor would be totally exposed; if all photons were attenuated (absorbed), the image receptor would be unexposed

3. As a result of photoelectric, Compton, and coherent interactions, x-ray photons are removed from the beam

4. Variances in the ability of tissues to absorb x-rays produce radiographic contrast

5. Generally, as density, atomic number, and electrons per gram of tissue increase, the number of absorbed photons increases; metallic dental restorative materials, enamel, dentin, cementum, and bone absorb photons to a great extent and produce radiopaque images; bone marrow spaces, sinuses, pulp chambers, and periodontal ligament spaces do not attenuate photons and produce radiolucent images

Interactions of Ionizing Radiation with Cells, Tissues, and Organs

A. Definitions

1. Whole-body exposure (total body)—each gram of tissue in the entire body absorbs equal amounts of radiation

2. Specific-area exposure (localized)—each gram of body tissue irradiated in the specific area absorbs equal amounts of radiation (e.g., skin exposure from four bitewing radiographs)

3. Direct effect—transfer of energy by ionization mechanism from an x-ray photon to a biologically critical molecule such as deoxyribonucleic acid (DNA)

4. Indirect effect—transfer of energy by the ionization mechanism from an x-ray photon to a noncritical molecule, which, in turn, delivers the energy to the biologically critical molecule

5. Genetic effect—causes mutations in future generations; results from the exposure of reproductive cells, yielding alterations in genetic coding

6. Somatic effect—injury in the person being irradiated

7. Latent period—time between the exposure and development of the biologic effect

8. Deterministic effect— when the severity of a biological response is dependent on the dose; for example: erythema (redness of the tissue) would be expected to increase in direct proportion to exposure to damaging radiation

9. Stochastic effect—a biologic response that is based on the probability of occurrence rather than its severity; for example: cancer may or may not occur with exposure to damaging radiation

10. Acute effects (short-term or early)—effects that may occur minutes, hours, or weeks after exposure; usually result from high doses of whole-body exposure

11. Chronic effects (long-term or late)—effects observed years after original exposure

B. Units of radiation measurement—two systems used to define radiation measurement: the metric equivalent system, or Systeme Internationale (SI), adopted in 1985, is preferred;[3] an older, traditional system may be found in the research literature published prior to 1985

1. Radiation exposure—measurement of ionization in air produced by x-rays

a. SI units of exposure—defined as electrical charge per unit mass of air or coulomb (C) per kilogram (kg)

b. The traditional unit of exposure is a roentgen—1 roentgen is the amount of x-radiation or gamma radiation that will produce 2.08×10^9 ion pairs in 1 cubic centimeter (cm^3) of air

2. Radiation absorbed dose—amount of radiation absorbed by tissue

a. SI unit—Gray (Gy)

b. Traditional unit—radiation absorbed dose (rad)

c. 1 Gy = 100 rad

3. Dose equivalent—measure of biologic effects produced by different types of radiation

a. SI unit—Sievert (Sv)

b. Traditional unit—roentgen-equivalent man (rem)

c. 1 Sv = 100 rem

d. Some radiations are more damaging than x-rays are; dose equivalent facilitates comparisons among the biologic effects of various radiations

C. Characteristics of dose–response relationships
   1. Linear—the response is directly proportional to the dose
   2. Nonthreshold—any dose, regardless of its size, is expected to produce a response
   3. Threshold—from zero to a particular point, no response would be expected; above the threshold point, any dose will produce a response

D. Biologic responses to irradiation
   1. Considerations
      a. Radiation exposure is harmful to all living tissues and should be used cautiously
      b. Injury to cells, tissues, and organs occurs at the time of exposure but may take hours, days, or generations to manifest
      c. Radiation injury is caused by ionization
         (1) The excitation of orbital electrons in an atom and the deposition of energy in the tissues
         (2) Occurs when atoms of a molecule are separated into charged atomic particles (e.g., table salt [NaCl] yields Na$^+$ Cl$^-$ when mixed in water [H$_2$O])
         (3) May cause a breakage in the molecule or a relocation of the atom in the molecule
         (4) Altered molecules may function improperly or cease to function altogether
   2. Radiation effects on cells
      a. Two types of cells in the human body:
         (1) Genetic cells—oogonium of the female; spermatogonium of the male
         (2) Somatic cells—all other cells
      b. Nucleus of proliferating somatic and genetic cells—area of the cell most sensitive to ionizing effects
         (1) Exposure to the nucleus results in cell inhibition
         (2) Most sensitive sites within the cell's nucleus—DNA and chromosomes
         (3) Chromosomal aberrations in somatic cells are observed during the metaphase stage of mitosis (cell division); changes in genetic material can occur during meiosis or reduction division
            (a) Chromosomes—control cell growth, development, and maintenance
            (b) Sufficient radiation damage to the DNA may yield visible or invisible chromosomal aberrations that may lead to cell death or malfunction
            (c) Tissue or organ destruction—occurs when several cells are damaged and not sufficiently repaired by the body's repair mechanism

(d) DNA damage can result in an uncontrolled, rapid proliferation of cells, the principal characteristic of radiation-induced malignant disease
(e) Genetic cell or germ cell injury—observed only in future generations (including increased susceptibility to disease, birth defects, and cancer)

c. Cells most sensitive to radiation exposure—young, rapidly dividing, nondifferentiated cells such as those of the developing fetus
d. Cell responses to irradiation
   (1) Cell death—the immediate or delayed death of a cell following exposure to a lethal dose
   (2) Swelling of the cell results from interference of fluid exchange through the cell wall
   (3) Alterations in specific cell function, such as the production of a protein or enzyme of changed chemical composition, can also occur following excessive exposure
   (4) Cellular aberration results from damage occurring during mitosis or meiosis

3. Radiolysis of water
   a. Yields radicals that combine to form hydrogen peroxide
   b. Hydrogen peroxide is toxic to living tissues; its formation is an indirect, damaging effect of ionizing radiation

4. Factors that determine tissue sensitivity
   a. The more mature the cell, the more resistant it is to radiation
   b. The younger the tissues and organs, the greater is their radiosensitivity
   c. The higher the metabolic activity of the cell, the higher is its radiosensitivity
   d. The higher the proliferation rate for cells and the growth rate for tissues, the higher is their radiosensitivity
   e. The more differentiated (or specialized in function) the cell, the more resistant it is to the biologic effects of radiation

5. Degree of tissue and organ sensitivity[4]
      (1) Radiosensitive
         (a) Lymphatic (most sensitive)
         (b) Erythrocytes
         (c) Reproductive
      (2) Radioresistant
         (a) Liver
         (b) Muscle
         (c) Nerve (most resistant)
   c. Organ tissues considered critical for dental radiography are skin, thyroid gland, lens of the eyes, and hemopoietic tissue

d. Continued low-dose exposure negatively affects the repair mechanism; overloading of the repair system by time or amount of exposure can result in somatic or genetic damage
6. Repair and accumulation of radiation effects
   a. Most injury resulting from low-dose radiation exposure is repaired within cells, tissues, and organs (depending on the relative biologic damaging ability of the radiation)
   b. Repeated exposure may lead to some unrepaired effects that accumulate in exposed tissues
   c. Accumulated radiation effects accelerate and increase the probability of inducing cancer and the normal aging process; high doses result in a more rapid expression of the effects

ETHICAL CONSIDERATIONS REGARDING THE USE OF IONIZING RADIATION

A. Regulatory and recommending agencies (see the unnumbered table "Web Site Information and Resources" at the end of this chapter)
   1. International Commission on Radiological Protection (ICRP)
   2. National Council on Radiation Protection and Measurements (NCRP)
   3. Federal and State Bureaus of Radiological Health
   4. American Dental Association (ADA)
   5. American Academy of Oral and Maxillofacial Radiology (AAOMR)
   6. State Bureau of Health and other local agencies
B. Assessment of need for radiographic procedures
   1. A licensed physician or dentist must prescribe radiographic services
   2. Dental hygiene assessment for recommendation of need for radiographs
      a. Must be based on a review of the client's health and dental histories; clinical examinations; client signs, symptoms, and complaints
      b. Radiographs are recommended only in the presence of reasonable expectation of client benefit[2]
      c. Recommendations based on U.S. Food and Drug Administration (FDA) selection criteria guidelines (Table 6-1)
      d. If no positive findings are noted in the clinical examination or the client's history, radiography should not be performed
         (1) The only exception to this rule may be the use of bitewing radiographs for caries detection when no clinical signs of early lesions exist[2]

(2) Posterior bitewing radiographs may be exposed when no clinical signs are present, according to FDA guidelines (see Table 6-1)
C. Radiation protection
   1. ALARA ("As Low As Reasonably Achievable") concept—individuals working with radiation should attempt to keep all radiation exposure as low as reasonably achievable
   2. Maximum permissible dose (MPD) (Table 6-2)
      a. "The maximum dose of radiation that in light of present knowledge would not be expected to produce significant radiation effects"[2]
      b. Possible occupational exposures received by oral health care personnel is small compared with other medical settings (Figure 6-5)
      c. Annual MPD for occupationally exposed workers is 50 mSv (or 5000 millirems [mrem])[5]
      d. Nonoccupational exposure (whole-body) is 10% of that for the radiation worker (5 mSv or 500 mrem per year)[5]
   3. Reduction of unnecessary client dose
      a. Eliminate unnecessary examinations
         (1) Base assessment of need for radiographs on client's needs
         (2) Use evidence-based selection criteria (see Table 6-1)
      b. Eliminate repeat examinations
         (1) Receive training and update skills to avoid retakes
         (2) Prepare the client correctly to gain adequate cooperation to perform the procedure
      c. Use proper exposure settings
         (1) Display exposure-setting guidelines and safety protocol near the control panel
         (2) Obtain a working knowledge of the exposure settings for kilovoltage, milliamperage, and exposure time to accurately adjust for proper image density and contrast
         (3) In children, reduce exposure time by one half
      d. Use safe equipment
         (1) Filtration
            (a) Removal of less penetrating x-rays from the beam
            (b) Inherent filtration—built into the x-ray unit, includes glass tube, insulating oil, and tube head
            (c) Added filtration—aluminum discs placed in the path of the x-ray beam at base of the position-indicating device (PID)

TABLE 6-1 Guidelines for Prescribing Dental Radiographs

TYPE OF ENCOUNTER	CHILDREN		ADOLESCENT		ADULT
	Primary Dentition (prior to eruption of first permanent tooth)	**Transitional Dentition (after eruption of first permanent tooth)**	**Permanent Dentition (prior to eruption of third molars)**	**Dentate or Partially Edentulous**	**Edentulous**
New Client* being evaluated for dental diseases and dental development	Individualized radiographic examination consisting of selected periapical views, occlusal views, or both; posterior bitewings if proximal surfaces cannot be visualized or probed Clients without evidence of disease and with open proximal contacts may not require a radiographic examination at this time	Individualized radiographic examination consisting of posterior bitewings with panoramic examination or posterior bitewings and selected periapical images	Individualized radiographic examination consisting of posterior bitewings with panoramic examination or posterior bitewings and selected periapical images. A full-mouth intraoral radiographic examination is preferred when the client has clinical evidence of generalized dental disease or a history of extensive dental treatment		Individualized radiographic examination based on clinical signs and symptoms
Recare Client* with clinical caries or at increased risk for caries**	Posterior bitewing examination at 6–12-month intervals if proximal surfaces cannot be examined visually or with a probe			Posterior bitewing examination at 6–18-month intervals	Not applicable
Recare Client* with no clinical caries and not at risk for caries**	Posterior bitewing examination at 12–24-month intervals if proximal surfaces cannot be examined visually or with a probe		Posterior bitewing examination at 18–36-month intervals	Posterior bitewing exam at 24-36-month intervals	Not applicable
Recare Client* with clinical periodontal disease	Clinical judgment as to the need for and type of radiographic images for the evaluation of periodontal disease. Imaging may consist of, but is not limited to, selected bitewing images, periapical images, or both, of areas where periodontal disease (other than nonspecific gingivitis) can be identified clinically				Not applicable
Client for monitoring of growth and development	Clinical judgment as to the need for and type of radiographic images for evaluation, monitoring, or both, of dentofacial growth and development		Clinical judgment as to the need for and type of radiographic images for evaluation, monitoring, or both, of dentofacial growth and development Panoramic or periapical exam to assess developing third molars.		Not usually indicated
Client with other circumstances, including, but not limited to, proposed or existing implants, pathology, needs, treated periodontal disease, and caries remineralization	Clinical judgment as to the need for and type of radiographic images for evaluation, monitoring, or both, in these circumstances				

TABLE 6-1 Guidelines for Prescribing Dental Radiographs—cont'd

TYPE OF ENCOUNTER	CHILDREN		ADOLESCENT		ADULT
	Primary Dentition (prior to eruption of first permanent tooth)	Transitional Dentition (after eruption of first permanent tooth)	Permanent Dentition (prior to eruption of third molars)	Dentate or Partially Edentulous	Edentulous

*Clinical situations for which radiographs may be indicated include, but are not limited to:

A. Positive historical findings
1. Previous periodontal or endodontic treatment
2. History of pain or trauma
3. Familial history of dental anomalies
4. Postoperative evaluation of healing
5. Remineralization monitoring
6. Presence of implants or evaluation for implant placement

B. Positive clinical signs and symptoms
1. Clinical evidence of periodontal disease
2. Large or deep restorations
3. Deep carious lesions
4. Malposed or clinically impacted teeth
5. Swelling
6. Evidence of dental or facial trauma
7. Mobility of teeth
8. Fistula involving sinus tract
9. Clinically suspected sinus pathology
10. Growth abnormalities
11. Oral involvement in known or suspected systemic disease
12. Positive neurologic findings in the head and neck
13. Evidence of foreign objects
14. Pain, dysfunction, or both, of the temporomandibular joint
15. Facial asymmetry
16. Abutment teeth for fixed or removable partial prosthesis
17. Unexplained bleeding
18. Unexplained sensitivity of teeth
19. Unusual eruption, spacing, or migration of teeth
20. Unusual tooth morphology, calcification, or color
21. Unexplained absence of teeth
22. Clinical erosion

**Factors increasing the risk for caries may include, but are not limited to:
1. High level of caries experience or demineralization
2. History of recurrent caries
3. High titers of cariogenic bacteria
4. Existing restoration(s) of poor quality
5. Poor oral hygiene
6. Inadequate fluoride exposure
7. Prolonged nursing (bottle or breast)
8. High-sucrose diet
9. Poor familial oral health
10. Developmental or acquired enamel defects
11. Developmental or acquired disability
12. Xerostomia
13. Genetic abnormality of teeth
14. Many multi-surface restorations
15. Chemotherapy or radiation therapy
16. Eating disorders
17. Drug or alcohol abuse
18. Irregular dental care

(Data from U.S. Department of Health and Human Services: The selection of patients for dental radiographic examinations, Revised 2004 by the American Dental Association: Council on Dental Benefit Program, Council on Dental Practice, Council on Scientific Affairs.)

TABLE 6-2 U.S. Nuclear Regulatory Commission Occupational Dose Limits

Tissue	Annual Dose Limit
Whole body	0.05 Sv
Any organ	0.5 Sv
Skin	0.5 Sv
Extremity	0.5 Sv
Lens of eye	0.15 Sv

Sv, Sievert.
(United States Nuclear Regulatory Commission: Standards for protection against radiation, Title 10, Part 20, of the Code of Federal Regulations. December 4, 2007: Available at http://www.nrc.gov/reading-rm/doc-collections/cfr/part020/part020-1201.html: Accessed Apr.11, 2010.)

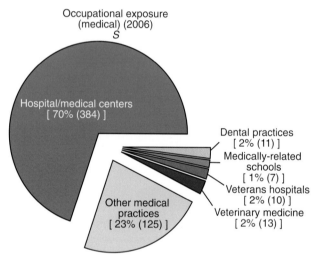

FIGURE 6-5 Occupational exposures by medical profession. This chart illustrates the approximate percentage of occupational exposures to medical radiations. *(Reprinted with permission of the National Council on Radiation Protection and Measurements, http://NCRPonline.org)*

    (2) Collimation
       (a) Lead disc placed in the path of the beam that controls the size and shape of the beam
       (b) Reduces scatter radiation
       (c) Reduces film fogging
    (3) Position-indicating device (PID)
       (a) Use only open-ended lead-lined cylinders
       (b) Rectangular collimated PID restricts client radiation exposure to size and shape of image receptor, significantly reducing exposure
       (c) A PID length that increases the focal-spot-to-object distance creates a less divergent beam

  e. Use the fastest image receptor system available
    (1) Currently the "F" speed intraoral film requires the least amount of radiation to produce a diagnostic image
    (2) Intraoral digital imaging systems that replace film with a solid state sensor or phosphor plate further reduce client radiation exposure
    (3) Rare-earth intensifying screens with corresponding green-light–sensitive extraoral film require less radiation than calcium tungstate intensifying screens with blue-light sensitive extraoral film
  f. Position client and image receptor properly
    (1) The client's head should be stabilized; place the client's head against the headrest
    (2) Image receptor holders should be used to stabilize intraoral receptors; never use the client's finger
  g. Shield specific areas from possible secondary radiation with 0.25-mm–thick lead or lead equivalent apron
    (1) Shield thyroid gland with lead or lead-equivalent collar when exposing intraoral radiographs
    (2) Use a cape-style lead or lead-equivalent drape when exposing panoramic or other extraoral radiographs
    (3) Shield reproductive tissues with lead or lead-equivalent apron

4. Reduction of occupational exposure
  a. Use protective shielding and apparel
    (1) The operator should remain behind a barrier during client exposure
    (2) Any part of the operator's body that will be in the path of the primary beam must be covered with 0.25 mm of lead or lead-equivalent protection
  b. Distance from the source of radiation, if structural shielding is not available
    (1) The operator should stand as far away as possible from source of radiation during exposure (a distance of 6 feet is considered the minimum safe distance)
    (2) The operator should be in a position of 90 to 135 degrees out of path of the primary beam[4] (Figure 6-6)
  c. Never hold the client, the image receptor, or the tube head during exposure
  d. Use personnel radiation-monitoring devices

D. Personnel radiation-monitoring devices[4]
  1. Film badge
    a. Specialized film packet sandwiched between metal filters contained inside a plastic holder or badge

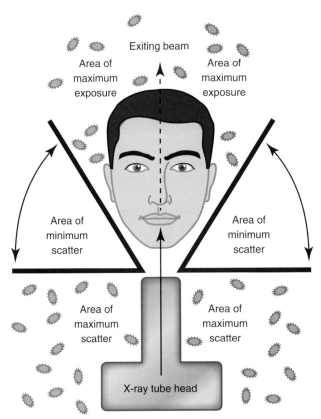

FIGURE 6-6 Illustration showing areas of minimum and maximum scatter.

b. Advantage—inexpensive, reliable technology
c. Limitation—cannot be worn for periods longer than 1 month
2. Thermoluminescent dosimeters (TLD)
   a. Plastic badge containing lithium fluoride crystals that absorb x-ray energy
   b. Advantage—more sensitive and accurate than film monitors
   c. Limitation—more costly than film monitors
3. Direct ion storage (DIS) monitor
   a. Miniature ion chamber absorbs radiation
   b. Advantage—instant reading with real time results
   c. Disadvantage—requires Internet connection and fee for service
E. Documentation of client's radiographic exposure
   1. The client's record should include appropriate space for listing radiographic services
   2. All radiographic exposures, both diagnostic and undiagnostic, should be entered sequentially and cumulatively
   3. Essential information for radiographic services
      a. Date of radiographic examination
      b. Number of radiographs
      c. Type of radiographs
      d. Number and type of retake radiographs
      e. Name of operator who exposed radiographs

F. Documentation of client's refusal of radiographic services
   1. The client must be informed of possible diagnostic information and possible risks from radiographic procedure
   2. The client should be informed of all protection procedures used (e.g., equipment standards, quality assurance, standard darkroom procedures, protective shielding, and operator competence)
   3. Having the client sign a refusal-of-radiographic-services form does not release the oral health care provider from responsibility

INFECTION CONTROL

See the section on "Prevention of Disease Transmission During Radiographic Procedures" in Chapter 10.
A. General considerations
   1. Infection control procedures established for the oral health care setting must include guidelines for dental radiographic procedures
   2. The client's health history must be reviewed and an oral examination performed before radiographic services
   3. All clients should be considered potentially infectious
B. Procedure
   1. Unit preparation
      a. Clean and disinfect the radiographic equipment (e.g., tube head and PID, tube-head support arm, control panel, countertop, treatment chair)
      b. Use the barrier technique and disposable plastic wrap to cover items likely to become contaminated (e.g., tube head and PID, tube-head support arm, control panel, countertop, treatment chair)
      c. Obtain radiographic supplies (e.g., image receptors, holding devices) *before* starting the procedure
      d. Disposable intraoral film packet barrier wraps may be used to minimize the possibility of disease transmission during the radiographic procedure and processing
      c. Digital sensors should be wiped with an Environmental Protection Agency (EPA)–accepted disinfectant before placing the protective sheath barrier and following removal; consult the manufacturers' recommendations
   2. While exposing intraoral radiographs, wear disposable client-care gloves
      a. Wipe the film packet with an EPA-accepted disinfectant after removal of the film from the

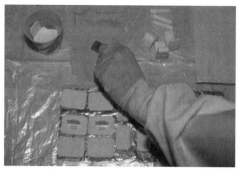

FIGURE 6-7 Excessive saliva is removed from the film packet by wiping it across a paper towel soaked with disinfectant. A disposable plastic barrier is in place, and film packets, film holders, and supplies have been assembled before the procedure. Note the cup used to contain contaminated film packets.

client's mouth and drop the film into a containment cup[6] (Figure 6-7)

b. If using a disposable intraoral film packet barrier wrap, after wiping the packet barrier wrap with an EPA-accepted disinfectant, aseptically tear open the wrap, allowing the protected film to drop aseptically into a containment cup; this same procedure is used for phosphor plates; allow the protected phosphor plates to drop into the light-tight containment box; consult the manufacturer's recommendations.

3. Process intraoral radiographs under safelight conditions
   a. Use disposable client-care gloves, and grasp the tab on the back the outer protective wrap and pull it open without touching the film inside
   b. Grasp the black paper tab, and pull it straight out, allowing the film to drop out onto a barrier such as a paper towel placed on the counter
   c. When all film packets are opened, remove and properly dispose of the client-care gloves
   d. Wash and dry hands
   e. With clean, dry hands, grasp the films by their edges and place them into the automatic film processor or onto manual film-processing racks
   f. Put on nitrile or neoprene utility gloves to remove the lead foils for proper disposal; properly dispose of other film packaging wastes and paper towels
   g. Clean and disinfect the countertop

4. Following radiographic procedures
   a. Use nitrile or neoprene utility gloves
   b. Remove and properly discard the contaminated plastic barriers

   c. Clean and disinfect the surfaces contaminated during procedure
   d. Dispose of or sterilize image receptor–holding devices

IMAGE RECEPTORS

A. Definition
   1. Mechanism for transferring information contained in an attenuated remnant x-ray beam into a visible image
   2. For dental radiography, the image receptor has traditionally been film
   3. Digital radiography requires the use of a sensor, or phosphor plate

B. Types
   1. Classified as direct-imaging and indirect-imaging systems
      a. Direct imaging—exposure of the film by the interaction of the x-ray beam and the photographic emulsion; exposure of a solid-state digital sensor by the interaction of the x-ray beam and a computer chip composed of a grid of x-ray sensitive cells[7]
      b. Indirect imaging—exposure of the film primarily by the light emitted from an intensifying screen and, to a lesser extent, by the x-ray beam; exposure of a polyester plate coated with phosphors that "store" the energy until stimulated by a laser to release light that is converted into an electronic signal[7]

Radiographic Film

A. Composition
   1. The base material (polyester) must possess the dimensional stability to withstand processing procedures
   2. An adhesive is applied evenly to the base to provide for uniform attachment of emulsion to the base
   3. The emulsion consists of gelatin and silver halide crystals; records information carried by the x-ray beam
   4. A protective coating is applied to protect the emulsion from being scratched

B. Classifications
   1. The terms *intraoral film* and *extraoral film* refer to the designated use of the film
      a. Intraoral film—placed within the oral cavity (e.g., bitewing, periapical, or occlusal)
      b. Extraoral film—placed outside the mouth for exposure of large areas (e.g., panoramic or cephalometric)

2. Screen film (used in indirect imaging)—a slower film, with a thinner emulsion layer; must be used with an intensifying screen (e.g., panoramic film)
3. Nonscreen film (used in direct imaging)—exposed by x-rays alone; has a thicker emulsion to increase its sensitivity to radiation
4. Film speed—the film's responsiveness to x-radiation; directly related to image visibility
   a. Fast film has larger silver halide crystals and decreased image resolution
   b. Slow film has smaller silver halide crystals and increased image resolution
   c. Speed ranges used in dental radiography are designated from "D" (slowest) to "F" (fastest)
   d. E-speed intraoral film requires only 50% of the exposure of D-speed intraoral film; F-speed film requires only 77% of the exposure of E-speed film[7]
5. Size—various sizes are available for both intraoral and extraoral films
   a. Intraoral film
      (1) No. 0—22 × 35 mm
      (2) No. 1—24 × 40 mm
      (3) No. 2—31 × 41 mm
      (4) No. 3—27 × 54 mm
      (5) No. 4—57 × 76 mm
   b. Extraoal film
      (1) 5 × 7 inches
      (2) 5 × 12 inches or 6 × 12 inches
      (3) 8 × 10 inches
6. Uses
   a. Intraoral films—used for periapical, bitewing, and occlusal radiographic exposures
   b. Extraoral films—used for extraoral projections, for example, panoramic and cephalometric exposures
7. Intraoral film is available in single-film or double-film packets; double-film packets provide a duplicate radiograph

C. Packet construction of intraoral films
1. Light-tight, leakproof wrapping protects film from light and moisture
2. Black protective paper is used for additional protection of the film from light
3. A lead foil is inserted between the black paper and the outer wrapping on the back side of the film packet; the purpose of the lead foil is to prevent backscatter from fogging the film
4. Double or single films are enclosed in the packet

D. Intensifying screens used with extraoral film
1. Housed inside a light-tight cassette
2. Used as a component of the indirect-imaging system to reduce client exposure to x-radiation for study of large anatomic areas

3. Screen construction
   a. Base material composed of polyester plastic
   b. Reflective layer, coated onto the base material, may be either magnesium oxide or titanium dioxide; redirects light toward the film to increase film efficiency
   c. Phosphor layer composed of phosphorescent crystals; calcium tungstate emits blue light to expose the film, but responds less efficiently to x-radiation; rare-earth crystals emit green light and respond more efficiently to reduce radiation exposure needed to produce the image
   d. Protective coating, applied to phosphor layer; prevents abrasion of the phosphor; must be transparent to light
4. Extraoral film identification methods
   a. Lead letter (R or L) attached to the tube-side surface of the cassette but positioned away from the structures of interest
   b. Commercially available light-flash identification machine used to record the client's name, date, and identification number onto the film emulsion before processing

E. Film care
1. Must be stored away from heat, moisture, chemical vapors, and radiation
2. Should be stored by expiration date so that the oldest films are used first

Digital Imaging Sensors

A. Solid state sensors
1. Charge-coupled device (CCD) and complementary metal oxide semiconductor (CMOS) replace film as the image receptor
2. CCD and CMOS sensors contain a silicone chip that detects and converts x-rays into an electronic signal, which is sent to a computer; the computer reconstructs the data into an image, which is displayed on a monitor
3. Usually wired via a Universal Serial Bus (USB) cable to a computer port; limited wireless systems available currently, but as wireless technology continues to improve may be used more in the future
4. Available in sizes that approximate film sizes #0, #1, and #2
   a. Actual image recording area is often smaller than that of film; may require additional exposures for a complete survey
   b. A packet that is thicker than the film packet and the presence of the USB cable may reduce client tolerance
5. Often referred to as *direct digital imaging*

B. Storage phosphor system

1. Photostimuable phosphor (PSP) plates replace film as the image receptor
2. PSP plates resemble film in appearance and in the method of capturing a radiographic image as analog data that is sent via a laser scanner to the computer for processing[4]
3. Not connected to a computer by wires
4. Requires a "processing" step where the plates must be placed into a scanner that stimulates the phosphors to emit light that is converted into an image by the computer
5. Available in sizes that approximate all film sizes #0, #1, #2, #3 and #4
   a. Actual image recording area is often smaller than that of film, so additional exposures may be required for a complete survey
   b. Requires multiple plates when exposing more than one radiograph
   c. Plates must be erased prior to reusing
6. Extraoral phosphor plates use a cassette without intensifying screens
7. Often referred to as *indirect digital imaging*

C. Radiation requirements and doses[7]

1. Can be acquired with the same intraoral x-ray machines that are used for film-based radiographs
   a. Direct current (DC) or constant potential intraoral x-ray machines purported to be best suited to producing digital images
   b. Low mA (5 mA) purported to be best suited to producing digital images
2. Radiation dose to the patient may be reduced by 0% to 50% of F-speed intraoral film
3. Digitally acquired extraoral radiographs may require the same or an increased radiation dose used for film-based extraoral radiographs
4. PSP systems have a wide range of exposures that will produce a diagnostic image, so careful attention is required to ensure that the lowest dose is used

D. Advantages of digital imaging over film-based radiography[7,8]

1. Generates an image on a computer monitor for immediate evaluation
2. Eliminates film and processing expenses and waste products

E. Limitations of digital imaging over film-based radiography[7,8]

1. The ease associated with retakes may result in excessive exposure of the patient to radiation[8]
2. Initial expense of computer equipment and sensors

ORAL RADIOGRAPHIC PROCEDURES

Radiographic Image Description

A. Definitions

1. Radiolucent—black to dark-gray areas on radiograph resulting from more exposure of the image receptor by radiation passing through less-dense anatomic structures
2. Radiopaque—white to light-gray areas on radiograph resulting from less exposure of the image receptor by radiation being absorbed by dense anatomic structures
3. Radiographic density—overall blackening of a radiograph; density is read with a densitometer
4. Radiographic contrast—differences in densities of adjacent areas of radiograph
   a. Long-scale contrast (also called *low contrast*)—scale with many shades of gray resulting from small differences in densities; obtained with a high-kVp technique
   b. Short-scale contrast (also called *high contrast*)—scale with few shades of gray resulting from large differences in densities; obtained with a low-kVp technique
5. Detail (definition)—degree of clarity of the image
6. Resolution—ability to record separate images of small objects placed close together; measured in line pairs, the number of distinct lines that can be detected within a 1 mm space
7. Sharpness—ability of the image to define an edge
8. Gray scale—the number of shades of gray within the image
9. Fog—overall gray appearance, yielding a lower image contrast; results from exposure by scatter radiation, unsafe illumination of the darkroom, use of expired film, or contaminated processing chemicals
10. Electronic noise—the digital image equivalent of film fogging

B. Factors affecting radiographic image

1. Exposure time
   a. Directly proportional to image density
   b. Increased exposure time results in more x-ray photons to interact with the image receptor
2. Milliamperage (mA)
   a. Directly proportional to image density
   b. Increased mA yields more heat in filament; produces more electrons by thermionic emission, which yields more x-ray photons to interact with the image receptor

c. To maintain image density when changing the mA, a corresponding change must be made to exposure time
   (1) Maintain milliampere-seconds (mAs)
   (2) mA × exposure time (in seconds) = mAs

3. Kilovolt potential
   a. Directly proportional to image density; a higher-kVp technique yields a more penetrating x-ray beam, and a greater number of x-ray photons are produced to interact with the image receptor
   b. Inversely proportional to image contrast; decreased kVp yields a high contrast image because the beam has less penetrating ability; increased kVp yields a low contrast image because the beam has more penetrating ability
   c. To maintain image density when changing the kV, a corresponding change must be made to exposure time
      (1) When kV is increased by 15, decrease exposure time by a factor of 2
      (2) When kV is decreased by 15, increase the exposure time by a factor of 2

4. Collimation
   a. Inversely proportional to image density; increased collimation of the x-ray beam decreases density because of the occurrence of a reduction in the number of scatter photons that cause fogging or electronic noise
   b. Directly proportional to image contrast; with fewer scatter photons causing fogging or electronic noise, the contrast is higher (short scale)

5. Filtration—inversely proportional to image density; the greater the filtration of the x-ray beam, the fewer photons available to penetrate the client and interact with the image receptor

6. Target–to–image receptor distance
   a. Inversely proportional to image density
   b. Based on the phenomenon of the inverse square law

$$\frac{\text{Original Intensity}}{\text{New Intensity}} = \frac{\text{New Distance}^2}{\text{Original Distance}^2}$$

   (1) States that the intensity of the x-ray beam is inversely proportional to the square of the distance
   (2) Rapid decrease in intensity results from the spreading out of the x-ray photons over a larger area as they move farther from the source; for example, if the intensity of an x-ray beam is 400 mSv at 36 inches, at 72 inches (double the distance) the intensity is only one fourth as great or 100 mSv
   c. To maintain image density when switching from a short target–to–image distance to a long target–to–image distance, exposure time must be increased

7. Client–object thickness or density—inversely proportional to image density; as the thickness increases, more of the beam is attenuated, yielding a decrease in image density

8. Type of image receptor
   a. Digitally acquired image resolution is less than that of film (film resolution equals 12 to 20 line pairs per millimeter (lp/mm), while digital imaging equals approximately 8 to 10 lp/mm[4]
   b. A digitally acquired image provides superior gray-scale resolution over film-based images, possibly leading to enhanced interpretation[7]

Radiographic Techniques

A. Shadow-casting principles
   1. Smallest focal spot (x-ray source) possible
      a. Yields more parallel x-ray photons
      b. Reduces penumbra
      c. Enhances image sharpness
   2. Longest focal spot (x-ray source-to-object [tooth] distance) possible
      a. Results in use of more parallel x-ray photons
      b. Decreases image magnification
      c. Enhances image sharpness
   3. Shortest object (tooth)-to-image receptor distance possible
      a. Decreases image magnification
      b. Enhances image sharpness
   4. Object (tooth) and image receptors should be in a parallel relationship; reduces image distortion (e.g., elongation and foreshortening)
   5. the x-ray beam should be perpendicular to the object (tooth) and the image receptor; reduces image distortion

B. Angulation of the x-ray beam
   1. Vertical angulation—the position of the x-ray tube head (PID) in the vertical plane
      a. Positive vertical angulation means that the PID is pointing downward
      b. Negative vertical angulation means that the PID is pointing upward
      c. Vertical angulation is noted in degrees (positive or negative) by the dial on the side of the tube head
   2. Horizontal angulation—position of the x-ray tube head (PID) in the horizontal plane

C. Intraoral procedures
　1. Paralleling technique
　　a. Theory
　　　(1) Yields radiographs with a minimum of image distortion
　　　(2) Minimizes the superimposition of adjacent oral structures
　　　(3) Commonly referred to as the *long-cone technique*, or *right-angle technique*
　　　(4) Applies shadow-casting principles 1, 2, 4, and 5 (see part A of this section, "Shadow-casting principles," parts 1-5)
　　b. Application (Figure 6-8)
　　　(1) The image receptor is placed parallel to the long axis of the tooth
　　　(2) The x-ray beam is directed perpendicularly to the long axis of the tooth and the image receptor
　　　(3) The x-ray beam is directed perpendicularly through interproximal spaces
　　　(4) The x-ray beam is centered over the anatomic structures and the image receptor
　2. Bisecting technique
　　a. Theory
　　　(1) Applies the rule of isometry—the accurate length of the tooth image is obtained if the x-ray beam is perpendicular to the imaginary bisector of the angle formed by the plane of the image receptor and the long axis of the tooth
　　　(2) Allows for ease of image receptor placement for certain clients (e.g., children, and those with a shallow palatal vault, large tori, or exaggerated gag reflex)
　　　(3) Commonly referred to as the *short-cone technique*

　　　(4) Does not follow shadow-casting principles 2, 4, and 5 (see part A of this section, "Shadow-casting principles," parts 1-5)
　　b. Application (Figure 6-9)
　　　(1) The image receptor is placed against teeth
　　　(2) The x-ray beam is directed perpendicular to the imaginary bisector of the angle formed by the plane of the image receptor and the long axis of the tooth
　　　(3) The x-ray beam is directed perpendicularly through the interproximal spaces
　　　(4) The x-ray beam is centered over the anatomic structures and the image receptor
　3. Intraoral radiographic techniques
　　a. Periapical radiograph demonstrates the entire tooth and surrounding structures (Figure 6-10)
　　　(1) Indications[9]
　　　　(a) Suspected periapical condition
　　　　(b) Evidence of periodontal disease

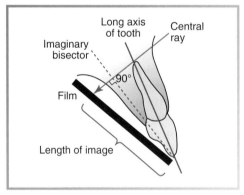

FIGURE 6-8 Paralleling technique. *(From Iannucci JM, Howerton LJ: Dental Radiography: Principles and Techniques, ed 4, St Louis, 2012, Saunders.)*

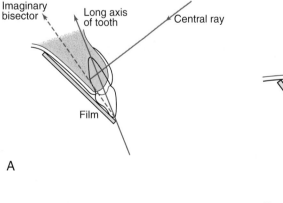

A

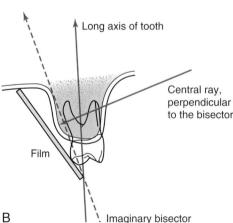

B

FIGURE 6-9 Bisecting technique. *(From Miles DA, Van Dis ML, Williamson GF, Jensen CW: Radiographic Imaging for the Dental Team, ed 4, St Louis, 2009, Saunders.)*

(c) Injury or trauma to teeth

(d) Endodontic therapy

(e) Deep or large caries

(f) Suspected impaction

(g) Unusual eruption, malposition, or unexplained missing teeth

(h) Unexplained sensitivity

(i) Unexplained tooth mobility

(j) Unusual tooth morphology or color

(k) Dental implant evaluation

(2) Anterior periapical image receptors are placed in the oral cavity with the long dimension positioned vertically

(3) Posterior periapical image receptors are placed in the oral cavity with the long dimension positioned horizontally

b. Bitewing radiographs demonstrate the anatomic crowns of maxillary and mandibular teeth as well as the height of alveolar bone (Figure 6-11)

(1) Indications[9]

(a) Suspected interproximal caries

(b) Defective restorations

(c) Suspected early periodontal disease

(d) Determination of local contributing factors for periodontal disease (e.g., calculus, overhanging restoration)

(2) Horizontal bitewings—the image receptor is placed in the oral cavity with the long dimension positioned horizontally; considered the traditional bitewing placement

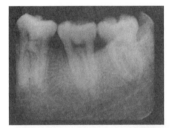

FIGURE 6-10 Periapical radiograph.

(3) Vertical bitewings—the image receptor is placed in the oral cavity with the long dimension positioned vertically; increases the image of alveolar bone, which is useful in imaging periodontal conditions

c. An occlusal radiograph demonstrates a large anatomic region or the entire arch (Figure 6-12)

(1) Indications[4]

(a) Image margins of large pathologic conditions

(b) Localization of objects (foreign or impactions)

(c) Injury or trauma to surrounding bone structure

(d) Suspected supernumerary teeth

(e) Unexplained swelling or growth abnormality

(f) Salivary stone detection

(g) When the client has limited jaw opening or cannot tolerate periapical image receptor placement

(2) Uses size #4 intraoral image receptor (size #2 may be used for children)

(3) Topographic occlusal radiograph—vertical angulation based on the bisecting technique, in which the x-ray beam is directed perpendicular to an imaginary bisector between the long axes of teeth being imaged and the image receptor; used to image either the maxilla or the mandible

(4) Cross-sectional occlusal radiograph—vertical angulation is such that the x-ray beam is directed perpendicular to the image receptor; most often used to image the mandible and to determine the relative buccal–lingual location of impactions or foreign bodies

d. Full mouth survey—combination of periapical and bitewing radiographs that image the entire dentition; the number of projections varies (Figure 6-13)

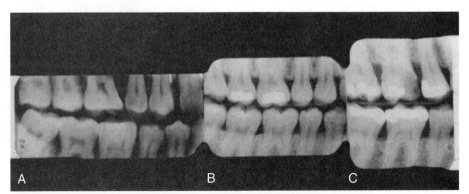

FIGURE 6-11 Bitewing radiographs. **A,** Long horizontal bitewing. **B,** Traditional horizontal bitewing. **C,** Vertical bitewing.

D. Extraoral radiographs—considered supplemental projections; used when evaluating a variety of maxillofacial conditions
   1. Panoramic radiograph (Figure 6-14)
      a. Single radiograph, either 5 × 12 inches or 6 × 12 inches, which records both maxillary and mandibular arches; all of the mandible (from condyle to condyle) and all of the maxilla (up to the middle third of the orbit) are imaged
      b. Most common extraoral exposure used to supplement oral hygiene care
      c. Indications[4]
         (1) Evaluation of growth and development (orthodontics)
         (2) Assessment of trauma to facial structures
         (3) Evaluation of dental anomalies
         (4) To image extensive pathologic conditions
         (5) While not an indication, images must be evaluated for possible carotid artery calcifications that may be an important marker for vascular risk
      d. Image production
         (1) Based on the principle of tomography, a radiographic technique that permits visualization of structures in a chosen plane or layer while intentionally blurring the images above and below the selected plane[10]
         (2) Tomography is accomplished by moving the image receptor and the x-ray source parallel to each other and in opposite directions while the client remains stationary
         (3) The layer or plane of interest is termed the *focal trough* (plane of acceptable focus)
         (4) Each manufacturer of panoramic x-ray units designs a curved, horseshoe-shaped focal trough to accommodate a wide range of client sizes
      e. Technique
         (1) Read the manufacturer's directions for specific positioning guidelines for determining the location of the focal trough

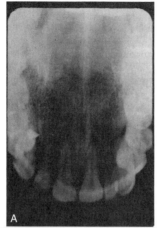
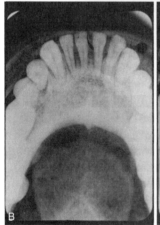
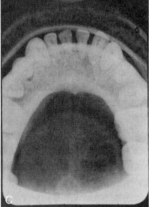

FIGURE 6-12 Occlusal radiographs. **A,** Topographic occlusal radiograph of the maxillary arch. **B,** Topographic occlusal radiograph of the mandibular arch. **C,** Cross-sectional occlusal radiograph of the mandibular arch.

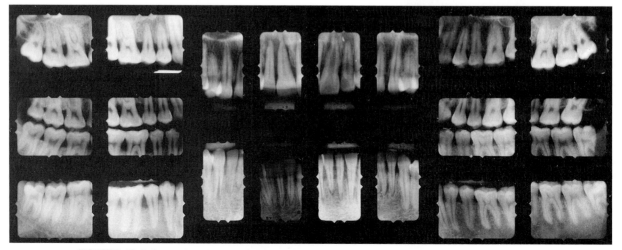

FIGURE 6-13 Full-mouth radiographic survey. *(From Bird DL, Robinson DS:* Modern dental assisting, *ed 10, St Louis, 2012, Saunders.)*

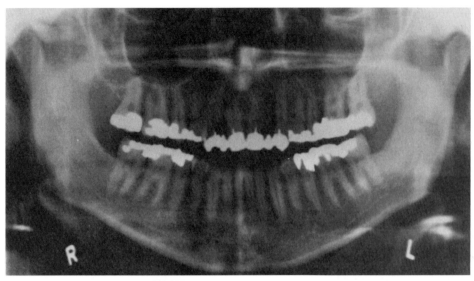

FIGURE 6-14 Panoramic radiograph.

(2) Load the image receptor and the cassette into the unit (film or phosphor plate)
(3) Position the client in the unit with the midsagittal plane perpendicular to the floor and the Frankfort plane parallel to the floor/ala-tragus line 5 degrees down
(4) Instruct the client to occlude on the bite rod or similar device
(5) Consult the unit manufacturer's instructions to select the appropriate exposure settings (mA and kVp); usually based on the width and density of the target object
(6) Maintain pressure on the exposure button until the procedure is completed, which usually takes 20 seconds
(7) Process the film; place the phosphor plate in a laser scanner; observe the digital image on a computer monitor

2. Lateral oblique mandible projection
   a. Images the mandible from the canine region posterior to the ramus
   b. Indications[4]
      (1) Evaluate the abnormalities seen on other projections
      (2) Image the third molars
      (3) Assess trauma-related conditions
3. Temporomandibular joint (TMJ)—transcranial projection
   a. Images the bony relationships in the TMJ
   b. Indications[4]
      (1) Evaluate the superior surface of the condyle
      (2) Evaluate the left and right joint spaces
      (3) Evaluate the joint in open and closed positions
4. Cephalometric projection
   a. Images lateral view of the skull
   b. Indications[4]
      (1) Evaluate growth and development
      (2) Orthodontic evaluation
      (3) Maxillofacial reconstructive surgical procedures
5. Water's projection
   a. Images maxillary sinuses with minimal superimposition of other anatomic structures
   b. Indications[4]
      (1) Assessment of trauma
      (2) Evaluation of abnormal conditions of the sinuses

Image Formation and Darkroom Techniques—Radiographic Film Processing and Duplication

A. Latent-image formation
   1. Film considerations
      a. Crystals within the emulsion composed of positive silver ions (Ag^+) and negative bromine (Br^-) and iodine (I^-) ions
      b. Crystals contain imperfections that trap recoil electrons to begin the process of latent-image formation
   2. Silver halide crystals are irradiated
   3. High-speed recoil electrons are trapped by latent-image sites (crystal imperfections); impart a negative charge to the site
   4. Free interstitial silver ions are attracted to the negatively charged latent image site

5. Accumulation of silver atoms at the latent-image sites (crystal imperfection sites) constitutes the latent (invisible) image
6. Crystals with metallic silver deposits are subjected to chemical reduction by the developer solution during film processing
7. Crystals not exposed to radiation are removed from emulsion by the fixer solution

B. Chemical solutions
  1. Developer
     a. Reducing agent (a hydroquinone and elon combination)—reduces the latent-image–containing silver bromide crystals to black metallic silver
     b. Alkalizer (sodium carbonate)—provides the required alkaline medium for the reducer to work; softens and swells the gelatin of the emulsion to allow the reducer to reach the silver bromide crystals
     c. Preservative (sodium sulfite)—slows the oxidation of the solution to prolong its lifespan
     d. Restrainer (potassium bromide)—slows down the action of chemicals
  2. Fixer
     a. Clearing or fixing agent (sodium or ammonium thiosulfate)—removes the unexposed or undeveloped crystals from the emulsion
     b. Acidifier (acetic acid)—provides the required acidity so that the fixing solutions can work; stops the action of the developer
     c. Preservative (sodium sulfite)—slows the oxidation of the solution to prolong its lifespan
     d. Hardener (potassium aluminum)—shrinks and hardens the emulsion
  3. Vehicle (distilled water)—used to mix the chemicals

C. Processing methods
  1. Basic film processing procedure
     a. Developing—reduces latent-image–containing silver bromide crystals to black metallic silver
     b. Rinsing—washes away excess developer solution to avoid contamination and neutralization of fixer
     c. Fixing—removes the unexposed or undeveloped crystals from the emulsion
     d. Washing—removes the fixer solution to avoid staining the film
     e. Drying—removes water from the emulsion; prepares the film for viewing
  2. Time-temperature method
     a. Recommended scientific method for film processing
     b. Optimal amount of reduction of silver bromide crystals occurs

TABLE 6-3 Time-Temperature Processing

Temperature of Developer	Time in Developer(minutes)
68°F (20°C)	5.0
70°F (21°C)	4.5
72°F (22°C)	4.0
76°F (24.5°C)	3.0
80°F (26.5°C)	2.5

From Carestream Health, Inc.

     c. The developer's activity is dependent on the solution's temperature
     d. Less activity occurs at lower temperatures; greater activity occurs at higher temperatures
     e. Optimal results are obtained at 68°F (20°C) for manual processing (Table 6-3)
  3. Manual method[11]
     a. Films are placed on racks and are hand dipped in solutions
     b. Advantage—Reliable (not subject to equipment malfunction)
     c. Limitation—Time-consuming process
  4. Automatic method[11]
     a. Films are carried from solution to solution to the dryer by a roller assembly or a conveyer
     b. Advantage—Increased volume of workload
     c. Limitation—Increased equipment maintenance
  5. Rapid processing method
     a. Accomplished by the use of high-temperature solutions or concentrated solutions at room temperature
     b. Completed in 1 minute or less
     c. Film quality is less than that obtained with standard methods
     d. Used for processing working films (i.e., endodontic or emergency procedures)
  6. Wet reading
     a. Immediate evaluation of a radiographic technique and oral disease
     b. Used in manual processing or as the fast ("endo") speed setting on an automatic processor
     c. Minimum manual fixing time of 3 minutes required before viewing radiographs under white-light conditions
     d. Films viewed as a wet reading must be returned to the fixer solution for the full normal time to convert to archival quality radiographs

D. Darkroom design and requirements[11]
   1. Location and size
      a. Located near rooms where x-ray units are placed
      b. Minimum of 16 square feet for one person to work
      c. Size-determining factors
         (1) Number of radiographs to be processed
         (2) Number of personnel using the darkroom
         (3) Processing method(s) used (manual, automatic, or both)
         (4) Space for storage of cleaning and maintenance supplies and for other radiographic processes such as film duplicating
      d. Light-tight room
      e. Revolving light-sealed door, or door with inside lock, to prevent accidental white-light exposure during processing
   2. Lighting
      a. Illuminating safelight
         (1) Ideal safelighting available commercially as an LED (light emitting diode) specifically designed for processing intraoral and extraoral dental radiographs[4]
         (2) A 15-watt bulb covered with a red filter placed four feet away from the working surface still is considered acceptable safelighting
         (3) Panoramic and other extraoral films are more sensitive to light than are intraoral films; therefore, extraneous light (e.g., from equipment dials, indicator lights, luminous watch faces) should be eliminated
      b. Overhead white light
         (1) Provides adequate illumination for the room
         (2) Light switches must be located out of easy reach to prevent accidental exposure to white light
      c. Viewing safelight—mounted on wall behind processing tanks for wet readings (after films have been in fixer solution for 3 minutes)
      d. Outside warning light
         (1) Prevents unintentional entry of other personnel during film processing procedures
         (2) When wired to safelight, both can be activated at the same time
   3. Plumbing
      a. Thermostatically controlled intake valve to maintain constant temperatures of solutions
      b. Adequate drainage
      c. Silver retrieval method for environmentally sound disposal of fixer
         (1) Used fixer solution contains silver thiosulphate complexes from interaction with the film emulsion[4]
         (2) Ethical responsibility to the environment to prevent release of this heavy metal into the waste stream
      d. Large sink with gooseneck faucet needed to accommodate cleaning procedures
   4. Record keeping
      a. Inventory of chemicals
      b. Dates of solution changes
      c. Film identification records
         (1) Client's name
         (2) Number of films
         (3) Rack numbers (manual) or slot numbers (automatic)
         (4) Date of film exposure and processing
E. Film duplication
   1. The purpose is to provide copies of radiographs for:
      a. Third-party payment
      b. A change to another oral health care practitioner
      c. Referrals to specialists
      d. Use in litigation
   2. Equipment
      a. Radiographic duplicating film
         (1) Base—blue-tinted polyester base
         (2) Solarized emulsion
            (a) Emulsion composed of gelatin and silver bromide crystals
            (b) Phenomenon in which more light exposure yields a decrease in image density, and less light exposure yields an increase in image density
         (3) Antihalation coating
            (a) Layer of gelatin containing a dye
            (b) Process of halation occurs when light passing through the film and into the air is reflected back toward the emulsion, causing blurred edges
            (c) The dye absorbs the reflected light to prevent image blurriness
            (d) The dye is washed away during processing
      b. Film-duplicating machine
         (1) Box-type device with a glass top, adjustable timer, and ultraviolet light source
         (2) Printing area of various sizes; depends on the manufacturer and the model type
   3. Procedure
      a. Original radiographs are positioned on the glass top
      b. The right and left sides are identified
      c. Under safelight conditions, the duplicating film is removed from the box; the solarized

emulsion side is placed down on top of original radiographs

d. The appropriate exposure time is selected; ultraviolet light passes through original radiographs to expose the duplicating film

e. The duplicating film is manually or automatically processed in the same manner as radiographic film

4. Duplication errors

a. A light duplicate image results from overexposure

b. A dark duplicate image results from underexposure

c. Poor definition of image results from loss of tight contact between the original radiograph and the duplication film

RADIOGRAPHIC ERRORS

A. Intraoral technique errors (Figure 6-15)

1. Typical packet placement errors involve improper positioning of the image receptor behind the teeth of interest and failure to achieve shadow-casting principles

2. Vertical angulation (Figure 6-16)

a. Typical vertical angulation errors with the paralleling technique evidenced by failure to record the apical or coronal portions of teeth

b. Typical vertical angulation errors with the bisecting technique evidenced by a foreshortened or elongated image

3. Horizontal overlap

a. Evidenced by an increased radiopacity or superimposition of adjacent interproximal tooth surfaces

b. Occurs when the x-ray beam is directed toward the image receptor from an excessively mesial or distal horizontal position

c. Occurs when the image receptor is not positioned parallel to the embrasures of the teeth of interest

4. Centering

a. Evidenced by a clear unexposed area (cone cut)

b. Results from not completely covering the image receptor within the x-ray beam

B. Exposure errors

1. Dark radiographs

a. Causes

(1) Exposure settings (mA, kV, time) too high

(2) Accidental white-light exposure

b. Corrective actions

(1) Place exposure-setting chart near the control panel for reference

(2) Apply working knowledge of the effects of exposure settings to achieve appropriate settings for the subject or object being imaged

(3) In the darkroom, position the overhead white-light switch away from the working area to prevent accidentally turning on the white light

2. Light radiographs

a. Causes

(1) Exposure settings (mA, kV, time) too low

(2) Increased distance between the open end of the PID and the object being imaged

(3) Reversed film packet placement intraorally (pattern of the lead foil evident)

(a) Wrong identification of the front side of the film packet because of lack of knowledge

(b) Disorganized placement of the film packet

(c) Use of an unfamiliar film-holding device

b. Corrective actions

(1) Place the exposure setting chart near the control panel for easy reference

(2) Apply working knowledge of the effects of exposure settings to achieve appropriate settings for the subject or object being imaged

(3) Maintain pressure on the exposure button until completion of the exposure

(4) Position the open end of the PID as close to the area being imaged as possible

(5) Place the white, unprinted side of the film packet facing the x-ray tube. (*Note*: The statement "opposite side toward tube" is printed on the back of some film packets.)

(a) Place film packets in an organized and systematic manner

(b) Learn the correct use of film-holding devices

3. Clear or blank radiographs

a. Causes

(1) No exposure to x-rays

(2) Not turning on power to the x-ray unit

(3) Placing film packet but not aligning PID toward film

(4) Positioning the back of the digital sensor or phosphor plate toward the x-ray source

b. Corrective actions

(1) Develop a systematic routine for exposing radiographs

(2) Develop working knowledge about the front and back sides of digital sensors or phosphor plates

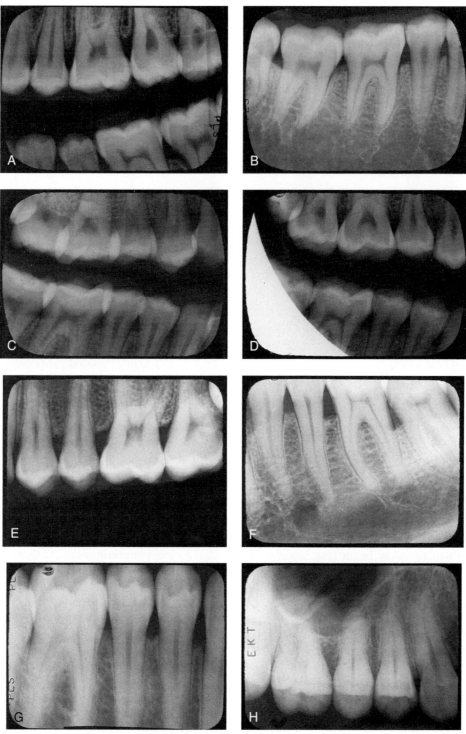

FIGURE 6-15 Errors in intraoral radiographic technique. **A,** Packet placement error: packet tilted. **B,** Packet placement error: third molar not fully recorded on film. **C,** Horizontal overlap. **D,** Conecut. **E,** Paralleling technique error: insufficient vertical angulation results in apices not imaged. **F,** Paralleling technique error: excessive vertical angulation results in occlusal edges not imaged. **G,** Bisecting technique error: insufficient vertical angulation results in an elongated image. **H,** Bisecting technique error: excessive vertical angulation results in a foreshortened image.

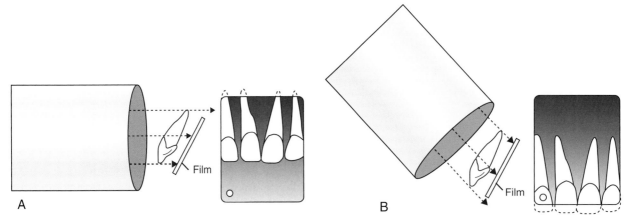

FIGURE 6-16 Incorrect vertical angulation when using the paralleling technique will result in incomplete recording of the entire tooth (crown edge to root tip). **A,** Insufficient vertical angulation. Vertical angulation that is too "flat" will cut off the root tips on the resulting radiograph. **B,** Excessive vertical angulation. Vertical angulation that is too "steep" will cut off the crown edges on the resulting radiograph.

4. Partially clear or blank image, or white artifacts
   a. Causes
     (1) Cone cut error
     (2) Leaving objects in the path of the beam, which will cause artifacts
     (3) Damaged or scratched digital sensor or phosphor plate
   b. Corrective actions
     (1) Center the image receptor to the path of beam
     (2) Use an image receptor holder with an external aiming device to aid in centering appropriately
     (3) Remove metal or dense objects from the path of the x-ray beam (e.g., eyeglasses, partial dentures, oral or facial piercings)
     (4) Handle digital sensors or phosphor plates carefully to avoid damage
5. Blurred images
   a. Causes—movement (client, image receptor, or tube head or PID assembly)
   b. Corrective actions
     (1) Maintain rapport with the client to obtain maximum cooperation during the radiographic procedure
     (2) Ensure that the image receptor is securely in place before the exposure
     (3) Never use the client's finger to hold the image receptor in place
     (4) Never activate the exposure until the tube head or the PID assembly is stabilized into position
C. Film processing or handling errors
   1. Fogged radiographs
     a. Causes
       (1) Improper safelighting in the darkroom

       (2) Exposure to scatter radiation, heat, humidity, chemical vapors
       (3) Contaminated processing chemicals
       (4) Old, expired, or damaged film
     b. Corrective actions
       (1) Check the darkroom for white-light leaks
       (2) Examine the safelight for correct wattage of bulb, distance from working surface, color and condition (not scratched) of filter
       (3) Store film protected from scatter radiation, heat, humidity, chemical vapors
       (4) Use caution when replenishing or changing processing chemicals to avoid contamination
       (5) Maintain the film inventory to ensure use of film before the expiration date
  2. Overdeveloped (dark) radiographs
     a. Causes
       (1) Temperature of developer solution too high
       (2) Excessive developing time used
       (3) Overactive developer solution (wrong water-to-concentrate ratio resulting in the mixture being too strong)
     b. Corrective actions
       (1) Check the developer temperature with a thermometer
       (2) Check the developing time with an accurate timing device
       (3) Check the chemistry of solutions and mixing procedures
  3. Underdeveloped (light) radiographs
     a. Causes
       (1) Temperature of developer solution too cool

(2) Insufficient developing time

(3) Developer solution

(4) Level of developer solution in the automatic processor tank too low

b. Corrective actions

(1) Check the developer temperature with a thermometer

(2) Check the developing time with an accurate timing device

(3) Replace the old developer solution

(4) Replenish the developer solution to the appropriate level

4. Clear (blank) radiographs

a. Causes

(1) Film placed in fixer solution first, which causes the removal of all silver bromide crystals

(2) Excessive washing, which causes the removal of emulsion

b. Corrective actions

(1) Label the solution tanks

(2) Display the correct processing procedures in the darkroom

(3) Remove films from wash after appropriate time

5. Dark-stained or light-stained radiographs

a. Developer, fluoride, glove powder, saliva (dark) or fixer (white) contamination

b. Corrected by keeping the work area clean to avoid dripping and splashing of processing chemicals; wipe dry the film packet immediately after removing it from the oral cavity; wash hands to remove contaminants

6. Brown-, yellow-, or green-stained radiographs

a. Insufficient fixing (yellow staining) or washing times (brown staining); a green color indicates intact emulsion that has not come in contact with the processing chemicals

b. Corrected by using appropriate film processing procedures; separate double film packets before placing the film into the processor

7. Automatic processor roller lines or marks

a. Dirty or contaminated processing chemicals cause dark lines to appear on automatically processed films

b. Corrected by periodic cleaning of automatic processor rollers and changing and replenishing chemical solutions appropriately

8. Static electricity artifacts

a. Caused by the rapid removal of the film from the packet or the cassette when the humidity level is very low (e.g., during winter); yields black artifacts in tree-shaped streaks, smudges, or dots

b. Corrected by the careful removal of the film from the packet or the cassette

9. White-light exposure

a. Causes

(1) Torn film packet covering

(2) Accidental opening of the film packet under white light

(3) Failure to cover the film-processing tanks during the procedure

(4) Failure to allow the film to be fully accepted by the automatic processor rollers before turning on the white light

(5) The cuffs of the daylight loader not tight enough around the arms; light enters during the unwrapping of the film packet

b. Corrective action

(1) Follow proper procedure for opening film packets and maintaining safelight conditions in the darkroom

(2) Examine the daylight loader cuffs for secure fit

D. Panoramic positioning errors (Figures 6-17 and 6-18)

1. When the dental arches are positioned too far back in the focal trough, anterior teeth will appear blurred and magnified in size; when positioned too far forward at the front of the focal trough, anterior teeth will appear narrowed and diminished in size

2. When the chin is tilted downward, the arches will appear to "smile," and the condyles will tilt inward; with the chin tilted upward, the arches will appear to "frown," and the dense bony palatal structures will absorb much of the beam, causing maxillary anterior teeth to be obscured or faintly imaged

3. When the midline is not centered but turned too far to the right or left, teeth on one side will appear narrowed and severely overlapped, while teeth on the other side will appear magnified; when turned too far to the right, it results in narrowed and severely overlapped teeth on the right; and when turned too far to the left, it results in narrowed and severely overlapped teeth on the left

Quality Assurance

A. Quality control—ensuring the production of diagnostic quality radiographs while minimizing radiation exposure through a plan of action; the means of testing and regulating x-ray equipment and procedures used to expose, process, and store radiographs[9]

B. Components of a quality control plan

1. Practitioner competence

a. Evaluation of radiographs for self-analysis of technique

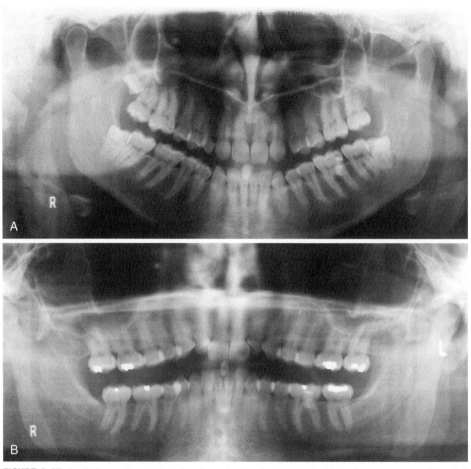

FIGURE 6-17 A, Chin positioned too far down in the focal trough. Note the exaggerated "smile" appearance. **B,** Chin positioned too far up in the focal trough. Note the exaggerated "frown" appearance.

    b. Peer review of radiographs for technique analysis

    c. Continuing education courses to maintain state-of-the-art practice

2. Equipment inspections by state and local radiation regulatory agencies

    a. Milliamperage, kilovoltage, timer accuracy

    b. Collimation and alignment of the x-ray beam

    c. Measures to avoid leakage radiation

    d. Mechanical support of the unit

    e. Penetrating quality of the beam tested by using the half-value layer (HVL); uses a material, usually aluminum, , which reduces exposure by one half when placed within path of radiation beam

3. Quality assurance procedures for film processing

    a. Periodic evaluation of the darkroom

      (1) Checks for light leaks

      (2) Coin test for safelight evaluation—placement of a coin on an unwrapped, unexposed film under a safelight for 2 to 3 minutes; if the coin's outline is present on the processed film, corrective action is necessary[11]

    b. Periodic cleaning, maintenance, and daily monitoring of processing equipment

      (1) Clean the automatic roller assembly and manual racks to prevent debris buildup and artifacts; schedule cleaning on the basis of usage

      (2) Schedule preventive maintenance for optimal equipment operation

      (3) Monitor solution temperatures daily

      (4) Replenish solutions in accordance with the volume of films processed

      (5) Evaluate films for consistency in density and contrast

RADIOGRAPHIC IMAGE INTERPRETATION

Film Mounting

A. Purpose—provides a systematic approach for viewing and evaluating radiographs, with

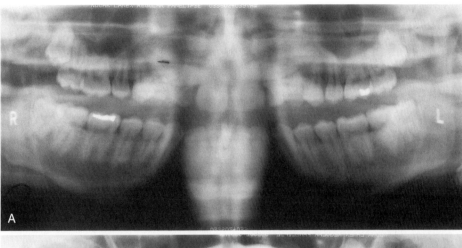

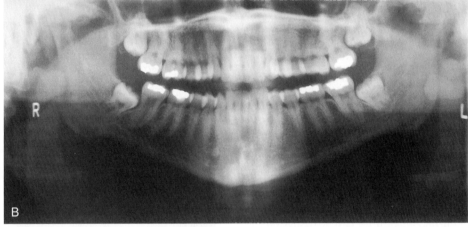

FIGURE 6-18 A, Dental arches positioned too far behind the focal trough. Note the magnified appearance of anterior teeth. **B,** Dental arches positioned too far forward of the focal trough. Note the diminished appearance of anterior teeth.

placement of radiographs in a holding device according to anatomic considerations
B. Mount construction—made of cardboard or plastic; available with windows for placement of radiographs in various number and size combinations
C. Mounting procedures
  1. Intraoral radiographs
    a. Labial mounting
      (1) Raised portion of the embossed dot is toward the viewer
      (2) The client's left side is the viewer's right side
      (3) The orientation is that of the viewer facing the client
    b. Lingual mounting
      (1) Raised portion of the embossed dot is away from the viewer
      (2) The client's left side is the viewer's left side
      (3) The orientation is that of the viewer behind the client

2. Extraoral radiographs
    a. During exposure, side(s) under examination should be identified with a metal letter (R or L) placed on the cassette
    b. A commercial film identification imprinter can be used to label after exposure but before processing

Radiographic Anatomy

A. General considerations
  1. Radiographic examination is an essential component of the total assessment of a client's oral health
  2. Radiographs play a key role in the identification of dental caries, periodontal disease, periapical inflammations, developmental disturbances, traumatic injuries, and neoplastic lesions
  3. Dental hygienists must be able to identify the anatomy of normal teeth as well as the common variations of normal teeth and supporting

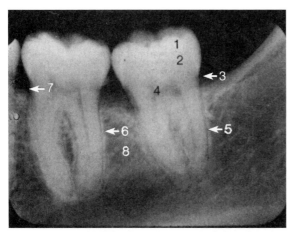

FIGURE 6-19 Tooth anatomy. *1,* Enamel. *2,* Dentin. *3,* Cementum. *4,* Pulp. *5,* Periodontal membrane. *6,* Lamina dura. *7,* Alveolar crest. *8,* Trabeculae.

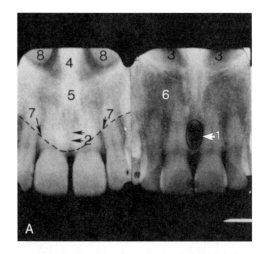

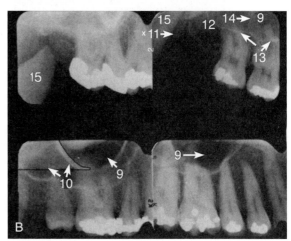

FIGURE 6-20 Maxillary anatomy. **A,** Maxillary anterior region. *1,* Incisive foramen. *2,* Median palatine suture. *3,* Nasal fossa. *4,* Nasal septum. *5,* Anterior nasal spine. *6,* Lateral fossa. *7,* Soft tissue outline of nose (dashed line). *8,* Nasal conchae. **B,** Maxillary posterior region. *9,* Maxillary sinus. *10,* Zygomatic process. *11,* Hamulus. *12,* Maxillary tuberosity. *13,* Floor of sinus. *14,* Sinus septum. *15,* Coronoid process.

structures before they can accurately identify deviations from the normal and signs of disease

4. Occasionally, a normal anatomic condition or a variation of a normal anatomic condition may be confused with oral disease; therefore, a clinical examination must accompany a thorough radiographic interpretation

B. Tooth anatomy
1. The radiographic appearance is distinguished by variations in radiographic densities
2. Dense tooth structures (e.g., enamel) appear radiopaque; less-dense tooth structures (e.g., pulp chamber) appear radiolucent
3. The radiographic appearance of a tooth and its supporting structures is illustrated in Figure 6-19

C. Radiographic anatomy of the maxilla (Figure 6-20)
1. Incisive foramen—oval radiolucency between maxillary central incisors; if superimposed over the apex of an incisor, should not be confused with periapical disease
2. Lateral fossa—diffuse radiolucency between the lateral incisor and the canine
3. Median palatine suture—radiolucent line extending vertically between maxillary incisors; should not be mistaken for a fracture line, nutrient canal, or fistula tract
4. Nasal fossae—two radiolucent densities observed superior to central incisors outlining the nasal passages; may appear less radiolucent when the angle of the x-ray beam images the nasal conchae (wafer-thin bone extending from the lateral walls of the nasal fossae)
5. Nasal septum—radiopaque density representing the bony division of the nasal cavities
6. Anterior nasal spine—increased radiopacity adjacent and superior to the incisive foramen

7. Inverted Y formation—Y-shaped radiopacity created by radiopaque lines that outline the nasal floor and the anterior portion of the maxillary sinus
8. Maxillary sinus—bilateral radiolucency originating at the canine region and extending posteriorly; outlined by a radiopaque wall
9. Nutrient canals—the thin radiolucent lines should not be confused with fracture lines; depending on the angle of the x-ray beam, the nutrient canal opening (foramen) may be imaged as a very small radiolucent dot
10. Zygomatic process (arch)—radiopaque structure observed superior to the maxillary posterior teeth, which joins the maxilla and frontal and temporal bones

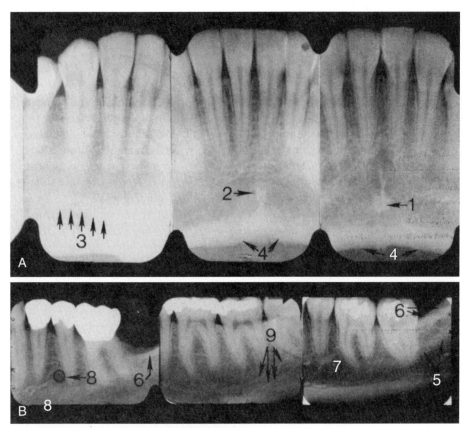

FIGURE 6-21 Mandibular anatomy. **A,** Mandibular anterior region. *1,* Genial tubercles. *2,* Lingual foramen. *3,* Mental ridge. *4,* Inferior border of mandible. **B,** Mandibular posterior region. *5,* Mylohyoid line. *6,* Oblique ridge. *7,* Submandibular fossa. *8,* Mental foramen. *9,* Mandibular canal.

11. Maxillary tuberosity—most posterior region of the maxilla; appears as a raised alveolar bony ridge
12. Hamulus—radiopaque spine located on the medial pterygoid plate observed only on the most posterior intraoral radiographs
13. Lateral pterygoid plate—radiopaque extension of sphenoid bone; distinguished as separate from the maxillary tuberosity; observed only on the most posterior intraoral radiographs
14. Maxillary torus—radiopaque density superior to the apices of maxillary teeth; recorded only if significantly large; not observed on all clients

D. Radiographic anatomy of the mandible (Figure 6-21)
 1. Genial tubercles—radiopaque spines (often imaged as a circle) located inferior to mandibular central incisors
 2. Lingual foramen—small radiolucency in the center of the genial tubercles for the passage of nerves and vessels
 3. Nutrient canals—narrow radiolucent lines often observed in the anterior mandibular regions; should not be confused with fractures; depending on the angle of the x-ray beam, the nutrient canal opening (foramen) may be imaged as a very small radiolucent dot

 4. Mental ridge—radiopaque density (lines) corresponding to raised bone along the anterior aspect of the mandible; often observed as an inverted "V" when both the right and left sides are imaged together on one radiograph
 5. Inferior border of the mandible—radiopaque density representing the dense cortical bone
 6. Mylohyoid line—radiopaque ridge of bone on the lingual surface; distinguished from the oblique ridge and mental ridges by its inferior and posterior location
 7. Oblique ridge—radiopaque line representing a raised bony surface on the facial side of the mandible; recorded on the radiograph superior to the mylohyoid line
 8. Submandibular fossa—large radiolucent area in the posterior body of the mandible, which represents the lingual depression corresponding to the location of the submandibular salivary gland
 9. Mental foramen—circular radiolucency on the facial aspect of the mandible; near the apex of the second premolar, for the exit of the mental

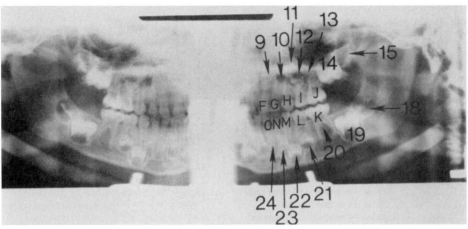

FIGURE 6-22 Developing dentition. Maxillary left side permanent teeth identified as: *9*, Central incisor; *10*, Lateral incisor; *11*, Canine; *12*, First premolar; *13*, Second premolar; *14*, First molar; *15*, Second molar. Mandibular left side permanent teeth identified as: *18*, Second molar; *19*, First molar; *20*, Second premolar; *21*, First premolar; *22*, Canine; *23*, Lateral incisor; *24*, Central incisor. Maxillary left side primary teeth identified as: *F*, Central incisor; *G*, Lateral incisor; *H*, Canine; *I*, First molar; *J*, Second molar; *K*, Second molar; *L*, First molar; *M*, Canine; *N*, Lateral incisor; *O*, Central incisor. *(Courtesy Dr. Henry Fields, Department of Pedodontics, University of North Carolina School of Dentistry, Chapel Hill, NC.)*

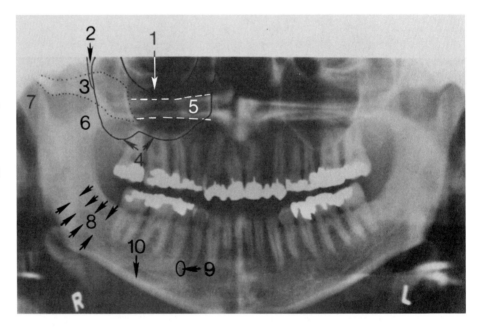

FIGURE 6-23 Panoramic anatomy. *1*, Orbital floor. *2*, Pterygoid maxillary fissure (solid lines). *3*, Zygomatic arch (*dotted outline*). *4*, Walls of maxillary sinus. *5*, Palate (dashed lines). *6*, Coronoid process. *7*, Mandibular condyle. *8*, Mandibular canal. *9*, Mental foramen. *10*, Inferior border of mandible.

nerve; should not be mistaken for a periapical pathologic condition of the premolars

10. Mandibular canal—radiolucent horizontal canal in the mandible through which the inferior alveolar nerve and artery pass; extends anterior from the mandibular foramen on the lingual aspect of the ramus through the body and terminates at the mental foramen; most often identified by two faint parallel radiopaque lines representing the canal walls

11. Mandibular torus—radiopacity superimposed over or imaged below the apices; recorded

only if significantly large; not observed on all clients

E. Radiographic appearance of tooth development—radiography of the developing dentition normally includes most of the 20 primary teeth and, depending on the age of the child, evidence of the development of the 32 permanent teeth (Figure 6-22)

F. Panoramic anatomy (Figure 6-23) and artifacts (Figure 6-24)

G. Restorative materials (Figure 6-25)
   1. Metallic (gold, amalgam, implants)
   2. Nonmetallic (e.g., composite, gutta-percha)

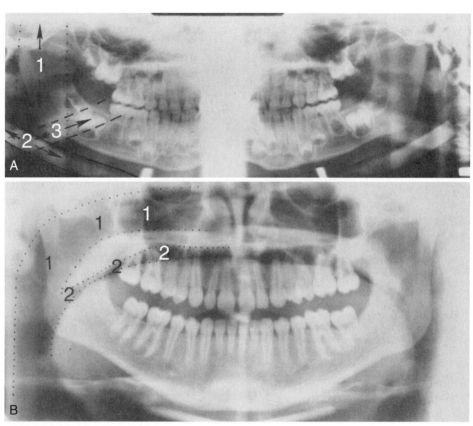

FIGURE 6-24 Panoramic artifacts. **A,** Split-image panoramic radiograph. *1,* Pancentric head positioner (*arrows, dotted lines*). *2,* Right side of chinrest. *3,* Shadow of left side of chinrest (*dashed lines*). **B,** Continuous-image panoramic radiograph. *1,* Nasopharyngeal air space. *2,* Palatoglossal air space. *(Courtesy Dr. Henry Fields, Department of Pedodontics, University of North Carolina School of Dentistry, Chapel Hill, NC.)*

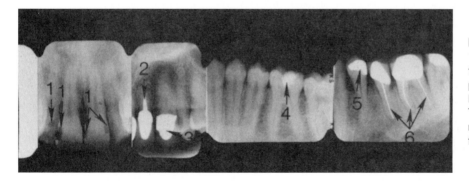

FIGURE 6-25 Restorative materials. *1,* Radiolucent composite restorations. *2,* Post and core with porcelain-fused-to-metal crown. *3,* Porcelain-fused-to-metal crown. *4,* Temporary restoration. *5,* Metallic restoration (amalgam). *6,* Endodontic filling material.

Interpretation and Identification of Dental Diseases

A. General considerations
  1. Use radiographs free of technical, processing, or handling errors
  2. Use magnification
  3. Dim the overhead lighting in the room
B. Film-based radiographs
  1. Mount the radiograph
  2. Use the illuminating viewbox
  3. Mask out extraneous light from around the mount
C. Digitally acquired radiographs
  1. Position the monitor to avoid the glare of ambient light[7]
  2. Use computer software and digital measurement tools to enhance and magnify the image
  3. Calibrate the density and contrast of the monitor, as recommended by the manufacturer[7]

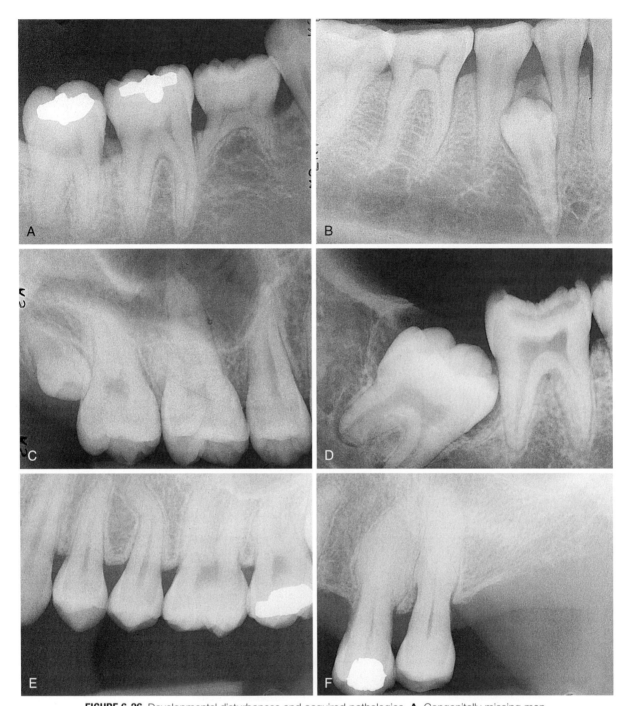

FIGURE 6-26 Developmental disturbances and acquired pathologies. **A,** Congenitally missing mandibular right second premolar. **B,** Supernumerary mandibular premolar. **C,** Microdontia of the maxillary right third molar. **D,** Impaction of the mandibular right third molar. **E,** Dilacerated root of the maxillary left second premolar. **F,** Hypercementosis of the maxillary left premolars.

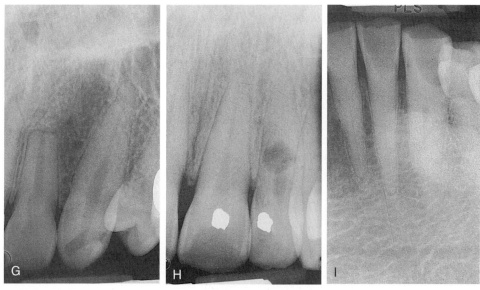

FIGURE 6-26, cont'd **G,** External root resorption of the maxillary left lateral incisor. **H,** Internal root resorption of the maxillary left lateral incisor. **I,** Attrition of the mandibular anterior teeth.

D. Systematic approach
  1. Evaluate the dentition
    a. Begin the assessment from the client's maxillary right third molar area, and continue examining through to the client's mandibular right third molar area
    b. Order of assessment
      (1) Presence or absence of teeth
      (2) Size of teeth
      (3) Shape of teeth
      (4) Eruption and location of teeth
      (5) Presence of restorative materials
      (6) Signs of pathoses (abnormal radiolucencies and radiopacities)
  2. Evaluate supporting structures
    a. Examine the:
      (1) Periodontal ligament space
      (2) Lamina dura
      (3) Bone trabecular pattern
      (4) Cortical plate of bone
      (5) Alveolar bone height
      (6) Sinuses (if imaged)
      (7) Orbits (if imaged)
      (8) Carotid artery (if imaged) for evidence of calcification
    b. Assess for deviations from normal
      (1) Developmental disturbances (Figure 6-26)
      (2) Periodontal disease (Figure 6-27)
      (3) Dental caries (see Figure 6-27)
      (4) Inflammatory responses (Figure 6-28)
      (5) Traumatic injuries (Figure 6-29)
      (6) Pathologic conditions (see Figure 6-29)

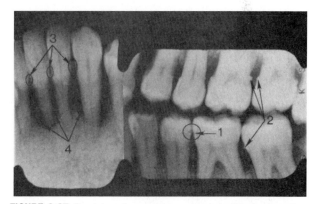

FIGURE 6-27 Dental caries and bone loss. *1,* Proximal surface caries. *2,* Calculus deposits. *3,* Heavy calculus deposits. *4,* Height of alveolar bone following resorption.

E. Using localization methods to aid interpretation
  1. Purpose—periapical and bitewing radiographs are two dimensional, imaging the teeth and bone in the superoinferior and anteroposterior dimensions; the relative buccal–lingual position of structures is often required for diagnosis and care planning in a variety of clinical situations[4]
  2. Indications
    a. Impacted teeth
    b. Supernumerary teeth
    c. Foreign objects
    d. Fractures or trauma
    e. Pathologic lesions
    f. Endodontic therapy
    g. Sialoliths

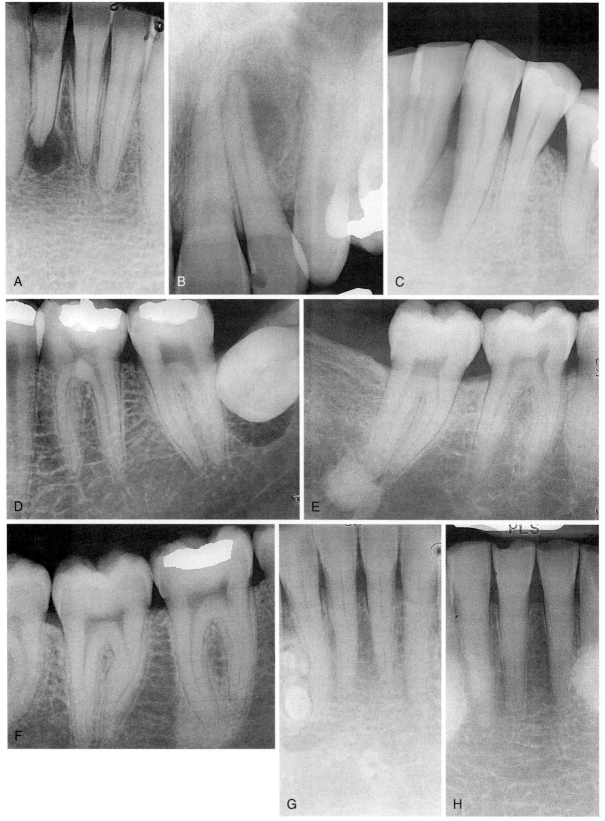

FIGURE 6-28 Inflammatory responses. **A,** Periapical pathology. **B,** Periodontal abscess. **C,** Lateral periodontal cyst. **D,** Dentigerous cyst. **E,** Condensing osteitis. **F,** Enostosis. **G,** Odontoma. **H,** Mandibular tori.

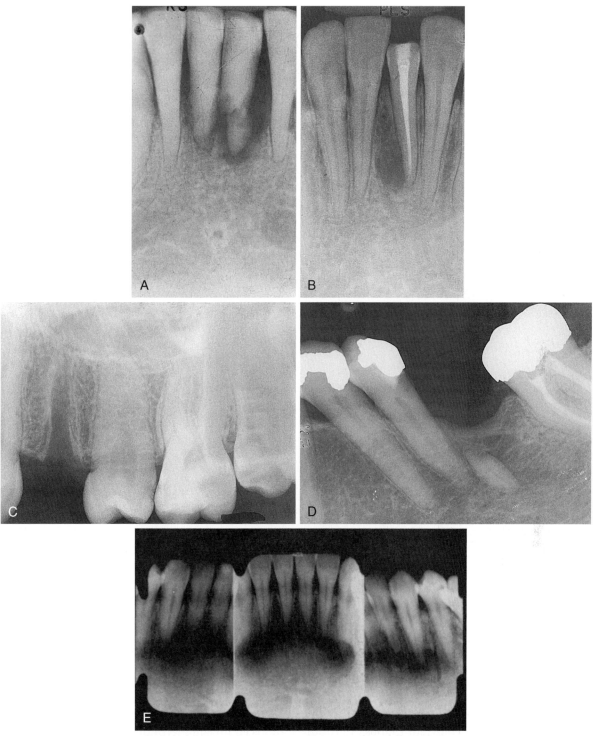

FIGURE 6-29 Traumatic injuries and neoplastic conditions. **A,** Fractured root of the mandibular right central incisor. **B,** Fractured crown of the mandibular left central incisor. **C,** Recent extraction site. **D,** Retained root tip. **E,** Periapical cemental dysplasia (PCD).

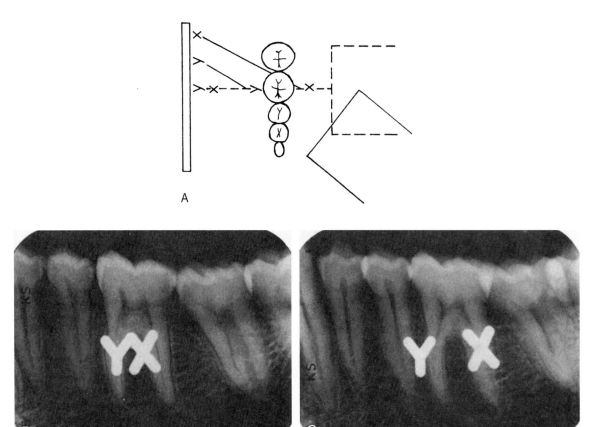

FIGURE 6-30 Localization using the buccal-object–rule technique. **A,** Dashed line, position-indicating device (PID) represents standard angulation. *Solid line,* Superimposes first molar and objects and represents mesial PID shift that yields visual separation of first molar and objects. **B,** Radiograph taken with standard angulation yielding visual superimposition of first molar and lead letters X and Y. **C,** Radiograph taken with mesial PID shift yielding visual separation of first molar and lead letters X and Y. X is facially positioned and appears to move in the direction opposite to the PID shift (distally). Y is lingually positioned and appears to move with the PID shift (mesially).

3. Buccal object rule (Figure 6-30)
   a. Also referred to as the *tube shift method* of localization
   b. Can be used to add the buccal–lingual dimension when viewing a full mouth or bitewing series because each of the periapical radiographs, the bitewing radiographs, or both may have been exposed with different vertical or horizontal angulations
   c. SLOB—the acronym stands for "same = lingual, opposite = buccal"
   d. When comparing two radiographs, a buccal object will appear to have moved in the direction opposite to the tube shift, whereas a lingual object will appear to have moved in the same direction as the tube shift

SUPPLEMENTAL TECHNIQUES AND SPECIALIZED IMAGING MODALITIES

While periapical, bitewing, and panoramic radiographs are the images most often used for assessing and evaluating oral diseases, innovative oral and maxillofacial imaging technologies are emerging that will influence dental hygiene practice.

A. Digital subtraction
   1. Computer-generated and stored images captured at different stages of treatment or disease progression are merged and "subtracted," leaving behind an image of the differences
   2. Computer software can match gray values between subsequent images to allow for comparison of digitally stored images to detect changes over time[8]

B. Computed tomography (CT)
1. Definition—method of selecting a single plane or "slice" of tissue to image, while extraneous structures in other planes are eliminated from the image; CT imagery uses radiation to expose sensors that generate computer images; originally called a CAT (computed axial tomography) scan
2. Indications for oral health care
   a. Diagnosis of soft tissue lesions, especially within salivary glands
   b. Evaluation and assessment for treatment planning for dental implants
   c. Evaluation of trauma and determination of the cause of pain

3. Radiation doses can be 600 times more than in panoramic radiography[12]
C. Cone beam volumetric imaging (CBVI), also called *cone beam computed tomography (CBCT)*
1. CT technology dedicated to oral and maxillofacial applications with significantly lower radiation exposures than with conventional medical CT scans[13]
2. Uses radiation to generate multi-planar images with no superimposed blurring of those structures outside the image layer[12,13]
3. Provides enhanced two-dimensional and three-dimensional digital images
4. Purported to become the gold standard for implant treatment planning[13]

@ WEB SITE INFORMATION AND RESOURCES

SOURCE	WEB SITE ADDRESS	DESCRIPTION
American Academy of Oral and Maxillofacial Radiology	http://www.aaomr.org	Promotes and advances the art and science of radiology in dentistry and provides a forum for communication among its members and to the health care community and to the public
International Commission on Radiological Protection (ICRP)	http://www.icrp.org	Provides recommendations and guidance on all aspects of protection against ionizing radiation
National Council on Radiation Protection and Measurements (NCRP)	http://www.ncrp.com	Dissemination of information and recommendations on protection against radiation
International Commission on Radiological Units and Measurements (ICRU)	http://www.icru.org	Develops and promulgates internationally accepted recommendations on radiation-related quantities and measurement procedures and references data for the safe and efficient application of ionizing radiation
U.S. Nuclear Regulatory Commission	http://www.nrc.gov	Regulates the nation's civilian use of radiation to ensure adequate protection of public health and safety and to protect the environment

REFERENCES

1. National Council on Radiation Protection and Measurements: *Report No 160 Ionizing radiation exposure of the population of the United States*, Bethesda, MD, 2009, NCRPM.
2. White SC, Pharoah MJ: *Oral radiology: Principles and interpretation*, ed 6, St Louis, 2008, Mosby.
3. Thompson A, Taylor BN: *Guide to the SI, with a focus on usage and unit conversions. Guide for the Use of the International System of Units (SI)*, National Institute of Standards and Technology Special Publication 811, 2008.
4. Thomson EM, Johnson ON: *Essentials of dental radiography for dental assistants and hygienists*, ed 9, Upper Saddle River, NJ, 2012, Pearson Education Prentice Hall.
5. United States Nuclear Regulatory Commission: Standards for protection against radiation, Title 10, Part 20, of the Code of Federal Regulations. Dec. 4, 2007: Available at http://www.nrc.gov/reading-rm/doc-collections/cfr/part020/part020-1201.html; Accessed April 11, 2010.
6. American Dental Association Council on Scientific Affairs. The use of dental radiographs: Update and recommendations, *J Am Dent Assoc* 137(9):1304–1312, 2006.
7. Horner K, Drage N, Brettle D: *21st century imaging*, London, UK, 2008, Quintessence Publishing Co., Ltd..
8. Van der Stelt PF: Better imaging: The advantages of digital radiography, *J Am Dent Assoc* 139:7S–13S, 2008.
9. American Dental Association and the U.S. Department of Health and Human Services: *The selection of patients*

for x-ray examinations, Rockville, MD, DHHS-FDA 88-8273, 1987, revised 2004.

10. Rushton VE, Rout J: *Panoramic radiography*, London, UK, 2006, Quintessence Publishing Co., Ltd.

11. Thomson EM: *Exercises in oral radiography techniques: A laboratory manual*, ed 3, Upper Saddle River, NJ, 2012, Pearson Education Prentice Hall.

12. Chau, ACM, Fung K: Comparison of radiation dose for implant imaging using conventional spiral tomography, computed tomography, and cone-beam computed tomography, *Oral Surg Oral Med Oral Pathol Oral Radiol Endod* 107:559–565, 2009.

13. Miles DA: Color atlas of cone beam volumetric imaging for dental applications, Chicago, 2008, Quintessence Publishing Co., Inc..

SUGGESTED READINGS

Frommer HH, Stabulas-Savage J: *Radiology for the dental professional*, ed 9, St Louis, 2011, Mosby.

Thomson EM, Johnson ON: Essentials of dental radiography for dental assistants and hygienists, ed 9, Upper Saddle River, NJ, 2012, Pearson Education Prentice Hall.

CHAPTER 6 REVIEW QUESTIONS

Answers and Rationales to Review Questions are available on this text's accompanying Evolve site. See inside front cover for details.
Use Case A to answer questions 1 to 11.

evolve

CASE A

This 54-year-old female is undergoing orthodontic therapy in response to temporomandibular disorder (TMD). The maxillary orthodontic appliances were placed 18 months ago after an examination revealed various issues with malocclusion that were contributing to her chief complaint of temporomandibular joint (TMJ) pain and "sore jaws." (See Figure 6-31.)

1. **Which of the following regions exhibits periodontal bone loss?**
   a. Maxillary right posterior quadrant
   b. Maxillary anterior sextant
   c. Mandibular left poster quadrant
   d. Mandibular anterior sextant
   e. Mandibular right quadrant

2. **What is the most likely reason for the shortened appearance of the roots of the maxillary central and lateral incisors?**
   a. Use of the bisecting instead of the paralleling technique
   b. External resorption possibly linked to the orthodontic movement of teeth
   c. A development anomaly that caused incomplete root formation
   d. Incorrect positioning that caused the roots to be located outside of the focus layer
   e. Supereruption that resulted when painful TMD impeded the client's ability to occlude normally

3. **To correct the error that rendered the right mandible premolar periapical radiograph undiagnostic, shift the tube head so that the x-ray beam intersects with the image receptor from the:**
   a. Mesial aspect
   b. Distal aspect
   c. Occlusal aspect
   d. Apical aspect

4. **Each of the following is a possible cause of the radiographic error noted in the left mandible premolar periapical radiograph EXCEPT one. Which is the EXCEPTION?**
   a. Movement of the tube head during exposure
   b. Image receptor not placed parallel to the embrasures of the teeth of interest
   c. Central ray of the x-ray beam not directed perpendicular to the image receptor
   d. Image receptor positioned too anteriorly
   e. Malpositioned or crowded teeth

5. **The radiographer considers the overlapping noted in the left maxillary molar periapical radiograph acceptable because it is the result of:**
   a. Bisecting technique
   b. Disto-oblique periapical technique
   c. Tube-shift method of localization
   d. Transcranial technique

6. **What restorative material is present on the mandibular right first molar?**
   a. Stainless-steel crown
   b. Full-metal crown
   c. Large MODBL amalgam
   d. Porcelain jacket crown
   e. Porcelain-fused-to-metal crown

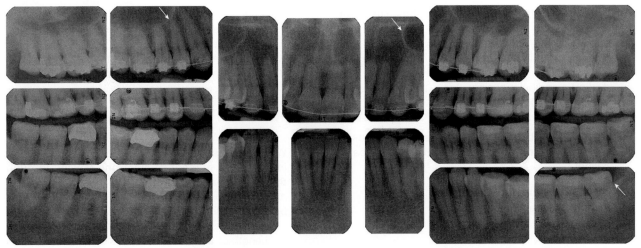

FIGURE 6-31 Case A: Full-mouth series of radiographs.

7. **Which one of the following lists correctly identifies all mandibular teeth restored with composite material?**
   a. Right first and second molars and right first and second premolars
   b. Right first and second molars and right first and second premolars, and left first, second, and third molars
   c. Left first and second molars and left first and second premolars
   d. Right first and second molars and left first, second, and third molars
   e. Right first and second molars and left first, second, and third molars, and left first and second premolars

8. **What is the most likely interpretation of the radiolucency near the apex of the maxillary left canine, as identified by the arrow?**
   a. Cyst
   b. Granuloma
   c. Periapical abscess
   d. Maxillary sinus
   e. Nasal cavity

9. **What is the most likely interpretation of the radiopaque line superimposed across the mandibular left third molar, as identified by the arrow?**
   a. Oblique ridge
   b. Mylohyoid line
   c. Buccal or lingual boney plate
   d. Cervical burnout
   e. Bent film

10. **What is the most likely interpretation of the small radiolucency near the apex of the maxillary right first premolar, as identified by the arrow?**
    a. Periapical abscess
    b. Periodontal abscess
    c. Incisive foramen
    d. Infraorbital foramen
    e. Nutrient canal and foramen

11. **Which of the following teeth exhibits suspected caries?**
    a. Right maxillary first molar
    b. Right maxillary canine
    c. Left maxillary first premolar
    d. Left mandibular canine
    e. Right mandibular second molar

12. **The process by which x-ray energy removes an orbital electron from an atom to yield an ion pair is called:**
    a. Diffraction
    b. Rectification
    c. Transformation
    d. Ionization
    e. Irradiation

13. **Which of the following is NOT a characteristic of x-radiation?**
    a. Penetrates tissues
    b. Affects photographic emulsions
    c. Made up of positively charged protons
    d. Causes ionization
    e. Travels in straight lines

14. **Which of the following constitutes the greatest percentage of overall exposure to the U.S. population?**
    a. Radon gas
    b. Terrestrial sources
    c. Cosmic radiation from outer space
    d. Medical or dental radiographs
    e. Consumer products

15. **What is the annual effective dose of radiation from all sources to a member of the U.S. population?**
    a. 3.2 millisieverts (mSv)
    b. 4.2 mSv
    c. 5.2 mSv
    d. 6.2 mSv
    e. 7.2 mSv

16. **Each of the following is required for the controlled production of x-radiation EXCEPT one. Which one is the EXCEPTION?**
    a. Target
    b. Source of free electrons
    c. High voltage
    d. Vacuum
    e. Radioactive material

17. **The cathode provides the source of electrons to the x-ray machine *because* the negative side of the vacuum tube is composed of a focusing cup and filament.**
    a. Both the statement and reason are correct and related
    b. Both the statement and reason are correct but *not* related
    c. The statement is correct, but the reason is *not*
    d. The statement is *not* correct, but the reason is correct
    e. *Neither* the statement *nor* the reason is correct

18. **When increased, which of the following would best increase the number of electrons flowing through the dental x-ray electrical circuit?**
    a. Impulses
    b. Kilovoltage
    c. Milliamperage
    d. Length of the position-indicating device (PID)

19. Decreasing the voltage decreases the force that moves the electrons along an electrical conductor BECAUSE amperage is the measurement of the number of electrons flowing in an electrical circuit.
    a. Both the statement and reason are correct and related
    b. Both the statement and reason are correct but *not* related
    c. The statement is correct, but the reason is *not*
    d. The statement is *not* correct, but the reason is correct
    e. *Neither* the statement *nor* the reason is correct

20. What is the duration of an impulse setting of 20?
    a. $\frac{1}{10}$ second
    b. $\frac{1}{5}$ second
    c. $\frac{1}{4}$ second
    d. $\frac{1}{3}$ second
    e. $\frac{1}{2}$ second

21. Which of the following best describes how x-rays are actually produced within the dental x-ray tube?
    a. Radioactive particulate matter undergoes controlled disintegration
    b. Electric current passes through an oil mixture releasing electrons
    c. Low-milliamperage current is transformed to high-kilovoltage current
    d. High-speed electrons collide with target material electrons

22. Which of the following terms describes the conversion of kinetic energy into x-ray energy by the sudden stopping or deceleration of a fast moving electron?
    a. α-radiation
    b. General (bremsstrahlung) radiation
    c. Characteristic radiation
    d. Particulate radiation

23. Each of the following is an interaction of x-rays with matter EXCEPT one. Which one is the EXCEPTION?
    a. The x-ray photon may be converted to a positive charge
    b. The x-ray photon may pass through without interaction
    c. The x-ray photon may be deflected from its path
    d. The x-ray photon may become scatter radiation
    e. The x-ray photon may be completely absorbed

24. What theory of radiation damage to cells results from free radicals combining to form toxins such as hydrogen peroxide?
    a. Molecular
    b. Primary
    c. Secondary
    d. Direct
    e. Indirect

25. The effect of radiation-induced biological changes in future generations resulting from excessive radiation exposure of reproductive cells is termed:
    a. Acute effect
    b. Chronic effect
    c. Genetic effect
    d. Latent effect
    e. Somatic effect

26. Whole body radiation induced biological damage is influenced by each of the following EXCEPT one. Which one is the EXCEPTION?
    a. Dose rate
    b. Dose amount
    c. Type of radiation
    d. Size of irradiated area
    e. Type of electrical current

27. For an occupationally exposed individual, the whole body annual maximum permissible dose is:
    a. 0.5 mSv
    b. 5 mSv
    c. 50 mSv
    d. 500 mSv
    e. 5,000 mSv

28. The principle of the National Committee on Radiation Protection to keep exposure low, based on the idea that all radiation, no matter how small the dose, may cause adverse biological effects is called:
    a. Coulomb per kilogram
    b. Nonstochastic effect
    c. Threshold policy
    d. ALARA concept
    e. Risk management

29. Tissues have the capacity to repair radiation damage to a certain degree. However, some damage cannot be repaired and remains weakened, especially with repeated exposures. This is called:
    a. A critical organ
    b. Radioresistant tissue
    c. Cumulative effect
    d. Stochastic effect
    e. Long-term effect

30. According to the factors that determine radiation injury, on the basis of age, who is the most radiosensitive?
    a. 6-year-old child
    b. 16-year-old adolescent
    c. 26-year-old young adult
    d. 46-year-old middle-aged adult
    e. 66-year-old senior adult

31. **On the basis of the Selection Criteria guidelines, what is the radiographic recommendation for bitewing radiographs on an adult recall patient with no clinical caries and no high-risk factors for caries?**
    a. Every 6 to 12 months
    b. Every 12 to 18 months
    c. Every 18 to 24 months
    d. Every 24 to 36 months
    e. Every 36 to 48 months

32. **Each of the following should be documented in the client's record when providing radiographic services EXCEPT one. Which one is the EXCEPTION?**
    a. Patient's informed consent
    b. X-ray unit used for the exposures
    c. Interpretative results
    d. Reason for exposure (assessment of need)
    e. Number and type of radiographs exposed

33. **In the darkroom, to aseptically remove films from a contaminated double-film packet, the clinician should tear open the packet and:**
    a. Hold the films by the edges to pull from the packet to carefully separate
    b. Grasp the black-paper tab and pull straight out, allowing the films to fall free of the packet onto a paper towel on the counter
    c. Remove the lead foil first to better access the films for removal from the packet
    d. Peel back the front and back sides of the packet exposing the films to allow for separation

34. **To maintain infection control following use intraorally, a digital sensor should be:**
    a. Packaged for steam sterilization and autoclaved
    b. Cleaned in an ultrasonic unit with detergent
    c. Decontaminated with soap and water
    d. Wiped with an Environment Protection Agency (EPA)–accepted disinfectant
    e. Immersed in a high-level disinfectant or chemical sterilant

35. **The purpose of the lead foil in the film packet is to:**
    a. Control latent image formation
    b. Protect the film from accidental light leaks
    c. Absorb back-scattered x-rays to reduce film fogging
    d. Eliminate the need for an intensifying screen

36. **Film speed is dependent on the:**
    a. Size and number of the crystals within the emulsion
    b. Number of films inside the packet
    c. Unit exposure settings selected
    d. Temperature of the developing solution
    e. Thickness of the gelatin

37. **A direct digital imaging system needs each of the following to produce an image EXCEPT one. Which one is the EXCEPTION?**
    a. Sensor
    b. Scanner
    c. Computer
    d. X-ray machine
    e. Specialized software

38. **Each of the following is true regarding digital radiography EXCEPT one. Which one is the EXCEPTION?**
    a. Initial setup costs can be expensive, but long-term costs may be less than for film-based radiography
    b. Provides an immediate image on a computer monitor, ready to be evaluated within seconds of exposure
    c. Requires that x-ray machines used with film-based radiography be digitized to be compatible
    d. Image sensors are available in sizes that correspond approximately to conventional film sizes
    e. Images may be manipulated through the use of computer software for enhanced interpretation

39. **Radiolucent images represent dense anatomy BECAUSE structures with a high atomic weight attenuate more energy from the x-ray beam.**
    a. Both the statement and reason are correct and related
    b. Both the statement and reason are correct but *not* related
    c. The statement is correct, but the reason is *not*
    d. The statement is *not* correct, but the reason is correct
    e. *Neither* the statement *nor* the reason is correct

40. **Using a milliampere (mA) setting of 10 with an exposure time of 1.5 seconds equals 15 milliampere-seconds (mAs). If you increase the mA setting to 15, to obtain an image of equal density, how many second(s) of exposure time should be used?**
    a. 0.25
    b. 0.5
    c. 1.0
    d. 2.0
    e. 2.5

41. **With all other variables remaining constant, an increase in kilovoltage will:**
    a. Decrease the radiographic density and decrease the radiographic contrast
    b. Increase the radiographic density and decrease the radiographic contrast
    c. Decrease the radiographic density and increase the radiographic contrast
    d. Increase the radiographic density and increase the radiographic contrast

42. At a distance of 2 feet from the x-ray tube head, the exposure intensity is 16 coulomb (C) per kilogram (kg). What would the intensity be at a distance of 4 feet away?
    a. 4 C/kg
    b. 8 C/kg
    c. 24 C/kg
    d. 32 C/kg
    e. 64 C/kg

43. An unsharp image results from each of the following EXCEPT one. Which one is the EXCEPTION?
    a. Large focal spot
    b. Long object-image receptor distance
    c. Short target–image receptor distance
    d. Movement of x-ray tube head during exposure
    e. Small silver halide crystal size within the film emulsion

44. Which of the following is true regarding the bisecting technique?
    a. Less likely to cause image distortion
    b. Decreased radiation exposure to the client
    c. Shorter exposure times required
    d. Increased client comfort during image receptor placement
    e. Easy standardization of subsequent radiographs taken at different appointments

45. The best rationale for taking vertical bitewing radiographs is that vertical bitewings:
    a. Result in less overlapping than horizontal bitewing radiographs
    b. Image more alveolar bone than horizontal bitewing radiographs
    c. Eliminate the need for periapical radiographs
    d. Are more easily tolerated by the client

46. In panoramic radiography, the horseshoe-shaped zone of sharpness where an object would be imaged in acceptable detail is called the:
    a. Rotation center
    b. Ghost image
    c. Scatter guard
    d. Focal trough
    e. Head positioner

47. Following irradiation, the latent-image–containing silver bromide crystals are converted to black metallic silver by:
    a. Water
    b. Acetic acid
    c. Sodium thiosulfate
    d. Potassium alum
    e. Hydroquinone

48. Until ready for use, unexposed radiographic films should be stored:
    a. In a cool and dry area in the original manufacture's packaging
    b. In the darkroom with the processing chemicals
    c. Near the x-ray unit where radiographs will be exposed
    d. In the sterilization room with other oral hygiene materials and supplies

49. The coin test is used to monitor darkroom safelight conditions. When an image of the coin appears on the radiograph, the safelight is effective.
    a. Both statements are true
    b. Both statements are false
    c. The first statement is true, and the second is false
    d. The first statement is false, and the second is true

50. When mounting intraoral radiographs according to the labial mounting method, which of the following is true?
    a. The embossed dot is convex. The viewer orientation is from behind the client
    b. The embossed dot is convex. The viewer orientation is facing the client
    c. The embossed dot is concave. The viewer orientation is from behind the client
    d. The embossed dot is concave. The viewer orientation is facing the client

CHAPTER 7 General Pathology

Joann R. Gurenlian

Concepts of general pathology relate to multiple facets of dental hygiene care. Inflammatory diseases significantly affect the oral cavity, and research continues to focus on the linkages among inflammatory processes, systemic diseases, and oral diseases.

Advances in genomics contribute to our understanding of the genetic basis of oral health conditions and their treatments. Individuals vary in their genetic makeup and hence their response to microbial challenges, injury, risk factors, and treatments. Dental hygienists use genomic information to assess clients for periodontal and other disease risks and will use genetics in planning effective care and evaluating therapeutic outcomes in the not-too-distant future.

This chapter reviews major concepts related to inflammation, wound healing, and repair; genetics; and the differential diagnostic process that enables dental hygienists to integrate the biologic basis of health and disease into client care and acquire skills in diagnostic decision making.

INFLAMMATION[2]

A. A host response to cellular injury that consists of vascular responses, migration and activation of leukocytes, and systemic reactions
B. Cellular injury may occur because of trauma, genetic defects, physical and chemical agents, tissue necrosis, foreign bodies, immune reactions, and infections
C. A protective response designed to rid the body of the initial cause of cell injury and the consequences of that injury
D. Inflammatory response consists of a vascular reaction and a cellular reaction
   1. Reactions are mediated by chemical factors derived from plasma proteins or cells
   2. Reactions are produced in response to or activated by the inflammatory stimulus
E. Cardinal signs of inflammation
   1. Rubor (redness)—caused by increased vascularity
   2. Tumor (swelling)—caused by exudation of fluid
   3. Calor (heat)—caused by a combination of increased blood flow and the release of inflammatory mediators
   4. Dolar (pain)—caused by the stretching of pain receptors and nerves by inflammatory exudates and by the release of chemical mediators
   5. Functio laesa (loss of function)—caused by a combination of the above effects
F. Types of inflammation
   1. Acute
      a. Characterized by rapid onset and short duration
      b. Manifests with exudation of fluid and plasma proteins and emigration of leukocytes, mainly neutrophils
   2. Chronic
      a. Longer duration
      b. Histologic manifestation identified by the presence of lymphocytes and macrophages, blood vessels, fibrosis, and tissue necrosis
G. Cells involved in inflammation (Figure 7-1)
   1. Neutrophil or polymorphonuclear leukocyte (PMN)
      a. First cell to emigrate to the site of injury
      b. Primary cell involved in acute inflammation
      c. Capable of phagocytosis
   2. Monocyte or macrophage
      a. Second white blood cell to emigrate to injured tissue, where it becomes a macrophage
      b. Capable of phagocytosis; helper during the immune response

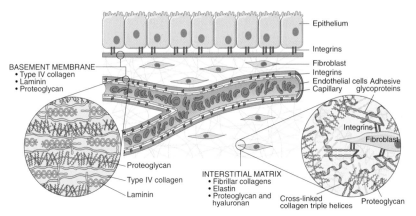

FIGURE 7-1 Components of acute and chronic inflammatory responses: circulating cells and proteins, cells of blood vessels, and cells and proteins of the extracellular matrix. *(From Kumar V, Abbas AK, Fausto N, Aster JC: Robbins and Cotran pathologic basis of disease, ed 8, Philadelphia, 2010, Saunders.)*

3. Lymphocytes and plasma cells
   a. Involved in both chronic inflammation and immune response
4. Eosinophil
   a. Involved in immune reactions and parasitic infections
5. Mast cells
   a. Involved in both acute and chronic inflammatory reactions (releasing chemical mediators) and in immune responses

Acute Inflammation

A. Vascular changes (Figure 7-2)
   1. Transient vasoconstriction of arterioles lasting several seconds
   2. Vasodilation
      a. First involves arterioles, and then results in the opening of new capillary beds
      b. Results in increased blood flow, which causes heat and redness
      c. Induced by chemical mediators such as histamine and nitric oxide on vascular smooth muscle
   3. Increased permeability of microvasculature
      a. An exudate of protein-rich fluid escapes into extravascular tissue, resulting in edema
      b. Proposed mechanisms that explain the leakage of endothelium in inflammation to allow this response are:
         (1) Formation of endothelial gaps in venules elicited by chemical mediators
            (a) Usually reversible
            (b) Lasts 15 to 30 minutes
         (2) Direct endothelial injury resulting in endothelial cell necrosis and detachment
            (a) Occurs in severe burns or lytic bacterial infections

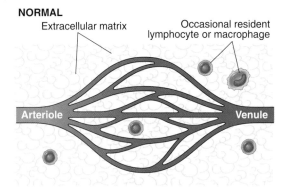

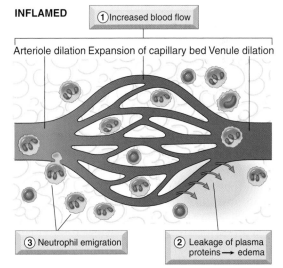

FIGURE 7-2 Major local manifestations of acute inflammation, compared with normal. *1,* Vascular dilation and increased blood flow (causing erythema and warmth). *2,* Extravasation and deposition of plasma fluid and proteins (edema). *3,* Leukocyte emigration and accumulation at the site of injury. *(From Kumar V, Abbas AK, Fausto N, Aster JC: Robbins and Cotran pathologic basis of disease, ed 8, Philadelphia, 2010, Saunders.)*

(b) Sustained for several hours

(c) Venules, capillaries, and arterioles affected

(3) Delayed prolonged leakage

(a) Begins after a delay of 2 to 12 hours

(b) Lasts for several hours or days

(c) Involves venules and capillaries

(d) Caused by thermal injury, radiation, and certain bacterial toxins

(4) Leukocyte-mediated endothelial injury

(5) Increased transcytosis across the endothelial cytoplasm

(6) Leakage from new blood vessels until new endothelial cells mature and form intercellular junctions

4. Concentration of red cells in small vessels and increased viscosity of blood, known as *stasis*

5. Leukocytes, mainly neutrophils, accumulate along the vascular endothelium (margination); the endothelium becomes lined by leukocytes (pavementing); leukocytes adhere to the endothelium and, soon after, migrate through the vascular wall into interstitial tissue (diapedesis or emigration)

a. Neutrophils predominate in the inflammatory infiltrate during the first 6 to 24 hours

b. Neutrophils are replaced by monocytes in 24 to 48 hours

B. Chemotaxis

1. Chemical attraction of leukocytes to emigrate in tissues

2. Exogenous agents are bacterial products

3. Endogenous chemoattractants

a. Components of the complement system, particularly C5a

b. Products of the lipoxygenase pathway such as leukotriene B4 (LTB4)

c. Cytokines, for example, interleukin 8 (IL-8)

C. Phagocytosis

1. Recognition and attachment

a. Mannose receptors and scavenger receptors bind and ingest microbes

b. Phagocytosis is greatly enhanced by opsonins, specific proteins such as immunoglobulin G (IgG) antibodies, fragments of the complement protein C3, and plasma lectins that are recognized by specific receptors on leukocytes

2. Engulfment

a. Extensions of the cytoplasm flow around the particle to be engulfed, resulting in the complete enclosure of the particle within a phagosome created by cell's plasma membrane

b. Neutrophils and monocytes become degranulated during this process

3. Killing and degradation

a. Eliminate infectious agents and necrotic cells

b. After the killing, acid hydrolases degrade the microbes within phagolysosomes

c. pH drops to between 4 and 5

4. Release of leukocyte products

a. Include lysosomal enzymes, reactive oxygen intermediates, and products of arachidonic acids such as prostaglandins and leukotrienes

b. These products may cause endothelial injury and tissue damage

c. If unchecked, this leukocyte infiltrate becomes harmful and is associated with many chronic systemic diseases

d. Also produce growth factors that aid in repair after tissue injury

5. Apoptosis-defined as programmed cell death used by the body to eliminate old cells

a. After phagocytosis, neutrophils undergo apoptotic cell death and are then ingested by macrophages

D. Chemical mediators (Table 7-1)

1. General principles

a. Originate from plasma proteins or from cells

(1) Plasma-derived mediators such as complement proteins and kinin are in precursor form and must be activated

(2) Cell-derived mediators such as histamine, prostaglandins, and cytokines come from mast cells, platelets, neutrophils, and monocytes or macrophages

b. Production of active mediators is triggered by microbial products or by host proteins

c. Mediators perform their activities by binding to specific receptors on target cells, having direct enzymatic activity, or mediating oxidative damage

d. Once activated, most mediators are short lived, but cause harmful effects

2. Vasoactive amines

a. Histamine

(1) Found in mast cells, blood basophils, and platelets

(2) Causes dilation of the arterioles and increases the permeability of venules; constricts large arteries

b. Serotonin

(1) Present in platelets and certain neuroendocrine cells

(2) Causes increased permeability during immunologic reactions

3. Plasma proteins

a. Complement system

(1) Consists of 20 component proteins found in greatest concentration in plasma

TABLE 7-1 Actions of the Principal Mediators of Inflammation

Mediator	Principal Sources	Actions
Cell-Derived		
Histamines	Mast cells, basophils, platelets	Vasodilation, increased vascular permeability, endothelial activation
Serotonin	Platelets	Vasodilation, increased vascular permeability
Prostaglandins	Mast cells, leukocytes	Vasodilation, pain, fever
Leukotrienes	Mast cells, leukocytes	Increased vascular permeability, chemotaxis, leukocyte adhesion and activation
Platelet-activating factor	Leukocytes, mast cells	Vasodilation, increased vascular permeability, leukocyte adhesion, chemotaxis, degranulation, oxidative burst
Reactive oxygen species	Leukocytes	Killing of microbes, tissue damage
Nitric oxide	Endothelium, macrophages	Vascular smooth muscle relaxation, killing of microbes
Cytokines (tumor necrosis factor [TNF], interleukin 1 [IL-1])	Macrophages, endothelial cells, mast cells	Local endothelial activation (expression of adhesion molecules), fever/pain/anorexia/hypotension, decreased vascular resistance (shock)
Chemokines	Leukocytes, activated macrophages	Chemotaxis, leukocyte activation
Plasma Protein-Derived		
Complement products (C5a, C3a, C4a)	Plasma (produced in liver)	Leukocyte chemotaxis and activation, vasodilation (mast cell stimulation)
Kinins	Plasma (produced in liver)	Increased vascular permeability, smooth muscle contraction, vasodilation, pain
Proteases activated during coagulation	Plasma (produced in liver)	Endothelial activation, leukocyte recruitment

(From Kumar V, Abbas AK, Fausto N Aster JC: Robbins and Cotran pathologic basis of disease, ed 8, Philadelphia, 2010, Saunders.)

(2) Causes increased vascular permeability, chemotaxis, and opsonization (the process by which certain cells are made more susceptible to phagocytosis)

(3) C3 and C5 are the most important inflammatory mediators of the complement components

    (a) Vascular phenomenon created by C3a, C5a, and to a lesser extent, C4a; stimulate histamine release from mast cells; called *anaphylatoxins* because they have similar effects in the reaction of anaphylaxis

    (b) Leukocyte adhesion, chemotaxis, and activation occur through C5a as a chemotactic agent for neutrophils, monocytes, eosinophils, and basophils

    (c) Phagocytosis enhanced by C3b, which acts as opsonin to facilitate foreign bodies being more efficiently engulfed by phagocytosis

b. Kinin system

    (1) Generates vasoactive peptides from plasma proteins called *kininogens* by the action of proteases known as *kallikreins*

    (2) Bradykinin increases vascular permeability; causes the contraction of smooth muscle, dilation of blood vessels, and pain

    (3) Is triggered by the activation of Hageman factor (factor XII of the intrinsic clotting pathway)

    (4) Is short lived; quickly inactivated by the enzyme kininase

c. Clotting system

    (1) Induces the formation of thrombin, fibrinopeptides, and factor XII, which have inflammatory properties

    (2) Activated by substances released during tissue destruction, such as collagen, proteinases, kallikrein, and bacterial endotoxins

    (3) Prevents the spread of infection and inflammation; localizes microorganisms

at the site of phagocytosis; helps clot formation to stop bleeding and for repair, chemotaxis of neutrophils, and increased permeability of vessels

4. Other mediators

    a. Arachidonic acid

        (1) A lipid mediator that is a short-range hormone; is formed rapidly and acts locally

        (2) Produces prostaglandins, leukotrienes, and lipoxins

            (a) Prostaglandins, including PGE_2, PGD_2, PGF_{2a}, PGI_2, and TxA_2, are most important in inflammation, causing increased permeability, the chemotactic effects of other mediators, and vasodilation resulting in edema as well as pain and fever in inflammation

            (b) Pathway initiating these prostaglandins occurs by two different enzymes, COX-1 and COX-2

                [1] COX-1 produces prostaglandins that are involved in inflammation and also maintains homeostasis

                [2] COX-2 stimulates the production of prostaglandins involved in the inflammatory reactions noted above and may play a role in normal homeostasis

            (c) Leukotrienes cause intense vasoconstriction, bronchospasm, and increased vascular permeability

                [1] Important in the pathogenesis of bronchial asthma

            (d) Lipoxins inhibit leukocyte recruitment, neutrophil chemotaxis, and adhesion to the endothelium and may play a role in resolving inflammation

            (e) Resolvins inhibit leukocyte recruitment and activation by inhibiting the production of cytokines

                [1] Aspirin may work by stimulating the production of resolvins

            (f) Platelet-activating factor (PAF) causes platelet stimulation, vasoconstriction, bronchoconstriction, vasodilation, and increased venular permeability; far more potent than histamine; increased leukocyte adhesion to endothelium; chemotaxis, degranulation, and oxidative burst; also boosts synthesis of other mediators

        (g) Tumor necrosis factor and interleukin 1

            [1] Two major cytokines that mediate inflammation and are produced primarily by macrophages

            [2] Responsible for endothelial activation, which induces the synthesis of endothelial adhesion molecules and chemical mediators; producing enzymes associated with matrix remodeling; and increasing the surface thrombogenicity of endothelium

            [3] Induces the systemic acute phase responses of infection and injury, including fever, loss of appetite, release of neutrophils, corticotropin, and corticosteroids

            [4] TNF—responsible for the hemodynamic effects of septic shock, regulates body mass, and contributes to cachexia (wasting away) that is part of some infections and diseases

        (h) Chemokines—small proteins that act as chemoattractants for leukocytes and control the normal migration of cells through various tissues

        (i) Nitric oxide (NO)—released from endothelial cells; causes vasodilation by relaxing vascular smooth muscle; microbicidal; a mediator of host defense against infection

        (j) Lysosomal components of leukocytes

            [1] Neutrophils and monocytes, contain lysosomal granules; granules contain a variety of enzymes used for phagocytosis (such as lysozyme, collagenase, alkaline phosphatase, elastase)

            [2] These enzymes are destructive, and if unchecked, can potentiate further inflammation and tissue damage

        (k) Oxygen-derived free radicals may be released from leukocytes following a phagocytic event and are potent mediators

            [1] Can be damaging to the host, causing endothelial cell damage and increased vascular permeability, inactivation of antiproteases, and injury to other cell types such as parenchymal cells and red blood cells

b. Neuropeptides, such as substance P and neurokinin A, play a role in the initiation and propagation of inflammatory response

E. Outcomes of inflammation
   1. Complete resolution
   2. Healing by connective tissue replacement
   3. Progression of tissue response to chronic inflammation

Chronic Inflammation

A. Causes
   1. Persistent infections
   2. Prolonged exposure to potentially toxic agents
   3. Autoimmunity
B. Characteristics
   1. Infiltration with macrophages, lymphocytes, and plasma cells
   2. Tissue destruction, a hallmark of chronic inflammation
   3. Attempts at healing by connective tissue replacement and fibrosis
C. Cells involved
   1. Macrophages, lymphocytes, plasma cells, eosinophils, and mast cells
   2. Produce granulomatous inflammation characterized by focal accumulation of activated macrophages that develops an epithelioid appearance
   3. Products of these cells eliminate injurious agents and help initiate repair but are also responsible for much of the tissue injury in chronic inflammation
D. Role of lymphatics
   1. Secondary line of defense that monitors the extravascular fluids
   2. Help drain edema from the extravascular space
E. Systemic effects of inflammation—acute phase response or the systemic inflammatory response syndrome
   1. Fever—produced in response to pyrogens that act by stimulating prostaglandin synthesis
   2. Acute phase proteins, including C-reactive protein (CRP), fibrinogen, and serum amyloid A protein (SAA) increase during the inflammatory process
      a. Bind to microbial cell walls and act as opsonin and fix complement
      b. Prolonged activation causes secondary amyloidosis in chronic inflammation
      c. Elevated CRP used as a marker for increased risk of myocardial infarction in persons with coronary artery disease

3. Leukocytosis
   a. Common feature in bacterial infections resulting in elevated to extremely high levels of different types of leukocytes, depending on the type of infection
   b. Normal count of white blood cells is 4000 to 10,000/mm^3 in blood
   c. In an inflammatory reaction, particularly with an infection, the white blood cell count can increase to 15,000 or 20,000 and sometimes to extremely high levels of well over 40,000/mm^3
4. Sepsis
   a. In severe bacterial infections, large quantities of cytokines, particularly TNF and IL-1, cause thrombosis and coagulation
   b. Eventually, hypoglycemia and cardiovascular failure occur, resulting in septic shock
   c. Multiple organs can be affected by inflammation and intravascular thrombosis, resulting in organ failure
F. Systemic disease affected by chronic inflammation
   1. Cardiovascular disease (CVD)
   2. Cancer
   3. Diabetes mellitus
   4. Asthma
   5. Chronic obstructive pulmonary disease (COPD)
   6. Alzheimer's disease
   7. Periodontal diseases

REGENERATION AND WOUND HEALING[2]

A. Definitions
   1. Regeneration—growth of cells and tissues to replace lost structures
   2. Healing—a tissue response to a wound, inflammatory process, or cell necrosis in organs that cannot regenerate; involves either regeneration or scar formation (Figure 7-3)
B. General concepts
   1. Involves a complex process that includes a number of steps
      a. An inflammatory response caused by the initial injury
      b. Proliferation of parenchymal and connective tissue cells
      c. Formation of new blood vessels (angiogenesis) and granulation tissue
      d. Synthesis of extracellular matrix (ECM) proteins and collagen deposition
      e. Tissue remodeling
      f. Wound contraction
      g. Acquisition of wound strength

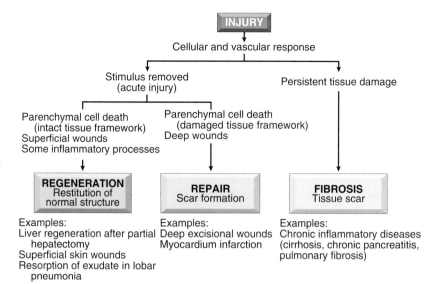

FIGURE 7-3 Repair responses after injury and inflammation. Repair after acute injury has several outcomes, including normal tissue restitution and healing with scar formation. Healing in chronic injury involves scar formation and fibrosis. *(From Kumar V, Abbas AK, Fausto N, Aster JC: Robbins and Cotran pathologic basis of disease, ed 8, Philadelphia, 2010, Saunders.)*

2. Repair process—a combination of regeneration and scar formation that is influenced by local and systemic factors that may inhibit or prolong the wound healing process
   a. Local factors
      (1) Size, location, and type of wound
      (2) Infection
      (3) Early movement
      (4) Foreign material
      (5) Ionizing radiation
   b. Systemic factors
      (1) Blood supply
      (2) Metabolic factors (e.g., diabetes)
      (3) Corticosteroids
      (4) Cytotoxic drugs
      (5) Nutrition
3. Generally, repair begins early in inflammation—formation of granulation tissue, which is a hallmark of healing
   a. Pink, soft, granular appearance on the surface of wounds
   b. Formation of new small blood vessels and the proliferation of fibroblasts
   c. New vessels tend to leak; edematous
   d. Amount of granulation tissue that forms depends on the size of the wound and the intensity of the inflammation
C. Angiogenesis
   1. Occurs from the branching and extension of adjacent blood vessels and the recruitment of endothelial progenitor cells (EPCs) from bone marrow
   2. Angiogenesis from adjacent blood vessels occurs through the vasodilation and increased permeability of existing vessels, degradation of ECM,

migration of endothelial cells, maturation of endothelial cells and remodeling into capillary tubes, and recruitment of periendothelial cells to support endothelial tubes and to form the mature vessel
3. Growth factors such as vascular endothelial growth factor (VEGF) support adult tissues undergoing angiogenesis
4. Directed migration of endothelial cells—controlled by ECM proteins, including integrins, matricellular proteins, and proteinases
D. Scar formation—three processes occur (emigration and proliferation of fibroblasts in the site of injury, deposition of ECM, and tissue remodeling)
   1. Fibroblast emigration and proliferation
      a. Migration of fibroblasts to the site of injury and their proliferation triggered by growth factors that come from platelets, inflammatory cells, and activated endothelium
   2. ECM deposition
      a. Fibroblasts deposit increased amounts of ECM
      b. Fibrillar collagens form a major portion of connective tissue in repair sites; help develop the strength of the healing wound
      c. Fibroblasts begin forming 3 to 5 days after injury and continue for several weeks
      d. Growth factors that stimulate fibroblasts also stimulate ECM synthesis
      e. Granulation tissue is converted into a scar composed of fibroblasts, dense collagen, fragments of elastic tissue, and other ECM components; richly vascularized granulation tissue transforms into a pale, avascular scar

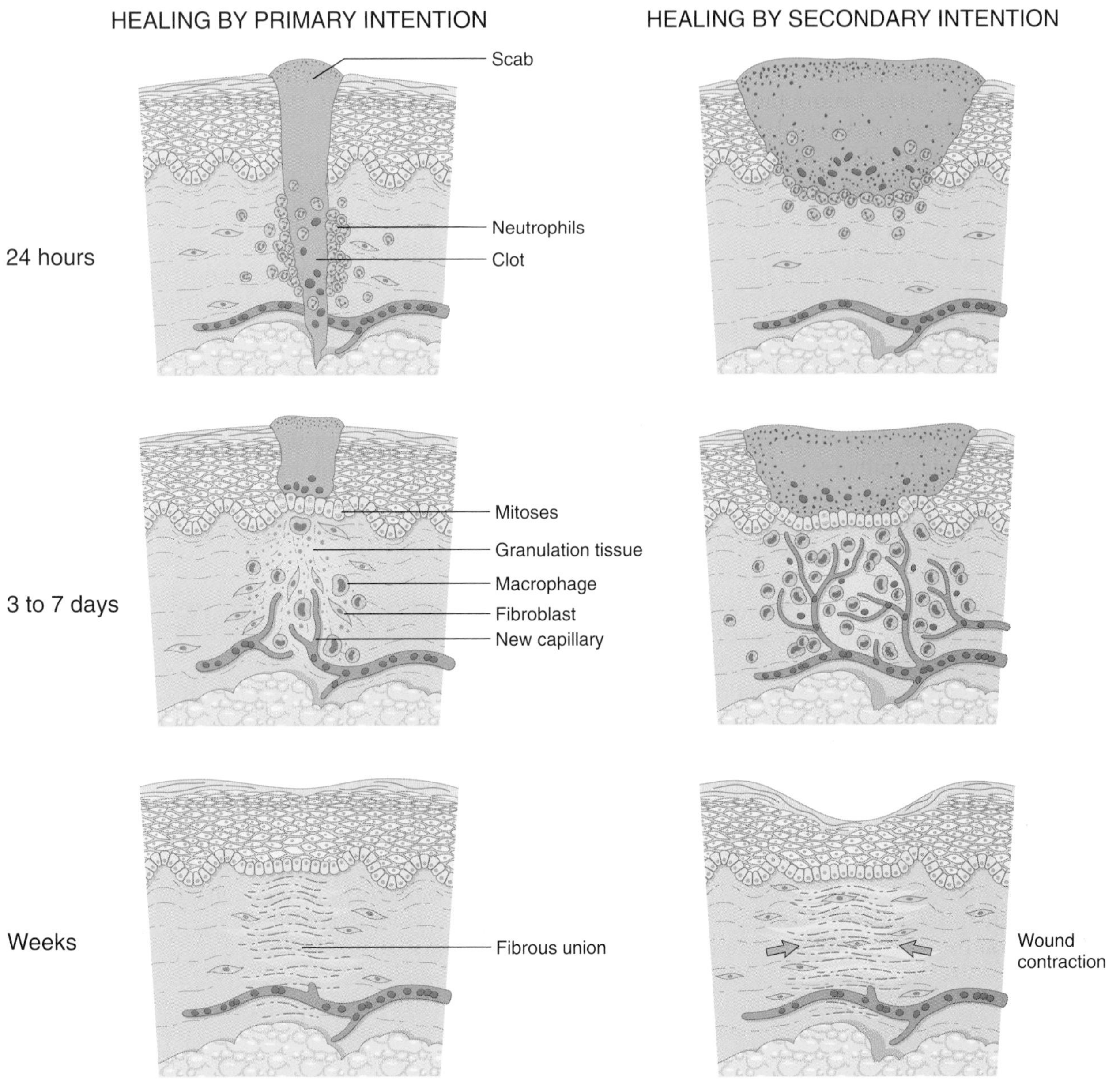

HEALING BY PRIMARY INTENTION   HEALING BY SECONDARY INTENTION

FIGURE 7-4 Steps in wound healing by primary intention (*left*) and secondary intention (*right*). Note large amounts of granulation tissue and wound contraction in healing by secondary intention. *(From Kumar V, Abbas AK, Fausto N Aster JC: Robbins and Cotran pathologic basis of disease, ed 8, Philadelphia, 2010, Saunders.)*

3. Tissue remodeling
   a. Degradation of ECM components causes tissue remodeling; achieved through matrix metalloproteinases (MMPs)
   b. MMPs are produced by fibroblasts, macrophages, neutrophils, synovial cells, and some epithelial cells; their secretion is induced by certain growth factors, physical stress, and phagocytosis; they are inhibited by steroids and other growth factors

E. Cutaneous wound healing (Figure 7-4)
   1. Healing by primary intention—primary union (e.g., surgical incision and placement of sutures)
      a. Narrow incisional space fills with clotted blood, a clot forms, and a scab covers the surface of the wound; the clot stops the bleeding and acts as a scaffold for migrating cells
      b. Within 24 hours, neutrophils appear at the margins of the incision and move toward the clot; in 24 to 48 hours, epithelial cells move

from the wound edges and fuse in the midline beneath the scab to close the wound; a basement membrane is formed

  c. Within 3 days, neutrophils are replaced by macrophages, and granulation tissue forms

    (1) Collagen fibers begin to form in the margins of the incision

    (2) Epithelial cells proliferate and thicken the epidermal layer

  d. By day 5, the incisional space is filled with granulation tissue

    (1) Collagen fibers become more abundant and start to bridge the incision

    (2) A mature epidermal architecture with surface keratinization appears

  e. During week 2, proliferation of collagen and fibroblasts continues

    (1) The inflammatory process has largely dissipated

    (2) Blanching begins as the incisional scar forms

  f. By week 4, the scar is composed of connective tissue and an intact epidermis; the tensile strength of the wound increases

  2. Healing by secondary intention—secondary union (e.g., wounds with separated edges)

    a. Abundant granulation tissue grows in from the margin to complete the repair

    b. The inflammatory reaction is more intense because of the presence of a larger clot and more necrotic debris and exudates that must be removed from the defect

    c. Wound contraction occurs in larger surface wounds because of myofibroblasts that have the characteristics of smooth muscle cells

    d. Substantial scar formation and thinning of the epidermis occurs

F. Wound strength

  1. Tissues recover approximately 70% to 80% of tensile strength over a 3-month period compared with intact skin

  2. Recovery of wound strength comes from an excess of collagen synthesis over collagen degradation during the first 2 months of healing and from structural modifications of collagen fibers after collagen synthesis is complete

G. Complications of cutaneous wound healing

  1. Deficient scar formation leading to wound dehiscence or ulceration—often seen after abdominal surgery or in lower extremity wounds with peripheral vascular disease

  2. Excessive scar formation

    a. Raised scar (hypertrophic scar)

    b. Scar grows beyond the boundaries of the original wound and does not regress (keloid)

  3. Contracture

    a. Exaggeration of the normal contraction process of wound healing, resulting in the deformity of the wound and surrounding tissues

    b. Common after serious burn injuries; can affect joint mobility

H. Fibrosis

  1. Processes that occur in cutaneous scar formation because of extensive deposition of collagen; similar to the fibrosis associated with chronic inflammatory diseases (rheumatoid arthritis, cirrhosis, etc.)

  2. Characterized by the persistence of initial stimuli for fibrosis or the development of immune and autoimmune reactions that sustain the synthesis and secretion of growth factors and other biologically active molecules

  3. May cause permanent dysfunction

REGENERATIVE MEDICINE[3]

A. Stem cells

  1. Characterized by self-renewal abilities and the capacity to generate differentiated cells

    a. Autogenous stem cells—derived from the individual being treated

    b. Allogenous stem cells—derived from other individuals

    c. May be totipotent, multipotent, or unipotent

    d. Process of differentiation is known as *plasticity* or *transdifferentiation*

  2. Types (Table 7-2)

    a. Embryonic stem cells (ES)

    (1) Pluripotent and can generate all tissue of the body

    (2) Isolated from inner cell mass of blastocytes

    (3) May be used in the future for the treatment of organs affected by diabetes, neurologic defects, myocardial infarction, and liver damage

    b. Adult stem cells or somatic stem cells

    (1) More restricted capacity to generate different cell types

    (2) Potential for adult stem cells to be reprogrammed into pluripotent cells similar to ES

    (3) Found in skin, lining of intestine, cornea, brain, and hematopoietic tissue (bone marrow, umbilical cord, etc.)

  3. Types of adult stem cells

    a. Induced pluripotent stem cells (iPs)

    (1) Adult cells that behave like embryonic cells

TABLE 7-2 Types of Stem Cells

Type of Stem Cell	May Differentiate to ...
Embryonic	Any type of cell
Amniotic fluid–derived	Cartilage cells Fat cells Bone cells Muscle cells Endothelial cells Neuron-like cells Liver cells
Umbilical cord	Liver cells Skeletal muscle cells Neural tissue Immune cells
Bone marrow–derived mesenchymal	Bone cells Cartilage cells Muscle cells Fat cells Neuron-like cells Pancreatic islet beta-cells
Tooth-derived	Neural cell lineages Bone cells Cartilage cells Muscle cells Fat cells Pancreatic islet beta-cells
Adipose-derived	Fat cells Cartilage cells Muscle cells Neuronal cells Bone cells
Induced pluripotent stem cells	Any type of cell, potentially

(From Mao JJ: Stem cells and the future of dental care, NY State Dent J 74(2):20–24, 2008.)

b. Amniotic fluid–derived stem cells (AFSCs)
   (1) Isolated from the aspirates of amniocentesis during genetic screening
   (2) Capacity to differentiate into multiple lineages such as chondrocytes, adipocytes, osteoblasts, myocytes, endothelial cells, neuron-like cells, and live cells
c. Umbilical cord blood stem cells (UCBSCs)
   (1) Derived from the blood of the umbilical cord
   (2) Differentiate into cells that resemble liver cells, skeletal muscle, neural tissue, pancreatic cells, immune cells, and mesenchymal stem cells
d. Bone marrow–derived stem cells (BMSCs)
   (1) Consists of both hematopoietic stem cells and stromal cells (mesenchymal stem

cells) that generate bone, cartilage, other connective tissues and fat
   (2) Most common commercially available stem cells
e. Adipose-derived stem cells (ASCs)
   (1) Derived from lipectomy or liposuction aspirates
   (2) Differentiate into adipocytes, chondrocytes, myocytes, and neuronal and osteoblastic lineages; may provide hematopoietic support
f. Dental stem cells
   (1) Develop from material created during the development of the nervous system and can differentiate into neural cell lines
   (2) Sources include primary teeth, permanent third molars, or extracted healthy permanent teeth and periodontal ligament
   (3) Have been transdifferentiated in the laboratory to form bone, nervous tissue, and pancreatic—beta islet cells that produce insulin
   (4) Current animal studies are exploring applications to regenerate bone, cartilage, skin, nerve and brain tissues, adipose, and heart and muscle tissues
   (5) Dental application may include tooth, root, jaw, and salivary gland regeneration and cranial bone repair

GENETICS[2]

A. General concepts
   1. Almost all health-related conditions (except trauma) have a genetic component; common diseases such as cardiovascular disease, dyslipidemia, diabetes, and cancer, as well as dental caries, periodontitis, oral cancer, cleft lip, and craniofacial abnormalities, are associated with genetic factors
   2. Draft sequencing of the human genome has been completed; provides information about biologic inheritance and health consequences
   3. Genome—all of the deoxyribonucleic acid (DNA) of a given organism
   4. Genomics—the study of all the genes in the genome, their extensive DNA sequences, and their interactions
   5. Gene—a segment of DNA that contains instructions for making a specific protein or proteins required by the human body; found in succession along the length of chromosomes; humans have 20,000 to 25,000 genes
   6. About 99.5% of DNA sequences are shared among human beings; the diversity of humans

is encoded in approximately 0.5% of human DNA; this 0.5% represents 15 million base pairs

7. Chromosomes—thread-like structures in the nucleus of a cell; made of DNA and structural proteins; human cells other than egg and sperm have 46 chromosomes (23 pairs); egg and sperm cells have 23 chromosomes

8. Molecular biology has resulted in the development of recombinant DNA technology that has allowed the isolation and characterization of genes through cloning, production of human biologically active agents, study of gene therapy, and development of molecular probes to aid in disease diagnosis

B. Mutations
  1. Mutations represent permanent changes in the DNA code; they can be beneficial, neutral, or harmful
     a. Four letters of the DNA code: A = adenine, T = thymine, C = cytosine, and G = guanine; one letter can be changed, deleted, or added; entire pieces of code can be spelled backward, cut and pasted, or cut short, which can change the form and function or the end protein product in the body
     b. The impact of a mutation is dependent on the environment in which it is expressed
     c. Classification of mutations
        (1) Genome mutations—involve the loss or gain of whole chromosomes resulting in monosomy or trisomy
        (2) Chromosome mutations—rearrangement of genetic material that gives rise to structural changes in the chromosome; most are incompatible with survival
        (3) Submicroscopic gene mutations—represent the vast majority of mutations associated with hereditary diseases; may result in a partial or complete deletion of a gene or may affect a single base

C. Single-gene disorders
  1. Autosomal dominant inheritance
     a. An affected person usually has an affected parent
     b. An affected person has a 50% chance of passing the trait to an offspring
     c. Both genders are equally likely to be affected, and both can transmit the condition
     d. Dominant traits are usually seen in multiple, successive generations
  2. Additional characteristics of autosomal dominant disorders
     a. Some affected persons do not have affected parents; the disorder is caused by new mutations involving either the egg or the sperm

and seems to occur in the germ cells of older fathers
     b. Some inherit the mutant gene but are phenotypically normal (called *reduced* or *incomplete penetrance*)
     c. If the trait is seen in all individuals but is expressed differently among them, the phenomenon is called *variable expressivity*; combinations of these traits can be less or more severe among individuals even within the same family
     d. In many conditions, onset is delayed, and symptoms do not appear until adulthood
     e. Biochemical mechanism is either loss-of-function mutations or gain-of-function mutations; the effects of these mutations depend on the nature of the enzyme protein affected
     f. Examples of autosomal dominant disorders
        (1) Huntington's disease
        (2) Neurofibromatosis
        (3) Polycystic kidney disease
        (4) von Willebrand disease
        (5) Marfan syndrome
        (6) Ehlers-Danlos syndrome
        (7) Osteogenesis imperfecta
        (8) Familial hypercholesterolemia
  3. Autosomal recessive inheritance
     a. Both genders equally likely to be affected
     b. Disease often found in siblings; affected individuals often have unaffected parents
     c. Offspring of the affected person are carriers of the gene mutation
     d. If a child is born to two carrier parents and is not affected, a two thirds chance of the child being a carrier is present
     e. Carriers are usually not clinically affected
     f. Two carrier parents have a 25% chance with each conception to have an affected child
     g. Onset is frequently early in life
     h. In many cases, enzyme proteins are affected by a loss of function
     i. Examples of autosomal recessive disorders
        (1) Cystic fibrosis
        (2) Phenylketonuria
        (3) Sickle cell anemia
        (4) Thalassemias
        (5) Congenital adrenal hyperplasia
        (6) Neurogenic muscular atrophies
        (7) Spinal muscular atrophy
  4. X-linked recessive inheritance
     a. Primarily affects males
     b. Sons of carrier females have a 50% chance of receiving the gene and expressing that trait or condition
     c. Carrier females may show no disease trait or mild symptoms only

d. No male-to-male transmission

e. Affected males transmit the genes to all daughters but not to their sons; all daughters are carriers

f. Uncles and cousins may also be affected

g. Examples of X-linked recessive disorders
  (1) Duchenne muscular dystrophy
  (2) Hemophilia A and B
  (3) Chronic granulomatous disease
  (4) Glucose-6-phosphate dehydrogenase (G6PD) deficiency
  (5) Agammaglobulinemia
  (6) Diabetes insipidus
  (7) Fragile-X syndrome

5. Biochemical and molecular basis of single gene disorders

a. The genetic defect may lead to the formation of an abnormal protein as reduction in the output of gene product

b. The pattern of inheritance is related to the kind of protein affected by the mutation

c. The mechanisms are classified into four categories:
  (1) Enzyme defects and their consequences
  (2) Defects in membrane receptors and transport systems
  (3) Alterations in structure, function or quality of nonenzyme proteins
  (4) Mutations resulting in unusual reactions to drugs—pharmacogenetics

6. Disorders with multifactorial inheritance

a. Result from the combined actions of environmental influences and two or more mutant genes having additive effects

b. The greater the number of inherited deleterious genes, the more severe is the expression of the disease

c. Risk is greater in siblings of persons having severe expressions of the disorder

d. Frequency of concordance for identical twins is between 20% and 40%

e. Examples of disorders with multifactorial inheritance
  (1) Cleft lip, cleft palate, or both
  (2) Congenital heart disease
  (3) Coronary heart disease
  (4) Hypertension
  (5) Gout
  (6) Diabetes mellitus
  (7) Pyloric stenosis

7. Diagnosis of genetic diseases—requires examination of genetic material through cytogenetic analysis or molecular analysis

a. Cytogenetic analysis involves karyotyping, an organized graphic representation of the chromosomes in a single cell
  (1) Normal human karyotypes show 23 pairs of chromosomes, numbered from larger to smaller
  (2) The twenty-third pair comprises the sex chromosomes (XX = female, XY = male)
  (3) Karyotypes are described using a shorthand notation, with the total number of chromosomes listed first, followed by the sex chromosome complement, and then a description of the abnormalities in ascending numerical order

b. Prenatal chromosome analysis should be offered to individuals at risk; can be performed on cells obtained by amniocentesis, on chorionic villus biopsy, or on umbilical cord blood

c. Postnatal chromosome analysis can be performed on peripheral blood lymphocytes in cases of multiple congenital anomalies, unexplained mental retardation or developmental delay, suspected genetic disorders such as Turner syndrome or fragile-X syndrome, infertility, or multiple spontaneous abortions

d. Recombinant DNA technology is also used for the diagnosis of inherited diseases, as it is highly sensitive; tests are not dependent on a gene product produced only in certain specialized cells
  (1) Testing performed through either direct gene diagnosis using polymerase chain reaction (PCR) analysis or indirect DNA diagnosis through linkage analysis, which involves studying several relevant family members
  (2) 0.1 μL of blood or cells scraped from the buccal mucosa is sufficient for PCR analysis
  (3) Salivary DNA-PCR used to evaluate periodontal status
    (a) MyPerioPathSM® identifies the type and quantity of 13 periodontopathic bacteria
    (b) MyPerioIDSM PST® determines if the patient is genetically predisposed to periodontal disease by evaluating IL-1 polymorphism

e. Identifying molecular genetic signatures for acquired diseases
  (1) Diagnosis and management of cancer
    (a) Detection of tumor-specific acquired mutations and cytogenic alterations that are hallmarks of specific tumors
    (b) Determination of clonality as an indicator of neoplastic condition

(c) Identification of specific gene alterations that can direct therapeutic choices

(d) Determination of treatment efficacy

(e) Determination of Gleeve-resistant forms of chronic myeloid leukemia or gastrointestinal stromal tumors

(2) Diagnosis and management of infectious diseases

(a) Detection of microorganisms and specific genetic material for definitive diagnosis (i.e., human immunodeficiency virus [HIV], human papilloma virus [HPV], herpes simplex virus [HSV])

(b) Identification of specific genetic alterations in the genomes of microbes that are associated with drug resistance

(c) Determination of treatment efficacy (e.g., assessing viral loads in HIV and hepatitis C virus)

f. Ribonucleic acid (RNA) analysis

(1) Not as stable as DNA-based diagnosis, but useful for the detection and quantification of RNA viruses such as HIV and hepatitis C virus

(2) Becoming an important tool for the molecular stratification of tumors

8. Referral for genetic counseling[4]

a. Clients who present with evidence of suspected or diagnosed genetic disorder should be referred to a genetics center for evaluation and counseling; any genetic health condition or risk that affects one individual can affect that person's biologic and extended family

b. Genetics professionals can be consulted through the National Society for Genetics Counselors (NSGC) Web site at http://www.nsgc.org

c. Document referrals are made to a physician, a genetics professional, or both by recording:

(1) Causes for concern

(2) Possible diagnosis (if known)

(3) Family history information obtained

(4) Relevant oral examination findings, radiographs, and records

d. Genetics consultation involves

(1) Confirming, diagnosing, or ruling out the genetic condition

(2) Identifying medical management issues

(3) Determining genetic risks

(4) Providing psychosocial support

DIFFERENTIAL DIAGNOSIS[1]

A. Diagnostic approaches

1. Appearance recognition—clinical manifestations of routine oral diseases can be recognized by their characteristic appearances because no other diseases produce these lesions (e.g., dental caries, gingivitis, periodontitis)

2. Differential diagnosis—determination of which of two or more diseases with similar signs and symptoms is the one manifested in the client

a. Requires a comparison of signs and symptoms and other pertinent details against the known features of all diseases that can produce the observed primary manifestation

b. Reflects a conceptual process and a listing of pathologic conditions in the order of most likely to least likely

c. Pathoses are ruled out on the basis of examinations, tests such as blood assays (see reference 5 for specific examples), urinalysis, biopsy, and so on.

B. Conceptual stages of the differential diagnosis process

1. Stage 1: Classification of the abnormality by primary manifestation—describe the general nature of the lesion that makes it different from normal tissue

a. A white mucosal discoloration without loss of mucosal integrity or enlargement

b. A dark discoloration without loss of mucosal integrity or enlargement

c. Loss of mucosal integrity or ulceration without enlargement

d. Enlargement of soft tissues

e. Radiographic manifestations of a lesion originating in bone

f. Concurrence of several dissimilar abnormalities suggestive of a syndrome

2. Stage 2: Listing of secondary features and contributing factors—objectively describe the secondary features of the lesion; reserve making judgments about the diagnosis based on information obtained

a. Visual examination

(1) Specific location of the lesion

(2) Shape of the lesion and contours of tissue

(3) Size of the lesion

(4) Occurrence of the lesion as isolated, multifocal, or diffuse

(5) Delineation of the borders of the abnormality from adjacent tissue

(6) Consistency of appearance as homogeneous or heterogeneous

(7) Surface color and texture

(8) Alteration of adjacent structures, such as displacement of teeth

b. Palpation

(1) Degree of compressibility

(2) Tenderness during compression

(3) Alteration in color during compression

c. Auscultation

(1) Wheezing

(2) Popping and clicking of the temporo-mandibular joint

(3) Clicking of ill-fitting dentures

d. Probing

(1) Tissue defects

(2) Exudates

e. Aspiration

(1) Pus

(2) Cysts and nodules

f. Evaluation of function

(1) Tear production

(2) Salivary glands

(3) Tongue

(4) Muscles of mastication

(5) Neurologic function

g. Client awareness

(1) Pain, discomfort, or altered function

(2) Duration

(3) Course as constant, healing with recurrence, or steady progression

(4) Response to factors such as stress and certain foods

h. Demographics

(1) Age

(2) Gender

(3) Race and ethnicity

i. Habits

(1) Alcohol use

(2) Tobacco use

(3) Oral

(4) Other (ask client)

j. Recent history

(1) Injury

(2) Infection

(3) Surgery

k. Medical conditions

(1) Chronic diseases

(2) Recent acute illnesses

l. Current medical treatment

(1) Medications

(2) Other treatment

3. Stage 3: Listing of conditions capable of causing primary manifestations

a. Consider the variety of abnormalities that cause the condition and compare them with the client's abnormality

b. Create a list of plausible diagnoses

4. Stage 4: Elimination of unlikely causes

a. Identify contradictions between the features of the lesion and the known characteristics of the diagnostic possibilities

b. The category of the lesion determines the secondary features that are most reliable; then eliminate those conditions that appear least likely

c. Elimination of malignant neoplasia as a possible cause is often more important than achieving a definitive diagnosis

5. Stage 5: Ranking of possible causes by probability

a. Rank the diseases that could explain the abnormality on the basis of the number of secondary features exhibited that correspond with the typical features of each possible diagnosis

6. Stage 6: Determination of a working diagnosis

a. The condition considered the most likely cause of the lesion is referred to as the *working, tentative,* or *preliminary diagnosis* or the *clinical impression*

b. Provides the basis for additional diagnostic testing and for the initial clinical management of the condition

c. When all of the diseases except one have been eliminated from the differential diagnosis, then that provides the definitive diagnosis

d. Re-evaluate to verify the correct diagnosis and that the client has responded to treatment without recurrence

@ WEB SITE INFORMATION AND RESOURCES

SOURCE	WEB SITE ADDRESS	DESCRIPTION
National Human Genome Research Institute/Talking Genetics Glossary	www.genome.gov/glossary.cfm	Talking glossary of genetic terms. Also available in Spanish
Centers for Disease Control/Office of Genomics and Disease Prevention	www.cdc.gov/genomics	Information about human genomic discoveries and how they can be used to improve health and prevent disease
National Library of Medicine/Genetics Home Reference	http://ghr.nlm.nih.gov/	Allows users to search for information on diseases, tutorials about basic concepts in genetics, and educational resources
GeneTests/University of Washington	http://www.genetests.org/	Medical genetics information, including PowerPoint presentations

REFERENCES

1. Coleman GC, Nelson JF: *Principles of oral diagnosis*, St Louis, 1993, Mosby.
2. Kumar V, Abbas AK, Fausto N, Aster JC: *Robbins and Cotran pathologic basis of disease*, ed 8, Philadelphia, 2010, Saunders.
3. Mao JJ, Giannobile WV, Helms JA, et al: *Craniofacial tissue engineering by stem cells, J Dent Res* 85(11):966–979, 2006.
4. National Coalition for Health Professional: *Education in Genetics (NCHPEG), Principles of genetics for health professionals, Genetic Primer*, June 2004: Available at http://www.nchpeg.org; Accessed December 23, 2004.
5. Pagana KD, Pagana TS: *Mosby's manual of diagnostic and laboratory tests*, ed 4, Philadelphia, 2010, Mosby.

SUGGESTED READINGS

Mariotti A: *A primer on inflammation, Compendium Cont Edu Dent* 25:7 (Suppl 1):7–15, 2004.
National Coalition for Health Professional *Education in Genetics (NCHPEG), Principles of genetics for health professionals, Genetic Primer June 2004*: Available at http://www.nchpeg.org: Accessed February 4, 2011.
Mao JJ, Collins FM. *Stem cells: Sources, therapies and the dental professions*, RDH 49–57, 2009.

CHAPTER 7 REVIEW QUESTIONS

Answers and Rationales to Review Questions are available on this text's accompanying Evolve site. See inside front cover for details

*e*volve

1. A host response to injury that consists of vascular responses, activation of white blood cells, and systemic reactions refers to:
   a. Inflammation
   b. Regeneration
   c. Autoimmune response
   d. Angiogenesis

2. The inflammatory response consists of a vascular reaction and a cellular reaction. These reactions are mediated by chemical factors derived from plasma proteins or cells.
   a. Both statements are true
   b. Both statements are false
   c. The first statement is true, and the second statement is false
   d. The first statement is false, and the second statement is true

3. Heat (calor) found during the inflammatory response is caused by:
   a. Vasoconstriction of blood vessels
   b. Exudation of fluid
   c. Increased blood flow
   d. Stretching of pain receptors

4. Acute inflammation is characterized by rapid onset and short duration. It is manifested by the presence of lymphocytes and macrophages, blood vessels, and fibrosis.
   a. Both statements are true
   b. Both statements are false
   c. The first statement is true, and the second statement is false
   d. The first statement is false, and the second statement is true

5. All of the following white blood cells are involved in the immune response EXCEPT one. Which one is the EXCEPTION?
   a. Macrophage
   b. Neutrophil
   c. Lymphocyte
   d. Eosinophil

6. The white blood cell that emigrates to injured tissue and converts to a macrophage is the:
   a. Neutrophil
   b. Mast cell
   c. Lymphocyte
   d. Monocyte

7. During the inflammatory response, neutrophils are replaced by monocytes in:
   a. 2 to 12 hours
   b. 6 to 12 hours
   c. 12 to 24 hours
   d. 24 to 48 hours

8. Phagocytosis is greatly enhanced by:
   a. Plasma lectins
   b. Complement proteins
   c. Opsonins
   d. All of the above

9. During which phase of phagocytosis does the pH drop?
   a. Engulfment
   b. Killing and degradation
   c. Release of leukocyte products
   d. Apoptosis

10. Chemical mediators bind to specific receptor on target cells. Most are short lived, and harmless.
    a. Both statements are true
    b. Both statements are false
    c. The first statement is true, and the second statement is false
    d. The first statement is false, and the second statement is true

11. Which chemical mediator produces prostaglandins, leukotrienes, and lipoxins?
    a. Arachidonic acid
    b. Bradykinin
    c. Complement
    d. Serotonin

12. Which complement protein enhances phagocytosis by acting as opsonin?
    a. C3a
    b. C3b
    c. C4a
    d. C5a

13. Two major cytokines that induce the systemic acute phase responses of infection and injury, including fever, loss of appetite and release of corticosteroids are:
    a. Histamine and serotonin
    b. Complement and bradykinin
    c. Tumor necrosis factor and interleukin-1
    d. Prostaglandins and leukotrienes

14. **Which chemical mediator is important in the pathogenesis of bronchial asthma?**
    a. Lipoxins
    b. Leukotrienes
    c. Prostaglandins
    d. Nitric oxide

15. **Outcomes of acute inflammation consist of:**
    a. Complete resolution
    b. Healing by connective tissue replacement
    c. Progression of tissue response to chronic inflammation
    d. All of the above

16. **In an inflammatory reaction, with infection, the white blood cell count can increase to:**
    a. 4,000 to 10,000/mm^3
    b. 10,000 to 15,000/mm^3
    c. 15,000 to 20,000/mm^3
    d. 20,000 to 25,000/mm^3

17. **Examples of acute phase proteins include:**
    a. C-reactive protein and fibrinogen
    b. Serum amyloid A and lipoxin
    c. Substance P and neurokinin A
    d. Hageman factor and fibrinogen

18. **Sepsis occurs in severe bacterial infections because large quantities of cytokines cause thrombosis and coagulation, which eventually lead to multiple organ failure.**
    a. Both the statement and the reason are correct and related
    b. Both the statement and the reason are correct but not related
    c. The statement is correct, but the reason is not correct
    d. The statement is not correct, but the reason is correct
    e. NEITHER the statement NOR the reason is correct

19. **Examples of systemic diseases affected by chronic inflammation include:**
    a. Cardiovascular disease and diabetes
    b. Cancer and asthma
    c. Alzheimer's disease and periodontal disease
    d. All of the above

20. **The formation of new blood vessels in wound healing is:**
    a. Angiogenesis
    b. Granulomatous tissue
    c. Granulation tissue
    d. Parenchymal cells

21. **Local factors that influence wound healing include all the following EXCEPT one. Which one is the EXCEPTION?**
    a. Size and location of wound
    b. Early movement
    c. Blood supply
    d. Infection

22. **Granulation tissue represents a hallmark of healing. The amount of granulation tissue that forms depends on the size of the wound and the intensity of the inflammation.**
    a. Both statements are TRUE
    b. Both statements are FALSE
    c. The first statement is TRUE, and the second statement is FALSE
    d. The first statement is FALSE, and the second statement is TRUE

23. **A wound with a narrow incisional space will heal by:**
    a. Primary intervention
    b. Primary intention
    c. Secondary intervention
    d. Secondary intention

24. **The inflammatory reaction is more intense with healing by secondary union because of the presence of a larger clot and the formation of more epidermis in the area.**
    a. Both the statement and the reason are correct and related
    b. Both the statement and the reason are correct but not related
    c. The statement is correct, but the reason is not correct
    d. The statement is not correct, but the reason is correct
    e. NEITHER the statement NOR the reason is correct

25. **A complication of wound healing commonly seen in serious burn injuries is:**
    a. Ulceration
    b. Hypertrophic scar
    c. Contracture
    d. Fibrosis

26. **A complication of wound healing commonly seen in lower extremity wounds with peripheral vascular disease is:**
    a. Ulceration
    b. Hypertrophic scar
    c. Contracture
    d. Fibrosis

27. Tissues recover approximately 70% of tensile strength over:
    a. 1 to 3 weeks
    b. 4 to 6 weeks
    c. 7 to 11 weeks
    d. 12 to 15 weeks

28. Allogenous stem cells are derived from the individual being treated. They may be multipotent or unipotent.
    a. Both statements are TRUE
    b. Both statements are FALSE
    c. The first statement is TRUE, and the second statement is FALSE
    d. The first statement is FALSE, and the second statement is TRUE

29. The process of a stem cell from one adult tissue generating to cell types of another tissue is known as:
    a. Unipotent
    b. Transdifferentiation
    c. Undifferentiation
    d. Biologic viability

30. The two main categories of stem cells are:
    a. Embryonic and pluripotent stem cells
    b. Primary and secondary stem cells
    c. Embryonic and adult stem cells
    d. Somatic and adult stem cells

31. The adult stem cells that are isolated from aspirates of liposuction are:
    a. Amniotic fluid stem cells
    b. Adipose-derived stem cells
    c. Bone marrow–derived stem cells
    d. Dental stem cells

32. The adult stem cells which are isolated from hematopoietic stem cells and stromal cells are:
    a. Amniotic fluid stem cells
    b. Adipose-derived stem cells
    c. Bone marrow–derived stem cells
    d. Dental stem cells

33. The adult stem cells that develop from material created during the development of the nervous system and can differentiate into neural cell lines are:
    a. Amniotic fluid stem cells
    b. Adipose-derived stem cells
    c. Bone marrow–derived stem cells
    d. Dental stem cells

34. Dental stem cells can be obtained from:
    a. Permanent third molars (wisdom teeth)
    b. Pulp of primary teeth
    c. Periodontal ligament
    d. All of the above

35. Stem cells that can differentiate into pancreatic islet beta-cells include:
    a. Bone marrow–derived and tooth-derived stem cells
    b. Amniotic fluid–derived and tooth-derived stem cells
    c. Umbilical cord and bone marrow–derived stem cells
    d. Amniotic fluid–derived and umbilical cord stem cells

36. All of the following stem cells may differentiate into fat cells EXCEPT one. Which one is the EXCEPTION?
    a. Amniotic fluid–derived stem cells
    b. Adipose-derived stem cells
    c. Tooth-derived stem cells
    d. Umbilical cord stem cells

37. Which of the following stem cells may differentiate into immune cells?
    a. Amniotic fluid–derived stem cells
    b. Adipose-derived stem cells
    c. Tooth-derived stem cells
    d. Umbilical cord stem cells

38. Which of the following are the most commercially available stem cells?
    a. Amniotic fluid–derived stem cells
    b. Bone marrow–derived stem cells
    c. Tooth-derived stem cells
    d. Adipose-derived stem cells

39. How many genes do humans have?
    a. 20,000 to 25,000
    b. 25,000 to 30,000
    c. 30,000 to 35,000
    d. 35,000 to 40,000

40. In approximately what percentage of human DNA is the uniqueness of humans encoded?
    a. 0.1%
    b. 0.5%
    c. 1%
    d. 5% percent

41. All of the following conditions have a genetic component EXCEPT one. Which one is the EXCEPTION?
    a. Cardiovascular disease
    b. Diabetes
    c. Cleft lip
    d. Trauma

42. Trisomy is an example of:
    a. Genome mutation
    b. Chromosome mutation
    c. Submicroscopic chromosome mutation
    d. Submicroscopic gene mutation

43. **With autosomal dominant disorders, when some persons inherit the mutant gene but are phenotypically normal, this refers to:**
    a. Variable expressivity
    b. Successive transmission
    c. Incomplete penetrance
    d. Autosomal inheritance

44. **Duchenne muscular dystrophy exemplifies:**
    a. Autosomal dominant inheritance
    b. Autosomal recessive inheritance
    c. X-linked recessive inheritance
    d. Multifactorial inheritance

45. **Sickle cell anemia exemplifies:**
    a. Autosomal dominant inheritance
    b. Autosomal recessive inheritance
    c. X-linked recessive inheritance
    d. Multifactorial inheritance

46. **Ribonucleic acid (RNA) analysis is not as stable as deoxyribonucleic acid (DNA)–based diagnosis. It cannot, as yet, be used to detect and quantify viruses such as human immunodeficiency virus (HIV) or hepatitis C virus.**
    a. Both statements are TRUE
    b. Both statements are FALSE
    c. The first statement is TRUE, and the second statement is FALSE
    d. The first statement is FALSE, and the second statement is TRUE

47. **Determining which of two or more diseases with similar signs and symptoms is the one the client is manifesting refers to:**
    a. Appearance diagnosis
    b. Differential diagnosis
    c. Definitive diagnosis
    d. Working diagnosis

48. **If all diseases except one are eliminated from the differential diagnosis, then that gives the:**
    a. Appearance diagnosis
    b. Preliminary diagnosis
    c. Definitive diagnosis
    d. Working diagnosis

49. **A client presents with an enlargement of soft tissue. Which conceptual stage of the differential diagnosis process does this represent?**
    a. Stage 1—classification of the abnormality by primary manifestation
    b. Stage 2—listing of secondary features and contributing factors
    c. Stage 3—listing of conditions capable of causing primary manifestations
    d. Stage 4—elimination of unlikely causes

50. **A client presents with an ulceration with a pattern of healing followed by recurrence. Which conceptual stage of the differential diagnosis process does this represent?**
    a. Stage 1—classification of the abnormality by primary manifestation
    b. Stage 2—listing of secondary features and contributing factors
    c. Stage 3—listing of conditions capable of causing primary manifestations
    d. Stage 4—elimination of unlikely causes

Oral Pathology

Olga A. C. Ibsen

Dental hygienists perform comprehensive extraoral and intraoral examinations, identify pathologic conditions, and communicate these findings to the dentist for diagnosis, treatment, or referral. Knowledge of oral pathology affects infection control, managing the risk of emergencies, and developing dental hygiene care plans congruent with the patient's health status and needs. The dental hygienist differentiates between normal and abnormal findings and relates significant health, dental, and cultural histories to clinical, radiographic, and histologic findings. Although the dental hygienist is not responsible for the dental diagnosis, skill in the use of the diagnostic process is essential for the dental hygiene diagnosis and collaborative practice.

BENIGN LESIONS OF SOFT TISSUE ORIGIN

General Characteristics

A. Etiology—unknown
B. Age and gender vary with the type of lesion
C. Clinical features
   1. Sharp line of demarcation outlines the lesion
   2. Sessile or pedunculated base
   3. Lesion is easily palpable
D. Histologic characteristics depend on the lesion (e.g., a lipoma is composed of fat cells)
E. Lesion grows slowly, or it may be encapsulated, which contributes to an evaluation of a benign state
F. Lesion is removed surgically and usually does not recur

Irritative Fibroma (or Traumatic Fibroma) (see Figure 8-1)

A. Etiology—chronic mild irritant; chronic trauma
B. Age and gender related—40 to 60 years; more common in females (2:1)
C. Location—most common on the buccal mucosa along the area of the occlusal plane and gingiva; also found on the tongue, lips, and palate
D. Clinical features
   1. Light pink
   2. Round or semi-circular shape
   3. Less than 1 cm in size
   4. Sessile or pedunculated base
   5. Exophytic lesion
E. Histologic characteristics
   1. Stratified squamous epithelium; surface may be keratinized or ulcerated (resulting from secondary trauma)
   2. Contains dense connective tissue and few blood vessels
F. Treatment—complete excision

Papilloma

A. Etiology—benign lesion of squamous epithelium; long duration; slow development
B. Age and gender related—may arise at any age, but there is a 50% incidence between ages 20 and 50 years; no gender predilection
C. Location—soft palate or tongue
D. Clinical features (Figure 8-2, A)
   1. Cauliflower-like appearance
   2. Usually grayish or white color; can also be pink; color depends on amount of keratin

3. Well-delineated, exophytic nodule with a pedunculated or sessile base
4. Under 0.5 cm in size
E. Histologic characteristics (see Figure 8-2, *B*)
   1. Composed primarily of long, finger-like projections of stratified squamous epithelium with

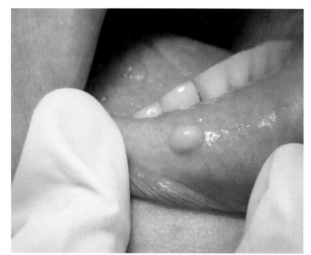

FIGURE 8-1 Fibroma with a sessile base. *(From Ibsen OAC, Phelan JA: Oral pathology for the dental hygienist, ed 5, Philadelphia, 2009, Saunders.)*

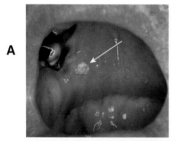

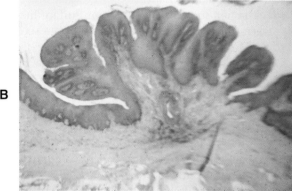

FIGURE 8-2 **A,** Clinical appearance of a papilloma on the palate showing a cauliflower-like appearance and rough surface resulting from finger-like projections. **B,** Microscopic appearance of a papilloma showing finger-like projections covered by a squamous epithelial layer and supported by thin cores of fibrous tissue. *(From Ibsen OAC, Phelan JA: Oral pathology for the dental hygienist, ed 5, Philadelphia, 2009, Saunders.)*

a core of fibrous connective tissue; surface keratin
2. Normal stratified squamous epithelium with a thick surface layer of keratin
F. Treatment and prognosis
   1. Surgical excision, including the base of the lesion
   2. Does not recur

Verruca Vulgaris (Wart)

A. Etiology—benign viral induced lesion of stratified squamous epithelium; caused by human papilloma virus (HPV)
B. Age and gender related—more common in children; but lesions have also been identified in adults; no gender predilection
C. Location—common skin lesion; lips are the most common intraoral site; can also be found on the tongue or mucosa
D. Clinical features (Figure 8-3, *A* and *B*)
   1. White, papillary exophytic lesion
   2. Can spread to other areas of a person's skin
   3. Self-inoculated (finger-to-mouth)
   4. Often sessile base
   5. Differs from a papilloma in that warts grow faster, are smaller, and develop in a shorter time
E. Histologic characteristics
   1. Hyperkeratotic stratified squamous epithelium with a prominent granular cell layer in the upper spinous layer of epithelium

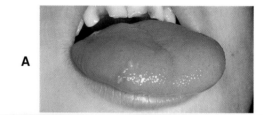

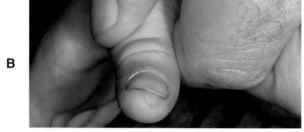

FIGURE 8-3 **A and B,** Verruca vulgaris on the tongue of a child, with a similar lesion on the thumb. *(Courtesy of Dr. Edward V. Zegarelli; from Ibsen OAC, Phelan JA: Oral pathology for the dental hygienist, ed 5, Philadelphia, 2009, Saunders.)*

2. Numerous koilocytes, cells with clear cytoplasm are located in the upper spinous layer of epithelium.

3. Central cores of fibrous connective tissue

F. Treatment and prognosis

1. Conservative surgical excision

2. Lesions may recur because of reinoculation

Hemangioma

A. Etiology—congenital or developmental origin; when found in adults, these lesions develop as a response to trauma during the healing stages; a benign proliferation of blood capillaries

B. Age and gender related—lesions present at birth or develop shortly thereafter; more common in females (3:1); occur in adults as a response to trauma

C. Location—most common on the tongue; also found on the buccal mucosa, labial mucosa, and the vermilion of lips

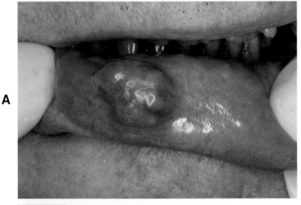

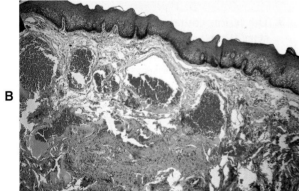

FIGURE 8-4 A, Clinical appearance of a hemangioma of the lower lip. **B,** Photomicrograph of a hemangioma. *(From Ibsen OAC, Phelan JA: Oral pathology for the dental hygienist, ed 5, Philadelphia, 2009, Saunders.)*

D. Clinical features (Figure 8-4, *A*)

1. Flat or raised, well-circumscribed lesion on the mucosa or tongue

2. Deep red or bluish-purple color

3. Lesions will blanch when pressure is applied

4. Two types:

a. Capillary—small to moderate size; soft texture

b. Cavernous—larger in size >2 cm in diameter; exhibits a significant protrusion of tissue; deep purple; soft or semi-firm texture

E. Histologic characteristics (see Figure 8-4, *B*)

1. Capillary—many small capillaries lined by a single layer of endothelial cells supported by a connective tissue stroma of varying density; endothelial cell proliferation

2. Cavernous—large, dilated blood sinuses with thin walls, each having an endothelial lining; sinusoidal spaces filled with blood and lymphatic vessels

F. Treatment and prognosis

1. Treatment is variable

a. Nonintervention in cases in which spontaneous remission has or can occurr

b. Surgical excision

c. Sclerosing agents injected into the lesion will cause the resolution of the lesion

d. Laser procedures

G. Prognosis is good

Lipoma

A. Etiology—unknown; rare; benign tumor of mature fat cells

B. Age and gender—over 40 years; no gender predilection

C. Location—most common on the buccal mucosa or in the mucobuccal fold

D. Clinical features (Figure 8-5, *A*)

1. Single or lobulated, well-defined, painless mass <3 cm in size

2. Sessile or pedunculated base

3. Soft to palpation

4. Yellowish color (if aspirated, a brown-yellow fluid is withdrawn)

E. Histologic characteristics (see Figure 8-5, *B*)

1. Circumscribed mass of mature fat cells with collagen strands and a few blood vessels

2. Thin epithelium covers lesion

3. If fibrous connective tissue forms a more significant part of the lesion, it is called a *fibrolipoma*

F. Treatment and prognosis

1. Conservative surgical excision

2. Recurrence is rare

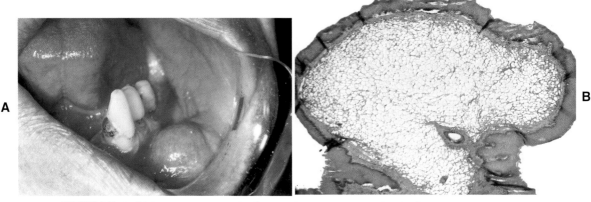

FIGURE 8-5 A, Clinical appearance of a lipoma. **B,** Photomicrograph of a lipoma showing mature fat cells. *(A, Courtesy of Dr. Edward V. Zegarelli; from Ibsen OAC, Phelan JA: Oral pathology for the dental hygienist, ed 5, Philadelphia, 2009, Saunders; B, from Regezi JA, Sciubba JJ: Oral pathology: Clinical-pathologic correlations, ed 5, Philadelphia, 2008, Saunders.)*

INFLAMMATORY TUMORS (GRANULOMAS)

General Characteristics

A. Growth or enlargement of tissue composed mainly of inflammatory cells
B. Account for the major portion of all oral tumors
C. Benign tumors

Pyogenic Granuloma

A. Etiology—an exuberant tissue response to chronic irritants or trauma (i.e., plaque biofilm, calculus, poor restorative margins, hormonal levels)
B. Age and gender related—children and young adults; more common in females (3:1), perhaps related to an increase in estrogen levels
C. Location—much more common on the maxillary labial gingiva than mandibular gingiva; can occur on the lips, tongue, and buccal mucosa
D. Clinical features (Figure 8-6)
　1. Protrusive mass; pedunculated, sessile, or lobulated base
　2. Deep red rather than pink surface
　3. Soft and spongy; freely movable; ulcerated, bleeds easily
　4. Lesions are a few millimeters to several centimeters
　5. In pregnancy, these lesions were formerly called *pregnancy tumors*
E. Histologic characteristics
　1. The epithelium, if present, is thin
　2. Rich in capillaries with proliferation of connective tissue; inflammatory cells

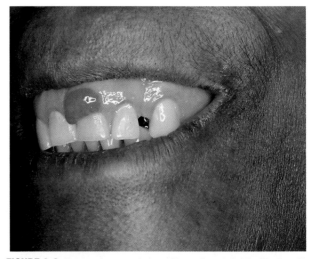

FIGURE 8-6 Pyogenic granuloma. *(From Ibsen OAC, Phelan JA: Oral pathology for the dental hygienist, ed 5, Philadelphia, 2009, Saunders.)*

　3. The lesion contains polymorphonuclear leukocytes (PMNLs), acute and chronic inflammatory cells, plasma cells, and lymphocytes
F. Treatment and prognosis
　1. Removal of the irritant
　2. Surgical excision of the lesion
　3. These lesions can recur if the irritant remains (e.g., calculus)
　4. The lesions that occur during pregnancy may resolve spontaneously

Papillary Hyperplasia of the Palate (Palatal Papillomatosis)

A. Etiology—type of denture stomatitis; chronic irritation to the vault of the hard palate related to an

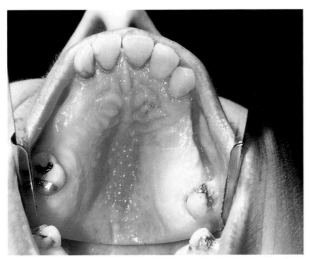

FIGURE 8-7 Papillary hyperplasia of the palate. *(Courtesy of Dr. Edward V. Zegarelli; from Ibsen OAC, Phelan JA: Oral pathology for the dental hygienist, ed 5, Philadelphia, 2009, Saunders.)*

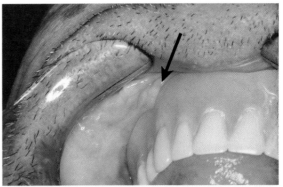
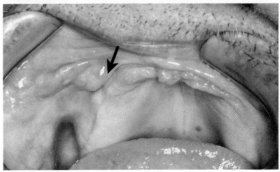

FIGURE 8-8 A, Denture-induced fibrous hyperplasia (epulis fissuratum) *(arrows)*, shown with denture in place, and **B,** denture removed. *(From Ibsen OAC, Phelan JA: Oral pathology for the dental hygienist, ed 5, Philadelphia, 2009, Saunders.)*

ill-fitting denture (full or partial); excessive pressure of an ill-fitting denture; poor denture hygiene (secondary); can also be associated with an orthodontic appliance; wearing the prosthetic device 24 hours a day

B. Age and gender related—no gender predilection
C. Location—especially—in vault of the hard palate in maxillary denture wearers (suction chamber area)
D. Clinical features (Figure 8-7)
  1. Closely clustered erythematous papillary projections, 1 to 4 mm in diameter
  2. Round, smooth, glistening red surface; granular appearance
  3. Varying degrees of inflammation present
E. Histologic characteristics
  1. Small vertical projections, each composed of stratified squamous epithelium and a central core of connective tissue
  2. Epithelial proliferation
  3. Infiltrated with inflammatory cells
F. Treatment
  1. Surgical excision of the hyperplastic tissue prior to construction of a new denture or a reline
  2. After surgery, emphasize denture care and removing the denture at night to rest the tissues
G. Prognosis—good

Denture-Induced Fibrous Hyperplasia (Epulis Fissuratum, Inflamatory hyperplasia)

A. Etiology—irritation caused by a denture flange, which produces a proliferation of tissue in the vestibule along the denture boarder

B. Age and gender related—denture wearers; no gender predilection
C. Location—vestibule along denture border; alveolar ridge in regions along the denture border
D. Clinical features (Figure 8-8)
  1. Exophytic folds of hyperplastic tissue in the vestibule under or around the denture flange
  2. Pink to red color (can have ulcerated areas)
  3. Firm to palpation
E. Histologic characteristics
  1. Dense fibrous connective tissue covered by stratified squamous epithelium
  2. Connective tissue composed of coarse bundles of collagen fibers
  3. Same type of tissue as seen in irritation fibroma
F. Treatment and prognosis
  1. Surgical removal of the excess tissue
  2. Construction of a new denture
  3. Prognosis is excellent

Peripheral Giant Cell Granuloma

A. Etiology—a reactive lesion caused by local irritants

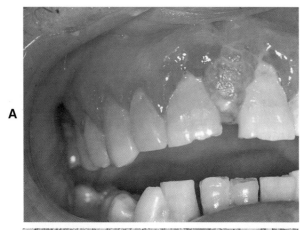

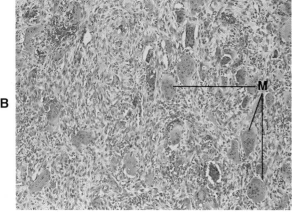

FIGURE 8-9 A, Peripheral giant cell granuloma. **B,** Microscopic appearance of a peripheral giant cell granuloma showing multi-nucleated giant cells (*M*), capillaries, and fibroblasts. *(From Ibsen OAC, Phelan JA: Oral pathology for the dental hygienist, ed 5, Philadelphia, 2009, Saunders.)*

B. Age and gender related—40 to 60 years; more common in females (2 : 1)
C. Location—gingiva or alveolar process, anterior to molars
D. Clinical features (Figure 8-9, *A*)
   1. Exophytic lesion 0.5 to 2.0 cm in diameter
   2. Deep red to bluish color
   3. Pedunculated or sessile base
   4. Arises from a deeper area in tissue than does a pyogenic granuloma or fibroma
E. Radiographic appearance—this soft tissue lesion can cause superficial destruction of alveolar bone
F. Histologic characteristics (see Figure 8-9, *B*)
   1. Composed of a delicate reticular and fibrillar connective tissue stroma containing a large number of ovoid or spindle-shaped, young, connective tissue cells
   2. Multi-nucleated giant cells
   3. Proliferation of blood vessels
   4. Appears to originate from the periodontal ligament or mucoperiosteum

G. Treatment and prognosis
   1. Surgical removal of the entire base to eliminate recurrence
   2. Usually does not recur

Central Giant Cell Granuloma

A. Etiology—occurs within bone; trauma caused by a fall, blow, or tooth extraction
B. Age and gender related—children and young adults; more common in females (2 : 1) age 10–30 years
C. Location—75% in the anterior segment of the mandible; also found in the maxilla
D. Clinical features
   1. Appears as a swelling or bulge resulting from the expansion of cortical plates
   2. No symptoms, so may be discovered by chance
   3. A similar lesion, often called "brown tumor," occurs in persons with hyperparathyroidism; resolves without treatment
E. Radiographic appearance (Figure 8-10, *A* and *B*)
   1. Usually a large radiolucent area with diffuse margins that are ill defined with faint trabeculae
   2. Displacement of teeth; divergence of the roots of teeth adjacent to the lesion
   3. Root resorption
F. Histologic characteristics
   1. Loose fibrillar connective tissue with many fibroblasts
   2. Rich vascularity
   3. Foreign-body multi-nucleated giant cells
G. Treatment and prognosis
   1. Curettage (perhaps more than one treatment)
   2. Surgical removal
   3. Radiotherapy is contraindicated
   4. Occasionally recurs

Chronic Hyperplastic Pulpitis (Pulpal Granuloma, Pulp Polyp)

A. Etiology—excessive proliferation of inflamed pulp tissue found in teeth with large open carious lesions; rapid caries; lesion projects from the pulp chamber
B. Age and gender related—children and young adults; no gender predilection
C. Location
   1. Usually in primary molars or permanent molars
   2. Can occur in any tooth with a large carious lesion

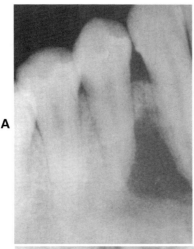

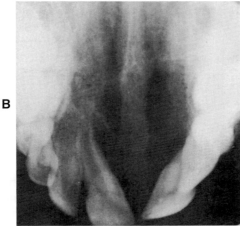

FIGURE 8-10 Radiographs of central giant cell granulomas showing multi-locular radiolucencies. **A,** The mandible. **B,** The maxilla. *(From Ibsen OAC, Phelan JA: Oral pathology for the dental hygienist, ed 5, Philadelphia, 2009, Saunders.)*

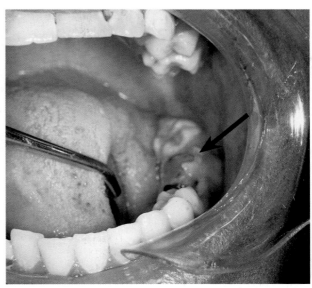

FIGURE 8-11 Chronic hyperplastic pulpitis (pulp polyp) *(arrow)*. *(From Ibsen OAC, Phelan JA: Oral pathology for the dental hygienist, ed 5, Philadelphia, 2009, Saunders.)*

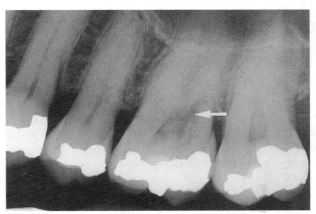

FIGURE 8-12 Radiograph showing an area of internal resorption on the maxillary first molar *(arrow)*. *(From Ibsen OAC, Phelan JA: Oral pathology for the dental hygienist, ed 5, Philadelphia, 2009, Saunders.)*

D. Clinical features (Figure 8-11)
  1. Red to pink outgrowth of pulp tissue protruding from the occlusal surface of the crown of a tooth that has a large, open, carious lesion
  2. Lesion is not painful because hyperplastic tissue contains few nerves
E. Histologic characteristics
  1. Originates from pulpal tissue
  2. Contains acute and chronic inflammatory cells, plasma cells, and lymphocytes
  3. Granulation tissue
F. Treatment and prognosis
  1. Extraction of the involved tooth
  2. Endodontic therapy
  3. Prognosis is good

Internal Resorption

A. Etiology—not clear; theories include:
  1. Inflammatory response in the pulp
  2. Trauma
  3. Caries-related pulpitis
B. Age and gender related—any age; no gender predilection
C. Location—usually found within a tooth in the permanent dentition
D. Clinical features
  1. Dentin immediately surrounding the pulp in the area of resorption is destroyed
  2. The crown may appear pink ("pink tooth") because of the vascularity of the lesion within (this is not easily observable on posterior teeth)
E. Radiographic appearance well defined, but radiolucent lesion in close proximity to the pulp canal (Figure 8-12)

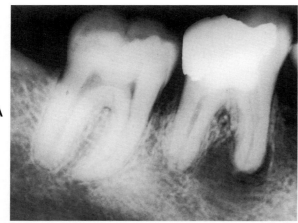
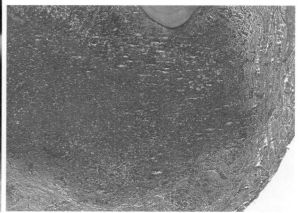

FIGURE 8-13 A, Radiograph of a periapical granuloma. **B,** Low-power microscopic appearance of a periapical granuloma. *(From Ibsen OAC, Phelan JA: Oral pathology for the dental hygienist, ed 5, Philadelphia, 2009, Saunders.)*

F. Histologic characteristics—highly vascularized chronic inflammatory tissue
G. Treatment—endodontic therapy if perforation of the root has not occurred; otherwise, extraction of the tooth is performed

Periapical Granuloma

A. Etiology—dental caries or deep restorations
B. Age and gender related—any age; no gender predilection
C. Location—apex of a nonvital tooth
D. Clinical features
　1. Nonvital tooth; asymptomatic
　2. Fistula or parulis may be present if the condition has been chronic
　3. The affected tooth can be sensitive to percussion
E. Radiographic appearance—varies from a well-defined, circular, radiolucent lesion at the apex of the involved tooth to a diffuse radiolucency or thickening of the periodontal ligament space (Figure 8-13, *A*)
F. Histologic characteristics (see Figure 8-13, *B*)
　1. Lymphocytes, plasma cells, macrophages
　2. Dense fibrous connective tissue
　3. Epithelial (Malassez) rests
G. Treatment—endodontic therapy or extraction of the affected tooth

BENIGN INTRAOSSEOUS NEOPLASMS

General Characteristics

A. Etiology—generally unknown
B. Onset—gradual, with slow development or enlargement

C. Early stages—asymptomatic
D. With expansion of the lesion, malocclusion may occur; bone tenderness on palpation; cortical bone may become thin

Osteoma

A. Etiology—asymptomatic benign tumor of compact bone; etiology generally unknown, but the cause may be irritation or inflammation; associated with a genetic condition called *Gardner syndrome*
B. Age and gender related—more common in young adults but can be found at any age; no gender predilection
C. Location—most common posterior mandible; mandibular condyle; craniofacial skeleton
D. Clinical features—the affected individual may be unaware of the lesion because it grows slowly; considerable growth must occur before cortical plates expand
E. Radiographic appearance—well-circumscribed radiopaque mass that is indistinguishable from scar bone; panoramic or lateral plate radiograph may be needed to view the lesion in its entirety (Figure 8-14)
F. Histologic characteristics—extremely dense, compact bone or coarse, cancellous bone
G. Treatment and prognosis
　1. Surgical excision
　2. Does not recur

Chondroma

A. Etiology—benign tumors of hyaline cartilage; cause unknown
B. Age and gender related—ages 30 to 40 years; no gender predilection

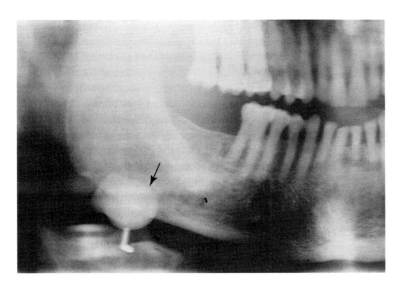

FIGURE 8-14 Radiograph of an osteoma showing a radiopacity (*arrow*) of the posterior mandible. *(Courtesy of Dr. Sidney Eisig; from Ibsen OAC, Phelan JA:* Oral pathology for the dental hygienist, *ed 5, Philadelphia, 2009, Saunders.)*

C. Location
  1. Maxilla—anterior area
  2. Mandible—posterior to canines
  3. May involve the body of the mandible or the coronoid or condylar process
D. Clinical features
  1. Painless
  2. Slow, progressive swelling of the jaw may loosen or malposition teeth
  3. Tendency to become malignant
E. Radiographic appearance—irregular radiolucent or mottled area in bone; may displace surrounding teeth or cause root resorption
F. Histologic characteristics
  1. Mass of hyaline cartilage with areas of calcification or necrosis
  2. Cartilage cells are small, and each has one nucleus
  3. Large biopsy sample must be obtained because the lesion is similar to a malignant chondrosarcoma (more common in men)
G. Treatment and prognosis
  1. Nonconservative surgical removal; tumor may be resistant to radiation therapy
  2. Periodic follow-up evaluation is necessary to detect recurrence or possibility of a chondrosarcoma

Odontogenic Myxoma

A. Etiology—unknown; benign; originates from mesenchymal tissue of the tooth germ
B. Age and gender related—most often in young adults (ages 10 to 30 years); no gender predilection
C. Location—mandible more often than maxilla
D. Clinical features—deeply situated lesion; small lesions asymptomatic

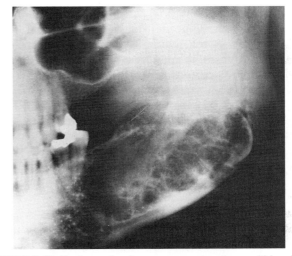

FIGURE 8-15 Radiograph of a myxoma showing multi-locular, honeycombed radiolucency. *(From Ibsen OAC, Phelan JA:* Oral pathology for the dental hygienist, *ed 5, Philadelphia, 2009, Saunders.)*

E. Radiographic appearance (Figure 8-15)
  1. May be unilocular or multilocular
  2. Several small radiolucencies occurring in groups, giving a "honeycomb" appearance
  3. May show displaced teeth, mandibular canal, and antrum (may also invade the antrum)
  4. Peripheral borders are irregular, diffuse, and not well defined
F. Histologic characteristics
  1. Loosely textured tissue containing delicate reticulin fibers and mucoid material
  2. Contains stellate, spindle-shaped cells
  3. The tumor is not encapsulated and may invade surrounding tissues
  4. Does not metastasize

G. Treatment and prognosis
1. Complete surgical excision
2. Recurrence is common (25%)

Exostosis

Torus Palatinus

A. Etiology—inherited, autosomal dominant; some believe the cause to be genetic or environmental factors
B. Age and gender related—usually seen by the age of puberty; rarely observed in children, but peak incidence occurs before 30 years; more common in females (2 : 1)
C. Location—midline of the hard palate
D. Clinical features (Figure 8-16, *A*)
1. Bony, hard protuberance in the midline in a variety of shapes—nodular; lobulated; smooth; spindle
2. Occurs in 20% to 35% of the U.S. population
3. Torus may appear ulcerated because of trauma to the thin overlying mucosa
E. Radiographic appearance—dense radiopaque area
F. Histologic characteristics—dense cortical bone
G. Treatment—usually none, but surgical removal if the lesion interferes with a prosthodontic appliance

Torus Mandibularis

A. Etiology—inherited, autosomal dominant; possibly genetic or environmental
B. Age and gender related—first observed in early teen years; slightly more common in males

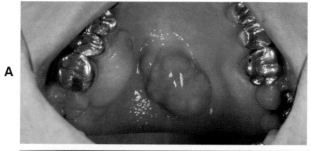
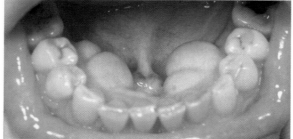

FIGURE 8-16 A, Clinical appearance of a lobulated torus palatinus. **B,** Clinical appearance of bilateral mandibular tori. *(From Ibsen OAC, Phelan JA: Oral pathology for the dental hygienist, ed 5, Philadelphia, 2009, Saunders.)*

C. Location—lingual surface of the mandible above the mylohyoid line in the area of premolars
D. Clinical features (see Figure 8-16, *B*)
1. Bony, hard protuberance varying in size and shape; common exostosis
2. Slow growing—usually unnoticed
3. Bilateral incidence more common (90%)
E. Radiographic appearance—dense radiopaque area
F. Histologic characteristics—dense cortical bone
G. Treatment—surgical excision if the lesion interferes with a prosthodontic appliance

Odontoma

A. Etiology—most common odontogenic tumor composed of all tooth structure and pulp but not considered a neoplasm
B. Age and gender related—usually seen in adolescents and young adults (mean age 14 years); no gender predilection
C. Location—more frequently seen in the maxilla (especially the anterior maxilla for the compound type) than in the mandible; usually between the roots of teeth or near apices; complex odontomas seen more often in the posterior of the mandible
D. Clinical features
1. Failure of a permanent tooth to erupt
2. Asymptomatic
E. Radiographic appearance—irregular mass of radiopacities ("tooth-like structures") surrounded by a narrow radiolucent halo
1. Two types
a. Compound—tooth structures are identified radiographically (Figure 8-17)
b. Complex—appears as a radiopaque mass (can be confused with other lesions in bone) (Figure 8-18)
2. Cyst involvement may occur with an odontoma
F. Histologic characteristics—tumor in which epithelial and mesenchymal cells show differentiation, resulting in abnormal enamel and dentin formation
G. Treatment and prognosis
1. Complete surgical removal (both forms are well encapsulated)
2. Prognosis is good

GINGIVAL FIBROMATOSIS

General Characteristics

A. Enlargement of gingival tissue, sometimes covering teeth
B. Contains a proliferation of dense fibrous connective tissue

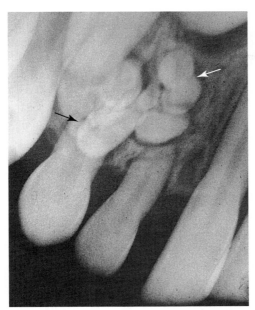

FIGURE 8-17 Radiograph of a compound odontoma, showing a collection of numerous, small, tooth-like radiopacities (*arrows*) surrounded by a radiolucent halo. *(From Ibsen OAC, Phelan JA: Oral pathology for the dental hygienist, ed 5, Philadelphia, 2009, Saunders.)*

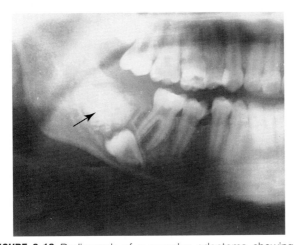

FIGURE 8-18 Radiograph of a complex odontoma showing a radiopaque mass surrounded by a radiolucent halo (*arrow*). *(From Ibsen OAC, Phelan JA: Oral pathology for the dental hygienist, ed 5, Philadelphia, 2009, Saunders.)*

C. Classification includes
　　1. Irritative fibromatosis—localized areas associated with extraneous irritants
　　2. Hereditary fibromatosis—generalized enlargement of gingival tissue
　　3. Chemical fibromatosis—caused by certain medications (drug-influenced gingival enlargement)

Irritative Fibromatosis

A. Etiology—irritant such as mouth breathing, orthodontic appliances, bacterial plaque biofilm, dental calculus, debris, overhanging restorations, or ill-fitting dental appliances
B. Age and gender related—any age; no gender predilection
C. Location—localized areas on interproximal papillae; in mouth breathers, on maxillary and mandibular anterior labial gingivae
D. Clinical features—solitary round, smooth-surfaced, pink enlargement of papillae; well attached to surrounding structures
E. Histologic characteristics—proliferation of dense, fibrous connective tissue with an increase in the number of fibroblasts
F. Treatment and prognosis
　　1. Removal of the irritant
　　2. Improved oral hygiene
　　3. Gingivectomy in severe cases
　　4. Prognosis is excellent

Hereditary Gingival Fibromatosis (Gingival Lesions of Genetic Origin)

A. Etiology (see the section on "Genetics" in Chapter 7)
　　1. Hereditary; believed to have genetic or developmental involvement or to be related to hormonal imbalances; a component of several syndromes (e.g., Zimmerman-Laband, Cross, Rutherfurd, Murray-Puretic-Drescher, and Cowden's syndromes)
　　2. Contributing factors include poor oral hygiene, food impaction, calculus, malocclusion
　　3. Other conditions associated with gingival fibromatosis may include growth hormone deficiency, hypothyroidism, epilepsy, and intellectual and developmental disabilities (IDD)
B. Age and gender related—appears during the eruption of primary or permanent teeth; slightly more common in females
C. Location—excessive enlargement of interproximal gingival tissues; can be localized
D. Clinical features
　　1. Gingival enlargement may be generalized or localized
　　2. Diffuse, smooth-surfaced, pink, firm tissue involving the interproximal papillae
　　3. Multiple protruding pink, stippled, firm masses; labial and buccal areas are most affected; teeth may be displaced; delays eruption of teeth
E. Histologic characteristics—bundles of fibrous connective tissue with fibroblasts and fibrocytes (depending on the formative stage)

F. Treatment and prognosis
  1. Gingivectomy
  2. Rigid adherence to home care
  3. Recurrence is common

Chemical Fibromatosis (Drug-influenced Gingival Enlargement)

A. Etiology—reaction to drugs, specifically phenytoin (Dilantin); calcium channel blockers including nifedipine (Procardia), amlodipine (Norvasc), diltiazem (Cardizem), and verapamil (Calan); cyclosporin, an immunosuppressant drug given in association with organ transplants
B. Age and gender—no gender predilection
C. Location—papillae and gingivae
D. Clinical features—smooth, pink, firm enlargement of the papillae (Figure 8-19)
E. Histologic characteristics—extensive proliferation of connective tissue
F. Treatment
  1. Change in the prescribed medication, if possible
  2. Gingivectomy
  3. Improved oral self-care

ULCERATIVE DISEASES

General Characteristics

A. Ulcer—formed by the destruction of the epithelium and some underlying tissue
B. Factors aiding in the diagnosis of ulcers occurring in the oral cavity
  1. Number and size
  2. Location
  3. Depth
  4. Borders
  5. Patient history (personal, health, cultural, and pharmacologic)
C. Etiology—not always known
D. Can be classified as an acute or chronic condition
  1. Acute ulcerative conditions include traumatic ulcers, aphthous ulcers, allergic reactions, and viral ulcerations
  2. Chronic ulcerative conditions include those caused by or associated with systemic diseases such as leukemia, colitis, malnutrition, tuberculosis, syphilis, sickle cell anemia, and drug toxicity

Traumatic Ulcer

A. Etiology—various types of trauma; history of lesion plays a significant role in the diagnosis

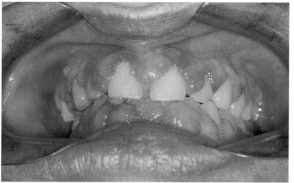

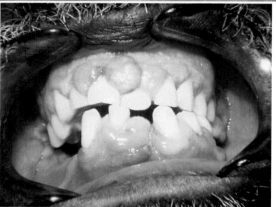

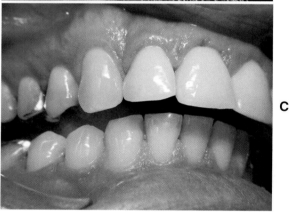

FIGURE 8-19 Drug-influenced gingival enlargement. **A,** Gingival enlargement caused by phenytoin (Dilantin). **B and C,** Gingival hyperplasia caused by nifedipine (Procardia). (**A,** Courtesy of Dr. Edward V. Zegarelli; **B and C,** Courtesy of Dr. Victor M. Sternberg; **A to C,** from Ibsen OAC, Phelan JA: Oral pathology for the dental hygienist, ed 5, Philadelphia, 2009, Saunders.)

  1. Physical—biting the mucosa, denture irritation, toothbrush injury, sharp tooth, fractured filling (Figure 8-20)
  2. Chemical—oral rinse, phenol, misuse of medication used to treat a toothache (e.g., misuse of asirin causes an aspirin burn) (Figure 8-21)
  3. Thermal—hot foods (i.e., soup) (Figure 8-22, *A*), crack cocaine (see Figure 8-22, *B*)
  4. Electrical

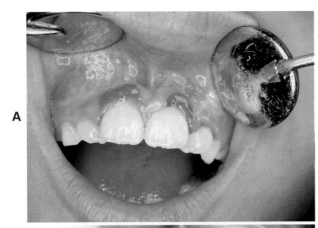

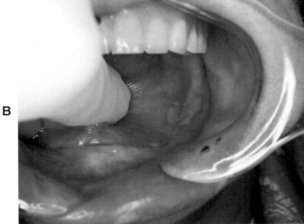

FIGURE 8-20 A, Traumatic ulceration caused by irritation of gingiva by fingernails. **B,** Traumatic ulcer caused by a denture. *(From Ibsen OAC, Phelan JA:* Oral pathology for the dental hygienist, *ed 5, Philadelphia, 2009, Saunders.)*

B. Age and gender related—any age; no gender predilection
C. Location—lateral border of the tongue, buccal mucosa, lips, palate (especially tori)
D. Clinical features
   1. Small, single, oval, round, or irregular shape
   2. Flat or slightly depressed
   3. Covered by necrotic membrane and surrounded by an inflammatory halo
   4. Painful for 2 to 5 days
   5. Heals within 7 to 14 days
E. Histologic characteristics
   1. Loss of continuity of surface epithelium
   2. Fibrinous exudate covering exposed connective tissue
   3. Infiltration of PMNLs in connective tissue
   4. Fibroblastic activity can be prominent
F. Treatment and prognosis
   1. Removal of the irritant or cause
   2. Application of benzocaine (e.g., Orabase) to relieve symptoms
   3. Corticosteroids (recommended by some, while others suggest these medications can delay healing)
   4. Topical dyclonine hydrochloride (HCl) for temporary relief
   5. In severe cases, systemic antibiotics are given to prevent secondary infection (these cases may also require surgical débridement depending on the extent of tissue damage)
   7. In cases of electrical burns, tetanus immunization is necessary
   8. Prognosis is good

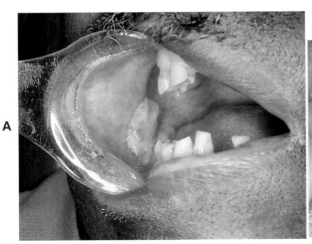

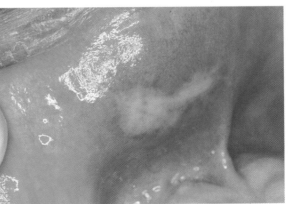

FIGURE 8-21 Mucosal burns. **A,** Burns caused by aspirin. **B,** Chemical burn caused by contact with caustic material during endodontic treatment. *(From Ibsen OAC, Phelan JA:* Oral pathology for the dental hygienist, *ed 5, Philadelphia, 2009, Saunders.)*

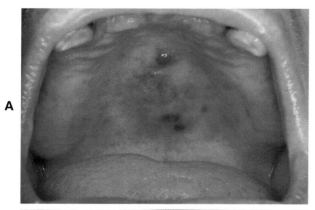

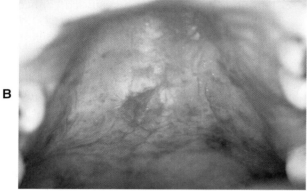

FIGURE 8-22 Mucosal burns. **A,** Thermal burn of palate caused by contact with hot soup. **B,** Ulcer of midline of palate caused by heat generated during the use of crack cocaine. (**A,** from Ibsen OAC, Phelan JA: Oral pathology for the dental hygienist, ed 5, Philadelphia, 2009, Saunders; **B,** from Mitchell-Lewis DA, Phelan JA, Kelly RB, Bradley JJ, Lamster IB: Identifying oral lesions associated with crack-cocaine use, J Am Dent Assoc 125:1104, 1994.)

Necrotizing Ulcerative Gingivitis (NUG, Vincent's Infection, Trench mouth)

A. Etiology
  1. Anaerobic bacteria—fusiform bacilli (*Bacillus fusiformis*)
  2. *Borrelia vincentii*, a spirochete
  3. Sophisticated technology has identified the involvement of other species as well
  4. Contributory factors
    a. Systemic—stress, fatigue, poor hygiene, malnutrition, suppressed immune system, recent illness
    b. Local—poor restorations, trauma, gingivitis, poor oral hygiene, heavy smoking
B. Age and gender related—any age, usually 17 to 35 years; no gender predilection
C. Location—free gingival margin, crest of gingiva, interdental papillae

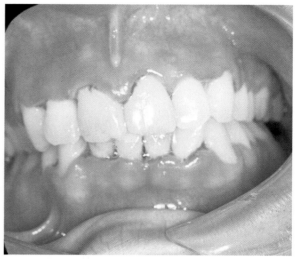

FIGURE 8-23 Necrotizing ulcerative gingivitis. (From Ibsen OAC, Phelan JA: Oral pathology for the dental hygienist, ed 5, Philadelphia, 2009, Saunders.)

D. Clinical features (Figure 8-23)
  1. Acute gingivitis with extensive necrosis
  2. Blunted, "punched-out," crater-like necrosis of interdental papillae
  3. Fetid mouth odor, pain, bleeding, bad taste
  4. Headaches, low-grade fever
  5. Regional lymphadenopathy
E. Histologic characteristics
  1. Ulcerated stratified squamous epithelium
  2. Thick fibrinous exudate containing PMNLs
  3. Significant bacterial colonization
  4. Connective tissue infiltrated by dense numbers of PMNLs
F. Treatment and prognosis
  1. Scaling and debridement (patient may need several visits)
  2. Use of ultrasonic instruments (except when contraindicated)
  3. Topical anesthetic or even local anesthetic may be necessary for the procedure
  4. Use of an oxygenating rinse four or more times daily for 1 to 2 weeks
  5. 0.12% chlorhexidine rinses
  6. Use of systemic antibiotics such as penicillin, tetracycline, or erythromycin, if patient has systemic symptoms such as a fever, lymphadenopathy, or both
  7. Home care to improve oral hygiene status (e.g., power toothbrush, interdental cleaning)
  8. Once treatment is completed, a 1-month follow-up appointment should be scheduled to evaluate therapy and reinforce oral self care; the patient should be encouraged to have recare visits every 4 months

9. Condition can recur if the individual lacks optimal oral self care or has associated risk factors

MINOR APHTHOUS ULCERS

Recurrent Ulcerative Stomatitis (RUS); Recurrent Aphthous Stomatitis

A. Etiology
1. Autoimmune response of oral epithelium
2. T cell–mediated immunologic response
3. Decrease of mucosal tissue barrier
4. Inherited predisposition
5. Risk factors
   a. Hormonal imbalance—premenstrual (incidence increases), pregnancy (incidence decreases)
   b. Psychological—anxiety, depression, acute emotional problems, stress
   c. Allergy—asthma, hay fever, food, drug, gluten
   d. Blood abnormalities
   e. Trauma
   f. Bacterial or viral agents (e.g., herpes simplex virus [HSV]; cytomegalovirus [CMV])
6. Systemic conditions associated with aphthous stomatitis
   a. Behçet syndrome
   b. Crohn disease
   c. Ulcerative colitis
   d. Cyclic neutropenia
   e. Sprue
   f. Intestinal lymphoma
B. Age and gender related—childhood to adolescence and young adults; more common in females
C. Location—buccal and labial mucosa, soft palate, pharynx, tongue; more common in the anterior regions
D. Clinical features (Figure 8-24)
1. Ulcerations—oval or round in shape with distinct borders; the center of the ulcer has a yellowish-white fibrous surface surrounded by a red halo
2. Range from 1 to 12 in number (3 to 10 most common)
3. Size—3 to 10 mm
4. Pain, tenderness, discomfort
5. Interference with functions—speech, eating
6. Prodromal period of 1 to 2 days; characterized by a burning sensation in the area where the ulcer will appear
7. Associated systemic factors can include low-grade fever and localized lymphadenopathy
E. Histologic characteristics
1. Superficial erosion of mucosal tissue covered by a membrane

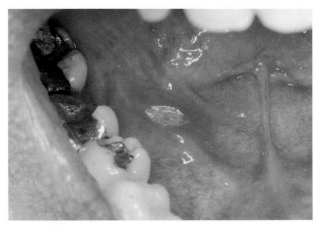

FIGURE 8-24 Example of a minor aphthous ulcer. *(From Ibsen OAC, Phelan JA: Oral pathology for the dental hygienist, ed 5, Philadelphia, 2009, Saunders.)*

2. Connective tissue shows increased vascularity
3. Increase in PMNLs, lymphocytes, and histiocytes
F. Treatment and prognosis
1. Self-limiting, healing in 10 to 12 days; recurrent episodes are common
2. Topical corticosteroids; 0.12% chlorhexidine rinse; topical tetracyclines
3. Betamethasone syrup (rinse and expectorate)

MAJOR APHTHOUS ULCERS

Recurrent Scarifying Ulcerative Stomatitis (RSUS); Periadenitis Mucosa Necrotica Recurrens; Mikulicz Aphthae; Sutton Disease

A. Etiology
1. Autoimmune response of oral epithelium
2. T cell–mediated immunologic response
3. Decrease of mucosal tissue barrier
4. Inherited predisposition
B. Age and gender related—usually young adults, onset after puberty; more common in females
C. Location—labial mucosa, buccal mucosa, soft palate, posterior fauces
D. Clinical features (Figure 8-25)
1. Multiple large ulcers, 1 to 10 in number and 1 to 3 cm in diameter
2. Crater-like formations with irregular shapes
3. Lesions heal in 3 to 6 weeks, producing scarring
4. Very painful
5. Occur at frequent intervals
E. Histologic characteristics
1. Fibrinopurulent membrane covering the ulcerated area

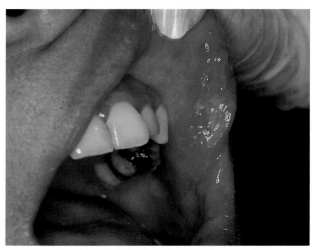

FIGURE 8-25 Example of major aphthous ulcers located on the labial mucosa. *(From Ibsen OAC, Phelan JA: Oral pathology for the dental hygienist, ed 5, Philadelphia, 2009, Saunders.)*

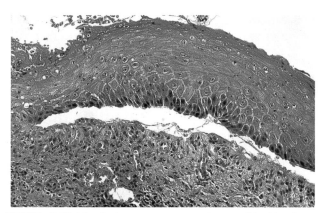

FIGURE 8-26 Histologic appearance of pemphigoid. *(Ibsen OAC, Phelan JA: Oral pathology for the dental hygienist, ed 5, Philadelphia, 2009, Saunders.)*

2. Necrotic epithelium
3. Intense inflammatory cell infiltration in connective tissue
4. Neutrophils and lymphocytes present
5. Granulation tissue at the base of the lesion
6. Microscopic picture is nonspecific; a conclusive diagnosis cannot be made without thorough clinical and historical data
F. Treatment and prognosis
  1. Corticosteroids
    a. Systemic
    b. Topical
  2. Inject the lesion with triamcinolone acetonide
  3. 0.05% halobetasol propionate ointment
  4. Recurrence is common

Mucous Membrane Pemphigoid, Cicatricial Pemphigoid, Benign Mucous Membrane Pemphigoid

A. Etiology—chronic benign autoimmune disease
B. Age and gender related—ages 50 to 65 years; more common in females (2 : 1)
C. Location
  1. Gingiva
  2. Oral mucous membranes
  3. Eyes, nasal, esophageal, and vaginal mucosa; skin
D. Clinical features
  1. Vesicles or bullous lesions; surface is "thick" and does not rupture easily
  2. After rupture, the surface is eroded and raw (desquamated)
  3. Desquamative appearance (not descriptive of this condition alone)

E. Histologic characteristics (Figure 8-26)
  1. Vesicles and bullae are subepithelial
  2. The epithelium appears to be detached from connective tissue
  3. No evidence of acantholysis—degeneration of cohesive elements of epithelial cells (as seen in pemphigus)
  4. Inflammatory infiltrate in connective tissue
  5. Direct immunofluorescence shows a linear pattern at the basement membrane in over 90% of cases
F. Treatment and prognosis
  1. Mild forms—topical corticosteroids
  2. With bullous eruptions or conjunctival involvement, high doses of systemic corticosteroids are needed
  3. Certain systemic antibiotics
  4. Once the diagnosis of cicatricial pemphigoid is made, the patient should be referred for an eye examination, since eye involvement can be severe but may not show any symptoms in the early stages
  5. Patients go through periods of remission; long-term disease or condition

Herpes

Primary Herpetic Gingivostomatitis
A. Etiology
  1. Virus—initial infection with herpes simplex virus (HSV)
  2. Member of the human herpesvirus (HHV) group
  3. Transmission—droplet infection; direct contact; highly contagious (the amount of virus is highest in the vesicle stage); patients can self-inoculate (especially the eyes)
B. Age and gender related—ages 6 months to 6 years; no gender predilection

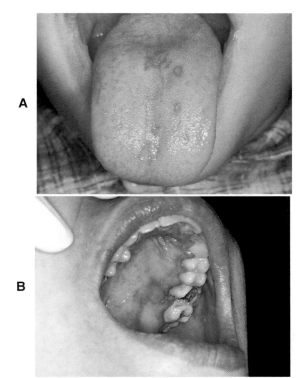

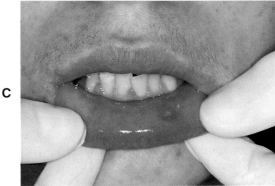

FIGURE 8-27 A, Example of primary herpetic gingivostomatitis in a child. **B and C,** Primary herpetic gingivostomatitis in an adolescent. (*A, Courtesy of Dr. Edward V. Zegarelli; **A to C,** from Ibsen OAC, Phelan JA: Oral pathology for the dental hygienist, ed 5, Philadelphia, 2009, Saunders.*)

C. Location—lips, gingiva, tongue, pharynx, floor of the mouth, buccal mucosa
D. Clinical features (Figure 8-27)
  1. Systemic symptoms
    a. Abrupt onset of fever
    b. Headache, irritability
    c. Pain on swallowing
    d. Regional lymphadenopathy
  2. Oral symptoms
    a. Hypertrophic gingivitis
    b. Initially, tiny vesicles (pinhead size) that develop into ulcerations

    c. Painful ulcers 1 to 3 mm in size; covered by a yellowish fibrinous surface
    d. Shallow craters covered by white or yellow plaque; bright erythematous margins ("halo")
    e. Most acute on days 3 to 7
E. Laboratory tests and findings
  1. Cytologic smear (noninvasive and inexpensive test)
  2. Blood test for HSV
  3. Viral isolation from tissue culture of intact vesicles (best diagnostic procedure but can take up to 2 weeks to obtain results)
F. Histologic characteristics
  1. Vesicle is an intraepithelial blister filled with fluid
  2. Degenerating cells show "ballooning"
  3. Displacement of chromatin around the nucleus
  4. Acantholysis of epithelium (Tzanck cells)
G. Treatment and prognosis
  1. Symptomatic therapy—bed rest, fluids
  2. Antiviral medications such as acyclovir ("swish and swallow") started within the first few days
  3. Ibuprofen to reduce pain and discomfort
  4. Self-limiting; healing in 7 to 14 days
  5. Recurrence most common in the form of herpes labialis

Herpes Labialis (Cold Sore or Fever Blister)
A. Etiology
  1. Residual form of HSV-1
  2. Recurrence of HSV from its latent stage
  3. Stimuli that can trigger the onset
    a. Exposure to sunlight
    b. Trauma
    c. Menstruation
    d. Emotional stress, anxiety, fatigue
    e. Allergic reactions
    f. Systemic diseases
B. Age and gender related—adults; no gender predilection
C. Location
  1. Lips—most common
  2. Intraorally—hard palate, attached gingiva, alveolar ridge
D. Clinical features (Figure 8-28, *A and B*)
  1. Prodromal period (any time up to 24 hours before the lesion erupts)—burning sensation, feeling of tightness, tingling, or soreness where the vesicle eventually appears
  2. Several fluid-filled papules may appear in clusters (most contagious state)
  3. Vesicles rupture, and crust forms on lips
  4. Intraoral lesions can appear on keratinized mucosa
  5. Do not confuse with angular cheilitis, a fungal infection.

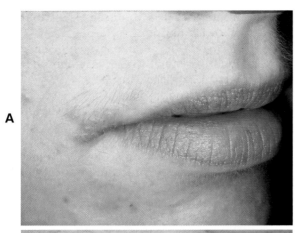

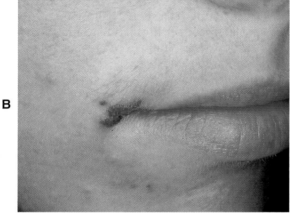

FIGURE 8-28 Herpes labialis. **A,** Twelve hours after onset. **B,** Forty-eight hours after onset. *(From Ibsen OAC, Phelan JA: Oral pathology for the dental hygienist, ed 5, Philadelphia, 2009, Saunders.)*

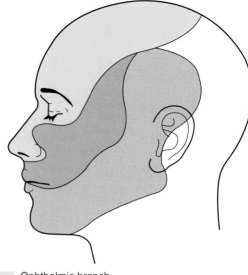

▨ Ophthalmic branch
▨ Maxillary branch
▨ Mandibular branch

FIGURE 8-29 The divisions of the trigeminal nerve. *(From Ibsen OAC, Phelan JA: Oral pathology for the dental hygienist, ed 5, Philadelphia, 2009, Saunders.)*

E. Histologic characteristics
  1. Ballooning degeneration
  2. Chromatin margination around the nucleus
  3. Isolation of HSV
F. Treatment and prognosis
  1. Antiviral drugs (e.g., acyclovir, valacyclovir) especially effective if given during the prodromal period
  2. Prophylactic treatment with antivirals prior to encountering a "risk factor," if possible
  3. Topical application of 10% n-docosanol cream has been effective
  4. Self-limiting; healing in 7 to 10 days
  5. Sunscreen to prevent the development of herpes labialis
  6. Chlorhexidine (0.12%) rinses, acyclovir suspension, or both can be helpful to treat intraoral recurrent HSV
  7. The condition does recur

Herpes Zoster (Shingles)

A. Etiology
  1. Reactivation of varicella zoster virus (VZV) from its latent stage; VZV also causes chickenpox, which is considered the primary infection with VZV
  2. Risk factors for the reactivation of VZV
    a. Systemic disease (malignancies, Hodgkin's disease, leukemia)
    b. Drug toxicity, radiation, alcohol abuse
    c. Advanced age
    d. Extreme fatigue
    e. Immunosupression
  3. Depression of cell-mediated immunity
B. Age and gender related—adults, usually over 50 years; no gender predilection
C. Location—skin or mucosa, supplied by the affected sensory nerve; any of the three branches of the trigeminal nerve (Figure 8-29)
D. Clinical features (Figure 8-30, *A* to *C*)
  1. Prodromal period of extreme pain 1 to 3 days prior to the eruption of the unilateral rash, which can be accompanied by systemic features such as fever, severe headaches, lymphadenopathy, and overall weakness
  2. The erythematous rash develops into vesicles; the pain becomes more intense with a burning, tingling, or stabbing sensation
  3. Clusters of these vesicles develop along the pathway of a sensory nerve

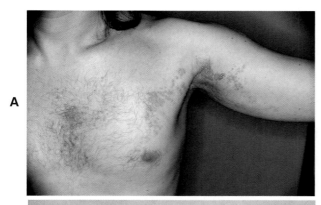

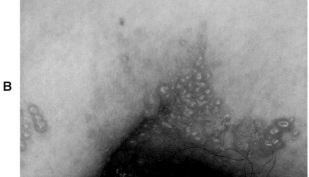

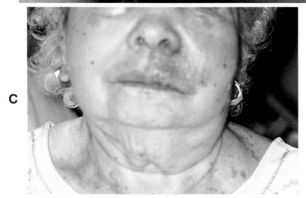

FIGURE 8-30 Herpes zoster. **A,** Unilateral distribution of vesicles along the distribution of a sensory nerve. **B,** Many vesicles coalesce to form large lesions. **C,** Unilateral facial lesions occurring along the distribution of the maxillary branch of the trigeminal nerve. *(From Ibsen OAC, Phelan JA: Oral pathology for the dental hygienist, ed 5, Philadelphia, 2009, Saunders.)*

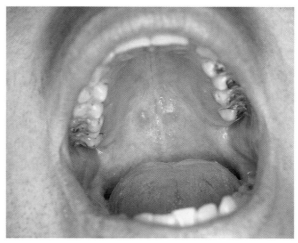

FIGURE 8-31 Herpangina. *(From Ibsen OAC, Phelan JA: Oral pathology for the dental hygienist, ed 5, Philadelphia, 2009, Saunders.)*

corticosteroids, anticonvulsants; biofeedback, and nerve block
3. Cutaneous lesions should be kept clean and dry to prevent secondary infection (antibiotics may have to be prescribed if the infection does occur)
4. Antibacterial oral rinses for intraoral lesions
5. A varicella vaccine is available; Zostavax, for people 60 years and older, is 14 times more effective than Varivax, the vaccine for chickenpox
6. Prognosis is good if trigeminal nerve involvement is present (healing in 2 to 3 weeks)
7. Postherpetic neuralgia can last for extended periods

Herpangina (Aphthous Pharyngitis)

A. Etiology—coxsackievirus
B. Age and gender related—children ages 6 months to 5 years; no gender predilection
C. Location—posterior hard or soft palate, fauces (pillars), uvula, tonsils; most likely seen in the summer
D. Clinical features
  1. Systemic symptoms
    a. Comparatively mild and of short duration
    b. Sore throat; dysphagia
    c. Fever
    d. Headache; vomiting
    e. No lymphadenopathy—differs from primary herpes, which has lymphadenopathy
    f. Transmission through fecal oral or droplets
  2. Oral symptoms (Figure 8-31)
    a. From erythematous macules to vesicles, to ulcers
    b. Vesicles are often overlooked

4. Intraoral lesions can appear as multiple vesicles with a white center, which eventually form shallow ulcerations. These lesions are also unilateral and can be on movable or attached mucosa
5. After the skin vesicles heal, a postherpetic neuralgia occurs
E. Treatment and prognosis
  1. Antiviral medications (acyclovir, valacyclovir, famciclovir)
  2. Postherpetic neuralgia is most difficult to control; several therapies, including analgesics, narcotics,

    c. Two to six small ulcers; ulcers appear with a gray base and inflamed periphery

    d. Slightly painful; the affected person has difficulty swallowing (dysphagia)

    e. Sudden onset

    f. Erythematous pharynx

E. Laboratory tests

    1. Viral isolation (throat culture during early stage)

    2. Stool specimens

F. Treatment and prognosis

    1. Self-limiting, with few complications

    2. Nonaspirin pain relievers

    3. Usually resolves within 7 days without treatment

Infectious Mononucleosis (Glandular Fever)

A. Etiology

    1. Epstein-Barr virus (EBV)

    2. Transmission—intimate oral exchange of saliva; "kissing disease"

B. Age and gender related—children (transmission through saliva on toys) and mostly young adults; no gender predilection

C. Clinical features

    1. Systemic symptoms (depending on age)

       a. Fever, chills, fatigue, malaise

       b. Sore throat, pharyngitis

       c. Headache

       d. Nausea, vomiting

       e. Lymphadenopathy

       f. Enlarged spleen

       g. Neurologic disorders, including seizures

    2. Oral symptoms

       a. Palatal petechiae

       b. NUG

       c. Inflamed attached gingiva

       d. Ulcerations similar to those of herpes or herpangina

       e. Purpuric spots beneath the epithelium (thrombocytopenia—a decrease in the number of platelets)

       f. Edema of the soft palate and uvula

D. Laboratory tests and findings

    1. Increased white blood cells with atypical activated lymphocytes; the presence of these atypical lymphocytes in peripheral blood is very characteristic

    2. Increased heterophil antibody titer; positive Paul-Bunnell test in young adults but not in children under 4 years old

    3. Indirect immunofluorescence test for EBV

E. Treatment and prognosis

    1. Bed rest

    2. Nonaspirin antipyretics

    3. Complications can include splenic, hepatic, and neurologic involvement

    4. Mononucleosis resolves in 4 to 6 weeks

    5. Benign and self-limiting; fatigue may last longer

SKIN DISEASES

General Characteristics

A. Characterized by various forms and sizes of ulcerative eruptions

B. Lesions may appear first or during the course of the disease

C. Reaction simulates an allergic-type reaction

Erythema Multiforme

A. Etiology

    1. Acute, self-limiting condition thought to be a hypersensitivity reaction

    2. May be triggered by HSV infection, tuberculosis, or histoplasmosis; drugs, e.g., barbituates and sulfonormides

    3. Immunologic response

B. Age and gender related—young adults ages 20 to 30 years; more common in males

C. Location

    1. Extremities—hands, feet, arms, legs

    2. Skin—macular, papular, or bullous eruptions; characteristic "target" or "bull's eye" lesions

    3. Oral findings—lips, buccal mucosa, tongue

D. Clinical features (Figure 8-32)

    1. Systemic symptoms

       a. Abrupt onset

       b. Fatigue, malaise, fever

       c. Previous occurrences

       d. Has been associated with systemic conditions

       e. The characteristic skin lesion is referred to as bull's eye, target, or iris

    2. Oral symptoms

       a. Generally lips, tongue, and buccal mucosa

       b. Red patches develop into multiple, painful ulcerations; onset is explosive

       c. Macules, papules, or vesicles ulcerate and bleed easily

       d. A raw tissue base with a grayish, necrotic slough

       e. Irregular shape; surrounded by a band of inflammation; encrustations

E. Laboratory tests—biopsy for differential diagnosis

F. Histologic characteristics

    1. Mixed inflammatory infiltrate

    2. Intraepithelial vesicle formation and thinning

    3. Absence of a basement membrane

    4. Dilation of capillaries and lymphatic vessels in the surface layer of connective tissue

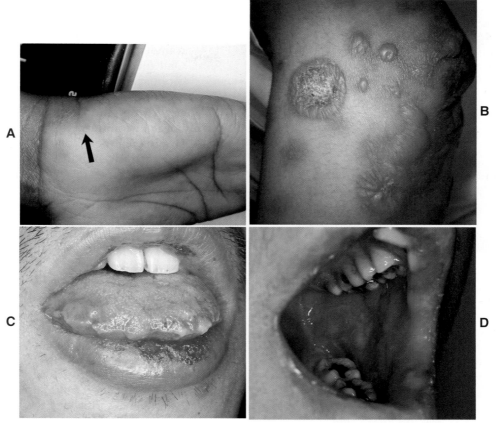

FIGURE 8-32 Skin lesions of erythema multiforme. **A,** Target lesion (*arrow*). **B,** Bullae. **C,** Crusted lip lesions with edema, ulceration, and erythema. **D,** Erythematous and ulcerated lesions of the lips and buccal mucosa. (*A, Courtesy of Dr. Edward V. Zegarelli; **A to D,** from Ibsen OAC, Phelan JA: Oral pathology for the dental hygienist, ed 5, Philadelphia, 2009, Saunders.*)

G. Treatment and prognosis
  1. Removal of the cause, if identified
  2. Topical or systemic applications of corticosteroids
  3. Mild antibacterial oral rinses; antibiotics if secondary infection develops
  4. If patient has significant oral pain, intravenous rehydration may be necessary
  5. Condition resolves in 2 to 4 weeks
  6. Recurrence is possible

Stevens-Johnson Syndrome

A. Severe bullous form of erythema multiforme
B. Etiology—unknown; usually triggered by a drug; the most severe form of erythema multiforme
C. Age and gender related—children and young adults under 25 years; more common in males; history of previous similar illness
D. Location—oral cavity, skin; lesions involving the eyes or genitalia must be present for the diagnosis to be made

E. Clinical features (Figure 8-33)
  1. Oral symptoms—bullae rupture, leaving ulcerations with a raw base; eating becomes impossible; lips are severely encrusted and bleed easily
  2. Skin lesions—severe, numerous; cover wide areas of the body (face, chest, abdomen)
  3. Eye involvement—severe conjunctivitis, photophobia, corneal ulceration, scarring, and blindness
F. Treatment and prognosis
  1. Antibiotics and corticosteroids to control severity
  2. Sometimes antiviral medications to reduce recurrent episodes if HSV recurs
  3. Duration of 1 to 4 weeks
  4. Some patients require hospitalization
  5. Prognosis is good

Behçet Syndrome

A. Etiology—chronic recurrent autoimmune disease
B. Age and gender related—young adults, no gender predilection

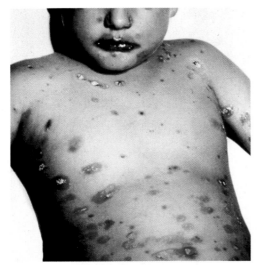

FIGURE 8-33 Stevens-Johnson syndrome. *(Courtesy of Dr. Sidney Eisig; from Ibsen OAC, Phelan JA: Oral pathology for the dental hygienist, ed 5, Philadelphia, 2009, Saunders.)*

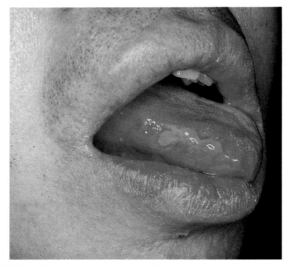

FIGURE 8-34 Oral lesion seen in Behçet syndrome. Aphthous-like oral mucosal ulcer. *(From Ibsen OAC, Phelan JA: Oral pathology for the dental hygienist, ed 5, Philadelphia, 2009, Saunders.)*

C. Location—although now considered a multisystem disorder, it is characterized by a triad of locations: Oral, ocular, and genital areas are involved. Two of the three areas must be involved for the diagnosis
  1. Oral cavity—in most cases, the first manifestation
  2. Eyes are involved in up to 85% of cases, with greater severity in men
  3. Genital lesions occur in 75% of cases (more involvement in men)
D. Clinical features (Figure 8-34)
  1. Oral lesions

  a. Painful ulcerations similar to aphthous ulcers
  b. Large ulcers with gray or yellow center surrounded by a red border,
  c. Oral ulcerations involve the soft palate and oropharynx
  2. Eye lesions
  a. Begin with photophobia and irritation
  b. Purulent conjunctivitis and uveitis
  c. Healing may be followed by scarification and, consequently, blindness
  d. Hypopyon (pus in the anterior chamber of the eye between the iris and the cornea) in severe cases; rare
  3. Genital lesions
  a. In females—painful ulcerations in the vulval folds and labia majora
  b. In males—painful ulcerations on the scrotum and the base of the penis
  4. Systemic symptoms
  a. Occasionally fever; pallor
  b. Complications can involve the central nervous, cardiac, and pulmonary systems
E. Laboratory tests and findings
  1. Cutaneous pathergy test is positive in many patients with Behçet syndrome
  2. Specific changes involving the neutrophils
F. Histologic characteristics
  1. Endothelial proliferation in lesions
  2. Other characteristics similar to those of aphthous stomatitis
G. Treatment and prognosis
  1. Systemic and topical corticosteroids
  2. Other immunosuppressive drugs are given for systemic and ocular involvement
  3. Lesions last 2 to 4 weeks
  4. Disease is long lasting with remission periods

Pemphigus Vulgaris

A. Etiology—severe, progressive autoimmune disease that affects skin and mucous membranes
B. Age and gender related—adults; usually between ages 40 and 55 years; no gender predilection; more common in Ashkenazic Jews
C. Location—anywhere on the oral mucosa; eyes, skin
D. Clinical features (Figure 8-35, *A* and *B*)
  1. In over 50% of cases, the oral lesions appear first. Skin lesions can erupt many months or even a year later
  2. Blisters (caused by an abnormal production of autoantibodies), vesicles, or bullae collapse as soon as they are formed
  a. Vary in shape and size (from several millimeters to several centimeters)

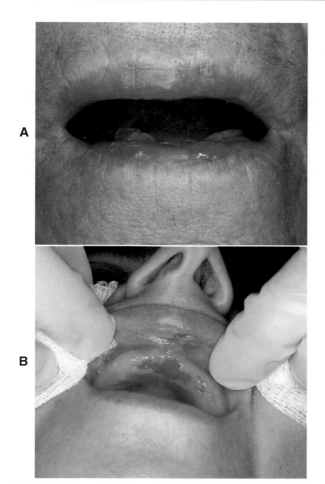

FIGURE 8-35 A and B, Examples of oral lesions in pemphigus vulgaris. *(B, Courtesy of Dr. Fariba Younai; **A and B,** from Ibsen OAC, Phelan JA: Oral pathology for the dental hygienist, ed 5, Philadelphia, 2009, Saunders.)*

    b. Ragged peripheral borders; flat or shallow; base intensely red and raw; may extend into the lips with crusting

  3. Filmy, necrotic slough of tissue can be detached from underlying tissue

  4. Neighboring soft tissue appears normal

  5. Nikolsky sign present—an intraoral bulla can form under light pressure from air syringe or tongue blade; same reaction can occur if pressure is applied to skin

  6. Pain may be severe, and the person is unable to eat

  7. Salivation is profuse; mouth odor

  8. Gingival desquamation

E. Laboratory tests and findings

  1. Biopsy and most conclusive microscopic analysis

  2. Direct immunofluorescence used to identify antibodies (intercellular)

  3. Indirect immunofluorescence is positive for 80% to 90% of patients with pemphigus vulgaris, showing circulating autoantibodies in the serum. It is also used to monitor the patient's therapy

F. Histologic characteristics

  1. The vesicle is entirely intraepithelial above the basal cell layer, producing a distinctive "split"; the basement layer stays attached to underlying connective tissue

  2. Intercellular bridges between epithelial cells disappear, with loss of cohesiveness; epithelial cells separate (acantholysis)

  3. Clumps of rounded epithelial cells, called *Tzanck cells*, are present

  4. Some inflammatory cell infiltration in connective tissue

G. Treatment and prognosis

  1. Systemic corticosteroids

  2. Other immunosuppressive drugs such as azathioprine and methotrexate are used in addition to corticosteroids

  3. Indirect immunofluorescence

  4. Patient may experience periods of remission; never a "cure"; mortality is under 10% and associated with complications from long-term corticosteroid therapy

▎WHITE LESIONS

General Characteristics

A. Often associated with hyperkeratosis; clinical term for leukoplakia

B. Vary from simple lesions to diffuse coverage; smooth to rough surfaces; elevated to flat

C. Attached to mucous membranes

D. Color—white, grayish white, yellowish white

E. Painless

F. Associated with a variety of conditions (including variants of normal, systemic disease, and premalignant lesions)

Nicotine Stomatitis

A. Etiology—heavy tobacco smoking using cigarettes, cigars, waterpipes (hookah), or pipes; commonly associated with pipes ("pipe smoker's palate")

B. Age and gender related—most common in male smokers over 40 years

C. Location—posterior hard and soft palates

D. Clinical features (Figure 8-36)

  1. Begins with erythema and inflammation of the palate; response to an irritant (heat)

  2. Over time, the palate becomes more keratinized and grayish white; thickened nodules surround the inflamed orifices of the minor salivary ducts

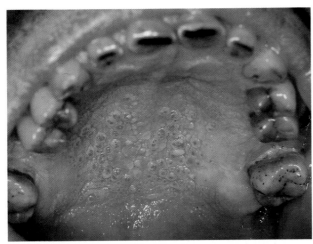

FIGURE 8-36 Nicotine stomatitis. *(From Ibsen OAC, Phelan JA: Oral pathology for the dental hygienist, ed 5, Philadelphia, 2009, Saunders.)*

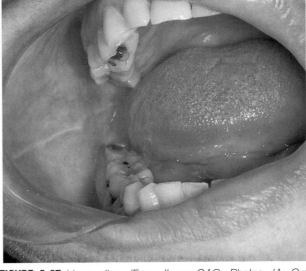

FIGURE 8-37 Linea alba. *(From Ibsen OAC, Phelan JA: Oral pathology for the dental hygienist, ed 5, Philadelphia, 2009, Saunders.)*

    3. Fissures or cracks around the nodules create an overall wrinkled appearance
E. Histologic characteristics
    1. Hyperkeratosis and acanthosis
    2. Thickening of the epithelium adjacent to the orifice
F. Treatment and prognosis
    1. If the cause is removed—smoking—the condition may be reversible
    2. The prognosis is good if the person permanently stops smoking and the tissues return to normal
    3. If tissues do not return to normal after smoking irritants are removed, biopsy may be necessary

Linea Alba

A. Etiology—pattern of occlusion; pressure of teeth on buccal mucosa
B. Age and gender related—any age; no gender predilection
C. Location—buccal mucosa along the occlusal plane; usually bilateral
D. Clinical features (Figure 8-37)
    1. "White line" on the buccal mucosa, anterior to posterior along the line of occlusion
    2. Localized, single line in thickness; usually bilateral
E. Histologic characteristics—hyperorthokeratosis; some localized intracellular edema
F. Treatment and prognosis—no treatment required

Leukoedema

A. Etiology—unknown; a variant of normal
B. Age and gender related—average age 45 years; no gender predilection; African Americans are more affected (85% of incidence) than other racial groups
C. Location—bilateral buccal and labial mucosa
D. Clinical features
    1. Soft, diffuse, velvety, filmy opalescence of buccal mucosa
    2. Later becomes grayish white with a coarsely wrinkled surface
    3. When the tissue is stretched, the white opalescence disappears (this clinical characteristic can help in the differential diagnosis)
    4. Some research shows it is more prominent in smokers
E. Histologic characteristics
    1. Intracellular edema of prickle cells (spinous layer)
    2. Increased thickness of epithelium with a superficial parakeratotic layer several cells thick
    3. Broad rete pegs that appear irregularly elongated
    4. Parakeratin on epithelial surface
F. Treatment and prognosis—no treatment required; considered a variant of normal

Systemic Lupus Erythematosus (SLE)

A. Etiology—acute and chronic inflammatory autoimmune disease involving several systems
    1. Cellular and humoral immunity are impaired

2. B lymphocytes increase function; T lymphocytes do not function properly

B. Age and gender related—much more common in females (8:1) during childbearing years; African American females more affected than white females (3:1)

C. Location
1. Buccal mucosa, palate, gingiva (25% to 30% of persons with SLE)
2. Skin—lesions occur in 85% of persons with SLE; a characteristic erythematous butterfly-shaped rash on the face (malar areas) and nose; chest, back, extremities; exposure to sunlight makes the rash worse

D. Systemic characteristics
1. Fever, weight loss, arthritis, muscle pain
2. Raynaud phenomenon is seen in up to 15% of persons with SLE
3. Central nervous system involvement, depression, and seizures
4. Ocular involvement; retinal nerve damage
5. Kidney involvement (complications can be fatal)
6. Cardiac involvement (endocarditis)

E. Clinical features (Figure 8-38)
1. Skin lesions—erythematous rash; scales form, scarring in the center; butterfly configuration on the malar areas of the face and nose
2. Among those with SLE, 25% to 30% have oral manifestations
3. Erythematous plaques with white striae; can resemble lichen planus but is less defined
4. Burning mouth; xerostomia

F. Laboratory tests and findings
1. Direct immunofluorescence of skin lesion (95% effective for SLE)
2. Direct immunofluorescence of normal skin showing a positive lupus band in 25% to 60% of persons with SLE
3. Anemia; leukopenia; thrombocytopenia
4. Positive identification of antinuclear antibodies (ANA); not very specific
5. Anti–double-stranded DNA antibodies, a specific finding in up to 80% of patients with SLE
6. A combination of these test findings, multi-organ involvement, skin lesions, and possible oral lesions can all play a role in the definitive diagnosis of this very complex disease

G. Histologic characteristics
1. Hyperkeratosis; alternating changes within the spinous layer of the epithelium
2. Necrosis of the basal cell layer
3. Inflammatory infiltrate around blood vessels in the connective tissue not in a subepithelial band as seen in lichen planus

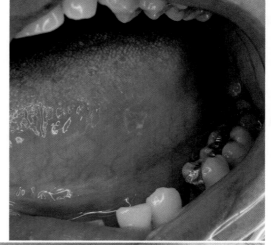
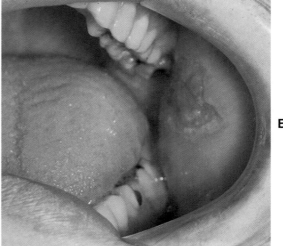

FIGURE 8-38 A and B, Oral lesions in lupus erythematosus. *(Courtesy of Dr. Edward V. Zegarelli; from Ibsen OAC, Phelan JA: Oral pathology for the dental hygienist, ed 5, Philadelphia, 2009, Saunders.)*

4. Deposits of a periodic acid–Schiff (PAS) material in the basement membrane
5. Subepithelial edema

H. Treatment and prognosis
1. Aspirin and nonsteroidal anti-inflammatory drugs (NSAIDs)
2. Antimalarial and corticosteroids combined with other immunosuppressive medications
3. Periods of remission; in mild cases, the prognosis is good; with significant organ involvement, the disease can be fatal
4. Consult with patient's physician before dental treatment; prophylactic antibiotic premedication may be necessary

White Sponge Nevus (Cannon Disease, Familial White Folded Dysplasia)

A. Etiology—hereditary; autosomal dominant trait; mutation in the mucosal keratin pair K4 or K13; complete penetrance with varying degrees of expressivity

B. Age and gender related—progressive from childhood to adulthood; no gender predilection

C. Location—bilateral buccal mucosa is always affected (sometimes soft palate or ventral tongue)

D. Clinical features
   1. White, velvety, thickened, and folded tissue of the buccal mucosa
   2. Diffuse, generalized, and bilateral
   3. Early years—the white mucosa is smooth and flat; becomes corrugated over time
   4. Adolescence—tissues become increasingly folded or corrugated; appear opalescent-white when the condition peaks

E. Histologic characteristics
   1. Thickened epithelium with hyperparakeratosis and acanthosis
   2. Perinuclear condensation of keratin tonofilaments in the superficial cells of the epithelium
   3. Cells of the spinous layer toward the surface exhibit vacuolation (space filled with fluid or air)

F. Treatment and prognosis
   1. No treatment required
   2. Prognosis is excellent

Lichen Planus

A. Etiology—benign, chronic disease; immunologically mediated disorder

B. Age and gender related—middle-aged adults; slight predilection for females

C. Location—skin; oral mucosa; especially buccal mucosa, dorsal tongue, gingiva, and palate

D. Clinical features—two forms: reticular and erosive
   1. Reticular lichen planus (most common) (Figure 8-39B)
      a. White, narrow, interconnecting, slightly elevated lines forming a mesh, net, or lace-like pattern (Wickham's striae); these lesions can also look like white papules; cannot be wiped off
      b. Mucous membrane between the white lines appears normal
      c. When the dorsal tongue is involved, the lesion may appear as a solid gray to white plaque-like area
      d. Usually asymptomatic
   2. Erosive or ulcerative form
      a. Lesions are symptomatic
      b. The condition begins as an erosive, flat lesion

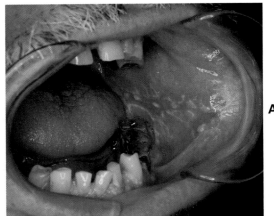
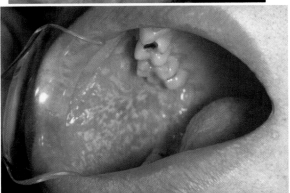
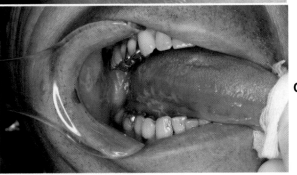

FIGURE 8-39 Lichen planus. **A,** Erosion of the mucosa appears as erythema adjacent to white striae. **B and C,** Two additional examples of the oral lesions of lichen planus. *(A, Courtesy of Dr. Edward V. Zegarelli; A to C, from Ibsen OAC, Phelan JA: Oral pathology for the dental hygienist, ed 5, Philadelphia, 2009, Saunders.)*

   c. This erythematous area is ulcerated and surrounded by fine white borders; painful
   d. Slight increased risk for squamous cell carcinoma in persons with erosive lichen planus; a 3-month recare appointment with thorough extraoral and intraoral examination should be scheduled
   e. Atrophy of the gingiva is described as desquamative (Figure 8-40); this feature can appear with other oral conditions

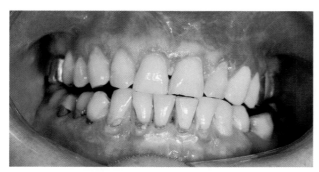

FIGURE 8-40 Lichen planus. The gingival lesions of lichen planus are described clinically as desquamative tissue. *(Courtesy of Dr. Edward V. Zegarelli; from Ibsen OAC, Phelan JA: Oral pathology for the dental hygienist, ed 5, Philadelphia, 2009, Saunders.)*

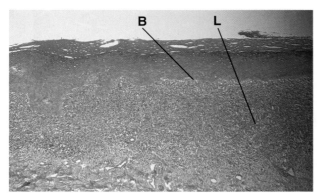

FIGURE 8-41 Lichen planus seen by low-power microscopy. Note the degeneration of the basal cell layer of the epithelium (*B*) and the band-like infiltrate of lymphocytes (*L*). *(From Ibsen OAC, Phelan JA: Oral pathology for the dental hygienist, ed 5, Philadelphia, 2009, Saunders.)*

E. Histologic characteristics (Figure 8-41)
  1. Hyperparakeratosis or hyperorthokeratosis on the surface epithelium
  2. Thickened spinous layer (acanthosis)
  3. Intracellular edema of cells in the spinous layer
  4. Necrosis or degeneration of the basal cell layer
  5. Band-like infiltrate of lymphocytes
F. Treatment and prognosis
  1. Treatment for symptomatic cases
  2. Corticosteroids to decrease ulcerations and inflammation (systemic only when absolutely necessary)
  3. Topical corticosteroids (e.g., fluocinonide) applied several times a day
  4. Meticulous oral hygiene
  5. Lesions are self-limiting; heal in a few weeks with topical corticosteroid therapy
  6. The condition does recur, and corticosteroids need to be reapplied

Hyperkeratosis

A. Etiology—local factors; constant, low-grade irritation (frictional keratosis; chronic tongue chewing, cheek biting, repetitive irritation)
B. Age and gender related—usually over age 40 years; more common in males
C. Location—anywhere in the oral cavity; alveolar ridge, buccal mucosa, lateral tongue
D. Clinical features (Figure 8-42, *A* and *B*)
  1. White, flat lesion with a diffuse boundary
  2. Three layers of epithelium affected; granular, prickle, and basal
  3. Fissures or ulcerations rare
E. Laboratory tests—incisional biopsy
F. Histologic characteristics (see Figure 8-42, *C*)
  1. Abnormal layer of keratin or parakeratosis where not normally found
  2. Increased thickness of keratin in areas where normally found (e.g., attached gingiva, palate)
  3. Normal underlying epithelial cells
  4. Scalpel biopsy necessary for microscopic evaluation
G. Treatment and prognosis
  1. Removal of the cause (irritant)
  2. Tissue should return to normal

NEOPLASIA

Squamous Cell Carcinoma

A. Etiology—chemicals, viruses, and radiation; secondary to genetic mutation; immunosuppression; risk factors include use of all forms of tobacco, alcohol abuse, and increasing age. A combination of these risks can be lethal. Iron-deficiency anemia is another factor that elevates the risk for squamous cell carcinoma in the posterior mouth and esophagus. Squamous cell carcinoma accounts for 90% to 95% of oral cancers
B. Age and gender related—young adults to adults in their 60s, 70s, and beyond; incidence increases with increasing age; sixth most common cancer in males and twelfth in females; ratio of incidence in males and females is 2 : 1; highest overall incidence in white males after 65 years; highest incidence in middle age is found in African American males
C. Locations
  1. Tongue—37% to 50% of all oral carcinomas, excluding cancer of the pharynx; posterior third, including the lateral borders and ventral surfaces, account for most of these. The tongue is, by far, the primary location for squamous cell carcinoma in the oral cavity

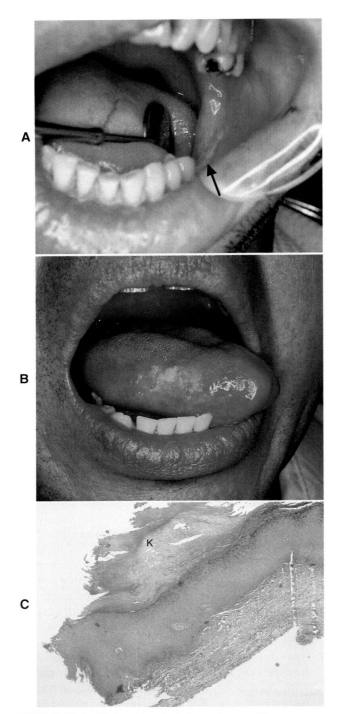

FIGURE 8-42 A, Frictional keratosis (*arrow*) caused by an opposing third molar. **B,** Caused by chronic tongue chewing. **C,** Low-power microscopic appearance of hyperkeratosis showing an increase in the amount of surface keratin (*K*). *(From Ibsen OAC, Phelan JA: Oral pathology for the dental hygienist, ed 5, Philadelphia, 2009, Saunders.)*

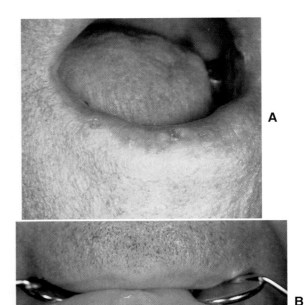

FIGURE 8-43 A and B, Clinical appearance of squamous cell carcinoma of the lower lip. *(Courtesy of Dr. Edward V. Zegarelli; from Ibsen OAC, Phelan JA: Oral pathology for the dental hygienist, ed 5, Philadelphia, 2009, Saunders.)*

2. Floor of the mouth—30% to 35%
3. Lips—22%; most of these occur on lower lip; pipe, cigar smokers, patients with fair skin, and persons with an outdoor occupation who are exposed to sunlight have a definite predilection for squamous cell carcinoma of the lower lip (Figure 8-43, *A* and *B*)
4. Buccal mucosa—6%
5. Gingiva—6%
6. Soft palate—4%; metastasis has already occurred by the time a diagnosis is made
7. The mandible is more common than the maxilla and is usually the result of metastasis from other areas

D. Clinical features (Figure 8-44, *A* to *C*)
   1. Exophytic, indurated, ulcerated, firm lesion in soft tissue; feels anchored to underlying tissue
   2. On lower lip, smaller crusted ulceration, indurated border; asymptomatic
   3. Sores or ulcerations that do not heal
   4. Stages—tumor node metastasis (TNM) staging system helps predict the patient's prognosis (Box 8-1)
      a. Stage I—early; asymptomatic; tumor <2 cm in diameter

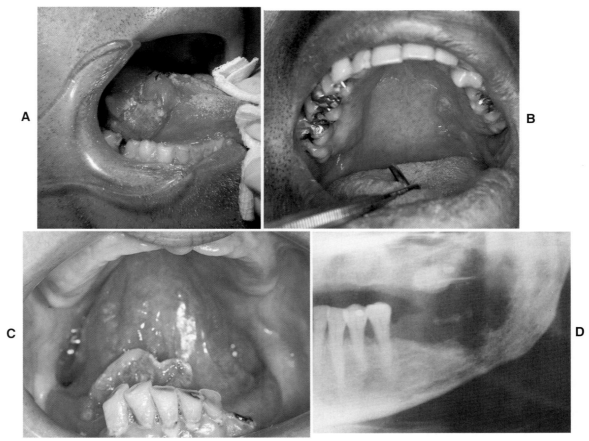

FIGURE 8-44 A, Clinical appearance of squamous cell carcinoma of the posterolateral tongue showing an exophytic, ulcerated mass. **B,** Clinical appearance of squamous cell carcinoma of the left side of the soft palate and fauces. **C,** Clinical appearance of squamous cell carcinoma on the floor of the mouth. **D,** Left side of a panoramic radiograph showing destruction of the mandible by squamous cell carcinoma. *(**C,** Courtesy of Dr. Edward V. Zegarelli; **A to D,** from Ibsen OAC, Phelan JA: Oral pathology for the dental hygienist, ed 5, Philadelphia, 2009, Saunders.)*

BOX 8-1 TNM Staging System for Oral Squamous Cell Carcinoma

T—Tumor
T1—Tumor <2 cm in diameter
T2—Tumor 2–4 cm in diameter
T3—Tumor >4 cm in diameter
T4—Tumor invades adjacent structures
N—Node
N0—No palpable nodes
N1—Ipsilateral (same side as primary tumor) palpable nodes (same side as tumor)
N2—Contralateral (opposite side from primary tumor) or bilateral nodes
N3—Fixed palpable nodes
M—Metastasis
M0—No distant metastasis
M1—Clinical radiographic evidence of metastasis

TNM, *tumor–node–metastasis.*
From Regezi JA, Sciubba JJ: Oral pathology: Clinical pathologic correlations, ed 5, Philadelphia, 2008, Saunders.

   b. Stage II—intermediate; tumor 2 to 4 cm in diameter
   c. Stage III—advanced; tumor >4 cm
   d. Stage IV—tumor metastasizes to other adjacent areas
E. Radiographic appearance (see Figure 8-44, *D*)
   1. Diffuse radiolucency with irregular borders after significant bone has been destroyed; penetration into the cortex
   2. Resorption of tooth roots; expansion in between roots
F. Laboratory tests and findings
   1. Biopsy- scalpel biopsy is the "gold standard"
      a. Incisional—removal of a segment or piece of the lesion
      b. Excisional—removal of the entire lesion in question
   2. Screening tools (see the section on "Diagnostic Tools for Oral Cancer Detection" in Chapter 16)
      a. Brush biopsy—a small circular brush is rotated about 10 times on the surface cells of

the lesion to obtain a transepithelial specimen from all layers of the epithelium to the basement membrane. Positive and atypical results require a scalpel biopsy for complete microscopic analysis and a definitive diagnosis; research needed to establish efficacy

   b. ViziLite—tissues are illuminated with a special light after patient rinses with acetic acid; areas that turn white are evaluated and, for those in question, a scalpel biopsy is performed. Subtle lesions that may appear "within normal limits" during the intraoral examination can clearly be identified with ViziLite, although some variants of normal may also become more obvious; research needed to establish efficacy

   c. VelScope—a hand held device that emits a fluorescent blue light into the oral cavity. Normal tissue reflects green; abnormal tissue reflects brown to black. "Abnormal" tissue may be linea alba. Clinician needs to be experienced with variants of normal prior to using VelScope; research needed to establish efficacy

G. Histologic characteristics
   1. Invasion of sheets of tumor cells into underlying connective tissue (neoplastic squamous cells)
   2. Presence of keratin pearls (cluster of concentrically layered keratinized cells)
   3. Neoplastic cells that contain large hyperchromatic nuclei and mitotic figures

H. Treatment and prognosis
   1. Surgical excision alone or excision with a combination of radiation and chemotherapy; sometimes radiation therapy alone
   2. Tumor size and location both influence the treatment protocol
   3. Adjunctive chemotherapeutic agents
   4. When metastasis has occurred (lymph node involvement), more radical procedures are performed
   5. Prognosis depends on the tumor stage

PLEOMORPHIC ADENOMA (BENIGN MIXED TUMOR)

A. Etiology—benign salivary gland tumor that accounts for 90% of all benign salivary gland tumors
B. Age and gender related—most common in adults ages 30 to 60 years; female predilection; can occur in children.
C. Location
   1. Parotid gland
   2. Posterior hard or soft palate (most common intra-oral site)

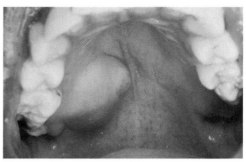

FIGURE 8-45 Benign salivary gland tumor of the palate (pleomorphic adenoma). *(From Ibsen OAC, Phelan JA:* Oral pathology for the dental hygienist, *ed 5, Philadelphia, 2009, Saunders.)*

D. Clinical features (Figure 8-45)
   1. Located on either side of the midline of the posterior palate
   2. Painless, slow-growing
   3. Smooth, dome-shaped mass, not ulcerated (unless traumatized)
   4. Size from a few millimeters to a few centimeters
E. Histologic characteristics
   1. An encapsulated tumor composed of epithelium and connective tissue
   2. Benign
F. Treatment and prognosis
   1. Surgical excision
   2. Sometimes partial or complete removal of the parotid gland in the area
   3. 5% risk of malignant transformation
   4. Conservative enucleation is not recommended because it leads to high recurrence rates
   5. Prognosis is excellent if proper surgical techniques are used
   6. Research reports that about 5% of tumors transform into malignancy

CYSTS

A. True cyst
   1. Cavity lined by epithelium and enclosed within a capsule of connective tissue
   2. Space often filled with fluid or fragments of tissues
B. Cysts are classified according to:
   1. Etiology, histologic components; location
   2. Odontogenic; nonodontogenic; inflammatory response

Radicular Cyst (Root-End Cyst, Periapical Cyst)

A. Etiology
   1. A true cyst; develops as an inflammatory response; associated with a nonvital tooth

2. Factors could include dental caries, trauma, deep restorations causing pulpitis

B. Age and gender related—any age, but common ages 30 to 60 years; slight predilection for males

C. Location—apex of a tooth or lateral to the tooth root

D. Clinical features
  1. Nonvital tooth
  2. Usually asymptomatic

E. Radiographic appearance
  1. Round or ovoid, well-defined radiolucent area attached to the apex or lateral to the root (Figure 8-46, *A*)
  2. Same radiographic appearance as periapical granuloma

F. Histologic characteristics
  1. Lined by stratified squamous epithelium; developing from epithelial rest of Malassez

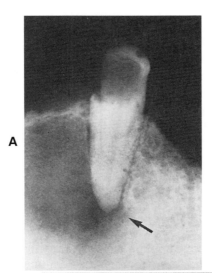

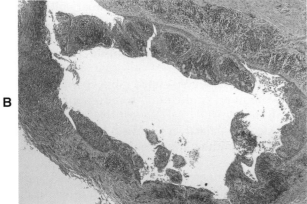

FIGURE 8-46 Radicular cyst. **A,** Radiograph showing a well-circumscribed radiolucency around the root of a tooth (*arrow*). **B,** Microscopic features of a radicular cyst. *(From Ibsen OAC, Phelan JA: Oral pathology for the dental hygienist, ed 5, Philadelphia, 2009, Saunders.)*

2. The wall is composed of well-vascularized dense fibrous connective tissue (see Figure 8-46, *B*)

3. Lumen is filled with cellular debris

G. Treatment
  1. Root canal therapy
  2. Extraction of the tooth and curettage of the socket and apical area to remove the cystic sac
  3. If radiolucency fails to resolve the condition, retreatment endodontically and possibly an apicoectomy is required

Residual Cyst

A. Etiology
  1. Radicular cyst that has not been removed after extraction of the involved tooth
  2. Open socket with debris acting as a stimulus

B. Age and gender related—usually adults who were treated for a radicular cyst

C. Location
  1. Apical area where a tooth had previously been extracted
  2. Within the socket area or on the alveolar ridge
  3. At the alveolar ridge where a tooth had previously been extracted

D. Clinical features—small and asymptomatic

E. Radiographic appearance
  1. Well-defined radiolucent area (Figure 8-47, *A* and *B*)
  2. Round or oval in shape
  3. In time, this radiolucency can become somewhat radiopaque because of histologic changes within the lumen

F. Histologic characteristics
  1. Stratified squamous epithelium lining the lumen
  2. Dense fibrous connective tissue wall

G. Treatment—surgical removal of the cyst

DEVELOPMENTAL CYSTS

Nonodontogenic Cysts

A. Etiology
  1. Median mandibular cyst—cyst in midline of the mandible; develops from an odontogenic origin, possibly a primordial cyst
  2. Globulomaxillary cyst—arises from the odontogenic epithelium between the maxillary lateral incisor and canine (not a fissural cyst)
  3. Nasolabial cyst—soft tissue cyst; develops from the inferior and anterior segments of the nasolacrimal duct; strong female predilection (4 : 1)
  4. Median palatine cyst—fissural cyst; posterior form of a nasopalatine canal cyst; young adults

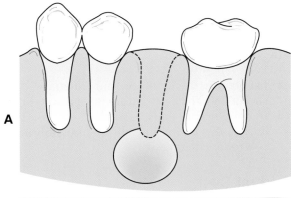

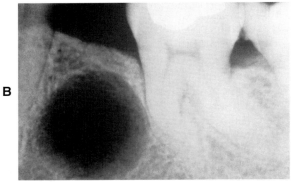

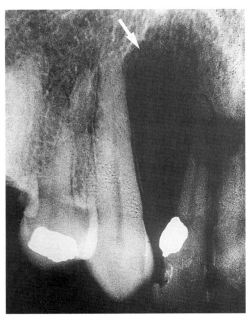

FIGURE 8-48 Radiograph of a globulomaxillary cyst showing a characteristic pear-shaped radiolucency between the maxillary lateral incisor and canine. *(From Ibsen OAC, Phelan JA: Oral pathology for the dental hygienist, ed 5, Philadelphia, 2009, Saunders.)*

FIGURE 8-47 A, Schematic of a residual cyst. **B,** Radiograph of a residual cyst showing a radiolucency at the site of a previously extracted tooth. *(Courtesy of Drs. Paul Freedman and Stanley Kerpel; from Ibsen OAC, Phelan JA: Oral pathology for the dental hygienist, ed 5, Philadelphia, 2009, Saunders.)*

5. Nasopalatine canal cyst (incisive canal cyst)—develops from the epithelial remnants of embryonal nasopalatine ducts; strong male predilection
B. Age and gender related—adults; no gender predilection, unless specified
C. Location—names are based on location
1. Median mandibular cyst—occurs at the midline of the anterior mandible
2. Globulomaxillary cyst—appears as a pear-shaped radiolucency between the roots of the maxillary lateral incisor and canine
3. Nasolabial cyst—upper lip, lateral to midline; in the mucolabial fold in the area of the maxillary canine and the floor of the nose
4. Median palatine cyst—arises at the midline of the hard palate
5. Nasopalatine canal cyst—appears within the nasopalatine canal or the incisive papilla
D. Clinical features
1. Cysts vary in size from no evidence of a lesion to a bulge or expansion of bone
2. All teeth are vital when associated with non-odontogenic cysts

E. Radiographic appearance—well-defined radiolucent area; some have particular shapes because of the anatomic location where they develop
1. Globulomaxillary cyst—located between the maxillary lateral incisor and canine; often pear shaped (Figure 8-48)
2. The nasopalatine canal (incisal canal) cyst is heart shaped
F. Histologic characteristics
1. Median mandibular cyst—most often lined by stratified squamous epithelium; few cases of pseudostratified ciliated columnar epithelium
2. Globulomaxillary cyst—lined by inflamed stratified squamous epithelium; can histologically resemble the components of several other cystic lesions
3. Nasolabial cyst—lined by pseudostratified columnar epithelium; some cuboidal epithelium
4. Median palatal cyst—lined by stratified squamous epithelium; chronic inflammation in cell wall
5. Nasopalatine canal cyst—several types of epithelium are found in this cyst; most often, stratified squamous epithelium
G. Treatment and prognosis
1. Enucleation of the cystic sac and curettage of surrounding bone
2. Prognosis is excellent

Thyroglossal Tract Cyst (Thyroglossal Duct Cyst)

A. Etiology—developmental; in the thyroglossal tract, which extends from the foramen cecum to the permanent position of the thyroid gland in the neck region; the embryonic thyroglossal tract; inflammation is the stimulus possibly associated with adjacent lymph tissue that reacts from a draining infection from the head and neck area

B. Age and gender related—usually young adults under 20 years; no gender predilection

C. Location—posterior tongue, anywhere from the foramen cecum to the suprasternal notch; 75% of these lesions are below the hyoid bone

D. Clinical features (Figure 8-49, *A* and *B*)
  1. Asymptomatic; painless; movable swelling; midline of the neck
  2. Bulge is of round or oval shape; usually <3 cm in diameter
  3. Fistulous tracts to the skin or mucosa can develop
  4. Swallowing becomes difficult (dysphagia)
  5. Inability to extend the tongue

E. Histologic characteristics
  1. Cysts below the hyoid bone are lined with ciliated columnar epithelium; squamous epithelium or other types of epithelial tissue above the hyoid bone
  2. Connective tissue wall may contain thyroid tissue

F. Treatment and prognosis
  1. Complete surgical excision of the cyst (after a thyroid scan)
  2. Surgical procedure will include removal of part of the hyoid bone and muscle tissue in the tract
  3. Prognosis is good
  4. Malignant transformation is rare

Lymphoepithelial Cyst (Branchial Cleft Cyst)

A. Etiology
  1. Epithelial remnants of the embryonic brachial arches
  2. 95% develop from the second branchial arch
  3. Epithelium entrapped in lymph nodes (another theory of development)

B. Age and gender related—young adults; no gender predilection

C. Location
  1. Intraorally—floor of the mouth and lateral borders of the tongue
  2. Usually close to the anterior border of the sternocleidomastoid muscle
  3. Area from the clavicle to the parotid gland

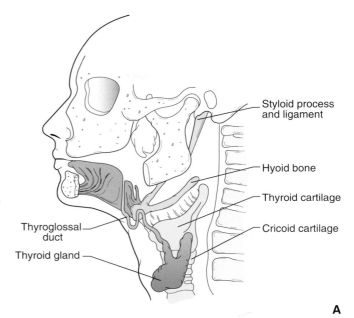

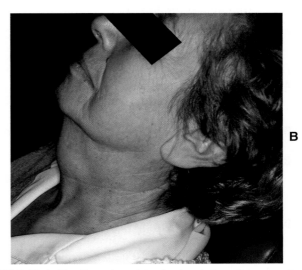

FIGURE 8-49 A, The thyroglossal tract extends from the area of the foramen cecum, lingual to the lower part of the neck. **B,** A thyroglossal tract cyst is the cause of enlargement at the midline of the neck. *(From Ibsen OAC, Phelan JA: Oral pathology for the dental hygienist, ed 5, Philadelphia, 2009, Saunders.)*

D. Clinical features
  1. Slow-growing, movable mass 1 to 10 cm in diameter; asymptomatic
  2. Can have a pink to yellowish color when found intraorally
  3. If trauma or infection is associated, pain may be present

E. Histologic characteristics (Figure 8-50)
  1. Lined by stratified squamous epithelium that may or may not be keratinized
  2. Lymphoid tissue in the wall

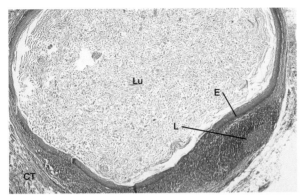

FIGURE 8-50 Low-power microscopic appearance of a lympho-epithelial cyst showing lumen (*Lu*), epithelial lining (*E*), surrounding lymphocytes (*L*), and connective tissue (*CT*). *(From Ibsen OAC, Phelan JA: Oral pathology for the dental hygienist, ed 5, Philadelphia, 2009, Saunders.)*

F. Treatment and prognosis
   1. Surgical removal
   2. Prognosis is good

Dermoid Cyst

A. Etiology—developmental from all three germ layers: ectoderm, endoderm, mesoderm; benign cystic form of teratoma
B. Age and gender related—present at birth or in young children; no gender predilection
C. Location
   1. In the oral cavity, anterior floor of the mouth
   2. Ovarian teratomas, or "dermoids," contain actual tooth structures
D. Clinical features
   1. Semi-firm, dough-like consistency
   2. Size—a few millimeters to several centimeters
   3. Midline of the floor of the mouth
E. Histologic characteristics
   1. Lined with orthokeratinized stratified squamous epithelium
   2. Keratin within the lumen
   3. A fibrous connective tissue wall
   4. May contain sebaceous glands, hair follicles, sweat glands, and occasionally teeth
F. Treatment and prognosis
   1. Surgical removal; approach depends on the location relative to the geniohyoid muscle
   2. Prognosis is good

ODONTOGENIC CYSTS

Lateral Periodontal Cyst

A. Etiology—developmental; odontogenic cyst; develops from the rests of the dental lamina

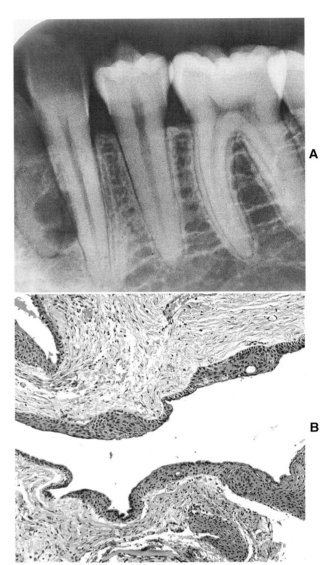

FIGURE 8-51 A, Radiograph of a lateral periodontal cyst. This biloculated, well-defined radiolucency is located lateral to the tooth root. **B,** Microscopic appearance of a lateral periodontal cyst showing a thin epithelial lining with focal epithelial thickenings. *(From Ibsen OAC, Phelan JA: Oral pathology for the dental hygienist, ed 5, Philadelphia, 2009, Saunders.)*

B. Age and gender related—adults over 30 years; common ages 50 to 70 years; male predilection
C. Location—most often lateral root surface of mandibular canine or premolar teeth (occasionally seen in the maxilla in the same areas)
D. Clinical features
   1. Tooth or teeth involved are vital
   2. Asymptomatic, no bulge
E. Radiographic appearance
   1. Small (<1 cm)
   2. Well-defined ovoid or elliptically shaped radiolucent area found lateral to a tooth root (Figure 8-51, *A*)

3. The odontogenic keratocyst and other inflammatory cysts can have the same radiographic features

F. Histologic characteristics (see Figure 8-51, *B*)
   1. Stratified squamous epithelial lining only a few cells thick; focal epithelial thickening
   2. Thin connective tissue wall

G. Treatment and prognosis
   1. Surgical enucleation of the cyst without damage to surrounding teeth
   2. Few cases of recurrence have been reported

Primordial Cyst

A. Etiology—neoplastic; arises from epithelium of the enamel organ or from primordial epithelium; history that a tooth was never present; the cyst develops in place of the tooth; sometimes histologically considered the same as an odontogenic keratocyst

B. Age and gender related—child to young adult; ages 10 to 40 years; slight male predilection

C. Location—posterior mandible; third molar area or posterior to an erupted third molar and up the ramus

D. Clinical features—no obvious clinical features; the affected person may be asymptomatic

E. Radiographic appearance—well-defined radiolucent oval lesion; can be multi-locular
   1. Tooth never present in the space occupied by the cyst (this history is essential to the diagnosis)
   2. An unerupted tooth can be involved in this cyst
   3. Size varies from a few millimeters to a centimeter
   4. Radiographic features not diagnostic

F. Histologic characteristics
   1. Four to eight cells of stratified squamous epithelium
   2. No rete pegs
   3. Cuboidal columnar epithelial cells are hyperchromatic and appear in the basal epithelial level

G. Treatment and prognosis
   1. Surgical removal of the cyst, biopsy, and histologic examination
   2. Recurrence depends on the histologic findings; odontogenic keratocysts recur in 30% of cases

Dentigerous Cyst (Follicular Cyst)

A. Etiology—from reduced enamel epithelium after the crown of the tooth is completely formed (unerupted or impacted tooth); accumulation of fluid between the crown and reduced enamel epithelium; cyst must be associated with a tooth; developmental or inflammatory origin

B. Age and gender related—ages 10 to 30 years; higher predilection for white males

C. Location
   1. Mandibular third molar area—around the crown of an unerupted third molar; often extending to the ramus
   2. Maxillary canine region—compromising the maxillary sinus

D. Clinical features
   1. Always associated with the crown of an unerupted tooth; asymptomatic
   2. Can be an aggressive lesion (causing expansion of bone and extreme displacement of teeth), fracture of the mandible, or both (in which case it would be painful)

E. Radiographic appearance (Figure 8-52, *A* and *B*)
   1. Smooth, unilocular radiolucency associated with the crown of an unerupted tooth
   2. At least 4 mm of radiolucency extending from the crown to the epithelium of the reduced enamel

F. Histologic characteristics
   1. Stratified squamous epithelium lining the lumen; not keratinized

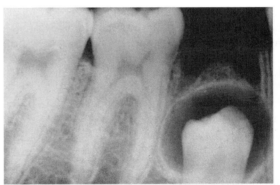
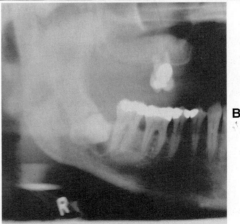

FIGURE 8-52 A, Radiographs of dentigerous cysts surrounding the crown of an unerupted premolar. **B,** Impacted third molar. *(From Ibsen OAC, Phelan JA: Oral pathology for the dental hygienist, ed 5, Philadelphia, 2009, Saunders.)*

2. Surrounded by a thin fibrous connective tissue wall
3. In the inflamed variety, the fibrous wall has an inflammatory infiltrate

G. Treatment and prognosis
1. Enucleation of the cystic sac, and sometimes the associated tooth
2. The tooth may be left in place, with orthodontic intervention to assist eruption
3. Rare transformation to the ameloblastoma
4. Prognosis is very good

Injuries to Oral Soft Tissue

Ranula

A. Etiology
1. Blockage or obstruction by a salivary "stone" (sialolith) in the duct of a major salivary gland (sublingual or submandibular); unilateral
2. Trauma to same area
3. Mucus spills into the adjacent connective tissue

B. Age and gender related—any age, but usually adults; no gender predilection

C. Location—unilaterally on the floor of the mouth

D. Clinical features (Figure 8-53)
1. Translucent, bluish, round, smooth-surfaced bulge 1 to 3 cm in diameter
2. Semi-firm, unilateral, fluctuant mass
3. Increases in size between meals; decreases immediately after a meal
4. Located lateral to the midline (helpful to the differential diagnosis)

E. Radiographic appearance—radiopaque sialolith in the duct area if it is present

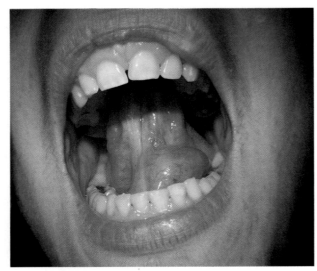

FIGURE 8-53 Ranula. *(From Ibsen OAC, Phelan JA: Oral pathology for the dental hygienist, ed 5, Philadelphia, 2009, Saunders.)*

F. Histologic characteristics
1. Epithelial lining is present; mucous fluid surrounded by granulation tissue
2. Inflammatory cells

G. Treatment and prognosis
1. Surgical excision
2. Removal of the obstruction, if present
3. May recur

Mucocele (Mucus Extravasation)

A. Etiology
1. Trauma to a minor salivary gland duct
2. Mechanical trauma to the salivary duct by lip biting or pinching

B. Age and gender related—all ages but most common in children and young adults; no gender predilection

C. Location—the most common site is the lower lip

D. Clinical features
1. Blister-like, raised, circumscribed vesicle; 1 to 4 mm in size; painless
2. Bluish hue if the mucocele is near the surface
3. Firm, movable on palpation
4. Vesicle ruptures and can leave fragments of epithelial tissue

E. Histologic characteristics
1. The lesion is not a true cyst because it is not lined with epithelium
2. Mucin surrounded by a granulation tissue response

F. Treatment and prognosis
1. Excision of the lesion and associated gland
2. Sometimes the vesicle breaks and the lesion resolves by itself
3. Recurrence is possible (and may occur in the same place)

Necrotizing Sialometaplasia

A. Etiology
1. Benign condition of salivary gland
2. Lack of blood supply to the area of the lesion
3. Trauma to the area that causes a blockage of blood supply

B. Age and gender related—adults

C. Location—most often found on the palate; however, it may be found in any site containing salivary glands

D. Clinical features (Figure 8-54)
1. Initial finding of tenderness and swelling in the area
2. Well-demarcated ulcer
3. Localized pain

E. Histologic characteristics
1. Necrosis of the salivary gland tissue involved
2. Squamous metaplasia of ductal epithelium
3. Islands of epithelium deep in connective tissue

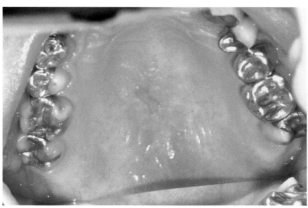

FIGURE 8-54 Necrotizing sialometaplasia. *(From Ibsen OAC, Phelan JA: Oral pathology for the dental hygienist, ed 5, Philadelphia, 2009, Saunders.)*

F. Treatment and prognosis
  1. Incisional biopsy may be performed to rule out other conditions
  2. May be self-limiting
  3. Prognosis is good

Pseudocysts

Aneurysmal Bone Cyst
A. Etiology—reactive cyst; etiologic theories include
  1. Arteriovenous shunt—a benign fibro-osseous lesion in the area alters blood vessels
  2. Trauma—trauma ruptures a blood vessel, and blood accumulates outside the wall
B. Age and gender related—under 30 years; no gender predilection
C. Location
  1. Long bones or vertebral column
  2. When the occurrence is in the jaws, the mandible is the more common site (2 : 1)
D. Clinical features
  1. May be asymptomatic or appear as a slightly to moderately well-defined bulge
  2. Tenderness, pain on motion ; may limit movement
  3. Mobility or migration of teeth
E. Radiographic appearance—hazy, gray, radiolucent area; appears cystic, with a "soap bubble" effect; multi-locular pattern can be present
F. Histologic characteristics
  1. No epithelial lining—a "pseudocyst"
  2. Walls of fibrous connective tissue
  3. Blood-filled spaces surrounded by multi-nucleated giant cells
G. Treatment and prognosis
  1. Surgical enucleation and thorough curettage (sometimes with cryosurgery—a freezing technique to help control bleeding)

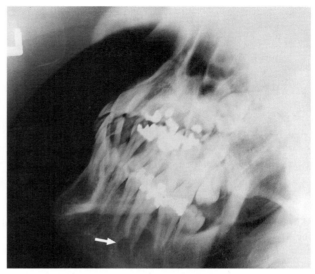

FIGURE 8-55 Extraoral radiograph showing a simple (traumatic) bone cyst *(arrow)* in the mandible, with its unique radiolucent characteristic scalloping around the roots. *(Courtesy of Dr. Edward V. Zegarelli; from Ibsen OAC, Phelan JA: Oral pathology for the dental hygienist, ed 5, Philadelphia, 2009, Saunders.)*

  2. Follow-up treatment, if necessary
  3. May sometimes recur

Simple Bone Cyst (Traumatic Bone Cyst, Idiopathic Bone)
A. Etiology—theories include:
  1. Intramedullary hemorrhage following trauma; altered bone prevents fibroblasts and endothelial cells from entering the hemorrhage; clotting does not occur; blood never organizes, leaving a void within the bone
  2. Ischemic marrow necrosis
  3. Degeneration of a benign tumor
  4. Bone did not develop in the area
B. Age and gender related—ages 10 to 20 years; male predilection
C. Location
  1. More common in the mandible than in the maxilla
  2. Most common in long bones
D. Clinical features—asymptomatic (discovered through radiographic examination)
E. Radiographic appearance (Figure 8-55)—well-defined radiolucent area 1 to 7 cm in diameter; round, oval; may be multi-locular; the radiolucent projections extend between roots of teeth defined as "scalloping around the roots"; borders are sometimes sharp or diffuse
F. Histologic characteristics
  1. Thin vascular fibrous connective tissue lining; no epithelium (not a true cyst)
  2. The center is a void

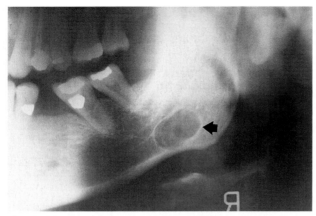

FIGURE 8-56 Part of a panoramic radiograph showing a lingual mandibular bone concavity (Stafne's bone cyst). Note the well-circumscribed radiolucency inferior to the mandibular canal (*arrow*). *(From Ibsen OAC, Phelan JA: Oral pathology for the dental hygienist, ed 5, Philadelphia, 2009, Saunders.)*

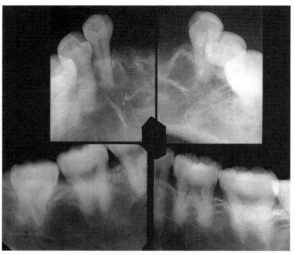

FIGURE 8-57 Sickle cell anemia. The radiograph shows abnormal trabeculation. *(Courtesy of Dr. Edward V. Zegarelli; from Ibsen OAC, Phelan JA: Oral pathology for the dental hygienist, ed 5, Philadelphia, 2009, Saunders.)*

G. Treatment and prognosis
   1. Surgical intervention to establish bleeding and clotting is often sufficient
   2. Lesion heals within a year
   3. Prognosis is excellent

Static Bone Cyst (Lingual Mandibular Bone Concavity, Stafne Bone Cyst)

A. Etiology—developmental; salivary gland extends laterally into the mandible
B. Age and gender affected—young persons; slightly more common in males
C. Location—posterior of the mandible, anterior to the angle of the ramus, inferior to the mandibular canal
D. Clinical features—asymptomatic; occasionally bilateral
E. Radiographic appearance (Figure 8-56)—sharp, well-defined ovoid radiolucency 1 to 3 cm in diameter, anterior to angle of the ramus, inferior to the mandibular canal
F. Histologic characteristics—lymphoid, fat, submaxillary salivary gland tissues; striated muscle (not a true cyst)
G. Treatment and prognosis
   1. Surgical intervention to determine contents; once diagnosed, no treatment necessary
   2. Prognosis is excellent; no complications

▌BLOOD DYSCRASIAS

General Characteristics

A. Disease with numerous variations
B. Important to know normal blood levels and chemistries in order to make differential diagnosis

C. Anemias are categorized according to etiology
   1. Blood loss
   2. Excessive destruction of red blood cells because of a congenital or hemolytic condition
   3. Decrease in production of red blood cells

Sickle Cell Anemia

A. Etiology—hereditary; severe genetic disorder involving hemoglobin; abnormal hemoglobin in red blood cells; decreased oxygen in red blood cells
B. Age and gender related—under 30 years; female predilection; 1 in 400 African Americans in the United States are affected
C. Clinical features
   1. Systemic symptoms
      a. Weakness, easily fatigued; pallor of tissues
      b. Shortness of breath; nausea, vomiting
      c. Pain in joints
      d. Sickle cell crisis involves severe systemic complications
      e. Infections—patients are prone to infection because of early destruction of the spleen
      f. Delayed growth and development in children
      g. Cardiac, kidney, and pulmonary involvement
   2. Oral symptoms
      a. Some radiographic findings
      b. Osteomyelitis of the mandible
      c. Prolonged paresthesia of the mandibular nerve
D. Radiographic appearance (Figure 8-57)
   1. Perpendicular trabeculations radiating outward, giving a "hair-on-end" appearance in the skull

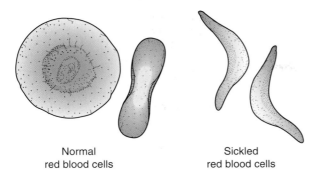

Normal
red blood cells

Sickled
red blood cells

FIGURE 8-58 Normal red blood cells compared with sickled red blood cells. *(From Ibsen OAC, Phelan JA: Oral pathology for the dental hygienist,* ed 3, *Philadelphia, 2000, Saunders.)*

2. Decrease in number of trabeculae in the jaws, with large marrow spaces
3. Lamina dura not affected
F. Laboratory tests and findings (Figure 8-58)
   1. Red blood cell count reduced to 1,000,000/mm³ (normal is 4,000,000 to 6,000,000/mm³)
   2. Decrease in the hemoglobin level in red blood cells (normal in males, 13.5 to 18 g/dL; in females, 12 to 16 g/dL)
   3. Blood smear showing sickle-shaped red blood cells
G. Histologic characteristics
   1. Crescent-shaped erythrocytes caused by hemoglobin S
   2. Atypical chromatin distribution
H. Treatment and prognosis
   1. Symptomatic management; oxygen and intravenous fluids
   2. Bone marrow transplantation has numerous complications and is a cure for a very low percentage of patients
   3. Hydroxyurea—drug treatment for adults, but it has several side effects
   4. Prognosis is unpredictable and depends on various aspects of disease activity

Pernicious Anemia (Primary Anemia, Addison Anemia, Biermer Anemia)

A. Etiology
   1. Autoimmune destruction of the parietal cells of the stomach
   2. Deficiency of intrinsic factor (produced by the parietal cells of the stomach lining) necessary to absorb vitamin B_{12} (cobalamin)
   3. Deficiency of vitamin B_{12} (extrinsic factor) necessary for deoxyribonucleic acid (DNA) synthesis
B. Age and gender related—older adults; rarely before age 30; no gender predilection

C. Clinical features
   1. Systemic symptoms
      a. General weakness, dizziness, pallor, anemia (caused by low oxygen in the blood)
      b. Numbness or tingling of extremities
      c. Gastrointestinal manifestations—nausea, vomiting, diarrhea, abdominal pain
      d. Loss of appetite and weight
      e. Shortness of breath
   2. Oral symptoms
      a. Sore, painful, burning tongue
      b. Shallow ulcers on the mucosa
      c. Atrophy of papillae; distorted perception of taste
      d. Pallor of the oral mucosa with focal patches of erythema
D. Laboratory tests and findings
   1. Diagnosis of pernicious anemia is made by laboratory testing; the Schilling test is also used to determine the body's inability to absorb an oral dose of vitamin B_{12}
   2. Achlorhydria—lack of gastric hydrochloric acid secretion
   3. Macrocytic anemia
E. Histologic characteristics
   1. Epithelial atrophy; no rete ridges
   2. Pale staining nuclei
F. Treatment and prognosis
   1. Injections of vitamin B_{12}
   2. Increased dietary intake of folic acid (leafy green vegetables, organ meats, wheat cereals)
   3. 1% to 2% of persons with pernicious anemia develop gastric carcinoma

Iron-Deficiency Anemia (Plummer-Vinson Syndrome)

A. Etiology—iron deficiency caused by:
   1. Chronic blood loss
   2. Inadequate dietary intake of iron
   3. Decreased iron absorption
   4. Increased iron requirements (e.g., infancy, pregnancy)
   5. Longstanding iron-deficiency anemia (symptoms include dysphagia and an increased predilection for squamous cell carcinoma)
B. Age and gender related—ages 40 to 50 years; more common in females (5% to 30% female incidence in the United States)
C. Clinical features
   1. Systemic symptoms
      a. Pallor of skin, weakness; fatigue
      b. Difficulty swallowing (dysphagia)
      c. Brittle fingernails
      d. Enlarged spleen (splenomegaly) (20% to 30% of cases)

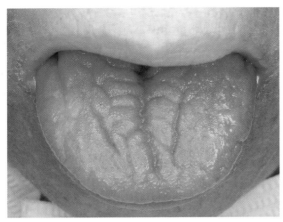

FIGURE 8-59 Iron-deficiency anemia. The tongue is devoid of filiform papillae. Angular cheilitis is also present. *(From Ibsen OAC, Phelan JA: Oral pathology for the dental hygienist, ed 5, Philadelphia, 2009, Saunders.)*

e. Absence of free hydrochloric acid in the stomach

f. Predisposition to development of oral cancer

  2. Oral symptoms (Figure 8-59)

    a. Angular cheilitis; pallor and atrophy of oral tissues

    b. Burning, painful tongue

D. Histologic characteristics

  1. Altered exfoliated squamous epithelial cells of the tongue and soft tissues

  2. Deficiency of keratinized cells

  3. Abnormal cell maturation; enlarged nuclei

E. Laboratory findings

  1. Complete blood count with red blood cell indices

  2. Hypochromatic microcytic red blood cells

  3. Low number of erythrocytes

  4. Low hemoglobin and hematocrit

F. Treatment

  1. Increased iron intake

  2. Parenteral iron occasionally

Aplastic Anemia

Primary Aplastic Anemia

A. Etiology—unknown; severe depression in bone marrow activity; rare life-threatening disease

B. Age and gender related—young adults; no gender predilection

C. Clinical features

  1. Oral symptoms

    a. Spontaneous bleeding

    b. Petechiae

    c. Purpuric spots

    d. Gingival infection

    e. Pallor of oral tissues

  2. Systemic symptoms

    a. Fatigue, weakness

    b. Tachycardia, dizziness

    c. Retinal and cerebral hemorrhages in most severe cases

    d. Predisposition to infection

D. Laboratory tests and findings establish the diagnosis

  1. Reduction in the number of all blood cells (pancytopenia)

  2. Reduction in the number of red blood cells (anemia)

  3. Reduction in the number of white blood cells (leukopenia)

  4. Reduction in the number of platelets (thrombocytopenia)

  5. Bone marrow changes

E. Treatment and prognosis

  1. Blood transfusions

  2. Antibiotic drugs to try to control infection

  3. Bone marrow transplantation

  4. Guarded prognosis, depending on the severity of the condition

  5. Rapid decrease in various blood cells usually fatal

Secondary Aplastic Anemia

A. Etiology

  1. Result of a drug or chemical substance; chemotherapy

  2. Exposure to radiant energy—x-rays, radium, or radioactive isotopes

B. Age and gender related—any age; no gender predilection

C. Clinical features—same as in primary aplastic anemia

D. Treatment and prognosis

  1. Remove the cause

  2. Supportive therapy

  3. Prognosis is good

Thalassemia (Cooley Anemia, Mediterranean Anemia)

A. Etiology—inherited; autosomal dominant

  1. Disorder of hemoglobin synthesis

  2. Ethnic predilection—high incidence in Mediterranean and African countries and India

B. Age and gender related

  1. Thalassemia major

    a. Affects individuals within the first year of life (homozygous type)

    b. Both X and Y chromosomes are involved

    c. Is a more severe type of anemia

2. Thalassemia minor
  a. The milder form appears in later childhood (heterozygous type)
  b. Only one gene at the locus is involved
3. No gender predilection
C. Clinical features
  1. Systemic symptoms for thalassemia major
    a. Yellow pallor of the skin
    b. Enlarged spleen (splenomegaly); enlarged liver (hepatomegaly)
    c. Mongoloid facial features
    d. Sunken nose bridge
    e. Protruding zygoma
    f. Slanting eyes
  2. Oral symptoms for thalassemia major
    a. Malocclusion; protrusion of the anterior maxillary teeth
    b. Pallor of the mucosa
  3. No significant clinical manifestations in thalassemia minor
D. Radiographic appearance
  1. Peculiar trabecular pattern of the maxilla and the mandible—"salt-and-pepper" or "hair on end" of the cranial bones
  2. Mild osteoporosis of the jaws
  3. Thinning of lamina dura
E. Laboratory tests and findings
  1. Elevated white blood cell count—10,000 to 25,000/mm^3
  2. Elevated serum bilirubin level
  3. Decreased hemoglobin level
F. Histologic characteristics—bone marrow shows cellular hyperplasia
G. Treatment and prognosis
  1. Blood transfusions (frequently administered every 2 weeks)
  2. Frequent transfusions cause a significant buildup of iron in tissues throughout the body; these toxic accumulations of iron may be fatal; treated with deferoxamine
  3. Bone marrow transplantation
  4. Prognosis is guarded; periods of remission can extend the lifespan to age 20

Polycythemia

General Characteristics
A. Abnormal increase in the number of circulating red blood cells
B. Increased hemoglobin level
C. Three forms:
  1. Relative polycythemia—temporary increase in the number of red blood cells; caused by shock, a severe burn, or excessive loss of body fluids
  2. Primary polycythemia (polycythemia vera)
  3. Secondary polycythemia

Primary Polycythemia (Polycythemia Vera)
A. Etiology—unknown; possibly familial; neoplastic proliferation of bone marrow stem cells
B. Age and gender related—ages 40 to 60 years; slightly more common in males
C. Clinical features
  1. Systemic symptoms
    a. Headache, dizziness, weakness
    b. Enlarged, painful spleen
    c. Gastric complaints; peptic ulcers
    d. Tips of fingers cyanotic
    e. Nose bleeds easily (epistaxis)
    f. Itching of skin (pruritus) without the presence of rash
  2. Oral symptoms
    a. Oral mucosa deep red to purple because of decreased hemoglobin level
    b. Gingivae edematous and spongy; bleed easily
    c. Submucosal petechiae; ecchymosis
D. Laboratory tests and findings
  1. Red blood cell count elevated to 10,000,000 to 12,000,000/mm^3 (significant increase)
  2. Increase in:
    a. Hemoglobin content
    b. Blood viscosity
    c. White blood cell counts
    d. Hematocrit value
E. Treatment and prognosis
  1. Medications and procedures to control platelets
  2. Intermittent phlebotomy
  3. Chemotherapeutic drugs

Secondary Polycythemia
A. Etiology—increased number of erythrocytes caused by a physiologic response to decreased oxygen
  1. Bone marrow anoxia (lack of oxygen) caused by:
    a. Pulmonary dysfunction
    b. Heart disease
    c. High altitudes
    d. Carbon monoxide poisoning
  2. Stimulatory factors such as drugs or chemicals
B. Other characteristics and features similar to those of primary polycythemia

Relative Polycythemia
A. Etiology—decreased plasma volume that may be caused by:
  1. Use of diuretics
  2. Vomiting, diarrhea
  3. Excessive sweating
B. Age and gender related—the chronic form of relative polycythemia (also called *stress polycythemia*) is more common in white, middle-aged men, who

are stressed, overweight, and hypertensive and who smoke

C. Treatment—related to the type of polycythemia and risk factors; attempt to remove risk factors

Agranulocytosis

A. Etiology—significant reduction in circulating neutrophils
   1. Primary form—unknown; immunologic disorder
   2. Secondary form—drug ingestion; chemotherapy; toxic effect of drugs or chemicals
B. Age and gender related—any age; more common in adults; female predilection
C. Clinical features
   1. Systemic symptoms
      a. Sudden onset
      b. High fever, chills, sore throat
      c. Malaise, weakness
      d. Skin is jaundiced
      e. Regional lymphadenopathy
   2. Oral symptoms
      a. Infection (clinical signs affecting the gingiva can be similar to NUG)
      b. Ulcerations of the pharynx, palate, buccal mucosa, and tongue
D. Laboratory tests and findings—confirm the diagnosis
   1. Severe decrease in or absence of granulocytes or polymorphonuclear cells
   2. Accelerated destruction of neutrophils; bone marrow has few or no granulocytes
   3. White blood cell count is reduced to less than 1000 cells/mm³
E. Histologic characteristics
   1. Necrosis of involved tissues
   2. Many bacterial microorganisms
F. Treatment
   1. Removal of the causative drug or agent, if possible
   2. Administration of antibiotics to control infection

Cyclic Neutropenia

A. Etiology—inherited; autosomal dominant; periodic episodes lasting 3 to 4 days with a significant decrease in circulating neutrophils
B. Age and gender related—infants and young children; no gender predilection
C. Clinical features
   1. Systemic symptoms
      a. General weakness, malaise
      b. Fever, sore throat, headache

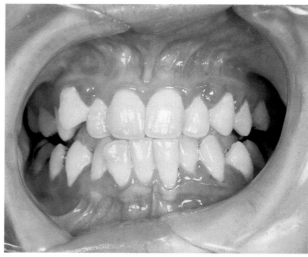

FIGURE 8-60 Marked gingivitis, with areas of gingival recession in a patient with cyclic neutropenia. *(From Ibsen OAC, Phelan JA: Oral pathology for the dental hygienist, ed 5, Philadelphia, 2009, Saunders.)*

    c. Cervical lymphadenopathy
    d. Gastrointestinal mucosal ulcerations
   2. Oral symptoms (Figure 8-60)
      a. Severe gingivitis, recession, and periodontitis
      b. Painful ulcerations
      c. Mild to severe loss of alveolar bone
      d. Dental treatment should be performed when circulating neutrophils are normal to reduce complications and secondary infections
D. Laboratory tests and findings
   1. Neutrophils may completely disappear in the acute stage
   2. Cycles occur at intervals of 21 to 27 days
   3. Sequential blood counts several times a week for several weeks are used to determine neutrophil cycling
E. Treatment and prognosis
   1. Optimal oral hygiene practices by the patient
   2. Treatment with granulocyte colony-stimulating factor (G-CSF) several times a week
   3. Antibiotics to control infections
   4. Premedication with antibiotics before dental hygiene or surgical procedures (which should be scheduled when neutrophils are at their highest peak)

Leukemia

General Characteristics

A. Malignant neoplastic disorder involving blood-forming cells; originates in the bone marrow
B. Excessive proliferation of white blood cells in the immature state

C. Etiology—combination of genetic and environmental factors; oncogenic viruses
  1. Chronic exposure to chemicals or ionizing radiation
  2. Higher incidence among persons with genetic disorders, including Down syndrome and other chromosomal abnormalities, neurofibromatosis, and Klinefelter syndrome(see the section on "Genetics" in Chapter 7)
D. A number of types and subtypes of this condition exist

Acute Leukemia

A. Two types:
  1. Acute myeloblastic leukemia (AML)
  2. Acute lymphoblastic leukemia (ALL)
B. Age and gender related—according to cell type; AML generally affects adolescents and young adults but can affect children; ALL almost always affects children; slight male predilection
C. Clinical features—onset is sudden
  1. Systemic symptoms
    a. Infection in lungs, urinary tract
    b. Weakness, fever, headache
    c. Swelling of lymph nodes
    d. Bruising of the skin and mucous membranes—caused by a decrease in the number of platelets
    e. Enlargement of organs—spleen, liver
    f. Bone and joint pain
  2. Oral symptoms (Figure 8-61)
    a. Purpuric spots; gingival hemorrhage
    b. Severe gingival enlargement—red, soft, spongy; spontaneous bleeding

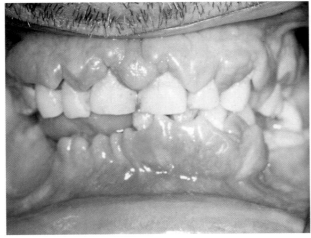

FIGURE 8-61 Generalized gingival hyperplasia in a patient with leukemia. *(Courtesy of Dr. Edward V. Zegarelli; from Ibsen OAC, Phelan JA: Oral pathology for the dental hygienist, ed 5, Philadelphia, 2009, Saunders.)*

    c. Gingiva sometimes similar to NUG—characterized by ulcerations, blunted papillae, necrosis, odor
    d. Pallor of tissues; nonulcerated edema
    e. Candidiasis, herpetic infection, or both
    f. Toothache caused by invasion and necrosis of the pulp
    g. Mobility of teeth caused by a breakdown of the periodontal membrane and supporting structures
D. Laboratory tests and findings
  1. Both anemia and thrombocytopenia present
  2. Prolonged bleeding and coagulation times
  3. White blood cell count elevated to $100,000/mm^3$ (many immature cells)
  4. Leukemic cells in bone marrow and peripheral blood
  5. Tests to identify certain enzymes can help classify the type
E. Treatment and prognosis
  1. Chemotherapy depending on the type and form of leukemia
  2. Antibiotics to control infection
  3. Drug and radiation therapy to the central nervous system (CNS)
  4. Transfusions with platelets or packed red blood cells
  5. Optimal oral hygiene care
  6. Prognosis depends on multiple factors (i.e., the type of leukemia, age)

Chronic Leukemia

A. Common forms
  1. Chronic myeloid leukemia (CML)—associated with the Philadelphia chromosome
  2. Chronic lymphocytic leukemia (CLL)—the most common form; asymptomatic for a long time
B. Age and gender related—adults; no gender predilection
C. Clinical features
  1. Systemic symptoms
    a. Very slow onset—disease may be present for weeks or months before symptoms lead to diagnosis
    b. Weight loss, fatigue
    c. Lymph node enlargement and enlarged spleen in the CLL type; not in the CML type
    d. Petechiae on the skin with nodules of leukemic cells
    e. Destructive bone lesions—result in bone fracture
  2. Oral symptoms
    a. Gingival tissues may appear normal for some time; become tender, enlarged, and bleed easily
    b. Pallor of the gingiva and lips

c. Purpuric spots; ecchymosis

d. Cervical lymphadenopathy may be an early sign (underlines the importance of the extra-oral clinical examination)

D. Laboratory tests and findings

1. Anemia and thrombocytopenia sometimes present

2. White blood cell count can increase to 500,000/mm^3 (95% of the total number of blood cells)

3. Shift to the left in the maturity of cells

4. Differential count elevated in the cell type involved

E. Treatment and prognosis

1. Chemotherapy

2. Bone marrow transplantation (especially for patients with CML—better survival rates)

3. Prognosis depends on the stage of the disease

Purpura

General Characteristics

A. Purplish discoloration of the skin and mucous membranes caused by the spontaneous escape of blood into tissues

B. Caused by:

1. Defect or deficiency in blood platelets (throm-bocytopenic purpura)

2. Unexplained increase in capillary fragility (vas-cular or nonthrombocytopenic purpura)

Thrombocytopenic Purpura

A. Etiology

1. Primary—idiopathic thrombocytopenic pur-pura; usually seen in young patients

2. Secondary—caused by a variety of conditions

   a. Drug toxicity

   b. Chemotherapy

   c. Infectious diseases

B. Age and gender related—primary form occurs in childhood before age 10; secondary form may appear at any age; no gender predilection

C. Clinical features

1. Systemic symptoms

   a. Spontaneous hemorrhagic skin lesions that vary in size (petechiae, ecchymosis, hemato-mas)

   b. Patient bruises easily

   c. Bleeding through the urinary tract (hematu-ria)

   d. Bleeding from the nose (epistaxis)

   e. Spleen not palpable

2. Oral symptoms

   a. Profuse gingival hemorrhage

   b. Clustered petechiae

D. Laboratory tests and findings

1. Severe reduction in the platelet count—below 50,000/mm^3 (normal is 150,000 to 400,000/mm^3)

2. Bleeding time prolonged to 1 hour or more

3. Positive capillary fragility test

E. Treatment

1. Discontinue causative drug, if known

2. Corticosteroid therapy

3. Blood transfusions (platelets, in particular)

4. Guarded prognosis

5. Consult patient's physician of record prior to any dental hygiene or surgical procedure

Nonthrombocytopenic Purpura

A. Etiology—results from a variety of conditions that produce capillary fragility

1. Defect in capillary walls

2. Disorder in capillary function (drugs)

B. Clinical features—platelet count normal; other symptoms similar to those of thrombocytopenic purpura

Hemophilia

A. Etiology—a genetic deficiency of a clotting factor in the blood; usually factor VIII or factor IX; bleeding disorder of blood coagulation

1. Inherited; X-linked disease; occurs mostly in males; occurs in females in extremely rare cases.

2. Defect carried by the X chromosome; females are carriers of the trait

3. Transmitted genetically from asymptomatic carrier mothers to sons

B. Age and gender related—usually present at birth; symptoms may not appear until later; males are most susceptible while females are carriers of the trait

C. Clinical features

1. Systemic symptoms

   a. Clotting deficiency produces persistent bleeding

   b. Massive hematomas; hemorrhage

   c. Three forms—differ in the deficiency of a blood clotting factor

      (1) Type A—most common type; factor VIII; X-linked recessive

      (2) Type B—or Christmas disease; factor IX; X-linked recessive

      (3) von Willebrand's disease—abnormal von Willebrand's factor; autosomal dominant

2. Oral symptoms

   a. Gingival hemorrhage

   b. Prolonged hemorrhage following tooth eruption, exfoliation, scaling, extraction, or surgery

D. Laboratory tests and findings—prolonged coagulation time (classic feature)

E. Treatment
1. Injections with clotting factor
2. Identify missing factors and replace them (complications can occur)
3. Genetic counseling
4. Optimal dental and dental hygiene care to prevent problems

HUMAN IMMUNODEFICIENCY VIRUS

A. Etiology—infectious disease; human immunodeficiency virus (HIV) (Box 8-2)

B. Syndrome includes HIV infection, cell lymphopenia, and reduced CD4 helper T lymphocyte function

C. Age—usually adults ages 20 to 40 years; infants of infected mothers; anyone to whom the virus is transmitted

D. Gender and ethnic characteristics
1. Male predilection; however, women comprise the fastest-growing group of infected persons
2. Homosexual or bisexual men
3. Overall increased incidence among intravenous drug users
4. Others at risk include sex workers, prison inmates, and children of infected mothers

E. Transmission
1. Sexual contact
2. Infected blood serum; in infected patients, the virus has been found in blood and bodily fluids, including saliva and tears
3. Infected mothers to newborn (breast milk); artificial insemination
4. IV drug users
5. Cofactors (e.g., other infections) may influence transmission

F. Clinical—oral (Box 8-3)
1. At the earliest stage of the disease, the oral findings can be subtle or totally asymptomatic

---

BOX 8-2 Definition of Acquired Immune Deficiency Syndrome*

Acquired immune deficiency syndrome (AIDS) is an illness characterized by one or more of the following diseases or conditions:

HIV Laboratory Tests Not Performed or Results Inconclusive and the Patient Has No Other Cause of Immunodeficiency
1. Candidiasis of the esophagus, trachea, bronchi, or lungs
2. Cryptococcosis, extrapulmonary
3. Cryptosporidiosis with diarrhea persisting longer than 1 month
4. Cytomegalovirus disease of an organ other than liver, spleen, or lymph nodes in a patient older than 1 month of age
5. Herpes simplex virus infection causing a mucocutaneous ulcer that persists longer than 1 month, or bronchitis, pneumonitis, or esophagitis for any duration affecting a patient older than 1 month of age
6. Kaposi's sarcoma affecting a patient <60 years of age
7. Lymphoid interstitial pneumonia or pulmonary hyperplasia, or both; affecting a child <13 years of age
8. *Mycobacterium avium* or *Mycobacterium kansasii* disease, disseminated
9. *Pneumocystis carinii* pneumonia
10. Progressive multi-focal leukoencophalopathy
11. Toxoplasmosis of the brain affecting a patient older than 1 month of age

With Laboratory Evidence for Human Immunodeficiency Virus (HIV) Infection
Less than 200 CD4+ T lymphocytes/mL, or a CD4+ T lymphocyte percentage of total lymphocytes of <14
Any of the diseases listed above or those that follow:
1. Multiple bacterial infections of certain types affecting a child <13 years of age
2. Coccidioidomycosis, disseminated
3. HIV encephalopathy (HIV dementia)
4. Histoplasmosis, disseminated
5. Isosporiasis with diarrhea persisting longer than 1 month
6. Lymphoma of the brain at any age
7. Kaposi's sarcoma at any age
8. Certain types of lymphoma
9. Mycobacterial disease, other than tuberculosis, disseminated
10. Extrapulmonary tuberculosis
11. Salmonella septicemia, recurrent
12. HIV wasting syndrome
13. Pulmonary tuberculosis
14. Recurrent pneumonia
15. Invasive cervical cancer
Even if HIV laboratory test results are negative, if other causes of immunodeficiency are not ruled out, a diagnosis of AIDS can be made if certain of these diseases are diagnosed.

*Adapted from Centers for Disease Control and Prevention: 1993 Revised classification system for HIV infection and expanded surveillance case definition for AIDS among adolescents and adults, *MMWR 41(RR-17), 1992.*

BOX 8-3 Oral Lesions Associated with Human Immunodeficiency Virus Infection

Candidiasis
Herpes simplex infection
Herpes zoster
Hairy leukoplakia
Human papillomavirus (HPV) lesions
Atypical gingivitis and periodontitis
Other opportunistic infections reported
   Mycobacterium avium
   Cytomegalovirus
   Cryptococcus neoformans
   Klebsiella pneumoniae
   Enterobacter cloacae
   Histoplasma capsulatum
Kaposi's sarcoma
Non-Hodgkin's lymphoma
Aphthous ulcers
Mucosal pigmentation
Bilateral salivary gland enlargement and xerostomia
Spontaneous gingival bleeding resulting from thrombocytopenia

From Ibsen OAC, Phelan JA: Oral pathology for the dental hygienist, ed 5, Philadelphia, 2009, Saunders.

2. Oral candidiasis occurs in more than 85% of cases (pseudomembranous, erythematous, hyperplastic, angular cheilitis)
3. History of herpes simplex; herpes zoster; aphthous ulcers
4. NUG; linear gingival erythema; necrotizing ulcerative periodontitis (NUP)
5. Petechiae on attached gingiva
6. Sudden onset of inflammation
7. A creamy white patch covering a raw, red base as seen in pemphigus
8. Distinct odor
9. Hairy leukoplakia
G. Clinical—general
  1. Opportunistic infections—candidiasis; infection by cytomegalovirus, herpes simplex viruses 1 and 2; pneumocystic pneumonia
  2. Susceptible to forms of cancer—squamous cell carcinoma, Kaposi sarcoma, and non-Hodgkin lymphoma
  3. Constitutional signs include sudden, unexplained weight loss, lymphadenopathy involving cervical and submandibular nodes
  4. Health history—past and present history of long-term illness, slow healing, vital signs (fever is especially significant), and patient profile
  5. Other characteristics—lymphadenopathy, fatigue, diarrhea, fever, gastrointestinal involvement, weight loss; oral lesions usually manifest last

6. Epstein-Barr virus (hairy leukoplakia involving corrugated white areas especially on the lateral tongue)
H. Laboratory
  1. Serologic testing for HIV infection using the enzyme-linked immunosorbent assay (ELISA) test twice
  2. Western blot test is performed after two positive ELISA tests
  3. The polymerase chain reaction (PCR) identifies the virus and the viral load rather than antibodies
I. Histologic findings—can be extremely variable, depending on the pathologic conditions involved
J. Treatment—symptomatic
  1. Antiretroviral drugs; nucleoside analogs, non-nucleoside reverse transcriptase inhibitors, protease inhibitors, and fusion inhibitors
  2. Drugs that prevent or treat opportunistic diseases (e.g., protease inhibitor)
K. Prognosis—depends on early diagnosis and current therapy

FIBROUS DYSPLASIA

General Characteristics

A. Etiology: unknown; abnormal mesenchymal function; rare diseases affecting bones
B. Swelling of bones with deformities in some forms of disease
C. Benign fibro-osseous lesion

Monostotic Fibrous Dysplasia

A. Etiology—unknown; theories include:
  1. Local infection
  2. Trauma
B. Age and gender related—children and young adults; no gender predilection
C. Location
  1. Ribs—most common site
  2. Mandible more often than maxilla
  3. Can affect any bone; most common form
D. Clinical features
  1. Painless swelling; enlargement of the jaw or expansion of the buccal plate
  2. Can cause malposition, tipping, or displacement of teeth
  3. In the maxilla, lesions are not clearly outlined because they extend into the sinus or the floor of the orbit
E. Radiographic features
  1. The lesion blends into surrounding bone
  2. Diffuse radiopacity; "ground glass" appearance

3. Sometimes a radiolucency with areas of radiopacity (depending on the degree of calcification)

F. Histologic characteristics
  1. Proliferating fibroblasts in the stroma of woven collagen fibers
  2. Irregularly shaped trabeculae; some are shaped like the letter "C"

F. Treatment and prognosis
  1. Surgical correction of the deformed bone
  2. Radiation therapy contraindicated because of possibility of malignant transformations

Polyostotic Fibrous Dysplasia

A. Etiology—unknown; involves more than one bone
B. Age and gender related—children; female predilection
C. Location
  1. Long bones (bowing); often unilateral
  2. Bones of the face and skull
  3. Clavicles
  4. Pelvic bones
D. Clinical features (depend on the type of polyostotic fibrous dysplasia)
  1. Systemic symptoms
    a. Café au lait; irregular light brown macules on the skin
    b. Painless to aching pain
    c. Bowing of long bones (pathologic fracture)
    d. Females may reach premature puberty at age 2 or 3 years
    e. Dysfunction of the endocrine system—pituitary, thyroid, and parathyroid glands
  2. Oral symptoms
    a. Expansion and deformity of the jaws
    b. Disturbed eruption pattern caused by endocrine dysfunction
  3. Types
    a. Craniofacial fibrous dysplasia—the maxilla is involved, and the lesion extends into the sinus and surrounding bones
    b. Jaffe-Lichtenstein type—lesions arise in multiple bones; café-au-lait skin lesions appear over the involved bone
    c. McCune-Albright syndrome—most severe form of polyostotic fibrous dysplasia
      (1) Severe endocrine abnormalities
        (a) Premature puberty in females before age 2
        (b) Stunted growth caused by early epiphyseal closure
        (c) Café-au-lait lesions
      (2) Other systemic complications (diabetes; hyperthyroidism)
E. Radiographic appearance—irregular bone trabeculae; expansion of cortical bone; sometimes a multi-locular cystic appearance with several radiolucencies
F. Laboratory tests and findings
  1. Serum alkaline phosphatase level sometimes elevated
  2. Moderately elevated basal metabolic rate
G. Histologic characteristics
  1. Fibrillar connective tissue
  2. Many trabeculae
  3. Irregularly shaped, coarse-woven fibers
  4. Osteocytes
H. Treatment and prognosis
  1. Surgical correction; postpone surgery as long as possible
  2. No treatment for minor involvement

Cherubism

A. Etiology—inherited; autosomal dominant gene; marked penetrance; gene 4p16
B. Age and gender related—onset at birth or early childhood (ages 2 to 5 years)
C. Location—only in the maxilla and the mandible (more common in the mandible)
D. Clinical features
  1. Painless bilateral enlargement of the posterior mandible; firm and hard when palpated
  2. Taut facial skin; downward pull of the eyelids; "cherubic" appearance
  3. Regional lymphadenopathy
  4. Has been mistaken for an ameloblastoma or multi-locular cyst
  5. Primary dentition may be prematurely shed at age three years
  6. Permanent dentition often defective; absence of teeth (hypodontia); lack of eruption of the teeth or delayed eruption
  7. Speech problems; distortion of alveolar ridge
E. Radiographic appearance
  1. Multi-locular radiolucencies
  2. Bilateral thinning of cortical plates
  3. Numerous unerupted or displaced teeth in cyst-like radiolucent spaces
F. Laboratory tests and findings—all blood levels normal
G. Histologic characteristics
  1. Similar to giant cell granuloma; fibrous tissue proliferation
  2. Numerous large multi-nucleated giant cells in a loose, delicate, fibrous connective tissue stroma
  3. Eosinophilic cuff-like deposits surround small blood vessels
H. Treatment and prognosis
  1. Self-limiting; remission at puberty
  2. Sometimes surgical intervention

3. Radiation contraindicated because of risk of sarcoma
4. Prognosis is good

Periapical Cemento-osseous Dysplasia (Cementoma)

A. Etiology—unknown; a common disease that affects periapical bone
B. Age and gender related—mid-thirties; more common in females (15:1) and African Americans (70%); these characteristics are critical to the diagnosis
C. Location
   1. Anterior mandible; rare in the maxilla
   2. Apex of teeth near the periodontal ligament
D. Clinical
   1. Asymptomatic and localized; teeth in the affected area are vital teeth (this feature is critical to the diagnosis, and is seen radiographically)
   2. Pulp testing must be part of the diagnostic process
E. Radiographic appearance—depends on the stage of development
   1. Early radiolucent lesion cannot be differentiated from several other principal pathologic (PAP) lesions
   2. Mature stage showing radiopacities surrounded by radiolucency
   3. Periodontal ligament remains intact
F. Histologic characteristics
   1. Increase in connective tissue cells of the periodontal ligament
   2. Normal bone replaced with a fibrous mass; varying amounts of calcified material within
G. Treatment and prognosis
   1. Self-limiting; no treatment necessary
   2. Prognosis is good

Paget Disease (Osteitis Deformans)

A. Etiology—unknown; non-neoplastic disease of bone; chronic metabolic disease of bone; theories include:
   1. Viral cause
   2. Inflammatory response
   3. Endocrine imbalance
B. Age and gender related—age over 50 years; male predilection
C. Location—especially in the pelvis and spine; more common in the maxilla than in the mandible
D. Clinical features
   1. Systemic symptoms
      a. Symptoms develop slowly

b. Enlargement of bones (bowing in long bones)—spine, femur, tibia; skull (change in hat size); pain in the involved bone
      c. Affected bones are warm to the touch as a result of increased vascularity
      d. Severe headaches, deafness, dizziness, bone neuralgia
      e. Joint pain with limited mobility
   2. Oral symptoms
      a. Enlarged maxilla; spread of the dentition
      b. No change in enamel or dentin; hypercementosis of the roots of teeth makes extractions more difficult
E. Radiographic appearance
   1. Initial decreased radiodensity
   2. Irregular radiolucent and radiopaque patches, giving a classic "cotton wool" appearance
   3. Root resorption; hypercementosis; lamina dura may be missing completely
F. Laboratory tests and findings
   1. Serum alkaline phosphatase level is significantly elevated (this is significant to the diagnosis)
   2. Serum calcium and phosphorus levels are normal
G. Histologic characteristics—characterized by both bone resorption and bone deposition
   1. Areas of resorption—osteoclast activity
   2. Areas of deposition—osteoblast activity
   3. Areas of both resorption and deposition—osteoclasts and osteoblasts present
   4. Vascular fibrous connective tissue replaces bone marrow
   5. Reversed bone lines—"mosaic bone"
H. Treatment and prognosis
   1. No treatment, if asymptomatic
   2. Bone pain—analgesics
   3. Neurologic complications (eyes, ears)

ENDOCRINE DISORDERS

General Characteristics

A. Associated with metabolic disturbances, deficiencies, or excesses
B. Excess or deficiency in hormone

Hyperparathyroidism

A. Etiology—excess secretion of parathyroid hormone (PTH)
   1. Primary hyperparathyroidism—parathyroid gland produces an excessive quantity of parathyroid hormone; results from parathyroid adenoma
   2. Secondary hyperparathyroidism—accompanies other systemic diseases such as renal

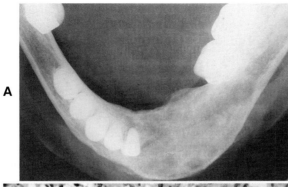

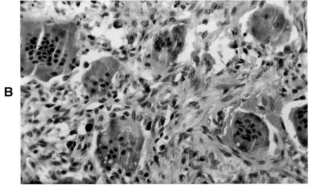

FIGURE 8-62 **A,** Radiograph of a mandibular lesion in a patient with hyperparathyroidism. **B,** Microscopic appearance of a jaw lesion occurring in a patient with hyperparathyroidism. The histologic appearance is identical to that of a central giant cell granuloma. *(**A,** Courtesy of Drs. Paul Freedman and Stanley Kerpel; **A and B,** from Ibsen OAC, Phelan JA: Oral pathology for the dental hygienist, ed 5, Philadelphia, 2009, Saunders.)*

disturbances in which calcium is excreted by the kidneys in abnormal amounts; rickets
B. Age and gender related—age over 60 years; female predilection (3 : 1)
C. Clinical features
  1. Systemic symptoms
    a. Joint and bone pain, joint stiffness, and resorption of bone with spontaneous fractures
    b. Urinary tract stones caused by increased calcium in urine (kidney stones)
    c. Weakness, fatigue, dementia
    d. Duodenal ulcers
  2. Oral symptoms
    a. Resembles a giant cell tumor or cyst
    b. Diffuse bone loss causing malocclusion and shifting or mobility of teeth
D. Radiographic appearance (Figure 8-62, *A*)
  1. Cyst-like radiolucencies found in posterior jaws; "ground glass" appearance
  2. Lamina dura lost or sketchy
  3. Mottled appearance
E. Laboratory tests and findings
  1. Loss of calcium replaced by fibrous tissue

  2. Serum calcium level elevated (hypercalcemia)
  3. Low levels of blood phosphorus (hypophosphatemia)
F. Histologic characteristics (see Figure 8-62, *B*)
  1. Osteoclastic resorption of trabeculae of spongiosa bone
  2. Fibrosis of marrow spaces
  3. Fibroblasts replace resorbed bone
  4. Indistinguishable from central giant cell granuloma
  5. Highly vascular granulation tissue
G. Treatment
  1. Correct the cause of increased hormone production (tumors, renal disease, vitamin D deficiency)
  2. Surgical removal of the hyperplastic functional parathyroid gland
  3. Parathyroidectomy
  4. Renal transplants

Osteomalacia

A. Etiology—deficiency of calcium over a long period of time
  1. Deficiency or impaired absorption of vitamin D (produces osteomalacia in adults and rickets in children)
  2. Urinary loss of calcium and phosphorus
  3. Fanconi syndrome—group of diseases related to renal tubular function
B. Age and gender related—adults; female predilection
C. Clinical features
  1. Loss of calcification in bone; soft bone
    a. Generalized weakness
    b. Bone pain and tenderness; fractures
    c. Affects gait
  2. Polyuria—urine output greatly increased
  3. Polydipsia—severe thirst
  4. No oral symptoms
D. Radiographic appearance
  1. Generalized demineralization of bone; milkman's syndrome
  2. Lamina dura of teeth may be absent
  3. Radiopaque renal calculi in the kidney
E. Laboratory tests and findings
  1. Low serum calcium and phosphorus levels
  2. Serum alkaline phosphatase level elevated
F. Treatment and prognosis
  1. Increased dosage of vitamin D; if malabsorption, water-soluble, synthetic vitamin D can be given
  2. Calcium supplements
  3. Pathologic fractures may occur in persons with osteomalacia

Rickets

A. Etiology
 1. Deficiency of vitamin D, phosphorus, and calcium
 2. Form of osteomalacia; failure of calcification of cartilage and bone
B. Age related—young children
C. Clinical features
 1. Systemic symptoms
  a. Pliable bones; bow legs, "knock knees"
  b. Muscle pain
  c. Enlarged skull, spinal curvature
  d. Enlarged liver and spleen
 2. Oral symptoms
  a. Retardation of tooth eruption
  b. Malposition of teeth
  c. Retardation of growth of the mandible; class II malocclusion
D. Treatment—increase dietary intake of vitamin D, calcium, and phosphorus; supplements

Langerhans' Cell Disease

General Characteristics

A. Etiology—unknown; a reactive process
B. Cells accumulate in granulomatous masses
C. Includes a group of three diseases characterized by proliferation of Langerhans' cells; a combination of histiocytic cells and eosinophils
D. Three forms:
 1. Letterer-Siwe disease (acute disseminated form)
  a. Age and gender related—first 2 years of life; infants; male predilection
  b. Clinical features
   (1) Skin rash on the trunk, scalp, and extremities
   (2) Persistent low-grade fever; malaise, irritability
   (3) Splenomegaly, hepatomegaly
   (4) Anemia
   (5) Oral lesions—not common because the disease is very rapid
   (6) Most severe form of Langerhans' cell disease
  c. Prognosis—invariably fatal; sometimes responds to chemotherapy
 2. Hand-Schüller-Christian disease (chronic disseminated form)
  a. Age and gender related—early life; more common in males
  b. Clinical features
   (1) Systemic symptoms—classic triad of symptoms:
    (a) Skull and jaws affected

   (b) Diabetes insipidus—result of pituitary dysfunction
   (c) Exophthalmos—bulging eyes caused by massive infiltration of reticulocytes
   (2) Oral symptoms
    (a) Sore mouth without lesions
    (b) Halitosis, unpleasant taste, gingivitis
    (c) Loose, sore teeth
    (d) Failure to heal after extractions
  c. Radiographic appearance—radiolucencies in the skull and jaws
  d. Treatment and prognosis
   (1) Curettage of the lesion
   (2) Radiation therapy
   (3) Cytotoxic drugs and adrenocortical hormones
   (4) Prognosis is poor; high fatality rate
 3. Eosinophilic granuloma (localized)
  a. Age and gender related—older children and young adults approximately age 20 years; male predilection (2 : 1)
  b. Clinical features
   (1) Most benign variety of Langerhans' cell disease
   (2) May be asymptomatic; local pain, swelling, tenderness
   (3) Sore mouth, fetid breath, loosening of teeth, swollen gingiva
   (4) Mandible more involved than maxilla
  c. Radiographic appearance—irregular radiolucencies, single or multiple; well defined, resembling a cyst (Figure 8-63)
  d. Treatment and prognosis
   (1) Curettage and conservative surgical excision
   (2) Radiation therapy
   (3) Prognosis is good; recurrence is rare

ABNORMALITIES OF TEETH

Loss of Tooth Structure

Attrition

A. Etiology—wearing away of tooth surfaces by active, physiologic forces
 1. Mastication
 2. Bruxism and chewing of tobacco accelerate attrition of teeth
 3. Occlusion—heavy biting forces
 4. Diet—chewing of coarse foods influences attrition
B. Age and gender related—occurs in primary and permanent dentition; the rate of attrition is higher in males

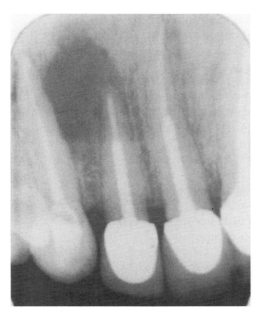

FIGURE 8-63 Radiograph of eosinophilic granuloma. *(Courtesy of Drs. Paul Freedman and Stanley Kerpel; from Ibsen OAC, Phelan JA: Oral pathology for the dental hygienist, ed 5, Philadelphia, 2009, Saunders.)*

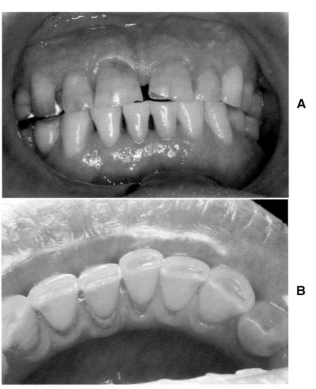

FIGURE 8-64 **A,** Attrition. **B,** Incisal view of attrition of the adult dentition. *(From Ibsen OAC, Phelan JA: Oral pathology for the dental hygienist, ed 5, Philadelphia, 2009, Saunders.)*

C. Clinical features (Figure 8-64, *A* and *B*)
1. Polished facets
2. Flat incisal edge
3. Discolored surface
4. Exposed dentin
5. Muscle tenderness (more associated with bruxism)

Abrasion
A. Etiology—wearing away of tooth structure through abnormal mechanical processes
1. Improper toothbrushing technique
2. Abrasive dentifrices
3. Repetitive oral habits
B. Clinical features (Figure 8-65)
1. U-shaped loss of tooth structure at the cervical margin; common in the canine and premolar areas
2. Recession of gingiva creates sensitivity
3. Pipe smoking abrades teeth where the pipe rests
4. Notching associated with carpenters and tailors who hold tacks, nails, and pins between their teeth

Abfraction
A. Etiology—biomechanical forces on teeth
B. Clinical features—a wedge-shaped or V-shaped loss of tooth structure at the cemento-enamel junction (CEJ); the tooth is more susceptible to toothbrush abrasion

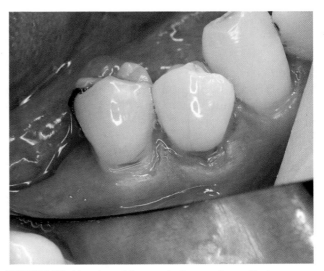

FIGURE 8-65 Abrasion of the cervical area of mandibular premolars caused by aggressive toothbrushing. *(From Ibsen OAC, Phelan JA: Oral pathology for the dental hygienist, ed 5, Philadelphia, 2009, Saunders.)*

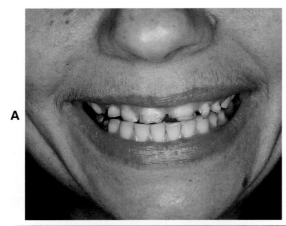

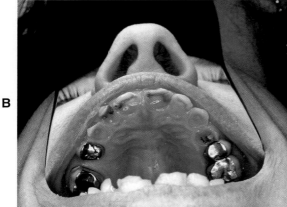

FIGURE 8-66 Erosion caused by bulimia. **A,** Decreased tooth size. **B,** Erosion of maxillary lingual surfaces. *(From Ibsen OAC, Phelan JA: Oral pathology for the dental hygienist, ed 5, Philadelphia, 2009, Saunders.)*

Erosion

A. Etiology—loss of tooth structure resulting from chemical action; when caused by gastric acids, it is known as *perimylolysis*
  1. Acid or low-pH fluid intake
  2. Acidic foods habitually used over long periods
  3. Eating disorders (bulimia)
B. Clinical features (Figure 8-66, *A* and *B*)
  1. Usually found on the labial or buccal surfaces; loss of enamel on the anterior maxillary lingual surfaces and mesial and distal surfaces may be indicative of bulimia
  2. "Wear" depressions or etchings on cervical or occlusal surfaces
  3. Hypersensitivity of affected teeth

Drugs Affecting Teeth

Methamphetamine Abuse and Addiction

A. Street names: Meth, Speed, Crystal, Ice, Glass, Fire
B. Etiology—a manmade psychostimulant that can be injected, snorted, inhaled, taken orally, or smoked.

Mood alterations depend on how it is taken. Smoking produces a high that can last from 10 to 24 hours
C. Gender related
  1. Majority are males ages 18 to 34
  2. Increased incidence in females
D. Clinical symptoms of use
  1. Inability to sleep
  2. Irritability
  3. Extreme anorexia (causes a decrease in appetite)
  4. Tremors
  5. Sensitivity to noise
  6. Increased craving for sweets
  7. Possession of drug paraphernalia
E. Clinical signs: oral
  1. "Meth mouth"; snorting or inhaling has the most severe effect on teeth
  2. Xerostomia; candidiasis
  3. "Rampant caries" caused by the acidic nature of the drug; smooth buccal or labial surfaces of teeth and interproximal surfaces of anterior teeth are especially affected
  4. Bruxism and clenching, leading to cracked teeth
  5. Advanced gingival problems and periodontal disease
  6. One report described the oral condition as "teeth rotted to the gumline"
  7. Dangerous interactions with common local anesthetics, nitrous oxide, and pain medications
F. Systemic
  1. Cardiovascular problems, including increased heart rate and blood pressure
  2. Toxic effects on the central nervous system
  3. Hyperthermia
  4. Irreversible stroke producing damage to the blood vessels in the brain
  5. Acute lead poisoning in intravenous (IV) drug abusers
  6. During pregnancy, congenital deformities, prenatal complications, and premature birth
  7. Rapid aging

Tetracycline Stain

A. Etiology—ingested medication during tooth development
B. Clinical—tooth staining that can be a yellow-green or a gray brown; endogenous stain

Developmental Defects Affecting Enamel and Dentin

Amelogenesis Imperfecta

A. Etiology—inherited condition affecting the enamel of teeth resulting from a malfunction of the tooth germ

B. Produces four types
1. Type 1: enamel hypoplasia—defect in the formation of the matrix
   a. Etiology—hereditary; environmental factors, nutritional deficiency, congenital syphilis, high fever, and birth injuries also can cause a hypoplastic response
   b. Clinically (Figure 8-67), the enamel of primary and permanent teeth appears pitted; vertical grooves, deficiency in thickness, yellow to dark-brown color, open contacts, and occlusal wear are noted; seven varieties of type 1 hypoplastic amelogenesis imperfecta; the pitted, autosomal variety is most common
   c. Radiographic appearance—enamel absent or very thin layer over tips of cusps and interproximal areas
   d. Histologic characteristics—thin, defective enamel; few enamel prisms; no lamellae
   e. Treatment—restorations; crowns; bonding; laminates
2. Type 2: enamel hypocalcification—defect in mineralization of the formed matrix; normal enamel thickness, but the enamel is poorly calcified
   a. Etiology—two varieties include autosomal dominant and autosomal recessive
   b. Clinically (Figure 8-68), the enamel appears yellow to dark brown and chalky; easily breaks down
   c. Radiographic appearance—the tooth shape is normal; enamel and dentin have the same radiodensity, which makes them difficult to differentiate; enamel appears "moth eaten" and is less radiopaque than dentin

d. Histologic characteristics—broadening of interprismatic substance; distinct enamel prisms; enamel low in mineral content
   e. Treatment—restorations; crowns; bonding; laminates
3. Type 3: enamel hypomaturation
   a. Etiology—X-linked recessive ("snowcapped") or autosomal dominant
   b. Clinical appearance (Figure 8-69)
      (1) Enamel is of normal thickness but appears mottled with large amounts of enamel matrix and is therefore softer
      (2) Occlusal third of teeth appear "white" with normal hardness
      (3) Enamel easily chips from crowns of teeth
      (4) Four varieties of this type (snowcapped type shown in Figure 8-69)
4. Type 4: hypoplastic—hypomaturation of enamel
   a. Etiology—characterized by association with taurodontic teeth
   b. Clinically, the enamel is thin, pitted, and appears yellow to brown in color

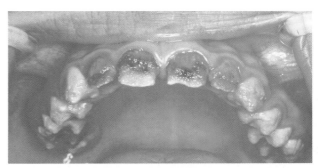

FIGURE 8-68 Note the loss of enamel in the teeth of a patient with hypocalcified amelogenesis imperfecta. *(From Ibsen OAC, Phelan JA: Oral pathology for the dental hygienist, ed 5, Philadelphia, 2009, Saunders.)*

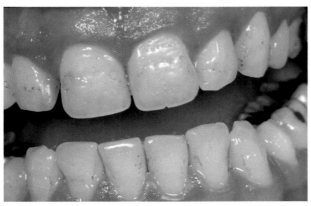

FIGURE 8-67 Pitted autosomal dominant amelogenesis imperfecta. Note the multiple pits on the labial surface of teeth. Some of the pits have been filled with composite. *(From Young WG, Sedano HO: Atlas of oral pathology, Minneapolis, MN, 1981, University of Minnesota Press.)*

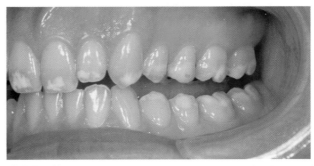

FIGURE 8-69 Note the uniform whitening of incisal edges and occlusal cusps in a case of "snowcapped" amelogenesis imperfecta. *(From Ibsen OAC, Phelan JA: Oral pathology for the dental hygienist, ed 5, Philadelphia, 2009, Saunders.)*

Dentinogenesis Imperfecta (Hereditary Opalescent Dentin)

A. Etiology
  1. Hereditary
  2. Disturbance of dentin formation
    a. Affects the mesodermal component
    b. Enamel remains normal
B. Clinical features (Figure 8-70, *A*)
  1. Teeth appear "opalescent," a translucent hue
  2. Gray to bluish-brown color
  3. Distinct constriction at the CEJ
C. Radiographic appearance (see Figure 8-70, *B*)
  1. Partial or total obliteration of pulp chambers and root canals
  2. Roots are short, blunted, and sometimes fractured
  3. Cementum, periodontal membrane, and alveolar bone appear normal
D. Histologic characteristics
  1. Disturbance of the mesoderm
  2. Dentin composed of irregular tubules; uncalcified matrix
  3. Tubules large in width; few in number
  4. Odontoblasts degenerate easily within the matrix
  5. Decrease in inorganic content

E. Treatment—cast-metal crowns; caution needed with partial appliances because of root fractures

Developmental Defects Affecting Tooth Shape

Dilaceration

A. Sharp bend or curve in the root of a formed tooth (Figure 8-71, *A*).
B. Etiology—trauma during tooth development
  1. Calcified area displaced
  2. Amount of tooth formed at the time of trauma will affect the angle or curve of the root; usually affects the apical third of the root
C. Radiographic appearance—sharp bend or curve in the root (see Figure 8-71, *B*)
D. Treatment—none

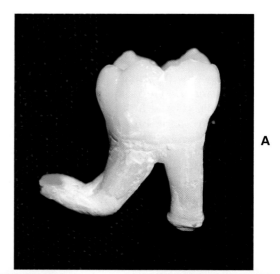

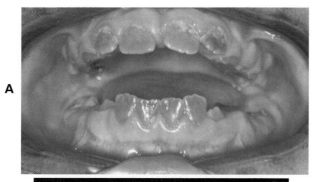

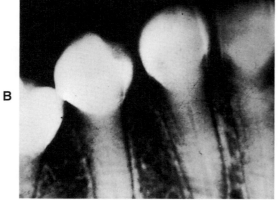

FIGURE 8-70 A, Clinical views of dentinogenesis imperfecta. **B,** Radiographic views. *(Courtesy of Dr. Edward V. Zegarelli; from Ibsen OAC, Phelan JA: Oral pathology for the dental hygienist, ed 5, Philadelphia, 2009, Saunders.)*

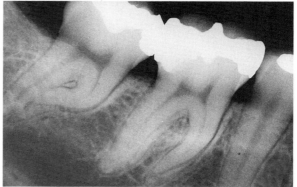

FIGURE 8-71 A, Dilaceration on the distal root of an extracted tooth. **B,** Mesial root dilaceration on a mandibular second molar. *(**A,** Courtesy of Dr. Rudy Melfi; **A and B,** from Ibsen OAC, Phelan JA: Oral pathology for the dental hygienist, ed 5, Philadelphia, 2009, Saunders.)*

Fusion

A. Union of two normally separated tooth germs
B. Etiology—physical force or external pressure; hereditary tendency
C. Clinical features (Figure 8-72)
   1. If the defect occurs early in development, one large tooth results
   2. If the defect occurs later, fusion of roots only
   3. Dentin always confluent (if true fusion)
   4. Can occur in both primary and permanent dentitions
   5. Can occur between two normal teeth or between one normal tooth and one supernumerary tooth
D. Location—anterior region; incisors are most often affected
E. Radiographic appearance—can have separate or fused root canals
F. Treatment—usually none; hemisection for a crown or bridge, if necessary

Gemination

A. Division of a single tooth germ by invagination; results in incomplete formation of two teeth (gemination means paired or occurring in twos)
B. Etiology—unknown; possibly trauma; hereditary tendency
C. Location—can affect the primary or permanent dentition, although it is slightly more common in the primary dentition (e.g., in mandibular incisors or in permanent maxillary incisors)
D. Clinically teeth usually have two completely or incompletely separate crowns with one root, or with one root canal (Figure 8-73)

Concrescence

A. Fusion that occurs after root formation is complete; roots united by cementum only

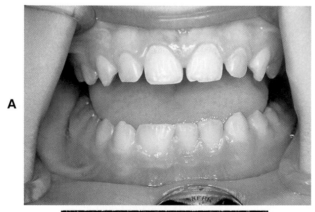

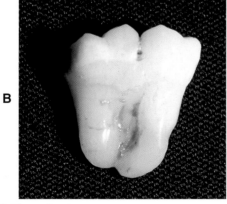

FIGURE 8-72 **A,** Clinical view of fusion involving a permanent mandibular lateral incisor. **B,** Fusion of mandibular molars. *(A, Courtesy of Dr. George Blozis; B, Courtesy of Dr. Rudy Melfi; from Ibsen OAC, Phelan JA: Oral pathology for the dental hygienist, ed 5, Philadelphia, 2009, Saunders.)*

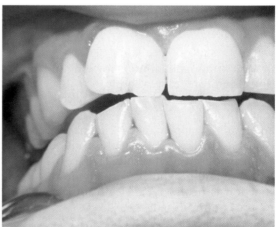

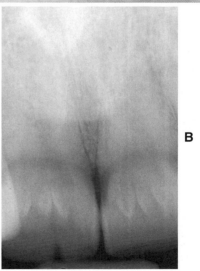

FIGURE 8-73 Clinical **(A)** and radiographic **(B)** views of gemination seen in the right maxillary central incisor. *(From Ibsen OAC, Phelan JA: Oral pathology for the dental hygienist, ed 5, Philadelphia, 2009, Saunders.)*

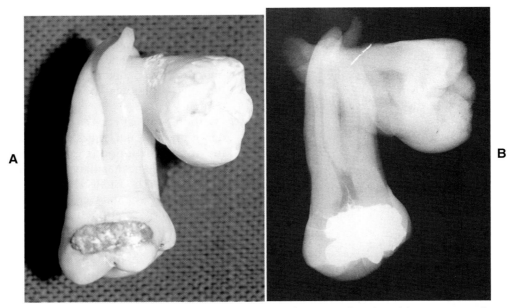

FIGURE 8-74 *A and B,* *Example of concrescence seen in extracted teeth and in a corresponding radiograph. (Courtesy of Dr. George Blozis; from Ibsen OAC, Phelan JA: Oral pathology for the dental hygienist, ed 5, Philadelphia, 2009, Saunders.)*

B. Etiology—traumatic injury; crowding of teeth with resorption of interdental bone
C. Location—most often seen in adjacent maxillary molars
D. Radiographic appearance—establishes diagnosis because teeth are joined at the root surfaces and cannot be observed clinically (Figure 8-74)
E. Treatment and prognosis—usually no treatment; if extraction is necessary, all teeth joined by cementum are compromised

Dens in Dente (Dens Invaginatus)
A. Tooth within a tooth
B. Etiology—increased localized external pressure; growth retardation
C. Location—maxillary lateral incisor (Figure 8-75)
D. Often bilateral
E. Radiographic appearance—small tooth within the pulp chamber (Figure 8-76)
F. Treatment—none, unless the pulp becomes inflamed or necrotic

Dens Evaginatus
A. An accessory cusp found on the occlusal surface
B. Etiology—rare developmental anomaly caused by proliferation of enamel epithelium
C. Location—most often mandibular premolars (tuberculated premolars)
D. Clinical appearance—small, round nodule of enamel found on the occlusal surface (Figure 8-77)
E. Treatment—usually none, unless the condition poses occlusal problems

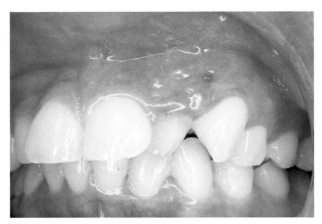

FIGURE 8-75 Clinical view of dens in dente in maxillary lateral incisor. *(Courtesy of Dr. George Blozis; from Ibsen OAC, Phelan JA: Oral pathology for the dental hygienist, ed 5, Philadelphia, 2009, Saunders.)*

Natal Teeth
A. Teeth present at birth
B. Etiology
  1. Develop from part of dental lamina before the deciduous bud or from bud of accessory dental lamina
  2. Neonatal teeth are those that erupt 30 days after birth
C. Location—usually found in the mandibular incisor area
D. Histologic characteristics—keratinized epithelial structures without roots (therefore not true teeth)

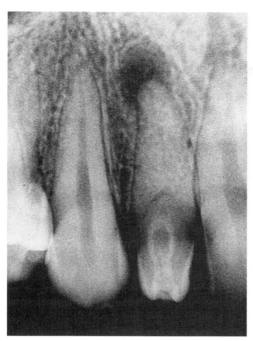

FIGURE 8-76 Radiograph of dens in dente in maxillary lateral incisor. *(From Ibsen OAC, Phelan JA: Oral pathology for the dental hygienist, ed 5, Philadelphia, 2009, Saunders.)*

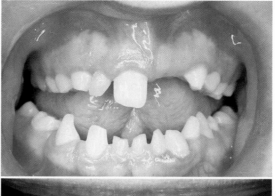

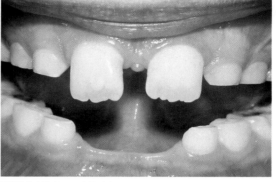

FIGURE 8-78 A and B, Hypodontia. The missing teeth were not extracted; they never developed. *(A, Courtesy of Dr. George Blozis; B, Courtesy of Dr. Margot Van Dis; from Ibsen OAC, Phelan JA: Oral pathology for the dental hygienist, ed 5, Philadelphia, 2009, Saunders.)*

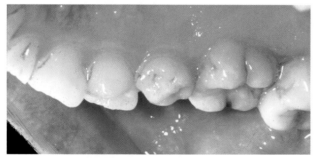

FIGURE 8-77 Dens evaginatus of maxillary premolar. *(Courtesy of Dr. Margot Van Dis; from Ibsen OAC, Phelan JA: Oral pathology for the dental hygienist, ed 4, Philadelphia, 2009, Saunders.)*

E. Treatment and prognosis
  1. Removal (after determining they are not prematurely erupted primary teeth)
  2. Prognosis is excellent; no complications

Developmental Defects Affecting the Number of Teeth

Anodontia
A. Missing teeth
B. Etiology—congenital lack of teeth; tooth germ did not develop
C. Two forms
  1. Total anodontia
    a. Rare condition—all teeth missing

    b. May involve both primary and permanent dentitions
    c. Usually associated with ectodermal dysplasia, a hereditary disturbance
  2. Hypodontia (partial anodontia) (Figure 8-78, *A* and *B*)
    a. Rather common
    b. Teeth usually affected include third molars and maxillary lateral incisors
    c. Familial or hereditary tendency
    d. Odontodysplasia, "ghost teeth" (Figure 8-79) (teeth in this condition are malformed and unerupted)
D. Treatment
  1. Space maintainers during childhood
  2. Crown and bridge work
  3. Prosthetic appliances
  4. Dental implants

Supernumerary Teeth
A. More than the normal number of teeth
B. Etiology—additional tooth buds arise from dental lamina; hereditary
C. Classification
  1. Mesiodent (mesiodens)—most common; cone-shaped crown; short root; located between maxillary centrals (Figure 8-80, *A* to *C*)

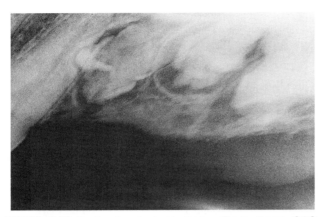

FIGURE 8-79 Regional odontodysplasia. *(From Ibsen OAC, Phelan JA: Oral pathology for the dental hygienist, ed 5, Philadelphia, 2009, Saunders.)*

2. Maxillary fourth molar—distal to the third molar; a mandibular fourth molar occasionally is found
3. Maxillary paramolar—usually a small molar; located buccally or lingually in the area of the maxillary molars
D. Treatment—none; observe for cystic transition; remove when interference occurs with normal dentition

Developmental Defects Affecting Tooth Size

Macrodontia
Abnormally large tooth; rare; possibly a result of fusion

Microdontia
Abnormally small tooth; maxillary lateral incisor and third molar most commonly affected (Figure 8-81)

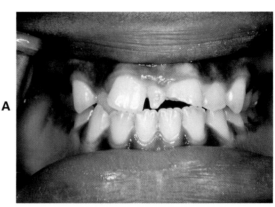

A

FIGURE 8-80 A, Mesiodens seen between maxillary central incisors. **B,** Radiograph of a mesiodens. **C,** Radiograph showing a pair of inverted, impacted mesiodens. **(A and B,** Courtesy of Dr. George Blozis; **A to C,** from Ibsen OAC, Phelan JA: Oral pathology for the dental hygienist, ed 5, Philadelphia, 2009, Saunders.)

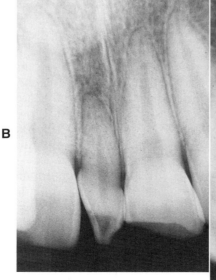

B

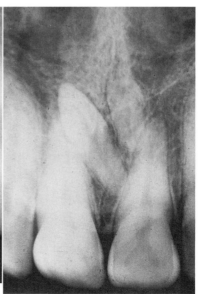

C

CONDITIONS OF ORAL SOFT TISSUES

Abnormalities Affecting Mucous Membranes or Skin

Amalgam Tattoo

A. Etiology—dust or particle of an amalgam restoration embedded in the mucosa or gingiva
B. Clinical features—blue to purplish area near an amalgam restoration (Figure 8-82, *A*)
C. Radiographic appearance—radiopaque if amalgam particles are present (see Figure 8-82, *B*)
D. Treatment

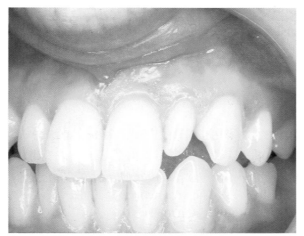

FIGURE 8-81 Peg-shaped lateral incisor. *(Courtesy of Dr. George Blozis; from Ibsen OAC, Phelan JA: Oral pathology for the dental hygienist, ed 5, Philadelphia, 2009, Saunders.)*

Melanin Pigmentation

A. Dark pigmentation of the gingiva or mucosa (Figures 8-83 and 8-84)
B. Etiology—hereditary; those with dark complexions are most commonly affected; can occur following inflammation from injury
C. Treatment—none, as tissue is healthy

Angular Cheilitis

A. Etiology (considered a form of candidiasis)
   1. Infection caused by *Candida albicans*
   2. Nutritional deficiency
   3. Denture-associated chelitis
B. Clinical features—inflammation and cracking at the corners of the lips; extend into facial skin (Figure 8-85)
C. Histologic characteristics—inflammatory cells
D. Treatment—depends on the etiology: improved diet; correction of the vertical dimension of the denture; applying antifungal ointment or cream three to four times per day for 5 to 7 days

Fordyce Granules

A. Etiology—developmental; aberrant sebaceous glands
B. Clinical features (Figure 8-86)
   1. Affects the vermilion of the lips and the buccal mucosa
   2. Yellow, slightly raised spots a few millimeters in size
C. Location—buccal mucosa; lips
D. Histologic characteristics—glandular tissue; not pathologic
E. Treatment—none

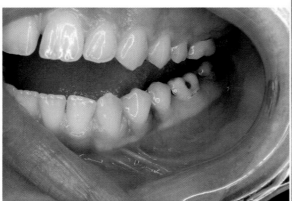
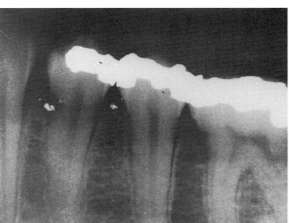

FIGURE 8-82 A, This blue-gray pigmentation on the gingiva is an amalgam tattoo. **B,** Periapical radiograph showing amalgam particles in the gingival tissue. *(From Ibsen OAC, Phelan JA: Oral pathology for the dental hygienist, ed 5, Philadelphia, 2009, Saunders.)*

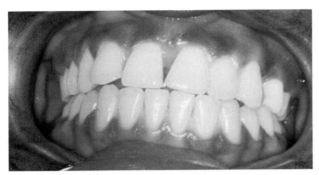

FIGURE 8-83 Melanin pigmentation of the gingiva. *(From Ibsen OAC, Phelan JA: Oral pathology for the dental hygienist, ed 5, Philadelphia, 2009, Saunders.)*

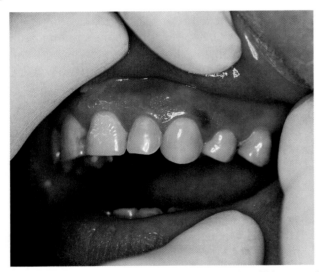

FIGURE 8-84 Post-traumatic melanin pigmentation. This area of melanin pigmentation on the gingiva occurred after the healing of an injury caused by trauma. *(From Ibsen OAC, Phelan JA: Oral pathology for the dental hygienist, ed 5, Philadelphia, 2009, Saunders.)*

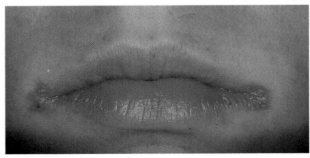

FIGURE 8-85 Angular cheilitis. *(From Ibsen OAC, Phelan JA: Oral pathology for the dental hygienist, ed 5, Philadelphia, 2009, Saunders.)*

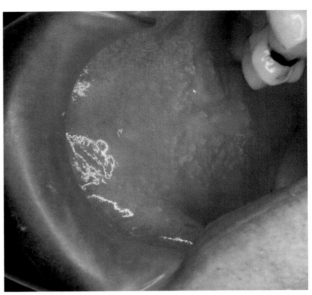

FIGURE 8-86 Fordyce granules on the buccal mucosa. *(From Ibsen OAC, Phelan JA: Oral pathology for the dental hygienist, ed 5, Philadelphia, 2009, Saunders.)*

Abnormalities Affecting the Tongue
(see Chapter 12, Table 12-4)

Geographic Tongue (Benign Migratory Glossitis)
A. Etiology—unknown; theories include:
  1. Nutritional deficiency
  2. Heredity
  3. Stress
  4. Psoriasis
B. Age and gender related—any age, but more common in children and young adults; no gender predilection
C. Clinical features (Figure 8-87)
  1. Fungiform papillae appear as red, mushroom-like projections
  2. Diffuse desquamation of filiform papillae
  3. Condition assumes variations in shape, giving a map-like appearance; remission in depapillated areas
  4. Discomfort occurs when the patient eats certain foods
D. Histologic characteristics—characteristic inflammatory cells; keratotic cells around the borders of the lesion
E. Treatment—none; variant of normal

Black Hairy Tongue
A. Etiology—irritation to filiform papillae caused by:
  1. Smoking
  2. Alcohol
  3. Hydrogen peroxide

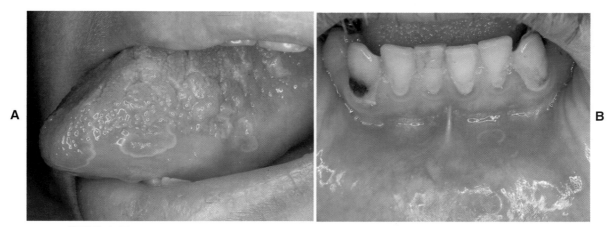

FIGURE 8-87 A, Geographic tongue. **B,** Ectopic geographic tongue observed in the anterior mandibular mucosa. *(From Ibsen OAC, Phelan JA: Oral pathology for the dental hygienist, ed 5, Philadelphia, 2009, Saunders.)*

4. Antacid liquids

5. Systemic antibiotic therapy

B. Clinical features—brownish to black appearance on the dorsal surface of the tongue (Figure 8-88)

C. Histologic characteristics—elongation of filiform papillae; characteristic inflammatory cells

D. Treatment and prognosis

   1. Gentle brushing or scraping of the tongue; toothpaste should not be used

   2. Removal of the cause

   3. Prognosis is good; the condition is totally reversible, but may recur

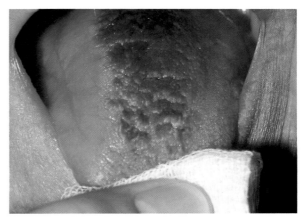

FIGURE 8-88 Black hairy tongue. *(From Ibsen OAC, Phelan JA: Oral pathology for the dental hygienist, ed 4, Philadelphia, 2004, Saunders.)*

@ WEBSITE INFORMATION AND RESOURCES

SOURCE	WEB SITE ADDRESS	DESCRIPTION
Doctor's Guide	http://www.pslgroup.com	Articles on medical industry and medical news
Electronic Doctor	http://www.edoc.co.za/dhw	Dental articles; also has a kids' corner
National Institute of Dental and Craniofacial Research	http://www.nidr.nih.gov	News and information related to dentistry and information about the Institute's research
Mayo Clinic Medicine Center	http://www.mayohealth.org	Information and links to health conditions and diseases
Clinical trials listing service	http://www.centerwatch.com	International listing of clinical research trials and medical centers that perform clinical research and drug therapies newly approved by the U.S. Food and Drug Agency (FDA)
National Cancer Institute	http://www.nci.nih.gov	Information about types of cancer, treatments, risk factors, screening, tests, and statistics
American Cancer Society	http://cancer.org	Information about cancers and leukemias from both professional and patient points of view

Continued

@ WEBSITE INFORMATION AND RESOURCES—cont'd

SOURCE	WEB SITE ADDRESS	DESCRIPTION
American Society of Pediatric Hematology and Oncology	http://www.aspho.org	Information for both professionals and patients about pediatric hematology and oncology
Support for People with Oral and Head and Neck Cancers	http://www.spohnc.org	Information and support for those suffering from oral and head and neck cancers
Leukemia and Lymphoma Society of America	http://www.leukemia.org	Information about blood-related cancers

SUGGESTED READINGS

Ibsen OAC, Phelan JA: *Oral pathology for the dental hygienist*, ed 5, Philadelphia, 2009, Saunders.

Neville BW, Damm DD, Allen CM, Bouquot JE: *Oral and maxillofacial pathology*, ed 3, Philadelphia, 2009, Saunders.

Regezi J, Sciubba J, Jordan RCK: Oral pathology: Clinical pathologic correlations, ed 5, Philadelphia, 2008, Saunders.

CHAPTER 8 REVIEW QUESTIONS

Answers and Rationales to Review Questions are available on this text's
accompanying Evolve site. See inside front cover for details.
Use Case A and Figure 8-89 to answer questions 1 to 11.

evolve

Synopsis of Patient History Case A

Age: _30_
Sex: _M_
Height: _6'3"_
Weight: _200 lb_

VITAL SIGNS
Blood pressure: _120/80_ mm Hg
Pulse rate: _60_
Respiration: _16_

1. Under the care of a physician   ____YES ✔NO
       Condition:
2. Hospitalization within the last five years   ____YES ✔NO
3. Has or had the following conditions:

   Rheumatic fever or rheumatic heart disease   ____YES ✔NO
   Congenital heart disease (bicuspid aortic valve)   ____YES ✔NO
   Heart attack   ____YES ✔NO
   Angina pectoris   ____YES ✔NO
   Hypertension   ____YES ✔NO
   Diabetes mellitus   ____YES ✔NO
   Hepatitis   ____YES ✔NO
   Bleeding disorder   ____YES ✔NO
   Fainting spells, seizures, or epilepsy   ____YES ✔NO
   Asthma   ____YES ✔NO
   Allergies (medication, food)   ____YES ✔NO

4. Current medications:

   Anticoagulants ___YES ✔NO   Nitroglycerin ___YES ✔NO
   Insulin ___YES ✔NO   High blood pressure medication ___YES ✔NO
   Antibiotics ___YES ✔NO   Corticosteroids ___YES ✔NO
   Aspirin ___YES ✔NO   Oral contraceptives ___YES ✔NO

   Other:_____

5. Smokes or uses tobacco products ____YES ✔NO

6. Is pregnant   ____YES ✔NO

MEDICAL HISTORY: *Patient is African-American and in good health.*

DENTAL HISTORY: *Patient is meticulous with his oral hygiene, but has a tendency to brush vigorously.*

SOCIAL HISTORY: *Patient lives with wife and 3 year old son.*

CHIEF COMPLAINT: *"I don't like the appearance of my gums pulling away from my teeth, and my teeth are sensitive around my upper canines."*

SUPPLEMENTAL ORAL EXAMINATION FINDINGS: *The patient has a generalized opalescent appearance of the buccal mucosa. The patient has generalized melanin pigmentation of the gingiva. A mucocele is noted.*

The gingiva is firm and stippled with no bleeding evident upon probing. There is gingival recession on teeth #6 & #11 and mandibular anterior facials, with a 1 mm zone of attached gingiva.

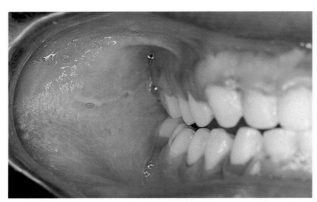

FIGURE 8-89 Leukoedema. *(From Regezi JA, Sciubba JJ, Jordan RCK: Oral pathology: Clinical pathologic correlations, ed 5, St Louis, 2008, Saunders.)*

1. **The generalized opalescence of the buccal mucosa is most likely:**
   a. Linea alba
   b. Leukoedema
   c. Lichen planus
   d. Leukoplakia

2. **In which layer of the stratified epithelium is the generalized opalescent condition in question 1 caused by significant intercellular edema?**
   a. Corneum
   b. Basal
   c. Prickle
   d. Granular

3. **What treatment does this condition require?**
   a. Nonsteroidal anti-inflammatory drugs
   b. Excision
   c. Antifungal drugs
   d. No treatment

4. **The patient has a 2-mm probing depth on the facial aspect of tooth #6, and he has 3 mm of recession. What is the attachment loss in this area?**
   a. 5 mm
   b. 2 mm
   c. 3 mm
   d. 1 mm

5. **The patient's sensitivity in this area is most likely related to:**
   a. Fluid entering the sulcular epithelium
   b. Fluid entering the rodless enamel
   c. Fluid entering the dentinal tubules
   d. Fluid entering the lacuna of cementum

6. **The tooth itself is capable of experiencing painful-nerve sensation from all of the following EXCEPT one. Which one is the EXCEPTION?:**
   a. Pressure
   b. Heat
   c. Cold
   d. Olfaction

The patient wants the areas of gingival recession treated to resolve issues of sensitivity and esthetic problems. The dental care plan includes covering the areas around the canines with soft tissue grafts. The periodontist explains that she will perform connective tissue grafts. She explains that the connective tissue taken from an area (donor site) will produce the same type of epithelium at the canine area (recipient site) as the tissue that exists at that donor site.

---

7. **The type of tissue normally present around the canine area is:**
   a. Keratinized, stratified squamous epithelium
   b. Nonkeratinized, stratified squamous epithelium
   c. Keratinized, simple squamous epithelium
   d. Pseudo-stratified columnar epithelium

8. **An appropriate connective tissue donor site would be the:**
   a. Buccal mucosa
   b. Soft palate
   c. Hard palate
   d. Sublingual area

9. **With this procedure, the ideal outcome would be for some of this tissue to form a fibrous attachment** to the tooth cementum. From which type of tissue would the cells come to remodel the cementum in this area in which root surfaces previously were exposed?
   a. Cellular cementum
   b. Bone
   c. Sulcular epithelium
   d. Periodontal ligament

10. **This patient also has a mucocele that is the result of trauma to a minor salivary duct. A mucocele is usually found on the:**
    a. Gingiva
    b. Lower lip mucosa
    c. Hard palate
    d. Dorsum of the tongue

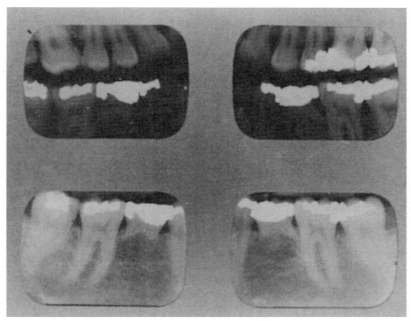

FIGURE 8-90 Bitewing radiographs.

11. To prevent further recession, what changes should this patient make in his oral self-care regimen?
   a. More frequent continued-care appointments
   b. Modifying flossing technique
   c. More frequent toothbrushing
   d. Modifying toothbrushing technique

12. The bitewing radiographs in Figure 8-90 indicate congenital absence of the:
   a. Maxillary right first premolar and the maxillary left first premolars
   b. Mandibular right first premolar and the mandibular left first premolar
   c. Mandibular left first premolar and the mandibular right second premolar
   d. Mandibular right second premolar and the mandibular left second premolar

13. A bony, hard developmental, benign asymptomatic area found on the midline of the hard palate that appears radiopaque on a radiograph is most likely a:
   a. Odontogenic myxoma
   b. Median palatal cyst
   c. Compound odontoma
   d. Torus palatinus

Use Figure 8-91 to answer questions 14 to 16.

14. On the panograph (see Figure 8-91), the bilateral radiolucent areas apical to the mandibular molars and identified by A are:
   a. Stafne bone cysts
   b. Periapical abscesses
   c. Submandibular fossae
   d. Traumatic bone cysts

15. The horizontal radiopaque structure identified by Figure 8-91, *B*, is the:
   a. Anterior coronoid process
   b. Maxillary tuberosity
   c. Mandibular condyle
   d. Zygomatic arch

16. The bilateral radiolucent areas identified by Figure 8-91, *C*, are:
   a. Nasal fossae
   b. Orbits
   c. Frontal sinuses
   d. Maxillary sinuses

17. Mixed tumors are most often found in the:
   a. Palate
   b. Mandible
   c. Buccal mucosa
   d. Lymph nodes

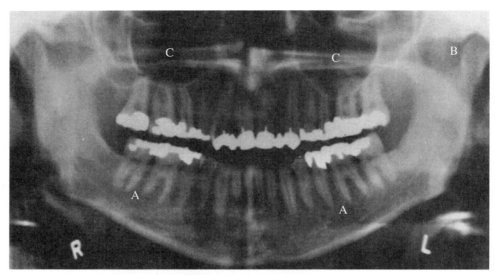

FIGURE 8-91 Panograph.

18. Which of the following cysts would create difficulty swallowing?
  a. Branchial cleft
  b. Thyroglossal
  c. Nasopalatine
  d. Mucocele

19. Which disease may have oral characteristics similar to those found in necrotizing ulcerative gingivitis (NUG)?
  a. Primary herpes
  b. Mononucleosis
  c. Leukemia
  d. Nonthrombocytopenic purpura

20. A ranula usually is found on the:
  a. Palate
  b. Inner lip
  c. Buccal mucosa
  d. Floor of the mouth

21. A definitive dental diagnosis of soft tissue oral cancer is made by:
  a. A complete radiographic survey
  b. Exfoliative cytology
  c. Scalpel biopsy
  d. Brush test

22. Figure 8-92 shows a periapical radiograph of the mandibular right quadrant, which was taken as part of a full-mouth radiographic series. The patient was 14 years of age and asymptomatic. The periapical radiolucency indicated by the arrow on tooth 31 is most likely:
  a. Resorption caused by a traumatic injury
  b. Periapical abscesses
  c. Incomplete root formation
  d. Hypercementosis

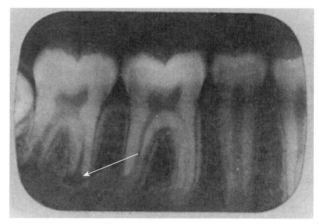

FIGURE 8-92 Periapical radiograph.

23. Primordial cysts are most often found radiographically:
  a. In the anterior maxillary regions
  b. Around a supernumerary tooth
  c. Posterior to erupted third molars or in place of a tooth that was never present
  d. In the mandibular canine and first premolar areas

24. The usual location of periapical cemento-osseous dysplasia (cementoma) is:
  a. Mandibular anteriors
  b. Maxillary anteriors
  c. The mandibular ramus
  d. Maxillary premolars

25. Which of the following is a rickettsial infection?
  a. Malaria
  b. Psittacosis
  c. Rocky Mountain spotted fever
  d. Tularemia

26. A slightly raised, noncoated, red, rectangular area in the midline of the tongue has been present as long as the patient can remember. It is associated with *Candida albicans*. This condition is most likely:
    a. Geographic tongue
    b. Pathologic tongue
    c. Median rhomboid glossitis
    d. Fissured tongue

27. Which of the following provides the most conclusive diagnostic evidence in distinguishing pemphigus from pemphigoid?
    a. Clinical picture
    b. History of the disease
    c. Biopsy and histology report
    d. Race and religion

28. An isolated radiopaque area in the periodontal ligament space is observed on a patient's radiographs. This radiopaque structure may be a(an):
    a. Epithelial rest
    b. Cementum spur
    c. Exostosis of alveolar bone
    d. Cementicle

29. A 30-year-old patient calls and complains of sudden swelling in both sides of his neck, which seems to be enlarging. His record indicates that he recently has cancelled two appointments. He needs to have restorative care completed on the mandibular second molars, which have extensive decay. The patient may have:
    a. Actinomycosis
    b. Mumps
    c. Syphilis
    d. Ludwig angina

30. Which of the following two diseases represent different forms of infection resulting from the same virus?
    a. Measles and German measles
    b. Chickenpox and smallpox
    c. Bacterial pneumonia and croup
    d. Shingles and chickenpox

31. A lesion is noted on the lips of a 40-year-old female patient. The lesion appears as several discrete vesicles; some have ulcerated. When questioned, the patient says she always gets a sore like that before she gets a cold. The patient most likely has:
    a. A chancre
    b. Perlèche
    c. An aphthous ulcer
    d. Herpes labialis

32. Which of the following statements most accurately describes the effect of pregnancy on the health of the mother's oral tissues?
    a. Pregnancy-associated gingivitis is caused by hormonal changes, and nothing can be done about it
    b. Pregnant women can often experience the growth of tumors in the mouth that relate to hormonal changes
    c. Hormonal changes during pregnancy result in increased bacteria and increased gingival response to plaque biofilm
    d. Pregnancy results in hormonal changes, but these changes do not affect the mother's oral tissues

33. The gingival enlargement shown in Figure 8-93 was caused by a calcium channel blocker drug. The condition was most likely caused by:
    a. Phenytoin (Dilantin)
    b. Enalapril (Vasotec)
    c. Fluoxetine (Prozac)
    d. Nifedipine (Procardia)

34. In Figure 8-94, the soft tissue lesion on the mandibular mucosa erupted suddenly, was filled with a clear fluid, and broke easily. The condition is most likely a:
    a. Ranula
    b. Mucocele
    c. Fibroma
    d. Fistula

35. Which of the following produce(s) no radiographic image?
    a. Dental caries
    b. Supernumerary teeth
    c. Odontoma
    d. Fibroma

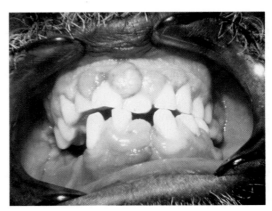

FIGURE 8-93 Gingival enlargement. *(Courtesy of Dr. Victor M. Sternberg; from Ibsen OAC, Phelan JA: Oral pathology for the dental hygienist, ed 5, Philadelphia, 2009, Saunders.)*

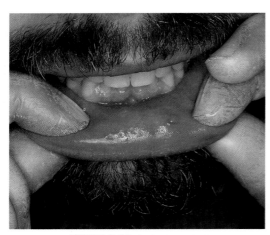

FIGURE 8-94 Soft tissue lesion.

36. **Which of the diagnostic methods listed below is most reliable and ensures the highest degree of accuracy when evaluating squamous cell carcinoma?**
    a. Surgical
    b. Microscopic
    c. Therapeutic
    d. Clinical

37. **Which of the following does not define the term *pathogenesis*?**
    a. How the lesion begins
    b. Behavior of the lesion
    c. Clinical picture of the lesion
    d. Development of the lesion

38. **A pyogenic granuloma is known to scar down to a(an):**
    a. Pregnancy tumor
    b. Fibrogranuloma
    c. Lipoma
    d. Osteoma

39. **The patient is a 28-year-old woman who is pregnant. A gingival lesion involving the interproximal papillae between teeth #7 and #8 on the labial surface is bright red, soft, and spongy; it bleeds easily. The histology report shows proliferation of inflammatory cells and thin epithelium. The lesion is most likely:**
    a. A fibroma
    b. A pyogenic granuloma
    c. Redundant tissue
    d. A papilloma

40. **Which one of the following cysts has the potential for developing into an ameloblastoma?**
    a. Lateral periodontal cyst
    b. Primordial cyst
    c. Stafne bone cyst
    d. Residual cyst

41. **The clinical oral examination of the patient reveals a possible leukoplakia. The first course of action should be to:**
    a. Perform a scalpel biopsy
    b. Perform a cytologic smear
    c. Give the client vitamin A therapy
    d. Have the patient return in 2 months to evaluate the growth

42. **Which one of the following tests is not used for pemphigus?**
    a. Pels-Macht
    b. Tzanck
    c. Enzyme-linked immunosorbent assay (ELISA)
    d. Nikolsky sign

43. **A palatal condition of an elderly patient that is primarily caused by chronic irritation from the suction chamber of a denture is clinically observed as:**
    a. A fibroma
    b. A papilloma
    c. Papillary hyperplasia
    d. A median palatal cyst

44. **A lesion found on the buccal mucosa of a 30-year-old white woman is pink, well defined, and soft to palpation. It has been slow-growing and histologically consists of collagenous fibers, fibroblasts, and fibrocytes, but with no fat cells or bone. It has a pedunculated base. The lesion is most likely a:**
    a. Sarcoma
    b. Fibroma
    c. Fibrolipoma
    d. Fibro-osteoma

45. **A radiolucent lesion in the posterior part of the mandible anterior to the angle has the radiographic features of a cyst. After surgical intervention, the histology report shows submaxillary salivary gland tissue; also, the lesion is not lined with epithelium. One may conclude that the lesion is most likely a(an):**
    a. Residual cyst
    b. Traumatic bone cyst
    c. Lingual mandibular bone concavity
    d. Ameloblastoma

46. **A cyst commonly found unilaterally in the floor of the mouth changes size between meals. Clinically, it has a bluish hue. It may be caused by:**
    a. A decayed tooth
    b. Blockage or trauma to a major salivary duct
    c. Failure of developmental fusion of the branchial arches
    d. Medications

47. The onset of this chronic, recurring autoimmune disease is at 30 years, with no gender predilection. A triad of symptomatic locations (oral, eye, and genital) is involved, and two of the three areas must be present to make the diagnosis. You suspect:
    a. Erythema multiforme
    b. Stevens-Johnson syndrome
    c. Behçet syndrome
    d. Recurrent ulcerative stomatitis (RUS)

48. For which one of the following is the etiology definitely known to be an irritant?
    a. Papilloma
    b. Torus
    c. Granuloma
    d. Lipoma

49. An intraoral examination of the gingiva reveals a clinical picture of punched-out papillae. The patient complains of pain and a bad taste. The history indicates that the patient's diet is poor, that he has been under stress, and that he has had little rest. What is the best course of action?
    a. Perform culture and laboratory studies
    b. Apply a therapeutic course, debride the mouth, and recommend hydrogen peroxide oral rinse and systemic antibiotics
    c. Immediately refer the patient to a periodontist
    d. Perform periodontal therapy, including extensive root planing and stain removal

50. Which one of the following is most important to the pathologist when a chondroma is suspected?
    a. A complete personal history of the patient
    b. Complete removal of the tumor in question
    c. Submission of a "large enough" sample of tissue for histologic study because a chondroma resembles a malignant chondrosarcoma
    d. Radiographs of all large bones

51. The clinical assessment of a patient's lesion is best described as a well-defined, yellowish, blister-like eruption. Straw fluid may be aspirated. It is a rare, benign neoplasm. The histology report shows a predominance of fat cells. The lesion is a (an):
    a. Papilloma
    b. Osteoma
    c. Lipoma
    d. Fibroma

52. A tooth involved in a cyst is discovered to be non-vital on pulp testing. The cyst is probably a:
    a. Residual cyst
    b. Lateral periodontal cyst
    c. Radicular cyst
    d. Dentigerous cyst

53. Which one of the following can be a characteristic of pemphigus vulgaris?
    a. Nikolsky sign
    b. Occurs predominantly in African American females

    c. Has an etiology of drug reaction
    d. Occurs predominantly in white males

54. The clinical assessment reveals an inflamed, palpable benign tumor in the anterior of the palate, lingual to the maxillary incisors. The tumor arises from deeper tissue and appears to originate from the periodontal ligament. The radiograph shows the lesion infiltrating bone but no metastasis. The client is a 35-year-old woman. A possible diagnosis is a:
    a. Peripheral giant cell granuloma
    b. Lipoma
    c. Torus palatinus
    d. Mixed tumor

55. Clinical assessment of a lesion reveals a severe hypersensitivity reaction, with the lips and tongue especially affected. Additionally, "bull's eye" or "target eye" skin lesions are present, and the onset of all lesions was abrupt or "explosive." The condition is most likely:
    a. Lichen planus
    b. Herpes
    c. Erythema multiforme
    d. Mononucleosis

56. Which one of the following cysts is the result of extracting a tooth without the cystic sac?
    a. Radicular cyst
    b. Residual cyst
    c. Lateral periodontal cyst
    d. Primordial cyst

57. The dental hygienist observes an adult patient with the following clinical feature: gingival fibromatosis resulting from a history of Zimmerman-Laband syndrome and phenytoin (Dilantin) therapy. Which one of the following statements is correct?
    a. The client should stop taking the drug
    b. An overgrowth of the connective tissue is present
    c. The epithelium remains the same
    d. A gingivectomy would "cure" the condition

58. Which one of the following diagnostic processes should be applied to establish the diagnosis of nicotine stomatitis?
    a. Surgical and microscopic
    b. Radiographic
    c. Laboratory
    d. Clinical and historical

59. Clinically, this benign white, cauliflower-like lesion usually on the palate is similar to a wart. The histology report indicates long, finger-like projections of epithelium. The etiology is human papilloma virus (HPV). What is the most likely condition?
    a. Verruca vulgaris
    b. Papilloma
    c. Aspirin burn
    d. Linea alba

60. In which of the following locations is a lateral periodontal cyst usually found?
   a. Between the roots of mandibular canines and premolars
   b. Between the roots of maxillary central incisors
   c. On the maxillary canine
   d. In the mandibular third molar area

61. A platelet count of 150,000 to 400,000/mm³ of blood and a normal bleeding time are not indicative of:
   a. Thrombocytopenia
   b. Anemia
   c. Leukemia
   d. Nonthrombocytopenic purpura

62. All of the following are characteristic of necrotizing ulcerative gingivitis (NUG) *except* one. Which one is the *exception*?
   a. Punched-out papillae and craters
   b. Hyperkeratinization
   c. Odor
   d. Pain and bleeding

63. Which of the following makes Behçet's syndrome different from recurrent ulcerative stomatitis?
   a. "Bull's eye" skin lesions
   b. A triad of locations of lesions (oral, eye, and genital)
   c. Exudate from lesions
   d. Mesenchymal proliferations

64. What is the causative agent of herpangina?
   a. Chickenpox virus
   b. Coxsackievirus
   c. Epstein-Barr virus
   d. Varicella zoster virus

65. In treating fibrous dysplasia, which one of the following would not be advised because it can trigger a malignancy?
   a. Radiation
   b. Surgery
   c. Chemotherapy
   d. Bone marrow depressants

66. Precocious puberty is most characteristic of:
   a. Jaffe syndrome
   b. Monostotic fibrous dysplasia
   c. Cherubism
   d. McCune-Albright syndrome

67. Achlorhydria, inability to absorb vitamin B₁₂, and burning, painful tongue are characteristics of:
   a. Thrombocytopenia
   b. Hypervitaminosis
   c. Pernicious anemia
   d. Hyperkeratosis

68. Bone marrow anoxia occurs in:
   a. Secondary polycythemia
   b. Pernicious anemia
   c. Thalassemia
   d. Aplastic anemia

69. Which one of the following is referred to as "Cooley anemia"?
   a. Acute anemia
   b. Thalassemia
   c. Primary aplastic anemia
   d. Thrombocytopenia

70. In which of the following cysts are nonvital teeth involved?
   a. Nasoalveolar cyst
   b. Lateral periodontal cyst
   c. Radicular cyst
   d. Cyst of the incisive papilla

71. Which of the following cysts could develop into an ameloblastoma?
   a. A residual cyst
   b. Primordial cyst
   c. Median mandibular cyst
   d. Lateral periodontal cyst

72. A radicular cyst is most often caused by:
   a. Deep restorations
   b. Trauma
   c. Primary occlusal traumatism
   d. Dental caries

73. Epulis fissuratum is caused by:
   a. A denture flange
   b. The suction chamber of a denture
   c. An allergic reaction to acrylic material
   d. Denture cleaners

74. Sickle cell anemia is of hereditary origin and occurs primarily in:
   a. Whites
   b. Native Americans
   c. Infants
   d. African Americans

75. Which one of the following characteristics does a person with achlorhydria have?
   a. A low blood glucose level
   b. A lack of hydrochloric acid
   c. Too much hydrochloric acid
   d. Xerostomia

76. Which one of the following characteristics does a person with leukopenia have?
   a. Decrease in the number of white blood cells
   b. Increase in the number of white blood cells
   c. Decrease in the number of red blood cells
   d. Decrease in the number of platelets

Microbiology and Immunology

Jessica C. Peek

Basic concepts of microbiology and immunology relate to transmissible diseases encountered in client care. Using standard precautions in the dental setting greatly reduces the transmission of pathogens. Dental hygienists must prevent and manage potential occupational exposures from infectious diseases.

GENERAL MICROBIOLOGY

MICROORGANISMS

General Considerations

A. Ubiquitous—found virtually everywhere
B. Only 3% are pathogenic (disease causing); 97% are nonpathogenic
C. Exhibit characteristics common to all biologic systems: reproduction, metabolism, growth, response to stimuli, adaptability, mutation, and organization
D. Medically important microorganisms
   1. Eukaryotes
      a. Protozoa—unicellular, nonphotosynthetic, heterotrophic
      b. Fungi—molds (multicellular) or yeast (unicellular)
         (1) Nonphotosynthetic, heterotrophic
         (2) Classified by type of spores produced, presence or absence of mycelia, mechanisms of sexual and asexual spore formation
         (3) Part of the fungi kingdom
         (4) Identification of infection is accomplished clinically and microbiologically
      c. Helminths
         (1) Multicellular, nonphotosynthetic, heterotrophic

(2) Generally macroparasites of the human alimentary tract or hemolymphatic system
(3) Part of the animal kingdom
(4) Identification of infection is accomplished on microbiologic and clinical grounds
   2. Prokaryotes (aerobic or anaerobic unicellular bacteria)
      a. Classified by shape
         (1) Cocci (round)
         (2) Bacilli (rod shaped)
         (3) Vibrio (comma shaped)
         (4) Spirochete (corkscrew shaped)
      b. Classified by Gram staining
         (1) Gram-positive (violet on Gram stain)
         (2) Gram-negative (pink on Gram stain)
      c. Classified into two taxa:
         (1) Eubacteria: "true" bacteria; most important bacteria in medicine
         (2) Archeobacteria: primitive bacteria; can occupy and inhabit extreme environments
   3. Viruses; classification based on:
      a. Type and properties of nucleic acid
      b. Morphology of nucleoproteins
      c. Presence and properties of envelopes—the envelope is the protein coat that protects the capsid and nucleic acid of the virus
   4. Prion
      a. Type of protein found in brain neurons; contains no genetic material
      b. Not bacterial, viral, or fungal
      c. Improper folding and inability to be degraded allows for accumulation and damage to the nervous system
      d. Transmissible (spongiform encephalopathies)
         (1) Creutzfeldt-Jakob disease
         (2) Mad cow disease

(3) Kuru

(4) Scrapie (in sheep)

e. Highly resistant to traditional sterilization methods because of the extreme stability of prion proteins

E. Nomenclature—the binomial system

   1. Two-word designation

      a. Genus and species

      b. First word capitalized and both words italicized (e.g., *Escherichia coli*)

   2. Devised by Carolus Linnaeus

Methods of Measurement and Observation

A. Types

   1. Macroscopic: measurable and observable by the naked eye

   2. Microsocopic: too small to be measured or observed by the naked eye. Requires a microscope or lens to see

B. Most commonly used units of measurement

   1. Centimeter (cm = 10^{-2} m)

   2. Millimeter (mm = 10^{-3} m)

   3. Micrometer or micron (μm = 10^{-6} m)

   4. Nanometer (nm = 10^{-9} m)

   5. Angstrom unit (Å = 10^{-10} m)

C. Light microscopes illuminate objects by visible light

   1. Bright-field microscopy

      a. Used to observe the morphologies of microorganisms

      b. Used with stained smears

      c. Cannot be used to observe microorganisms <0.2 μm, such as viruses and spirochetes

      d. Compound microscopes have at least two lens systems

         (1) Objective

            (a) Magnifies the specimen and is close to it

            (b) Four powers—×4, ×10, ×40, and oil immersion (×100)

         (2) Ocular

            (a) Eyepiece

            (b) Magnifies the image produced by the objective lens

   2. Darkfield microscopy

      a. Specimens seen as bright objects against a dark background

      b. Used for the examination of unstained microorganisms and spirochetes and hanging-drop preparations

      c. Advantage—allows a view of living bacteria not visible by Gram stain; undisturbed in size or shape by fixing and staining techniques

3. Phase-contrast microscopy

   a. Useful in examining transparent, living cells, including their internal structure, and in determining motility in a fluid medium; can show dense structures

   b. Variations in density between the microbes and the surrounding medium are capitalized on to increase the contrast between the two

4. Fluorescence microscopy

   a. Used to visualize objects that fluoresce or emit light when exposed to light of different wavelengths

   b. Ultraviolet light, fluorescent chemicals, and special filter systems required

   c. Commonly used in the medical field to track antigen–antibody reactions and as a diagnostic technique (immunofluorescence)

5. Confocal-scanning laser microscopy

   a. A conventional light microscope uses a laser light source to illuminate planes of a fluorochrome-stained specimen

   b. Confocal images combine fluorescent and reflected images

   c. Successive planes are scanned until the entire specimen is scanned

   d. Useful in creating three-dimensional pictures of biofilms

6. Specimen preparation

   a. Viewing living organisms

      (1) Methods

         (a) Hanging drop

         (b) Temporary wet mount

      (2) Advantages

         (a) Maintains the shape of organisms

         (b) Is useful to determine organisms' size, shape, motility, and reactions to chemicals or immune sera

   b. Staining

      (1) Procedure

         (a) Thin films of microorganisms are spread on a glass slide and allowed to dry (smear)

         (b) Films are fixed, either by a chemical fixative or by passing through a flame; this denatures the proteins and kills the cell

         (c) Dyes or stains are applied to the smear to allow for greater visualization; allows for some differentiation of species

         (d) Fixation process tends to reduce the sizes of cells; dye addition tends to increase the sizes of cells

      (2) Types of dyes

         (a) Acidic, or negative, dye is used to stain basic components of the cell (e.g., glycoproteins, matrix)

TABLE 9-1 Comparison of Gram-Positive and Gram-Negative Bacteria

	Gram-Positive Bacteria	Gram-Negative Bacteria
Color after Gram's stain procedure	Blue to purple	Pink to red
Peptidoglycan layer in cell walls	Thick	Thin
Teichoic acid in cell walls	Present	Absent
Lipopolysaccharide in cell walls	Absent	Present

(b) Basic, or positive, dye is used to stain acidic components of the cell (e.g., nucleic acid and polysaccharides)

(3) Simple staining procedures
  (a) Use a single dye (e.g., carbolfuchsin, crystal violet, methylene blue, or safranin)
  (b) Are used to show shapes, sizes, and arrangements of bacterial cells

(4) Differential staining procedures (Table 9-1)
  (a) More than one dye preparation used
  (b) Used for initial bacterial grouping
  (c) Most common methods
    [1] Gram stain—differentiates microorganisms based on color as gram positive (blue to purple) or gram negative (pink to red); certain characteristics of microorganisms appear correlated with their staining reactions: cell wall thickness, chemical composition, and sensitivity to penicillin; useful in the diagnosis of infectious diseases
    [2] Acid-fast stain—differentiates between acid-fast and non–acid-fast bacteria; differentiates mycobacteria (e.g., *Mycobacterium leprae* and *Mycobacterium tuberculosis*) from other bacteria by indicating the presence or absence of special lipids in the cell wall; organisms resist decolorization with an acidic solution of alcohol after being stained with a basic dye

(5) Special staining procedures—used to color and isolate specific parts of microorganisms
    (a) Negative staining for capsules—determines if organism is encapsulated
    (b) Schaeffer-Fulton spore stain (e.g., *Bacillus, Clostridium*)—determines if organism is a spore former
    (c) Flagellar staining—determines if organism has flagella
    (d) Toluidine blue-O staining—determines prions, proteoglycans, and glycosaminoglycans in tissues

D. Electron microscopy
  1. Electrons used as a source of illumination
  2. Higher magnification and better resolving power available than with a light microscope, but because specimens must be dead, dynamic processes cannot be examined
  3. Types
    a. Transmission electron microscope—used to visualize the ultrastructures of cells and viruses
    b. Scanning electron microscope—used to visualize three-dimensional images of surface features of cells and viruses

Prokaryotic (Bacterial) Cell Structure and Function

A. Bacterial morphology
  1. Cocci (*singular*, coccus)
    a. Spherical or ovoid shape
    b. Occur in pairs (diplococci), chains (streptococci), four-in-a-square arrangement (tetrad), eight cells in a cubic arrangement (sarcinae), and irregular clusters (staphylococci)
  2. Bacilli (*singular*, bacillus)
    a. Cylindrical or rod-like
    b. Occur in pairs (diplobacilli); chains (streptobacilli); small, rounded rods (coccobacilli); and with tapered ends (fusiform bacilli)
  3. Spirilla (*singular*, spirillum)
    a. Spiral or curved
    b. Vary in number and fullness of turns
    c. Vibrios are portions of a spiral
  4. Palisade arrangement (bacterial cells form weird angles to one another)
    a. Fence post appearance
    b. *Cornynebacterium diphtheriae*
  5. Pleomorphic (no defined cell shape)
    a. Variable in shape
    b. *Mycoplasma pneumoniae*

B. External cell structures
  1. Appendages
    a. Provide motility
      (1) Flagella (*singular*, flagellum)
        (a) Threads of protein that extend from the cell surface and move in a whip-like motion

(b) Vectored motility must be distinguished from brownian movement, which is caused by bacteria randomly hitting molecules in the surrounding medium; flagella enable bacteria to move toward favorable environments and away from adverse ones (chemotaxis)

(2) Axial filaments

b. Allow for movement—spirochetes (e.g., *Treponema pallidum*, *Borrelia burgdorferi*) move by this method

c. Provide attachments
  (1) Pili (singular, pilus)
    (a) —Hair-like structures often found on gram-negative bacteria; not associated with motility
    (b) Longer and fewer in number
    (c) Sex pili join bacterial cells in preparation for deoxyribonucleic acid (DNA) transfer (conjugation)
  (2) Fimbriae (singular, fimbria)
    (a) Shorter and numerous
    (b) Enable a cell to adhere to surfaces (e.g., *Neisseria gonorrhoeae*, *Escherichia coli*)

2. Surface coating (glycocalyx)
  a. Capsules
    (1) Condensed and well-defined masses of polysaccharides or polypeptides firmly attached to the cell wall
    (2) Encapsulation protects pathogenic organisms from drugs, phagocytosis, and bactericidal factors
    (3) Some bacteria need capsules to maintain virulence (e.g., *Streptococcus pneumoniae*, *Streptococcus mutans*)
  b. Slime layer (glycocalyx)
    (1) Unorganized, soluble mass of polysaccharides or polypeptides loosely attached to the cell wall; polymeric material (glycoprotein)
    (2) Protects microorganisms; aids in adherence and gliding motility of organism

3. Cell wall
  a. Functions
    (1) Determines and maintains the shape of the microorganism
    (2) Provides support for flagella
    (3) Prevents rupture of the cell resulting from osmotic pressure differences on either side of the cell wall
  b. Composed of the macromolecule peptidoglycan
  c. Comparison of gram-negative and gram-positive cell walls

    (1) Gram-positive cell walls consist of many layers of peptidoglycan and contain teichoic acids
    (2) Gram-negative bacteria have a lipoprotein–lipopolysaccharide–phospholipid outer membrane surrounding a thin peptidoglycan layer
    (3) Outer membrane protects gram-negative cells from phagocytosis, penicillin, lysozymes, and other chemicals
    (4) Gram-negative cell walls are more easily broken by mechanical forces; susceptible to lysis by antibody, complement, and streptomycin

4. Cytoplasmic (plasma) membrane
  a. Structure—consists of a phospholipid bi-layer interspersed with proteins in a mosaic pattern (fluid mosaic)
  b. Functions
    (1) Barrier that regulates movement of materials in and out of the cell
    (2) Active transport
    (3) Excretion of hydrolytic exoenzymes
    (4) Bears enzymes and carrier molecules
    (5) Bears receptors and other proteins of the chemotactic and other sensory transduction systems
  c. Lies adjacent to and beneath the cell wall and encloses the cytoplasm of the cell

5. Cell envelope
  a. Includes all external structures and appendages, including the capsule, pili, flagella, cell wall, and cytoplasmic membrane
  b. May play a role in protection from degradation, maintenance of cell shape, and cell adhesion
  c. Properties confer staining characteristics
  d. Organization and structure different in gram-positive and gram-negative bacteria

C. Internal cell structure
  1. Cytoplasm (protoplasm)
    a. Fluid compartment inside the cytoplasmic membrane
    b. Prominent site for many of the cell's biochemical and synthetic activities
    c. Contains chromatin body, ribosomes, and granules
  2. Mesosomes—irregular folds of the cytoplasmic membrane resulting from dehydration of cells in preparation for electron microscopy; considered artifacts
  3. Genetic material or genome (nucleoid)
    a. Prokaryotes lack the distinct nucleus of eukaryotes
    b. Single chromosome is composed of a single molecule of DNA, existing as a closed loop

not enclosed by the nuclear membrane; located in the nucleoplasm of the cell

c. Additional genetic material is found in plasmids, which are extrachromosomal DNA molecules; they often carry information that determines drug resistance or sensitivity

4. Ribosomes
   a. Function in protein synthesis
   b. Composed of ribosomal protein and ribosomal ribonucleic acid (RNA)
   c. Distributed throughout the cytoplasm
5. Photosynthetic apparatus
6. Inclusions
   a. Accumulations of reserve storage materials
   b. Include polysaccharide granules, metachromatic granules, sulfur granules, lipid inclusions, carboxysomes, and gas vacuoles

D. Endospores (spores)
   1. Dormant structures formed within gram-positive bacterial cells as a means of survival
   2. Formed during a process called *sporulation*: disintegration of parent cell releases endospore; then called *exposure* or *free spore*
   3. Can remain in a spore state for years; exhibit unusual resistance to heat, drying, chemical disinfection, and radiation
   4. Can transform back into a vegetative cell through a process called *germination*
   5. Ability of bacteria to produce endospores restricted mainly to the genera *Bacillus* and *Clostridium*

Eukaryotic Cell Structure and Function

See Tables 9-2 and 9-3.

A. More complex than a prokaryotic cell; has a distinct nucleus bounded by a nuclear membrane, a nucleolus, and membrane-bound organelles

B. Animal cells
   1. Cell membrane

TABLE 9-2 Eukaryotic Organelles and Their Functions

Cell Part or Organelle	Associated Functions and Activities
Cell membrane	Transport of substances into and out of cells (selective permeability)
	In some cells, engulfment of foreign material (phagocytosis)
	Pinocytosis
Cell wall	Found only in plants and certain bacteria; imparts shape and strength to the cell
	Protection against certain osmotic imbalances
Centrioles	Involved in cell division
Chloroplast	Photosynthesis
Cilium	Motion, or movement of substances, past the ciliated cell
Endoplasmic reticulum	Protein synthesis
	Transport of nutrients to the nucleus
Flagellum and cilium	Propulsion
Golgi complex	Transfer of proteins and other cellular components to exterior of a secretory cell
	Storage and packing structure for cellular products
Lysosomes	Contain lysozymes and other digestive enzymes
	Break down foreign material and worn out cell parts
Microbody, or peroxisome	Enzymatic activities
Microtubule	Cell transport
	Development and maintenance of cell shape
	Cell division
	Ciliary and flagellar movement
Mitochondrion	Synthesis of the energy-rich compound adenosine triphosphate (ATP)
Nucleolus	Major site for the formation of ribosomal components

Continued

TABLE 9-2 Eukaryotic Organelles and Their Functions—cont'd

Cell Part or Organelle	Associated Functions and Activities
Nucleus	Control of cellular physiologic process
	Contains chromosomes
	Transfer of hereditary factors to subsequent generations
Plastids	Contain photosynthetic pigments
	Sites of photosynthesis
	Found in plant cells
Ribosome	Protein synthesis
	Attach to outer surface of rough endoplasmic reticulum
Vacuoles	Locations of water
	Storage site for certain amino acids, carbohydrates, and proteins
	Dumping ground for cellular wastes

TABLE 9-3 Major Characteristics of Eukaryotes and Prokaryotes

	EUKARYOTES		PROKARYOTES
Characteristic	Plants	Animals	
Major Groups	Plants, algae, fungi	Animals, protozoa	Bacteria
Size (approximate)	>5 μm	>5 μm	1–3 μm
Nuclear Structures			
Nucleus	Classic membrane	Classic membrane	No nuclear membrane
Chromosomes	Strands of deoxyribonucleic acid (DNA) and protein	Strands of DNA and protein	Single, closed strand of DNA
Cytoplasmic Structures			
Mitochondria	Present	Present	Absent
Golgi complex	Present	Present	Absent
Endoplasmic reticulum	Present	Present	Absent
Ribosomes (sedimentation coefficient)	80S	80S	70S
Cytoplasmic membrane	Contains sterols	Contains sterols	Does not contain sterols
Cell wall	Composed of cellulose or chitin	Absent	Complex structure containing protein, lipids, and peptidoglycans
Reproduction Movement	Sexual or asexual	Sexual or asexual	Asexual (binary fission)
	Flagella or cilia (complex and similar to centrioles)	Flagella or cilia (complex and similar to centrioles)	Flagella, if present, are simple twisted proteins (no cilia)
Respiration	Via mitochondria	Via mitochondria	Via cytoplasmic membrane
Photosynthesis	Present (absent in fungi)	Absent	Present in cyanobacteria and some others

a. Surrounds the cell and interconnects with the cell's internal membrane systems
b. Functions
   (1) Regulates the passage of substances in and out of the cell through active and passive transport

   (2) Involved in phagocytosis, tumor formation, drug sensitivity, and immune response
2. Nucleus
a. Controls the cell's physiologic and reproductive processes

b. Composition
  (1) Nuclear membrane
  (2) Nucleoli (involved in RNA synthesis)
  (3) Chromosomes (composed of DNA)
  (4) Nucleoprotein (chromatin)
3. Internal structures
  a. Mitochondria are sites of adenosine triphosphate (ATP), or energy, production
  b. Endoplasmic reticulum
    (1) Network of membranes involved in chemical reactions, storage, and transportation
    (2) Rough endoplasmic reticulum has ribosomes attached
  c. Golgi complex-storage and packaging structure for cellular components
  d. Lysosomes—contain digestive enzymes
  e. Microtubules
  f. Vacuoles

Microbial Growth and Cultivation

A. Definitions
  1. Culture media—nutrient preparations used to cultivate microorganisms
  2. In vitro techniques—procedures using nonliving materials in a culture vessel
  3. In vivo techniques—procedures using living cells or entire animals or plants
  4. Colony—accumulation of bacteria on a medium
B. Conditions that affect growth
  1. Physical
    a. Thermal conditions
      (1) Most bacteria grow best over a range of temperatures
        (a) Psychrophiles—$0°C$ to $15°C$
        (b) Mesophiles—$20°C$ to $40°C$
        (c) Thermophiles—$45°C$ to $60°C$
      (2) Minimal, maximal, and optimal requirements are the organisms' cardinal temperatures
      (3) $30°C$ is the optimal temperature for many free-living organisms
    b. Acidity or alkalinity (pH)—most bacteria prefer a neutral pH, between 7.0 and 7.4
      (1) Acidophiles—pH 0 to 4
      (2) Neutrophiles—pH 5 to 9
      (3) Alkalinophiles—pH >9
    c. Osmotic pressure
      (1) Most microorganisms must be grown in an aquatic medium
      (2) Halophilic organisms require high salt concentration
      (3) Osmophilic organisms require high osmotic pressure

2. Chemical
  a. Gaseous requirements
    (1) Aerobes require oxygen
    (2) Micro-aerophilic organisms require low concentrations of oxygen
    (3) Anaerobes do not require oxygen
    (4) Obligate (strict) anaerobes cannot tolerate any free oxygen
    (5) Facultative anaerobes can metabolize aerobically if oxygen is present or anaerobically if it is absent
    (6) Aero-tolerant anaerobes metabolize substances anaerobically but are not harmed by oxygen
  b. Nutrition available
    (1) Heterotrophic organisms
      (a) Require organic compounds for growth; obtain carbon from glucose
      (b) Most commonly cultured on a medium of glucose
    (2) Autotrophic organisms
      (a) Do not require organic nutrients for growth
      (b) Use inorganic compounds such as carbon dioxide
      (c) Thrive in soils and bodies of water
    (3) Hypotrophic organisms
      (a) Obligate intracellular parasites; grow only within a living host cell
      (b) Include viruses and rickettsiae
    (4) Phototrophic organisms
      (a) Use light for energy
    (5) Chemotrophic organisms
      (a) Oxidize chemical compounds for energy
    (6) Nutrients needed include sulfur and phosphorus
    (7) Nitrogen is derived from proteins and their products
    (8) Certain vitamins and growth factors required
C. Types of culture media
  1. Synthetic defined media—exact chemical composition is known
  2. Rich complex media—exact chemical composition varies slightly from batch to batch (e.g., addition of blood or beef extract); contain digested extracts from animal organs, meats, fish, yeasts, and plants
  3. Differential media
    a. Contain combinations of nutrients and pH indicators to produce visual differentiation between several microorganisms
    b. Examples
      (1) Blood agar is an enriched medium that allows streptococci to leave different signs

on the medium; green discoloration around colonies indicates α-hemolytic streptococci, clear zone signifies β-hemolysis, and no effect denotes γ-hemolysis

    (2) Chocolate agar is even more enriched than blood agar

4. Selective media

  a. Allow interference with or prevention of the growth of certain microorganisms while permitting others to grow

  b. Dyes and antibiotics make the media selective

  c. Examples

    (1) Sabouraud dextrose agar is selective for fungi

    (2) Thayer-Martin agar is selective for *N. gonorrhoeae*

5. Selective and differential media

  a. Combine properties of the preceding two types of media

  b. Examples—mannitol, salt agar, and MacConkey agar

6. Enriched media—similar to selective media but designed to increase the numbers of particular microbes to detectable levels

7. Reducing media

  a. Contain ingredients that chemically combine with and deplete oxygen in the culture medium

  b. Used for anaerobes

D. Pure culture techniques

1. Used to isolate and identify a bacterial species

2. Methods

  a. Pour-plate technique

    (1) Cool the melted agar-containing medium

    (2) Inoculate the medium

      (a) Use the loop or needle to transfer the organism

      (b) Pass the loop through the flame and heat to redness

      (c) Flame the edges of tubes from which cultures are taken before and after removal of the organism

    (3) Pour the inoculated medium into a sterile Petri dish

    (4) Allow the medium to solidify

    (5) Incubate at the desired temperature

  b. Streak-plate technique

    (1) Spread a loopful of material containing organisms over the surface of the solidified agar

    (2) Various streaking directions or patterns are possible

E. Bacterial growth

1. Most bacteria reproduce via binary fission (i.e., two new cells are produced by one parent cell)

2. Growth on the culture medium

  a. Typical growth curve results

  b. Phases

    (1) Lag phase—period of intense metabolic activity but no increase in cell number

    (2) Log phase or exponential growth phase—cell number increases in an exponential manner; generation time is the average time for the cell to divide; phase when cells are most metabolically active

    (3) Stationary phase—total number of viable cells is constant; metabolic activity slows

    (4) Phase of decline (death phase)—number of viable cells decreases

3. Measurement of growth

  a. Population growth curve—made by observing an increase in mass or numbers over time

  b. Cell mass can be measured by dry weight, chemical analysis, and turbidity

  c. Population counts—cell numbers can be measured by viable platlet counts; estimates are expressed as colony-forming units (CFU) for bacteria or plaque-forming units (PFU) for viruses

Microbial Metabolism and Cell Regulation

A. Metabolism

1. Definition—set of chemical reactions by which cells maintain life

2. Phases

  a. Anabolism—biosynthetic reactions that use energy (ATP);

    (1) Energy-consuming phase in which macromolecules such as nucleic acids, proteins, lipids, and polysaccharides are synthesized

  b. Catabolism—degradative reactions that release energy (ATP)

    (1) energy-releasing phase in which complex compounds are broken down, creating energy in the form of ATP

3. Energy storage and transfer

  a. Chemical energy is stored as ATP

  b. May be generated through the transport of electrons (electron transport system)

  c. Energy produced through oxidation–reduction reactions

    (1) Aerobic oxidation (respiration)

    (2) Anaerobic oxidation (fermentation)

4. Metabolic pathways
   a. Series of steps to complete biochemical process
   b. Glycolytic pathway (glycolysis)
      (1) Most important way carbohydrates are metabolized
      (2) Converts glucose to pyruvic acid
      (3) Anaerobic fermentation process
      (4) Tricarboxylic acid (Krebs) cycle
   c. Occurs inside mitochondria
      (1) Follows the glycolytic pathway
      (2) Responsible for further oxidation of glucose and the production of other biochemically important intermediates
      (3) Important to aerobic bacteria
5. Protein synthesis
   a. DNA directs the formation of proteins aided by various types of RNA
   b. Transcription—synthesis of messenger RNA (mRNA) from a DNA template
   c. Translation—synthesis of protein from an mRNA template
   d. Three stages of protein synthesis occurring at the ribosome:
      (1) Initiation
      (2) Elongation
      (3) Termination
B. Metabolic control
   1. Largely by enzymatic control
   2. Types of regulation
      a. Feedback inhibition
         (1) Allosteric enzymes—end product binds to the enzyme and lowers its affinity for its substrate, thus preventing further product formation
         (2) When more end product is needed, the enzyme is released
      b. Genetic regulation—regulated by a specific unit of DNA called an *operon*
         (1) Enzyme repression—when the level of end product is sufficient, the genetic synthesis of the enzyme is suppressed
         (2) Enzyme induction—enzymes are genetically synthesized only when substrates are present

Microbial Genetics

A. Eukaryotic genome
   1. Almost all of the eukaryotic genome is diploid
   2. Gene expression can be recessive or dominant
   3. Mitochondria and chloroplasts have a single circular DNA; function of DNA is related to that organelle

B. Prokaryotic genome
   1. Most prokaryotes have a single circular chromosome
   2. Additional genes are present on plasmids (small circles of DNA)
C. Some viruses (phage) multiply in bacteria
D. Genetic recombination (see the section on "Genetics" in Chapter 7)
   1. Conjugation
      a. Transfer of genetic material between two living bacteria that are in physical contact
      b. Plasmids are most frequently transferred
   2. Transduction—a bacterial virus (bacteriophage) transfers genetic material
   3. Transformation—the direct uptake of donor DNA by a recipient cell
E. Genetic rearrangement—transposons are small segments of DNA that can move from one region of a chromosome to another region of the genome
F. Mutations
   1. Result in changes in DNA sequence
   2. Can be caused by agents such as ultraviolet light, radiation, nitrous acid, and carcinogens

Microbial Relationships

A. Syntrophism
   1. Organisms are not intimately associated with each other but benefit from each other
   2. Examples—yogurt production, organisms feeding in soil where decaying plant material is found
B. Competition
   1. Interaction between organisms resulting from a demand for a finite supply of nutrients and other resources
   2. Example—molds such as *Penicillium* compete by secreting substances toxic to other organisms
C. Predation—interaction that controls the population by predators feeding on another species; the prey
D. Symbiosis—interaction in which two different species live in a mutually beneficial coexistence
E. Commensalism—interaction in which only one organism benefits and the other neither benefits nor is harmed
F. Parasitism—interaction in which one organism benefits at the expense of the other

Bacteria

See Table 9-4.
A. Firmicutes—gram-positive eubacteria
B. Gracilicutes
   1. Gram-negative eubacteria
   2. Largest group of bacteria

TABLE 9-4 Major Categories and Groups of Bacteria That Cause Disease in Humans*

Category	Bacteria
I. Gram-Negative Eubacteria That Have Cell Walls Group 1: The spirochetes	*Treponema* *Borrelia* *Leptospira*
Group 2: Aerobic or micro-aerophilic, motile, helical, or vibroid gram-negative bacteria	*Campylobacter* *Helicobacter* *Spirillum*
Group 3: Nonmotile (or rarely motile), curved bacteria	None
Group 4: Gram-negative, aerobic, or micro-aerophilic rods and cocci	*Alcaligenes* *Bordetella* *Brucella* *Francisella* *Legionella* *Moraxella* *Neisseria* *Pseudomonas* *Rochalimaea* *Bacteroides* (some species)
Group 5: Facultatively anaerobic gram-negative rods	*Escherichia* (and related coliform bacteria) *Klebsiella* *Proteus* *Providencia* *Salmonella* *Shigella* *Yersinia* *Vibrio* *Haemophilus* *Pasteurella*
Group 6: Gram-negative, anaerobic, straight, curved, and helical rods	*Bacteroides* *Fusobacterium* *Prevotella* *Tannerella*
Group 7: Dissimilatory sulfate-reducing or sulfur-reducing bacteria	None
Group 8: Anaerobic gram-negative cocci	None
Group 9: Rickettsiae and chlamydiae	*Rickettsia* *Coxiella* *Chlamydia*
Group 10: Anoxygenic phototrophic bacteria	None
Group 11: Oxygenic phototrophic bacteria	None
Group 12: Aerobic chemolithotrophic bacteria and assorted organisms	None
Group 13: Budding or appendaged bacteria	None
Group 14: Sheathed bacteria	None
Group 15: Nonphotosynthetic, nonfruiting gliding bacteria	*Capnocytophaga*
Group 16: Fruiting gliding bacteria: the myxobacteria	None
II. Gram-Positive Bacteria That Have Cell Walls Group 17: Gram-positive cocci	*Enterococcus* *Peptostreptococcus* *Staphylococcus* *Streptococcus*
Group 18: Endospore-forming gram-positive rods and cocci	*Bacillus* *Clostridium*

TABLE 9-4 Major Categories and Groups of Bacteria That Cause Disease in Humans—cont'd

Category	Bacteria
Group 19: Regular, nonsporing gram-positive rods	*Erysipelothrix* *Listeria*
Group 20: Irregular, nonsporing gram-positive rods	*Actinomyces* *Corynebacterium* *Mobiluncus*
Group 21: Mycobacteria	*Mycobacterium*
Groups 22–29: Actinomycetes	*Nocardia* *Streptomyces* *Rhodococcus*
III. Eubacteria That Do Not Have Cell Walls: Mycoplasmas or Mollicutes Group 30: Mycoplasmas	*Mycoplasma* *Ureaplasma*
IV. Archaeobacteria Group 31: Methanogens	None
Group 32: Archaeal sulfate reducers	None
Group 33: Extremely halophilic archaeobacteria	None
Group 34: Archaeobacteria without cell walls	None
Group 35: Extremely thermophilic and hyperthermophilic sulfur metabolizers	None

Used as an identification scheme in Bergey's Manual of Determinative Bacteriology, *ed 9.*
From Holt JG, Krieg NR, Sneath PHA, et al: Bergey's manual of determinative bacteriology, *ed 9, Baltimore, Williams & Wilkins, 1998; and Sakamoto M, Suzuki M, Umeda M, et al: Reclassification of* Bacteroids forsythus (Tanner et al. 1986) *as* Tannerella forsythensis *corrig., gen., nov., comb., nov,* Int J Syst Evol Microbiol *52:841–849, 2002.*

3. Contain many medically significant microorganisms

C. Tenericutes (mycoplasmas)
   1. Eubacteria lacking cell walls—because they lack cell walls, they are highly pleomorphic
   2. Enclosed by the plasma membrane—plasma membranes have lipids called *sterols* that aid in resisting lysis
   3. Mycoplasmas are the smallest self-replicating microorganisms

D. Mendosicutes (archaeobacteria)
   1. Conventional peptidoglycan in the cell wall is replaced with pseudomurein
   2. Often live in extreme environments
   3. Carry out atypical metabolic processes
   4. No known medically significant species

Fungi

A. Description
   1. Eukaryotic
   2. Nonphotosynthetic
   3. Heterotrophic saprophytes—use preexisting organic products, either living or dead
   4. Grow well in dark, moist environments
   5. Few species are pathogenic to humans

B. Forms
   1. Molds (mycelial forms)
      a. Long filaments are structural units called *hyphae;* multicellular hyphae result in a cobweb-like growth called a *mycelium*
      b. Reproduce by sexual or asexual spores
   2. Yeasts
      a. Oval or spherical single cells
      b. Produce moist, shiny colonies
      c. Reproduce asexually by producing new buds or daughter cells
   3. Dimorphic fungi—some fungi exhibit characteristics of both molds and yeasts, depending on growth conditions

C. Classification of medically important fungi
   1. Zygomycota (the phycomyces)—include the common bread molds *Rhizopus* and *Mucor*
   2. Ascomycota (sac fungi)—include *Histoplasma, Microsporum, Aspergillus, Trichophyton, Penicillium* (a source of antibiotics), and *Saccharomyces* (leavened bread and fermented beer and wine)
   3. Basidiomycota—include *Cryptococcus neoformans*
   4. Deuteromycota (the imperfect fungi)—include *Candida, Pneumocystis, Coccidioides, Sporothrix,* and *Epidermophyton;* do not produce sexual spores

D. Fungal diseases (mycoses)
1. Generally long-lasting infections
2. Classification
   a. Systemic—involving a number of tissues and organs
   b. Subcutaneous—beneath the skin
   c. Cutaneous (superficial)—involving only the epidermis, hair, and nails
      (1) Tinea infections caused by *Microsporum*, *Trichophyton*, and *Epidermophyton*
   d. Opportunistic—generally harmless; can become pathogenic in a debilitated host

Protozoa

A. Description
1. Unicellular
2. Eukaryotic
3. Heterotrophic

4. Most have a motile feeding stage called *trophozoite*
5. Many can form cysts
   a. Protective resting stage
   b. Can serve as a site for division or spreading of pathogenic protozoans (e.g., *Entamoeba histolytica*, which causes amoebic dysentery)
6. Reproduce asexually by fission, budding, or schizogony (multiple fission); reproduce sexually by conjugation

B. Four phyla (Table 9-5)

Helminths (Worms) as Human Parasites

A. Nematodes (roundworms)
1. Hookworm infection (*Necator americanus, Ancylostoma duodenale*)
   a. Adult worm lives in the small intestine

TABLE 9-5 Some Representative Parasitic Protozoa

Phylum and Subphylum	Human Pathogens	Distinguishing Features	Disease	Source of Human Infections
Sarcomastigophora Sarcodina (amoebas)	*Acanthamoeba*	Pseudopods	Keratitis	Water
	Entamoeba histolytica	Pseudopods	Amoebic dysentery	Fecal contamination of drinking water
	Naegleria fowleri	Some flagellated forms	Meningoencephalitis	Water in which people swim
Mastigophora (flagellates)	*Giardia lamblia*	Two nuclei, eight flagella	Giardial enteritis	Fecal contamination of drinking water
	Trichomonas vaginalis	No encysting stage	Urethritis; vaginitis	Contact with vaginal–urethral discharge
	Trypanosoma cruzi	Undulating membrane	Chagas' disease	Bite of *Triatoma* (kissing bug)
	T. brucei gambiense, *T.b. rhodesiense*		African trypanosomiasis	Bite of tsetse fly
Ciliophora	*Balantidium coli*	Only parasitic ciliate of humans	Balantidial dysentery	Fecal contamination of drinking water
Apicomplexa	*Babesia microti* *Cryptosporidium*	Complex life cycles may require more than one host	Babesiosis Diarrhea	Domestic animals, ticks humans, other animals, water
	Cyclospora	—	Diarrhea	Water
	Isospora	—	Coccidiosis	Domestic animals
	Plasmodium	—	Malaria	Bite of *Anopheles* mosquito
	Toxoplasma gondii	—	Toxoplasmosis	Cats, other animals; congenital
Microspora	*Nosema*	Unknown	Diarrhea, keratoconjunctivitis, conjunctivitis	Other animals

From Tortora GJ, Funke BR, Case CL: Microbiology: An introduction, *ed 8, Menlo Park, CA, 2003, Benjamin/Cummings.*

b. Transmitted through contaminated soil, skin, or contaminated water

c. Symptoms include iron-deficiency anemia, abdominal pain, and protein deficiency; mild infections are asymptomatic

2. Pinworm (*Enterobius vermicularis*)
   a. Adult worm lives in the large intestine
   b. More common in children
   c. Tickling or intense itching in the perianal area
   d. Transmission
      (1) Ingestion of larvae
      (2) Handling of fomites (infected bedding and clothes)
      (3) Contaminated hands
      (4) Inhalation of eggs

3. Trichinosis (*Trichinella spiralis*)
   a. Adult worm lives in the muscles
   b. Transmitted by eating improperly cooked or inadequately processed pork
   c. Symptoms include diarrhea, muscular pain, and nervous disorders; many light infections are asymptomatic

B. Platyhelminthes (flatworms)
1. Tapeworms (cestodes)—*Taenia saginata, Taenia solium, Echinococcus granulosus*
   a. Adult worm lives in the small intestine, lung, liver, or brain
   b. Transmitted by eating contaminated or inadequately cooked beef, pork, lamb, or fish
   c. Symptoms include nausea and abdominal discomfort; many cases are asymptomatic or have poorly defined symptoms

2. Flukes (trematodes)—*Paragonimus westermani, Schistosoma* spp.
   a. Adult worms can live in the liver, lungs, bladder, or large intestine, causing various diseases
   b. Transmitted by eating inadequately cooked or contaminated fish, vegetation, or crayfish; also by swimming or working in contaminated water

Viruses

A. Properties of a mature virus particle or virion
1. Has a single type of nucleic acid, RNA or DNA, that contains genetic material, or a genome
2. Nucleic acid is surrounded by an outer protein coat, the capsid; nucleic acid and capsid compose the nucleocapsid
3. Capsids may or may not be covered by an envelope
4. Viral nucleic acid contains the necessary information for programming an infected host cell
5. Absence of cellular structures

6. Lack components for energy production and protein synthesis
7. Obligate intracellular parasites

B. Bacteriophages (bacterial viruses)
1. Contain either RNA or DNA
2. Life cycles: lytic and lysogenic
   a. Lytic cycle: virus enters a host cell, takes over cell replication mechanism, makes viral DNA and protein, then lyses (breaks open) the cell. This allows newly produced viruses to leave host cell and infect other cells. (destroys host cell.)
   b. Lysogenic cycle: virus attaches to host cell's DNA and replicates when host cell divides. Once integrated, the virus is referred to as a prophage, and a stable association is established between the host cell and the virus (no harm done to host cell.)

C. Plant viruses (most contain RNA)—viroids
1. Small, single-stranded, circular RNA molecules
2. Found mainly in plants

D. Human viruses (Table 9-6)
1. Classified by structure and type of nucleic acid, mode of replication, and morphology
2. Destructive effects on cells are termed *cytopathic*
3. Prions
   a. Proteinaceous infectious particles believed to cause kuru and Creutzfeldt-Jakob disease (CJD)
   b. Organization, replication, and how they cause disease are unknown

E. Viral replication
1. Uses biosynthetic mechanisms of the host cell
2. Phases
   a. Attachment, penetration, and uncoating
   b. Synthesis of viral components
   c. Morphogenesis and release

F. Modes of viral transmission
1. Direct transmission from person to person
2. Transmission from animal to animal
3. Transmission by an arthropod vector

G. Role of virus in cancer
1. Oncogenous viruses can induce various types of cancers (RNA-type or DNA-type viruses)
2. Proto-oncogenes are highly conserved, "friendly" transforming genes
3. Mechanisms of oncogene activation
   a. Transduction by a virus
   b. Insertional mutagenesis
   c. Translocation
   d. Gene amplification
   e. Mutation
4. Role oncogenes play in the development of cancer is unclear

TABLE 9-6 Selected Important Groups of Viruses and Viral Diseases

Virus Type	Viral Characteristics	Virus	Disease
Poxviruses	Large brick shape with envelope, double-stranded segment of deoxyribonucleic acid (DNA)	Variola	Smallpox
		Vaccinia	Cowpox
Polyoma-papilloma	Polyhedral, d.s. DNA	Papillomavirus	Warts
		Polyomavirus	Some tumors, some cancers
Herpesvirus	Polyhedral with envelope, d.s. DNA	Herpes simplex I	Cold sores or fever blisters
		Herpes simplex II	Genital herpes
		Herpes zoster	Shingles
		Varicella	Chickenpox
Adenovirus	Icosahedral, with envelope, d.s. DNA		Respiratory infections, pneumonia, conjunctivitis, some tumors
Picornaviruses ("means small ribonucleic acid [RNA] viruses")	Tiny icosahedral, with envelope, single-stranded (s.s.) RNA	Rhinovirus	Colds
		Poliovirus	Poliomyelitis
		Hepatitis types A and B	Hepatitis
		Coxsackievirus	Respiratory infections, meningitis
Reoviruses	Icosahedral, with envelope, d.s. RNA	Enterovirus	Intestinal infections
Myxoviruses	Helical with envelope, RNA	Orthomyxoviruses types A and B	Influenza
		Myxovirus parotidis	Mumps
		Paramyxovirus	Measles (rubeola)
		Rhabdovirus	Rabies
Arbovirus	Cubic, arthropodborne RNA	Mosquitoborne type B	Yellow fever
		Mosquito-borne type A and B	Encephalitis (many types)
		Tickborne coronavirus	Colorado tick fever
Retrovirus	Helical with envelope, d.s. RNA	RNA tumor virus	Tumors
		Human T lymphotropic virus (HTLV)	Leukemia
		Human immunodeficiency virus (HIV)	Acquired Immunodeficiency syndrome (AIDS)

From Burton GRW, Engelkirk PG: Microbiology for the health sciences, ed 7, Philadelphia, 2004, Lippincott Williams & Wilkins.

MICROBIAL VIRULENCE AND DISEASE TRANSFER

A. Bacteria that produce disease or pathologic changes in humans (Table 9-7)
B. Definitions
   1. Pathogen—agent producing disease or pathologic changes

   2. Opportunist—commensal bacterium that invades the host under favorable conditions
   3. Virulence—the degree of pathogenicity; properties that determine pathogenicity of an organism include invasiveness (transmissibility), ability to multiply in the host, and toxin production
   4. Infection—invasion of the tissue by a pathogenic microorganism and multiplication of the organism

TABLE 9-7 Bacteria of Human Importance

Organism	Diseases	Other Features
Gram-Positive Cocci		
Staphylococcus aureus	Boils, carbuncles, septicemia, food poisoning, pneumonia	Common skin commensal; phage typing identifies virulent strains; enterotoxin causes food poisoning
Streptococcus pyogenes	Tonsillitis, scarlet fever, erysipelas, septicemia, strep throat, rheumatic fever	Also causes glomerulonephritis and rheumatic fever, with immunopathologic basis
Streptococcus viridans group (Streptococcus sanguis, etc.)	Infective endocarditis	Oral commensals settle on abnormal heart valves during bacteremia
Streptococcus mutans	Dental caries	Regular inhabitant of mouth; initiates plaque on tooth surface
Streptococcus pneumoniae	Pneumonia, otitis, meningitis	Normal upper respiratory tract commensal; can spread to infected or damaged lungs
Gram-Negative Cocci		
Neisseria gonorrhoeae	Gonorrhea	Obligate human parasite
Neisseria meningitidis	Meningitis, nasopharyngitis	Obligate human parasite; increased upper respiratory carriage in epidemics
Gram-Positive Bacilli		
Corynebacterium diphtheriae	Diphtheria	Natural host humans; noninvasive disease caused by toxin
Bacillus anthracis	Anthrax	Pathogen of herbivorous animals that ingest spores; occasional human infection
Clostridium spp.	Tetanus, gas gangrene, botulism	Widely distributed in soil and intestines
Gram-Negative Bacilli		
Escherichia coli	Urinary tract infections, infantile gastroenteritis	Normal intestinal inhabitant (humans and animals); many antigenic types
Salmonella spp.	Enteric fever, food poisoning, gastroenteritis	Salmonella typhi—natural host is humans; invasive; other Salmonella—1000 species, mainly animal pathogens
Shigella spp.	Bacillary dysentery (shigellosis)	Obligate parasites of humans; local invasion only
Proteus spp.	Urinary tract infection, gastroenteritis, wound infection	Common in soil, feces; occasionally pathogenic
Klebsiella spp.	Urinary tract and wound infection, otitis, meningitis, pneumonia	Present in vegetation, soil, sometimes feces; pathogenic when host resistance lowered
Pseudomonas aeruginosa	Urinary tract, respiratory and wound infection	Common human intestinal bacteria; resists many antibiotics
Haemophilus influenzae	Pneumonia, meningitis	Human commensal; invades damaged lung
Bordetella pertussis	Whooping cough	Specialized human respiratory parasite
Yersinia pestis	Plague	Fleaborne pathogen of rodents; transfer to humans as greatest infection in history
Brucella spp.	Undulant fever, brucellosis	Pathogens of goats, cattle, and pigs with secondary human infection
Acid-Fast Bacilli		
Mycobacterium tuberculosis	Tuberculosis	Chronic respiratory infection in humans; 10 to 15 million active cases in the world; enteric infection with bovine type via milk
Mycobacterium leprae	Leprosy (Hansen's disease)	Obligate parasite of humans; attacks skin, nasal mucosa, and nerves; 15 million people with leprosy in the world

Continued

TABLE 9-7 Bacteria of Human Importance—cont'd

Organism	Diseases	Other Features
Miscellaneous *Vibrio cholerae*	Cholera	Obligate parasite of humans; noninvasive intestinal infection
Treponema pallidum	Syphilis	Obligate human parasite; sexual transmission; related nonvenereal human bacteria
Actinomyces israelii	Actinomycosis	Normal inhabitant of the human mouth
Leptospira spp.	Leptospirosis (Weil's disease, etc.)	Mostly pathogens of animals; human infection from urine of rats, etc.
Legionella pneumophila	Legionnaire's disease	Respiratory pathogen of humans, often acquired from contaminated air conditioning units

a. Localized—organism remains in a particular area of the body
b. Generalized or systemic—microorganism invades the bloodstream and the lymphatic system
c. Acute—runs a rapid course; terminates abruptly (<6 months)
d. Chronic—slow onset; infection of long duration
e. Primary—original infection
f. Secondary—infection that follows a primary infection and is often caused by an opportunistic organism
g. Toxemia—presence of toxin in the blood
h. Subclinical—lacking recognizable symptoms
i. Focal—localized in one area and spreading elsewhere in the body from that point
j. Bacteremia—presence of bacteria in the bloodstream
k. Latent—causative agent remains inactive for a time but then becomes active to produce symptoms of the disease
l. Sequelae—long-term or permanent damage to diseased tissues or organs
m. Nosocomial—acquired during a hospital stay
n. Sign—objective changes that a health care provider can observe and measure
o. Symptom—subjective changes in body experienced by the patient or client

5. Infectious disease—interference with the normal functioning of the host; proof by Koch's postulates:
a. Microorganisms are present in every case of disease
b. Microorganisms grow in pure culture from the diseased host
c. Same disease is reproduced when pure culture is inoculated into a healthy host
d. Microorganism is recovered from the inoculated host

C. Transmission of disease
1. Reservoir of infection—contains potential sources of the disease-causing agent
   a. Human
      (1) Active cases of infectious disease
      (2) Carriers—persons (asymptomatic) harboring infectious agents potentially pathogenic for other members of the population
      (3) Endogenous infection—the causative organism is derived from the host's own microflora
   b. Animal—zoonosis; disease transmitted from animal to human
   c. Insects and arthropods—flies, mosquitoes, fleas, lice, ticks, and mites
   d. Nonliving—water, food, soil, and dust
2. Portals of exit are sources of infectious body fluids
   a. Gastrointestinal tract
   b. Genitourinary system
   c. Oral region
   d. Respiratory tract
   e. Blood and blood derivatives
   f. Skin lesions
   g. Conjunctiva
3. Routes of transmission
   a. Contact
      (1) Direct
      (2) Indirect—involves nonliving reservoir (fomite)
      (3) Droplet transmission (short distance)
   b. Vehicles
      (1) Waterborne transmission
      (2) Foodborne transmission
      (3) Airborne transmission
   c. Vectors—insects and arthropods

4. Basic path of an infectious disease
   a. Exposure to the pathogen
   b. Incubation period
   c. Prodromal period
   d. Appearance of the signs and symptoms of the disease
   e. Outcome of the disease (e.g., convalescence, disability, or death)

Microbial Virulence Factors

A. Capsules (*S. pneumoniae*)—resist the host's defenses by impairing phagocytosis
B. Enzyme production—includes coagulases, kinases, hyaluronidases, collagenases, mucinases, lecithinases, leukocidins, and hemolysins
C. Toxin production
   1. Exotoxins
      a. Soluble substances secreted by gram-positive bacteria
      b. Clinically significant exotoxins are associated with botulism, tetanus, diphtheria, gas gangrene, scarlet fever, staphylococcal food poisoning, toxic shock syndrome, and traveler's diarrhea
   2. Endotoxins
      a. Heat-stable lipopolysaccharides—toxic component associated with cell wall
      b. From gram-negative bacteria
      c. Pathologic effects
         (1) Fever
         (2) Interference with hemostatic mechanisms of blood
         (3) Activation of the complement system
         (4) Leukopenia
         (5) Hypotension and shock
         (6) Organ dysfunction
         (7) Activation of complement system
         (8) Death

Disease Barriers

See Table 9-8.
A. Normal or indigenous flora
   1. Most highly specialized bacteria; highly adapted to commensal life; cause minimal damage under normal conditions
   2. Includes beneficial microorganisms and pathogens
   3. When ecologic balance is disturbed, infection can occur (e.g., antibiotic therapy may result in *Candida albicans* infection)
B. Nonspecific immunity
   1. Physical and chemical barriers (see Table 9-8)
      a. Intact skin
      b. Mucous membranes and their secretions
      c. Gastric acid barrier

TABLE 9-8 Constitutive Defenses: Barriers to Infection

PHYSICAL		
System or Organ	Cell Type	Clearing Mechanism
Skin	Squamous	Desquamation
Mucous membranes	Columnar nonciliated (e.g., gastrointestinal tract)	Peristalsis
	Columnar ciliated (trachea)	Mucociliary movement
	Cuboidal ciliated (e.g., nasopharynx)	Tears, saliva, mucus, sweat
	Secretory (various)	Antimicrobial compounds, flow of liquids

CHEMICAL		
	Source	Substance
Skin	Sweat, sebaceous glands	Organic acids from skin bacteria
Mucous membranes	Parietal cells of stomach	Hydrochloric acid, low pH
	Secretions	Antimicrobial compounds
	Neutrophils	Lysozyme, peroxidase, lactoferrin
Lung	A cells	Pulmonary surfactant
Upper alimentary tract	Salivary glands	Thiocyanate
	Neutrophils	Myeloperoxidase
		Cationic proteins
		Lactoferrin
		Lysozymes
Small bowel and below	Liver via biliary tree	Bile acids
	Gut flora	Low-molecular-weight fatty acids

From Schaechter M, Engleberg NC, Einstein BI, Medoff G: Mechanisms of microbial disease, ed 3, Baltimore, 1998, Williams & Wilkins.

   2. Blood and lymphatics
      a. Leukocytes—proportionate number changes in response to infection
         (1) Granulocytes (basophils, eosinophils, and neutrophils [polymorphonuclear leukocytes])
         (2) Agranulocytes (lymphocytes and monocytes)

b. Lymphatic system transports white blood cells and removes foreign cells and tissue debris
   (1) Consists of lymphatic vessels, lymph fluid, nodes, and lymphocytes
   (2) Mononuclear phagocyte system—mononuclear phagocytic cells that remove particulate matter from bloodstream and lymph (e.g., Kupffer cells in the liver)
3. Phagocytosis
   a. Digestion of the invading matter
   b. Accomplished by neutrophils and mature monocytes, or macrophages
4. Inflammation
   a. Produced by disease agents or irritants such as chemicals, heat, or mechanical injury
   b. Cardinal signs include heat, pain, redness, swelling, and loss of function
   c. Pus formation possible
5. Fever
   a. Bacterial endotoxins and interleukin 1 (IL-1) can induce fever

b. Intensifies the effect of interferon (IFN)
c. Inhibits the growth of some microorganisms
6. Antimicrobial substances
   a. Complement system—a defense system consisting of serum proteins that participate in lysis of foreign cells, inflammation, and phagocytosis
   b. Interferons (IFNα, β, and γ)—interfere with viral replication
C. Specific immunity—the immune system (Figure 9-1 and Box 9-1)
   1. Humoral immunity—β-lymphocyte production and release of specific antibodies into the circulating blood or body fluids; antibodies then interact with foreign antigens; defends primarily against bacteria, toxins, and viruses; antibodies protect the host as follows:
      a. Recognize an organism or its toxin by binding to it
      b. Opsonize or coat bacteria, which enhances ingestion by macrophages or natural killer (NK) cells

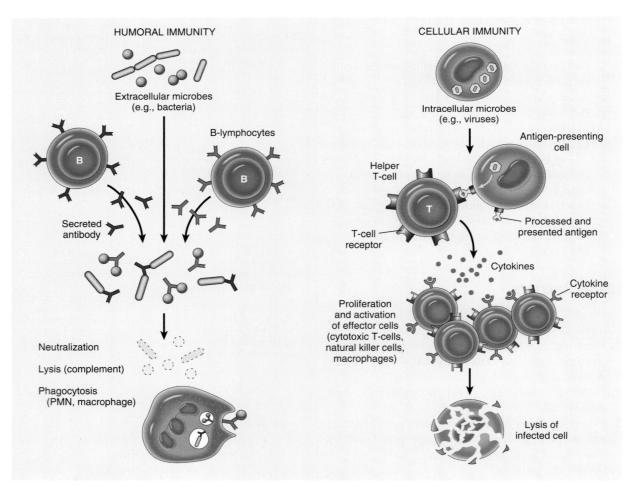

FIGURE 9-1 The duality of the immune system. *Left,* humoral immunity mediated by soluble antibody proteins produced by B lymphocytes. *Right,* cellular immunity mediated by T-lymphocytes. *(Modified from Kumar V, Cotran R, Robbins S:* Basic Pathology, *ed 7, Philadelphia, 2005, Saunders.)*

BOX 9-1 Immunology Terms

Anaphylatoxin: a substance produced by complement activation (especially C3a, C5a) that results in increased vascular permeability through release of pharmacologically active mediators from mast cells

Antibody (Ab): a protein that is produced as a result of the introduction of an antigen and has the ability to combine with the antigen that stimulated its production

Antigen (Ag): a substance that can induce a detectable immune response when introduced into an animal

B cell (also B lymphocyte): strictly, a bursa-derived cell in avian species and, by analogy, a cell derived from the equivalent of the bursa in non-avian species; B-cells are the precursors of plasma cells that produce antibody

Chemotaxis: a process whereby phagocytic cells are attracted to the vicinity of invading pathogens

Complement: a system of serum proteins that is the primary mediator of antigen–antibody reactions

Cytokine: a factor such as a lymphokine or monokine produced by cells that affect other cells (e.g., lymphocytes and macrophages) and have multiple immunomodulating functions; cytokines include interleukins and interferons

Cytolysis: the lysis of bacteria or of cells such as tumor cells or red blood cells by the insertion of the membrane attack complex derived from complement activation

Hapten: a molecule that is not immunogenic by itself but can react with a specific antibody

Histocompatible: sharing transplantation antigens

Hypersensitivity reactions: these occur in four types: Antibody-mediated hypersensitivity:

Type I. Anaphylactic ("immediate"): immunoglobulin E (IgE) antibody is induced by allergen and binds via its Fc receptor to mast cells and basophils; after encountering the antigen again, the fixed IgE becomes cross-linked, inducing degranulation and release of mediators, especially histamine (e.g., in asthma, hay fever, hives, anaphylactic shock)

Type II. Cytotoxic: antigens on a cell surface combine with antibody, which leads to complement-mediated lysis (e.g., transfusion or Rh reactions) or other cytotoxic membrane damage (e.g., in autoimmune hemolytic anemia)

Type III. Immune complex: antigen–antibody immune complexes are deposited in tissues, complement is activated, and polymorphonuclear cells are attracted to the site, causing tissue damage (e.g., in serum sickness, arthus reactions)

Cell-mediated hypersensitivity:

Type IV. Delayed: T lymphocytes, sensitized by an antigen, release lymphokines on second contact with the same antigen; the lymphokines induce inflammation and activate macrophages (e.g., in contact dermatitis, poison ivy, graft rejection, tuberculin skin reaction)

Immune response: development of resistance (immunity) to a foreign substance (e.g., infectious agent); it can be antibody mediated (humoral), cell mediated (cellular), or both

Immunoglobulin: a glycoprotein composed of H and L chains that functions as an antibody. All antibodies are immunoglobulins, but not all immunoglobulins have an antibody function

Immunoglobulin class: a subdivision of immunoglobulin molecules based on unique antigenic determinants in the Fc region of the H chains; the five immunoglobulin classes in humans are:

1. IgG: principal immunoglobulin of the secondary immune response. The only immunoglobulin capable of crossing placental barriers
2. IgM: first immunoglobulin to appear in a given immune response
3. IgA: principal immunoglobulin in external secretions of mucosal surfaces, tears, saliva, bile, urine, and colostrum
4. IgD: thought to activate the B cell
5. IgE: plays important role in immediate hypersensitivity reactions and parasitic infections

Interferon: one of a heterogeneous group of low-molecular-weight proteins elaborated by infected host cells that protect noninfected cells from viral infection; interferons, which are cytokines, also have immunomodulating functions

Interleukin (IL): a cytokine that stimulates or otherwise affects the function of lymphocytes and some other cells

IL-1: induces T helper cell synthesis of IL-2; activates T cells; induces chemotaxis for neutrophils

IL-2: stimulates antibody synthesis, T cytotoxic cells, and natural killer cells

IL-3: stimulates hematopoiesis

IL-4: induces isotype switching

IL-5: promotes the growth and differentiation of B cells

IL-6: stimulates B cell differentiation; activates T cells

IL-7: promotes pre–B cell growth and pre–T cell growth

IL-8: stimulates chemotaxis of neutrophils

IL-9: promotes T cell growth; enhances mast cell

IL-10: inhibits T helper cell 1 (TH1) and cytokine release; stimulates mast cell growth

IL-11: stimulates development of B cells; stimulates hematopoiesis

IL-12: activates T cells; stimulates TH1 cell development

IL-13: anti-inflammatory activity; B cell growth and differentiation

IL-14: induces proliferation of activated B cells

IL-15: stimulates growth of intestinal epithelium, T cells, and natural killer cells

IL-16: lymphocyte chemoattractant factor

Lymphocyte: a mononuclear cell 7 to 12 μm in diameter containing a nucleus with densely packed chromatin and a small rim of cytoplasm; lymphocytes include T cells and B cells, which have primary roles in immunity

Lymphokine: a cytokine that is a soluble product of a lymphocyte; lymphokines are responsible for multiple effects in a cellular immune reaction

Continued

BOX 9-1 Immunology Terms—cont'd

Macrophage: a phagocytic mononuclear cell derived from bone marrow monocytes and found in tissues and at the site of inflammation; macrophages serve accessory roles in cellular immunity

Major histocompatibility complex (MHC): a cluster of genes located close to each other; this determines the histocompatibility antigens of the members of a species

Membrane attack complex: the end product of activation of the complement cascade, which contains C5, C6, C7, and C8 (and C9); the membrane attack complex makes holes in the membranes of gram-negative bacteria, killing them and, in red blood cells or other cells, resulting in lysis

Monocyte: a circulating phagocytic blood cell that develops into tissue macrophages

Opsonin: a substance capable of enhancing phagocytosis; antibodies and complement are the two main opsonins

Opsonization: the coating of an antigen or particle (e.g., infectious agent) by substances such as antibodies, complement components, fibronectin, and so on, that facilitate uptake of the foreign particle into a phagocytic cell

Polymorphonuclear cell (PMN): also known as a *neutrophil* or *granulocyte*; a PMN is derived from a hematopoietic cell of bone marrow and is characterized by a multi-lobed nucleus; PMNs migrate from the circulation to a site of inflammation by chemotaxis and are phagocytic for bacteria and other particles

T-cell (also T lymphocyte): a thymus-derived cell that participates in a variety of cell-mediated immune reactions

TH1 (helper) or CD4 cell—activates macrophages and cytotoxic and other T cells

TH2 (helper) or CD4 cell—activates B cells to secrete immunoglobulin

TC (cytotoxic) or CD8 cell—destroys target cells

TD (delayed hypersensitivity) cell—causes inflammation associated with allergic reactions and tissue transplant rejection

TS (suppressor) or CD8 cell—regulates the immune response

Modified from Stites DP, Stobo JD, Wells JV, editors: Basic and clinical immunology, *ed 8, East Norwalk, CT, 1994, Appleton & Lange.*

    c. Cause antigens to clump or agglutinate, which enhances phagocytosis

    d. Activate complement system, resulting in cell lysis

  2. Cell-mediated (cellular) immunity—stimulation of T lymphocytes to activate a variety of effector T cells in response to foreign organisms or tissues (antigens); defends primarily against bacteria, viruses, fungi, protozoa, helminths, foreign tissue, and cancerous cells

  3. Acquired immunity

    a. Natural

      (1) Active—person is exposed to an antigen and the body produces antibodies

      (2) Passive—antibodies of a mother are passed to her infant

    b. Artificial

      (1) Active—vaccination with killed, inactivated, or attenuated microorganisms or toxoid

      (2) Passive—injection of immune serum or γ globulin

D. Hypersensitivity or allergy is an exaggerated response to specific substances; the inciting agent is the allergen (Figure 9-2; see Box 9-1)

Immunodeficiency

See the section on "Human immunodeficiency virus" in Chapter 8.

A. Inability of the immune system to perform normally; properly functioning system recognizes and destroys all that is foreign or non-self

B. Results in increased susceptibility to infection

C. Autoimmune disease (autoallergic)

  1. Self-antigens stimulate the production of antibodies or sensitized lymphocytes; antigen–antibody complex

  2. Mechanisms

    a. May be caused by the release of sequestered antigens; escape of tolerance to the "self" antigen at the T cell level; diminished suppressor T cell function

    b. Intolerance of "self" antigen because of cross-reactions

    c. Decreased function of suppressor T cells

  3. Includes systemic lupus erythematosus, rheumatoid arthritis, myasthenia gravis, and Graves' disease

D. Immunodeficiencies in B cells or T cells

  1. Hypergammaglobulinemias—overabundance of immunoglobulin

  2. Hypogammaglobulinemias—decreased catabolism, or loss of immunoglobulins

  3. Thymic aplasia (DiGeorge syndrome)—congenital absence of thymus gland

E. Drug-induced immunosuppression

  1. Used as an adjunct to organ transplantation and other organ grafts; also used for the treatment of immunologically mediated disease

2. Examples of drugs used include corticosteroids, rapamycin (now sirolimus), 15-deoxy-spergualin trihydrochloride (now gusperimus trihydrochloride), and cyclosporine; common complication is infection

F. Acquired immune deficiency syndrome (AIDS)

    1. Definition—disease that occurs because of a defect in cell-mediated immunity; cellular immunity is profoundly suppressed, allowing development of opportunistic infections and cancers; the Centers for Disease Control and Prevention (CDC) surveillance case definition includes all human immunodeficiency virus (HIV)–infected persons with a CD4+ T-lymphocyte count of less than 200 cells/μL or a CD4+ percentage of <14% percent. This definition includes the following clinical conditions and is to be used by all states for AIDS case reporting effective January 1993:

        a. Candidiasis of bronchi, trachea, or lungs

        b. Candidiasis, esophageal

        c. Cervical cancer, invasive

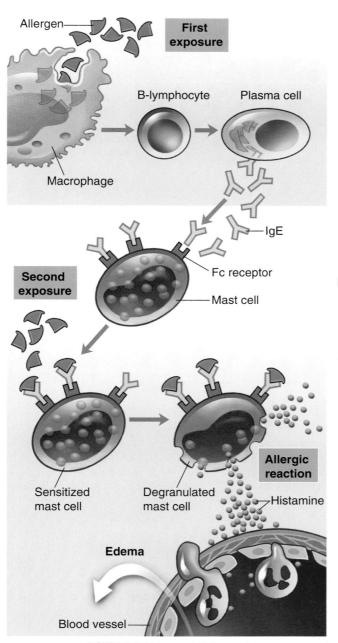

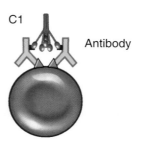

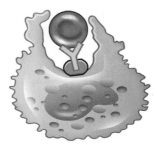

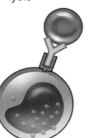

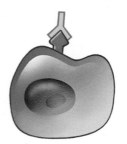

FIGURE 9-2 Hypersensitivity reactions are secondary responses to antigens that occur in an exaggerated or inappropriate form. These reactions have been classified into four major types: **A,** Type I reaction (antibody-mediated). **B,** Type II reaction (antibody-mediated)

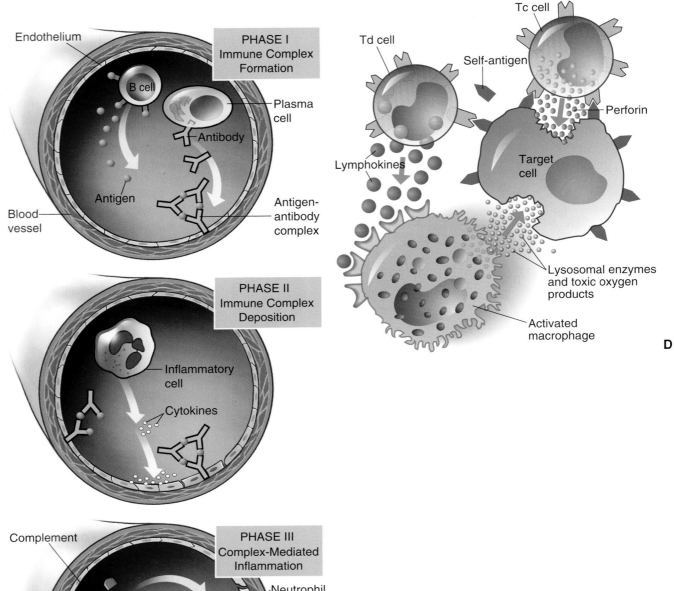

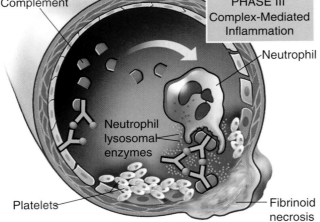

FIGURE 9-2, cont'd C, Type III reaction (antibody-mediated). **D,** Type IV reaction (cell-mediated). *(Modified from Huether SE, McCance KL: Understanding pathophysiology, ed 4, St Louis, 2008, Mosby.)*

d. Coccidioidomycosis, disseminated or extrapulmonary

e. Cryptococcosis, extrapulmonary

f. Cryptosporidiosis, chronic intestinal (more than 1 month in duration)

g. Cytomegalovirus (CMV) disease (other than liver, spleen, or nodes)

h. CMV retinitis (with loss of vision)

i. Encephalopathy, HIV related

j. Herpes simplex: chronic ulcer(s) (more than 1 month in duration); or bronchitis, pneumonitis, or esophagitis

k. Histoplasmosis, disseminated or extrapulmonary

l. Isosporiasis, chronic intestinal (more than 1 month in duration)

m. Kaposi sarcoma

n. Lymphoma, Burkitt (or equivalent term)

o. Lymphoma, immunoblastic (or equivalent term)

p. Lymphoma, primary, of brain

q. *Mycobacterium avium* complex or *M. kansasii*, disseminated or extrapul-monary

r. *M. tuberculosis*, any site (pulmonary or extrapulmonary)

s. *Mycobacterium*, other species or unidentified species, disseminated or extrapulmonary

t. *Pneumocystis carinii* pneumonia

u. Pneumonia, recurrent

v. Progressive multi-focal leukoencephalo-pathy

w. *Salmonella* septicemia, recurrent

x. Toxoplasmosis of brain

y. Wasting syndrome caused by HIV

2. Irreversible acquired defect

3. Etiology

a. Lentivirus subfamily of human retroviruses

b. Infects lymphocytes, macrophages, promyelocytes, and epidermal Langerhans' cells

4. High fatality rate

5. Virus isolated from blood, semen, vaginal secretions, saliva, tears, breast milk, cerebrospinal fluid, amniotic fluid, and urine

6. Transmission

a. Susceptible exposure to infected blood (e.g., intravenous drug use, blood transfusion)

b. Sexual contact

c. Mother to newborn (perinatal)

d. Co-factors (e.g., genital herpes) may influence transmission

7. CDC classification system for HIV-infected adolescents and adults categorizes persons based on CD4+ T lymphocyte counts and clinical conditions associated with HIV infection

a. CD4+ T lymphocyte categories

　(1) Three CD4+ T lymphocyte categories

　　(a) Category 1: 500 or more cells/μL

　　(b) Category 2: 200 to 499 cells/μL

　　(c) Category 3: less than 200 cells/μL

　(2) These categories correspond to CD4+ T lymphocyte counts per microliter of blood and guide clinical and therapeutic actions in the management of HIV-infected adolescents and adults; the revised HIV classification system also allows for the use of the percentage of CD4+ T cells

　(3) Classification of HIV-infected persons should be based on existing guidelines for the medical management of HIV-infected persons; thus, the lowest accurate but not necessarily the most recent CD4+ T-lymphocyte count should be used for classification purposes

b. Clinical categories of HIV infection

　(1) Category A—consists of one or more of the conditions listed below in an adolescent or adult (at least 13 years old) with documented HIV infection; conditions listed in categories B and C must not have occurred

　　(a) Asymptomatic HIV infection

　　(b) Persistent generalized lymphadenopathy

　　(c) Acute (primary) HIV infection with accompanying illness or history of acute HIV infection

　(2) Category B—consists of symptomatic conditions in an HIV-infected adolescent or adult that are not included among conditions listed in clinical category C and that meet at least one of the following criteria: the conditions are attributed to HIV infection or are indicative of a defect in cell-mediated immunity, or the conditions are considered by physicians to have a clinical course or to require management that is complicated by HIV infection. Examples of conditions in clinical category B include, but are not limited to:

　　(a) Bacillary angiomatosis

　　(b) Candidiasis, oropharyngeal (thrush)

　　(c) Candidiasis, vulvovaginal; persistent, frequent, or poorly responsive to therapy

　　(d) Cervical dysplasia (moderate or severe) or cervical carcinoma in situ

　　(e) Constitutional symptoms such as fever (38.5°C) or diarrhea lasting longer than 1 month

　　(f) Hairy leukoplakia, oral

(g) Herpes zoster (shingles), involving at least two distinct episodes or more than one dermatome

(h) Idiopathic thrombocytopenic purpura

(i) Listeriosis

(j) Pelvic inflammatory disease, particularly if complicated by tubo-ovarian abscess

(k) Peripheral neuropathy

(3) For classification purposes, category B conditions take precedence over those in category A; for example, someone previously treated for oral or persistent vaginal candidiasis (and in whom a category C disease has not developed) but who is now asymptomatic should be classified in category B

(4) Category C—includes the clinical conditions listed in the AIDS surveillance case definition; for classification purposes, once a category C condition has occurred, the person will remain in category C

8. Secondary neoplasms

   a. Kaposi's sarcoma—skin lesions; may be oral; multiple small reddish blue, purple, or hyperpigmented brown papules, plaques, or nodules; associated with human herpesvirus 8 (HHV-8) (Figure 9-3)

   b. B cell lymphomas

9. Opportunistic infections

   a. Cytomegalovirus (CMV)—frequently involves the eye, causing retinal lesions

   b. Tuberculosis

   c. *P. carinii*

   d. Oral and esophageal infection from *C. albicans*

   e. Herpes simplex viruses 1 and 2

10. Incidence and prevalence

   a. Approximately 1.1 million people live with AIDS in the United States

   b. Leading cause of death among men (25 to 44 years) and the fifth leading cause of death among women (15 to 44 years) in the United States

   c. Risk factors

     (1) Unsafe sexual practices

     (2) Exposure to blood or blood products

     (3) Intravenous drug use

     (4) Infant of infected individual

   d. Transmission to health care personnel providing care to infected individuals is rare

11. Treatment (see the section on "Antiviral agents" in Chapter 11)

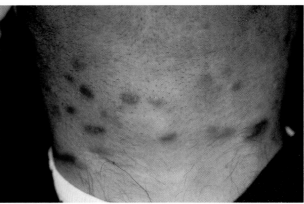
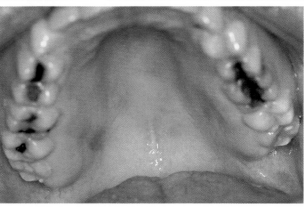

FIGURE 9-3 Kaposi's sarcoma of the neck (*top*); presenting as a dark macule in the right posterior palate (*bottom*). *(From Regezi JA, Sciubba JJ, Jordan RCK: Oral pathology: Clinical pathologic correlations, ed 5, St Louis, 2008, Saunders.)*

   a. No known cure or vaccine yet

   b. Vaccine will have to be targeted both to free virus in bloodstream and to virus present in infected host cells

   c. Food and Drug Administration approved antiretroviral drugs used for the treatment of HIV:

     (1) Multi-class combination products. (e. g., Atripila)

     (2) Nucleoside reverse transcriptase inhibitors (NRTIs) (e.g., Zidovudine [AZT], Didanosine [ddI], Stavudine [d4T], Lamivudine [3TC])

     (3) Nonnucleoside reverse transcriptase inhibitors (NNRTIs) (e.g., Nevirapine [NVP], efavirenz [EFV])

     (4) Protease inhibitors (PIs) (e.g., Amprenavir [AP], Indinavir [IDV], Darunavir, Atazanavir sufate [ATV])

     (5) Fusion inhibitors (e.g., Enfuvirtide [T-20])

(6) Entry inhibitors
(e.g., maraviroc [Selzentry, Celsentri])
(7) HIV integrase strand stransfer inhibitor
(e.g., Raltegravir)
12. Oral manifestations
a. Hairy leukoplakia
b. Herpetic lesions
c. Oral and esophageal candidiasis
d. Kaposi sarcoma
e. Linear gingival erythema and necrotizing ulcerative periodontitis
f. Human papillomavirus
g. Lymphoma
h. Recurrent aphthous ulcers

Infections of the Skin, Nails, and Hair

A. Bacterial infections
1. Tetanus
a. Etiology—*Clostridium tetani*
b. Pathogenesis and transmission—by spores that germinated in the wound and produce tetanus-causing toxin
c. Clinical findings and symptoms
(1) Trismus (stiff jaw); eventually, locked jaw
(2) Spasms of facial muscles
(3) Dysphagia
(4) Difficulty breathing
2. Leprosy
a. Etiology—*M. leprae*
b. Pathogenesis and transmission—transmitted via prolonged direct contact or inhalation of organisms
c. Clinical findings and symptoms
(1) Skin lesions
(2) Oral lesions are tumor-like masses of tissue that involve the oral lining, tongue, lips, or palate
3. *Pseudomonas aeruginosa* infections
a. Pathogenesis
(1) Low pathogenicity for humans, except in debilitated persons (e.g., burn victims or those taking antibiotics or immunosuppressive drugs)
(2) Ubiquitous in nature
b. Clinical findings and symptoms
(1) *Pseudomonas* dermatitis—self-limiting rash associated with swimming pools, hot tubs, and saunas
(2) Otitis externa—infection of the external ear canal
4. Staphylococcal infections
a. Etiology—*Staphylococcus aureus* and *Staphylococcus epidermidis*
b. Pathogenesis—determined by extracellular factors and invasive properties of the strain

c. Clinical findings and symptoms
(1) Most *S. aureus* strains are resistant to penicillin
(2) Causes furuncles (boils), carbuncles, impetigo, and cellulitis
5. Streptococcal infections
a. Etiology—*Streptococcus pyogenes* (group A β-hemolytic)
b. Pathogenesis
(1) Determined by portal of entry
(2) Diffuse and rapidly spreading infection
c. Clinical findings and symptoms
(1) Scarlet fever
(a) Acute inflammation of the upper respiratory tract
(b) Generalized rash caused by erythrogenic exotoxin
(c) Oral mucosa is red; "strawberry tongue"
(d) Sequelae from group A streptococcal infection include rheumatic fever and hemorrhagic glomerulonephritis
(2) Erysipelas
6. Acne
a. Etiology—*Propionibacterium acnes*
b. Pathogenesis—*P. acnes* metabolizes sebum trapped in hair follicles and sets up an inflammatory response
7. Lyme disease
a. Etiology—*Borrelia burgdorferi* (spirochetes)
b. Pathogenesis
(1) Transmitted by ticks (zoonotic)
(2) Antigen–antibody complexes may be responsible for arthritic or neurologic difficulties
c. Clinical findings and symptoms
(1) Initial phase—rash, headache, fever, and myalgia
(2) Secondary phase—possible cardiac involvement
(3) Recurring neurologic symptoms, arthritis, or both
B. Fungal infections
1. Ringworm infections (tinea)
a. Etiology—dermatophytes most important; *Microsporum, Trichophyton, Epidermophyton*
b. Pathogenesis—grow only within dead keratinized tissue
c. Clinical findings and symptoms—inflammatory response, especially at the border of lesions; patching; scaling
2. Candidiasis
a. Etiology—*C. albicans*
b. Pathogenesis
(1) Dissemination and sepsis in compromised patients (opportunistic infection)

(2) Normal inhabitant of the skin and mucosal surfaces

(3) Predisposing factors include diabetes mellitus, pregnancy, obesity, vitamin deficiency, use of broad-spectrum antibiotics, and immunologic defects

c. Clinical findings and symptoms—vary with site

3. Sporotrichosis

a. Etiology—*Sporothrix schenckii*

b. Pathogenesis—organisms enter the skin of an extremity; subsequent nodular lesions form in the subcutaneous tissue; gardeners and farmers at increased risk for accidental infection

c. Clinical findings and symptoms—nodules ulcerate at the surface and discharge pus

C. Viral infections

1. Herpes simplex

a. Etiology—herpes simplex virus (HSV)

b. Pathogenesis

(1) Transmission through oral and ocular secretions

(2) Virus is present in saliva even in apparent good health

(3) Indirect contact (e.g., fomites)

(4) Infects epithelial cells

(5) Establishes a latent infection from retroviruses

c. Clinical findings and symptoms

(1) Types

(a) HSV-1—generally above the waist; commonly found in and around the mouth

(b) HSV-2—herpes genitalis

(2) Frequently asymptomatic

(3) Most commonly acute gingivostomatitis; usually in children—fever, malaise, irritability, local lymphadenopathy, and anorexia; red, edematous gingiva and adjacent mucosa; lesions are vesicles with yellowish contents that rupture and ulcerate; bright margin of erythema; sharply defined; pain may be severe; duration of about 7 days; self-limiting

(4) Herpetic whitlow infection of fingers; can be caused by HSV-1 or HSV-2; abrupt onset; local irritation; tenderness, edema, erythema, and vesicles; difficult to differentiate from bacterial pyoderma caused by staphylococci

(5) Recurrent secondary infections by HSV-1

(a) Virus now latent but permanently established in nerve ganglia (carrier)

(b) Infections may be induced by stress, sun, or colds

(6) Herpes labialis is the most common clinical manifestation of recurrent infection

(a) Cold sores, fever blisters

(b) Vesicles on an erythematous base

(c) Prodromal burning and hyperesthesia

(d) Swollen lymph nodes

(7) Intraoral lesions

(a) Usually found on the mucosa or hard palate overlying bone

(b) Small, discrete lesions; vesicles of clear fluid; ulcerate with a red base

2. Chickenpox

a. Etiology—varicella zoster virus

b. Pathogenesis

(1) Route of infection through the mucosa of the upper respiratory tract

(2) Highly infectious

(3) Virus probably circulates in the blood and localizes on the skin

(4) Incubation period 2 weeks

(5) Vaccine available

c. Clinical findings and symptoms

(1) Earliest symptoms are malaise and fever, followed by a rash and formation of vesicles

(2) Oral lesions may occur throughout the mouth and appear like small canker sores or aphthae; vesicles rupture quickly

3. Shingles

a. Etiology—varicella zoster virus

b. Pathogenesis

(1) Reactivation of latent virus in dorsal root ganglion

(2) Closely follows area of innervation

(3) Chickenpox and shingles represent different forms of infection by the same agent

(4) Virus resides in ganglia; usually affects sensory nerves (thoracic area is the most often involved; ophthalmic division of the trigeminal nerve is the next most involved)

(5) Vaccine available

c. Clinical findings and symptoms

(1) Mostly found in adults

(2) Malaise, fever, followed by severe pain in area

(3) Rash and vesicles along the nerve trunk

4. Warts

a. Etiology—papillomaviruses

b. Pathogenesis—affects epithelial cells of skin and mucous membranes

c. Clinical findings and symptoms

(1) Skin warts, plantar warts, flat warts, genital condylomas, laryngeal papillomas

(2) Oral warts are papular or nodular lesions covered with papilliferous projections; also may look like common warts

5. Measles
  a. Etiology—rubeola virus
  b. Pathogenesis
   (1) Transmission through the respiratory tract
   (2) Spreads to regional lymphoid tissue
   (3) Primary viremia disseminates the virus
   (4) Secondary viremia seeds the epithelial surfaces of the body
  c. Clinical findings and symptoms
   (1) Koplik's spots
     (a) Small bluish white spots with a red surrounding zone; cannot be wiped off
     (b) Occur on the buccal mucosa opposite the molars
   (2) Followed by a diffuse skin rash and fever
   (3) Bacterial secondary infections occur, such as middle ear infections or pneumonia

6. German measles
  a. Etiology—rubella virus
  b. Pathogenesis:
   (1) Occurs through the upper respiratory tract
   (2) Incubation period 2 to 3 weeks
  c. Clinical findings and symptoms
   (1) Malaise, low-grade fever, rash, and lymphadenopathy
   (2) Rash starts on face; extends to trunk and extremities

7. Erythema infectiosum (also called *fifth disease*)
  a. Etiology—human parvovirus B19
  b. Pathogenesis
   (1) Children most affected by the virus
   (2) Virus transmitted through the upper respiratory tract
  c. Clinical findings and symptoms
   (1) Low-grade fever, malaise, and bright red rash on cheeks spreading to the rest of the body
   (2) Sequelae include arthritis in adulthood

Infections of the Respiratory Tract

Upper Respiratory System Infections
A. Bacterial infections
  1. Diphtheria
   a. Etiology—*Corynebacterium diphtheriae*
   b. Pathogenesis
    (1) Droplets or by contact with susceptible individuals
    (2) Bacilli grow on mucous membranes or in skin abrasions

   (3) Damage caused by the systemic distribution of toxin
   c. Clinical findings and symptoms
    (1) Enlarged lymphadenopathy of the neck; possibly edema
    (2) Pseudomembrane forms on tonsils
  2. Streptococcal pharyngitis ("strep" throat)
   a. Etiology—*S. pyogenes* (group A)
   b. Pathogenesis—transmitted by the respiratory route and contaminated food, water, and milk
   c. Clinical findings and symptoms: severe inflammation of the throat and tonsils; fever
B. Viral infections—common cold (Table 9-9)

Lower Respiratory System Infections
A. Bacterial infections
  1. Pneumococcal pneumonia
   a. Etiology—most common agent is *S. pneumoniae*
   b. Pathogenesis
    (1) Spread by droplets from nasal or pharyngeal secretion
    (2) Person may contract the disease or become an asymptomatic carrier
    (3) Predisposing factors include age, impaired resistance, and bacteremia
   c. Clinical findings and symptoms: symptoms include sudden onset of high fever, chills, chest pain, dry cough, and rust-colored sputum
  2. Bacterial pneumonia
   a. Etiology—several species—*S. pyogenes, S. aureus, Klebsiella pneumoniae, Haemophilus influenzae*
   b. Pathogenesis is similar to that caused by *S. pneumoniae*
   c. Inflammation of the lungs
  3. Legionnaire's disease
   a. Etiology—*Legionella pneumophila*
   b. Pathogenesis
    (1) Inhalation of bacteria from aerosols
    (2) Bacteria multiply in lungs and produce pneumonia
   c. Clinical findings and symptoms
    (1) Influenza-like illness with pneumonia
    (2) Complications include renal failure, gastrointestinal (GI) hemorrhage, and respiratory failure
  4. Tuberculosis
   a. Etiology—*M. tuberculosis*
   b. Pathogenesis
    (1) Transmitted by inhalation of droplets, ingestion, or direct inoculation; disseminated by coughing, sneezing, or contaminated dust

TABLE 9-9 Viral Infections of the Respiratory Tract

		MOST COMMON VIRAL CAUSES		
Syndrome	Main Symptoms	Infants	Children	Adults
Common cold	Nasal obstruction, nasal discharge	Rhinovirus	Rhinovirus	Rhinovirus
		Adenovirus	Adenovirus	Coronavirus
Pharyngitis	Sore throat	Adenovirus	Adenovirus	Adenovirus
		Herpes simplex virus	Coxsackievirus	Coxsackievirus
Laryngitis/croup	Hoarseness, "barking" cough	Parainfluenza virus	Parainfluenza virus	Parainfluenza virus
		Influenza virus	Influenza virus	Influenza virus
Tracheobronchitis	Cough	Parainfluenza virus	Parainfluenza virus	Influenza virus
		Influenza virus	Influenza virus	Adenovirus
Bronchiolitis	Cough, dyspnea	Respiratory syncytial virus	Rare virus	Rare virus
		Parainfluenza virus		
Pneumonia	Cough, chest pain	Respiratory syncytial virus	Influenza virus	Influenza virus
		Influenza virus	Parainfluenza virus	Adenovirus

From Brooks GF, Butel JS, Morse SA: Jawetz, Melnick & Adelberg's medical microbiology, ed 23, Columbus, OH, 2004, McGraw-Hill.

(2) Predisposing factors include advanced age, chronic alcoholism, poor nutrition, diabetes mellitus, and prolonged stress

(3) Incubation period is generally 28 to 47 days; can be as long as 6 months

c. Clinical findings and symptoms

(1) Symptoms vary but include fever, general discomfort, weight loss, tubercle formation (nodule in lung tissue), night sweats, and persistent cough

(2) Oral lesions may appear as an ulcerated lesion on the tongue or mucosa (rare)

(3) Diagnosis by a skin test and a radiograph

5. Whooping cough (pertussis)

a. Etiology—*Bordetella pertussis*

b. Pathogenesis—transmitted by inhalation of droplets; produce toxins

c. Clinical findings and symptoms—spasmodic coughing and gasping noise with inhalation

6. Psittacosis

a. Etiology—*Chlamydia psittaci*

b. Pathogenesis—humans infected by inhaling dust contaminated with excreta of infected birds

c. Clinical findings and symptoms—symptoms in humans include fever and pneumonitis; spread from the lungs to the spleen, brain, or other organs; mild, cold-like illness; may be asymptomatic

7. Mycoplasmal pneumonia

a. Etiology—*Mycoplasma pneumoniae*

b. Pathogenesis—transmitted in airborne droplets; binds respiratory epithelium and inhibits ciliary action

c. Clinical findings and symptoms—mild symptoms of low fever, cough, and headache that persist for 3 weeks or longer

B. Fungal infections

1. Histoplasmosis

a. Etiology—*Histoplasma capsulatum*

b. Pathogenesis—transmitted by inhalation of spores, especially in excreta of wild birds, poultry, and bats

c. Clinical findings and symptoms

(1) Skin lesions are common

(2) Meningitis

2. Pneumocystis pneumonia

a. Etiology—*Pneumocystis jiroveci*

b. Pathogenesis—inhalation of spores; disease more common among immunosuppressed persons, especially those with AIDS

c. Clinical findings and symptoms—nonspecific; fever; dry, nonproductive cough

3. Coccidioidomycosis

a. Etiology—*Coccidioides immitis*

b. Spores in desert soils are inhaled along with dust (common in the southwest)

c. Clinical findings and symptoms—chest pain, fever, cough, weight loss

C. Viral infections
1. Influenza virus infection
   a. Etiology—orthomyxoviruses
   b. Pathogenesis
      (1) The genome can undergo sudden genetic reassortment
      (2) Spread by airborne droplets or contact with contaminated objects
      (3) Virus attaches to the respiratory epithelium
   c. Clinical findings and symptoms
      (1) Chills, headache, dry cough, fever, malaise, muscular ache, and inflammation of the soft palate
      (2) Secondary infection by *S. aureus*, *H. influenzae*, *S. pyogenes*, and *S. pneumoniae*; may result in bronchitis and pneumonia
      (3) Reye syndrome may be a complication
2. Hantavirus pulmonary syndrome
   a. Etiology—hantavirus
   b. Pathogenesis—inhalation of excreta of deer mice
   c. Clinical findings and symptoms—severe cold followed by an internal hemorrhage of blood plasma in the lungs

Infections of the Gastrointestinal Tract

A. Bacterial infections
1. Cholera
   a. Etiology—*Vibrio cholerae*
   b. Pathogenesis
      (1) Transmitted as a result of unsanitary living conditions and through ingestion of the organisms
      (2) Organisms attach to microvilli of epithelial cells; produce toxin
   c. Clinical findings and symptoms: dehydration, nausea, vomiting, profuse diarrhea, and abdominal and leg cramps
2. Salmonellosis
   a. Etiology—several species of *Salmonella*
   b. Pathogenesis—organisms enter by the oral route usually via contaminated food or drink
   c. Clinical findings and symptoms—organisms cause enteric fevers, bacteremia, followed by focal lesions or endocarditis
3. Shigellosis (bacillary dysentery)
   a. Etiology—*Shigella dysenteriae*, *Shigella flexneri*, *Shigella boydii*, and *Shigella sonnei*
   b. Pathogenesis
      (1) Transmitted through contaminated food or water
      (2) The organism invades the mucosal epithelium

   c. Clinical findings and symptoms—abdominal pain, fever, and watery or bloody diarrhea
4. Enteric infections caused by *E. coli*
   a. Etiology
      (1) Enterotoxigenic *E. coli* (ETEC)—traveler's diarrhea
      (2) Enteroinvasive *E. coli* (EIEC)
      (3) Enteropathogenic *E. coli* (EPEC)
      (4) Enterohemorrhagic *E. coli* (EHEC)—serotype O157: H7
      (5) Enteroaggregative *E. coli* (EaggEC)
   b. Pathogenesis
      (1) Acquired by ingestion of contaminated food or water or through contact with contaminated persons
      (2) Factors responsible for the different ways in which *E. coli* produces disease vary with strain
   c. Clinical findings and symptoms—abdominal pain, malaise, loss of appetite, diarrhea, and dehydration; diarrhea may be watery or bloody, depending on the strain of *E. coli*
5. Typhoid fever
   a. Etiology—*Salmonella typhi*
   b. Pathogenesis—transmitted through contaminated food or water
   c. Clinical findings and symptoms
      (1) Fever, severe headache, abdominal pain, and abdominal rash
      (2) Complications include carrier state, relapses, inflammation of the gallbladder, and intestinal bleeding
6. *Helicobacter* peptic disease syndrome
   a. Etiology—*Helicobacter pylori*
   b. Pathogenesis—*H. pylori* produces ammonia, which neutralizes stomach acid, allowing the bacteria to colonize the stomach mucosa
   c. Clinical findings and symptoms—peptic ulcers
7. *Campylobacter* gastroenteritis
   a. Etiology—*Campylobacter jejuni*
   b. Pathogenesis—infection acquired by ingestion of contaminated food or water; organisms invade the intestinal mucosa and release toxins
   c. Clinical findings and symptoms—sudden onset of abdominal pain, nausea, fever, headache, and muscle pain
8. *Yersinia* enterocolitis
   a. Etiology—*Yersinia enterocolitica*
   b. Pathogenesis—infection acquired by ingestion of contaminated food or water
   c. Clinical findings and symptoms—diarrhea, fever, and abdominal pain suggestive of acute appendicitis in children younger than 7 years

9. Food poisoning
   a. Botulism
      (1) Etiology—*Clostridium botulinum*
      (2) Pathogenesis
         (a) Regularly contaminates human, plant, and animal food products
         (b) Produces a deadly toxin that acts on nerves
         (c) Transmitted through improperly preserved foods and uncooked fish and meats; foods do not appear contaminated
      (3) Clinical findings and symptoms
         (a) Difficulty speaking, blurred vision, inability to swallow, heart failure, and respiratory paralysis
         (b) Infant botulism may be one of the causes of sudden infant death syndrome
   b. Staphylococcal food poisoning
      (1) Etiology—toxin produced by staphylococci (usually *S. aureus*) in unrefrigerated foods such as dairy products, custard, cream-filled products, fish, or processed meats
      (2) Pathogenesis
         (a) Caused by ingestion of preformed enterotoxin
         (b) Incubation period is from 1 to 8 hours
         (c) Symptoms include nausea, violent vomiting, diarrhea; no fever
         (d) Rapid convalescence; self-limiting
   c. *Perfringens* poisoning
      (1) Etiology—*Clostridium perfringens*
      (2) Pathogenesis
         (a) The precise mechanism is unknown
         (b) The organism produces an enterotoxin
         (c) The incubation period is 8 to 16 hours
      (3) Clinical findings and symptoms
         (a) Symptoms are similar to those of staphylococcal food poisoning
         (b) Usually self-limiting

B. Viral infections
   1. Hepatitis A (Tables 9-10 and 9-11)
      a. Etiology—hepatitis A virus (HAV)
      b. Pathogenesis
         (1) Oral–fecal route in unsanitary conditions; contaminated food and water; close intimate contact with infected person
         (2) Rarely through the blood
         (3) The incubation period is 15 to 50 days
         (4) Usually occurs in children and young adults
      c. Clinical findings and symptoms
         (1) Preicteric (before jaundice appears)—similar to influenza; fever, headache,

TABLE 9-10 Characteristics of the Various Types of Viral Hepatitis

Characteristic	Hepatitis A	Hepatitis B	Hepatitis C	Hepatitis D	Hepatitis E	Hepatitis G*
Transmission	Fecal–oral (ingestion of contaminated food, ice, and water)	Parenteral (injection of contaminated blood or other body fluids)	Parenteral	Percutaneous, permucosal, or parenteral (host must be co-infected with hepatitis B or as a superinfection in persons with chronic HBV infection)	Fecal–oral (contaminated drinking water most common)	Bloodborne and co-infection with HCV
Agent	Hepatitis A virus (HAV); single- stranded ribonucleic acid (RNA); no envelope	Hepatitis B virus (HBV); double- stranded deoxyribonucleic acid (DNA); envelope	Hepatitis C virus (HCV); single- stranded RNA; envelope	Hepatitis D virus (HDV); defective single-stranded RNA, envelope from HBV	Hepatitis E virus (HEV); single-stranded RNA; no envelope	Hepatitis G virus, although causal association remains to be confirmed
Incubation period	15–50 days	45–160 days	2–26 weeks	Uncertain	15–60 days	Acute disease spectrum unknown

TABLE 9-10 Characteristics of the Various Types of Viral Hepatitis—cont'd

Characteristic	Hepatitis A	Hepatitis B	Hepatitis C	Hepatitis D	Hepatitis E	Hepatitis G*
Manifestations or symptoms	Children under age 6 years may not have signs of illness; severe cases: fever, headache, malaise, jaundice, fatigue, loss of appetite, nausea, dark urine	Clinical manifestations are age dependent; anorexia, nausea, malaise, vomiting, jaundice, dark urine, clay-colored stools, abdominal pain, and more likely to progress to severe liver damage	Similar to HBV	Severe liver damage; high mortality rate	Similar to HAV, but pregnant women may have high mortality rate; less common symptoms include arthralgia, diarrhea, pruritus, urticaria	
Chronic liver disease	No	Yes	Yes	Yes	No	No
Vaccines	A sterile suspension of inactivated virus	Genetically engineered	None	HBV vaccine is protective because co-infection is required	None	None

*Information on hepatitis G, from the Centers for Disease Control and Prevention, Guidelines for viral hepatitis surveillance and case management, Atlanta, 2005: Available at http://www.cdc.gov/ncidod/diseases/hepatitis/resource/PDFs/revised_GUIDELINES_formatted5.pdf: Accessed May 11, 2011.
From Tortora GJ, Funke BR. Case DL: Microbiology: An introduction, ed. 8, Menlo Park, CA, 2003, Benjamin/Cummings.

TABLE 9-11 Viral Hepatitis: Abbreviations, Terms, and Their Meanings

Abbreviations	Term	Significance
Hepatitis A		
HAV	Hepatitis A virus	Causative agent for hepatitis A
Anti-HAV	Antibody to hepatitis A virus	Acute or resolved infection
		Protective immune response to infection
		Passively acquired antibody
		Response to vaccination
IgM anti-HAV	Immunoglobulin M (IgM) antibody to hepatitis A virus	Recent HAV infection
HAV-RNA	Ribonucleic acid (RNA) of HAV	Detected by nucleic acid amplification, hybridization, or both
Hepatitis B		
HBV	Hepatitis B virus (Dane particle)	Causative agent for hepatitis B
		Current HBV infection
HBsAg	Hepatitis B surface antigen	Surface marker in acute disease and carrier state
		Antigen used in hepatitis B vaccine
Anti-HBs	Antibody to hepatitis B surface antigen	Indicates
		(1) Active immunity to HBV (past infection)
		(2) Passive immunity from HBIg
		(3) Immune response from HB vaccine

Continued

TABLE 9-11 Viral Hepatitis: Abbreviations, Terms, and Their Meanings—cont'd

Abbreviations	Term	Significance
HBeAg	Hepatitis B e antigen	High-titer HBV in serum indicates high infectivity
		Persists into carrier state
Anti-HBe	Antibody to hepatitis B e antigen	Low-titer HBV
		Low-degree infectivity
HBcAg	Hepatitis B core antigen	Indicates acute, chronic, or resolved HBV infection
		Not elicited by vaccination
Anti-HBc	Antibody to hepatitis B core antigen	Indicates prior HBV infection
IgM anti-HBc	IgM class antibody to hepatitis B core antigen	Indicates recent HBC infection
HBV-DNA	Deoxyribonucleic acid (DNA) of HBV	Detected by nucleic acid amplification, hybridization, or both
Hepatitis C HCV	Hepatitis C virus (formerly parenterally transmitted non-A, non-B)	Causative agent for hepatitis C
Anti-HCV	Antibody to hepatitis C virus	Indicates acute disease and chronic state
		Resembles hepatitis B
HCV-RNA	RNA of HCV	Defines viremia; detected by nucleic acid amplification
Hepatitis D HDV	Hepatitis delta virus	Causative agent for hepatitis D
		Only infectious in presence of acute or chronic HBV infection
HDV-Ag	Delta antigen	Detectable during early acute HDV infection
Anti-HDV	Antibody to hepatitis D virus	Indicates acute, resolved, or chronic infection
IgM anti-HDV	IgM-class antibody to HDV	Indicates either acute or chronic infection with active viral replication
HDV-RNA	RNA of HDV	Detected by nucleic acid amplification, hybridization, or both
Hepatitis E HEV	Hepatitis E virus (formerly enterically transmitted non-A, non-B)	Causative agent for hepatitis E
Anti-HEV	Antibody to hepatitis E virus	Indicates acute or resolved infection
IgM anti-HEV	IgM-class antibody to hepatitis E virus	Indicates acute infection
Non-ABCDE Parenterally transmitted (HSG)	Diagnosis of exclusion	Epidemiologic evidence of parenteral or sexual transmission
Enterically transmitted (HSF)	Diagnosis of exclusion	Epidemiologic evidence of fecal–oral transmission
Immunoglobulins Ig	Immunoglobulin	Contains antibodies to HAV and low-titer HBV antibodies
HBIg	Hepatitis B immunoglobulin	Contains high-titer antibodies to HBV

From Wilkins EM: Clinical practice of the dental hygienist, ed 10, Philadelphia, 2009, Lippincott Williams & Wilkins.

nausea, vomiting, fatigue, abdominal pain, loss of appetite, dark urine

(2) Icteric—jaundice (rare in children); other symptoms continue

(3) Anicteric—without jaundice; two or three times more prevalent than the icteric state; symptoms resemble those of influenza

(4) Recovery and immunity

    (a) Antibody to HAV (anti-HAV) is usually in the blood 2 weeks after onset

    (b) Most individuals recover completely in 4 to 6 weeks

    (c) Immunity develops after recovery

    (d) No carrier state develops

    (e) Usually self-limiting

d. Active immunization

(1) Hepatitis A vaccine (Havrix) at least 2 weeks before expected exposure; booster dose recommended 6 to 12 months later for adults

(2) The vaccine may be administered concomitantly with immunoglobulin in persons exposed to HAV

2. Hepatitis B (see Tables 9-10 and 9-11)

a. Etiology—hepatitis B virus (HBV)

b. Pathogenesis

(1) Infected blood or serum through parenteral inoculation (e.g., blood transfusions, contaminated dental or medical instruments, needles and syringes used by drug abusers, and accidental self-inoculation by health care professionals)

(2) Other body fluids, including saliva, semen, tears, urine, sweat, and nasopharyngeal secretions

(3) Oral or sexual contact or other close personal contact

(4) Coughing, sneezing, and aerosols

(5) Salivary transmission by way of hands, instruments, and other equipment is an important consideration in the practice of dental hygiene

c. Incubation

(1) Between 45 and 160 days

(2) Presence of hepatitis B surface antigen (HBsAg) indicates potential to be infective

d. Symptoms

(1) Similar to hepatitis A

(2) Slower onset; longer duration

(3) Asymptomatic to severe and debilitating

(4) The patient may have subclinical disease and remain undiagnosed

(5) May result in chronic liver disease; strong evidence for link between chronic HBV infection and hepatocellular carcinoma (liver cancer)

e. Recovery

(1) Development of antibody to HBsAg (anti-HBs) indicates immunity

(2) Approximately 5% to 10% of those infected develop a chronic carrier state; HBsAg still present after 6 months; carriers are usually asymptomatic and often remain undetected

f. Risk factors

(1) Exposure to virus at birth (e.g., infants born to mothers infected with HBV)

(2) Exchange of blood or blood products (e.g., during hemodialysis, blood transfusions, or intravenous drug use)

(3) Exposure to blood or blood products (e.g., in the case of health care workers)

(4) Close intimate contact with infected person

(5) Unsafe sexual practices

(6) Institutionalization (e.g., in the case of some individuals with Down syndrome and prisoners)

(7) Immunosuppressive therapy

g. Immunization

(1) Two types of HBsAg vaccines

    (a) Obtained from HBsAg-positive carriers (Heptavax)

    (b) Obtained from recombinant DNA in yeast cells (Recombivax)

(2) Passive immunization results from hepatitis B immune globulin (HBIg); used for postexposure prophylaxis; preferably within 24 to 48 hours; partially effective

(3) Given as a series of 3 or 4 shots

3. Hepatitis type C (see Tables 9-10 and 9-11)

a. Etiology—hepatitis C virus

b. Pathogenesis

(1) Originally named non-A, non-B hepatitis virus

(2) Risk factors include blood transfusion, intravenous drug use, and heterosexual transmission

c. Clinical findings and symptoms

(1) Mild symptoms; most asymptomatic

(2) Development of chronic hepatitis in 50%; may develop into cirrhosis and hepatocellular carcinoma

4. Hepatitis D (formerly *delta hepatitis*) (see Tables 9-10 and 9-11)

a. Etiology—hepatitis D virus

b. Pathogenesis

(1) Similar to HBV

(2) Infection dependent on HBV replication

c. Clinical findings—may produce acute exacerbations of chronic HBV and fulminant hepatitis

5. Hepatitis type E (see Tables 9-10 and 9-11)
   a. Etiology—hepatitis E virus
   b. Pathogenesis
      (1) Originally named non-A, non-B hepatitis virus
      (2) Enteric transmission
      (3) Epidemic outbreaks occurring in developing countries

6. Hepatitis G (see Table 9-10)
   a. Etiology—hepatitis G virus
   b. Pathogenesis
      (1) Bloodborne transmission and co-infection with HCV
      (2) Acute disease spectrum unknown

7. Rotavirus
   a. Pathogenesis—disease spread via the fecal–oral route; the virus replicates in the epithelial cells on the tips of the villi in the small intestine
   b. Clinical findings and symptoms—acute onset of vomiting, watery diarrhea, fever, and abdominal pain in children younger than 2 years

8. Norwalk virus and Norwalk-like virus
   a. Pathogenesis—disease spread via the fecal–oral route
   b. Clinical findings and symptoms—nausea, vomiting, abdominal cramps, lethargy, and diarrhea in older children and adults

Infections of the Circulatory System

Diseases of the Heart

A. Rheumatic fever
   1. Etiology—β-hemolytic group A streptococcal infection
   2. Pathogenesis
      a. Rheumatic fever—hypersensitivity state developing after streptococcal infection; associated with β-hemolytic group A streptococci
      b. Heart valves become inflamed; subsequent abnormal growths of connective tissue; scarring of valves occurs, resulting in rheumatic heart disease
   3. Clinical findings and symptoms
      a. Fever, malaise, polyarthritis, inflammation of the heart
      b. Defective heart valves are a result of carditis
      c. Heart valve damage
         (1) Stenosis—narrowing of the valve opening
         (2) Valvular insufficiency—failure of the valve to close completely

4. Prophylactic antibiotic premedication is necessary before dental and dental hygiene treatments

B. Infective endocarditis
   1. Etiology—most often associated with the normal flora of the respiratory or intestinal tract
   2. Pathogenesis
      a. Inflammatory condition of the heart; microbial colonization of the endothelial membrane that covers the inner surface of the heart and the heart valves
      b. Predisposing factors
         (1) Artificial heart valves
         (2) Congential heart defects
         (3) History of endocarditis
         (4) Damaged heart valves
         (5) History of IV illegal drug use
      c. Dental and dental hygiene procedures may allow bacteria to enter the bloodstream (bacteremia) and lodge in the heart valves
   3. Clinical findings and symptoms
      a. Fever, anemia, weakness, and heart murmur
      b. Inflammation of the heart
      c. May result in death

Other Microbial Diseases of the Circulatory System

A. Bacterial infections
   1. Tularemia
      a. Etiology—*Francisella tularensis*
      b. Pathogenesis—transmitted by biting arthropods, contact with infected tissue, aerosols, and ingestion of contaminated food or water
      c. Clinical findings and symptoms
         (1) Enlargement of lymph nodes
         (2) Fever, malaise, headache, regional pain
   2. Rickettsial infections
      a. Etiology—obligate intracellular parasites
      b. Pathogenesis
         (1) Transmitted by arthropods such as fleas, lice, mites, and ticks
         (2) Rocky Mountain spotted fever (tick vector)
         (3) Typhus (fleaborne, common in rats)
         (4) Rickettsialpox (mouse-mite vector)—usually involves fever, rash, and vasculitis

B. Protozoan infections
   1. Malaria—*Plasmodium* spp.
      a. Spread by mosquitoes
      b. Symptoms—shaking, chills, fever, headache, and nausea, which appear at 2- to 3-day intervals

2. Babesiosis—*Babesia microti*
   a. Spread by ticks
   b. Symptoms similar to those of malaria
   c. Symptoms more serious in immunocompromised host
C. Viral infections
   1. Infectious mononucleosis
      a. Etiology—Epstein-Barr virus (EBV)
      b. Pathogenesis
         (1) Transmitted by kissing or sharing drinking glasses with an infected person
         (2) Involves lymph nodes and the spleen; increase in lymphocytes
      c. Clinical findings and symptoms
         (1) Acute leukemia-like infection
         (2) Primarily found in young adults
         (3) Symptoms include mild jaundice, fever, enlarged and tender lymph nodes, sore throat, bleeding gingiva, and general weakness
   2. Cytomegalovirus (CMV) infections
      a. Etiology—cytomegalovirus
      b. Pathogenesis
         (1) Cytomegalic inclusion disease is caused by intrauterine or perinatal infection
         (2) Virus may persist in organs in a latent state or as a chronic infection
         (3) CMV mononucleosis occurs spontaneously or through blood transfusions
         (4) The route of infection in older infants, children, and adults is unknown
      c. Clinical findings and symptoms
         (1) May result in death in infants
         (2) Prematurity, jaundice, pneumonitis, central nervous system damage, and mental or motor retardation can occur in infants
         (3) Acquired infection in children results in hepatitis, pneumonitis, and anemia
         (4) CMV mononucleosis produces a mononucleosis-like disease

Infections of the Reproductive and Urinary Systems

Reproductive System Infections

A. Bacterial infections
   1. Gonorrhea
      a. Etiology—*N. gonorrhoeae*, a gram-negative aerobic bacterium; often co-infection with *Chlamydia trachomatis*
      b. Pathogenesis
         (1) Risk of infection is 20% to 30% from a single exposure for men; higher percentage for women

(2) Grows primarily in the genitourinary tract; possesses pili that allow attachment to mucosal cells and resist phagocytosis; can infect the eye, rectum, and throat
(3) Type of host epithelium influences invasiveness
   (a) Columnar and transitional epithelia highly susceptible
   (b) Stratified squamous epithelium highly resistant
   c. Clinical findings and symptoms
      (1) Sometimes found in the pharynx; localized yellow or gray-white raised patches or generalized lesions with a gray membrane; the membrane sloughs, leaving a bright area; seen on the gingiva, tongue, and soft palate; may have itching or burning
      (2) Gonococcal glossitis (Figure 9-4)
      (3) The newborn's eyes may be infected while the baby is passing through the birth canal (ophthalmia neonatorum); use of silver nitrate or antibiotic after birth alleviates the condition
      (4) Men experience painful and frequent urination and discharge containing mucus and pus
      (5) Women often do not have symptoms; may have urethral or vaginal discharge, backache, or abdominal pain (pelvic inflammatory disease)
      (6) Oral infection results in pharyngitis, glossitis, or stomatitis, including some areas of ulceration
      (7) Complications include sterility, disseminated infection, and meningitis

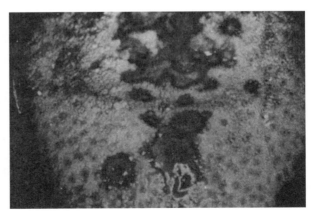

FIGURE 9-4 Gonococcal glossitis. *(Courtesy of Beverly Entwistle Isman, formerly with the Department of Applied Dentistry, University of Colorado School of Dentistry, Denver.)*

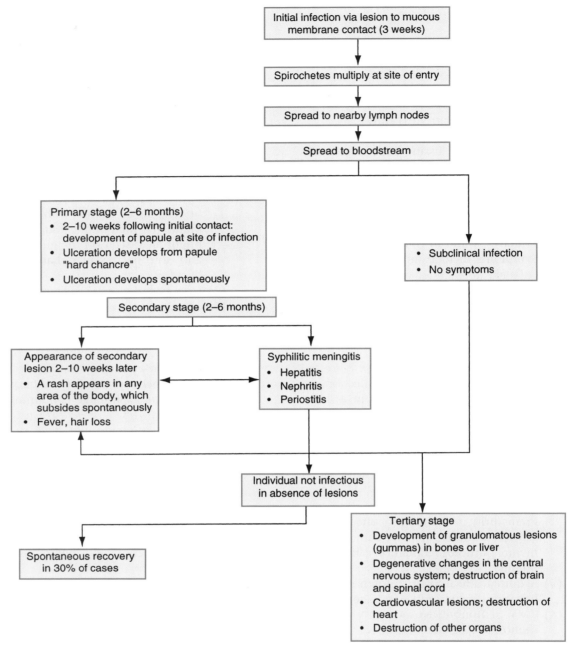

FIGURE 9-5 Primary, secondary, and tertiary stages of syphilis.

2. Syphilis (Figure 9-5)
  a. Etiology
    (1) *T. pallidum*
    (2) Spirochete, anaerobic
  b. Pathogenesis
    (1) Usually transmitted by sexual contact with skin or mucous membrane lesions of an infected person
    (2) Infection limited to the human host
    (3) Congenital syphilis occurs when the organism crosses the placenta

    (4) *T. pallidum* can pass through abraded skin and can probably pass through intact mucous membranes
    (5) If the organisms gain access to the circulatory system, they can affect all organs and spread rapidly to the lymphatic system and bloodstream
  c. Clinical findings and symptoms (Figure 9-6)
    (1) Primary stage—chancre, a single granulomatous lesion; often asymptomatic; common on the lips; may involve the

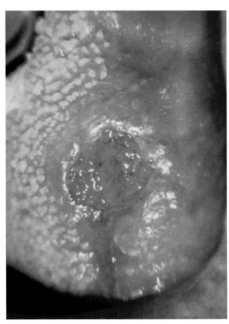

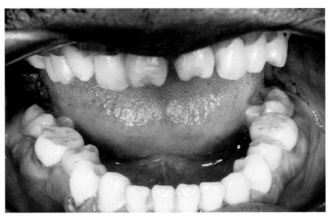

FIGURE 9-7 Congenital syphilis. The patient exhibits anomalously shaped teeth, consisting of incisors with screwdriver-shaped crowns and notched incisal edges and molars with constricted crowns and a lack of cuspal development (mulberry molars). *(From Sapp JP, Eversole LR, Wysocki GP:* Contemporary oral and maxillofacial pathology, *ed 2, St Louis, 2004, Mosby.)*

FIGURE 9-6 Chancre lesion of primary syphilis. *(From Sapp JP, Eversole LR, Wysocki GP:* Contemporary oral and maxillofacial pathology, *ed 2, St Louis, 2004, Mosby.)*

tongue and oral mucosa; highly contagious; occurs 2 to 3 weeks after exposure and lasts 3 to 5 weeks; red, small, elevated nodule; heals spontaneously; no scarring

(2) Secondary stage

    (a) Appears 6 to 8 weeks after exposure; the patient can be asymptomatic for 2 to 6 months, and then secondary lesions appear

    (b) Flu-like symptoms

    (c) Skin rashes—maculopapular rash on the face, hands, and feet

    (d) Mucous patches on the lips, soft palate, and tongue—painless shallow ulcers; grayish white areas may be removed, leaving red areas of erosion; highly contagious

    (e) Swollen lymph nodes

(3) Tertiary stage

    (a) Gumma—inflammatory granulomatous lesion with a central zone of necrosis; may be on the tongue, palate (perforation), or facial bones; soft, swollen areas or tumors; not contagious and usually asymptomatic

    (b) Often takes 5 to 20 years to develop

    (c) Involvement of the central nervous system and spinal cord leads to paresis, loss of fine-muscle coordination, and personality changes

    (d) Involvement of the cardiovascular system—major cause of death

(4) Congenital syphilis

    (a) Hutchinson's incisors—notched, bell shaped (Figure 9-7)

    (b) "Mulberry molars"—first molars are irregular with poorly developed cusps (see Figure 9-8)

    (c) Skin, mucous membrane lesions

    (d) High mortality

3. Nongonococcal urethritis

  a. Etiology—*C. trachomatis*

  b. Pathogenesis—via sexual contact

  c. Clinical findings and symptoms

    (1) Symptoms in men are similar to those of gonorrhea but less severe

    (2) Women have a muco-purulent cervical discharge; the disease may extend to the fallopian tubes or the endometrium and lead to infertility

4. Toxic shock syndrome (TSS)

  a. Etiology—*S. aureus*

  b. Pathogenesis

    (1) Short incubation period of 1 to 8 hours

    (2) The toxin is produced by the microorganism

  c. Clinical findings and symptoms

    (1) Rash, nausea, violent vomiting, and diarrhea, but no fever

    (2) Rapid convalescence

    (3) Often occurs within 5 days of the onset of menses

    (4) Can recur

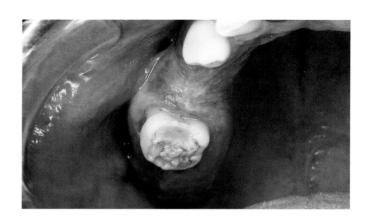

FIGURE 9-8 "Mulberry molars" of congenital syphilis. *(Courtesy of Beverly Entwistle Isman, formerly with the Department of Applied Dentistry, University of Colorado School of Dentistry, Denver.)*

B. Viral infections
   1. Genital herpes
      a. Etiology
         (1) Herpesvirus
         (2) HSV-2—herpes genitalis (genital herpes)
      b. Pathogenesis—transmitted by sexual contact
      c. Clinical findings and symptoms
         (1) Lesions appear 2 to 7 days after exposure
         (2) Lesions appear in or on the genitalia and skin
         (3) Lesions may ulcerate early and be painful or crust over
         (4) Fever, lymphadenopathy, malaise, anorexia
         (5) Initial lesions subside and heal in 2 to 3 weeks
         (6) Recurrent lesions have a milder course
         (7) Highly infectious
         (8) Primary and recurrent infections
            (a) Most (90%) primary infections are subclinical
            (b) Recurrent infections in women often serve as a source of neonatal herpes

Urinary Tract Infections
A. Etiology—primarily caused by *E. coli*
B. Pathogenesis—predisposing conditions
   1. Diabetes mellitus
   2. Neurologic diseases (e.g., polio and spinal cord injury)
   3. Lesions (e.g., kidney stones) interfering with urine flow
   4. Eclampsia of pregnancy
C. Clinical findings and symptoms
   1. Blood in urine
   2. Accumulation of fluid in tissue
   3. Pain

Infections of the Central Nervous System

A. Bacterial infections
   1. Meningitis
      a. Etiology
         (1) Aseptic meningitis—caused by a variety of agents including viruses, spirochetes, bacteria, mycoplasmas, or chlamydias
         (2) Meningococcal meningitis—caused by *Neisseria meningitidis*
      b. Pathogenesis—meningococcal meningitis is transmitted by droplet inhalation
      c. Clinical findings and symptoms
         (1) Aseptic meningitis produces an acute onset, fever, headache, and stiff neck
         (2) Meningococcal meningitis produces headache, vomiting, stiff neck, and coma within a few hours
B. Viral infections
   1. Poliomyelitis
      a. Etiology—poliomyelitis virus
      b. Pathogenesis—virus transmitted through the mouth and intestines
      c. Clinical findings and symptoms
         (1) Flaccid paralysis; destruction of motor neurons in the spinal cord
         (2) Acute inflammation of the meninges
         (3) May range from mild illness to paralysis
   2. Rabies
      a. Etiology—rabies virus
      b. Pathogenesis
         (1) Transmitted to humans through the bite of a rabid animal
         (2) Incubation period is 4 to 6 weeks or longer
      c. Clinical findings and symptoms—include visual difficulties, painful throat spasms, convulsions, and respiratory paralysis

3. Viral encephalitis
   a. Etiology—commonly caused by arboviruses
   b. Pathogenesis—virus replicates in, and is spread by, arthropods, usually mosquitoes or ticks
   c. Clinical findings and symptoms
      (1) Causes extensive nervous tissue damage and encephalitis
      (2) Symptoms—include fever, chills, nausea, fatigue, drowsiness, pain, stiff neck, general disorientation, blindness, deafness, and paralysis
C. Protozoan infection—toxoplasmosis
   1. Etiology
      a. *Toxoplasma gondii*
      b. Sources include infected cat feces, contaminated raw meat and soil, and rodents (cats may eat infected mice)
   2. Pathogenesis
      a. Inhaling or ingesting cysts when handling cat litter or sandboxes frequented by the infected cat
      b. Eating raw meat
      c. Through the placenta (pregnant women must not eat raw or undercooked meat and handle litter boxes)
   3. Clinical findings and symptoms
      a. Resembles infectious mononucleosis in adults
      b. Congenital infection can lead to stillbirth, psychomotor dysfunction, blindness, and other congenital defects
D. Fungal infection—cryptococcosis
   1. Etiology—*C. neoformans*
   2. Pathogenesis
      a. The organism tends to reside in pigeon droppings
      b. Transmitted by inhalation of dehydrated yeasts
   3. Clinical findings and symptoms
      a. Meningitis most common; often associated with immunocompromised patients
      b. Disseminated disease can affect skin, lungs, or other organs

Infections of the Eye

A. Bacterial infections
   1. Conjunctivitis
      a. Etiology—*Haemophilus aegyptius*
      b. Clinical findings
         (1) Purulent conjunctivitis
         (2) Epidemic in warmer climates
   2. Trachoma-inclusion conjunctivitis
      a. Etiology—*C. trachomatis*

   b. Pathogenesis—transmitted through person-to-person contact; associated with poor sanitation and poor personal hygiene
   c. Clinical findings and symptoms
      (1) Inflammation of conjunctiva; scarring of eyelids or cornea; can lead to secondary infection; can lead to partial or complete blindness
      (2) "Swimming pool conjunctivitis," which results in conjunctival inflammation; is usually self-limiting
B. Viral infections
   1. Adenovirus infection
      a. Etiology—adenoviruses
      b. Pathogenesis
         (1) Hand-to-eye contact is the most significant factor
         (2) "Swimming pool conjunctivitis" most likely transmitted by the waterborne route
      c. Clinical findings and symptoms—inflammation of the conjunctiva, excessive lacrimation, periorbital edema
   2. Enterovirus type 70 is one of the causes of acute hemorrhagic conjunctivitis
   3. Herpetic keratitis
      a. Etiology—primarily caused by HSV-1; occasionally by HSV-2
      b. Pathogenesis—cytolytic, herpetic infection of the cornea
      c. Clinical findings and symptoms
         (1) Severe keratoconjunctivitis; corneal ulcers or vesicles on the eyelids
         (2) May recur
         (3) May cause blindness

Chemotherapeutic Agents

See Tables 9-12 and 9-13.

MICROBIOLOGY OF THE ORAL CAVITY

NORMAL ORAL FLORA

A. Composition and distribution—different types of surfaces create distinct habitats within the mouth, so the distribution of microflora is not uniform throughout the mouth (Table 9-14)
   1. Lips—predominantly facultatively anaerobic streptococci; *Streptococcus vestibularis* found in the vestibule
   2. Palate—predominantly *Actinomyces* spp. and *Streptococcus* spp.

TABLE 9-12 Choice of Antibacterial Agents for Therapy

Causative Organism	Disease	Agent(s) of First Choice
Gram-Negative Cocci		
Neisseria gonorrhoeae	Gonorrhea	Ceftriaxone
Neisseria meningitidis	Meningitis	Penicillin
Gram-Positive Cocci		
Enterococcus spp.	Endocarditis	Ampicillin or vancomycin ± gentamicin
	Urinary tract infection	Ampicillin, amoxicillin
Staphylococcus aureus	Furuncles, abscesses, pneumonia, meningitis, osteomyelitis, bacteremia, endocarditis	
Non–penicillinase producing		Penicillin
Penicillinase producing		Methicillin, oxacillin
Methicillin resistant		Vancomycin
Streptococcus pneumoniae	Pneumonia	Penicillin*
Streptococcus		
Group A	Strep throat, scarlet fever, postpartum fever, erysipelas	Penicillin
Group B	Neonatal meningitis, bacteremia	Penicillin, ampicillin
V rindans group	Endocarditis	Penicillin ± gentamicin
Other (including anaerobic) streptococci		Penicillin
Gram-Positive Bacilli		
Actinomyces spp.	Actinomycosis	Penicillin
Bacillus anthracis	Anthrax	Ciprofloxacin, doxycycline
Clostridium perfringens	Gas gangrene	Penicillin ± clindamycin
Clostridium tetani	Tetanus	Metronidazole
Corynebacterium diphtheria	Diphtheria	Erythromycin
Listeria monocytogenes	Meningitis, bacteremia	Ampicillin
Nocardia spp.	Nocardiosis	Trimethoprim–sulfamethoxazole
Gram-Negative Bacilli		
Prevotella	Anaerobic infections	
– Mouth strains		Penicillin
– Gastrointestinal strains		Metronidazole
Brucella spp.	Brucellosis	Doxycycline ± rifampin or gentamicin
Enterobacter spp.	Urinary tract infection	Imipenem
Escherichia coli	Urinary tract infection	A cephalosporin
Francisella tularensis	Tularemia	Streptomycin, gentamicin
Haemophilus influenzae	Meningitis, epiglottitis	Cefotaxime, ceftriaxone
Klebsiella spp.	Pneumonia, urinary tract infection	A cephalosporin
Legionella spp.	Pneumonia	Erythromycin ± rifampin
Proteus mirabilis	Urinary tract infection	Ampicillin
Proteus, Providencia spp.	Urinary tract infection	Cefotaxime, ceftizoxime, ceftriaxone
Pseudomonas aeruginosa	Urinary tract infection	A fluoroquinolone
	Other infections	Ticarcillin, mezlocillin ± an aminoglycoside

TABLE 9-12 Choice of Antibacterial Agents for Therapy—cont'd

Causative Organism	Disease	Agent(s) of First Choice
Salmonella spp.	Typhoid, paratyphoid, enteritis	Ceftriaxone, a fluoroquinolone
Shigella	Dysentery	A fluoroquinolone
Vibrio cholera	Cholera	Tetracycline
Yersinia pestis	Plague	Streptomycin, gentamicin
Acid-Fast Bacilli		
Mycobacterium tuberculosis	Tuberculosis	Isoniazid ± rifampin ± pyrazinamide
Mycobacterium leprae	Hansen's disease (leprosy)	Dapsone ± rifampin ± clofazimine
Spirochetes		
Borrelia burgdorferi	Lyme disease	Ceftriaxone, doxycycline, amoxicillin
Borrelia recurrentis	Relapsing fever	Tetracycline
Leptospira interrogans	Leptospirosis	Penicillin
Treponema pallidum	Syphilis	Penicillin
Other Bacteria		
Mycoplasma pneumoniae	Pneumonia	Erythromycin, azithromycin, clarithromycin, tetracycline
Rickettsia spp.	Rocky Mountain spotted fever, typhus and other fevers	Tetracycline
Chlamydia psittaci	Psittacosis	Erythromycin
Chlamydia trachomatis	Inclusion conjunctivitis, pneumonia	Doxycycline or azithromycin
	Urethritis, cervicitis	Tetracycline
	Lymphogranuloma venereum	
Chlamydia pneumoniae	Pneumonia	Doxycycline

Penicillin-allergic patients are often treated with erythromycin or clarithromycin. Resistant strains are treated with vancomycin ± rifampin.
Modified from Morello JA, Mizer HE, Granato PA: Microbiology in patient care, ed 6, Boston, 1998, WCB/McGraw-Hill.

TABLE 9-13 Antimicrobial Agents for Fungi, Parasites, and Viruses

Agent	Mechanism of Action	Susceptible Microorganisms	Comments
Antifungal Agents			
Amphotericin B	Binds to sterols in fungal cell membranes, increasing their permeability and causing leakage of cellular constituents	Systemic fungi, including *Paracoccidioides brasiliensis, Coccidioides immitis, Cryptococcus neoformans, Histoplasma capsulatum, Sporothrix schenckii, Blastomyces dermatitidis, Candida* spp., *Aspergillus fumigatus*	Toxic for mammalian cells that contain sterols, such as certain kidney cells and erythrocytes; used only for severe systemic fungal infections; may have activity against some protozoa (*Leishmania, Naegleria*)
Flucytosine	Degrades in cell to an antimetabolite; also inhibits deoxyribonucleic acid (DNA) synthesis	Some *Cryptococcus, Candida* spp.	Used only for serious infections caused by susceptible strains of *Cryptococcus* and *Candida*, or topically in ophthalmic preparations

Continued

TABLE 9-13 Antimicrobial Agents for Fungi, Parasites, and Viruses—cont'd

Agent	Mechanism of Action	Susceptible Microorganisms	Comments
Griseofulvin	Interrupts fungal cell mitosis; causes defective DNA production	Ringworm fungi, including species of *Trichophyton*, *Microsporum*, and *Epidermophyton*	Used to treat ringworm infections of the hair, skin, and nails only; may need treatment for a year or longer for fungal nail infections
Ketoconazole*	Alters cellular membranes and increases cell permeability	Active against a wide range of systemic and ringworm fungi (see above) and *Candida* spp.	Given orally for systemic and superficial fungal infections; not recommended for fungal meningitis; topical preparation available; may cause liver toxicity
Miconazole	Alters cellular membranes and interferes with intracellular enzymes	Same as ketoconazole	Given orally or intravenously for severe systemic fungal infections and intravenously for fungal meningitis; may be effective for eye infections caused by the parasite *Acanthamoeba*
Nystatin	Binds to sterols in fungal cell membranes and alters their permeability	*Candida* spp.	Used orally or topically for local, but not systemic, *Candida* infections
Terbinafine	Kills fungal cells by inhibiting an enzyme important for synthesis of the fungal cell wall and membrane	Ringworm fungi, yeasts	Used to treat ringworm infections, especially of the nails; requires 6 weeks of therapy for fingernail infections and 12 weeks for toenail infections; may cause liver dysfunction and skin reactions
Anti-parasitic Agents			
Albendazole	Kills worms and their larvae by interfering with adenosine triphosphate (ATP) production and thus causing depletion of energy	Larval forms of *Taenia solium* and *Echinococcus granulosus*	The first drug approved in the United States for treating neurocysticercosis and hydatid cyst disease, the infections caused by these organisms; effective in 70%–80% of patients
Chloroquine	Binds to nucleoproteins and interferes with protein synthesis	*Plasmodium* spp.	Effective against circulating forms of malarial parasites, but not *P. falciparum* gametocytes; many *P. falciparum* strains now resistant
Emetine	Causes nuclear degeneration; interferes with trophozoite multiplication	*Entamoeba histolytica* trophozoites	Used in severe amebic dysentery only; used in combination with iodoquinol to completely eradicate disease
Iodoquinol	Unknown	*Entamoeba histolytica*	Used alone for treating mild or asymptomatic intestinal disease; or in combination with emetine for severe disease
Mebendazole	Inhibits uptake of glucose by helminths, depleting glycogen stores and interfering with absorptive and secretory functions	Pathogenic roundworms, including hookworm, pinworm, whipworm, threadworm; some tapeworms (beef, pork, dwarf), *Echinococcus* larvae (hydatid cyst)	Highly effective in curing infection caused by susceptible worms
Niclosamide	Inhibits mitochondrial oxidative phosphorylation in worms	Most tapeworms, pinworm	Does not act on larval or tissue stage of tapeworm infection (cysticercosis)
Piperazine	Causes paralysis of the worm by inhibiting nerve transmissions at neuromuscular junctions	*Ascaris lumbricoides* (roundworm), *Enterobius vermicularis* (pinworm)	Effective only when given in multiple doses

TABLE 9-13 Antimicrobial Agents for Fungi, Parasites, and Viruses—cont'd

Agent	Mechanism of Action	Susceptible Microorganisms	Comments
Praziquantel	Unknown, but result is paralysis of the worm's suckers, causing the worm to dislodge from the intestine	*Schistosoma* spp., flukes, some tapeworms, larval stage of *T. solium*	Highly effective against susceptible worms
Primaquine	Interferes with DNA function of malarial parasites	*Plasmodium* spp.	Active against tissue forms of malarial parasites and *P. falciparum* gametocytes; not active against other erythrocytic forms, therefore must be used in conjunction with chloroquine to eradicate all parasite forms
Pyrimethamine	Folic acid inhibitor similar to the antibacterial trimethoprim	*Toxoplasma gondii, Plasmodium* spp.	Used with a sulfonamide to treat toxoplasmosis; less effective against malarial parasites than other drugs
Quinacrine	Unclear, but may inhibit nucleic acid synthesis in *Giardia lamblia*	*G. lamblia*, tapeworms, blood forms of malarial parasites (*Plasmodium* spp.)	Drug of choice for giardiasis; used for chemoprophylaxis against malaria; not effective for circulating gametocytes of *P. falciparum*
Thiabendazole	Unclear, but may deprive worm of energy source by decreasing formation of ATP	Most intestinal roundworms	Drug of choice for *Strongyloides* infections; variable results against other roundworms
Antiviral Agents Acyclovir	Interferes with DNA synthesis and inhibits viral replication of herpes simplex and varicella zoster viruses; others unknown	Herpes virus family (including herpes simplex virus, varicella zoster virus, Epstein-Barr virus, cytomegalovirus)	Used for treating initial and recurring herpes simplex infections in immunocompromised children and adults; in the immunocompetent host, used only against severe genital herpes; some herpes viruses now resistant
Amantadine[†]	Prevents the virus from penetrating the host cell or inhibits uncoating so that the virus cannot replicate	Influenza A virus only	Virustatic drug; effective primarily for prophylaxis or symptomatic treatment of early influenza A; most effective when given on exposure before symptoms develop
Didanosine	Competitively inhibits reverse transcriptase enzyme; causes premature termination of viral replication	Retroviruses, including human immunodeficiency virus (HIV)	Used for the treatment of patients with advanced HIV infection (acquired immune deficiency syndrome, AIDS) who cannot tolerate zidovudine therapy or who deteriorate clinically and immunologically during zidovudine therapy
Ganciclovir	Competes with guanosine compound for uptake into viral DNA, interferes with DNA synthesis	Herpesvirus family	Used almost exclusively to treat human cytomegalovirus infections, especially in immunosuppressed organ or bone marrow transplant patients; some viruses already resistant
Lamivudine	Interferes with viral DNA synthesis by acting as a competitive inhibitor of the viral reverse transcriptase enzyme	HIV	Approved for use in combination with zidovudine; may delay viral development of resistance to zidovudine or improve its effectiveness

Continued

TABLE 9-13 Antimicrobial Agents for Fungi, Parasites, and Viruses—cont'd

Agent	Mechanism of Action	Susceptible Microorganisms	Comments
Ribavirin	Interferes with ribonucleic acid (RNA) and DNA synthesis, inhibiting protein synthesis and replication	In vitro, many RNA and DNA viruses	Available in the United States only for aerosol therapy; used in infants to treat severe lower respiratory infections caused by respiratory syncytial virus
Saquinavir	Blocks the action of a protease vital to the final stages of viral replication; the first of a type of drug known as a protease inhibitor to gain the U.S. Food and Drug Administration (FDA) approval	HIV	Approved for use in combination with zidovudine; does not work well alone; ritonavir and indinavir are newer such drugs now in use in combination with zidovudine and other anti-HIV drugs
Zalcitabine	Same as didanosine	HIV	Approved for use only in combination with zidovudine for adults with full-blown AIDS
Zidovudine	Inhibits reverse transcriptase enzyme in retroviruses	Retroviruses, including HIV	An "orphan" drug used only to treat symptomatic HIV infections (AIDS)

*A number of anti-fungal imidazole drugs that are similar to ketoconazole in mechanisms of action and spectra of antifungal activity are available as topical preparations. These agents, which include clotrimazole, econazole, and terconazole, are not used to treat serious systemic disease.
†Rimantadine, a similar agent for prophylaxis of influenza A, may produce fewer side effects than does amantadine.
Modified from Morello JA, Mizer HE, Granato PA: Microbiology in patient care, ed 6, Boston, 1998, WCB/McGraw-Hill.

3. Cheek—predominantly *Streptococcus* spp. and *Haemophilus* spp.; 5 to 25 bacteria per epithelial cell
   a. Majority of streptococci are *S. oralis* and *S. mitis*, and fewer are *S. sanguis*
   b. *Simonsiella* spp. isolated primarily from human cheek cells
4. Tongue (100 bacteria per tongue epithelial cell)—papillae allow for a large surface area for colonization, resulting in higher bacterial density and diverse microflora
   a. Predominantly *S. oralis*, *S. mitis*, and *Streptococcus salivarius*
   b. *Stomatococcus mucilagenosus* is found exclusively on the tongue
   c. *Veillonella* spp., *Actinomyces naeslundii*, *Actinomyces odontolyticus*, and *Haemophilus* spp. also isolated
   d. Increased numbers of *Porphyromonas*, *Prevotella*, *Fusobacterium*, and *Treponema* spp. lead to halitosis resulting from an increase in volatile sulfur compound production
5. Saliva—108 to 109 bacteria/mL of saliva; normal salivary flow ensures that bacteria do not multiply in saliva; so saliva does not contain resident flora but rather bacteria from other surfaces—primarily from the dorsum of the tongue and dental plaque

6. Tooth surfaces (plaque)
   a. Pits and fissures
      (1) Morphologic condition allows for proliferation
      (2) Predominantly *S. mutans* and *A. naeslundii*
      (3) Common sites for caries
   b. Interproximal surfaces
      (1) Inaccessible to routine oral hygiene care
      (2) Bacteria in biofilm can proliferate in microcolonies undisturbed
      (3) Predominantly *A. naeslundii*, *Actinomyces israelii*, *Streptococcus* spp., *Veillonella* spp., and *Prevotella* spp.
      (4) Majority of streptococci are *S. sanguis*
      (5) Common site for caries
   c. Smooth coronal surfaces
      (1) Can be covered with plaque if oral hygiene is not practiced
      (2) Plaque formation limited by the cleaning action of saliva, the movement of soft tissue, and the action of food particles
      (3) Oral bacteria colonize in a predictable succession
B. Factors that influence microbial composition
   1. Temperature 35°C to 36°C
      a. Temperature may influence proportions of bacterial species

TABLE 9-14 Bacterial Genera Found in the Oral Cavity

	Gram-Positive	Gram-Negative
Cocci	Abiotrophia	Moraxella
	Enterococcus	Neisseria
	Peptostreptococcus	Veillonella
	Staphylococcus	
	Stomatococcus	
	Streptococcus	
Rods	Actinomyces	Aggregibacter
	Bifidobacterium	Campylobacter
	Corynebacterium	Cantonella
	Eubacterium	Capnocytophaga
	Lactobacillus	Centipeda
	Propionibacterium	Desulfovibrio
	Pseudoramibacter	Desulfobacter
	Rothia	Eikenella
		Fusobacterium
		Haemophilus
		Johnsonii
		Leptotrichia
		Porphyromonas
		Prevotella
		Selenomonas
		Simonsiella
		Tannerella
		Treponema
		Wolinella

  b. Periodontal pockets with active disease have higher temperatures—up to 39°C
2. Nutrient sources
  a. Exogenous sources include the host's diet, especially dietary sugar, which is needed for acid and polysaccharide production
  b. Endogenous sources
   (1) Saliva
   (2) Gingival exudate
   (3) Epithelial cells and leukocytes
   (4) Continuing existence of flora even when humans and animals are fed by a stomach tube
   (5) Certain bacteria use metabolic byproducts from other bacteria

3. pH requirements
  a. The pH of most surfaces regulated by saliva (pH 6.75–7.25)
  b. Dietary sugars provide a selective force favoring predominance of certain organisms that tolerate an acidic medium (pH 5)
  c. Strains of *S. mutans*, related streptococci, and lactobacilli are both acidogenic (produce acid) and aciduric (tolerate low pH values)
  d. Dairy products can elevate pH
  e. The pH of the gingival sulcus becomes alkaline during the host inflammatory response in periodontal disease (pH 7.2–7.8)
  f. Alkaline pockets favor the growth of the pathogen *Porphyromonas gingivalis*
4. Oxygen concentration
  a. Distribution of microorganisms in the mouth is related to the redox potential at a particular site
  b. The majority of organisms are microaerophilic, facultative, or obligate anaerobes
5. Microbial interactions
  a. Microbial aggregation
   (1) Certain species undergo reactions between host cell surfaces (adhesion–receptor)
   (2) Bacterial cells can attach to each other (co-aggregation)
   (3) Some bacteria produce extracellular polysaccharides (glucans, fructans, heteropolysaccharides) that provide structural and energy sources for plaque
  b. Interspecies antagonisms
   (1) Competition for host receptors
   (2) Competition for endogenous nutrients
   (3) Production of inhibitory substances (e.g., hydrogen peroxide by *S. mitis* and *S. sanguis*; bacteriocin by streptococci; formation of acid by *S. mutans*, *S. salivarius*, and lactobacilli)
6. Saliva
  a. Nonspecific factors
   (1) The flow of saliva removes planktonic bacteria from oral surfaces
   (2) The flow rate bears some relationship to caries susceptibility
   (3) The rate of secretion is correlated to buffering capacity
   (4) Proteins and glycoproteins form acquired pellicles on teeth; bacteria can attach to the pellicle
   (5) Proteins and glycoproteins act as nutrient source for microflora
   (6) Proteins and glycoproteins can aid in co-aggregation of bacteria, thus facilitating their clearance

(7) Antibacterial components include lysozymes, lactoperoxidase, lacto-ferrin, salivary thiocyanate, and peptides
   b. Specific factors—secretory immunoglobulin A inhibits microbial attachment
7. Host factors that affect microflora
   a. Oral hygiene—antimicrobial agents in toothpaste and mouthrinses; mechanical force of toothbrush and interdental care
   b. Gender and race
   c. Age
   d. Alterations in the food web
   e. Long-term use of antibiotics and the development of antimicrobial resistance
   f. Scratches and grooves on tooth surfaces or restorations, or margins between dental restorations and tooth surface that enhance biofilm formation
   g. Genetics

Development of Oral Microflora

A. The oral cavity is usually sterile at birth
B. Initial colonization of the infant's mouth by the microflora of the mother, milk, water, and saliva of those in close contact
   1. Oral microflora consist of aerobic and facultatively anaerobic gram-positive species
   2. *S. salivarius*, *S. oralis*, and *S. mitis* predominate by the first month of the infant's life
C. The microflora diversify in the next few months with several gram-negative anaerobes—*Prevotella melaninogenica*, *S. nucleatum*, and *Veillonella* spp.
D. At 12 months, most children have the following organisms:
   1. Streptococci
      a. *S. salivarius*, *S. oralis*, and *S. mitis* predominate
      b. *S. mutans* and *S. sanguis* are not established until tooth eruption
      c. *S. mutans* disappears when full-mouth extractions occur; reappears with dentures
   2. Staphylococci
   3. *Veillonella* spp.
   4. *Neisseria* spp.
   5. *Actinomyces* spp.
   6. Lactobacilli
   7. *Nocardia* spp.
   8. *Fusobacterium* spp.
E. Preschool-age child
   1. Adult-like microflora
   2. *Prevotella melaninogenica* and spirochetes not common at age 5 years, but increase in numbers by age 13 years
F. Relatively stable oral microflora in healthy adults

G. Age-related changes in oral microflora
   1. Increase in numbers of yeast (*C. albicans*) may be associated with increased denture wear, changes in the oral mucosa, blood glucose level, and malnutrition
   2. Increased use of medications common with aging; may decrease salivary flow

BACTERIAL PLAQUE

See the section on "Bacterial plaque biofilm" in Chapter 14.
A. Definition
   1. Deposit formed by the colonization of teeth by members of the normal oral flora
   2. Complex of bacteria in the matrix mainly of bacterial polysaccharides; biofilm
   3. Bacteria embedded in an exopolymeric matrix that provides a protective environment for bacteria
B. Stages of formation
   1. Cell-free pellicle
      a. High-molecular-weight salivary glycoproteins
      b. Quickly colonized by bacteria
   2. Supragingival plaque formation
      a. Phase I: Initiation
         (1) Begins in 1–2 days of plaque accumulation
         (2) Gram-positive cocci and short rods show early dominance
         (3) Streptococci (aerobe)
      b. Phase II:
         (1) 2–4 days of plaque accumulation
         (2) Cocci still dominate, but gram-positive rods and gram-negative cocci begin to appear
         (3) *S. sanguis*, *S. oralis*, or *S. mitis* usually first colonizer but *Haemophilus* and *Neisseria* spp. may also be early colonizers
      c. Phase III
         (1) 4–7 days of plaque accumulation
         (2) After 7 days, streptococci remain the dominant organism, but by day 8, their numbers decrease
         (3) Filamentous bacteria (*Veillonella* and *Actinomyces* spp.) appear in 7 to 14 days
         (4) Respiration becomes increasingly anaerobic; rods and filaments predominate (increase in *Tannerella*, *Actinomyces*, *Capnocytophaga*, *Treponema*, *P. melaninogenica*, and *Fusobacterium*)
         (5) Composition of mature plaque biofilm varies with site, oxygen and nutrient sources, and level of protection

3. Subgingival plaque formation
   a. Microbiota
      (1) Vibrios and spirochetes prevalent. Anaerobic, gram-negative, motile, asaccharolytic
   b. Types
      (1) Tooth associated (attached)
      (2) Tissue associated
      (3) Unattached subgingival
C. Factors that affect adherence and retention
   1. Salivary glycoprotein
      a. Affinity for hydroxyapatite
      b. Causes bacteria to aggregate
   2. Specific bacterial attachment mechanisms
      a. Electrostatic forces
      b. Bacterial surface components (adhesions) bind specific sites of the pellicle (receptors)
      c. Hydrophobic interactions
   3. Bacterial competition
      a. Relative numbers of a species may affect colonization patterns
      b. *S. sanguis* has a stronger affinity for enamel than does *S. mutans*; fewer numbers of *S. mutans* are in saliva to compete for tooth sites
   4. Bacterial interactions—some evidence that *S. mutans* and *S. sanguis* are antagonistic
   5. Natural local cleansing activity and retentive areas
   6. Diet
D. Plaque polysaccharides
   1. Extracellular glucans—structural component of plaque
      a. Synthesized from sucrose
      b. Properties
         (1) Insoluble
         (2) May mediate attachment of bacteria to dental tissues
         (3) May entrap bacterial enzymes or metabolic products
         (4) Ability of *S. mutans* to produce glucans appears essential for cariogenicity
   2. Levans (fructans and heteropolysaccharides)—produced by *S. mutans, S. sanguis, S. salivarius, Lactobacillus* spp., *Rothia* spp., *Eubacterium* spp., and *A. naeslundii*
      a. Soluble
      b. Reserve nutrients
      c. Can be used as sources of energy in bacterial metabolism
E. Microbial composition of plaque
   1. Bacterial composition of supragingival (supramarginal) plaque
      a. Thin layer; 1 to 20 cells thick
      b. Mostly gram-positive facultative anaerobic organisms

   c. Most predominant organisms are *S. sanguis* and *A. naeslundii*
   d. Other species found include *A. israelii, S. mutans, Veillonella* and *Fusobacterium* spp., *Treponema* spp., and *Capnocytophaga* spp.
   2. Bacterial composition of normal gingival crevicular plaque
      a. Gingival crevice—an area of stagnation and bacterial proliferation—environmental influences include an increase in crevicular fluid, desquamation of epithelial cells, and bacterial acid products
      b. Quantity of species relatively constant; proportions of species vary among people and even within the same mouth
      c. Predominant organisms are *S. mitis, S. sanguis, A. naeslundii, A. odontolyticus, A. meyeri, A. georgiae, Rothia dentocariosus, Eubacterium* spp., *Fusobacterium* spp., and *Treponema* spp.
   3. Calculus
      a. Inorganic salts, 70% to 90%
      b. Microbes similar to those of the gingival crevicular area
      c. Main role in periodontal disease is to serve as a collection site for more bacteria

DENTAL CARIES

A. Prerequisites for caries development
   1. Cariogenic bacteria
   2. Supply of substrate for acid production
   3. Susceptible host
B. Cariogenic bacteria
   1. Essential properties
      a. Acidogenic and aciduric; acid must be produced and a low pH maintained for a long period
      b. Ability to attach to tooth surfaces
      c. Formation of a protective matrix
   2. Streptococci
      a. *S. mutans*
         (1) Most strongly cariogenic bacteria in animals
         (2) Hard surfaces are a prerequisite for its presence; the organisms disappear if teeth are extracted and reappear with dentures
         (3) Homo-fermentive lactic acid former
         (4) Produces insoluble and soluble glucans
         (5) A high-sucrose diet is generally associated with an increase in the *S. mutans* population
         (6) Usually found in the early stages of plaque formation

b. *S. sobrinus*
(1) A mutans streptococci
(2) Possible roles in caries are still evolving
c. *S. sanguis*
(1) Produces glucans
(2) Some strains cariogenic in animals
(3) Colonizes tooth enamel
(4) Is present in plaque and sometimes cheek
d. *S. mitis*
(1) Cariogenic in animals
(2) Found on oral soft tissues
e. *S. salivarius*
(1) Produces fructans
(2) Usually has a strong affinity for oral soft tissues, especially the tongue
(3) Some strains cariogenic in animals
3. Lactobacilli
a. Present in small numbers in plaque
b. Increase in number in the mouth when the sugar content in the diet is high
(1) Present in the mouth where sugar is retained
(2) Carious lesions act as retention sites
c. Strongly acidogenic and aciduric
d. May have important role in the progression of caries
4. Actinomyces
a. *A. naeslundii* primary cause of root-surface caries
b. Plaque-forming organisms
c. Ferment glucose to produce mostly lactic acid
d. *A. naeslundii* present on tongue, tooth surfaces, and plaque
C. Acid production in plaque
1. Decalcification of teeth caused by acids produced through bacterial fermentation
2. Cariogenic plaque, when exposed to sugar, shows a decrease in pH that is low enough to decalcify enamel within minutes; pH returns to resting levels after approximately 40 minutes; even though sugar is washed away by saliva, pH can remain at a low level for 20 minutes
3. Important features of the acid production process
a. Amount of plaque
b. Predominant microflora
c. Rate of salivary flow
d. Substrate characteristics
e. Location of plaque
4. More lactic acid present than any other acid
D. Bacterial substrates and diet
1. Sucrose
a. Main substrate for cariogenic bacteria
b. Important in the formation of smooth-surface caries
c. Metabolized to form acids and glucans

d. Essential for caries production in animals
e. Epidemiologic evidence has established its role in human caries
f. Increase in the frequency of sucrose consumption is associated with an increase in caries
g. High cariogenic effect when retained on teeth for a long period
2. Starches
a. Low cariogenicity
b. Probably influences plaque microflora
E. Host factors
1. Tooth surface
a. Caries formation influenced by tooth morphology and arch form
b. Enamel surfaces are probably more caries resistant than the subsurface
2. Saliva
a. Functions that affect the carious process
(1) Clearance of food
(2) Buffer activity
(3) Bacterial aggregation
(4) Antibacterial function (e.g., immunoglobulin A, lysozymes, salivary peroxidase)
b. Amount of ambient calcium, phosphate, and fluoride ions in the saliva for remineralization of tooth structure
c. Rate of flow and buffering abilities
(1) As flow rate increases, pH rises
(2) High salivary flow rates and buffering are associated with low caries activity

PERIODONTAL DISEASES

See the section on "Diseases of the periodontium" in Chapter 14.
A. Classification of periodontal diseases
1. Gingival diseases
a. Dental plaque–induced gingival diseases
(1) Early gingivitis
(a) Plaque is thicker (100 to 300 cells thick) and more complex than in healthy tissue
(b) Proliferation of *Fusobacterium nucleatum* and *Actinomyces* organisms
(c) Mostly gram-positive organisms
(2) Chronic gingivitis (Box 9-2)
(a) Anaerobic, gram-negative organisms increase; rods form 75% of the subgingival flora
(b) Presence of *A. naeslundii*, *Fusobacterium nucleatum*, *Prevotella intermedia*, and *Veillonella parvula*
(c) Spirochetes are elevated at affected sites

BOX 9-2 Predominant Bacteria of Experimental Gingivitis in Young Adults

GRAM-POSITIVE BACTERIA	GRAM-NEGATIVE BACTERIA
Actinomyces israelii	Prevotella oris
Actinomyces naeslundii	Prevotella intermedia
Actinomyces odontolyticus	Campylobacter spp.
Propionibacterium acnes	Veillonella parvula
Lactobacillus spp.	Fusobacterium nucleatum
Streptococcus anginosus	Treponema spp.
Streptococcus mitis	Wolinella spp.
Peptostreptococcus micros	
Eubacterium spp.	

From Marsh P, Martin MV: Oral microbiology, ed 4, Boston, 1999, Wright.

BOX 9-3 Some Bacterial Species that Have Been Commonly Implicated in Chronic Periodontitis

GRAM-POSITIVE	GRAM-NEGATIVE
Eubacterium brachy	Tannerella forsythensis
Eubacterium nodatum	Dialister pneumosintes
Eubacterium timidium	Fusobacterium nucleatum
Peptostreptococcus anaerobius	Porphyromonas gingivalis
Peptostreptococcus micros	Prevotella intermedia
	Prevotella loescheii
	Prevotella oralis
	Campylobacter rectus
	Treponema spp.
	Aggregibacter actinomyetemcomitans

b. Plaque-induced gingival disease is modified by systemic factors
  (1) Endogenous sex-steroid–hormone gingival disease (pubertal-associated gingivitis, pregnancy-associated gingivitis, menstrual gingivitis)
  (2) Diabetes mellitus–associated gingivitis
  (3) Hematologic (leukemic) gingival disease
  (4) Drug-influenced gingival enlargement
  (5) Gingival disease associated with nutrition
c. Non–plaque-induced gingival disease
  (1) Gingival disease of specific bacterial, viral, fungal, or genetic origin
  (2) Gingival manifestations of systemic conditions
  (3) Traumatic lesions, foreign-body reactions, and nonspecific gingival lesions
2. Periodontal diseases
  a. Necrotizing periodontal diseases
    (1) Necrotizing ulcerative gingivitis (NUG)
      (a) Anaerobic infection of gingival margins causes ulceration; if allowed to progress, destruction of gingivae and underlying bone occurs; onset is sudden and acute
      (b) The interproximal areas are affected first
      (c) Appears to be an opportunistic infection based on predisposing factors (e.g., plaque formation, depression of polymorphonuclear [PMN]

function, stress, poor diet, immunocompromised)
      (d) Predominant microflora include *P. intermedia*, spirochetes, and fusiform bacteria
    (2) Necrotizing ulcerative periodontitis
      (a) Appearance—necrosis of gingival tissues, periodontal ligaments, and alveolar bone
      (b) Indications—the client presents with pain and excessive necrosis
      (c) Severe and rapid periodontal destruction; lack of deep-pocket formation
      (d) Occurs in persons infected with HIV and those undergoing immunosuppressive therapies
      (e) Predominant microflora include *C. albicans*, *Haemophilus actinomycetemcomitans*, *F. nucleatum*, and *Porphyromonas gingivalis*
  b. Chronic periodontitis (slight or early; moderate; severe or advanced) (Box 9-3)
    (1) Extension of inflammatory changes into deeper periodontal structures, with resulting bone loss
    (2) May indicate multiple diseases that share similar characteristics
    (3) Pockets provide a favorable environment for bacterial growth
    (4) Different bacterial populations associated with destructive periodontitis have been described (Boxes 9-4 and 9-5)
    (5) Periodontitis can be a manifestation of systemic diseases such as hematologic or genetic disorders
    (6) Associated with abscesses of the periodontium and endodontic lesions

---

BOX 9-4 Species of Bacteria for Which Proportions in Plaque Rise with Increasing Severity of Periodontal Disease

GRAM-POSITIVE	GRAM-NEGATIVE
Eubacterium alactolyticum	*Aggregatibacter actinomycetemcomitans*
Eubacterium brachy	*Bacteroides gracilis*
Eubacterium nodatum	*Campylobacter concisus*
Eubacterium. saphenum	*Campylobacter rectus*
Eubacterium timidium	*Campylobacter curvus*
Eubacterium spp.	*Filifactor alocis*
Atopobium *rimae*	*Fusobacterium nucleatum*
Peptostreptococcus. *anaerobius*	*Prevotella denticola*
	Prevotella intermedia
	Prevotella nigrescens
	Prevotella melaninogenica
	Prevotella oris
	Prevotella tannerae
	Prevotella veroralis
	Porphyromonas gingivalis
	Selenomonas flueggei
	Selenomonas infelix
	Selenomonas noxia
	Selenomonas sputigena

BOX 9-5 Principal Bacteria Associated with Periodontal Disease

Chronic periodontitis	*Porphyromonas gingivalis, Prevotella intermedia, Campylobacter rectus, Fusobacterium nucleatum, Tannerella forsythensis*
Aggressive periodontitis	*Aggregibacter actinomycetemcomitans, P. intermedia, Eikenella corrodens, Capnocytophaga sputigena*
Necrotizing periodontal diseases	*P. gingivalis, A. actinomycetemcomitans, F. nucleatum, P. intermedia, Streptococcus* spp., *C. albicans, Treponema, Selenomonas*

---

(7) Causative organisms include *P. intermedia, Aggregatibacter actinomycetemcomitans, P. gingivalis, Eubacterium* spp., *F. nucleatum,* spirochetes, *Tannerella forsythensis,* and *Campylobacter rectus*

c. Aggressive periodontitis
  (1) Onset occurs before age 35 years and is associated with a rapid rate of progression of tissue destruction, host defense defects, and composition of subgingival flora

---

BOX 9-6 Identification of the Bacterial Cause in Periodontal Diseases

1. Large numbers of the bacteria are associated with the disease state, and absence or reduced numbers are associated with health.
2. Elimination or suppression of the organism reverses or reduces the disease.
3. Elevated host responses are associated with the disease.
4. Animal pathogenicity similar to periodontal disease occurs on implantation of the organism(s) into germ-free animals.
5. Bacteria possess potentially pathogenic mediators that could contribute to the disease process.

From Newman MG, Nisengard R: Oral microbiology and immunology, *ed 2, Philadelphia, 1994, Saunders.*

---

(2) Subclassifications are identified as:
  (a) Prepubertal periodontitis
  (b) Juvenile periodontitis—localized and generalized forms
(3) Primary organism—*Aggregatibacter actinomycetemcomitans*
(4) Clinical findings and symptoms
  (a) Periodontitis as a manifestation of systemic diseases such as hematologic or genetic disorders
  (b) Abscesses of the periodontium
  (c) Periodontitis associated with endodontic lesions
  (d) Developmental or acquired deformities and conditions

B. Bacterial plaque biofilm and periodontal disease
  1. Factors that determine the severity of periodontal disease
    a. Level of oral hygiene
    b. Type of bacteria in plaque biofilm
    c. Host resistance and immunity
  2. Evidence supports microbial cause of periodontal disease (Box 9-6)
    a. Gram-negative microorganisms are the principal bacteria associated with disease
    b. Plaque associated with gingivitis and periodontitis has different bacterial populations
  3. Pathogenic mechanisms of plaque bacteria
    a. Attachment mechanisms—attachment to the tooth surface may depend on early colonizers of tooth surface and pellicle (e.g., *Streptococcus* and *Actinomyces,* which are gram-positive organisms)
    b. Products of bacteria
      (1) Bacteria themselves may invade tissue
      (2) Products may cause tissue destruction

(a) Endotoxins

(b) Enzymes (collagenase, lysozyme, and hyaluronidase)

c. Survival mechanism—slime layer and biofilm formation

4. Immunologic aspects of periodontal disease

a. Bacteria in biofilm are antigenic in varying degrees; present a challenge to the immune system

b. Immune responses are just as likely to be protective as they are injurious to tissue

c. Mechanisms of tissue destruction may involve anaphylactic, cytotoxic, immune complex, and cell-mediated or delayed hypersensitivity reactions

d. Participation of the humoral immune system

(1) Lymphocytes and plasma cells are the predominant cells in the gingiva in the vicinity of plaque

(2) Antibody production is stimulated

(3) Complement system is activated

(a) Mediates inflammatory response and immunologic reactions

(b) Complement is activated by plaque bacteria, either by endotoxin (lipopolysaccharide) or by bacterial antigen–antibody complexes

(c) Involved in chemotaxis (directed migration of inflammatory cells)

e. Participation of the cell-mediated immune system

(1) Cell-mediated immunity leads to release of lymphokines (e.g., osteoclast-activating factor)

(2) Reports on the relationship between cell-mediated reactivity and the severity of periodontal disease are conflicting

(3) Clinically not possible to distinguish between cell-mediated immunity (resistance) and delayed hypersensitivity (damaging) reactions in humans; both reactions depend on the same cellular participants

PERIAPICAL INFECTIONS AND ORAL–FACIAL TISSUE INFECTIONS

A. Infections

1. Abscesses (periodontal and periapical)
2. Postsurgical and post-extraction wound infections
3. Endodontically involved infections
4. Sinus tract infections

5. Cellulitis
6. Traumatic injuries
7. Osteomyelitis
8. Post-extraction alveolar osteitis (dry socket)
9. Pericoronitis
10. Periodontally involved infections

B. Bacteria cultivated from such infections

1. Polymicrobial and opportunistic in nature
2. Obligate anaerobic bacteria predominate in acute endodontic infections

C. Ludwig's angina

1. Mixed infection

a. *Fusobacterium* spp., *Prevotella* spp., *Porphyromonas* spp., and streptococci

b. Often caused by the normal oral flora gaining access through the infected tooth

2. Symptoms

a. Rapidly spreading, diffuse bilateral cellulitis of the floor of the mouth and neck

b. Swelling that may block air passages

c. Fever and malaise

3. Predisposing factors

a. Infected mandibular molars

b. Thin lingual cortical plate of the mandible

OPPORTUNISTIC INFECTIONS OF THE ORAL CAVITY

A. Definition—organisms that take advantage of a compromised situation in the host and subsequently invade and cause infections of the oral cavity

B. Actinomycosis

1. Etiology

a. *A. israelii* most common

b. *A. naeslundii* and *Arachnia propionica* found in some lesions

2. Pathogenesis

a. Gram-positive bacteria; member of the normal oral flora

b. Infection may follow injury with introduction of contaminated debris into tissue

3. Clinical findings and symptoms

a. Facial swelling, most commonly in soft tissue below the angle of the jaw

b. Small, chronic, superficial mass

c. Abscess with sinus and chronic discharge develops

C. Oral candidiasis—four clinically distinct forms:

1. Pseudomembranous candidiasis

a. A removable soft, creamy, white plaque; red or bleeding base

b. Predominantly found on the buccal and labial mucosa, tongue, hard and soft palates

2. Erythematous candidiasis
   a. A smooth, flat, red lesion on the dorsum of the tongue; associated with loss of papillae
   b. Can also be found on the hard palate
3. Angular cheilitis—cracking or redness around the corners of the mouth
4. Hyperplastic candidiasis
   a. A raised, white, nonremovable plaque
   b. Appears on the buccal mucosa, hard palate, or dorsum of the tongue
D. Staphylococci
   1. Etiology—*S. aureus* and *S. epidermidis*
   2. Pathogenesis—normal flora of the skin, oral cavity, and anterior nares
   3. Clinical manifestations
      a. Mandibular osteomyelitis
      b. Acute suppurative parotitis
E. Other oral diseases
   1. Mumps
      a. Etiology—mumps virus
      b. Clinical findings and symptoms
         (1) Painful, swollen parotid or submaxillary glands
         (2) Fever and malaise
         (3) Red and swollen papilla of Stensen's duct
      c. Prevention through vaccine
   2. Herpangina (vesicular pharyngitis)
      a. Etiology—coxsackievirus A

b. Pathogenesis
   (1) Transmitted by ingestion of contaminated materials
   (2) Primarily occurs in children
c. Clinical findings and symptoms—fever and vomiting; vesicles and later ulcers on the mucous membrane of the throat, palate, or tongue
d. Recovery in 7 to 10 days; complications rare
3. Recurrent aphthous ulcers
   a. Etiology—unknown; evidence suggests immunologic etiology
   b. Clinical findings and symptoms
      (1) Canker sore, small ulcer
      (2) Covered by pseudomembrane
      (3) Surrounding erythematous halo
      (4) Occur on nonkeratinized mucosa
4. Hand-foot-and-mouth disease
   a. Etiology—coxsackievirus A
   b. Pathogenesis
      (1) Highly infectious
      (2) Typically affects many children, particularly in schools
   c. Clinical findings and symptoms
      (1) Vesicular stomatitis and rash
      (2) Affects the buccal mucosa, tongue, gingiva, lips, hands, and feet
      (3) Pain

@ WEB SITE INFORMATION AND RESOURCES

SOURCE	WEB SITE ADDRESS	DESCRIPTION
Bergey's Taxonomic Outline	http://www.bergeysoutline.com	Online publication, updated approximately six times per year and is free to registered users
Centers for Disease Control and Prevention (CDC)	http://www.cdc.gov/	One of the 13 major operating components of the Department of Health and Human Services (HHS), which is the principal U.S. government agency for protecting the health and safety of all Americans and for providing essential human services, especially for persons who are least able to help themselves
Organization for Asepsis and Safety Procedures (OSAP)	http://www.osap.org/	Promotes infection-control and related science-based health and safety policies and practices through quality education and information dissemination
Morbidity and Mortality Weekly Report (MMWR)	http://www.cdc.gov/mmwr/	The MMWR series is prepared by the CDC and provides data regarding a variety of health and safety concerns

Jessica C. Peek and the publisher acknowledge the past contributions of Marie Collins to this chapter.

CHAPTER 9 REVIEW QUESTIONS

Answers and Rationales to Review Questions are available on this text's accompanying Evolve site. See inside front cover for details.

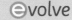

1. **What cellular structure is directly involved in protein synthesis?**
   a. Golgi complex
   b. Ribosome
   c. Mitochondrion
   d. Nucleus

2. **The type of microscopy used to observe living cells is:**
   a. Phase-contrast microscopy
   b. Fluorescence microscopy
   c. Bright-field microscopy
   d. Darkfield microscopy

3. **Identify the type of staining procedure used to determine if an organism is a spore former.**
   a. Flagellar stain
   b. Acid-fast stain
   c. Gram stain
   d. Schaeffer-Fulton stain

4. **What is the correct morphological name for cocci that appear in chains?**
   a. Staphylococci
   b. Diplococci
   c. Sarcinae
   d. Streptococci

5. **All of the following are functions of the cell wall EXCEPT one. Which one is the EXCEPTION?**
   a. Aid in adherence and gliding motility of an organism
   b. Maintains the shape of the microorganism
   c. Provides support for flagella
   d. Prevents rupture of the cell

6. **A barnacle must attach to a hard surface such as rocks, shells, or whales. When the barnacle attaches to the whale, it benefits by having a place to stay, while the whale is unaffected. This is an example of what type of relationship?**
   a. Symbiosis
   b. Predation
   c. Commensalism
   d. Parasitism

7. **In which phase of metabolism is energy consumed?**
   a. Catabolism
   b. Anabolism
   c. Glycoysis
   d. Protein synthesis

8. **An agent producing disease of pathologic change is called a (an):**
   a. Antibody
   b. Leukocyte
   c. Phagocyte
   d. Pathogen

9. **All of the following are prerequisites for the development of dental caries EXCEPT one. Which one is the EXCEPTION?**
   a. Family history of dental caries
   b. Susceptible host
   c. Supply of substrate for acid production
   d. Cariogenic bacteria

10. **A chancre is present during which stage of a syphilis infection?**
    a. Primary
    b. Secondary
    c. Tertiary
    d. Quaternary

11. **The incubation period for hepatitis A is:**
    a. 28-47 days
    b. 45-160 days
    c. 8-16 hours
    d. 15 to 50 days

12. **The structure responsible for regulating movement of materials in and out of a cell is the:**
    a. Ribosome
    b. Plastids
    c. Cytoplasmic membrane
    d. Vacuole

13. **In prokaryotic organisms, respiration occurs via what cellular structure?**
    a. Cytoplasmic membrane
    b. Mitochondria
    c. Ribosomes
    d. Lysosomes

14. **The type of media designed to increase the numbers of particular microbes to detectable levels is:**
    a. Reducing media
    b. Enriched media
    c. Selective media
    d. Differential media

15. **Which of the following pairs is mismatched?**
    a. Prokaryotes—nuclear membrane
    b. Eukaryotes—mitochondria present
    c. Prokaryotes—mitochondria absent
    d. Eukaryotes—nuclear membrane

16. **What microorganisms metabolize substances aerobically if oxygen is present or anaerobically if oxygen is absent?**
    a. Obligate aerobes
    b. Aerotolerant anaerobes
    c. Microaerophilics
    d. Facultative anaerobes

17. **Which immunoglobulin is the first to appear in a given immune response?**
    a. IgG
    b. IgE
    c. IgM
    d. IgD

18. **German measles is caused by this virus:**
    a. Rubella virus
    b. Human parvovirus B19
    c. Varicella zoster virus
    d. Papilloma virus

19. **All of the following are bacterial infections EXCEPT one. Which one is the EXCEPTION?**
    a. Conjunctivitis
    b. Toxoplasmosis
    c. Meningococcal meningitis
    d. Syphillis

20. **The bacteria primarily responsible for root caries are:**
    a. *Streptococcus mitis*
    b. *Streptococcus sanguis*
    c. *Streptococcus salivarius*
    d. *Actinomyces naeslundii*

21. **A toxemia is indicative of which type of infection?**
    a. Latent
    b. Systemic
    c. Local
    d. Opportunistic

22. **The type of immunity acquired when a mother passes antibodies to her infant is called:**
    a. Natural—Active
    b. Artificial—Active
    c. Natural—Passive
    d. Artificial—Passive

23. **The transfer of genetic material between two living bacteria that are in physical contact is called:**
    a. Transformation
    b. Mutation
    c. Transduction
    d. Conjugation

24. **Most primary herpetic infections are subclinical. Recurrent herpetic infections cannot be passed from mother to child during birth.**
    a. Both statements are true.
    b. Both statements are false.
    c. First statement is true. Second statement is false.
    d. First statement is false. Second statement is true.

25. **Severe and rapid periodontal destruction with a lack of deep-pocket formation is indicative of:**
    a. Chronic periodontitis
    b. Necrotizing ulcerative periodontitis
    c. Gingivitis
    d. Aggressive periodontitis

26. **Herpes simplex viruses are responsible for the formation of:**
    a. Cold sores
    b. Warts
    c. Chickenpox
    d. Shingles

27. **Meningococcal meningitis is caused by *Neisseria meningitidis*. The route of transmission of meningococcal meningitis is by direct contact.**
    a. Both statements are TRUE.
    b. Both statements are FALSE.
    c. First statement is TRUE. Second statement is FALSE.
    d. First statement is FALSE. Second statement is TRUE.

28. **The primary organism in aggressive periodontitis is:**
    a. *S. mutans*
    b. *A. actinomycetemcomitans*
    c. *C. albicans*
    d. *P. intermedia*

29. **Periodontal disease is caused by calculus. Calculus serves as a collection site for bacteria.**
    a. Both statements are TRUE.
    b. Both statements are FALSE.
    c. First statement is TRUE. Second statement is FALSE.
    d. First statement is FALSE. Second statement is TRUE.

30. **The causative agent of Lyme disease is:**
    a. *Chlamydia psittaci*
    b. *Treponema pallidum*
    c. *Borrelia burgdorferi*
    d. Mycobacterium tuberculosis

31. **All of the following are factors that place a person at risk of acquiring HIV EXCEPT one. Which one is the EXCEPTION?**
    a. Unsafe sexual practices
    b. Kissing someone already infected
    c. Intravenous drug use
    d. Exposure to blood or blood products

32. Trismus is a clinical symptom of what disease?
 a. Tetanus
 b. Leprosy
 c. Lyme
 d. Ringworm

33. All of the following are gram-positive bacilli EXCEPT one. Which one is the EXCEPTION?
 a. *Bacillus anthracis*
 b. *Clostridium perfringens*
 c. *Listeria monocytogenes*
 d. *Escherichia coli*

34. Exotoxins are soluble substances secreted by gram-positive bacteria. A few clinically significant exotoxins are associated with botulism, tetanus, diptheria, gas gangrene, and scarlet fever.
 a. Both statements are TRUE.
 b. Both statements are FALSE.
 c. First statement is TRUE. Second statement is FALSE.
 d. First statement is FALSE. Second statement is TRUE.

35. The causative agent of whooping cough is:
 a. *Yersenia pestis*
 b. *Bacillus anthracis*
 c. *Escherichia coli*
 d. *Bordatella pertussis*

36. In which phase of bacterial growth is there an exponential increase in cell number?
 a. Lag phase
 b. Log phase
 c. Stationary phase
 d. Phase of decline

37. In vivo culturing techniques involve using non-living materials in a culture vessel. In vitro culturing techniques involve using living cells.
 a. Both statements are TRUE.
 b. Both statements are FALSE.
 c. First statement is TRUE. Second statement is FALSE.
 d. First statement is FALSE. Second statement is TRUE.

38. The antibacterial agent used to treat syphilis is:
 a. Doxycycline
 b. Erythromycin
 c. Penicillin
 d. Metronidazole

39. The virus responsible for hand, foot, and mouth disease is:
 a. Mumps virus
 b. Herpes virus
 c. Coxsackievirus
 d. Orthomyxovirus

40. All of the following are clinical findings and symptoms of the mumps EXCEPT one. Which one is the EXCEPTION?
 a. Dehydration
 b. Swollen parotid gland
 c. Papilla of Stenson's duct is red and swollen
 d. Fever

41. Erythematous candidiasis is associated with loss of papillae. Pseudomembranous candidiasis is a smooth, flat, red, lesion on the dorsum of the tongue.
 a. Both statements are TRUE.
 b. Both statements are FALSE.
 c. First statement is TRUE. Second statement is FALSE.
 d. First statement is FALSE. Second statement is TRUE.

42. Angular cheilitis is caused by:
 a. Candida
 b. Herpes virus
 c. Coxsackie virus
 d. Papillomavirus

43. A person presents with a small ulcer on the right buccal mucosa. Upon further examination, the dental hygienist observes a small erythematous halo surrounding the ulcer. The ulcer is MOST likely called:
 a. Herpetic whitlow
 b. Recurrent aphthous ulcer
 c. Hyperplastic candidiasis
 d. Ludwig's angina

44. Necrotizing ulcerative periodontitis is associated with severe and rapid periodontal destruction. Aggressive periodontitis occurs prior to age 35 and is associated with a rapid rate of progression of tissue destruction.
 a. Both statements are TRUE.
 b. Both statements are FALSE.
 c. First statement is TRUE. Second statement is FALSE.
 d. First statement is FALSE. Second statement is TRUE.

Use the following case study to answer questions 46–50

A 45-year old man with a full dentition presents for a continued dental hygiene care appointment. The extraoral examination reveals multiple reddish blue and brown skin lesions in the neck area. The intraoral examination reveals a dark macule in the right posterior palate and a few creamy white raised lesions on the left buccal mucosa. The client's health history reveals a previous addiction to heroin.

46. **The extraoral and intraoral findings are MOST likely indicative of what disease?**
    a. Syphilis
    b. Hepatitis B
    c. AIDS
    d. Shingles

47. **The reddish blue and brown skin lesions on the neck and the dark macule in the right posterior palate are indicative of what secondary neoplasm?**
    a. Kaposi's sarcoma
    b. B-cell lymphoma
    c. Herpes simplex virus
    d. Cytomegalovirus

48. **Which of the following infections is the MOST likely cause of the white creamy lesions on the left buccal mucosa?**
    a. Candida
    b. Herpes
    c. Influenza
    d. Cytomegalovirus

49. **What term BEST describes the type of infection presented by the white creamy lesions on the left buccal mucosa?**
    a. Nosocomial
    b. Systemic
    c. Opportunistic
    d. Latent

50. **What is the BEST practice for preventing the transmission of this client's disease in the dental practice?**
    a. Wear personal protective equipment
    b. Use preprocedural mouthrinse
    c. Refer to another dentist to treat
    d. Treat the patient using standard precautions

Prevention of Disease Transmission in Oral Health Care

Darnyl M. Palmer

Preventing disease transmission in dental hygiene practice requires an understanding of the control of microbial contamination, infection, and disease in the oral health care environment. Implementing and practicing protective measures from the perspective of standard precautions is essential.

DISEASE TRANSMISSION

See the section on "Microbial Virulence and Disease Transfer" in Chapter 9.

A. Development of an infectious disease
   1. Source of microorganism or pathogen (microorganism capable of causing infectious disease)
      a. Primarily originating from a person's mouth
      b. May originate from a dental team member (this mode less likely than from a client's mouth)
      c. Microbes may be present in saliva, blood, respiratory secretions, and other bodily fluids
   2. Escape of microorganism from the source
      a. Coughing, sneezing, and talking
      b. Contaminated dental equipment, instruments, and supplies used in a client's mouth
      c. Spatter droplets and aerosol particles generated by using power instrumentation, low-speed and high-speed handpieces, and air/water syringe
         (1) Spatter droplets—large, visible particles that settle quickly, contaminating the clinician and the surfaces of the treatment area
         (2) Aerosol particles—small, invisible particles that may be inhaled or remain airborne for an extended period
   3. Spread of microorganisms to another person
      a. Direct contact with microorganisms in a client's mouth that penetrate through nonintact skin
      b. Indirect contact with items contaminated by a client's microorganisms, including sharps (all items that can puncture skin), instruments, surfaces, hands, and equipment
      c. Droplet infection from spatter that contacts nonintact skin or mucous membranes (oral, nasal, ocular)
      d. Airborne infection from inhaling aerosols
      e. Waterborne infection from contaminated dental unit waterlines (DUWL)
   4. Entry of a microorganism into the person
      a. Inhalation—breathing aerosol particles
      b. Ingestion—swallowing droplets of saliva or blood spattered into the mouth
      c. Through mucous membranes—droplets of saliva or blood spattered into the eyes, nose, or mouth
      d. Through breaks in the skin—by touching contaminated objects, spattering of microorganisms onto nonintact skin, or punctures with contaminated sharps
         (1) Percutaneous injury—injury that penetrates the skin
         (2) Parenteral—piercing mucous membranes or skin
   5. Infection
      a. The infectious agent has a portal of entry into a susceptible host
      b. Establishment and survival of microorganism in the body
   6. Damage to the body—the disease occurs when microorganisms multiply to a harmful level
   7. Pathogenic agents and diseases associated with oral health care (Table 10-1)

TABLE 10-1 Pathogenic Agents Important in Oral Health Care

Disease	Pathogen
Bloodborne Diseases	
Viral	
Hepatitis B	Hepatitis B virus (HBV)
Hepatitis C	Hepatitis C virus (HCV)
Hepatitis D	Hepatitis D virus (HDV)
Acquired immune deficiency syndrome (AIDS)	Human immunodeficiency virus (HIV)
Oral Diseases	
Bacterial	
Gonococcal pharyngitis	*Neisseria gonorrhoeae*
Streptococcal pharyngitis and scarlet fever	*Streptococcus pyogenes*
Syphilis	*Treponema pallidum*
Viral	
Primary herpetic gingivostomatitis	Human herpesvirus 1 or 2
Recurrent herpes (e.g., herpes labialis)	Human herpesvirus 1 or 2
Hand-foot-and-mouth disease	Coxsackievirus
Herpangina	Coxsackievirus
Hairy leukoplakia	Human herpesvirus 4
Fungal	
Candidiasis (thrush)	*Candida albicans*
Denture stomatitis	*Candida albicans*
Systemic Diseases with Oral Lesions	
Bacterial	
Secondary syphilis	*Treponema pallidum*
Viral	
Chickenpox	Human herpesvirus 3 (varicella zoster virus)
Infectious mononucleosis	Human herpesvirus 4 (Epstein-Barr virus)
Other Diseases Spread by Respiratory or Oral Fluids	
Bacterial	
Tuberculosis	*Mycobacterium tuberculosis*
Diphtheria	*Corynebacterium diphtheriae*
Pneumonia	*Streptococcus pneumoniae, Staphylococcus aureus, Mycoplasma pneumoniae, Chlamydia pneumoniae, Moraxella catarrhalis, Haemophilus influenzae*
Meningitis, sinusitis, conjunctivitis	*Haemophilus influenzae* type B
Meningitis	*Neisseria meningitidis*
Bronchitis	*Haemophilus influenzae, Moraxella catarrhalis*
Legionnaires' disease	*Legionella pneumophila*
Viral	
Common cold	Rhinoviruses and several others
Influenza	Influenza viruses
Bronchitis	Influenza A, parainfluenza virus, coronavirus
Pneumonia	Influenza virus, adenovirus, respiratory syncytial virus
Cytomegalovirus (CMV) disease	Cytomegalovirus

TABLE 10-1 Pathogenic Agents Important in Oral Health Care—cont'd

Disease	Pathogen
Other Diseases Spread by Respiratory or Oral Fluids	
Infectious mononucleosis	Human herpesvirus 4 (Epstein-Barr virus)
Erythema infectiosum (fifth disease)	Human parvovirus B19
Measles	Rubeola (measles) virus
Rubella	Rubella virus
Mumps	Mumps virus
Severe acute respiratory syndrome (SARS)	SARS-CoV

Modified from Miller CH, Palenik CJ: Infection control and management of hazardous materials for the dental team, *ed 4, St Louis, 2010, Mosby.*

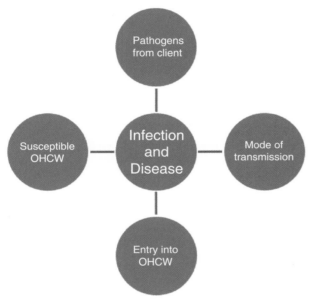

FIGURE 10-1 Factors related to infection and disease transfer.

B. Infection control
1. Reducing the numbers of microorganisms that may be transmitted from individual to individual or from individuals to contaminated surfaces, and vice versa
2. Infection control protocol to reduce or eliminate the likelihood of disease transmission by eliminating one or more factors required for disease transfer (Figure 10-1)
   a. Asepsis—absence of infectious materials; achieved by removing or killing microorganisms
   b. Disinfection—reducing the number of pathogenic organisms in or on an object, thereby minimizing the potential for disease transmission
      (1) Disinfectants are applied to inanimate objects
      (2) Antiseptics are applied to living tissues

   c. Engineering controls—devices that reduce the risk of exposure to potentially infectious materials (e.g., self-sheathing needles)
   d. Personal protective equipment (PPE)—items designed to protect oral health care workers (OHCWs) from exposure to bloodborne and other pathogens (e.g., gloves, masks, safety glasses, face shields, and barrier gowns)
   e. Standard precautions—treating all blood and bodily fluids (including secretions and excretions, except sweat), nonintact skin, and mucous membranes as potentially infectious in all clients; in the oral health care setting, saliva is an important source of contamination, as it is invisible but capable of containing infectious agents that can survive on surfaces for a long period
   f. Sterilization—the destruction or removal of all microorganisms in or on an object
   g. Work practice controls—procedures that reduce the chance of exposure to potentially infectious materials (e.g., using a one-handed "scoop" technique to recap needles)
   h. OHCW-related controls
      (1) Maintaining a healthy lifestyle and immune status
      (2) Receiving appropriate vaccinations
      (3) Abiding by the recommended U.S. Public Health Service work restrictions for OHCWs in the case of certain infections and after exposure to some diseases
   i. Client-related controls
      (1) Prophylactic antibiotic premedication to reduce the possibility of infection in immunocompromised individuals and others with various conditions
      (2) Pre-procedural rinse to decrease the microbial load in spatter and aerosols and to help protect against autogenous (self-derived) infection

(3) Avoiding treatment of clients with known communicable illnesses (i.e., influenza) or contagious lesions (i.e., herpes)
3. Designed to reduce or prevent the spread of pathogens from:
   a. Client to OHCW
   b. OHCW to client
   c. Client to client
   d. Dental office to community, including families of OHCWs
   e. Community to client
4. Table 10-2 outlines the mechanisms of the spread and the prevention of diseases

TABLE 10-2 Mechanisms of Disease Spread and Prevention

Pathway of Cross-Contamination	Source of Microorganism	Mode of Disease Spread	Mechanism or Site of Entry into Body	Infection-Control Procedure
Patient to OHCW	Patient's mouth	Direct contact	Through breaks in skin of dental team	Gloves or handwashing Immunizations
		Droplet infection	Inhalation by OHCW	Mask Rubber dam Mouthrinsing
			Through breaks in skin of OHCW	Gloves or handwashing Protective clothing Face shield Rubber dam Mouthrinsing
			Through mucosal surfaces of OHC team	Mask Eyewear Face shield Rubber dam Mouthrinsing Immunizations
		Indirect contact	Cuts, punctures, or needlesticks in member of dental team	Needle safety and waste management
				Heavy gloves for cleanup
				Ultrasonic cleaning rather than handscrubbing
				Instrument cassettes to reduce direct handling during cleaning
				Antimicrobial holding solution
				Antimicrobial cleaning solution
			Through breaks in skin of OHC team member	Heavy gloves for cleanup Protective clothing Immunizations
	Patient's skin lesions	Direct contact	Through breaks in skin of OHC team member	Gloves or handwashing Immunizations
OHCW to patient	OHCW's hands (lesions or bleeding)	Direct contact	Through mucosal surfaces of patient	Gloves or handwashing Care in handling sharp objects Immunizations
		Indirect contact	Bleeding on items used in patient's mouth	Gloves or handwashing Instrument sterilization Surface disinfection Immunizations
	OHCW's mouth (oral or respiratory fluids)	Droplet infection	Inhalation by patient	Mask Face shield
			Through oral mucosal surfaces of patient	Mask Face shield

TABLE 10-2 Mechanisms of Disease Spread and Prevention—cont'd

Pathway of Cross-Contamination	Source of Microorganism	Mode of Disease Spread	Mechanism or Site of Entry into Body	Infection-Control Procedure
Patient to patient	Patient's mouth	Indirect contact (instruments, surfaces, hands)	Through oral mucosal surfaces of patient	Instrument and handpiece sterilization Sterilization monitoring Surface covers Surface disinfection Handwashing and proper gloving Changing mask Decontaminating protective eyewear Changing protective clothing when needed Use of sterile or clean supplies Flushing dental unit water lines Monitoring water-line anti-retraction valves Use of disposable items
Office to community	Patient's mouth	Indirect contact	Cuts, punctures, breaks in skin of dental laboratory worker, waste disposal, or laundry personnel	Waste management Disinfection of impressions and appliances Proper management of contaminated laundry Handwashing
OHCW's family	OHCW's body fluids	Direct or indirect contact	Intimate contact	Immunization
Community to patient	Municipal water	Direct contact	Patient's mouth	Use of new and separate water source Periodically disinfecting inside of dental unit water lines Use of water containing an approved antimicrobial agent Filtering the water

OHCW, *Oral healthcare worker;* OHC, *oral healthcare.*
Data from US Department of Labor, Occupational Safety and Health Administration: Controlling occupational exposure to bloodborne pathogens, *Washington, D.C., 1996, 2001, OSHA 3127 (revised).*

INFECTION CONTROL PROCEDURES FOR ORAL HEALTH CARE WORKERS

A. Health history
  1. Obtain, review, and update clients' health histories at all visits
  2. Address specific questions related to present health status, physician care, hospitalizations, surgery, diseases, medications, allergies, current or chronic illness, review of major organ systems, and recent overseas travel
  3. Be aware that obtaining health histories will not identify all infectious clients; clients may suppress information purposely or unknowingly (many persons with hepatitis B virus [HBV], hepatitis C virus [HCV], and human immunodeficiency virus [HIV] are asymptomatic)

  4. Health history may identify conditions requiring:
    a. Diagnostic evaluation and laboratory testing
    b. Medical consultations
    c. Prophylactic antibiotic premedication to reduce the incidence of autogenous infections, that is, conditions caused by introducing the microflora of clients into injured tissues (e.g., bacteremia, abscess)
  5. The Centers for Disease Control and Prevention (CDC) recommends conducting a tuberculosis risk assessment for an oral health care setting and then formulating a prevention program appropriate for its designated risk category; most dental settings will be low or very low risk

B. Immunizations are recommended for OHCWs
  1. Essential component of an infection control program

2. Most effective method to prevent contracting a vaccine-preventable disease

3. Immunizations are recommended for the following diseases, unless evidence of past infection and immunity: hepatitis B, varicella zoster, influenza, measles, mumps, polio, rubella, tetanus, influenza A (H1N1); consult with a primary care physician before vaccination, as some vaccines are contraindicated for immunocompromised and pregnant persons

4. The Occupational Safety and Health Administration (OSHA) policies regarding hepatitis B vaccination

   a. The OSHA requires employers to make hepatitis B vaccine available at no cost to employees who are or may be exposed by occupation to bloodborne pathogens and within 10 working days

   b. Employers must provide information about the vaccine and ensure that all medical records concerning the vaccination are kept confidential

   c. Employees have the right to refuse vaccination but must read and sign an OSHA declination statement

   d. Employers cannot demand that employees be serologically prescreened before vaccination

5. Hepatitis B vaccine

   a. Two single antigen vaccines available

     (1) Recombivax HB (Merck & Co., Inc.)

     (2) Engerix-B (GlaxoSmithKline)

   b. Process

     (1) Serologic screening for antibodies to hepatitis B surface antigen before vaccination is not recommended, unless infection is suspected

     (2) Pregnancy is not a contraindication for vaccination

     (3) A series of three injections in the deltoid muscle given at 0, 1, and 6 months

     (4) Seroconversion rates are 95% to 97% in healthy younger adults; lower rates (approximately 70%) in persons over 40 years old, smokers, overweight persons, and those receiving injections in the buttocks

     (5) Genetic factors may influence seroconversion rates

     (6) Testing for antibody (anti-HBsAg) is recommended after vaccination to ensure protection against HBV; testing should be conducted 1 to 2 months after the final injection

     (7) With successful seroconversion, protective antibodies have been sustained for at least 20 years

     (8) Failure to seroconvert requires a second series of three injections

     (9) Continued failure to seroconvert could signal chronic HBV infection in a person who is unable to produce antibodies; nonresponders should be evaluated by a medical provider

    (10) The CDC currently does not recommend a booster injection until further research is conducted on past recipients of vaccine

    (11) Minimal side effects of vaccine include injection site soreness, headache, and fever

    (12) Individuals with allergies to yeast or iodine (vaccine preservatives) must consult a physician before the vaccination

6. Recommended screenings for OHCWs

   a. OHCWs should know their HBV status

   b. Mantoux tuberculin skin test for tuberculosis should be administered annually according to the CDC risk level of dental setting

C. Hand hygiene

   1. Extremely important disease prevention practice in oral health care

   2. Hands are a primary source of microorganisms capable of disease transmission

   3. Rationale

     a. Handwashing reduces both resident and transient flora on skin

      (1) Resident flora are permanent residents that colonize several skin layers and cannot be completely removed. This type is less important and less likely to transmit disease than are transient flora

      (2) Transient flora contaminate hands when hands touch contaminated surfaces. This type colonizes the outer layers of skin, only survive for a limited time, and can be easily removed by routine handwashing

     b. Protects clients and OHCWs by reducing the spread of microorganisms and subsequent infections via the hands

     c. Unwashed hands can contaminate sterile instruments, dental equipment, and environmental surfaces

   4. Use of gloves is not a substitute for routine handwashing

   5. Hands must be washed before gloves are put on to minimize organisms that can multiply rapidly when enclosed in a moist, warm environment; bacteria and yeast growth can cause skin irritation

6. Hands must be washed after removal of gloves because defects, tears, and punctures may occur in gloves, permitting microorganisms to be transferred to hands; this also helps remove glove powder, which contains latex protein and other glove chemicals that can elicit irritant contact dermatitis or an allergic reaction in sensitized individuals

7. Watches, bracelets, and rings must be removed to prevent harboring of microorganisms; also, rings may perforate glove materials

8. Nails must be kept short and clean and the cuticles well maintained; artificial nails and nail jewelry are not recommended, since current research has implicated them in disease transmission in hospitals

9. Intact skin is the best protection against infection; this can be achieved by:
   a. Minimizing trauma to hands (e.g., cuts and scrapes) while outside the dental setting
   b. Protecting hands from drying and chapping during cold weather
   c. Frequent use of lubricating hand lotions

10. OHCWs who have open or weeping lesions or dermatitis on hands should not provide client care until the condition resolves, since dermatitis reduces the effectiveness of handwashing and nonintact skin provides a portal of entry for microorganisms

11. Hand hygiene procedures for routine dental hygiene care include:
   a. Vigorous lathering of hands using an interlacing finger motion with either an antimicrobial or plain soap for 15 seconds
      (1) Disposable soap containers should not be refilled, and when empty should be discarded and replaced
      (2) Soap dishes accumulate microorganisms and are not recommended
      (3) Sinks and soap dispensers should be electronically operated or have foot controls; if not, paper towels should be used to turn off sink faucet
   b. Rinsing with cool to lukewarm water while rubbing hands together for 10 seconds
   c. Drying hands with single-use paper towels
   d. Using alcohol-based hand rubs as an alternative to handwashing
      (1) Used when no visible soil appears on the hands
      (2) Have been shown to be effective, sometimes reducing bacterial counts more effectively than soap and water
      (3) May increase the frequency of hand hygiene because of ease of use

      (4) According to manufacturer's directions, place an adequate amount of alcohol-based hand rub in hand and then vigorously rub hands until dry
      (5) Alcohol-based hand sanitizers may cause dry skin (choose ones that contain emollients)
   e. Washing hands between clients, before and after lunch, before and after restroom visits, or any time hands become contaminated
   f. Maintaining asepsis by touching only sterile instruments or disinfected surfaces

12. For surgical procedures, an antimicrobial soap with substantivity (prolonged anti-microbial effect) is recommended; chlorhexidine digluconate or triclosan

D. Personal protective equipment (PPE)
   1. Protective barriers used to reduce exposure of mucous membranes, hands, and body of OHCWs to microorganisms and also to prevent injury from chemicals and particles of debris
   2. Used during client care, laboratory, disinfection, and sterilization procedures
   3. PPE includes gloves, masks, protective eyewear, and protective clothing
   4. Sequence for donning PPE: protective clothing, then mask and eyewear, and finally, after handwashing, gloves
   5. The employer is responsible for providing and maintaining appropriate PPE for employees
   6. Gloves
      a. The use of gloves provides a high level of protection for both OHCWs and clients
         (1) Prevents direct contact with microorganisms in the client's mouth and on contaminated surfaces (bare hands often will have areas of nonintact skin providing portals of entry for pathogenic microorganisms)
         (2) Prevents saliva and blood from being retained under fingernails; saliva and blood have been shown to persist for several days even with handwashing
         (3) Protects against contact with disinfecting and cleaning chemicals and x-ray solutions
         (4) Protects clients from the microorganisms on the hands of the OHCW
         (5) Examination gloves provide little protection against sharps injuries; utility gloves provide more protection; however, injuries still can occur
      b. Risks associated with not routinely wearing gloves
         (1) OHCW exposure to potentially infectious client tissues and contaminated

surfaces—most likely route by which OHCWs have acquired HBV from clients

(2) Client exposure to infectious agents originating from the OHCW

(a) Documented source of transmission of HBV from ungloved dentist to clients

(b) Documented case in which an ungloved hygienist transmitted herpes to 20 of her clients

(3) Skin irritation from contact with disinfecting chemicals

(4) Burns resulting from contact with hot items from sterilizer

c. Protocol for glove use

(1) Wear during intraoral procedures and when in contact with contaminated items or surfaces (e.g., contaminated laundry or waste)

(2) If it is necessary to leave the chairside during client care, remove gloves, and after hand hygiene, don a new pair on returning (prevents contamination of additional surfaces one may touch and also prevents contamination of the client with microorganisms that already may be present on those surfaces)

(3) Ensure that gloves cover the cuff of a long-sleeved gown

(4) Change gloves between clients and during long appointments because defects in gloves increase with use beyond 60 minutes

(5) Do not wash or disinfect gloves; may cause "wicking" or enhanced penetration of liquids through undetected defects in gloves

(6) Remove torn or punctured gloves as soon as possible. Wash hands and don new gloves

(7) Do not apply petroleum-based hand lotion prior to wearing gloves because it degrades latex gloves; for the same reason, do not apply petroleum-based lubricants to client's lips

d. Types of gloves—See Table 10-3 for glove materials

(1) Nonsterile, ambidextrous gloves in sizes extra-small, small, medium, and large are adequate for most procedures; proper glove fit is important to ensure efficient instrumentation and to prevent hand fatigue and possibly carpal tunnel syndrome

(2) Sterile gloves are recommended for surgical procedures

TABLE 10-3 Types of Gloves Used in Oral Health Care

Nonsterile (examination) gloves	Latex Nitrile Neoprene Vinyl Polyurethane Styrene-based co-polymer Butadiene methyl methacrylate
Sterile (surgical) gloves	Latex Nitrile Neoprene Polyurethane Styrene-based co-polymer Synthetic polyisoprene
Utility gloves	Latex Nitrile Neoprene Butyl rubber Fluoroelastomer Polyethylene and ethylene vinyl Alcohol co-polymer
Overgloves	Thin co-polymer Thin plastic ("food handlers")

(3) Use puncture-resistant and chemical-resistant utility gloves to prepare chemicals, handle contaminated instruments, and clean and disinfect surfaces

(a) Utility gloves are reusable and can be disinfected or sterilized in an autoclave

(b) Replace utility gloves when they show any signs of wear (e.g., cracks, punctures, discoloration)

(4) Overgloves are worn over treatment gloves to prevent cross-contamination of items and surfaces such as pens, charts, and drawers

(5) Heat-resistant gloves are worn when handling hot items (e.g., unloading sterilizers)

e. Dermatitis and latex allergy

(1) Irritant contact dermatitis

(a) Nonimmunologic (nonallergic) reaction of skin to chemicals used in glove manufacturing

(b) Skin on hands becomes dry, red, itchy, and cracked

(c) The condition is aggravated by soaps, not rinsing or drying hands completely, perspiration, or cornstarch powder

(d) Most skin reactions from wearing gloves are caused by irritant contact dermatitis and are not true allergic reactions

(2) Allergic contact dermatitis
  (a) Type IV or delayed hypersensitivity occurring within hours or days because of allergy to glove chemicals
  (b) Limited to area of contact, causing itching, redness, and vesicles to appear within 24 to 48 hours followed by dry skin, fissures, and sores
  (c) Patch test identifies sensitivity to specific chemical

(3) Latex allergy
  (a) Type I or immediate hypersensitivity within minutes or hours
  (b) Allergy to naturally occurring latex proteins
  (c) Symptoms: skin (hives, swelling, burning, tightness, itching, redness, tingling), lungs (asthma, wheezing, constriction, coughing, sneezing, rhinitis, angioedema), and other (nausea, vomiting, diarrhea, cramps, hypertension, tachycardia, shock)
  (d) Anaphylactic shock and death can occur with subsequent exposures to latex
  (e) High-risk individuals for latex allergy include: persons who have had multiple surgeries and persons with spina bifida, urogenital anomalies, spinal cord injuries, and allergies to bananas, kiwis, chestnuts, or avocados
  (f) Reductions in exposure to latex proteins are known to decrease sensitivity (important for OHC team to reduce their daily exposure to airborne latex proteins by wearing powder-free, reduced-protein latex or latex-free gloves)
  (g) The CDC indicates that OHCWs need to be educated about skin problems that can occur with frequent hand hygiene and the use of gloves
  (h) Latex-free environment should be provided to clients and OHCWs with a latex allergy

(4) Procedures for management of persons with latex allergy
  (a) Include questions in health history appropriate for identifying possible latex allergy
  (b) Document latex allergy in health history record in a way that will ensure observation by OHCWs
  (c) Schedule allergic clients for the first appointment of the day when airborne latex proteins are at their lowest levels (still risky)
  (d) Ensure that OHC team uses latex-free gloves for treatment area preparation and for touching all items that will come in contact with the client
  (e) Use latex-free gloves and dental materials during client care

7. Masks
  a. Purpose
    (1) Worn to protect the mucous membranes of the nose and mouth from spatter of oral fluids
    (2) Provide a lesser degree of protection from inhalation of aerosol particles
      (a) Surgical masks will not provide protection from airborne infections (e.g., SARS)
      (b) The N-95 respirator is needed to protect against airborne infections
    (3) May provide some protection to client from nasal or oral secretions of OHCWs
  b. Composed of synthetic material that should filter at least 95% of small particles
  c. Types of masks
    (1) Dome mask with elastic band
    (2) Tie-on or ear-loop mask
  d. Should have a seal against the face to minimize leakage around the margins
  e. Maximizing effectiveness and minimizing cross-contamination
    (1) Use a new mask for each client
    (2) Change the mask if it becomes moist. Moistness compromises its effectiveness by increasing the passage of unfiltered air around the edges of the mask and may wick contaminants through the mask
    (3) Don a new mask every 20 to 30 minutes to maintain high filterability
    (4) Adjust the mask so that it fits snugly against the face
    (5) Avoid touching the mask during the appointment
    (6) Keep the mask on after completing the procedure to reduce inhalation of aerosols
    (7) When removing the mask, handle it by its strings or elastic

(8) Do not leave the mask on the head, dangling around neck, or in your pocket

8. Protective eyewear
   a. Purpose—protect the mucous membranes of the eye from microbial invasion, chemicals, and physical projectiles
   b. Risks for unprotected eyes
      (1) Conjunctivitis
      (2) Ocular herpes (can cause blindness)
      (3) Hepatitis B (eye as portal of entry)
      (4) Eye injury (physical or chemical)
   c. Types of eyewear
      (1) Regular glasses offer limited side or top protection and are not recommended
      (2) Safety glasses, goggles, or loupes
         (a) Cover entire eye orbit (providing protection on all sides)
         (b) Some may be worn over prescription glasses
         (c) Are more shatter resistant than regular glasses
         (d) Provide minimal visual distortion
         (e) Are able to withstand disinfection (should be cleaned and disinfected between clients)
         (f) Should meet American National Standards Institute (ANSI) guidelines
      (3) Face shields
         (a) An alternative to safety glasses
         (b) Should be chin-length and provide top and side protection
         (c) Masks should still be worn to reduce inhalation of aerosols
         (d) Provide maximum coverage of face for high-spatter procedures (e.g., air polishing or power scaling)
         (e) Face shields made of thin plastic may have limited impact resistance
      (4) Protective eyewear should be provided to clients
         (a) Orange tinted to protect against damage from ultraviolet (curing) light
         (b) Protection against physical and chemical injury to the client's eyes during treatment

9. Protective (barrier) clothing
   a. Purpose
      (1) Protects nonintact skin from contamination by microorganisms
      (2) Reduces the risk of bringing contaminants beyond dental setting on unprotected clothing
      (3) May protect client from microorganisms on street clothing or may provide protection against disease transmission when soiled protective clothing is changed between clients (fomites—clothing and paper that can absorb and transmit infectious agents)
      (4) Microorganisms adhere to clothing; however, lack of evidence exists to support the extent to which barrier clothing protects against disease transmission
   b. Characteristics of protective clothing
      (1) Reusable or disposable
      (2) Gowns, aprons, laboratory coats, or uniforms used as a covering for street clothing or scrub uniforms
      (3) High collar that fits closely around the neck
      (4) Long-sleeved garments with fitted cuffs allow gloves to extend over them for complete coverage
   c. To maximize effectiveness and minimize cross-contamination
      (1) Use fabric made of synthetic material, which is more fluid-resistant
      (2) Do not wear protective clothing outside treatment area (remove before going out [e.g., to lunch] or leaving the dental setting)
      (3) Change protective clothing daily or when visibly soiled
      (4) Avoid touching clothing during client care and throughout the day
      (5) Roll protective clothing inside out to minimize contact with exposed surface

10. Additional barrier protection used when cleaning or performing surgery
    a. Plastic aprons or other fluid-proof garments
    b. Head covers
    c. Shoe covers

11. Laundering of reusable clothing
    a. Laundered in the office following the manufacturer's instructions
    b. Sent to a laundry service in a leak-proof bag labeled with the biohazard symbol
    c. It is against OSHA regulations for OHCWs to take contaminated protective clothing home for laundering

ORAL HEALTH CARE ENVIRONMENT AND PROMOTION OF INFECTION CONTROL

A. Design and equipment selection emphasizes
   1. Smooth construction—eliminates knobs, hooks, and crevices

2. Design of client chairs and operator stools that:
   a. Minimize buttons and seams
   b. Use vinyl upholstery instead of cloth
   c. Provide foot-control operation
3. Avoidance of fabric-covered, coiled, or mechanically retracted tubings
4. Sink faucets and soap dispensers with foot or electronic controls
5. Paper-towel dispenser that is designed to avoid touching hardware or is electronically controlled
6. Plastic-lined waste containers recessed under cabinet, with opening on countertop
7. Surfaces that are compatible with disinfectants and detergents
8. Plastic laminate instead of wood for cabinets and countertops
9. Vinyl flooring and walls that are smooth and seamless
10. Carpeting or wallpaper not recommended
11. Dental unit water lines (DUWLs) that provide:
    a. Anti-retraction valves to prevent the aspiration of microorganisms into water lines
    b. Equipment, devices, and treatments for DUWLs
       (1) Filtration unit
       (2) Sterile-water delivery system
       (3) Flushing the lines with antimicrobial agents
       (4) Independent water reservoirs
12. Reduction of airborne microbes
    a. Air circulation exchange system or single-room filtration units
    b. Ventilation systems to control noxious sterilization and laboratory vapors
    c. Prevention of recirculation of contaminated air or transport of microbes
    d. Cooling and heating system filters that prevent transfer of microbes
13. Housekeeping surfaces (e.g., walls, cabinets, and floors) should be cleaned and disinfected routinely with detergent and water or with detergents or low-level hospital disinfectants
    a. Clean mops and cloths after use and allow to dry before reuse, or use single-use items
    b. Clean walls, blinds, and window treatments in client-care areas when they are visibly soiled
    c. Perform cleaning with a wet cloth or mop to prevent distribution of microorganism-laden dust particles
14. Keep treatment area free of unnecessary or seldom-used equipment and items

Maintaining Asepsis in the Oral Health Care Environment

A. Items associated with oral health care are classified as:
   1. Critical—instruments that penetrate oral soft tissue or bone, enter the bloodstream, or enter other sterile tissues of the mouth (e.g., curet); must be heat sterilized or be single-use (disposable) devices (SUDs)
   2. Semi-critical—items that come in contact with mucous membranes (used in the mouth) but will not penetrate soft tissue, contact bone, enter the bloodstream, or enter other sterile tissues of the mouth (e.g., radiographic film holders)
      a. Should be heat sterilized or be SUDs (disposable)
      b. If heat sensitive, decontaminate using a chemical sterilant or a high-level disinfectant, or cover the device with a barrier to prevent contamination (e.g., digital radiography sensors)
   3. Noncritical—items that contact intact skin (e.g., blood pressure cuff)
      a. If contamination is possible, cover the device to prevent contamination, or otherwise just maintain cleanliness
      b. If the device is contaminated, clean and disinfect
         (1) If contaminated by blood, use intermediate-level disinfectant
         (2) If not contaminated by blood, use low-level disinfectant
B. Maintaining asepsis with the use of chemicals and surface covers
   1. Categories of disinfecting or sterilizing chemicals (Table 10-4)
      a. Sterilant—destroys all microorganisms, including high numbers of bacterial spores
      b. High-level disinfectant—destroys all microorganisms but may not destroy bacterial spores (depending on contact time, can be either a disinfectant or sterilant)
      c. Intermediate-level—destroys vegetative bacteria, most fungi, and most viruses; inactivates *Mycobacterium tuberculosis* var. *bovis*
      d. Low-level—destroys vegetative bacteria, some fungi and viruses; does not inactivate *M. tuberculosis* var. *bovis* (Figure 10-2)
C. Surface disinfection of clinical contact surfaces
   1. Any surface that is touched by contaminated hands, instruments, devices, or other items during the provision of oral health care (e.g., light handles, dental equipment)
   2. Identify and list surfaces that will be contaminated during treatment

TABLE 10-4 Categories of Disinfecting or Sterilizing Chemicals

Category	Definition	Examples	Use
Sterilant*	Destroys all microorganisms, including high numbers of bacterial spores	Glutaraldehyde, glutaraldehydephenate, hydrogen peroxide, hydrogen peroxide with peracetic acid, peracetic acid	Heat-sensitive reusable items: immersion only
High-level disinfectant*	Destroys all microorganisms, but not necessarily high numbers of bacterial spores	Glutaraldehyde, glutaraldehydephenate, hydrogen peroxide, hydrogen peroxide with peracetic acid, peracetic acid, orthophthaldehyde	Heat-sensitive reusable items: immersion only
Intermediate-level disinfectant	Destroys vegetative bacteria, most fungi, and most viruses; inactivates *Mycobacterium tuberculosis* var. *bovis* (is tuberculocidal)	Environment Protection Agency (EPA)–registered hospital disinfectant† with label claim of tuberculocidal activity (e.g., chlorine-based products, phenolics, iodophors, quaternary ammonium compounds with alcohol, bromides)	Clinical contact surfaces, noncritical surfaces with visible blood
Low-level disinfectant	Destroys vegetative bacteria, some fungi, and some viruses; does not inactivate *Mycobacterium tuberculosis* var. *bovis* (is not tuberculocidal)	EPA-registered hospital disinfectant with no label claim of tuberculocidal activity (e.g., quaternary ammonium compounds)	Housekeeping surfaces (e.g., floors, walls); noncritical surfaces without visible blood; clinical contact surfaces‡

*Some, but not all, of these products can serve as high-level disinfectants and sterilants, depending on the immersion time used.
†A hospital disinfectant is one that has been shown to kill Staphylococcus aureus, Pseudomonas aeruginosa, and Salmonella choleraesuis.
‡The Centers for Disease Control and Prevention (CDC) indicates that low-level disinfectants can be used on clinical contact surfaces if the product has a label claim of killing human immunodeficiency virus (HIV) and hepatitis B virus (HBV) in addition to being an EPA-registered hospital disinfectant.
Modified from Centers for Disease Control and Prevention: Guidelines for infection control in dental health-care settings, Morbidity and Mortality Weekly Report 52(RR-17):1–66, 2003.

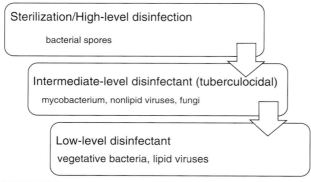

FIGURE 10-2 Decreasing order of resistance of microorganisms to germicidal chemicals. *(Adapted from Centers for Disease Control and Prevention: Guidelines for infection control in dental health-care settings,* Morbidity and Mortality Weekly Report 52(RR-17):1–68, 2003.)

3. Post the list in the treatment area to increase effectiveness and efficiency of decontamination procedures
4. Approaches to clinical contact surface asepsis
  a. Avoid unnecessarily contaminating surfaces during treatment by:
    (1) Using unit doses of materials to avoid contamination of multiple-use containers
    (2) Using prearranged tray setups and cassettes containing a complete selection of instruments needed for a particular procedure
    (3) Gathering the needed supplies and equipment at the beginning of treatment to eliminate the need to open drawers and cabinets or to leave the treatment area to retrieve supplies during client care
    (4) Having sterile pliers, overgloves, gauze, and paper towels available for use as barriers between contaminated gloved hands and uncontaminated objects (e.g., drawer handle, dental record)
  b. Prevent contamination by using a surface cover or barrier protection (single-use, disposable)
    (1) Surface covers protect surfaces that are difficult to preclean adequately
    (2) May be less time-consuming than precleaning or disinfecting surfaces before and after client care
    (3) Surface covers include clear plastic wrap, bags, and tubing
    (4) May be placed using bare hands on cleaned and disinfected surfaces

(5) Should be placed to protect the entire surface and to ensure that the barrier protection will not come off when the surface is touched

(6) Reduce the use of chemicals that may stain or corrode and are hazardous to OHCWs and the environment

c. Clean and disinfect the surface after contamination and before reuse

(1) Requires purchase and proper use of disinfecting chemicals

(2) Chemical use requires that Material Safety Data Sheets (MSDS) be filed on site and that OHCWs be provided information and training on the hazards and proper use of chemicals

(3) Cleaning and disinfection are best reserved for surfaces that are difficult to cover, smooth surfaces, and those not involving electricity

d. A dual approach consisting of both barrier protection and cleaning or disinfection with chemicals is most often used in oral health care settings

5. Clinical contact surfaces to be covered or cleaned or disinfected

a. Countertops, cabinets, mobile cart, tray table, and radiographic equipment; digital intraoral sensors should be covered because they cannot be heat sterilized, and some cannot be disinfected with chemicals

b. Air–water syringe, high-volume and low-volume evacuators (parts of these may be sterilized or disposable, which is preferred because these items come in contact with mucous membranes)

c. Hoses, tubing, and controls attached to handpieces

d. Supports for handpieces, air–water syringe, and suction devices

e. Chairs, including switches and levers

f. Control switches

g. Light handles

h. Faucet handles and soap dispenser (if manually operated)

i. Instrument tray (if it cannot be sterilized)

j. Stethoscope earpieces

k. Floss dispenser, hand mirror, pens, pencils

l. Chairside computers and keyboards

m. Phones, intercoms

6. Factors influencing effectiveness of surface disinfection with chemicals

a. Numbers and types of organisms present; some organisms have a higher resistance to destruction by chemicals (e.g., *Mycobacterium* species)

b. Amount of bioburden (blood, saliva, and microorganisms)

(1) Organic materials in blood and saliva insulate microorganisms from chemicals

(2) May partially inhibit the active ingredient in the disinfectant

c. Selection of an Environmental Protection Agency (EPA)–registered disinfectant that is tuberculocidal (sterilant or high-level disinfectant should not be used for clinical contact surfaces)

d. Use of a water-based disinfectant is reported to clean organic material better than alcohol-based disinfectants

e. Performing procedures carefully and following manufacturer's instructions by using appropriate disinfectant concentration, use life, and contact time

f. Clean surfaces with a combination of a detergent and a disinfectant to maximize the removal of bioburden before the disinfection step

(1) The detergent or disinfectant used for the cleaning step must contain a surfactant

(a) Surfactant—an agent that loosens, emulsifies, and holds soil in suspension, allowing for easier removal of debris and for more thorough cleaning

(2) An advantage to using a combination agent is that a chemical disinfectant starts the killing process during the cleaning step and reduces the opportunity for contaminants to spread to other surfaces

7. Cleaning or disinfection technique for clinical contact surfaces

a. Exercise care when using disinfectants, and wear PPE, including utility gloves

(1) To prevent irritation or injury to eyes, mucous membranes, and skin

(2) To avoid breathing in noxious vapors

b. Step 1—Clean; spray the detergent or disinfectant, or apply with a premoistened cloth

c. Step 2—Wipe; vigorously wipe surfaces with a paper towel to remove stuck-on debris

d. Step 3—Reapply the disinfectant

(1) Leave surfaces undisturbed for a specified contact time

(2) Wipe any remaining wet areas with a paper towel

(3) Rinse off any residual disinfectant with water (if the surface will come in contact with clients' skin or mouth)

TABLE 10-5 Chemical Agents for Surface Disinfection

Chemical Classification	Advantages	Disadvantages
Chlorines	Rapid-acting Broad spectrum Economical	Prepare solution daily Diminished activity by organic matter Corrosive Strong odor
Iodophors	Broad spectrum Few reactions Residual biocidal activity	Unstable at high temperatures Dilution and contact time critical Prepare solution daily Discoloration of some surfaces Inactivated by hard water
Synthetic phenolics	Broad spectrum Residual biocidal activity Compatible with most metals	Degrades certain types of plastic over time Difficult to rinse Film accumulation Alcohol-based products are only fair-to-poor in cleaning ability
Dual or synergized quaternaries	Broad spectrum Contains detergent for cleaning	Easily inactivated by anionic detergents and organic matter Damaging to some materials

8. Chemical disinfectants for surface disinfection (Table 10-5)—selection criteria
   a. EPA-registered intermediate-level disinfectant that is tuberculocidal (kills *M. tuberculosis* var. *bovis*)
   b. Effective within 10 minutes or less
   c. Does not have an offensive odor
   d. Reasonable cost
   e. Provides residual effect (called *substantivity*) on treated surfaces
   f. Retains stability and effectiveness in the presence of bioburden, preferably water based
   g. Good penetrating and cleaning ability
   h. Compatible with and innocuous to equipment and clinical surfaces (consult product manufacturer for recommendations)
   i. The CDC does not recommend alcohol, household bleach, or early-generation quaternary ammonium compounds as surface disinfectants

D. DUWL asepsis
   1. High concentrations of bacteria have been found in untreated DUWLs (e.g., power instrumentation, air-polishing units, high-speed handpieces, and air–water syringes)
      a. Municipal water entering the dental unit is not sterile and contains 0 to 500 colony-forming units per milliliter (CFU/mL) of heterotrophic bacteria
      b. Water exiting untreated DUWLs may contain more than 100,000 CFU/mL
         (1) Consists of waterborne bacteria of low pathogenicity or opportunistic pathogens, which pose the greatest risk to immunocompromised individuals
         (2) Organisms of greatest concern are *Pseudomonas*, *Legionella*, and *Mycobacterium* species
   2. Microorganisms attach to and accumulate on the inside of the water line tubing, creating biofilm colonies (an organized, protected, and highly resistant colony of live microorganisms attached to a surface) (see the section on "Bacterial Plaque Biofilm" in Chapter 14); formation of biofilm:
      a. Biofilm includes naturally occurring waterborne bacteria and may include microorganisms from the oral cavities of clients treated before the current client
      b. Stagnation of water and small-diameter tubing in DUWLs encourages biofilm formation
      c. Incoming water brings a continuous source of nutrients to bacteria
      d. As water flows past the biofilm in the waterline, it picks up detached bacteria before exiting through dental equipment
   3. Dental unit water and infection control
      a. No epidemiologic evidence of a widespread public health problem caused by dental unit water
      b. However, using water that does not meet the standards for drinking water, increases client and OHCW exposure to microorganisms
      c. Oral health care facilities should use water that meets the EPA drinking water standard and the American Dental Association (ADA) recommendation (no more than 500 CFU/mL of heterotrophic bacteria) for routine dental care
      d. Dental unit water from a municipal supply should not be used for oral surgery or in the treatment of immunocompromised persons (sterile water delivery systems must be used)
      e. Boil water notices in the community
         (1) Do not use dental unit or faucet water until the notice is lifted

(2) After the notice is lifted, flush all the water lines, and disinfect them following manufacturer's recommendations

4. Improving the quality of dental unit water
   a. Routinely check anti-retraction valves (valves can get stuck in the open position with age)
   b. Flush water lines for 3 to 5 minutes at the beginning of each day; flush for 30 seconds between clients
      (1) Flushing does not remove biofilm but may temporarily reduce planktonic (free-floating) microbes
      (2) Flushing may help remove client materials that have entered the turbine, air, and water lines
   c. Use an independent water reservoir—a bottle that supplies nonmunicipal water to dental unit
   d. Chemical treatment of DUWLs is still necessary to control biofilm formation, even when an independent water reservoir is used

Maintaining the Treatment Area During Client Care

A. Spatter and aerosol management to reduce the number of microorganisms escaping from the source
   1. Use a pre-procedural, antimicrobial rinse containing chlorhexidine, essential oils, or iodophor to reduce microbial counts in spatter and aerosols
   2. Use air and water separately instead of a combination spray
   3. Use high-volume evacuation, whenever possible; when using the saliva ejector, do not allow the client to close the lips around the tip creating a seal. Research has shown that in one in five cases, previously suctioned fluids might enter a client's mouth by way of a reverse flow in the vacuum line
   4. Use of a rubber dam will not only reduce spatter and aerosols but also will lessen the chance of a client's saliva retracting into the dental handpiece and the air–water syringe

B. Reducing the risk of contamination and disease transmission
   1. Limit the areas of contamination; use overgloves when touching clinical contact surfaces
   2. Disinfect anything not covered with barriers when touched by contaminated hands
   3. Avoid accessing drawers, cabinets, and other storage areas with contaminated gloves; ask for assistance if additional supplies are needed

4. Protect dental records from contamination
   a. Ask for the help of a hygiene assistant or other personnel to record
   b. Use overgloves
   c. Record data on audio, and make manual entries in client record after glove removal
   d. Generate client record with voice-activated computer software

5. Eating, drinking, smoking, applying of cosmetics or lip balm, and handling of contact lenses are prohibited in client-care areas

6. Food and drink cannot be stored in refrigerators, freezers, or cabinets or on shelves and countertops where blood or saliva is present

C. Waste disposal during treatment
   1. Immediately discard blood-soaked items in a small biohazard bag taped to the cart or the cabinet
   2. Do not allow contaminated waste to accumulate on trays

D. Precautions and care in handling syringes or sharp instruments
   1. Needlestick injuries are a major cause of disease transmission to health care personnel
      a. Never permit "sharps" to be directed toward the body
      b. Do not allow uncovered needles to remain on tray
      c. Never recap a needle using a two-handed technique
         (1) Use the "scoop" technique, in which the cap is scooped up from the tray with one hand
         (2) Use the sheath holder
         (3) Use self-sheathing disposable needles
      d. Never bend, break, or otherwise manipulate a needle
      e. OHCWs giving an injection should appropriately recap the needle to eliminate the danger of passing an uncovered needle to another worker for recapping
   2. Instrument sharpening
      a. Sharpening contaminated instruments poses risk of disease transmission
         (1) Avoid sharpening during a procedure
         (2) Instead, include duplicates of most-used instruments in the cassette for difficult cases
      b. The ideal method involves sharpening sterile instruments and then resterilizing them before use
   3. Avoid injury with contaminated instruments during client care (i.e., curettes and scalers)
      a. Avoid fulcruming on the same tooth that is being worked on

BOX 10-1 Recommendations for the Contents of the Occupational Exposure Report

Date and time of exposure

Details of the procedure being performed, including where and how the exposure occurred; if related to a sharp device, the type and brand of device and how and when in the course of handling the device the exposure occurred

Details of the exposure, including the type and amount of fluid or material and the severity of the exposure (e.g., for a percutaneous exposure, depth of injury and whether fluid was injected; for a skin or mucous membrane exposure, the estimated volume of material and the condition of the skin [e.g., chapped, abraded, intact])

Details about the exposure source (e.g., whether the source material contained hepatitis B virus (HBV), hepatitis C virus (HCV), or human immunodeficiency virus (HIV); if the source is HIV infected, the stage of disease, history of anti-retroviral therapy, viral load, and anti-retroviral resistance information, if known)

Details about the exposed person (e.g., hepatitis B vaccination and vaccine-response status)

Details about counseling, postexposure management, and follow-up

From Centers for Disease Control and Prevention: Updated U.S. Public Health Service guidelines for the management of occupational exposures to HBV, HCV and HIV and recommendations for postexposure prophylaxis, U.S. Government Printing Office, Morbidity and Mortality Weekly Report 50 (RR-11): 1–42, 2001.

    b. Never wipe instruments on gauze held in your hand or wrapped around your finger

    c. Never grab instruments by the working end

    d. Avoid holding more than one instrument in each hand

E. Exposure incident protocol (Box 10-1)

  1. Includes all needlesticks, puncture wounds, cuts, and scrapes with contaminated instruments and all nonintact skin and mucous membrane exposure to blood and saliva

  2. Immediately wash the injured area with antimicrobial soap and water

  3. Inform the employer about the incident

  4. If the source individual can be identified, request his or her consent for blood testing for hepatitis B virus (HBV), hepatitis C virus (HCV), and human immunodeficiency virus (HIV) as soon as possible (if the source individual's disease status is not already known)

  5. Results of the source individual's tests are confidential and are revealed only to the exposed employee, not to the employer

  6. The employer is responsible for providing to the exposed employee laboratory testing for HBV, HCV, and HIV status, medical evaluation, and counseling by a preselected, qualified, licensed health care provider

  7. Medical care for the exposed employee should be sought as soon as possible, ideally within 2 hours of exposure, in order to give postexposure prophylaxis (PEP) with an immunoglobulin or antiviral, if indicated, and allow for the greatest chance of success in preventing disease transmission (seroconversion)

    a. PEP may reduce the risk of infection by 80%

    b. PEP may fail because of resistant virus, increased viral load or dose of blood, or host factors

  8. If the employee declines testing, a blood sample from the employee may be preserved for 90 days in case the employee later consents to testing

  9. The employee is informed of both his or her own test results and the source client's test results by the health care provider and is informed of any conditions that require further evaluation and treatment

  10. The employer receives a written report from the health care provider confirming that the employee was tested, counseled, and informed of results, and the report also recommends any further evaluation or treatment needed; the report notes if hepatitis B vaccine was administered; the report does not include test results or diagnoses because this information is kept confidential between health care provider and employee

  11. OSHA requires that an exposure incident report be completed and filed in the employee's medical record

F. Prevention of disease transmission during radiographic procedures (see the section on "Infection Control" in Chapter 6)

  1. Although radiographic procedures are generally noninvasive, the potential for disease transmission does exist

  2. The use of barriers on equipment will prevent contamination and promote efficiency

    a. Plastic bag to cover position-indicating device (PID), tube head, and swivel arms

    b. Plastic cover for exposure-control switch

    c. Cover for headrest and chair controls

  3. If contamination occurs, clean and disinfect

    a. Use EPA-registered intermediate-level disinfectant

    b. Disinfect all touched surfaces that are unprotected by barriers

c. Do not directly spray disinfectant on the control panel because it has electrical components

4. Radiographic film holders; use reusable film holders that can be heat sterilized, or use disposable items (SUDs)

5. Radiographic film options
   a. Digital radiographs (no film processing necessary for some methods)
   b. Film in plastic covering or pouch (best option when using film)
   c. Film without plastic covering (during processing, special handling is necessary when removing the film from the packet to avoid contaminating the film)

6. Aseptic procedure for imaging and processing dental radiographs in plastic pouches
   a. Drape the client with lead apron and thyroid shield, and position the client's bib to act as a barrier; if shields become contaminated, disinfect with an intermediate-level disinfectant
   b. Wear PPE
   c. After exposing the film, drop it into a disposable cup
   d. Remove the plastic pouches, and drop the film packet into another noncontaminated cup without contaminating the film packet or the outside of the cup
   e. Remove gloves, and wash hands before transporting the film to the processing area
   f. With ungloved hands, unwrap the film and put it into the automatic processor

7. Aseptic procedure for processing dental radiographs without plastic covering
   a. After exposure, contaminated film should be placed in a plastic cup without contaminating the outside of the cup
   b. Don a new pair of gloves before transporting the film to the darkroom
   c. Open the film packet, and drop the film on a paper towel (proceed carefully to avoid contaminating the film)
   d. Remove gloves, wash hands, and with bare hands, feed the film into the automatic processor

G. Infection control for the dental laboratory
   1. Prevention of disease transmission between the treatment area and the dental laboratory
   2. OSHA regulations include measures for the protection of dental laboratory personnel from bloodborne pathogens
   3. Impression materials, prostheses, and appliances are contaminated
   4. Protective attire and barrier techniques
      a. When performing laboratory procedures, PPE should be worn; use caution with lathes because gloves can get caught and cause injury
      b. Masks and eyewear protect against chemicals, aerosols, spatter, and projectiles

   5. Preparation of materials and transport to laboratory
      a. Clean and disinfect impressions, prostheses, and casts before transport
      b. Always disinfect prostheses before sending them to another location or returning to the client
      c. Use new packing material every time the prosthesis is transported between the laboratory and the oral health care facility to prevent contamination of shipping materials
      d. Communicate the infection control protocol to the laboratory and the OHC team

   6. Minimizing contamination of common areas in laboratory
      a. Use paper covers on countertops
      b. Place plastic barriers on frequently touched areas
      c. Procedures for using the lathe
         (1) Use fresh pumice each time
         (2) Use disposable trays
         (3) Use sterile or disposable ragwheels

   7. Use a shielding device and air-suction motor with the polishing lathe, model trimmer, or grinding bench to minimize aerosol spray

   8. An EPA-registered intermediate-level disinfectant should be used to disinfect contaminated laboratory materials (e.g., impressions, fixed and removable prostheses, retainers, crowns)
      a. Spray the chemical or, preferably, immerse the material in the chemical using minimal effective exposure time (at least 15 minutes) to prevent damage to the material
      b. Consult with the manufacturer to determine which chemicals are compatible with the item to be disinfected and the immersion time required

   9. Professional cleaning of removable prostheses
      a. Use of denture-cleaning solutions is not a substitute for disinfection
      b. To prevent microbial contamination:
         (1) Use self-sealing disposable bags
         (2) Do not reuse the denture-cleaning solution
         (3) Place sealed bags in a disinfected beaker in the ultrasonic unit
         (4) Sterilize the equipment used in cleaning (e.g., brushes)
      c. Rinse the prosthesis with water to remove any residual chemical, and place it in a mouthwash solution to ensure a pleasant taste for the client

Maintaining the Oral Health Care Environment After Client Care

A. Decontamination of the treatment area
   1. Wear PPE, including utility gloves
   2. Seal and transport the biohazard bag (that is taped to the mobile cart) containing blood-soaked gauze to the biohazard waste container
   3. Remove all disposable surface barriers carefully to avoid touching the surfaces underneath
   4. Flush all of the water lines for 30 seconds between clients
   5. Close the instrument cassette or cover the procedure trays to control airborne microorganisms while transporting the instruments to the instrument processing area
   6. If instrument sterilization is delayed, place the instruments in a holding solution to prevent bioburden from drying on the instruments
   7. Discard the disposable and single-use items (e.g., saliva ejectors)
   8. Flush high-volume and low-volume suction tubing with a cleaning and disinfecting solution; periodically clean the trap of the evacuation system or preferably replace with a disposable trap using PPE
B. Regulated infectious waste
   1. Medical waste that has the potential for disease transmission and requires special handling and disposal
   2. The OSHA regulates the handling of infectious waste; the EPA regulates the disposal of infectious waste for three categories:
      a. Sharps (e.g., needles, scalpel blades, instruments)
      b. Tissue and extracted teeth; the CDC allows extracted teeth to be returned to the client
      c. Blood, items soaked or caked with blood, or items that could release potentially infectious materials when compressed; the CDC considers saliva as infectious material but not as regulated medical waste
   3. Unregulated medical waste—solid waste that is generated, including all disposable items other than sharps, tissues, extracted teeth, and blood-soaked items (e.g., gloves, saliva ejectors, cups, surface barriers); unregulated medical waste may be potentially infectious; however, it is unregulated and may be disposed of as common trash unless restricted by state and local laws
   4. Contact state and local governments for regulations on the disposal of regulated and unregulated medical waste

C. Waste management
   1. Line trash receptacles with plastic bags
   2. Sharps containers should be placed in each treatment area
D. Waste disposal
   1. Regulated infectious waste must be separated from other waste, put in a color-coded ("red bagged") container, and labeled with the biohazard symbol (Figure 10-3)
      a. Sharps must be in a closed, leakproof, and puncture-resistant sharps container
      b. Nonsharp items must be placed in a leakproof container (e.g., biohazard bag)
   2. Disposal options
      a. Sterilization on site and disposal according to local and state regulations
         (1) Do not process instruments and waste in same load
         (2) Properly perform biologic monitoring during sterilization
         (3) Extracted teeth with amalgam restorations must not be heat sterilized because

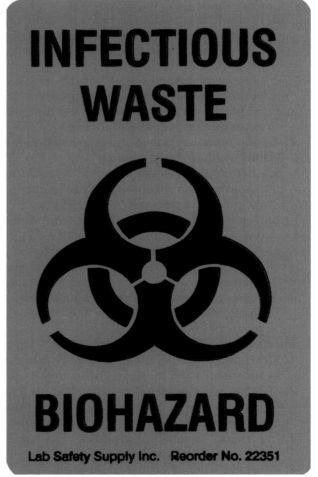

FIGURE 10-3 Biohazard symbol: Courtesy of Lab Safety Supply, Inc., Janesville, WI.

this will generate toxic vapors; use a chemical sterilant instead
  b. Hazardous waste removal service by an EPA-approved waste hauler
    (1) The oral health care facility is ultimately responsible for the proper disposal of infectious waste; therefore, the waste hauler's credentials should be checked carefully
    (2) A manifest should be provided by the waste hauler indicating the method by which the waste would be treated and its final disposal site
E. Instrument processing
  1. Organization of sterilization area
    a. For efficiency, the instrument-processing area should be centrally located
    b. The area is designed to allow for linear progression of instrument processing and for the separation of contaminated and clean or sterile items
    c. The area should be divided into three designated areas:
      (1) Decontamination area—receiving area for contaminated instruments (soaking and waste disposal), ultrasonic cleaning, rinsing, and drying
      (2) Packaging area—instruments are arranged in sets; chemical and biologic indicators are added; instruments are wrapped or bagged, sealed, and labeled
      (3) Sterilization and storage area—instruments are processed and stored
  2. Decontamination area procedures
    a. Use PPE, including utility gloves
    b. If a delay occurs before decontamination, soak instruments in a holding solution to prevent the drying of saliva and blood
      (1) Extended soaking is not recommended because it can damage the instruments
      (2) The holding solution can be water, enzyme solution, or detergent
    c. Cleaning instruments in an ultrasonic unit or instrument washer is an important step; otherwise, stuck-on blood or other organic material will remain on the instruments even after sterilization
    d. Ultrasonic cleaning
      (1) Vibrations dislodge and dissolve organic material
      (2) The safest and most efficacious method of cleaning
      (3) Eliminates the need for hand scrubbing and potential for injury with contaminated instruments

(4) Procedure for using ultrasonic instrument cleaner
  (a) Use solution specifically designed for ultrasonic cleaners; may contain antimicrobial properties
  (b) Time—4 to 16 minutes, depending on the unit, the instruments, and the amount of material on the instruments (instruments in cassettes require longer exposure time)
  (c) Keep the unit covered to prevent exposure to aerosols
  (d) Rinse the instruments and let excess water drain from the cassettes
  (e) Replenish the ultrasonic solution and disinfect the unit daily
  (f) Periodically test the unit (aluminum foil test)
e. Manual scrubbing technique—not recommended; used only if ultrasonic exposure would damage the equipment or if no ultrasonic cleaner is available
  (1) Scrub with a long-handled, stiff brush; wear utility gloves
  (2) Scrub the instruments, holding them low in the sink to minimize spatter
  (3) Scrub only a few instruments at a time
  (4) Manual scrubbing poses an increased risk for injury
f. Asepsis for high-speed and low-speed dental handpieces
  (1) Refer to the manufacturer's instructions for cleaning, lubrication, and sterilization
  (2) Some handpieces can be cleaned ultrasonically; all handpieces must be able to withstand heat sterilization (the CDC recommends heat sterilization, even though handpieces are semi-critical items)
  (3) Flush the water lines of high-speed handpieces for 30 seconds after use
g. Prophylaxis angles; should be heat sterilized or SUDs (disposable); consult the manufacturer's instructions for cleaning, lubrication, and sterilization
3. Packaging area procedures
  a. The instruments to be bagged should be dry to avoid penetrating the autoclave bag
  b. Packaging materials vary according to the type of sterilization method (Table 10-6)
  c. Packaging materials include plastic or paper pouches, plastic tubing, cassettes, or trays to be wrapped with paper or cloth, sealed with appropriate tape, labeled, and dated

TABLE 10-6 Comparison of Heat Sterilization Methods

Method	Sterilizing Conditions*	Packaging Materials	Advantages	Precautions
Steam Autoclave		Paper wrap Nylon "plastic" tubing	Time-efficient Good penetration	No closed containers Damage to plastic and rubber
Standard cycles	20–30 minutes at 250°F	Paper or plastic peel pouches Thin cloth Wrapped, perforated cassettes		Non–stainless steel items corrode Use of hard water may leave deposits Items may be wet after cycle
Flash cycles	3–10 minutes at 273°F	No packaging (unwrapped)		Unwrapped items quickly contaminated after processing
Unsaturated Chemical Vapor	20 minutes at 270°F	Paper wrap Paper or plastic peel pouches Wrapped, perforated cassettes	Time-efficient No corrosion Items dry quickly after cycle	No closed containers Damage to plastic and rubber Must use special solution Pre-dry instruments Provide adequate ventilation Cannot sterilize liquids No cloth wrap (absorbs too much chemical vapor)
Dry Heat	60–120 minutes at 320°F	Paper wrap	No corrosion	Some paper may get charred Pre-dry instruments
Oven-type (static-air)		Appropriate nylon "plastic" tubing Closed containers Wrapped, perforated cassettes	Can use closed containers[‡] Low cost Items are dry after cycle	Long sterilization time (oven-type) Damage to plastic and rubber Door cannot be opened during cycle Cannot sterilize liquids
Rapid heat transfer (forced-air)	12 minutes at 375°F (wrapped) 6 minutes at 375°F (unwrapped)	Aluminum foil[†]	No corrosion Short cycle Items are dry after cycle	Unwrapped items quickly contaminated after processing

These conditions do not include warm-up or cool-down time, and they may vary, depending on the contents and volume of the load and brand of the sterilizer.
[†]*Tears or punctures easily.*
[‡]*BI must be used to assure sterility.*
Modified from Miller CH, Palenik CJ: Infection control and the management of hazardous materials for the dental team, *ed 4, St Louis, 2010, Mosby.*

  d. To maintain package integrity, do not seal the package using staples, pins, or paper clips
  e. The packaging materials used must not:
    (1) Melt or get charred
    (2) Prevent the sterilizing agent from penetrating
    (3) Be easily torn by sharp instruments
  f. Instruments should be packaged loosely to allow for maximum contact with steam or chemical vapors; overloaded packages can lead to incomplete sterilization
  g. Biologic and chemical indicators are added during packaging procedures
4. Sterilization area procedures
5. Sterilization methods (see Table 10-6)
  a. Steam autoclave (moist heat under pressure)
    (1) Moist heat denatures and coagulates microbial proteins; pressure serves to elevate temperature

    (2) Steam must be able to penetrate the instrument package; pack loosely to allow for free passage of steam
    (3) Packages and cassettes should be placed on their edges, not laid flat
    (4) No more than two layers of packs should be placed on each shelf. The upper layer is placed perpendicular and crosswise to the one below
    (5) Avoid the package coming in contact with chamber walls
    (6) Use distilled or deionized water to prevent deposits on instruments
  b. Dry heat
    (1) Sterilizes by oxidizing cell parts
    (2) Keeps air spaces between packages
    (3) If the sterilizer is opened, timer must be restarted
  c. Unsaturated chemical vapor; alcohols, formaldehyde, ketone, acetone, and water are

heated under pressure to produce the gas that permeates and destroys microbes

d. Ethylene oxide gas sterilization
  (1) Used mostly in hospitals and large clinics
  (2) Operation
      (a) Sterilize at room temperature, 75°F (25°C), for 10 to 16 hours
      (b) Alternatively, sterilize at 120°F (49°C) for 2 to 3 hours
      (c) Aerate plastic and rubber materials for at least 16 hours after sterilization to remove stuck-on gas molecules
      (d) Warning: Residual gas can cause tissue burns

e. Liquid chemical sterilants
  (1) Used for heat-sensitive, semi-critical items when ethylene oxide gas is not available
      (a) Should not be used as a substitute for heat sterilization of semi-critical items that are not heat sensitive
      (b) Should be avoided because mostly heat-tolerant or SUDS are available
      (c) Biologic monitoring is not possible, so this method cannot ensure sterility
  (2) Follow the manufacturer's instructions for dilution, temperature, and contact time
  (3) Ensure that the instruments are dry to avoid diluting the solution
  (4) Remove the instruments with sterile forceps, rinse with sterile water, and package or cover with sterile towel
  (5) Chemicals used for sterilization (see Table 10-4); the disadvantages of chemicals are:
      (a) They produce toxic fumes and are irritating to tissues
      (b) Biologic indicators (BIs) are not available with the use of chemical sterilants; therefore, the sterility of items cannot be verified
      (c) When removed from chemicals, items are exposed to the environment and can easily become contaminated because of lack of packaging
      (d) Chemical sterilization requires an extended contact time of 3 to 12 hours, depending on the chemical

6. Verification of sterilization
  a. Failure of sterilization can occur as a result of operator or mechanical failure
    (1) Overloading—the reason for failure in the majority of cases
    (2) Improper packaging
    (3) Improper timing
    (4) Improper unit operation
    (5) Unit malfunction
    (6) Improper maintenance of equipment
  b. The CDC recommends routine use of BIs (spore tests) for verification of sterility
    (1) *Biologic monitoring* is a process in which highly resistant spores are passed through the sterilizer and then cultured to determine whether they have been killed
        (a) If spores have been killed, then all the less-resistant microorganisms exposed to the same conditions will also have been destroyed
        (b) Primary method to ascertain sterility
        (c) Biologic monitoring with BIs can be done in the dental setting or in a processing facility
    (2) Types of BIs
        (a) Spore strips—paper strips containing either one or two types of spores enclosed in a glassine envelope
            [1] After sterilization, remove the spore strip aseptically, place it in a culture medium, and incubate for 7 days
            [2] If spores are present, they will grow and change the color of the growth medium indicating sterilization failure
            [3] Strips can be used for all methods of heat sterilization
        (b) Self-contained vial—contains spore strip with an ampoule of growth medium in a plastic vial
            [1] After sterilization, squeeze the vial to break the internal ampoule, which would mix the growth medium with the spores
            [2] Incubate the vial; if spores are present, they will multiply and change the color of the growth medium, indicating sterilization failure
            [3] Vials can only be used in a steam autoclave
        (c) Specific bacterial endospores used in BIs
            [1] Steam autoclave and chemical vapor sterilizer
                [a] Spores of *Geobacillus stearothermophilus*
            [2] Dry heat and ethylene oxide gas sterilizer; spores of *Bacillus atrophaeus*

(3) Use of BIs
    (a) Place a strip inside one of each type of package (e.g., autoclave bag, cassette)
    (b) Incubate a control BI that has not been sterilized, along with the test BI
    (c) Growth of spores from the control BI confirms that live spores were present
    (d) No growth from the test BI indicates that sterilization has been achieved
(4) Test sterilization equipment weekly and when:
    (a) The equipment has been repaired
    (b) New packaging material is used
    (c) A new sterilizer is operated
    (d) Training new staff
    (e) The loading procedure is changed
(5) Sterilization failure (growth on the BI test, or positive spore test)
    (a) Review the procedures to determine any operator error
    (b) Take the sterilizer out of operation, and retest with mechanical, chemical, and biologic monitors
    (c) If the repeat BI test is negative, put the sterilizer back in service
    (d) If the repeat BI test is positive, determine the cause of failure, and repeat the BI test three times before putting the sterilizer back into service
    (e) Withdraw the instruments, and repeat the process
(6) Documentation
    (a) Record the results of biologic monitoring in a log book
    (b) Necessary for compliance with federal regulations
    (c) Serves quality assurance and risk-management purposes
c. Chemical monitoring
  (1) Chemical indicators—items containing heat-sensitive chemicals that change color when exposed to certain temperatures to assess conditions during the sterilization process (e.g., autoclave tape, special markings on autoclave bags, chemical indicator strips)
  (2) Chemical monitoring does not provide proof of sterilization
  (3) Types of chemical indicators
    (a) Integrated indicator—changes color slowly when exposed to a combination of time, temperature, and steam; placed inside each instrument package to confirm whether instruments have been exposed to sterilizing conditions
    (b) External chemical indicator—changes color after a certain temperature has been reached (e.g., autoclave tape)
      [1] Distinguishes those instruments that have been in the sterilizer from those that have not, preventing accidental use of unprocessed items
      [2] Should be present on packaging material or applied on the outside of every instrument package and cassette
d. Mechanical monitoring
  (1) Observation of sterilizer gauges, including temperature, pressure, and exposure time
  (2) Incorrect reading indicates a functional problem
7. Storage area procedures
  a. Instruments must not be stored unwrapped or unpackaged (unpackaged instruments are immediately contaminated when exposed to the environment)
  b. Packaged instruments should be stored away from treatment areas to lessen chances of contamination
  c. After sterilization, allow the instrument packages to cool and dry before storage
    (1) Microorganisms and instrument tips can penetrate wet packaging material and thereby compromise sterility
    (2) Microorganisms on contaminated surfaces can wick through wet packaging
  d. Sealed packages should be kept on shelves protected by glass doors for dry, low-dust storage
  e. Sealed instrument packages can maintain sterility for up to 30 days
  f. Instrument packages should be rotated so that the oldest dated instrument pack is used first
  g. Packages that are dropped on the floor, punctured, torn, or wet are considered contaminated
  h. Wrapped cassettes are ideal for storing and then serving as sterile instrument trays

THE OSHA AND OCCUPATIONAL EXPOSURE TO BLOODBORNE PATHOGENS

A. Protection of OHCWs against exposure to bloodborne pathogens requires employers to provide a safe working environment; the Web sites listed in the table below provide the oral health care professional with immediate access to current recommendations and regulations concerning infection control

1. OSHA Bloodborne Pathogens Standard
   a. The most important infection-control regulation in dentistry for the protection of OHCWs
   b. The final Bloodborne Pathogen Standard was published in 1991 and became effective in 1992
   c. The Needlestick Safety and Prevention Act was added to the Standard in 2001
      (1) On an annual basis, employers must solicit input from OHCWs to identify, evaluate, and select safer medical devices to minimize or eliminate occupational exposures (e.g., self-sheathing needles)
   d. Employers are responsible for staff compliance with the Standard; this includes:
      (1) Review of the Standard and ensuring that a copy is available on site
      (2) Formulation of a written exposure control plan that contains:
         (a) Clarification of which employees face a potential risk for occupational exposure and will be covered under the Standard
         (b) Description of how and when provisions will be implemented (i.e., communication of the hazards to employees, hepatitis B vaccination, postexposure evaluation and follow-up, record keeping, use of PPE, engineering and work practice controls, and housekeeping)
         (c) Evaluation of exposure incidents
         (d) Prevention of sharps injuries
      (3) Training of employees
         (a) Training that provides information about the hazards and preventive measures related to occupational exposure to bloodborne pathogens
         (b) Training to be completed at the initial time of assignment and annually thereafter
         (c) Person conducting the training shall be qualified and knowledgeable about the subject matter
         (d) Training must provide an opportunity for interactive questions and answers with the person conducting the training
      (4) Providing employees with necessary materials to comply with the Standard
         (a) Offer and pay for hepatitis B vaccination
         (b) Provide, maintain, and ensure use of PPE and engineering controls
         (c) Establish appropriate work practices and decontamination procedures in the oral health care setting to ensure the safety of OHCWs (appropriate decontamination, laundry handling, and infectious waste disposal)
         (d) Establish and provide postexposure medical evaluation and follow-up without any cost to employees
         (e) Provide appropriate biohazard communication by posting signs, biohazard-waste labels, and red containers that indicate infectious waste on site
      (5) Maintain appropriate records
         (a) Training sessions (participants, trainers, summary of content, evaluations)
         (b) Employee medical records (HBV immunization status, incident exposure reports, postexposure evaluation and follow-up)
2. Inspections conducted by OSHA
   a. Initiated by employee complaints
   b. Programmed inspections of randomly selected worksites employing 11 or more people
   c. Noncompliance with any provision in the Standard can result in the imposition of fines

Evaluation of Infection Control Programs (see Table 10-7)

TABLE 10-7 Evaluating Infection Control Programs

Program Element	Evaluation Activity
Appropriate immunization of dental health care personnel (DHCP)	Conduct annual review of personnel records to ensure up-to-date immunization
Assessment of occupational exposures to infectious agents	Report occupational exposures to infectious agents. Document the steps that occurred around the exposure and plan how such exposure can be prevented in the future

Continued

TABLE 10-7 Evaluating Infection Control Programs—cont'd

Program Element	Evaluation Activity
Comprehensive postexposure management plan and medical follow-up program after occupational exposures to infectious agents	Ensure the postexposure management plan is clear, complete, and available at all times to all DHCP. All staff should understand the plan, which should include toll-free phone numbers for access to additional information
Adherence to hand hygiene before and after patient care	Observe and document circumstances of appropriate or inappropriate handwashing. Review findings in a staff meeting
Proper use of personal protective equipment to prevent occupational exposures to infectious agents	Observe and document the use of barrier precautions and careful handling of sharps. Review findings in a staff meeting
Routine and appropriate sterilization of instruments using a biologic monitoring system	Monitor paper log of steam cycle and temperature strip with each sterilization load, and examine results of weekly biologic monitoring. Take appropriate action when failure of sterilization process is noted
Evaluation and implementation of safer medical devices	Conduct an annual review of the exposure control plan and consider new developments in safer medical devices
Compliance of water in routine dental procedures with current drinking U.S. Environmental Protection Agency water standards (fewer than 500 colony-forming units [CFU] of heterotrophic water bacteria)	Monitor dental water quality as recommended by the equipment manufacturer using commercial self-contained test kits, or commercial water-testing laboratories
Proper handling and disposal of medical waste	Observe the safe disposal of regulated and nonregulated medical waste and take preventive measures if hazardous situations occur
Health care–associated infections	Assess the unscheduled return of patients after procedures and evaluate them for an infectious process. A trend might require formal evaluation

From Centers for Disease Control and Prevention: Guidelines for infection control in dental health-care settings, Morbidity and Mortality Weekly Report 52(RR-17):1–68, 2003.

Legal and Ethical Issues in Disease Prevention (see Box 10-2)

BOX 10-2 Legal and Ethical Issues in Disease Prevention

Treat all clients regardless of disease status
Practice infection control according to the standard of care
   Adhere to the Centers for Disease Control and Prevention (CDC) and the Occupational Safety and Health Administration (OSHA) guidelines
   Adhere to state and federal laws
   Use evidence-based protocols
   Follow state board of dentistry laws and regulations
   Follow expert opinion related to infection control
   Stay current of new protocols and guidelines
Abide by U.S. Public Health Service guidelines for employee work restrictions

@ WEB SITE INFORMATION AND RESOURCES

SOURCE	WEB SITE ADDRESS	DESCRIPTION
Association for Professionals in Infection Control and Epidemiology (APIC)	http://www.apic.org	Infection control organization for health care
Centers for Disease Control and Prevention (CDC)	http://www.cdc.gov	U.S. government agency that provides resources and recommendations for numerous health and safety topics
Organization for Safety, Asepsis, and Prevention (OSAP)	http://www.osap.org	Organization that promotes infection control and safety policies to the dental community
Occupational Safety and Health Administration (OSHA)	http://www.osha.gov	U.S. government agency responsible for ensuring the health and safety of employees at workplaces
National Institutes for Occupational Safety and Health (NIOSH)	http://www.cdc.gov/niosh	U.S. government agency that provides national and world leadership to prevent illness and injury

SUGGESTED READINGS

Centers for Disease Control and Prevention: Guidelines for disinfection and sterilization in healthcare facilities, *Morbidity and Mortality Weekly Report* 52(RR-17):1–68, 2008.

Centers for Disease Control and Prevention: Guidelines for infection control in dental health-care settings, *Morbidity and Mortality Weekly Report* 52(RR-17):1–68, 2003.

Miller CH, Palenik CJ: *Infection control and management of hazardous materials for the dental team*, ed 4, St Louis, 2010, Mosby.

Molinari JA, Harte JA: *Cottone's practical infection control in dentistry*, ed 3, Baltimore, 2010, Lippincott Williams & Wilkins.

United States Department of Labor, Occupational Safety and Health Administration: *Controlling occupational exposure to bloodborne pathogens*, Washington, DC, 1996, 2001, OSHA 3127 (revised).

CHAPTER 10 REVIEW QUESTIONS

Answers and Rationales to Review Questions are available on this text's accompanying Evolve site. See inside front cover for details.
Use Case A to answer questions 1 to 6.

*e*volve

CASE A

Maria, a dental hygienist, is air polishing Kyle's teeth. Kyle is a 9-year-old boy currently undergoing phase I orthodontics. The air temperature in the office is warm today because of a malfunctioning air conditioning unit. Because of this situation, Maria has opted not to use a face mask. She feels that the face shield she is wearing will be adequate protection; she also thinks that a face mask will make it difficult for her to breathe normally and will make her feel more uncomfortably hot. She finishes the treatment and dismisses her client. Two weeks later, vesicles break out all over her skin. Maria visits her health care provider and is diagnosed with chickenpox.

1. **Which of the following pathways of cross-contamination is depicted in this case?**
   a. Client to dental team
   b. Dental team to client
   c. Client to client
   d. Office to community

2. **Which of the following modes of disease spread is depicted in this case?**
   a. Direct contact
   b. Indirect contact
   c. Droplet infection
   d. Airborne infection

3. **What is the source of the microbes in this case?**
   a. Client's mouth
   b. Hygienist's hands
   c. Contaminated instrument
   d. Clinical contact surface

4. **In this case, which of the following infection-control procedures likely would have prevented disease transmission?**
   a. Using barriers
   b. Cleaning the environmental surfaces
   c. Processing the instruments in cassettes
   d. Wearing proper PPE

5. **Which of the following microorganism type is responsible for chickenpox?**
   a. Bacterium
   b. Prion
   c. Virus
   d. Fungus

6. **Which of the following pathogens is responsible for the acquisition of chickenpox?**
   a. Treponema pallidum
   b. Coxsackievirus
   c. Varicella zoster virus
   d. Epstein-Barr virus

CASE B

While hand-scaling tenacious calculus, a dental hygienist's curette slips off the client's tooth and penetrates the hygienist's fulcrum finger. He sees a small spot of blood forming under his glove. Use Case B to answer questions 7 to 12.

7. **After removing his glove, what should the hygienist do next?**
   a. Scrub the finger using a stiff brush
   b. Squeeze the finger to let out the contaminants
   c. Wash the finger with antimicrobial soap
   d. Immerse the finger in bleach for 1 minute

8. **The employee has sustained a percutaneous injury and may have been exposed to a blood-borne pathogen. In this situation, what is the responsibility of the employer according to the OSHA?**
   a. None, an employee works at his own risk
   b. Pay for the treatment of any acquired disease

   c. Give the employee the following day off with pay
   d. Arrange for a consultation with a qualified health care provider

9. **The client's blood was tested and she was found to have hepatitis C virus (HCV). Postexposure prophylaxis (PEP) of the exposed employee (dental hygienist) is not recommended because HCV cannot be transmitted in the dental setting.**
   a. Both the statement and the reason are TRUE
   b. Both the statement and the reason are FALSE
   c. The statement is true; the reason is FALSE
   d. The statement is false; the reason is TRUE

10. **The dental hygienist elects to be tested for HCV, and he is informed of the results. Which of the following actions is he then required to take?**
    a. Inform his employer of the results
    b. Document the results on the incident report
    c. Inform the CDC and the OSHA
    d. None of the above is required

11. **All the following information should be included in the incident exposure report EXCEPT one. Which one is the EXCEPTION?**
    a. Date and time of exposure
    b. How the exposure occurred
    c. Presence of HCV in blood
    d. Client's Social Security Number

12. **What is the level of risk related to the transmission of HCV from this exposure?**
    a. High
    b. Moderate
    c. Low
    d. Very low

13. **All of the following viruses are bloodborne pathogens EXCEPT one. Which one is the EXCEPTION?**
    a. Human immunodeficiency virus
    b. Hepatitis B virus
    c. Hepatitis C virus
    d. Varicella zoster virus

14. **Which term is used for the practice of treating a client's blood, bodily fluids, nonintact skin, and mucous membranes as potentially infectious?**
    a. Standard precautions
    b. Pervasive precautions
    c. Universal precautions
    d. Protective precautions

15. **Glutaraldehyde is a high-level disinfectant, so it can be used to sterilize heat-sensitive items.**
    a. Both statements are true
    b. Both statements are false
    c. The first statement is true; the second is false
    d. The first statement is false; the second is true

16. **An unvaccinated OHCW with weeping dermatitis of her hands touches a drawer pull contaminated with HBV and later contracts the disease. Which of the following modes of disease spread would be involved in this situation?**
    a. Direct contact
    b. Indirect contact
    c. Droplet infection
    d. Airborne infection

17. **Which of the following methods will achieve sterilization?**
    a. Dry heat at 320°F for 50 minutes
    b. Steam autoclave at 200°F for 30 minutes
    c. Chemical vapor at 270°F for 20 minutes
    d. Ethylene oxide gas for 5 hours

18. **The CDC recommends disinfecting clinical contact surfaces with an intermediate level disinfectant that is tuberculocidal because *Mycobacterium tuberculosis* var. *bovis* is a resistant microbe and all other less resistant microbes would also be killed.**
    a. Both the statement and the reason are true
    b. Both the statement and the reason are false
    c. The statement is true; the reason is false
    d. The statement is false; the reason is true

19. **What is the ultimate goal of infection control in the oral health care setting?**
    a. Prevent all pathogens from entering the client treatment area
    b. Sterilize clinical contact surfaces between clients
    c. Reduce the dose of microbes that may be shared
    d. Eliminate all microbes emanating from the source

20. **Alcohol-based hand rubs may be used instead of handwashing between clients because the rubs have been found to be more effective than handwashing, especially when visible soil is present.**
    a. Both the statement and the reason are true
    b. Both the statement and the reason are false
    c. The statement is true; the reason is false
    d. The statement is false; the reason is true

21. **All of the following are true related to using instrument cassettes EXCEPT one. Which one is the EXCEPTION?**
    a. Unwrap the cassette in view of the client
    b. Unwrap with clean hands
    c. Exposure to bioburden is decreased
    d. The use of cassettes is less time efficient

22. **Many OHCWs experience skin problems on their hands related to the use of gloves. In most cases, these problems are caused by an allergic response to latex proteins in gloves.**
    a. Both statements are true
    b. Both statements are false
    c. The first statement is true; the second statement is false
    d. The first statement is false; the second statement is true

23. **Which of the following indicators is used to determine sterility?**
    a. External indicator
    b. Integrated indicator
    c. Biologic indicator
    d. Chemical indicator

24. **Which of the following is the OSHA primarily concerned with protecting?**
    a. Employee
    b. Employer
    c. Client
    d. Community

25. **Which of the following characteristics is an advantage of chemical-vapor sterilization?**
    a. A ventilation system is not required
    b. It can sterilize closed containers
    c. Extra drying time is not needed
    d. It is the least costly method of sterilization

26. **All of the following are vaccine preventable illnesses EXCEPT one. Which one is the EXCEPTION?**
    a. Hepatitis B virus (HBV)
    b. Hepatitis A virus (HAV)
    c. Hepatitis C virus (HCV)
    d. Varicella zoster virus (VZV)

27. **Which of the following statements best characterizes the resident flora on hands?**
    a. They colonize the deeper layers of the skin
    b. They are less resistant to removal by handwashing
    c. They are the primary source of disease transmission
    d. They are associated with allergic contact dermatitis

28. **Which of the following statements is true regarding the handling of regulated infectious waste?**
    a. Containers of infectious waste must be identified with the biohazard symbol
    b. Infectious waste can be disinfected and then combined with the regular trash
    c. Infectious waste must be sterilized before leaving the oral health care setting
    d. Infectious waste does not require any special handling in some states

29. **Gloves to be used intraorally should be donned:**
    a. Prior to operatory setup
    b. Prior to unwrapping the cassette
    c. Prior to taking the blood pressure
    d. Prior to entering the client's mouth

30. **Which of the following packaging materials should not be used with chemical-vapor sterilization?**
    a. Paper wrap
    b. Paper pouches
    c. Plastic pouches
    d. Cloth wrap

31. **Which of the following characteristics best describes the use of protective barriers for clinical contact surfaces?**
    a. They need to be changed only when visibly soiled
    b. They should not replace disinfection between clients
    c. They are ideally used for surfaces that are difficult to disinfect
    d. They decrease the cost of maintaining asepsis

32. **All of following characteristics describe EPA-registered intermediate-level disinfectants EXCEPT one. Which one is the EXCEPTION?**
    a. Must inactivate *Mycobacterium tuberculosis* var. *bovis*
    b. Will kill vegetative bacteria and most viruses
    c. Must be used on surfaces with visible blood
    d. Will achieve sterilization if long contact time is used

33. **All practitioners who are vaccinated for hepatitis B will become immune to the virus. Therefore, the CDC does not recommend booster injections.**
    a. Both statements are true
    b. Both statements are false
    c. The first statement is true; the second statement is false
    d. The first statement is false; the second statement is true

34. **Face shields provide maximum coverage for the face and protection from spatter during oral health care procedures. Therefore, wearing a facemask is not required when using a face shield.**
    a. Both statements are true
    b. Both statements are false
    c. The first statement is true; the second statement is false
    d. The first statement is false; the second statement is true

35. **Which of the following pathogens has been identified in the biofilm that accumulates inside dental unit water lines?**
    a. *Pseudomonas aeruginosa*
    b. *Neisseria meningitidis*
    c. *Candida albicans*
    d. *Treponema pallidum*

36. **Which of the following individuals may file a complaint with the OSHA regarding an oral health care facility?**
    a. Dentist (employer) at the facility
    b. Employee at facility
    c. Client at facility
    d. Dentist at another facility

37. **An individual should be tested for antibodies to HBV 1 to 2 months after receiving the last dose of the hepatitis B vaccine. The reason for this testing is that not all individuals will seroconvert.**
    a. Both statements are true
    b. Both statements are false
    c. The first statement is true; the second statement is false
    d. The first statement is false; the second statement is true

38. **In which of the following methods are biologic monitors containing spores of *Geobacillus stearothermophilus* used to verify sterilization?**
    a. Steam autoclave
    b. Dry-heat oven
    c. Ethylene oxide gas
    d. Rapid-heat transfer

39. **The primary reason for routinely wearing powder-free gloves is to:**
    a. Reduce airborne latex proteins
    b. Help with glove donning
    c. Eliminate skin problems
    d. Reduce glove costs

40. **Sterilization failure is most often caused by:**
    a. The autoclave not working properly
    b. Improper packaging materials used
    c. Overloading the steam autoclave sterilizer
    d. Not reaching the effective temperature

41. **A chemical indicator is used on the outside of packaging to identify the items that have been processed through the sterilizer. The chemical indicator changes color when the packages are sterile.**
    a. Both statements are true
    b. Both statements are false
    c. The first statement is true; the second statement is false
    d. The first statement is false; the second statement is true

42. **Dental handpieces are considered critical items and must be sterilized using:**
    a. The heat sterilization method
    b. A chemical sterilant
    c. Ethylene oxide gas sterilization
    d. A high-level disinfectant

43. **What is the maximum level of bacteria that the EPA allows in dental unit water?**
    a. 100 CFU/mL (colony-forming unit per milliliter)
    b. 300 CFU/mL
    c. 500 CFU/mL
    d. 800 CFU/mL

44. **In most cases, what is the number of bacteria in the water exiting from an untreated dental unit water line?**
    a. Lower than in drinking water
    b. The same as in drinking water
    c. Higher than in drinking water
    d. Depends on municipal water

45. **All of the following materials are considered regulated infectious waste EXCEPT one. Which one is the EXCEPTION?**
    a. Extracted tooth
    b. Blood-soaked gauze
    c. Anesthetic needle
    d. Saliva-coated gloves

46. **The primary reason for clients to perform a pre-procedural rinse before undergoing oral health care is to:**
    a. Give the client fresh breath
    b. Eliminate food particles
    c. Reduce the microbes in aerosols
    d. Prevent infection in the client's mouth

47. **Which of the following methods or materials is the most effective for preventing transmission of hepatitis B in the oral health care setting?**
    a. Vaccination with HBV surface antigen
    b. Disinfecting surfaces contaminated with HBV
    c. Wearing double gloves for HBV carriers
    d. Screening clients for active HBV infection

48. **How often should biologic indicators be used to test sterilizing equipment? Biologic monitors should be used once every:**
    a. Day
    b. Week
    c. Month
    d. Quarter

49. **All of the following methods inhibit the formation of biofilm in dental unit waterlines (DUWLs) EXCEPT one. Which one is the EXCEPTION?**
    a. Flushing waterlines for 2 minutes
    b. Independent water reservoir
    c. Chemical disinfection of waterlines
    d. Sterile water delivery systems

50. **To prevent cross-contamination, the practice of using a cotton roll taped to the bracket tray for wiping debridement instruments instead of a gauze square wrapped around the finger is considered:**
    a. Standard bioburden control
    b. Safe practice control
    c. Engineering control
    d. Work practice control

Elena Bablenis Haveles

As a health care provider responsible for client assessment and care, the dental hygienist must understand drugs, the conditions for which these drugs are used, and the actions, range of effects, and interactions of the drugs. The health, dental, and pharmacologic histories are the foundation on which decisions regarding client care rest. For example, some clients may need prophylactic antibiotic premedication before dental and dental hygiene care. Therefore, before care is planned, the client's medical conditions and the medications used to manage them are assessed and recorded in the client's permanent record. Contraindications or cautions to professional care concerning these drugs are determined using appropriate references and consultations. Through this knowledge, medical emergencies may be prevented; and, if an emergency occurs, the oral health care team can act within the standard of care.

GENERAL CONSIDERATIONS

Definitions

A. Pharmacology—the study of drugs and their effects on living organisms
B. Pharmacotherapy—the use of medications to treat different disease states
C. Pharmacodynamics—the action of drugs on living organisms
D. Pharmacokinetics—what the body does in response to the drugs (e.g., absorption, distribution, metabolism, excretion)
E. Pharmacy—the practice of compounding, preparing, and dispensing drugs and of counseling clients about their medications
F. Toxicology—the study of the harmful effects of drugs on living organisms
  1. Drugs—biologically active substances that can modify cellular function; used in the prevention,

diagnosis, treatment, and cure of disease or in the prevention of pregnancy
  2. Nomenclature—each drug has several names
    a. Chemical name—based on the drug's chemical formula (e.g., N-acetyl para-amino phenol)
    b. Trade (proprietary) name—each drug company makes up its own product trade name (e.g., Tylenol, Peridex, Atridox, Arestin)
    c. Brand name—technically, the name of the drug company itself, but often used interchangeably with the trade name (e.g., either Astra [company that makes Xylocaine] or Xylocaine can be considered the brand name)
    d. Generic name—official name of the drug determined by the U.S. Adopted Names Council that is used by all manufacturers of a particular drug (e.g., acetaminophen, chlorhexidine gluconate)
G. Table 11-1 lists the Latin abbreviations used in prescription writing

References

A. Books
  1. *Physicians' Desk Reference (PDR)*[1]—provides an index of drug manufacturers, brand and generic names of drugs, product categories, drug identification and information guide, and diagnostic information; updated yearly; most commonly used reference in the oral health care environment; inclusion of a drug in this reference is paid for by the manufacturer (seldom-used products not listed); information about the drug is similar to that found in the package insert, but this information is not updated regularly
  2. *Facts and Comparisons*[2]—drugs organized by pharmacologic classes; complete listing; updated monthly; contains both prescription and

TABLE 11-1 Common Latin Abbreviations Used in Prescription Writing

Abbreviation	Interpretation
a., ante	Before
a.c., ante cibum	Before meals
A.D., auris dextra	Right ear
A.L., auris laeva	Left ear
b.i.d., bis in die	Twice per day or twice daily
gt., gutta	Drop (plural gtt.)
h., hora	Hour
h.s., hora somni	At bedtime
o.d., oculus dexter	Right eye
o.s., oculus sinister	Left eye
o.u., oculus uterque	Each eye
p.c., post cibum	After meals
p.o., per os	By mouth
p.r.	By rectum
p.r.n., pro re nata	As needed
q.d., quaque die	Once per day or once daily
q.i.d., quater in die	Four times per day
q.o.d.	Every other day
q.h.	Every 6 hours
sl.	Sublingual
supp.	Suppository
t.i.d., ter in die	Three times per day
u.d.	As directed

over-the-counter (OTC) drugs; prepared by independent editors

3. *Applied Pharmacology for the Dental Hygienist;*[3] *Oral Pharmacology for the Dental Hygienist;*[4] *Basic Principles of Pharmacology with Dental Hygiene Applications*[5]—basic pharmacology textbooks for the dental hygienist; all three focus on dental hygiene considerations and provide the necessary information to avoid adverse reactions and drug interactions

4. *Mosby's Dental Drug Reference*[6]—provides comments on a limited number of drugs specifically related to dentistry; includes dental drug interactions, oral side effects, and dental considerations

5. *Drug Information Handbook for Dentistry*[7]—provides an alphabetical listing of drugs and their effects on dental therapy; sections on

managing medically compromised clients and treating specific oral conditions; information on dental office emergencies; comprehensive appendix on dental drug interactions and OTC dental products

6. *Drug Information for the Health Care Professional,* Volume 1, and *Advice for the Patient,* Volume 2;[8] published yearly and updated quarterly by U.S. Pharmacopoeia; includes basic information regarding pharmacology, pharmacokinetics, adverse reactions, drug interactions, doses, and advice to the patient

B. CD-ROM sources—more titles are becoming available; it is important to preview CD-ROMs before purchasing them because the ease of computer access ("user-friendliness") varies considerably; many can be purchased with quarterly updates included

C. Internet sites—extensive and growing volume of information; use a search engine to explore sites related to dental hygiene (see the table titled "Web Site Information and Resources" at the end of this chapter)

Agencies and Legislation

A. U.S. Food and Drug Administration (FDA)—determines drugs to be marketed in the United States; after considering safety, efficacy, and physical and chemical data, the FDA requires quality control of manufacturing facilities, determines what drugs are sold by prescription, and regulates the advertising and labeling of prescription drugs

B. U.S. Drug Enforcement Administration (DEA)—branch of the Department of Justice; determines the degree of control for substances with abuse potential; controlled substances used in dentistry are classified under Schedules I to V (Table 11-2)

Drug Action

A. Log dose–response curve—as the dose of a drug increases (x axis), the percentage of maximum response increases (y axis) until increasing the dose further produces no increase in the percentage of response (the effect of the drug reaches a plateau) (Figure 11-1)

B. Definitions
1. Effective dose (ED) 50—dose that produces 50% of the maximum response, or the dose of a drug that produces a specific response in 50% of the subjects

2. Lethal dose (LD) 50—dose that is lethal to (kills) 50% of the subjects; laboratory animals are used to derive LD

TABLE 11-2 Drug Enforcement Administration Schedules Used in Dentistry (I Through V)

Schedule	Abuse Potential	Examples	Handling
I	High	Heroin, phencyclidine (PCP)	Prescriptions may not be sent by telephone
II	High	Morphine, meperidine, oxycodone mixtures (Percodan, Percocet)	Prescriptions must be signed by the prescriber; may not be telephoned to pharmacist; emergency prescriptions may be phoned; however, signed original prescription order must be delivered to the pharmacy within 72 hours of the phone order; no refills
III	Some	Codeine mixtures (Tylenol and codeine), hydrocodone mixtures (Vicodin), "weaker" stimulants and sedatives	Prescriptions may be telephoned to pharmacy; may be refilled five times within 6 months
IV	Low	Dextropropoxyphene (Darvon), diazepam (Valium)	Same as schedule III
V	Very low	Some cough syrup containing codeine	Same as schedule III

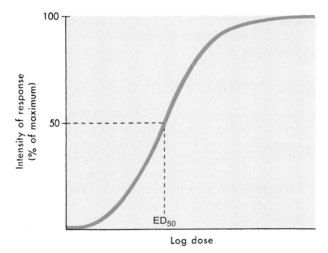

FIGURE 11-1 Log dose-effect curve. *ED*, effective dose.

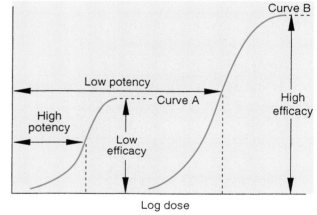

FIGURE 11-2 Potency and efficacy of a drug. Curve A has high potency and low efficacy; Curve B has low potency and high efficacy.

3. Therapeutic index (TI)—LD50 divided by ED50; a measure of the safety of a drug
4. Onset—time required for a drug's effect to begin; onset is short if the drug is given intravenously, longer if administered orally
5. Duration—length of time a drug's effect lasts; related to a drug's half-life
6. Half-life $(t\frac{1}{2})$—time required for a drug's serum concentration to decrease by 50%; five half-lives are required for a drug to be eliminated from the body
7. Potency—amount of drug (e.g., in milligrams) needed to produce an effect; the more potent an agent is, the lower is the dose needed to produce an effect (Figure 11-2)
8. Efficacy—the desired effect elicited by a drug, independent of dose (see Figure 11-2)

9. Tolerance—physiological response to the same dose produces less effect, or a higher dose is required to achieve the same effect
10. Therapeutic effect—desired pharmacologic effect
C. Routes of administration
   1. Oral (PO)—by mouth; easiest to use; good client acceptance; however, a latency period exists
   2. Rectal—administration by suppository or enema; produces either local or systemic effect
   3. Parenteral—a route other than an oral route; usually refers to an injection
   4. Intravenous (IV)—administration into a vein; shortest onset of action and higher risk of adverse events compared to other routes of administration

5. Intramuscular (IM)—administration into the muscle; sometimes painful
6. Subcutaneous (SC, SQ)—injected beneath the skin (e.g., insulin)
7. Intradermal—injected into the dermis (e.g., skin test for tuberculosis produces a bleb [bump]; progesterone implants are administered intradermally)
8. Intrathecal—administered into the spinal fluid (e.g., to treat meningitis)
9. Intraperitoneal—injected into the peritoneal cavity (abdomen)
10. Oral or nasal—particles, volatile liquids, or gasses that are inhaled (e.g., nitrous oxide-oxygen (N_2O–O_2) analgesia; as are some medications used to treat allergies and asthma)
11. Topical—ointments or creams applied to the skin or mucous membranes (e.g., hydrocortisone)
12. Sublingual—a tablet that dissolves or a solution that is sprayed under the tongue (for systemic effect)

D. Dosage forms
1. Capsule—gelatin shell
2. Tablet—compressed or molded dosage form
3. Ointment or cream—semi-solid for topical application
4. Suppository—penile, rectal, or vaginal; systemic or local
5. Solution—single-phase system consisting of more than one constituent
6. Suspension—insoluble particles in liquid (e.g., milk of magnesia)
7. Emulsion—two immiscible (not mixable) liquids (e.g., oil and water)
8. Elixir—sweetened and hydroalcoholic (water and alcohol mixture)
9. Tincture—usually alcoholic

E. Dosage
1. Varies depending on the client's:
   a. Age—older adults may require lower doses because they may metabolize and excrete drugs more slowly
   b. Weight—total body weight, muscle-to-fat ratio, and body size can affect drug absorption
   c. Condition (disease)—many different disease states can affect drug absorption, metabolism, or excretion (e.g., congestive heart failure slows down metabolism; hyperthyroidism speeds up metabolism)
   d. Route of administration
2. Pediatric dose
   a. Less than the adult's dose
   b. Based on:

(1) Manufacturer's recommendations—best method
(2) Surface area—good method
(3) Weight—adequate method
(4) Age—very poor method

Adverse Reactions

Side Effect

A. Side effect on a nontarget organ—effect on an organ other than that intended to be altered (e.g., insomnia resulting from a β_2-agonist or theophylline); dose-related and often predictable
B. Toxic reaction—predictable and dose-related effect on a target organ (e.g., insulin can lower blood glucose levels to the point of hypoglycemia)
C. Allergic reaction—varies from mild rash to anaphylaxis; involves an antigen–antibody reaction (e.g., rash from penicillin); can include urticaria, soft tissue swelling, and difficulty breathing; not predictable and not dose related
D. Idiosyncrasy—abnormal drug response that is genetically related
E. Interference with natural defense mechanisms—body is less able to fight infection (e.g., steroids weaken the immune system)
F. Teratogenic effect—adverse effect on a fetus (e.g., alcohol intake during pregnancy produces fetal alcohol syndrome)
G. Safety—related to the therapeutic index; therapeutic index: LD50/ED50. The measure of a drug's safety can be determined using this formula; the larger the number of this ratio, the safer is the drug

Pharmacokinetics

Pharmacokinetics is the way in which the body responds to drugs through the four processes of absorption, distribution, metabolism, and excretion (ADME)

A. Absorption depends on:
1. Degree of ionization—the more ionized (charged) the drug, the less it will be absorbed; conversely, the less ionized the drug, the more it will be absorbed; with weak acids or bases, this is a function of pH
2. Lipid solubility—the more lipid soluble the drug, the more readily it will be absorbed; the less lipid soluble it is, the less readily it will be absorbed
3. Factors that affect absorption
   a. Client compliance
   b. Age
   c. Gender
   d. Other disease states
   e. Genetic variations
   f. Placebo effect

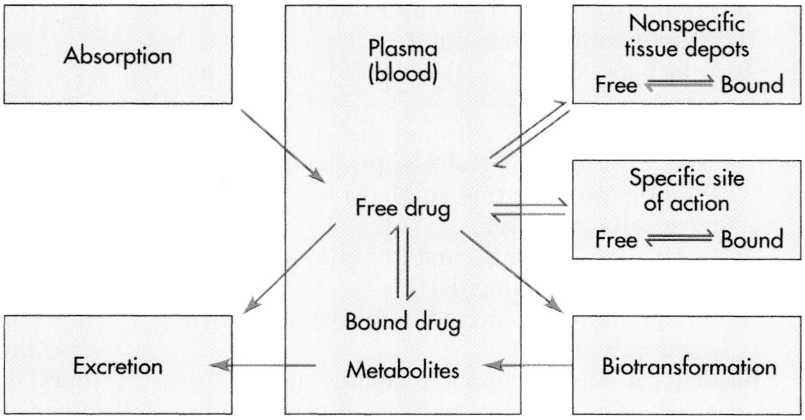

FIGURE 11-3 Absorption and outcome of a drug. *(Modified from Holroyd SV, Wynn RL, Requa-Clark B: Clinical pharmacology in dental practice, ed 4, St Louis, 1989, Mosby.)*

B. Distribution of the drug (Figure 11-3)[9]
   1. Drugs are transported to the site of action
   2. Only the free, or unbound, drug can cross cell membranes (indicated by arrows between boxes in Figure 11-3)
   3. In each cellular compartment, equilibrium is reached between the bound and unbound (free) drug
   4. Redistribution—the drug moves from one tissue (where it exerts an effect) to another tissue (where it is inactive); this is one method of terminating a drug's effect
   5. Protein binding—drugs bind to protein receptors to varying degrees; once the drug binds to a protein receptor, it cannot exert its pharmacologic effect; when more than one drug is present in the system, the drugs may compete for the same receptor site; the drug with the stronger affinity will bind to the receptor site, and the drug with the weaker affinity will then exert its pharmacologic effect
   6. Tissue binding—some drugs can also bind to body tissues and cause significant chemical effects (e.g., tetracycline has an impact on developing bones and teeth of the fetus and of a young child)
C. Metabolism (biotransformation)—takes place mainly in the liver by hepatic microsomal enzymes; metabolites are more polar, less protein bound, and more easily excreted; drugs metabolized by microsomal enzymes can affect their own metabolism or that of other drugs (e.g., either increasing [as with barbiturates] or decreasing [as with cimetidine, erythromycin] the rate of metabolism); biotransformation is a source of drug interactions
D. Excretion—usually by way of kidneys (urine); can also occur through feces (enterohepatic circulation), sweat, tears, or lungs (e.g., N_2O is exhaled)

Receptors

An area in the body to which a drug binds
A. Agonist—a drug that has an affinity for a receptor site and binds to it, producing an effect (e.g., opioid [narcotic] analgesic agent)
B. Antagonist—a drug has an affinity for a receptor site and binds to it but produces no effect; competitively blocks the effect of an agonist (e.g., naloxone, an opioid [narcotic] antagonist blocks the effect of the agonist, an opioid)

AUTONOMIC NERVOUS SYSTEM AGENTS

Agents affecting the autonomic nervous system are divided into four groups: parasympathetic (P) nervous system stimulation (P+) and inhibition (P−), and sympathetic (S) nervous system stimulation (S+) and inhibition (S−).

Sympathetic (Adrenergic) Agents

A. Mimic the action of the sympathetic autonomic nervous system (SANS); act like norepinephrine (NE) in the SANS, producing stimulation of the SANS; epinephrine produces the same effect (Figure 11-4)
B. Adrenergic agonists
   1. The SANS is activated by fear (the "fight-or-flight" response)
   2. Catecholamine—chemical structure of some adrenergic agents
   3. Receptors in the SANS include:
      a. α_1-Receptors—produce constriction of smooth muscles and blood vessels (vasoconstriction)

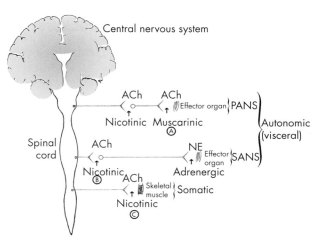

FIGURE 11-4 Typical neurons with neurotransmitters (*ACh*, acetylcholine; *NE*, norepinephrine), and the typical parasympathetic nervous system (PANS); the sympathetic nervous system (SANS); somatic nerves; and muscarinic (*A*), and nicotinic (*B* and *C*) receptors.

TABLE 11-3 Adrenergic Agents and Their Use

Adrenergic Agent	Receptor Stimulated	Comments
Epinephrine (Adrenalin)	αβ	Endogenous catecholamine; local anesthetic additive
Methylphenidate (Ritalin)	α	Attention deficit hyperactivity disorder (ADHD)
Phenylephrine (Neo-Synephrine)	α	Nasal decongestant
Levonordefrin (Neo-Cobefrin)	α > β	Local anesthetic additive
Amphetamine	αβ	Diet pill (abused)
Pseudoephedrine (Sudafed)	αβ	Orally active nasal decongestant

b. β-Receptors
  (1) β$_1$-Receptors—stimulate the heart, increase heart rate (HR), increase the contractility and conduction velocity of the heart, and cause bronchodilation
  (2) β$_2$-Receptors—relax smooth muscles, causing dilation of the blood vessels of skeletal muscle (vasodilation) and bronchodilation
C. Pharmacologic effects and adverse reactions
  1. The central nervous system (CNS)—stimulation produces increased alertness; may also cause anxiety, anorexia
  2. Stimulation of the heart—S+, produces
    a. Positive chronotropic effect (increased HR)
    b. Positive inotropic effect (increased strength of contraction of the heart)
    c. Arrhythmias, with higher doses
    d. α-Receptor stimulation—decreases HR because of the indirect (reflex vagal) effect
  3. Vascular effects (on the arterial tree) result from
    a. α-Receptors—causing vasoconstriction of blood vessels
    b. β-Receptors—causing vasodilation of skeletal muscle blood vessels
    c. Total peripheral resistance (TPR)—force against which the heart works to circulate blood
      (1) α-Receptors—increased TPR
      (2) β-Receptors—decreased TPR
  4. Mydriasis (pupil dilation) and reduced intraocular pressure; useful in treating glaucoma
  5. Bronchodilation (by action of β$_2$-agonist); useful in treating clients with asthma

  6. Alterations in the blood glucose level; persons with diabetes mellitus must be observed for adverse reactions
  7. Production of thick, viscous saliva
D. Drug interactions—examples of interactions caused by adrenergic agents are listed below:
  1. Tricyclic antidepressants (e.g., amitriptyline [Elavil], imipramine [Tofranil])—interaction increases blood pressure; produces dysrhythmias
  2. β-Blockers (e.g., propranolol [Inderal])—produce hypertension and bradycardia (slowed HR)
  3. Antidiabetic agents (e.g., insulin, glipizide [Glucotrol], glyburide (DiaBeta)—increase the blood glucose level
  4. Monoamine oxidase inhibitors (MAOIs)—no problem with epinephrine; indirect-acting amines (e.g., pseudoephedrine) must be avoided
  5. General anesthetics—halogenated hydrocarbons (e.g., halothane [Fluothane]) sensitize the myocardium to catecholamines; epinephrine is a catecholamine; increase the chance of arrhythmia/dysrhythmias
E. Dental hygiene considerations—the client's pulse and blood pressure must be checked; all of these medications can increase heart rate and blood pressure
F. Therapeutic uses (Table 11-3)
  1. Medical purposes—treatment of:
    a. Anaphylaxis
    b. Cardiac arrest
    c. Nasal congestion—decongestant
    d. Asthma (β$_2$-agonist)

e. Attention deficit hyperactivity disorder (ADD or ADHD)

f. Glaucoma

2. Dental purposes

a. Local anesthetic additive (vasoconstrictor)

b. Hemostatic additive to reduce bleeding; provides adequate tissue retraction (cord)

G. Adrenergics as vasoconstrictors are contained in local anesthetic solutions

1. Examples

a. Epinephrine (Adrenalin)

b. Levonordefrin (Neo-Cobefrin)

2. Advantages of adrenergic vasoconstriction

a. Prolongs duration of anesthesia

b. Reduces systemic toxicity

c. Provides hemostasis

d. Reduces absorption (vasoconstriction)

e. Increases concentration of anesthetic at the nerve membrane

3. Disadvantages of adrenergic vasoconstriction

a. Excessive amount produces systemic toxicity

b. In persons with cardiovascular disease:

(1) Reasonable amounts can be used in local anesthetic additives for clients whose cardiovascular conditions are stable

(2) Avoid using epinephrine-impregnated retraction cords

(3) Maximum (safe) dose (MD) varies for normal and clients with cardiovascular disease

(a) Epinephrine—dose for normal clients, 0.2 mg; for clients with cardiovascular disease, 0.04 mg

(b) Levonordefrin (Neo-Cobefrin)—dose for normal clients, 1 mg; for clients with cardiovascular disease, 0.2 mg (some sources state 1.0 mg)

c. Hyperthyroidism—vasoconstrictors may produce a thyroid storm in clients who have not received treatment and in those receiving drug therapy; thyroid storm or thyroid crisis is characterized by an acceleration of all body processes (e.g., increases in heart rate, blood pressure, respiration, body temperature, and pulse); pulmonary edema and congestive heart failure can occur

4. Minimize toxicity by:

a. Injecting slowly

b. Aspirating before injecting

c. Calming the client

d. Using the lowest effective dose

5. Dental hygiene considerations

a. Use is contraindicated in clients with uncontrolled cardiovascular disease

b. Check blood pressure and pulse

α-Adrenergic Blockers (α-Blockers)

See the section on "Cardiovascular Agents" for a more detailed discussion.

A. Mechanism of action—block α-receptors, which block action of the SANS

B. Used to treat hypertension (e.g., Raynaud's disease)

C. Examples (note generic names ending with "sin")

1. Prazosin (Minipress)

2. Terazosin (Hytrin)

3. Doxazosin (Cardura)

β-Adrenergic Blocker (β-Blocker) Antagonists

See the section on "Cardiovascular Agents" for more information.

A. Mechanism of action—drug blocks SANS action (β-receptors); some β-blockers are more selective for the β_1-receptor than β_2-receptor; some drugs are formulated to target β_1-receptors, others to β_2-receptors; other drugs target both β_1 and β_2 receptors

B. Used to treat hypertension, angina, arrhythmias; also congestive heart failure, anxiety, and glaucoma; and used to prevent myocardial infarction (MI, heart attack)

C. Examples (note generic names ending with "olol")

1. Propranolol (Inderal)

2. Metoprolol (Lopressor)

3. Atenolol (Tenormin)

D. Dental hygiene considerations

1. Check the client's blood pressure and pulse—these medications can increase or decrease the heart rate

2. Raise the dental chair slowly, and allow the client to remain seated for a few minutes to minimize the risk of orthostatic hypotension

Adrenergic Neuronal Agonists and Antagonists

A. Pharmacologic effects—affect the release of norepinephrine from nerve endings and the level of adrenergic activity; influence α-receptor and β-receptor activities

B. Therapeutic use—treatment of hypertension; use is limited by adverse effects (e.g., can cause xerostomia and sedation)

C. Examples

1. Reserpine (Serpasil)

2. Guanethidine (Ismelin)

3. Methyldopa (Aldomet)

4. Clonidine (Catapres)

Parasympathomimetic (Cholinergic) Agents

A. Cholinergic agonists—mimic the action of the parasympathetic autonomic nervous system (PANS); stimulation of the PANS

   1. Receptors—see Figure 11-4 for an illustration of a typical cholinergic nerve

   a. Muscarinic—receptor stimulated by the compound found in the poisonous mushroom *Amanita muscaria* (see Figure 11-4, *A*)

   (1) Areas affected (*A*)

   (a) Smooth muscle

   (b) Cardiac muscle

   (c) Gland cells

   (2) Neurotransmitter—acetylcholine (ACh)

   (3) Location—the synapse between the postganglionic fiber and the neuroeffector organ in the PANS

   (4) Stimulated by muscarine

   (5) Blocked by atropine

   b. Nicotinic—receptor stimulated by nicotine; found in cigarettes (see Figure 11-4, *B* and *C*)

   (1) Areas affected

   (a) Postganglionic neurons (*B*)

   (b) Skeletal muscle end plates (*C*)

   (2) Neurotransmitter—acetylcholine (ACh)

   (3) Location—autonomic ganglia (*B*) and neuromuscular junction (*C*)

   (4) Stimulated by nicotine

   (5) Blocked by hexamethonium (autonomic, *B*) and d-tubocurarine at the neuromuscular junction (*C*)

   2. Acetylcholine—the following diagram illustrates synthesis and inactivation of ACh

A   Ch   Choline   ACh

acetyltransferase

Acetyl + Choline ⇌ Acetylcholine

(CoA)   Acetylcholinesterase
                (AChE)

   3. Classification and mechanism of action

   a. Direct-acting drugs—act just like acetylcholine at the receptor site, such as:

   (1) Choline derivatives

   (2) Pilocarpine (Salagen)

   b. Indirect-acting drugs—increase the amount of acetylcholine indirectly; block acetylcholine inactivation by inhibiting acetylcholinesterase (AChE, the enzyme that normally destroys acetylcholine)

   (1) "Reversible" cholinesterase inhibitors—drugs that block action of AChE, but whose action is terminated (ACh is then destroyed)

   (a) Edrophonium (Tensilon)

   (b) Physostigmine (Eserine)

   (c) Neostigmine (Prostigmin)

   (2) "Irreversible" cholinesterase inhibitors—drugs that attach to and inactivate AChE (e.g., organophosphates used as insecticides [malathion, parathion])

   4. Pharmacologic effects—similar to stimulation of the PANS

   a. Smooth muscle stimulation

   (1) Increase in gastrointestinal (GI) motility—diarrhea may result; advantageously used to treat postoperative GI and genitourinary (GU) retention

   (2) Bronchoconstriction—causes constriction of bronchial smooth muscle, an adverse reaction

   b. Glands—increased secretion of saliva; used to treat dry mouth (xerostomia)

   c. Eye—decreased intraocular pressure; used to treat glaucoma

   5. Toxic reactions—symptoms of overdose are extensions of the pharmacologic effects; the "too much" effect

   a. SLUD—excessive salivation, lacrimation (tearing), urination, and defecation

   b. Treatment of overdose

   (1) Pralidoxime (2-PAM, Protopam)—regenerates acetylcholinesterase

   (2) Atropine—antimuscarinic; blocks the muscarinic effects of acetylcholine excess (not nicotinic effects)

   6. Dental hygiene considerations

   a. Oral forms can cause increased salivation and may cause hypotension and bradycardia

   b. Clients should maintain good oral hygiene

   c. Have client rise slowly from the dental chair to minimize orthostatic hypotension

   7. Dental use—treatment of xerostomia; pilocarpine tablets may increase salivary flow

B. Anticholinergic agents—block muscarinic actions of the PANS

   1. Basic principles

   a. Decreased salivary flow; used advantageously to dry up saliva

   b. Many drugs can have an anticholinergic, atropinic, or atropine-like effect

   c. Anticholinergic agents block the muscarinic receptors

   2. Pharmacologic effects on the:

   a. Heart—tachycardia (increased HR; useful during general anesthesia when HR may fall too low)

TABLE 11-4 Xerostomia-Producing Drug Groups with Examples

Drug Group	Examples
Antiacne	Isotretinoin
Anticholinergics* (P-)	Atropine
Anticonvulsants	Carbamazepine, felbamate, gabapentin, lamotrigine
Antidepressants	Amitriptyline, imipramine, fluoxetine, fluvoxamine
Antihistamines	Astemizole, brompheniramine, chlorpheniramine, loratadine
Antihypertensives*	Clonidine, guanethidine, methyldopa, captopril
Antinauseants	Cyclizine, diphenhydramine, meclizine
Antiparkinson drugs	Benztropine mesylate, biperiden, carbidopa, levodopa, trihexyphenidyl
Antipsychotics	Chlorpromazine, clozapine, fluphenazine, haloperidol, thioridazine
Antispasmodics	Dicyclomine, propantheline
Antidiarrheal	Diphenoxylate, loperamide
Benzodiazepines	Diazepam, alprazolam, lorazepam
Decongestants	Pseudoephedrine
Diuretics	Hydrochlorothiazide, furosemide
Muscle relaxants	Baclofen, orphenadrine
Nonsteroidal anti-inflammatory drugs (NSAIDs)	Diflunisal, ibuprofen, naproxen

More likely to produce xerostomia; effect still dose related.

b. Eye—produces:
   (1) Mydriasis—dilation of pupils; results in photophobia
   (2) Cycloplegia—paralysis for distant vision; client cannot focus or read up close
   (3) Avoid repeated doses in clients who have narrow-angle glaucoma (this is the only autonomic drug group relatively contraindicated in certain forms of glaucoma)
c. Salivary secretions—salivary flow reduced; useful in dentistry (Table 11-4 lists several drug groups that produce xerostomia)
d. CNS—can cause sedation or excitation
3. Adverse reactions and toxicity—contraindications to use

a. Xerostomia, dry skin, and dry eyes—caution in persons wearing contact lenses; reduces lactation in nursing mothers
b. Eyes—blurred vision; avoid use in clients with narrow-angle glaucoma; careful use of eyedrops in persons with wide-angle glaucoma is usually acceptable
c. Urinary retention—avoid use in persons with prostatic hypertrophy (enlarged prostate)
d. Dizziness and fatigue—toxic levels can cause delirium, hallucinations, coma, and convulsions
e. Tachycardia—monitor persons with cardiovascular disease
f. Reduced GI motility—avoid in persons with gastric retention or intestinal obstruction
4. Clinical uses—effects offer advantageous treatment in:
a. GI activity—has antispasmodic properties (reduced GI overactivity) and reduces secretions (e.g., stomach acid)
b. Ophthalmology—dilates eyes and paralyzes the muscles of accommodation (the person can see only distant objects); used for eye examinations
c. Parkinson's disease
d. Drug-induced Parkinson's disease
e. Dental
   (1) Used before general anesthesia to dry up saliva and to prevent vagal slowing of the heart
   (2) Used to prepare the mouth for procedures that require a drier field
5. Dental hygiene considerations
a. Xerostomia—instruct the client to drink plenty of water, suck on tart sugarless gum or candy with xylitol or ice chips, avoid products containing alcohol and caffeine, and avoid juices and soft drinks to reduce the risk of dental caries; saliva substitutes (Xero-lube, Salivart) can also be recommended
b. Tachycardia—check the client's blood pressure and pulse
c. Sedation—an increased risk of sedation exists if combined with other sedating agents; client should be instructed to avoid driving or operating heavy machinery or anything that requires thinking or concentration
6. Examples of anticholinergic agents
a. Atropine
b. Benztropine mesylate (Cogentin)
c. Dicyclomine (Bentyl)
d. Methantheline (Banthine)
e. Propantheline (Pro-Banthine)
f. Trihexyphenidyl hydrochloride (Artane)

NEUROMUSCULAR BLOCKING AGENTS

A. Pharmacologic effects—paralysis of voluntary skeletal muscles; can include muscles of respiration; these are not autonomic nervous system (ANS) agents

B. Therapeutic use—paralyzing skeletal muscles at the start of general anesthesia to facilitate intubation (insertion of an orotracheal or nasotracheal tube)

C. Examples
   1. Tubocurarine—active constituent of curare (the poison used on arrows)
   2. Succinylcholine (Anectine)

Local Anesthetic Agents

See the section on "Management of Pain and Anxiety" in Chapter 18.

A. Properties of the ideal local anesthetic (LA) agent
   1. Potent
   2. Reversible
   3. No systemic anesthesia
   4. No local, systemic, or allergic reactions
   5. Rapid onset
   6. Satisfactory duration
   7. Adequate tissue penetration
   8. Low cost
   9. Stable in solution (long shelf life)
   10. Can be sterilized by autoclave
   11. Metabolized and excreted easily

B. Chemistry
   1. Three components common to LAs
      a. Aromatic lipophilic group—contains a benzene ring
      b. Intermediate chain—either ester or amide
      c. Hydrophilic amino group—secondary or tertiary amine
   2. Intermediate chain
      a. Composed of esters
         (1) Tetracaine (Pontocaine)
         (2) Procaine (Novocain)
         (3) Propoxycaine (in Ravocaine)
      b. Composed of amides
         (1) Articaine (Septocaine)
         (2) Lidocaine (Xylocaine)
         (3) Mepivacaine (Carbocaine)
         (4) Prilocaine (Citanest)
         (5) Bupivacaine (Marcaine)

C. Mechanism of action by:
   1. Nerve fiber susceptibility—nerves and sensations generally are affected in this order: autonomic, cold and warmth, pain, touch pressure, vibration, proprioception, and motor; sensations and nerve functions are regained in reverse order

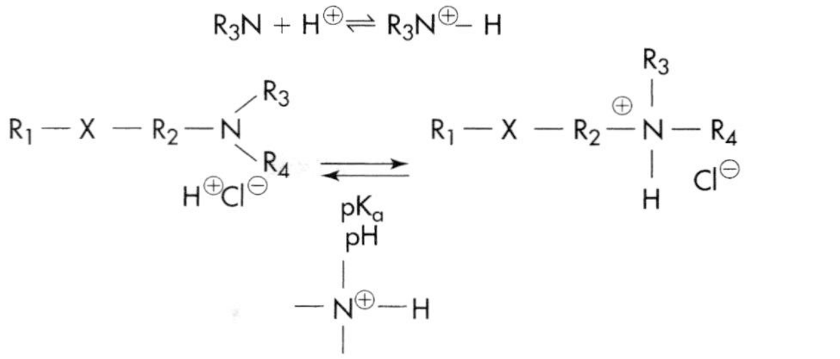

$$R_3N + H^{\oplus} \rightleftharpoons R_3N^{\oplus} - H$$

Free base
Uncharged, un-ionized
Fat soluble (lipophilic)
Penetrates nerve tissue

Salt
Charged, cation (ionized)
Water soluble (hydrophilic)
Form present in dental cartridge (pH 4.5-6.0)
Infection, doesn't penetrate

FIGURE 11-5 Base and salt forms of local anesthetics. The pH determines the amounts on each side (in equilibrium).

   2. Specific receptor theory—the anesthetic agent binds to receptors on the sodium channel; permeability to sodium ions is decreased, and nerve conduction is interrupted
   3. Base and salt forms of LAs (Figure 11-5)—both forms are needed; the base penetrates the lipid membranes, and the salt traverses the cellular fluid
   4. Inflammation—reduces LA effect
      a. Acid environment (pH 5.5) of inflammation increases the ionized form and reduces the anesthetic effect
      b. Edema—dilutes the LA because an increase in fluids is present
      c. Increased tissue vasculature—increased blood supply carries away the LA; the duration of action is shortened

D. Pharmacokinetics
   1. Absorption
      a. Effect on the vasculature—LAs produce vasodilation (except cocaine); vasoconstrictors are added to counteract dilation
      b. Absorption and distribution of LAs are determined by the pH of the environment, as shown in the equation below:

Inflammation $\rightarrow\downarrow$ pH $\rightarrow\uparrow$ [H$^+$] $\rightarrow\uparrow$ charged form
(more acid) (more hydrogen ions)
S $\rightarrow\downarrow$ un-ionized form B $\rightarrow\updownarrow$; charged distribution

      c. Solubility
         (1) Lipid-soluble—the nonionized form penetrates membranes
         (2) Water-soluble—the ionized form crosses the cell membrane and exerts its effect at the nerve

d. Rate of absorption
  (1) The faster the rate of absorption, the greater is the chance of systemic toxicity and the shorter is the duration of action
  (2) Route of administration alters the rate of absorption; the topical anesthetic agent can be absorbed quickly
2. Distribution—the level of the LA in the blood is determined by movement of the LA around the body; side effects occur if the LA reaches a high enough level in other organs (e.g., CNS, heart); blood level is determined by:
  a. Rate of injection
  b. Speed of absorption (depends on proximity to blood vessels)
  c. Speed of distribution to other tissues
  d. Speed of metabolism and excretion
3. Metabolism (biotransformation)
  a. Esters—hydrolyzed by plasma pseudocholinesterases
    (1) Procaine—metabolized to para-aminobenzoic acid (PABA)—allergenic
    (2) Congenital cholinesterase deficiency—LAs containing esters are absolutely contraindicated
  b. Amides—metabolized in the liver
    (1) Liver dysfunction—LAs containing amides should be given cautiously; they may be metabolized more slowly; toxic levels can build up if repeated doses are administered
    (2) Prilocaine—metabolized to orthotoluidine, which can produce methemoglobinemia, a condition in which excess methemoglobin in the blood results in lowered oxygen-carrying capacity; not usually a problem in healthy clients
4. Excretion capacity
  a. Esters are almost completely metabolized before they are excreted
  b. Amides are mostly metabolized before they are excreted
  c. The presence of significant renal disease can cause all LA metabolites to accumulate
E. Adverse reactions
  1. Factors influencing toxicity
    a. Drug
    b. Concentration
    c. Route
    d. Tissue inflammation
    e. Vasoconstriction
    f. Body weight
    g. Rate of metabolism and excretion
  2. Symptoms of LA toxicity—the CNS and the cardiovascular system (CVS) are affected most; the severity of effects is related directly to the amount of the LA in blood
    a. CNS response—stimulation followed by depression
      (1) CNS stimulation (excitatory)—produces restlessness, shivering, tremors, convulsions
      (2) CNS depression—results in sedation, drowsiness, respiratory and cardiovascular depression, coma; can occur without previous excitation
    b. CVS response
      (1) Antidysrhythmic action—lidocaine used intravenously to treat dysrhythmias
      (2) Vasodilation produces hypotension; releases vascular smooth muscle; lowers resistance
  3. Toxicity—the higher the number, the more likely it is that an LA agent is toxic; "absolute" toxicity considers only the drug, whereas "relative" toxicity considers the concentration (percent) available in the bloodstream; a comparison of LAs is provided in Table 11-5
  4. Malignant hyperthermia—life-threatening complication associated with the administration of general anesthesia, characterized by tachycardia, tachypnea, cardiac dysrhythmia, muscle rigidity, and extreme increase in body temperature; LA agents containing amide administered in standard doses in oral health care appear to be safe for individuals susceptible to malignant hyperthermia (Box 11-1)
  5. Allergic reactions
    a. Range of reactions—mild rash to anaphylaxis
    b. Esters—much more allergenic than amides; note that the presence of true allergic reactions to amides is still debated; it is unclear whether or not people are actually allergic to amides

TABLE 11-5 Toxicity of Local Anesthetic Agents

Drug	TOXICITY	
	Absolute	Relative
Lidocaine (Xylocaine, Octocaine)	2	2
Mepivacaine (Carbocaine, Isocaine)	1.5	1.5
Prilocaine (Citanest)	1+	2+
Tetracaine (Pontocaine—topical)	10	5
Bupivacaine (Marcaine)	4	3+
Articaine (Septocaine)	1	1.5

    c. Skin testing—a poor method of testing for allergic response because of false-positive and false-negative results; need emergency equipment and trained personnel on hand in case a severe allergic reaction occurs in clients

    d. Other ingredients may produce allergic reactions (preservatives, antioxidants); see the section on "Composition of LA solutions" below

    e. Administer LAs containing amides to clients allergic to esters, and vice versa

F. Drug interactions

    1. Esters administered in the presence of sulfonamides—esters may interfere locally with the sulfonamides' anti-infective action

    2. Lidocaine administered in the presence of cimetidine (Tagamet)—cimetidine prolongs the metabolism of lidocaine in the liver; levels of lidocaine in blood may increase with repeated doses; not important to dentistry

G. Dental hygiene considerations

    1. CNS stimulation—calm client with a soothing voice and manner

      a. Administer a lower dose of the LA

      b. Switch to another LA

    2. Sedation

      a. Have someone drive the client home

      b. Have the client sit in the reception area until he or she no longer feels tired

      c. Use caution while using opioid analgesics, antianxiety drugs, or other sedating drugs if sedation persists

    3. Have the client refrain from imbibing very hot and very cold foods or drinks

H. Vasoconstrictors and cardiovascular disease

    1. Clients with controlled cardiovascular disease (e.g., hypertension, angina, arrythmias) can receive LAs

    2. Do not exceed the maximum dose of a vasoconstrictor in clients with cardiovascular disease; use caution

    3. Check the client's pulse rate and blood pressure before administering an LA that contains a vasoconstrictor

I. Composition of LA solutions

    1. Other ingredients

      a. Vasoconstrictors—epinephrine (Adrenalin), levonordefrin (Neo-Cobefrin)

      b. Preservatives (antiseptics)—methylparabens and propylparabens are no longer present in dental anesthetic cartridges

      c. Antioxidant—sodium bisulfite or sodium metabisulfite; the antioxidant is present if the LA contains a vasoconstrictor; may precipitate asthma attacks in susceptible persons. Sulfite, sulfa, and sulfur are not cross-allergenic.

      d. Alkalinizing agent—sodium hydroxide; adjusts pH; maintains the LA in salt form so that it will be soluble in water

      e. Sodium chloride—makes the solution isotonic

    2. LAs in dental cartridges (see Table 11-6)

J. Topical LAs and injection-free local anesthesia

    1. Cocaine—high potential for abuse; never indicated for dental use

    2. Benzocaine—ester-based anesthetic; used topically because it cannot be used systemically; some sensitization occurs; use gloves to avoid skin contact with the drug, rash, and sensitization

    3. Lidocaine—topically effective

TABLE 11-6 Local Anesthetic Agents in Dental Cartridges*

Local Anesthetic	Concentration (%)	Vasoconstrictor	
Amides			
Lidocaine (Xylocaine, Octocaine)	2	Epinephrine	1:100,000
	2	Epinephrine	1:50,000
Mepivacaine (Carbocaine, Isocaine)	2	Levonordefrin (Neo-Cobefrin)	1:20,000
	3	None	
Prilocaine (Citanest, Forte Citanest)	4	Epinephrine	1:200,000
	4	None	
Bupivacaine (Marcaine, Sensorcaine)	0.5	Epinephrine	1:200,000
Articaine (Septocaine)	4	Epinephrine	1:100,000
			1:200,000

*Cartridge = 1.8 mL.

4. Tetracaine—avoid use because of toxicity and slow onset

5. Lidocaine and prilocaine (injection-free local anesthesia)

   a. Used in adults who require limited pain control during root debridement or in those who fear injections

   b. Gel applied into the periodontal pocket to provide pain relief during scaling and root planing procedures (e.g., Oraqix)

   c. Amide-type topical anesthetic agent

6. Dental hygiene considerations

   a. Use the smallest volume and the lowest concentration to avoid adverse effects

   b. Limit area of application

   c. Instruct the client not to swallow the topical LA

   d. Instruct the client to avoid very hot and very cold foods; he or she may not be able to sense temperature changes because of the topical LA

LOCAL ANESTHETIC REVERSAL AGENT

General Considerations

A. Dental use—for reversal of soft tissue anesthesia (lip, tongue, and functional deficits resulting from an intraoral submucosal injection of an LA with a vasoconstrictor; reduces recovery time of normal sensation

B. Contraindications—not recommended for use in children <6 years of age or weighing <15 kg (33 lb)

C. Mechanism of action—expands blood vessels and increases blood flow, thereby accelerates the reversal of soft tissue numbness

D. Adverse effects

   1. Transient pain at injection site

   2. Tachycardia and arrhythmia may occur with parenteral administration but are uncommon after submucosal administration

E. Example—phentolamine mesylate (OraVerse)

GENERAL ANESTHETICS

General Considerations

A. Dental use—in extensive oral surgery and in an anxious client, a mentally challenged client who cannot cooperate, and any client who cannot control his or her behavior during dental care

B. Stages and planes of anesthesia

   1. Stage I—analgesia; divided into three planes

   2. Stage II—excitement and delirium; avoid, if possible

   3. Stage III—surgical anesthesia; divided into four planes

   4. Stage IV—respiratory paralysis (medullary paralysis); death ensues without intervention

C. Routes of administration

   1. Intravenous anesthetics—fixed anesthetics (cannot be removed by respiration)

      a. Barbiturates (e.g., thiopental [Pentothal])

      b. Dissociative—ketamine (Ketalar, Ketaject)

      c. Neuroleptanalgesic—fentanyl (Sublimaze) plus droperidol (Inapsine, Innovar)

   2. Inhalation gases

      a. N_2O combined with oxygen

      b. Cyclopropane

   3. Inhalation volatile liquids

      a. Diethyl ether

      b. Halogenated hydrocarbons (e.g., halothane [Fluothane])

Specific Agents

A. Nitrous oxide–oxygen (N_2O–O_2) analgesia

   1. Incomplete anesthetic; if used alone, the client cannot reach stage III

   2. Usual concentration maintained at 30% to 50% to prevent O_2 deprivation

   3. Administration

      a. Begin with 100% O_2 for 2 to 3 minutes

      b. Then add N_2O in 5% to 10% increments until the desired state of sedation is reached (usually 3 to 5 minutes)

      c. Once the procedure is terminated, the client should receive O_2 for 5 minutes

   4. Advantages

      a. Rapid onset and recovery

      b. Least toxic; safe when used appropriately

      c. May be used in children

      d. Nonflammable

      e. Nonirritating to the GI tract

      f. Good analgesic properties; anxiolytic (antianxiety) effect

   5. Disadvantages

      a. "Misuse" potential exists with both clients and oral health care professionals

      b. Reduces fertility

      c. Associated with high rate of miscarriages

      d. Improper use (without concomitant LA block injection) gives N_2O a "bad name"; analgesia from N_2O–O_2 still requires the use of an LA agent

      e. Nausea—most common complaint; caused by rapid changes in N_2O concentration of inspired air, change levels slowly

f. Diffusion hypoxia—low level of O_2 in lungs because of diffusion of O_2 into the blood supply rarely occurs; administer 100% oxygen at the end of the procedure to prevent this

6. Adverse effects
   a. Misuse or faulty installation of equipment
   b. Nausea, vomiting
   c. Headache, if oxygen is not given at the end of the procedure
   d. N_2O abuse

7. Drug interactions—occur with any drug that can cause CNS depression or sedation

8. Contraindications
   a. Respiratory problems
      (1) Upper respiratory tract infection (URI)—difficult to administer N_2O–O_2 analgesia when nasal passages are congested
      (2) Chronic obstructive pulmonary disease (COPD), such as emphysema or bronchitis
         (a) Administering O_2 at the usual concentration with N_2O could produce apnea (cessation of respiration)
         (b) The client's respiration is driven by carbon dioxide (CO_2) levels
   b. Pregnancy—the first trimester is the most critical; the greatest number of spontaneous abortions occur at this stage (especially in oral health care personnel); teratogenic effect unknown, but not probable
   c. Lack of communication
      (1) Psychological—clients with psychological problems may respond inappropriately
      (2) Language—when the client cannot comprehend the practitioner's language or speaks a foreign language
   d. Contagious disease—danger of transmitting diseases (e.g., tuberculosis, hepatitis) if the tube is not completely sterilized
   e. Epilepsy
   f. Emotional instability
   g. Multiple sclerosis
   h. Previous negative experience

9. Dental hygiene considerations
   a. The client's emotional and psychiatric history
   b. Clients may have fanciful dreams while under the effects of N_2O–O_2; male dental personnel should ensure that female dental personnel are always present with female clients to avoid unfounded accusations

B. Diethyl ether—unpopular because it is:
   1. Explosive
   2. Slow in onset and recovery
   3. Proven to cause GI upset; nausea and vomiting are common

C. Halogenated hydrocarbons
   1. Examples
      a. Halothane (Fluothane)
      b. Enflurane (Ethrane)
      c. Isoflurane (Forane)
      d. Desflurane
      e. Sevoflurane
   2. Does not cause irritation of the mucosal membrane; not explosive; poor muscle relaxation; no analgesia; little nausea or vomiting
   3. The myocardium is sensitized to catecholamines (epinephrine)—can produce dysrhythmias
   4. Hepatotoxic—greater with more exposures
   5. Drug interaction—can occur if administered with drugs that cause CNS depression or sedation (e.g., opioid analgesics, barbiturates, benzodiazepines, antipsychotic drugs, antidepressants, and antihistamines)
   6. Dental hygiene considerations
      a. Sedation and amnesia—the client should have someone to drive him or her home after the procedure
      b. The client should be instructed to avoid driving or operating heavy machinery or anything that requires thinking or concentration

D. Ultrashort-acting barbiturates
   1. Examples
      a. Thiopental (Pentothal); also known as "truth serum"
      b. Methohexital (Brevital)
      c. Thiamylal (Surital)
   2. Rapid onset; short duration secondary to re-distribution to brain, muscles, and adipose tissue
   3. Used to induce general anesthesia; the client advances rapidly to stage III
   4. Adverse reaction—laryngospasm
   5. Contraindicated in porphyria and status asthmaticus

E. Ketamine (Ketalar, Ketaject) produces dissociative anesthesia
   1. Not a complete anesthetic
   2. The client is not asleep and does not respond to stimuli in the environment (trance-like state)
   3. Reactions—bad dreams, may be described by the client as "bad trip"; more likely to occur in adults
   4. Can produce hyperactive reflexes such as coughing, gagging, or tongue movements

F. Neuroleptanalgesia—anesthetic, analgesic (Innovar)
   1. Fentanyl (opioid) plus droperidol (tranquilizer)
   2. Adverse reaction—produces "board-like" chest, which requires ventilatory action; performing cardiopulmonary resuscitation (CPR) is difficult

SEDATIVE–HYPNOTIC MEDICATIONS

General Considerations

A. Used to treat anxiety disorder, situational anxiety, and insomnia
B. Other drugs, in addition to sedative–hypnotics, can cause sedation; all can increase a client's risk for sedation when used together
C. Dental concerns
   1. Additive CNS depressant effects when taken with alcohol, opioid analgesics, or other CNS depressants
   2. The client should be instructed to avoid driving or operating heavy machinery or anything that requires thinking or concentration

Benzodiazepines

A. Mechanism of action—more specific anxiolytic (antianxiety) action than barbiturates; potentiates the inhibitory neurotransmitter γ-aminobutyric acid (GABA); GABA-ergic neurotransmission increases sedation
B. Wide therapeutic index when ingested alone; much safer than barbiturates
C. Adverse reactions
   1. Sedation—the client should be instructed to avoid driving or operating heavy machinery or anything that requires thinking or concentration
   2. Addiction potential—some potential exists but less than that for barbiturates
   3. Teratogenicity—increased incidence of birth defects if taken during the first trimester; this is an FDA (U.S. Food and Drug Administration) category D or X drug
   4. Thrombophlebitis—when administered intravenously; local irritation may occur with diazepam because of the use of propylene glycol as diluent; midazolam (Versed) is soluble in water, so no propylene glycol is used
   5. Overdose—treated with flumazenil (Mazicon), a benzodiazepine antagonist
D. Specific agents
   1. Examples of benzodiazepines and typical doses are provided in Table 11-7 (see also Table 11-3)
   2. Differences between benzodiazepines
      a. Equivalent dose—usual dose varies with agent
      b. Duration—varies from a few hours to a few days
      c. Metabolism
         (1) Most benzodiazepines are metabolized by oxidation to active metabolites
         (2) Oxazepam, lorazepam, and temazepam are inactivated by glucuronidation

TABLE 11-7 Examples of Benzodiazepines

Drug	Usual Dose (oral) (mg/day)
Alprazolam (Xanax)	0.5–4.0
Chlordiazepoxide (Librium)	15.0–100.0
Diazepam (Valium)	2–10
Flurazepam (Dalmane)	15–30
Lorazepam (Ativan)	2–6
Midazolam (Versed)	Intravenous
Oxazepam (Serax)	15–30
Temazepam (Restoril)	15–30
Triazolam (Halcion)	0.125–0.5

         (3) The client's age is a factor that can reduce the metabolism of oxidized benzodiazepines
      3. Drug interactions—the presence of cimetidine reduces the metabolism of oxidized benzodiazepines; clients who smoke experience less sedation (smoking induces liver enzymes)
E. Dental hygiene considerations
   1. Can cause anterograde amnesia (limited to events occurring after drug administration); clients should be cautioned about making life-changing decisions after taking a benzodiazepine
   2. All other dental hygiene considerations are the same as the general considerations

Barbiturates

A. Pharmacologic effects
   1. Continuum with increasing doses—from sedation and anxiety relief, to sleep, and then anesthesia
   2. Anticonvulsant—long-acting agents are usually the most useful
   3. Muscle relaxation—this action is inseparable from CNS sedation effects
   4. No analgesic action—in the presence of pain, agitation may result if an analgesic is not given concurrently
B. Adverse reactions
   1. CNS depression—drowsiness and impaired performance and judgment; the client should be instructed to avoid driving or operating heavy machinery, or anything that requires thinking or concentration. (See Box 11-1 for drugs that produce sedation)
   2. Abuse—euphoria, habituation, withdrawal, increased tolerance

3. Acute overdose—causes depression of respiratory system and respiratory arrest
4. Barbiturates—contraindicated in porphyria; stimulate liver microsomal enzymes (drugs metabolized by the liver disappear more quickly)
C. Therapeutic uses
  1. Medical uses—treatment of epilepsy, sedation, or anxiety
  2. Dental uses
    a. Preoperative anxiety reduction—oral or intramuscular administration
    b. Induction of general anesthesia—intravenous barbiturates
D. Dental hygiene considerations—same as general considerations under earlier section titled "Sedative–hypnotic medications"
E. Examples—barbiturates
  1. Ultrashort-acting—for induction of general anesthesia
    a. Thiopental (Pentothal)
    b. Methohexital (Brevital)
  2. Short-acting—for insomnia; most abused form
    a. Pentobarbital (Nembutal)
    b. Secobarbital (Seconal)
  3. Intermediate-acting—for insomnia or daytime sedation; frequently abused
    a. Amobarbital (Amytal)
    b. Butabarbital (Butisol)
  4. Long-acting—treatment of seizure disorders, anticonvulsant; seldom abused
    a. Phenobarbital (Luminal)
    b. Primidone (Mysoline)

Nonbarbiturate Nonbenzodiazepines

A. Chloral hydrate (Noctec)
  1. Produces GI irritation
  2. Used in children
B. Nonbenzodiazepine—benzodiazepine receptor agonists
  1. Zolpidem (Ambien)
  2. Zaleplon (Sonata)
  3. Eszopiclone (Lunesta)
C. Melatonin receptor agonist—ramelteon (Rozerem); used to treat insomnia characterized by difficulty falling asleep
  1. Centrally acting muscle relaxants
    a. Carisoprodol (Soma)
    b. Chlorzoxazone (Paraflex)
    c. Methocarbamol (Robaxin)
    d. Orphenadrine (Norflex)
  2. Miscellaneous
    a. Baclofen (Lioresal)
    b. Tizanidine (Zanaflex)
    c. Dantrolene (Dantrium)

D. Dental hygiene considerations—same as general considerations

Analgesics

See Table 11-8.

General Considerations
A. Pain is characterized by:
  1. Perception—experienced uniformly through the nerve (signal from the site of pain to the CNS)
  2. Reaction—varies greatly from person to person (interpretation of the signal within the CNS)
B. Variables—client's age, gender, race, ethnic group, fatigue, pain threshold
C. Placebo effect—occurs when inert ingredient produces a perceived pharmacologic effect; clinical trials must include a placebo; expressing confidence in the medication often makes it more effective in the perception of the client

Salicylates (Aspirin)

A. Mechanism of action—primarily peripheral; prostaglandin synthesis inhibitor functions by inhibiting the enzyme cyclooxygenase or prostaglandin synthetase
B. Pharmacologic effects—"the three As"
  1. Analgesic—reduces pain
  2. Antipyretic—therapeutic dose reduces elevated body temperature
  3. Anti-inflammatory—higher dose reduces inflammation
C. Adverse reactions
  1. GI upset—minimized by ingesting the drug with food, water, or antacids
  2. Alteration in bleeding
    a. Platelet adhesiveness—reduced platelet adhesion for the life of the platelet (4 to 7 days); normal clotting reappears 72 hours after ingestion; reduced clotting effect requires only a low single dose; useful in low doses to prevent clotting
    b. Hypoprothrombinemia—reduced prothrombin levels; requires several consecutive doses to reduce prothrombin levels
  3. Salicylate toxicity ("salicylism")—symptoms include tinnitus, hyperthermia (increased body temperature), electrolyte and glucose problems, and altered sensorium
  4. Allergic reactions—true allergy is uncommon; if person is allergic, some cross-reactivity exists with other agents (e.g., nonsteroidal anti-inflammatory drugs [NSAIDs]); can produce an acute asthma attack; persons with asthma and nasal polyps are more susceptible

TABLE 11-8 Analgesic Summary

Pharmacologic Effects and Adverse Reactions	Aspirin	NSAIDs	Acetaminophen	Opioids (Narcotics)
Analgesic	+	++	+	++++
Antipyretic	+	+/0	+	0
Anti-inflammatory	+	++	0	0
Central nervous system (CNS) effects (drowsiness)	++[a]	++	0[b]	++
Gastrointestinal (GI) effects	++[c]	+[c]	0	+[d]
Bleeding	++	+[e]	0	0
Hepatotoxic	+[f]	+	+[g]	0
Nephrotoxic	+[e]	+[e]	+[e]	0
Addicting effects	0	0	0	++++

[a]Poisoning—salicylism.
[b]Very high doses.
[c]Upset stomach, ulcers, pain.
[d]Nausea, constipation.
[e]Aspirin or nonsteroidal anti-inflammatory drugs (NSAIDs) and acetaminophen.
[f]Hepatitis in persons with systemic lupus erythematosus or rheumatoid arthritis.
[g]With acute overdose.
+very low; ++low; +++moderate; ++++high; 0 = no effect.

5. Reye's syndrome—children with chickenpox or influenza should not be given aspirin; avoid aspirin in children and adolescents up to 18 years of age
D. Drug interactions—adverse reactions occur with aspirin used in conjunction with:
1. Warfarin (Coumadin)—used as an anticoagulant; bleeding or hemorrhage
2. Probenecid (Benemid)—used to treat gout; acute attack of gout
3. Tolbutamide (Orinase)—used to control diabetes; altered blood glucose level
4. Methotrexate (MTX)—used to treat cancer or control arthritis; MTX toxicity in bone marrow
5. Alcohol—can increase bleeding or hemorrhage
6. Other anti-inflammatory drugs—can increase bleeding or hemorrhage
E. Dental hygiene considerations
1. Avoid drugs that can cause GI upset or prolong bleeding time
2. Check for aspirin allergies
3. If taken prior to procedure, client may experience more bleeding than normal

Nonsteroidal Anti-inflammatory Agents (NSAIAs) and Drugs (NSAIDs)

A. Mechanism—similar to that of aspirin, drug inhibits prostaglandin synthesis (cyclooxygenase)

B. Pharmacologic effects—"the three As" (similar to aspirin)
1. Analgesic
2. Antipyretic
3. Anti-inflammatory
C. Adverse reactions
1. GI—more severe than aspirin; abdominal problems range from discomfort to ulcers; treated or managed with prostaglandin—misoprostol (Cytotec)
2. CNS—dizziness, sedation; the client should be instructed to avoid driving or operating heavy machinery, or anything that requires thinking or concentration
3. Blood coagulation—reduction in platelet aggregation and possible prolongation of bleeding time; alteration is reversible, unlike the effect of aspirin, which is not reversible
4. Oral—can produce stomatic gingival ulceration and xerostomia
5. Renal—can result in renal failure or cystitis
6. Hypersensitivity—ranges from mild rash to anaphylaxis
D. Drug interactions
1. Lithium—can increase lithium levels
2. Digoxin—can increase the effects of digoxin
3. MTX—can increase the effects of MTX
4. Antihypertensives—can reduce the antihypertensive effects of diuretics, angiotensin-converting enzyme (ACE) inhibitors, and β-blockers

5. Other inflammatory drugs—can increase bleeding and hemorrhage

6. Alcohol—can increase bleeding or hemorrhage

E. Contraindications

  1. Contraindicated in patients that have experienced asthma or allergic reaction to aspirin therapy

  2. Fluid-retention problems

  3. Coagulation problems

  4. Peptic ulcer disease

  5. Ulcerative colitis

F. Dental hygiene considerations

  1. Same as aspirin

  2. CNS sedation—the client should be instructed to avoid driving or operating heavy machinery or anything that requires thinking or concentration

G. Therapeutic uses

  1. Pain control—analgesic; stronger than aspirin, equal to or stronger than some opioids; strength of effect is dose dependent; anti-inflammatory effect makes NSAIDs especially useful in dentistry

  2. Arthritis—anti-inflammatory action

  3. Dysmenorrhea (painful menstruation)—effective because the mechanism of action is specific for the problem of excess prostaglandins caused by excessive uterine contractions

H. Examples

  1. Ibuprofen (Motrin-IB, Rufen, Nuprin, Advil); naproxen sodium (Anaprox; Aleve); available without a prescription

  2. Naproxen (Naprosyn)

  3. Indomethacin (Indocin)—prescription only

  4. Celecoxib (Celebrex)—prescription only

    a. Caution should be exercised as COX II inhibitors can increase the risk of a heart attack

    b. Caution should be exercised because of an increased risk for significant GI bleeding

Acetaminophen (N-Acetyl-p-Aminophenol [NAPAP]; Tylenol [Available Over the Counter; OTC])

A. Pharmacologic effects—"the two As"

  1. Analgesic

  2. Antipyretic

  3. Not an anti-inflammatory

B. Adverse reactions

  1. Analgesic nephropathy—adversely affects the kidneys; more likely to occur if used chronically in combination with aspirin or NSAIDs

  2. Hepatotoxicity—may occur with acute overdose or chronic use; delayed reaction; treated with N-acetylcysteine; may be fatal without liver transplantation

C. Drug interactions—alcohol increases the risk of acetaminophen toxicity

D. Contraindications

  1. Hepatotoxicity

  2. Renal toxicity

  3. Clients with alcohol-abuse problems

E. Dental hygiene considerations—avoid use in clients with hepatotoxicity, renal toxicity, or alcohol-abuse problems

Opioid (Narcotic) Analgesic Agents

A. Pharmacologic effects—proportional to the "strength" of the opioid

  1. Analgesia

  2. Sedation (anxiety relief)

  3. Euphoria

  4. Dysphoria

  5. Cough suppressant

  6. GI effects

  7. Respiratory effects

B. Examples of agonists (combine with opioid receptor and produce an effect) are provided in Table 11-9)

  1. Agonist–antagonist agents

    a. Example—pentazocine (Talwin-NX)

    b. Principle

      (1) Maintain analgesic properties

      (2) Have lower abuse potential

    c. Can precipitate withdrawal in opiate addicts

  2. Antagonists

    a. Example—Naloxone (Narcan), Naltrexone (Vivitrol), Nalmefene (Revex)

    b. Combine with opioid receptor; produces no effect; reverses opioid overdose

    c. Therapeutic uses

      (1) Treat opioid overdose

      (2) Counteract respiratory depression

      (3) Include in any dental emergency kit

TABLE 11-9 Examples of Agonists

Drug	Usual Dose (Oral) (mg/day)	"Strength"
Morphine	10–30 po q4h	Stronger
Hydromorphone (Dilaudid)	1–6 q4–6h	
Meperidine (Demerol)	50–150 po q4h	
Oxycodone (in Percodan)	5 q6h	
Hydrocodone (in Vicodin)	5–10 po q4–6h	
Codeine (in Tylenol no. 3, Empirin no. 3)	30–60 q4–6h	Weaker

po, *by mouth;* q4h, *every 4 hours;* q4–6h, *every 4–6 hours;* q6h, *every 6 hours.*

C. Adverse reactions—proportional to the "strength" of the opioid
  1. CNS effects—sedation, euphoria, dysphoria
  2. Respiratory depression—dose related; overdose can result in death; reversed with naloxone
  3. GI—nausea, vomiting, constipation; diphenoxylate can be useful therapeutically
  4. Abuse—can occur with all opioid analgesics; tolerance develops to all pharmacologic effects except miosis (pupillary constriction) and constipation; withdrawal produced if the drug is abruptly stopped
  5. Miosis
  6. Urinary retention
  7. Cardiovascular effects—orthostatic hypotension
D. Therapeutic uses
  1. Pain relief—this is the central mechanism; agent affects a person's perception of pain; some opioids can relieve severe pain
  2. Sedation and anxiety relief—not the main use of opioids; used preoperatively
  3. Cough suppression—antitussive action (cough suppressant); low dose needed (e.g., codeine-containing cough syrups)
  4. Diarrhea—symptomatic relief only; reduce GI motility by increasing tone and spasm; diphenoxylate (in Lomotil)
E. Drug interactions
  1. Increase sedation when used with other CNS-depressant drugs
  2. Increase constipation when combined with anticholinergic drugs
F. Dental hygiene considerations
  1. Decrease the dose in hypertensive clients because of associated urinary retention caused by opioids
  2. Increased risk for sedation—as with other CNS-depressant drugs
  3. Increased risk for xerostomia—as with anticholinergic drugs

Drugs Used for Gout

A. Disease—gout is a metabolic condition involving increased serum uric acid, with episodes of acute attacks of pain in joints (big toe, knee) and severe inflammation caused by deposition of monosodium urate
B. Prevention
  1. Probenecid (Benemid)—uricosuric (promotes uric acid excretion); aspirin interferes with this effect of probenecid
  2. Allopurinol (Zyloprim)—xanthine oxidase inhibitor (inhibits uric acid synthesis); also used in clients with cancer before chemotherapy or radiation therapy when many cells are killed and

release their amino acids, which leads to accumulation of uric acid and attacks of gout
C. Treatment
  1. Colchicine—binds to microtubular protein tubulin (prevents leukocyte migration and phagocytosis); inhibits formation of leukotriene; GI toxicity—nausea, vomiting, diarrhea are endpoints of treatment and adverse reactions
  2. NSAIDs—anti-inflammatory action ameliorates symptoms (e.g., indomethacin)

ANTI-INFECTIVES (ANTIBIOTICS)

General Considerations

A. Prevention of infection (see the section on "Disease Transmission" in Chapter 10)
  1. Sterilization measures prevent infection
  2. Many infections—treat with local measures (e.g., incision and drainage), antibiotics are often not needed; the client's resistance and the development of resistant strains of bacteria must be considered
  3. Antibiotic administration carries risks
  4. Prophylaxis is rarely indicated except for decreasing the likelihood of infective endocarditis in persons who have the highest risk, prosthetic joint infection, or when client is immunosuppressed[10] (see Chapter 15, Table 15-2).
B. Definitions
  1. Antimicrobial—agents that act against microbes
  2. Anti-infective—agents that act against the organisms that cause infections
  3. Antibacterial—agents that act against bacteria
    a. Bactericidal—kills bacteria
    b. Bacteriostatic—retards or incapacitates bacteria (reversible)
  4. Antiviral—agents that act against viruses
  5. Antifungal—agents that act against fungi
  6. Antibiotic—agents that are effective in low concentrations; produced by microorganisms; kill or suppress growth of other organisms
  7. Spectrum—range of an antibiotic's anti-infective properties; can be narrow (acting on few organisms) to wide or broad (acting on many organisms); may include effectiveness against gram-positive and gram-negative bacteria
  8. Resistance—the organism is unaffected by an anti-infective agent; the resistance may be natural (always has been resistant) or acquired (resistance has developed); prolonged exposure to antibiotics allows for the organism to develop resistance towards the antibiotic.

9. Suprainfection (superinfection)—onset of a new infection from an organism other than the original organism; occurs after taking an anti-microbial agent; the new infection is usually more difficult to treat, and commonly occurs when the spectrum is the widest; for example, *Candida* infection may arise in person taking tetracycline
10. Synergism—agent's effect is more than additive (1 + 1 > 2)
11. Antagonism—agent's effect is less than additive (1 + 1 < 2)

C. General side effects
1. GI side effects—variable, depending on antibiotic; includes nausea, vomiting, diarrhea, dyspepsia
2. Suprainfection from antibiotic-resistant bacteria is possible, usually in the form of a vaginal yeast infection
3. Drug interactions
   a. Oral contraceptives—antibiotics may reduce effectiveness; warn the client
   b. Warfarin (Coumadin)—antibiotics alter the GI flora that make vitamin K, which then can potentiate warfarin's effect
   c. Bacteriostatic and bactericidal antibiotics mixed—the "static" stops the bacteria from growing and therefore the "cidal" cannot work properly to kill bacteria

D. Treatment versus prophylaxis
1. Treatment—the anti-infective is used to treat an infection that is present
2. Prophylaxis—used to prevent some potential future infection; only proven beneficial in a few instances

E. General dental concerns for all antibiotics—make sure that the client:
1. Knows the name of the antibiotic and how to take it
2. Understands the need to complete the full course of therapy
3. Understands the rationale for prophylactic antibiotic medication
4. Takes all antibiotics with a full glass of water
5. Takes antibiotics on an empty stomach; if the medicine causes nausea, it should be taken with food

Penicillins

A. Mechanism—inhibit cell wall synthesis; bactericidal
B. Spectrum—three penicillin subgroups:
1. Penicillin G, penicillin V
2. Penicillinase-resistant penicillin

3. Extended-spectrum penicillins
   a. Ampicillin-like
   b. Carbenicillin-like
C. Stability
1. Acid labile—degrades in stomach acid; therefore administered parenterally (e.g., penicillin G, methicillin, carbenicillin)
2. Acid stable—may be used orally (e.g., penicillin VK, amoxicillin)
D. Pharmacokinetics
1. Peak—penicillin blood levels peak between 30 minutes and 1 hour when administered by the oral or intramuscular route; peak immediately when administered intravenously
2. Half-life ($t\frac{1}{2}$)—between 30 minutes and 1 hour
3. Excretion very rapid, actively secreted; duration prolonged by concomitant probenecid (Benemid) administration
E. Adverse effects
1. GI—mild GI upset to nausea and vomiting
2. Allergic reactions—range from mild rash to anaphylaxis
3. Nephrotoxicity—occurs occasionally; kidney damage more likely with broader-spectrum penicillins

Penicillin G and Penicillin V

A. Examples
1. Penicillin G potassium
2. Penicillin G procaine (Wycillin, Crysticillin)
3. Penicillin G benzathine (Bicillin)
4. Penicillin VK (V-Cillin K, Pen-Vee K)
B. Spectrum—potent against many gram-positive aerobic organisms, such as *Streptococcus* and *Staphylococcus*, certain gram-negative aerobic cocci, such as *Neisseria gonorrhoeae*, and some anaerobic organisms; not resistant to penicillinase
C. Penicillin G—parenteral administration
1. Dose specified in units (e.g., 5 million units [MU])
2. Intramuscular salts (procaine and benzathine) provide longer duration of action than do sodium and potassium salts
D. Penicillin V—more acid stable than penicillin G, thus, can be used orally; potassium salt better absorbed; therefore, penicillin VK is the most frequently used antibiotic in dentistry; 400,000 units (U) =250 mg

Penicillinase (β-Lactamase)-Resistant Penicillins

A. Examples
1. Methicillin (Staphcillin)
2. Nafcillin (Unipen, Nafcil)
3. Oxacillin (Prostaphlin, Bactocill)
B. Therapeutic use—limited; used against penicillinase-producing staphylococci

Extended-Spectrum ("Broader-Spectrum" or "Wider-Spectrum") Penicillins

A. Ampicillin-like
  1. Examples
    a. Ampicillin (Omnipen, Totacillin, Polycillin)
    b. Amoxicillin (Amoxil, Larotid, Polymox)
  2. Spectrum—effective against many gram-positive and some gram-negative bacteria such as *Haemophilus influenzae, Escherichia coli*, and *Proteus mirabilis*
  3. Not penicillinase resistant
  4. Augmentin—amoxicillin combined with clavulanic acid (CA); CA binds with penicillinase, so amoxicillin is not inactivated; can be used with penicillinase-producing organisms
B. Extended-spectrum penicillins
  1. Examples
    a. Ticarcillin (Ticar)
    b. Carbenicillin (Geopen, Pyopen)
    c. Piperacillin (Pipracil)
  2. Spectrum—provides coverage against gram-negative bacteria such as *Pseudomonas aeruginosa, Proteus*, and organisms resistant to ampicillin-like drugs
  3. Administered parenterally (in hospitalized clients) for systemic action

Macrolides

A. Mechanism—interfere with protein synthesis by binding to the 50S ribosomal subunit; provide bacteriostatic action
B. Spectrum
  1. Erythromycin
    a. Effective primarily against gram-positive microorganisms; ineffective against anaerobes
    b. Used against certain strains of *Rickettsia, Chlamydia*, and *Actinomyces*; drug of choice for treating infections caused by *Mycoplasma pneumoniae* and *Legionella pneumophila*
  2. Azithromycin (Zithromax)
    a. Recently recommended by the American Heart Association (AHA) for use in the prevention of bacterial endocarditis before certain dental procedures, in persons who are allergic to penicillin[10]
    b. Adverse effects—stomatitis, candidiasis, angioedema (allergic reaction), heart palpitations, chest pain, nausea, vomiting, diarrhea, abdominal pain, hepatotoxicity, heartburn, flatulence
    c. Alternative drug of choice for mild infection caused by susceptible organisms in persons allergic to penicillin

  3. Clarithromycin (Biaxin)
    a. Recently recommended by the AHA for use in the prevention of bacterial endocarditis prior to certain dental procedures in persons who are allergic to penicillin[10]
    b. Adverse effects—abnormal taste, candidiasis, stomatitis, nausea, abdominal pain, diarrhea, hepatotoxicity, heartburn, anorexia, vomiting, vaginitis, moniliasis, urticaria, rash, pruritus
    c. Alternative drug of choice for mild infection caused by susceptible organisms in persons allergic to penicillin
C. Pharmacokinetics of erythromycin
  1. Erythromycin—high acid lability (instability) requires enteric coating (does not dissolve in the stomach; dissolves in the intestine) or formulation as an ester to protect against stomach acid (e.g., ethylsuccinate, erythromycin ethylsuccinate [EES])
  2. Effect peaks in 2 to 4 hours
D. Adverse effects
  1. GI upset is very common; must be taken with food to decrease
  2. Cholestatic jaundice is primarily associated with the estolate ester
E. Drug interactions—theophylline and erythromycin; increase theophylline levels
F. Examples—erythromycin
  1. Erythromycin base (E-mycin)
  2. Erythromycin estolate (Ilosone)
  3. Erythromycin ethylsuccinate (EES, Pedia-mycin)
  4. Erythromycin stearate (Erythrocin)
G. Therapeutic uses
  1. Treatment of dental infections in persons allergic to penicillin
  2. Specific suspected infections (see "Spectrum")

Cephalosporins

A. Mechanism—similar to penicillins; inhibits cell wall synthesis; bactericidal
B. Chemistry similar to penicillins
C. Spectrum—effective against many gram-positive and gram-negative bacteria; the third-generation cephalosporins and the newest fourth-generation cephalosporins have the widest spectrum of action
D. Adverse reactions
  1. GI upset common (33%)
  2. Other—similar to those of the broader-spectrum penicillins (e.g., nephrotoxicity, suprainfection)
  3. Allergy—some cross-hypersensitivity (10%) with penicillin allergy (possess a similar chemical structure)

E. Examples
   1. Cefuroxime (Ceftin)
   2. Cephalexin (Keflex)
   3. Cephradine (Velosef, Anspor)
F. Suggested oral antibiotic regimen for the client with joint prosthesis less than 2 years after surgery[10]

Clindamycin (Cleocin)

A. Mechanism—inhibits protein synthesis (binds to the 50S ribosomal subunit); bacteriostatic protection
B. Spectrum—effective against gram-positive organisms and many anaerobes such as *Bacteroides*
C. Adverse reactions
   1. GI—diarrhea; pseudomembranous colitis (PMC) or antibiotic-associated colitis (AAC, incidence up to 10%); drug must be discontinued if bloody stools with mucus occur
   2. The FDA states that this agent should be "reserved for serious anaerobic infections"
D. Dental use—used against certain anaerobic infections thought to be caused by *Bacteroides* species, jaw infections, and periodontal infections; and for the prophylaxis of infective endocarditis[10]

Tetracyclines

A. Mechanism—inhibit protein synthesis by binding to the 30S ribosome; provide bacteriostatic action
B. Spectrum—truly broad spectrum; effective against many gram-positive and gram-negative bacteria
C. Pharmacokinetics
   1. Tetracyclines—divalent and trivalent cations (e.g., calcium [Ca^{++}; in dairy products], magnesium [Mg^{++}] and aluminum [Al^{+++}] [in antacids], iron [Fe^{++}]); inhibit the absorption of tetracycline by chelation
   2. Doxycycline (Vibramycin) and minocycline (Minocin)—less affected by food or dairy products than is tetracycline; avoid taking antacids or Ca^{++} supplementation concomitantly
D. Resistance—cross-transference can occur; organisms can become resistant without being exposed to drug
E. Adverse effects
   1. GI upset—relatively common
   2. Suprainfection—very common because of the wide spectrum of action; drug alters normal flora (e.g., may result in vaginal candidiasis)
   3. Photosensitivity—exaggerated sunburn with exposure to ultraviolet (UV) light
   4. Teeth—both hypoplasia and intrinsic stain can occur if the drug is taken during enamel development; primary teeth affected from the last half of the pregnancy to age 4 to 6 months;

permanent teeth are affected from age 2 months to 7 to 12 years
F. Examples
   1. Doxycycline (Vibramycin, Atridox)
   2. Minocycline (Minocin, Arestin)
   3. Tetracycline (Achromycin-V)
   4. Tetracycline fibers (Actisite)
G. Therapeutic uses
   1. Medical—treatment of acne, respiratory tract infections in clients with COPD (emphysema or bronchitis), certain sexually transmitted diseases (STDs)
   2. Dental—management of periodontal diseases; drug placed in periodontal pocket (e.g., tetracycline fibers [Atridox, Actisite, and Arestin])
H. Dental hygiene considerations
   1. Must be taken 1 hour before or 2 hours after eating
   2. Should be taken with crackers if stomach upset occurs
   3. Should not be taken with antacids or dairy products
   4. Clients must be counseled about photosensitivity

Quinolones

A. Mechanism—inhibition of bacterial gyrase so that the daughter segment of deoxyribonucleic acid (DNA) cannot acquire the proper configuration to divide
B. Spectrum—effective against gram-negative bacteria, including *Enterobacter* species, *Escherichia coli*, and *Morganella morganii*
C. Adverse reactions—abdominal pain, nausea, vomiting, diarrhea, rash, urticaria, angioedema
D. Dental concerns—the client must avoid direct light (e.g., dental light); offer the client dark glasses to be worn during dental procedures; the client must also avoid direct sun exposure
E. Examples
   1. Ciprofloxacin (Cipro)
   2. Enoxacin (Penetrex)
   3. Ofloxacin (Floxin)

Aminoglycosides

A. Mechanism—inhibit protein synthesis by binding to the 30S ribosomal subunit; provide bactericidal action (the only group that combines the inhibition of protein synthesis with "cidal" action)
B. Spectrum—effective against some gram-positive and many gram-negative bacteria
C. Pharmacokinetics—not effective systemically when administered orally; must be administered

parenterally, intravenously, or by intramuscular injection

D. Adverse reactions—toxicity usually results from excessive levels in blood
  1. Ototoxicity—adverse effect on cranial nerve VIII; both vestibular (balance) and auditory functions are affected
  2. Nephrotoxicity—adverse effect on kidney

E. Examples
  1. Gentamicin (Garamycin)
  2. Kanamycin (Kantrex)
  3. Neomycin (Mycifradin)
  4. Tobramycin (Tobrex)

Sulfonamides ("Sulfa" Drugs)

A. Mechanism—competitive antagonist of para-aminobenzoic acid (PABA); prevents the use of PABA to make the folic acid needed in an organism

B. Adverse reactions
  1. Allergic reactions—rash
  2. Photosensitivity

C. Examples
  1. Sulfisoxazole (Gantrisin)
  2. Trimethoprim sulfamethoxazole (Bactrim, Septra)

D. Therapeutic uses
  1. Urinary tract infections
  2. Otitis media (children's ear infections)
  3. Respiratory infections
  4. Dental use unclear; probably not useful

Metronidazole (Flagyl)

A. Mechanism—breaks DNA structure, which inhibits protein synthesis; provides bactericidal action

B. Spectrum
  1. Trichomonicidal (effective against *Trichomonas vaginalis*)
  2. Bactericidal (effective against anaerobes such as *Bacteroides* species)

C. Adverse reactions
  1. GI—anorexia, nausea, vomiting, headache, dizziness
  2. CNS—disulfiram (Antabuse)–like reaction; concurrent alcohol ingestion produces nausea and vomiting
  3. Carcinogenic in animals; mutagenic in bacterial organisms; however, significance with regard to cancer is unknown

D. Dental use—management of periodontal clients with anaerobic infections; effective against organisms; inexpensive

E. Dental hygiene considerations

1. Clients must avoid alcohol-containing products, including beverages, foods cooked with alcohol, colognes, aftershaves, perfumes
2. Clients must avoid mouthrinses with alcohol; recommend alcohol-free mouthrinses

Antituberculosis Agents

A. Tuberculosis (TB)—a chronic disease
  1. Resistant organisms develop easily
  2. Treatment is difficult, so drug combinations are frequently required; multidrug-resistant (MDR) organisms are common
  3. Requires drug treatment regimen of 6 to 9 months

B. Drugs
  1. Isoniazid (INH)—used alone as prophylaxis; used in combination with other agents; hepatitis is an adverse side effect
  2. Rifampin (Rifadin, Rimactane)
  3. Pyrizinamide
  4. Ethambutol (Myambutol)

C. Dental implications—use standard precautions; affected persons are treated for 6 weeks to 2 months; the client is generally not contagious if compliant with TB treatment regimen; direct observation and monitoring of the client are needed

Antifungal Agents

A. Disease—candidiasis (*Candida albicans*), called *thrush* in infants

B. Nystatin (Mycostatin, Nilstat)—dosage forms: oral suspension or pastille (rubbery lozenge)

C. Clotrimazole (Mycelex)—lozenges available

D. Ketoconazole (Nizoral)
  1. Tablets—dose: once per day
  2. An acid stomach environment is required for adequate absorption—be alert to histamine (H_2)-blockers
  3. Adverse reactions
    a. Nausea and vomiting
    b. Hepatocellular dysfunction
    c. Teratogenic potential
    d. Drug interactions

E. Fluconazole (Diflucan)
  1. Tablets, oral suspension, and intravenous administration
  2. Therapeutic use—systemic fungal infections
  3. Adverse reactions—headache, abdominal pain, nausea, diarrhea, hepatic toxicity

F. Itraconazole (Sporanox)
  1. Capsules
  2. Therapeutic use—indicated for the treatment of certain fungal infections in both immunocompromised clients and those who are not

3. Adverse reactions—nausea, vomiting, diarrhea, abdominal pain, anorexia, edema, rash, fatigue, fever, malaise

Antiviral Agents

A. Acyclovir (Zovirax)
  1. Topical, oral, and intravenous forms available
  2. Therapeutic uses
    a. Treatment of initial genital herpes in clients who are not immunocompromised
    b. Treatment of recurrent genital herpes in immunocompromised clients
    c. Oral administration is recommended with continuous use as a prophylactic
B. Docosanol (Abreva)
    a. Treatment of oral herpes simplex labialis (cold sores)
    b. Available without a prescription
    c. Adverse effects—stinging at the site of application
C. Ganciclovir (Cytovene)
  1. Inhibits replication of most herpesviruses
  2. Therapeutic use—prevention and treatment of cytomegalovirus (CMV) in persons with acquired immune deficiency syndrome (AIDS)
  3. Adverse effects—fever, coma, chills, confusion, abnormal thoughts, dizziness, bizarre dreams, headaches, psychosis, tremors, paresthesia, dysrhythmia, hypertension, hypotension, hemorrhage, anorexia, blood dyscrasia
D. Anti-retroviral drugs—indications: HIV-positive clients and those with AIDS
  1. Zidovudine (AZT, Retrovir)
  2. Didanosine (ddI, Videx)
  3. Zalcitabine (ddC, Hivid)
E. Dental hygiene considerations—use standard precautions

CARDIOVASCULAR AGENTS

See Chapters 8 and 19 for contraindications and cautions involving dental treatment in persons with cardiovascular disease[11]

Digitalis Glycosides

A. Pharmacologic effects—heartbeats are stronger (positive chronotropic effect) but usually slower (bradycardia), therefore efficiency is increased
B. Adverse reactions
  1. GI disturbances—nausea, vomiting
  2. Cardiovascular—arrhythmias and dysrhythmias
  3. CNS—yellow-green vision, halos around lights

C. Therapeutic uses—heart failure, certain arrhythmias
D. Dental hygiene considerations
  1. Hypokalemia—decreased potassium levels because of diuretics; digitalis toxicity may exacerbate dysrhythmias; epinephrine exacerbates dysrhythmias
  2. Epinephrine—use of epinephrine may increase the risk for arrhythmias (dysrhythmias)
  3. Pulse rate must be monitored
  4. Tetracycline and erythromycin can increase the levels of digoxin in blood, causing digoxin toxicity (signaled by nausea, vomiting, and copious salivation)
E. Example—digoxin (Lanoxin)

ANTIDYSRHYTHMICS

A. Pharmacologic effects—suppress dysrhythmias
B. Dental considerations—in clients with cardiac problems, use caution when administering local anesthetics with epinephrine
C. Examples
  1. Lidocaine (Xylocaine)—local anesthetic agent can be used parenterally as an antidysrhythmic agent
  2. Procainamide
  3. Propranolol (Inderal)
  4. Quinidine
D. Dental hygiene considerations
  1. Review health history to determine the client's state of health
  2. Check blood pressure and pulse

Antianginal Agents

A. Pharmacologic effects—reduce the "work" of the heart because these agents function as nonspecific vasodilators, thereby reducing the amount of blood returning to the heart
B. Adverse reactions—hypotension and severe headache are common; client should be in the sitting position to take nitroglycerin (NTG)
C. Therapeutic use—angina pectoris
D. Dental hygiene considerations
  1. Storage—unstable products; must be stored properly; heat, light, and moisture cause further degradation; discard opened containers after 2 months or on the basis of the expiration date on the original vial, whichever comes first
  2. Acute anginal attack—administer NTG sublingually (SL)
  3. Routes of NTG administration
    a. Sublingual—tablets or spray

TABLE 11-10 Selected Antihypertensives: Examples, Mechanisms, and Adverse Reactions

Drug Group	Examples	Mechanism	Adverse Reactions
Diuretics–thiazides	Hydrochlorothiazide (HCTZ)	Inhibits sodium (Na) resorption, direct vasodilator, moderate potency	Hypokalemia Hyperuricemia Hyperglycemia NSAIDs* ↓ effect
Loop diuretic Thiazides combined with potassium (K++) sparing	Furosemide (Lasix) Maxzide Dyazide	Loop of Henle, high potency K-sparing, low potency	Similar to thiazides Hyperkalemia
α Selective blockers	Terazosin (Hytrin) Doxazosin (Cardura) Prazosin (Minipress)	Blocks α_1-receptor in arterioles/venules	Sedation D/C* gradually Also used for benign prostatic hypertrophy
β-Blockers (Selected drugs)	Propranolol (Inderal) Atenolol (Tenormin) Metoprolol (Lopressor)	Blocks sympathetic effect on heart (↓ CO*); ↓ PVR,* inhibits stimulation of rennin	NSAIDs ↓ effect
Angiotensin-converting enzyme (ACE) inhibitor	Captopril (Capoten) Lisinopril (Zestril) Enalapril (Vasotec) Quinapril (Accupril)	Inhibits ACE,* angiotensin II (vasoconstriction; aldosterone secretion) production inhibited	Neutropenia Bone marrow depression Cough Dysgeusia (altered taste) NSAIDs* ↓ effect
Angiotensin Receptor Blocker	Irbesartan (Avapro) Losartan (Cozaar) Valsartan (Diovan)	Blocks the binding of angiotensin I to angiotensin II receptors; blocks vasoconstriction and aldosterone-secreting effects of angiotensin II	Oral lesions, nausea, vomiting, dyspepsia
Calcium channel blocking agents	Verapamil (Isoptin, Calan) Diltiazem (Cardizem) Nifedipine (Procardia) Nisoldipine (Sular) Isradipine (Dynacire)	Blocks calcium channel: relaxes vascular smooth muscle, decreases myocardial contractility (force)	Gingival enlargement Hyperkalemia Renal failure Dysgeusia
Adrenergic blockers Centrally acting antiadrenergic agents	Clonidine (Catapres) Methyldopa (Aldomet)	Stimulates arteriolar and the central nervous system (CNS; medulla) α receptors	Transdermal patch Xerostomia
Postganglionic sympathetic blockers	Guanethidine (Ismelin) Reserpine (Serpasil)	Inhibits release of NE,* replaces NE (false neurotransmitter) Blocks uptake and storage of amines	Postural hypotension Diarrhea Impaired ejaculation Mental depression Sedation
Vasodilators	Hydralazine (Apresoline) Minoxidil (Loniten)	Relaxes smooth muscles of arterioles	Combined with sympathetic blockers, β-blockers, and diuretics Hirsutism

NSAIDs, nonsteroidal anti-inflammatory drugs; CO, cardiac output; PVR, peripheral vascular resistance; D/C, discontinue; NE, norepinephrine.

   b. Transdermal—patches applied to chest or arm
   c. Ointment—in ointment applied to skin
 4. Anxiety about the dental appointment may cause the angina attack; the client can take tablet prophylactically
E. Examples
 1. Nitroglycerin (Nitrostat), SL tablet or spray (Nitrolingual SL spray)
 2. Isosorbide dinitrate (Isordil) or mononitrates

Antihypertensives

See Table 11-10.
A. Pharmacologic effects—reduce elevated blood pressure
B. Adverse reaction—CNS depression, fatigue, xerostomia, orthostatic hypotension, constipation and diarrhea, sexual dysfunction, upset stomach
C. Therapeutic use—treatment of hypertension

D. Dental hygiene considerations
  1. Take blood pressure to ensure that it is normal
  2. Xerostomia—instruct the client to drink plenty of water; suck on tart sugarless gum or candy that contains xylitol, or ice chips; avoid products containing alcohol and caffeine; and avoid juices and soft drinks to reduce the risk of dental caries; saliva substitutes (Xero-lube, Salivart) can also be recommended
  3. Have the client rise slowly from the dental chair
  4. Some calcium channel blockers can cause drug-influenced gingival enlargement; clients should perform meticulous oral hygiene and obtain frequent periodontal maintenance care
  5. CNS sedation—several antihypertensive medications can cause sedation; the client is at an increased risk for sedation if an opioid analgesic or benzodiazepine is prescribed; the client should be instructed to avoid driving or operating heavy machinery, or anything that requires thinking or concentration
  6. GI effects—several antihypertensives can cause GI irritation; NSAIDs may increase the risk of GI irritation; these agents must be taken with food, milk, or an antacid
  7. Constipation—may be further aggravated by the addition of an opioid analgesic; have the client drink plenty of water and eat fruits, vegetables, and other high-fiber foods

Diuretics

A. Pharmacologic effects—remove excess water and sodium by way of the kidneys; direct vasodilating action on blood vessels lowers total peripheral resistance and blood pressure
B. Adverse reactions
  1. Hypokalemia (low potassium)—the client may need to take a potassium replacement
  2. Hyperglycemia, hyperuricemia
  3. The client may urinate more frequently after taking the medicine (usually in the morning)
C. Therapeutic uses—treatment of hypertension, edema
D. Dental hygiene considerations—hypokalemia (reduced potassium level) potentiates epinephrine-induced arrhythmias; pulse rate must be monitored
E. Examples
  1. Thiazide diuretics—hydrochlorothiazide (HCTZ, HydroDIURIL)
  2. Loop diuretics—furosemide (Lasix)
  3. Combinations of thiazide diuretics with potassium-sparing diuretics—Dyazide, Maxzide; reduce the side effect of hypokalemia

Anticoagulants[11]

A. Mechanism—interfere with vitamin K–dependent clotting factors (II, VII, IX, X)
B. Pharmacologic effects—reduce the ability of blood to clot; latent time required before full effect is seen (several days); a certain amount of time is required for the effect to subside after discontinuation of treatment
C. Adverse reactions—bleeding, hemorrhage
D. Therapeutic uses—used after myocardial infarction, thrombophlebitis, atrial fibrillation, emboli, valve replacement (any condition in which too much blood clotting occurs)
E. Dental hygiene considerations
  1. Excessive bleeding may result; assess health history at every appointment
  2. Monitoring—performed using international normalized ratio (INR);[11,12] older test is prothrombin time (PT)—clients with INRs ≤3 can safely receive periodontal debridement
F. Examples—warfarin (Coumadin)
G. Drug interactions—occur with warfarin given with:
  1. Aspirin or NSAID—potentiates bleeding problems; do not use concomitantly; alternative is acetaminophen
  2. Vitamin K—helps blood clot; used to treat overdose or to reduce the latent period for improving the clotting status; antibiotics may reduce vitamin K levels by altering the intestinal flora that would potentiate the angicoagulant's effect

Anticonvulsants

A. General properties of anticonvulsants (Table 11-11)
  1. Pharmacologic effects—reduction of frequency or elimination of seizures (see Table 11-11)
  2. GI upset—common side effect
  3. Teratogenicity—variable teratogenic potential (pregnant women with epilepsy need to be treated)
  4. Sedation—tolerance to sedative effect occurs without tolerance to anticonvulsant effect
  5. Blood dyscrasias—sudden and drastic drops in either white blood cell count or red blood cell count, or both, which can be serious; laboratory monitoring is important
  6. Dental hygiene considerations
    a. Sedation—client should be instructed to avoid driving or operating heavy machinery, or anything that requires thinking or concentration
    b. GI upset—need to avoid NSAIDs and aspirin because they increase the risk of GI upset
    c. Increased risk for sedation with CNS depressants or sedating drugs

TABLE 11-11 Anticonvulsant Agents of Choice for Seizures

Seizure Type	First-Choice Agent—FDA Approved	Alternatives—FDA Approved
Generalized Seizures		
Absence (petit mal)	Ethosuximide (Zarontin)	Clonazepam (Clonopin)
	Valproate (Depakote)	
Tonic–clonic (grand mal)	Carbamazepine (Tegretol)	Phenobarbital (Luminal)
	Phenytoin (Dilantin) Valproate (Depakote)	Primidone (Mysoline) Lamotrigine (Lamactil) Topiramate (Topamax)
Status epilepticus	Diazepam (Valium) Phenytoin (Dilantin) Phenobarbital (Luminal)	
Partial Seizures		
Simple Complex Secondarily generalized	Carbamazepine (Tegretol) Or phenytoin (Dilantin) Or lamotrigine (Lamactil) Or oxcarbazepine (Trileptal)	Valproate (Depakote) Gabapentin (Neurontin) Topiramate (Topamax) Tiagabine (Gabitril) Zonisamide (Zonegran) Levetiracetam (Keppra) Primidone (Mysoline) Phenobarbital (Luminal) Pregabalin (Lyrica) Felbamate (Felbatol)

FDA, *U.S. Food and Drug Administration.*

d. CNS stimulant effects—may be difficult to treat a client who cannot sit still

e. Xerostomia—instruct the client to drink plenty of water; suck on tart sugarless gum or candy containing xylitol, or ice chips; avoid products containing alcohol and caffeine; and avoid juices and soft drinks to reduce the risk of dental caries; saliva substitutes (Xero-lube, Salivart) can also be recommended

B. Barbiturates—CNS adverse effects: sedation, hyperactivity in children, confusion, excitation, or depression in older adults

C. Phenytoin (Dilantin)—adverse effects
   1. Drug-influenced gingival enlargement—meticulous oral hygiene reduces the enlargement
   2. Vitamin deficiencies—may induce deficiency in vitamins D and folate
   3. Fetal hydantoin syndrome—associated with teratogenic conditions

D. Valproic acid (Depakene, Depakote)—adverse effects
   1. Hepatic failure—liver function tests are required to monitor the client's liver status
   2. Thrombocytopenia—bleeding; use caution when combining with aspirin, NSAIDs, or warfarin
   3. GI—nausea, vomiting
   4. CNS—sedation, drowsiness; hyperactivity, aggressiveness in children

E. Carbamazepine (Tegretol)—adverse effects
   1. Induces metabolism of itself and other drugs
   2. CNS—drowsiness, dizziness
   3. GI—nausea and vomiting
   4. Hematologic—can cause agranulocytosis; frequent monitoring of white blood cell count is necessary; signs and symptoms of a low count include fever, chills, aches, and pains
   5. Hepatic—liver function tests are necessary
   6. Indications—various seizures and trigeminal neuralgia
   7. Drug interactions—carbamazepine increases the metabolism of warfarin, theophylline, and doxycycline; the drug's metabolism is inhibited by erythromycin, verapamil, and diltiazem; increases the effect of lithium

F. Benzodiazepines
   1. Diazepam (Valium)—used for status epilepticus and emergency treatment of seizures
   2. Clonazepam (Clonopin)—taken orally for absence seizures (nonconvulsive seizures characterized by "staring off") and psychiatric conditions; oral adverse effects include coated tongue, xerostomia, encopresis, abnormal thirst, tender gums

G. Ethosuximide
   1. Used to treat absence seizures
   2. GI—anorexia, GI upset, nausea, vomiting
   3. CNS—drowsiness, dizziness, lethargy, hyperactivity
   4. Oral adverse drug reactions—drug-influenced gingival enlargement, swollen tongue

H. Newer agents
   1. Gabapentin—no reported drug interactions
   2. Felbamate—increased risk for developing aplastic anemia, severe liver disease

3. Lamotrigine
4. Topiramate
5. Tiagabine
6. Fosphenytoin—parenteral use only
7. Levetiracetam
8. Oxcarbazepine
9. Pregabalin—a schedule V drug, because of reported euphoria in some clinical trials
10. Zonisamide

PSYCHOTHERAPEUTIC AGENTS

Antipsychotics

A. Pharmacologic effects
   1. Antipsychotics—used in the management of psychoses; the client may perceive comments as threats (paranoia)
   2. Sedation and drowsiness—additive CNS depression with other CNS depressants
   3. Antiemetics—depress the chemoreceptor trigger zone (CTZ); reduce nausea and vomiting
B. Adverse reactions
   1. Orthostatic hypotension—dizziness or fainting on rising from a supine position
   2. Extrapyramidal effects—areas in the brain affecting bodily movements
      a. Dyskinesia—uncontrollable movements of the tongue or face
      b. Tardive dyskinesia—abnormal involuntary movements that occur with prolonged use of conventional antipsychotic agents
      c. Parkinsonian symptoms—tremors and rigidity resembling Parkinson's disease
      d. Akathisia—motor restlessness (e.g., swinging legs)
      e. Acute dystonic reaction—difficulty in opening the mouth; jaw muscles are contracted; dislocation of the jaw might occur
   3. Anticholinergic—xerostomia increases the risk of dental caries
C. Drug interactions—occur with antipsychotic agent given with:
   1. CNS depressants—additive CNS depression
   2. Anticholinergic—additive anticholinergic toxicity
D. Dental hygiene considerations
   1. Dyskinesia, akathisia, and tardive dyskinesia—the client may not be able to perform self-care
   2. Acute dystonic reaction—can occur during a procedure; the client needs to be treated with an anticholinergic drug
   3. Orthostatic hypotension—raise the dental chair slowly; have the client remain seated for a few minutes before standing to prevent a fall

TABLE 11-12 Selected Antipsychotic Drugs

Group	Drug
Conventional Antipsychotics High potency	Haloperidol (Haldol)
Medium potency	Trifluoperazine (Stelazine) Thiothixene (Navane)
Low potency	Chlorpromazine (Thorazine) Thioridazine (Mellaril)
Atypical Antipsychotics	Clozapine (Clozaril) Risperidone (Risperdal) Olanzapine (Zyprexa)

   4. Xerostomia—instruct the client to drink plenty of water; suck on tart sugarless gum or candy containing xylitol, or ice chips; avoid products containing alcohol and caffeine; and avoid juices and soft drinks to reduce the risk of dental caries; saliva substitutes (Xero-lube, Salivart) can also be recommended
E. Therapeutic uses
   1. Treatment of psychosis (e.g., schizophrenia)
   2. Antiemetic—for nausea or vomiting
   3. Opioid potentiation—combined with an opioid to potentiate analgesia and sedation; reduce the dose of the opioid if an antipsychotic is added
F. Examples of selected antipsychotic agents are provided in Table 11-12

Antidepressants

A. Pharmacologic effects
   1. Pharmacologic effect—affect norepinephrine and serotonin levels in the brain (require 4 to 6 weeks to be effective)
   2. Adverse reactions
      a. Cardiotoxic in overdose—dysrhythmias (mainly with tricyclic antidepressants); usual cause of death when used in a suicide attempt
      b. Xerostomia (anticholinergic action)
      c. Sedation
      d. GI—nausea resulting from selective serotonin reuptake inhibitors (SSRIs)
      e. Orthostatic hypotension
B. Drug interactions—occur with tricyclic antidepressants given with:
   1. Epinephrine—results in hypertension (increased vasopressor response); low doses contained in local anesthetic solutions can be used safely in normotensive persons (those with normal blood pressure)

2. Anticholinergic—results in additive anticholinergic action and excessive xerostomia

C. Therapeutic uses
  1. Treatment of depression
  2. Migraine headache prophylaxis
  3. Treatment of nocturnal enuresis (bed wetting) in children
  4. Chronic pain treatment adjuvant

D. Drugs
  1. Selected tricyclic antidepressants
    a. Amitriptyline (Elavil)
    b. Imipramine (Tofranil)
  2. MAOIs—Phenelzine (Nardil); tranylcypromine (Parnate)
    a. Infrequently used for depression
    b. Potential for numerous severe drug–food interactions (e.g., wine, sausage, cheese; indirect-acting adrenergic agents, meperidine)
  3. Dopamine–norepinephrine reuptake inhibitors
    a. Bupropion (Wellbutrin, Zyban)
    b. Bupropion, sustained-release (Wellbutrin SR)
    c. Bupropion, extended release (Wellbutrin ER)
  4. Selected SSRIs
    a. Fluoxetine (Prozac)
    b. Sertraline (Zoloft)
    c. Paroxetine (Paxil)
    d. Citalopram (Celexa)
  5. Serotonin and norepinephrine reuptake inhibitors
    a. Venlafaxine (Effexor)
    b. Venlafaxine, extended release (Effexor XR)
  6. Serotonin modulators
    a. Nefazodone (Serzone)
    b. Trazodone (Desyrel)
  7. Norepinephrine–serotonin modulator— mirtazapine (Remeron)

Other Psychotherapeutic Agents

A. Lithium—for treating bipolar–affective disorder (manic depression); blood level is difficult to maintain; NSAIDs increase serum lithium levels

B. Carbamazepine, valproate—these drugs are also used to treat seizure disorders; drug interactions and dental concerns are the same as those in the treatment of seizure disorders

ENDOCRINE AGENTS

Adrenocorticosteroids (Steroids)

A. Classification
  1. Glucocorticoids—regulate glucose metabolism and have an anti-inflammatory effect

  2. Mineralocorticoids—regulate sodium (minerals) and water

B. Pharmacologic effect—anti-inflammatory, antiallergenic, involved in carbohydrate metabolism, and have catabolic effects

C. Adverse reactions
  1. Cushing's syndrome—long-term, high-dose steroids produce symptoms including:
    a. Metabolic effects—"moon face," "buffalo hump," truncal obesity
    b. Peptic ulcers—exacerbation or stimulation of stomach acid secretion
    c. Skin conditions—bruising, striae, delayed healing
    d. Mental changes—euphoria, depression, psychosis, mood swings
    e. Infection—caused by suppression of immunity, symptoms may be masked; close observation and aggressive treatment are necessary
    f. Osteoporosis—bones break more easily
    g. Hypertension—elevated water and sodium retention (mineralocorticoid action)
    h. Hyperglycemia—exacerbation of diabetes
  2. Adrenal crisis (thyroid storm)—abrupt withdrawal or stress (e.g., a dental appointment) can precipitate a crisis; can be prevented by premedicating with additional steroids; potentially serious situation

D. Contraindications and cautions
  1. Ulcers—ulcerogenic
  2. Cardiovascular disease—can precipitate congestive heart failure, edema (result of mineralocorticoid effect)
  3. Acute psychoses
  4. Infection—increased susceptibility to bacterial, fungal, or viral infections
  5. Diabetes—hyperglycemia is induced

E. Dental hygiene considerations
  1. Check blood pressure prior to procedure or administration of a vasoconstrictor
  2. Avoid NSAIDs, aspirin, and opioid analgesics because of the increased risk of GI upset
  3. Steroids can delay wound healing and mask the symptoms of infection; consider administration of prophylactic antibiotic before procedure
  4. Osteoporosis may be evident on dental radiographs
  5. The steroid-dependent client may need short-term increase in steroid dose before a dental procedure to avoid an adrenal crisis

F. Therapeutic uses
  1. Medical—treatment of many inflammatory conditions (e.g., arthritis, asthma, dermatitis)
  2. Dental—treatment of:
    a. Aphthous lesions—palliative treatment; topical or intralesional therapy

TABLE 11-13 Steroids and Their Uses

Steroid	Comments	Equivalent Dose (mg/day)
Hydrocortisone	Some mineralocorticoid action	20–240
Prednisone	Most commonly used orally	5–60
Triamcinolone (Kenalog)	Used topically and injected into joints	2–20
Dexamethasone (Decadron)	Very potent, thus lower dose used	0.75–9.0

   b. Oral lesions secondary to collagen vascular diseases—respond to topical, intralesional, or systemic therapy
   c. Temporomandibular joint (TMJ) disease—intra-articular injection (into the joint) if the patient has arthritis
G. Examples of steroid agents are listed in Table 11-13

Agents for Diabetes Mellitus

See also the section on "Diabetes Mellitus" in Chapter 19.
A. Definition
   1. Symptoms
      a. Polyuria—increased urination
      b. Polydipsia—increased thirst
      c. Polyphagia—increased hunger
      d. Weight loss
      e. Xerostomia
   2. Classifications
      a. Type 1 diabetes (insulin-dependent diabetes mellitus)—circulating insulin is absent; usually is a result of autoimmune destruction of pancreatic β-cells; requires insulin therapy
      b. Type 2 diabetes (non–insulin-dependent diabetes mellitus)—decreased tissue sensitivity to insulin and impaired β-cell response to glucose; controlled by diet, oral hypoglycemic agents, and insulin, alone or in combination
   3. Microvascular and macrovascular complications
      a. Cardiovascular problems—circulation and heart problems, myocardial infarction, stroke
      b. Retinopathy—vision problems, cataracts, blindness
      c. Neuropathy—reduced sensations in the extremities
      d. Renal failure—nephropathy (kidney problems)
      e. Immunity—reduced ability to fight infections
      f. Healing—slower or delayed

   g. Oral manifestations—reduced immunity caused by white blood cell dysfunction; reduced vascular supply (small vessel disease), and other alterations in immune system function predispose the client to periodontal disease; loss of alveolar bone is characteristic
B. Dental hygiene considerations
   1. Reinforce the importance of good oral hygiene to minimize the risk of xerostomia, candidiasis, and dental caries
   2. Keep at hand a source of glucose that will act quickly (e.g., tube of cake frosting or orange juice) in case the client experiences hypoglycemia
   3. Clients with diabetes are at increased risk for periodontal disease and disease progression
   4. These clients are at a higher risk for delayed wound healing and infection; those with poorly controlled diabetes may require prophylactic antibiotic premedication
   5. Epinephrine, steroids, and opioid analgesics can decrease insulin release or increase insulin requirements; must therefore be used with caution in clients with diabetes
C. Adverse reactions
   1. Hypoglycemia—too much drug or too little food (intakes are not balanced)
      a. Symptoms—nervousness, sweating, tremulousness, compulsive talking, mental confusion, nausea, convulsions, coma
      b. Treatment—administer glucose orally if the client is conscious and able to swallow; if the client is unconscious, administer glucose intravenously, or administer glucagon subcutaneously or intramuscularly
   2. Hyperglycemia—less common cause of problems in the person with diabetes; treated in the emergency room with insulin and fluids
   3. Lipodystrophy occurs when insulin is injected into the same site for a prolonged period of time.
D. Examples of hypoglycemic agents
   1. Insulin
      a. Rapid-acting—insulin lispro, insulin aspart
      b. Short-acting—regular insulin (Humulin R, Novolin R) and prompt insulin zinc suspension (Semilente, Semilente Insulin, Semitard)
      c. Intermediate-acting—insulin time suspension (Lente, Humulin L); isophane insulin suspension (Humulin, WPH, Novolin N)
      d. Long-acting—extended insulin zinc suspension (Ultralente, Humulin U Ultralente)
      e. Mixed preparations—isophane insulin suspension and regular insulin injection (Humulin 70/30)

2. Use and sources
  a. Combined regular and neutral protamine Hagedorn (NPH) insulin—given one to two times per day
  b. Human insulin—from gene splicing (made from *E. coli*) or altered pork insulin
3. Oral hypoglycemic agents (sulfonylureas)
  a. First-generation agents
    (1) Tolbutamide (Orinase)
    (2) Chlorpropamide (Diabinese)
  b. Second-generation agents
    (1) Glyburide (DiaBeta, Micronase)
    (2) Glipizide (Glucotrol)
    (3) Glimepiride (Amaryl)
4. Other, newer agents
  a. Biguanides—metformin (Glucophage)
  b. α-Glucosidase inhibitors—acarbose (Precose); miglitol (Glyset)
  c. Thiazolidinediones—pioglitazone (Actos); rosiglitazone (Avandia)
  d. Non–sulfonylurea secretagogues—nateglinide (Starlix); repaglinide (Prandin)

Thyroid Agents

A. Hypothyroidism—also hypothyroidosis, athyroidosis, hypothyrosis, thyroid insufficiency; deficient thyroid activity results in lowered metabolism, fatigue, lethargy; more common in women than in men; can lead to cretinism in infants
  1. Thyroid replacements used; leads to a euthyroid condition (normal thyroid)
  2. Examples of hypothyroidism agents
    a. Levothyroxine (Synthroid, Levothroid)
    b. Liotrix (Euthroid, Thyrolar)
  3. The client requires no special handling if the dose is adequate
  4. Dental hygiene considerations
    a. Carefully examine children suspected of having hypothyroidism and children diagnosed with hypothyroidism; the client with hypothyroidism must maintain good oral health
    b. Clients with hypothyroidism are more sensitive to medications that depress the CNS; lower doses may therefore be necessary; counsel the client about the CNS side effects
B. Hyperthyroidism—also Graves' disease; various causes lead to the excessive production of thyroid hormones; produces goiter, cardiopulmonary dysfunction (atrial fibrillation, palpitations, widened pulse rate), skin and behavioral conditions (tremor, excessive sweating, heat intolerance, nervousness, fatigue), and ocular symptoms (exophthalmos)
  1. Partial thyroidectomy (treated surgically or with radioactive iodine [^{131}I]) ablates part of the thyroid gland—the client requires supplemental thyroid hormone therapy; no unusual dental considerations if the client is taking drug treatment
  2. Clients awaiting surgery or those who are poor surgical candidates are maintained on a regimen of thyroid suppressants
    a. Drugs suppress thyroid function—propylthiouracil (PTU)
    b. β-Blockers are given to bring down elevated heart rate (e.g., propranolol)
    c. Dental hygiene considerations—avoid epinephrine because it can trigger a thyroid storm; clients have a lower pain threshold and may require higher doses of local anesthetic agents or higher doses of CNS-depressing medications

Estrogens and Progesterone

Estrogen

A. Responsible for female sex characteristics, reproduction development, and preparing for conception
B. Adverse reactions
  1. Nausea, vomiting
  2. Uterine bleeding, vaginal discharge
  3. Edema
  4. Thrombophlebitis
  5. Weight gain
  6. Headache
  7. Hypertension
C. Dose forms
  1. Oral tablets
  2. Creams
  3. Transdermal patches
D. Clinical uses include treatments for:
  1. Symptoms of menopause
  2. Menstrual disturbances
  3. Osteoporosis

Progesterone

A. Responsible for preparing the uterus for implantation of the fertilized egg
B. Adverse reactions
  1. Abnormal menstrual bleeding
  2. Breakthrough bleeding
  3. Spotting between menstrual periods
  4. Change in amount of menstrual blood flow
  5. Amenorrhea
C. Dose forms
  1. Oral
  2. Parenteral
D. Clinical uses include treatments for:
  1. Dysfunctional uterine bleeding
  2. Endometriosis

3. Dysmenorrhea

4. Premenstrual tension

Oral Contraceptives

A. Pharmacologic activity—inhibits the release of follicle-stimulating hormone (FSH) and luteinizing hormone (LH), which prevent ovulation and pregnancy

B. Contain either progesterone alone or a combination of estrogen and progesterone; both come in varying doses

C. Adverse reactions

1. Nausea, dizziness, weight gain, headache, breast tenderness

2. Hypertension, liver damage, thrombophlebitis, thromboembolism

3. Oral—increased gingival fluid, susceptibility to gingivitis, gingival inflammation, increased risk of dry socket after extraction (newer formulations contain less hormone and therefore are less likely to cause these conditions)

D. Dental hygiene considerations

1. Review with the client the importance of good oral hygiene because of the potential for gingivitis

2. Extractions should be performed on days 23 to 28 of the oral contraceptive cycle to reduce the risk of dry socket

3. Check blood pressure at each appointment because of the risk of hypertension

4. During long procedures, have scheduled breaks to minimize risk of thrombophlebitis; have the client stretch the legs and walk around, if possible

5. Instruct clients to use a contingent method of birth control if they require antibiotic therapy

RESPIRATORY SYSTEM AGENTS

Agents for Asthma

A. Disease—dyspnea, cough, and wheezing, secondary to bronchospasm (hyperirritable bronchioles), inflammation of bronchioles with secretions

B. Drugs

1. Adrenergic agonists (sympathomimetics)—see the section on the ANS

a. Dose forms—oral inhalers, tablets, liquid

b. Inhalers—β_2-adrenergic agonists

(1) Short-acting β_2-agonists

(a) Albuterol (Proventil, Ventolin)

(b) Metaproterenol (Alupent, Metaprel)

(2) Long-acting β_2-agonists

(a) Salmeterol (Serevent)

(b) Formoterol (Foradil Aerolizer)

c. Epinephrine—administered intravenously for an acute attack

d. Used for maintenance and prophylactic therapy

e. Adverse reactions—nervousness, tachycardia, insomnia, xerostomia with oral inhalers

f. Dental hygiene considerations for short-acting and long-acting β_2-agonists

(1) Measure the client's blood pressure and pulse rate before the procedure because of the potential for tachycardia

(2) Have the client "rinse, swish, and expectorate" after each inhaler use to reduce xerostomia

(3) Instruct the client to maintain good oral hygiene, especially with the use of oral inhalers

2. Methylxanthines

a. Examples

(1) Aminophylline (theophylline, ethylenediamine)

(2) Caffeine—relative of theophylline

(3) Theophylline (Theo-dur, Slo-bid)

b. Pharmacologic effects

(1) Bronchodilation (smooth muscle relaxation) helps reduce the symptoms of asthma

(2) CNS stimulation—alertness, insomnia

(3) Diuresis—increased urination

3. Cromolyn sodium (Intal, Nasalcrom)

a. Used for asthma prophylaxis by inhalation, for allergic rhinitis, and for maintenance therapy for asthma

b. Adverse reactions—nausea, vomiting, restlessness, anxiety

c. Dental concerns—same as with β_2-adrenergic agonists

4. Ipratropium bromide (Atrovent)

a. Anticholinergic bronchodilator; used mainly to treat emphysema

b. Adverse reactions—xerostomia and bad taste

c. Dental concerns

(1) Counsel the client to rinse well and expectorate after each use

(2) Counsel the client about the importance of good oral hygiene

5. Adrenocorticosteroids

a. Used for acute and maintenance therapy

b. Dose forms—oral, parenteral, metered-dose inhalers (MDI), tablets

c. Adverse reactions with MDIs—dysphonia (hoarseness), xerostomia, cough, and candidiasis

d. Dental hygiene considerations

(1) MDIs—same as with other oral inhalers

e. Examples
(1) Flunisolide (Aerobid)
(2) Fluticasone (Flovent)
(3) Triamcinolone (Azmacort)

C. Dental hygiene considerations
  1. Disease considerations
    a. Degree of control—avoid elective treatment if the asthma is poorly controlled
    b. The client's anxiety may precipitate an acute attack; an antianxiety agent may be useful (e.g., benzodiazepine)
  2. Analgesic choice—sometimes difficult to make
    a. Aspirin-containing compounds—may precipitate an attack
    b. NSAIDs—if aspirin causes bronchospasm, NSAIDs are contraindicated
    c. Opioids—produce bronchoconstriction (histamine release) and respiratory depression; can be used with care in lower doses or strengths
    d. Acetaminophen—best choice; may be used in combination with a weak opioid (e.g., Tylenol no. 3)

GASTROINTESTINAL AGENTS

Agents Affecting Gastrointestinal Motility

A. Laxatives—increase GI motility; symptomatically used to treat constipation (e.g., milk of magnesia)

B. Antidiarrheals—reduce GI motility; symptomatically used to treat diarrhea (e.g., Lomotil, Imodium, any opioid)

C. Dental hygiene considerations
  1. Central nervous system sedation—the client should be instructed to avoid driving or operating heavy machinery, or anything that requires thinking or concentration
  2. Xerostomia—instruct the client to drink plenty of water; suck on tart sugarless gum or candy containing xylitol, or ice chips; avoid products containing alcohol and caffeine; and avoid juices and soft drinks to reduce the risk of dental caries; saliva substitutes (Xero-lube, Salivart) can also be recommended

Agents for Gastroesophageal Reflux Disease—Histamine (H₂)-Blockers

A. Mechanism of action—block stomach acid secretion; pain subsides and no further damage occurs from esophageal exposure to stomach acid

B. Examples (all available OTC [over the counter])
  1. Cimetidine (Tagamet HB)
  2. Famotidine (Pepcid AC)
  3. Nizatidine (Axid AR)
  4. Ranitidine (Zantac 75)

C. Dental hygiene considerations
  1. These agents interfere with the absorption of drugs that need acid for absorption (e.g., ketoconazole [Nizoral])
  2. Avoid ulcerogenic medications unless absolutely necessary (e.g., aspirin, NSAIDs, and glucocorticoids)
  3. Cimetidine
    a. Reduces hepatic blood flow
    b. Inhibits the metabolism of certain drugs (diazepam, warfarin)

Proton Pump Inhibitors

A. Mechanism—irreversibly bind to the proton pump, resulting in acid suppression lasting more than 24 hours

B. Examples
  1. Omeprazole (Prilosec)
  2. Lansoprazole (Prevacid)
  3. Esomeprazole (Nexium)

C. Adverse reactions
  1. Esophageal candidiasis
  2. Mucosal atrophy of the tongue
  3. Xerostomia

D. Dental hygiene considerations
  1. Evaluate for adverse oral reactions
  2. Xerostomia—instruct the client to drink plenty of water; suck on tart sugarless gum or candy that contains xylitol, or ice chips; avoid products containing alcohol and caffeine; and avoid juices and soft drinks to reduce the risk of dental caries; saliva substitutes (Xero-lube, Salivart) can also be recommended

Emetics and Antiemetics

A. Emetics—induce vomiting; used to treat most poisonings (e.g., syrup of ipecac, which is available without a prescription); abused by persons with bulimia

B. Antiemetics
  1. Reduce nausea or vomiting
  2. Examples
    a. Benzquinamide (Emete-Con)
    b. Prochlorperazine (Compazine)
    c. Trimethobenzamide (Tigan)

C. Dental hygiene considerations
  1. CNS sedation—the client should be instructed to avoid driving or operating heavy machinery

or doing anything that requires thinking or concentration

2. Xerostomia—instruct the client to drink plenty of water; suck on tart sugarless gum or candy containing xylitol, or ice chips; avoid products containing alcohol and caffeine; and avoid juices or soft drinks to reduce the risk of dental caries; saliva substitutes (Xero-lube, Salivart) can also be recommended

ANTINEOPLASTIC AGENTS

A. Mechanism—interfere with the metabolism or reproductive cycle of malignant cells; also affect normal cells

B. Drugs
  1. Alkylating agents
    a. Nitrogen mustards
      (1) Cyclophosphamide (Cytoxan)
      (2) Chlorambucil (Leukeran)
      (3) Melphalan (Alkeran)
    b. Nitrosoureas—carmustine (BiCNU)
    c. Busulfan (Myleran)
  2. Antimetabolites
    a. Folic acid analog—methotrexate (MTX)
    b. Purine antagonists
      (1) Mercaptopurine (6-MP)
      (2) Thioguanine (6-TG)
    c. Pyrimidine antagonists
      (1) 5-Fluorouracil (5-FC)
      (2) Cytarabine (Cytosar-U, ara-C)
  3. Other antineoplastics
    a. Plant alkaloids
      (1) Vinblastine (Velban)
      (2) Vincristine (Oncovin)
    b. Antibiotics
      (1) Dactinomycin (actinomycin D, Cos-megen)
      (2) Daunorubicin (Cerubidine)
      (3) Doxorubicin (Adriamycin)
      (4) Mitomycin (Mitocin-C)
    c. Hormones
      (1) Adrenocorticosteroids
      (2) Androgens
      (3) Estrogens
      (4) Progestin
      (5) Tamoxifen (Nolvadex)—antiestrogen
    d. Aminobisphosphonates
      (1) Alendronate (Fosamax)
      (2) Ibandronate (Boniva)
      (3) Pamidronate (Aredia)
      (4) Risedronate (Actonel)
      (5) Zoledronic acid (Zometa)
    e. Miscellaneous
      (1) Asparaginase (Elspar)
      (2) Bleomycin (Blenoxane)
      (3) Cisplatin (Platinol)
      (4) Hydroxyurea (Hydrea)

C. Adverse reactions
  1. Lack of specificity against tumor cells because normal cells are also destroyed; cells with the fastest life cycle are affected first
  2. Bone marrow activity suppression
    a. Leukopenia—lowered white blood cell count; infections are more likely
    b. Thrombocytopenia—lowered platelets; the risk of bleeding is increased
    c. Anemia
  3. GI—stomatitis, mucosal sloughing
  4. Infection—reduced immunity and ability to fight infection
  5. Skin and hair—rash, alopecia (baldness)
  6. Oral effects
    a. Symptoms—pain, ulcers, dryness, impaired taste, gingival hemorrhage, sensitivity of teeth and gingivae
    b. Treatment—avoid mouthrinses with alcohol; substitute saline or sodium bicarbonate; avoid alcohol
    c. Candidiasis—use antifungal agents (e.g., Nystatin)
    d. Xerostomia—instruct the client to drink plenty of water; suck on tart sugarless gum or candy with xylitol, or ice chips; avoid products containing alcohol and caffeine; and avoid juices and soft drinks to reduce the risk of dental caries; saliva substitutes (Xero-lube, Salivart) can also be recommended
  7. Osteonecrosis of the jaw (ONJ)
    a. In cancer patients receiving intravenous bisphosphonates, 94% of cases with ONJ have been reported; the incidence is much lower in patients taking oral bisphosphonates for osteoporosis
    b. Prolonged use may suppress bone turnover—leads to microdamage
    c. Most cases of ONJ occur after tooth extractions or other procedures that cause trauma to the jawbone
    d. Very difficult to treat once it occurs
    e. Oral health examinations and other dental procedures should be performed before starting bisphosphonate therapy and continued every 3 months thereafter
    f. Any dental procedures that are performed should involve minimal trauma to the jaw and adjacent tissue
    g. Necrotic bone should be removed in those with ONJ
    h. If clinically necessary, 0.12% chlorhexidine gluconate rinses, systemic antibiotics, and analgesics can be used

D. Dental hygiene considerations
1. Have clients improve their oral hygiene before chemotherapy, if possible
2. Avoid elective procedures during chemotherapy; timing is important; the best time for procedures is the day on which chemotherapy begins (period of highest blood counts)
3. Check the coagulation status before any emergency surgery
4. Use of prophylactic antibiotic premedication is controversial
5. If xerostomia is a problem, client will need custom-fitted mouth trays for at-home, self-administered fluoride therapy

SUBSTANCE ABUSE

See the section on "Chemical Dependency" in Chapter 19.

Definitions

A. Tolerance—increasingly higher doses are required to produce the same effect; the same dose produces less effect; occurs with repeated administration
B. Physical dependence—symptoms of withdrawal occur if the drug is abruptly discontinued
C. Psychological dependence—craving occurs if the drug is stopped; no physical withdrawal syndrome; however, psychological dependence is just as likely to result in relapse (e.g., cocaine)
D. Abuse—improper or excessive self-administration of a drug that results in an adverse outcome
E. Addiction—pattern of abuse that continues despite medical or social complications
F. Withdrawal—a physical reaction attributable to physical dependence
G. Abstinence—drug-free state
H. Enabling—a pattern of coping methods (e.g., making excuses for absences) used by the associates of those addicted, which allows the addicted person to continue the drug use

Drugs of Abuse

A. Depressants
1. Alcohol—impaired judgment, slurred speech, ataxia, seizures, coma, death; withdrawal produces autonomic hyperactivity, hallucinations, or seizures; cirrhosis with chronic use
2. Opioids (heroin, codeine, morphine)—euphoria, abscesses, constipation, respiratory depression; withdrawal produces "cold turkey" syndrome; methadone maintenance and naltrexone (acts like orally active naloxone) used to suppress a "high"
3. Barbiturates—secobarbital, pentobarbital
4. Volatile solvents—glue sniffing and paint solvent inhaling; called "huffing"
5. Benzodiazepines—diazepam
6. Anesthetics—nitrous oxide–oxygen (N_2O–O_2) analgesia

B. Stimulants
1. Amphetamines—methamphetamine; highly addictive; street name "ice"
2. Cocaine—most psychologically addicting drug; produces euphoria, hyperactivity, paranoia, acute MI; street names "coke," "crack"
3. Nicotine—in cigarettes, chewing tobacco, and cigars
4. Caffeine—in soft drinks, coffee, tea

C. Psychedelics
1. Lysergic acid diethylamide (LSD)—flashbacks occur (without the drug); called "bad trip"
2. Psilocybin—hallucinogen derived from mushrooms of the genus *Psilocybe*
3. Phencyclidine (PCP)—disorientation, seizures; treatment consists of "talking down"
4. Marijuana (cannabis)—active ingredient is tetrahydrocannabinol (THC); causes silliness, relaxation, euphoria, paranoia, confusion, chronic amotivational syndrome; entrance drug (used first before trying other addictive drugs)

D. Dental hygiene considerations
1. Cocaine—cardiac stimulant effect; causes addictive effect on heart with local anesthetic agents with vasoconstrictors
2. N_2O—sense of euphoria; incidence of dental personnel abuse (unsupervised use); abuse produces neuropathy (sometimes irreversible); without adequate O_2, hypoxia is produced
3. Addicts—"shopper" clients attempt to obtain prescriptions for controlled substances from several dental offices; feign dental pain but refuse definitive treatment; suspicion is warranted
4. Caffeine—increased heart rate and blood pressure with excessive caffeine intake
5. Nicotine—check for oral manifestations of tobacco use (e.g., nicotine stomatitis, periodontal disease, oral leukoplakia, precancerous lesions, hairy tongue, halitosis)

DRUG USE DURING PREGNANCY

A. General—pregnant women must:
1. Avoid any unnecessary drugs
2. Consult with an obstetrician

B. Pregnancy and professional oral health care
   1. First trimester—period of highest risk for drug effects on the fetus; negative organogenic effects possible
   2. Second trimester—best for elective dental treatment
   3. Third trimester—use of any unnecessary drugs must be avoided because of client comfort and proximity to delivery
C. Drugs used in dental practice that are probably safe
   1. Amoxicillin
   2. Penicillin
   3. Erythromycin
   4. Lidocaine
   5. Epinephrine (limit dose)
D. Drugs used in dental practice that must be avoided
   1. Aspirin
   2. NSAIDs
   3. Metronidazole
   4. N_2O—dental personnel who are pregnant should be especially careful. Women exposed to high levels of nitrous oxide (>5 hours/week) were significantly less fertile than unexposed women. Levels of exposure vary from state to state. Dental practices should improve room air circulation and cleaning procedures and use an air evacuation system all in an effort to reduce adverse outcomes.[13,14] (http://www.osha.gov/dts/osta/anestheticgases/index.html#C1)

Smoking Cessation

A. Nicotine reduction systems
   1. Nicotine is a ganglionic cholinergic-receptor agonist
   2. Nicotine reduction (also known as *replacement*) therapies reduce the withdrawal symptoms associated with smoking cessation
   3. Smoking cessation reduces the risk of oral and lung cancers, heart disease, and other lung diseases
B. Types of nicotine reduction systems
   1. Chewing gum—Nicorette 2 or 4 mg; available without a prescription
   2. Transdermal system—all available without a prescription
      a. Habitrol
      b. Nicoderm

   c. Nicotrol
   d. Prostep
   3. Nasal spray—Nicotrol NS
   4. Adverse effects
      a. Chewing gum—sore mouth, hiccups, dyspepsia, jaw ache, nausea
      b. Chewing gum can stick to dentures and dental work
      c. Transdermal systems—nausea, hypersalivation, abdominal pain, vomiting, diarrhea, perspiration, headache, dizziness, hearing and visual disturbances, confusion, weakness
      d. Nasal spray—runny nose, throat irritation, watery eyes, sneezing, cough
   5. Dental hygiene considerations
      a. Evaluate the client who smokes for oral benign and malignant changes
      b. Stress the importance of tobacco cessation
      c. Evaluate clients who use the chewing gum for any problems, for example, if the gum is sticking to dentures or dental work; recommend using another form of smoking cessation aid
C. Bupropion (Zyban)
   1. Antidepressant used to reduce nicotine cravings
   2. Concomitant treatment modalities are encouraged (behavior modifications)
   3. Recommended dosing—150 mg once a day for 3 days, followed by 150 mg two times a day for 2 to 3 months if the client is experiencing success
D. Varenicline (CHANTIX)
   1. Nicotine receptor blocker; amount of dopamine released into the brain is reduced; thereby blocking the feelings of pleasure associated with tobacco use
   2. Dosing—once daily for the first 3 days, two times daily thereafter for the full course of therapy (usually 12 weeks)
   3. Taken after meals and with a full glass of water
   4. Adverse effects include nausea, sleep problems, constipation, gas, vomiting, changes in mood and behavior
   5. Cannot be used in conjunction with other smoking cessation products

WEB SITE INFORMATION AND RESOURCES

SOURCE	WEB SITE ADDRESS	DESCRIPTION
RxList, The Internet Drug Index	http://www.rxlist.com	A HealthCentral.com Network site providing information about medications, indications, contraindications, dosages, and client information

@ WEB SITE INFORMATION AND RESOURCES—cont'd

SOURCE	WEB SITE ADDRESS	DESCRIPTION
Drug Topics	http://www.drugtopics.modernmedicine.com	Current news on drug-related topics
Center for Drug Evaluation and Research	http://www.fda.gov/cder/index.html	Information on new drug development and regulatory issues
Med Watch	http://www.fda.gov/medwatch/safety.htm	Safety information
Alternative Medicine Foundation	http://www.amfoundation.org	Current information on alternative therapies
American Herbal Products Association	http://www.ahpa.org	Current information on herbal remedies
Malignant Hyperthermia Association of the United States	http://www.mhaus.org	Online brochures, including an explanation of malignant hyperthermia as a concern in dentistry and oral and maxillofacial surgery

REFERENCES

1. *Physician's desk reference*, ed 69, Oradell, NJ, 2010, Medical Economics.
2. Olin BR, Hebel SK, Dombek CE, editors: *Drug facts and comparisons*, St Louis, 2010, Facts and Comparisons Inc.
3. Bablenis-Haveles E: *Applied pharmacology for the dental hygienist*, ed 6, St Louis, 2010, Mosby.
4. Pickett FA, Terézhalmy GT: *Dental drug reference with clinical implications*. ed 2, Baltimore, 2009, Wolters Kluwer Health–Lippincott Williams & Wilkins.
5. Weinberg MA, Westphal C, Fine JB: *Oral pharmacology for the dental hygienist*, ed 1, Upper Saddle River, 2008, Pearson–Prentiss Hall.
6. Jeske AH: *Mosby's dental drug reference*, ed 10, St Louis, 2012, Mosby.
7. Wynn RL, Meiller TF, Crossley HL: *Drug information handbook for dentistry*, Hudson, OH, 2010, Lexi-Comp
8. U.S. Pharmacopeia Drug Information (USP DI): *Drug information for the health care professional*, Volume 1; *Advice for the patient*, Volume 2, ed 21, Montvale, NJ, 2010: Available at www.usp.org: Accessed 10 January 2010.
9. Holroyd SV: *Clinical pharmacology in dental practice*, ed 4, St Louis, 1989, Mosby.
10. Wilson W, Taubert KA, Gewitz M, et al: Prevention of infective endocarditis: Guidelines from the American Heart Association, *Circulation* 116:1736.11, 2007.
11. Hirsh J, Dalen J, Guyatt G, editors: The sixth (2000) ACCP guidelines for antithrombotic therapy for prevention and treatment of thrombosis. American College of Chest Physicians, *Chest* 119(1 Suppl):1S–2S, 2001.
12. American Hospital Formulary Service: Drug information, Bethesda, MD, 2010, American Society of Hospital Pharmacists.
13. Crawford JS, Lewis M: Nitrous oxide in early pregnancy, *Anaesthesia* 41:900, F186.
14. Little JW, Falace DA, Miller CS, Rhodus NL: Dental management of the medically compromised patient, St Louis, Mosby, 2008.

CHAPTER 11 REVIEW QUESTIONS

Answers and Rationales to Review Questions are available on this text's
accompanying Evolve site. See inside front cover for details.
Use Case A to answer questions 1 to 10.

℮volve

SYNOPSIS OF PATIENT HISTORY	Age	16	VITAL SIGNS	
	Sex	M	Blood pressure	102/60 mmHg
	Height	5'9"	Pulse rate	70 bpm
			Respiration rate	22 rpm
CASE	A	Weight	162 lbs	
			73.6 kgs	

1. Under Care of Physician
   Yes No
   ☒   ☐   Condition: _____asthma_____
2. Hospitalized within the last 5 years
   Yes No
   ☐   ☒   Reason: _____
3. Has or had the following conditions
   _____ – _____
   _____ – _____
4. Current medications
   Albuterol inhaler: as needed
   Montelukast (Singulair) 10mg: one tablet daily
   Fluticasone/salmeterol (Advair HFA) inhaler:
   one inhalation twice daily
   Multivitamin: once daily
   Doxycycline
   Cetirizine (Zyrtec) 10 mg daily
5. Smokes or uses tobacco products
   Yes No
   ☐   ☒
6. Is pregnant
   Yes No N/A
   ☐   ☐   ☒

MEDICAL HISTORY:
Patient has a history of asthma and is under the care of his pediatrician. Patient also has acne for which he is being treated by his pediatrician.

DENTAL HISTORY:
Visits the dental office for regular examinations and cleanings.

SOCIAL HISTORY:
He lives with his mother, father, and brother
He enjoys golf, soccer, movies, and traveling
He is a junior at a local high school.

CHIEF COMPLAINT:
I have a sore and dry throat.

---

1. **Which of the following drugs could be causing the sore throat and dry mouth?**
   a. Albuterol
   b. Montelukast
   c. Multivitamins
   d. Doxycycline

2. **Albuterol is a bronchodilator that can be administered via a metered dose inhaler. It is recommended for treating an acute asthma attack.**
   a. Both statements are TRUE
   b. Both statements are FALSE
   c. The first statement is TRUE; the second is FALSE
   d. The first statement is FALSE; the second is TRUE

3. **Which one of the following drugs can result in oral candidiasis?**
   a. Cetirizine
   b. Ibuprofen
   c. Acetaminophen
   d. Fluticasone

4. **All of the following are recommendations that you should make to patients with asthma EXCEPT one. Which one is the EXCEPTION?**
   a. Bring your inhaler (albuterol) to the dental appointment
   b. Rinse after using corticosteroid inhaler
   c. Avoid erythromycin
   d. Avoid aspirin
   e. Avoid acetaminophen

5. **Though this teenager with asthma does not have emphysema, several of the drugs used to treat asthma are also used to treat emphysema. Which of the following drugs is the better choice for treating emphysema?**
   a. Albuterol
   b. Zileuton
   c. Ipratropium
   d. Cetirizine

6. **Which of the following orally inhaled drugs should the patient bring with him to each appointment in case of an acute asthma attack?**
   a. Salmeterol
   b. Albuterol
   c. Flunisolide
   d. Ipratropium bromide

7. **Which of the following is the BEST recommendation you could make to your patient if he required oral prednisone (steroid therapy)?**
   a. Continue to rinse, swish, and spit after taking your oral tablet
   b. Rinse, swish, and swallow after taking your oral tablet
   c. Check for any signs of infection, since this medication can mask the signs of infection and can delay wound healing.
   d. Be careful, since this drug can cause significant dry mouth

8. **Patients using the fluticasone–salmeterol inhaler should be instructed about all of the following EXCEPT one. Which one is the EXCEPTION?**
   a. Rinse, swish, and spit after each use of the inhaler
   b. The inhaler must be discarded 1 month from the date of first use
   c. It is a good idea to brush your teeth after each inhaler use
   d. This inhaler can be used for acute attacks

9. **Patients taking doxycycline should be counseled about all of the following EXCEPT one. Which one is the EXCEPTION?**
   a. Esophageal irritation
   b. Photosensitivity
   c. Gastrointestinal upset
   d. Sedation

10. **Histamine 1 (H_1) blocking drugs such as cetirizine are preferred over drugs such as diphenhydramine because they are less sedating. Cetirizine is a non-sedating H_1-blocking drug.**
    a. Both statements are TRUE
    b. The first statement is TRUE; the second statement is FALSE
    c. The first statement is FALSE; the second statement is TRUE
    d. Both statements are FALSE

Use Case B to answer questions 11 to 25.

SYNOPSIS OF PATIENT HISTORY		
Age	55	
Sex	M	
Height	5'10"	
CASE	B	
Weight	220 lbs / 100 kgs	

VITAL SIGNS
Blood pressure   145/85 mmHg
Pulse rate   75 bpm
Respiration rate   25 rpm

1. Under Care of Physician
   Yes ☒ No ☐   Condition: Hypertension, high cholesterol, type 2 diabetes, coronary artery disease, depression
2. Hospitalized within the last 5 years
   Yes ☒ No ☐   Reason: rule out MI
3. Has or had the following conditions
   _ _____
   _ _____
4. Current medications
   Lisinopril (Zestril)
   Hydrochlorothiazide
   Baby aspirin
   Atorvastatin (Lipitor)
   Glipizide (Glucotrol) 10 mg bid
   Metformin (Glucophage)
   Citalopram (Celexa) 40 mg qd
   Sublingual nitroglycerin as needed
5. Smokes or uses tobacco products
   Yes ☐ No ☑
6. Is pregnant
   Yes ☐ No ☐ N/A ☑

MEDICAL HISTORY:
Client has a history of cardiovascular disease, type 2 diabetes, depression, and high cholesterol. Patient being treated by his cardiologist and general physician.

DENTAL HISTORY:
Visits the dental office for regular examinations and dental hygiene care.

SOCIAL HISTORY:
Married with 3 children
He enjoys golf, football, television, and good meals
Currently employed as a government contractor

CHIEF COMPLAINT:
I am here for my routine oral health examination.

11. **What is meant by the term *essential hypertension*?**
    a. Hypertension of unknown cause
    b. Iatrogenic hypertension
    c. Hypertension precipitated by another disorder
    d. Developing form of hypertension, requiring aggressive therapy

12. **Eating a banana or drinking a glass of orange juice when taking a thiazide diuretic will:**
    a. Deplete calcium
    b. Prevent diuresis
    c. Replenish potassium
    d. Inhibit the drug's metabolism

13. **A myocardial infarction 9 months before an office visit would be considered a CONTRAINDICATION to dental treatment. After 9 months, if treatment is provided, the client should receive prophylactic antibiotic premedication.**
    a. Both statements are TRUE
    b. The first statement is TRUE; the second statement is FALSE
    c. The first statement is FALSE; the second statement is TRUE
    d. Both statements are FALSE

14. **One of the main differences between angiotensin-converting enzyme (ACE) inhibitors and angiotensin receptor blockers is that ACE inhibitors cause a dry, nonproductive cough. Angiotensin receptor blockers do not cause a dry, nonproductive cough.**
    a. Both statements are TRUE
    b. The first statement is TRUE; the second statement is FALSE
    c. The first statement is FALSE; the second statement is TRUE
    d. Both statements are FALSE

15. **Clients taking antihypertensive agents who have been supine for some time should rise from that position slowly. They should dangle their legs over the side of the chair and wiggle them before rising to the standing position.**
    a. Both statements are true
    b. Both statements are false
    c. The first statement is true; the second is false
    d. The first statement is false; the second is true

16. **Which of the following drugs inhibits hydroxymethylglutaryl coenzyme A (HMG CoA) reductase?**
    a. Pravastatin
    b. Ramipril
    c. Nifedipine
    d. Ezetimibe

17. **Which agent reduces serum cholesterol by increasing its use for bile acid synthesis?**
    a. Niacin
    b. Atorvastatin
    c. Gemfibrozil
    d. Cholestyramine

18. **Which class of drugs is recommended in persons with diabetes?**
    a. Beta adrenergic blockers
    b. Ca^{++} channel blocker
    c. Angiotensin-converting enzyme (ACE) inhibitors
    d. Anticholinergic agents

19. **All of the following drugs inhibit platelet function EXCEPT one. Which one is the EXCEPTION?**
    a. Clopidogrel
    b. Dipyridamole
    c. Ticlopidine
    d. Aspirin

20. **Patients taking nitroglycerine (NTG) sublingual tablets should be instructed to:**
    a. Store their NTG in plastic
    b. Keep their NTG in the refrigerator
    c. Use NTG once every 5 minutes until the anginal attack has stopped
    d. Bring their NTG to the dental appointment and make it available to the practitioner in the event that the patient experiences an acute anginal attack

21. **Your patient complains of chest pain while sitting in the dental chair. Even though the information is not recorded on his health history or pharmacologic history form, it is a good idea for you to ask if he has taken sildenafil (Viagra) within the last 24 hours. The use of nitroglycerine is contraindicated if sildenafil has been taken within 24 hours because the nitroglycerine–sildenafil combination can precipitate a hypertensive crisis.**
    a. Both statements are TRUE
    b. Both statements are FALSE
    c. The first statement is TRUE; the second statement is FALSE
    d. The first statement is FALSE; the second statement is TRUE

22. **Which oral antidiabetic agent produces lactic acidosis as a significant adverse effect?**
    a. Tolbutamide
    b. Metformin
    c. Repaglinide
    d. Acarbose

23. **Patients taking glipizide should be instructed to:**
    a. Schedule their dental appointments after mealtimes and take their medicine on time
    b. Schedule their dental appointments around the time they take their medicine
    c. Schedule their dental appointments around mealtimes only
    d. Schedule their dental appointment any time, as the timing of the appointment is not a significant factor

24. Which antidepressant is LEAST likely to cause xerostomia?
a. Bupropion
b. Citalopram
c. Chlorpromazine
d. Amitriptyline

25. Selective serotonin reuptake inhibitors (SSRIs) tend to produce central nervous system (CNS) stimulation rather than CNS depression. Therefore, SSRIs are less sedating.
a. Both statements are TRUE
b. The first statement is TRUE; the second statement is FALSE
c. The first statement is FALSE; the second statement is TRUE
d. Both statements are FALSE

Use Case C to answer questions 26 to 40.

SYNOPSIS OF PATIENT HISTORY		
Age	49	
Sex	F	
Height	5'2"	
CASE	C	
Weight	125 lbs	
	57 kgs	

VITAL SIGNS
Blood pressure _95/68 mmHg_
Pulse rate _65 bpm_
Respiration rate _20 rpm_

1. Under Care of Physician
   Yes ☑ No ☐   Condition: _menopause_
2. Hospitalized within the last 5 years
   Yes ☐ No ☒   Reason: _____
3. Has or had the following conditions
   –
   –
4. Current medications
   LoEstrin 24
   Occasional over-the-counter
   ibuprofen and acetaminophen
5. Smokes or uses tobacco products
   Yes ☐ No ☐
6. Is pregnant
   Yes ☐ No ☐ N/A ☐

MEDICAL HISTORY:
Menopausal, otherwise healthy

DENTAL HISTORY:
Visits the dental office for regular examinations and dental hygiene care
Predental anxiety, requires pretreatment with a benzodiazepine

SOCIAL HISTORY:
Married with two children
She enjoys golf, gardening, scrapbooking, reading and traveling
She is a pharmacist.

CHIEF COMPLAINT:
I need a crown

ANTICIPATED MEDICATIONS
Lorazepam 2mg the night before the appointment
Nitrous oxide and oxygen conscious sedation during the procedure
Acetaminophen with codeine post procedure

26. Patients should be warned that an acute overdose with acetaminophen can result in damage to the:
a. Eyes
b. Liver
c. Spleen
d. Kidney

27. Alcohol consumption in combination with acetaminophen stimulates the breakdown of acetaminophen, thereby increasing the toxic potential of acetaminophen use.
a. Both statements are TRUE
b. Both statements are FALSE
c. The first statement is TRUE; the second statement is FALSE
d. The first statement is FALSE; the second statement is TRUE

28. Approximately 90% of dental pain is BEST managed with:
a. Codeine 60 mg
b. Ibuprofen 400 mg
c. Acetaminophen 650 mg
d. Aspirin 650 mg

29. Which of the following drugs should you avoid recommending to a person taking lithium?
a. Aspirin
b. Ibuprofen
c. Acetaminophen
d. Oxycodone

30. Patients taking ibuprofen should be counseled about all of the following EXCEPT one. Which one is the EXCEPTION?:
    a. Gastrointestinal upset
    b. Heartburn
    c. Sedation
    d. Increased risk for bleeding

31. Both opioid and nonopioid analgesics relieve pain by raising the pain threshold. Raising the pain threshold increases one's reaction to pain.
    a. Both statements are TRUE
    b. The first statement is TRUE; the second statement is FALSE
    c. The first statement is FALSE; the second statement is TRUE
    d. Both statements are FALSE

32. Following the dental procedure, the patient developed itching and urticaria after taking her acetaminophen with codeine. This response MOST likely represents:
    a. A pharmacologic action of codeine
    b. A hypersensitivity reaction to codeine
    c. A placebo effect from receiving codeine
    d. A reaction unrelated to codeine administration

33. Which of the following is the major symptom of opioid overdose?
    a. Miosis
    b. Respiratory depression
    c. Urticaria
    d. Mydriasis

34. For pain control, often an opioid analgesic is combined with a nonopioid analgesic. This combination produces an additive analgesic effect with fewer adverse reactions.
    a. Both statements are TRUE
    b. The first statement is TRUE; the second statement is FALSE
    c. The first statement is FALSE; the second statement is TRUE
    d. Both statements are FALSE

35. Which of the following is an adverse reaction to codeine?
    a. Diarrhea
    b. Miosis
    c. CNS excitation
    d. Hepatotoxicity

36. Antianxiety agents are most commonly administered as the oral dose form because the blood levels achieved from the oral administration of the antianxiety agent are very predictable.
    a. Both statements are TRUE
    b. Both statements are FALSE
    c. The first statement is TRUE; the second statement is FALSE
    d. The first statement is FALSE; the second statement is TRUE

37. Once a benzodiazepine is absorbed into the systemic circulation, all of the following contribute to the rate at which it reaches its site of action EXCEPT one. Which one is the EXCEPTION?
    a. Lipid solubility
    b. Protein binding
    c. Ionization
    d. Client's gender

38. The patient has begun to inhale nitrous oxide and oxygen (N_2O–O_2) as part of conscious sedation. The BEST way to determine her level of sedation under N_2O–O_2 is:
    a. Response to a painful stimulus
    b. Percent N_2O being delivered
    c. Response to questions
    d. Muscle tone

39. Conscious sedation with N_2O–O_2 is CONTRAINDICATED in a patient with:
    a. Diabetes
    b. Emotional instability
    c. Hypertension
    d. Glaucoma

40. N_2O–O_2) is often combined with a halogenated inhalational anesthetic because it:
    a. Increases the minimum alveolar concentration (MAC)
    b. Decreases the MAC
    c. Typically precipitates a toxic reaction
    d. Inhibits the metabolism of the halogenated anesthetic

Use Case D to answer questions 41 to 50.

SYNOPSIS
OF PATIENT
HISTORY

Age _76_
Sex _F_
Height _5'3"_

CASE _D_

Weight _140_ lbs
_63.6_ kgs

VITAL SIGNS
Blood pressure _115/75 mmHg_
Pulse rate _70 bpm_
Respiration rate _22 rpm_

1. Under Care of Physician
Yes ☒ No ☐ Condition: _arthritis, seizures, hypertension_

2. Hospitalized within the last 5 years
Yes ☐ No ☒ Reason: _____

3. Has or had the following conditions
____ – ____
____ – ____

4. Current medications
Ibuprofen 400mg tid
Hydrochlorothiazide 25mg qd
Phenytoin (Dilantin)

5. Smokes or uses tobacco products
Yes ☐ No ☐

6. Is pregnant
Yes ☐ No ☒ N/A ☐

MEDICAL HISTORY:
Patient has a history of arthritis, seizure disorders, and hypertension. She is being treated by a general physician for all three. She often complains of GI upset after taking ibuprofen. She is also one year post-joint replacement surgery on her right knee.

DENTAL HISTORY:
Visits the dental office for regular examinations and dental hygiene

SOCIAL HISTORY:
She is widowed and lives alone.
She enjoys volunteering, reading, gardening and traveling

CHIEF COMPLAINT:
I need my teeth scaled

ANTICIPATED MEDICATIONS
Requires antibiotic prophylaxis – Amoxicillin 2 gms one hour prior to procedure.

41. The distribution of a drug across biologic membranes is determined by all of the following EXCEPT one. Which one is the EXCEPTION?
a. Blood flow to the organ
b. Presence of certain barriers
c. Plasma-protein binding capacity
d. Half-life

42. A drug effect that is NEITHER predictable NOR dose related is called a:
a. Therapeutic effect
b. Toxic reaction
c. Side effect
d. Allergic reaction

43. Prophylaxis for infective endocarditis with an anti-infective agent is indicated for patients who have had:
a. Coronary artery bypass surgery
b. Joint replacement
c. Functional murmur
d. Cardiac pacemaker

44. Which drug should be used as an antibiotic pre-medication before invasive dental or dental hygiene care for a patient who has a history of congenital heart disease, artificial heart valves, and an allergy to penicillin?
a. Amoxicillin
b. Tetracycline
c. Clindamycin
d. Cephalexin

45. Which of the following drugs can result in a severe drug interaction with alcohol?
a. Erythromycin
b. Tetracycline
c. Metronidazole
d. Aminoglycosides (e.g., streptomycin)

46. Which organ is involved in the "first pass" effect after oral administration of a drug?
a. Kidney
b. Lungs
c. Liver
d. Spleen

47. **All of the following are true with regard to cytochromes P450 EXCEPT one. Which one is the EXCEPTION?**
    a. Cytochromes P450 are located in the endoplasmic reticulum
    b. Cytochromes P450 exist as numerous isozymes
    c. Cytochromes P450 are involved in the first-pass effect
    d. Cytochromes P450 inactivate drugs through conjugation reactions

48. **The effects of which of the following antihypertensive medications are antagonized by nonsteroidal anti-inflammatory drugs (NSAIDs) such as ibuprofen?**
    a. ACE inhibitors
    b. alpha blockers
    c. Calcium channel blockers
    d. angiotensin receptor blocker

49. **Which anticonvulsant medication has been documented to cause osteomalacia?**
    a. Carbamazepine
    b. Phenytoin
    c. Ethosuximide
    d. Gabapentin

50. **Alopecia may be an adverse effect of phenytoin. Carbamazepine can cause hirsutism.**
    a. Both statements are TRUE
    b. Both statements are FALSE
    c. The first statement is TRUE; the second statement is FALSE
    d. The first statement is FALSE; the second statement is TRUE

CHAPTER 12 Biochemistry, Nutrition, and Nutritional Counseling

Lisa F. Harper Mallonee

Humans, as multicellular organisms, require specific chemicals or nutrients from food to grow, maintain homeostasis, and achieve optimal health. An understanding of cellular biochemistry and nutrition is essential for preventing and treating disease and for promoting health. Nutrition science includes the intake of food and the processes involved in digestion, absorption, transportation, metabolism of nutrients, and excretion. As an applied science, it involves counseling people to adapt food patterns to nutritional needs within the cultural, economic, and psychosocial environment. Nutritional assessment counseling, when performed effectively, motivates individuals to modify eating behaviors so that optimal health can be achieved.

This chapter reviews the six major nutrient groups and their metabolic activities in mammalian cells, dietary modifications for diseases, nutritional diseases and disorders, and oral manifestations of nutritional deficiencies and toxicities. The effects of nutrients on oral tissues and the dietary assessment tools and techniques available for counseling individuals with various types of oral diseases are also described. Because nutritional problems in the developed countries are a result of overeating and undereating, a review of energy balance and weight control is included. Cellular biochemistry is fundamental to the study of nutrition; therefore, the reader is referred to the "General Histology" section in Chapter 2 for a review of structural and functional similarities in cells.

SIX MAJOR CLASSES OF ESSENTIAL NUTRIENTS

Carbohydrates

A. Definition—polyhydroxy aldehydes or ketones that serve as the body's primary sources of quick energy; carbohydrates (CHO) are composed of monosaccharides, basic units that contain carbon, hydrogen, and oxygen

B. Basic chemical structure
   1. The ratio of carbon, hydrogen, and oxygen is $1:2:1$
   2. The reactive portion of the molecule may be in a ketose form or an aldose form

Ketose	Aldose
H_2COH	$HC = O$
$\mid$	$\mid$
$C = O$	$HCOH$
$\mid$	$\mid$
R	R

   3. The position of the hydroxyl (–OH) groups determines properties such as sweetness and absorbability

C. Classification
   1. Simple carbohydrates
      a. Monosaccharides
         (1) Trioses (C3) and tetroses (C4)—usually formed during intermediary metabolism and are not important dietary components
         (2) Pentoses (C5)—important in nucleic acids and coenzymes; do not occur in free form (uncombined); not important dietary components (e.g., ribose)
         (3) Hexoses (C6)—most important group physiologically
            (a) Glucose—blood sugar; primary energy source
            (b) Galactose—seldom found free; but found in lactose

(c) Fructose—fruit sugar; sweetest tasting sugar; found in honey and fruits

b. Disaccharides—composed of two monosaccharide units
  (1) Sucrose—glucose plus fructose (e.g., cane and beet sugar)
  (2) Lactose—glucose plus galactose (e.g., milk sugar)
  (3) Maltose—glucose plus glucose (intermediate of starch hydrolysis [digestion])

c. Oligosaccharides—composed of two to six monosaccharide units

2. Complex carbohydrates
  a. Homopolysaccharides—made up of more than six identical monosaccharide units
    (1) Starch—plant storage form of glucose; source of half of dietary carbohydrates
      (a) Amylose—straight chain
      (b) Amylopectin—branched chain
    (2) Glycogen—animal storage form of glucose; found in the liver and muscle of living animals; insignificant source of dietary carbohydrates
    (3) Cellulose—chief constituent of the framework of plants; glucose units are in β-linkages, not capable of being hydrolyzed by human digestive enzymes; provides bulk and fiber in the diet
  b. Heteropolysaccharides—carbohydrates associated with noncarbohydrates or carbohydrate derivatives
    (1) Pectin, lignin—important contributors to fiber in the diet

(2) Glycoproteins—carbohydrate and protein in a specific, functional arrangement (e.g., blood group substances and many hormones)
(3) Glycolipids—carbohydrate and lipid, as in gangliosides
(4) Mucopolysaccharides—protein and carbohydrate in a loose binding
  (a) Hyaluronic acid—vitreous humor and joint lubricant
  (b) Heparin—anticoagulant
  (c) Chondroitin sulfate—cartilage, skin, bone, and teeth
  (d) Keratin sulfate—nails and teeth

D. Digestion, absorption, and transport
  1. Digestion (Table 12-1)
    a. Mouth
      (1) Teeth and tongue—mechanical breakdown and mixing of food
      (2) Saliva—hydration and lubrication of food
      (3) Salivary amylase (ptyalin)—initial enzymatic hydrolysis of starch
    b. Stomach—no digestive enzymes for carbohydrates; initial enzymatic hydrolysis of starch by salivary amylase may continue
    c. Small intestine
      (1) Pancreatic juices—pancreatic amylases
      (2) Intestinal villi (brush border) enzymes—disaccharidases
        (a) Sucrase—converts sucrose to glucose and fructose
        (b) Lactase—converts lactose to glucose and galactose

TABLE 12-1 Digestive Action at Various Points Along the Gastrointestinal Tract

	Carbohydrates	Proteins	Fats
Mouth	Salivary amylase: starch → maltose	No action	No action
Stomach	Salivary amylase:* starch → maltose	Pepsin: proteins → smaller peptides Hydrochloric acid (HCl): activates pepsin and denatures proteins	Gastric lipase:[†] short- and medium-chain triglycerides→ fatty acids + monoglycerides
Small intestine Pancreatic enzymes	Pancreatic amylase: starch → maltose	Trypsin, chymotrypsin, carboxypeptidase: proteins, polypeptides → dipeptides, amino acids	Pancreatic lipase: triglycerides → fatty acids + monoglycerides
Bile salts	No action	No action	Bile salts: emulsification of fats
Brush border enzymes	Disaccharidases: disaccharides → monosaccharides	Aminopeptidases, dipeptidases: dipeptides → amino acids	Lecithinase: lecithin → monoglyceride + fatty acid + PO_4 + choline
Large intestine	Some fermentation of undigested nutrients but with negligible absorption of the fermentation products		

*A small amount of action within the bolus of swallowed food.
[†]A minor role in total fat digestion.

(c) Maltase—converts maltose to glucose

d. Large intestine—bacterial "fermentation" of some undigested carbohydrates
   (1) No significant contribution to absorbable carbohydrates
   (2) May be the cause of gas production and bloating during primary or secondary disaccharidase deficiency (e.g., "lactose intolerance")

2. Absorption (Figure 12-1)
   a. Factors affecting absorption
      (1) Intestinal motility
      (2) Type of food mixture

   (3) Integrity of intestinal mucosa
   (4) Endocrine activity

b. Mechanism
   (1) Passive diffusion along the osmotic gradient—when the intestinal concentration of carbohydrates is greater than the level of carbohydrate in the blood
   (2) Facilitated diffusion—only certain molecules allowed to pass across a membrane using an ion channel or a carrier protein
   (3) Active transport—requires energy and allows molecules to pass against a concentration gradient with the aid of an ion

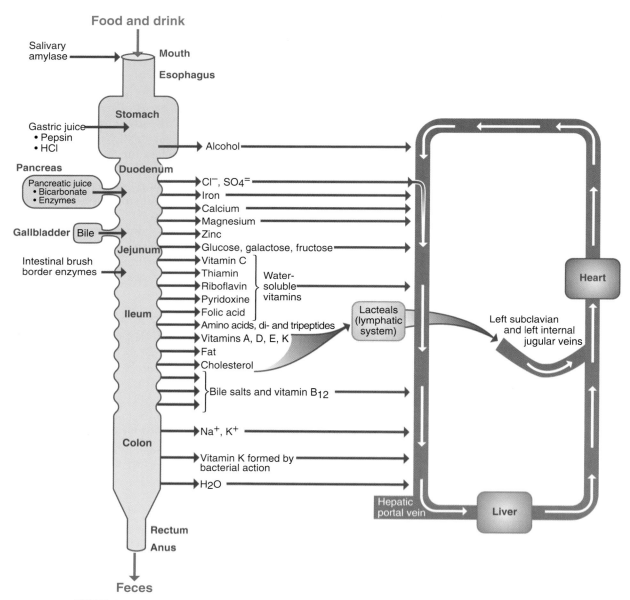

FIGURE 12-1 Absorption of major nutrients, vitamins, and minerals. *(From Mahan LK, Escott-Stump S: Krause's food and nutrition therapy, ed 12, St Louis, 2008, Saunders.)*

channel or a carrier protein at the brush border
c. Route
  (1) Carbohydrates are water soluble and are absorbed directly into the capillaries of the intestinal mucosa
  (2) Carried by the portal circulation to the liver
E. Metabolism—glucose is the main immediate source of energy for the body; a glucose level of 70 to 120 mg/100 mL blood is maintained by most healthy persons (Figure 12-2)
  1. Sources of blood glucose
    a. Dietary carbohydrates—sugars, starches
    b. Stored liver glycogen breakdown—glycogenolysis
    c. Synthesis from intermediary metabolites such as pyruvic acid—glyconeogenesis
    d. Synthesis from noncarbohydrate sources—gluconeogenesis

  (1) Deaminated (glucogenic) amino acids
  (2) Glycerol portion of lipids
2. Reactions of blood glucose—"burned" (oxidized) for energy
  a. Glycolysis—end product is pyruvate or lactic acid in the absence of oxygen (anaerobic conditions) or acetyl–coenzyme A (acetyl-CoA) in the presence of oxygen (aerobic conditions)
  b. Tricarboxylic acid cycle (TCA) or Krebs cycle—oxidation of acetyl-CoA with the release of carbon dioxide (CO_2)
  c. Oxidative phosphorylation and electron transport—production of adenosine triphosphate (ATP, a high-energy molecule) and water
3. Storage for reserve use
  a. Glycogenesis—glycogen is the short-term storage form of glucose in the liver and muscle (6 to 18 hours)

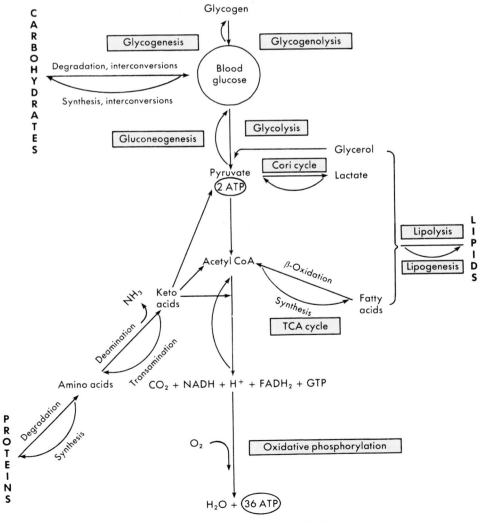

FIGURE 12-2 An overview of metabolism.

b. Lipogenesis—excess carbohydrate in the diet is converted to fat to be stored in adipose tissue as a long-term energy storage form

4. Conversion to other molecules, such as:
   a. Other carbohydrates needed for structural or functional roles
   b. Keto acids to be used in protein synthesis

F. Metabolic regulators
   1. Anabolic hormones—lower the blood glucose level (e.g., insulin)
      a. Increase the entry of glucose into cells
      b. Increase glycogenesis
      c. Increase lipogenesis
   2. Catabolic hormones—raise the blood glucose level
      a. Glucagon—stimulates glycogenolysis
      b. Steroid hormones—stimulate gluconeogenesis
      c. Epinephrine—stimulates glycogenolysis
      d. Growth hormone and adrenocorticotropic hormone (ACTH)—act as insulin antagonists
      e. Thyroxine—increases insulin breakdown, intestinal absorption of glucose, and epinephrine release
   3. Coenzymes—B-complex vitamins are important precursors of the coenzymes involved in the catabolism of carbohydrates

G. Fiber
   1. Definition—substance, usually nonstarch polysaccharide, found in plants; not broken down by human digestive enzymes; some of it is digested by bacteria in the gastrointestinal (GI) tract
      a. Insoluble fiber—substance (e.g., cellulose, hemi-cellulose, and lignin) that gives structure to plant cell walls; adds bulk and softness to stools; reduces contact with possible carcinogens by decreasing transit time through the colon; foods high in insoluble fiber include wheat bran, raw fruits, and vegetables
      b. Soluble fibers—substances (e.g., gums, mucilages, pectin, and oat bran) that dissolve to become gummy or viscous; lower blood cholesterol; regulate the use of sugars and slow down gastric emptying; foods high in soluble fiber include legumes, raw apples, and whole oats
   2. Epidemiologic studies indicate that individuals whose diets include a significant amount of fiber have a low incidence of chronic "Western" diseases, for example, coronary heart disease, diabetes, atherosclerosis
   3. Specific fibers are believed to play roles in decreasing the incidence of obesity, irregularity, hemorrhoids, appendicitis, diverticulosis, colon cancer, hyperlipidemia, and fluctuations in blood glucose (Table 12-2)

4. Excessive dietary fiber
   a. For persons with a limited intake, diets high in fiber bulk may cause nutritional deficiency
   b. Use of large doses of purified fiber may inhibit absorption of calcium, potassium, zinc, and iron
   c. Phytic acid, often found in high-fiber foods such as cereal grains, can bind and prevent absorption of minerals such as iron, calcium and zinc
5. Recommended fiber intake—for adults, 20 to 30 grams per day (g/day); an upper limit of 35 to 40 g/day is recommended for individuals with a family history of diet-implicated cancer; a limit of 50 g/day is recommended for diabetics

H. Biologic role and functions of carbohydrates
   1. Provide precursors of structural and functional molecules (e.g., gangliosides)
   2. Energy source (4 kilocalories [kcal]/g)
   3. Spare protein
   4. Provide bulk and palatability to the diet

I. Role in oral biology
   1. Pre-eruptive effect on teeth
      a. Energy source for growth and development
      b. Protein-sparing nutrient
   2. Post-eruptive effect on teeth
      a. Energy source for oral cariogenic bacteria (e.g., *Streptococcus mutans*)
      b. Acidogenic bacteria metabolize monosaccharides and disaccharides, particularly sucrose, for the production of energy through glycolysis that results in the formation of lactic acid, pyruvate, and other acetyl–CoA–dependent on the conditions
      c. *S. mutans* synthesizes polysaccharides (glucans, levans, and glycogen) from sucrose
         (1) Polysaccharides are used for energy when sucrose is unavailable
         (2) Glucans form insoluble complexes with *S. mutans* and have a strong affinity for enamel, thus enhancing bacterial plaque formation
         (3) The organic acids are liberated into the interface between the bacterial plaque and surface enamel
         (4) At pH 5.5, decalcification and demineralization begin
      d. The firm texture of some complex carbohydrates, as found in raw fruits and vegetables, can help to remove food debris retained between teeth; the chewing action can also stimulate salivary flow
   3. Dietary sweeteners (see Table 12-2)
      a. Nutritive sweeteners are used by the body as an energy source; they provide calories

TABLE 12-2 Dietary Sweeteners

Common Category	Chemical Structure and Category	Examples	Caries Promoting Potential	Relative Sweetness in Comparison to Sucrose*	Food Sources
Sugars	Monosaccharide	Glucose, dextrose	Yes	0.7	Most foods
		Fructose, high fructose corn syrup	Yes	1.4–1.8	Fruits, honey, condiments, soft drinks
		Galactose	Yes	0.6	_____
	Disaccharide	Sucrose, granulated, powdered or brown sugar, turbinado, molasses	Yes	1.0	Fruits, vegetables, table sugar
		Lactose	Yes	0.2	Milk
		Maltose	Yes	0.4	Beer
Other carbohydrates	Polysaccharide	Starch	Yes	N/A	Potatoes, grains, rice, legumes, bananas, cornstarch
	Fiber	Cellulose, pectin, gums, β-glucans, fructans	No	N/A	_____
Sugar alcohols	Polyol-monosaccharide	Sorbitol, mannitol, xylitol, erythritol	No	0.5–1.0	Grains, fruits, vegetables
	Polyol-disaccharide	Lactitol, isomalt, maltitol	No	0.3–0.9	Fruit, seaweed, exudates of plants or trees
	Polyol-polysaccharide	Hydrogenated starch, hydrolysates (HSH) or maltitol syrup	No	0.7	Derived from lactose, maltose, or starch
Non-nutritive sweeteners	Aspartame	Nutrasweet, Equal	No	188	_____
	Saccharin	Sweet' n Low	No	300	Derived from monosaccharides
	Acesulfame-K	Sunett	No	130	_____
	Sucralose	Splenda	No	600	_____

NA, *not applicable.*
*Sucrose = 1.
Adapted from Hubrich B, Nabors LO. Glycemic Response. *In Formulating Glycemic Strategies, a supplement to* Food Product Design. *July 2006, pp 3–17. July 2006, pp. 3–17.*

(1) Sugar alcohols (xylitol, sorbitol, and mannitol) are noncariogenic nutritive sweeteners that are slowly fermented through anaerobic metabolism by oral bacteria; excessive intake of these polyols can cause diarrhea because of the osmotic transfer of water into the bowel

(2) Xylitol is found naturally in plants and is equal to or sweeter than sucrose. Consumption of xylitol-containing products following consumption of food has been shown to interfere with the metabolism of *S. mutans* and decrease the demineralization of enamel

b. Nonnutritive sweeteners are calorie free and have no nutritive value; aspartame, saccharin, and acesulfame-K are nonnutritive sweeteners approved by the U.S. Food and Drug Administration (FDA); are noncariogenic

c. Aspartame should be avoided by patients who have phetylketonuria, a genetic disorder characterized by an inability to metabolize the amino acid phenylalanine

d. Food labels often list sugar content in its various forms (e.g., invert sugars, dextrose, fructose, corn sweeteners) to give an appearance of lower sugar content

4. Cariogenicity factors of diet habits (from most to least important)
   a. Intake frequency of simple sugars—the more frequent the exposure to sugar, the more cariogenic is the diet; six candy bars eaten at six different times during the day are more harmful in terms of acid and bacterial plaque formation than six candy bars consumed at the same time
   b. Form of simple sugars (liquid or retentive)—liquid sweets clear the oral cavity faster than solid or retentive sweets do and therefore are less cariogenic
   c. Time of ingestion of simple sugars—combining sweets with liquids and other noncariogenic foods during a meal is less cariogenic than a concentrated exposure to sweets between meals as a snack
   d. Total intake of simple sugars—average daily intake of sugar is 22 teaspoons; the majority of our simple sugar intake comes from soft drinks, fruit drinks, desserts, candies, and ready-to-eat cereals. The American Heart Association (AHA) recommends 6 teaspoons per day for women and 9 teaspoons for men[1]
   e. Starch-rich foods that are retained on the teeth for prolonged periods are ultimately degraded to organic acids and can contribute to the production of dental caries
   f. Combining cariogenic foods with noncariogenic foods—recent studies indicate that certain cariogenic foods (e.g., canned pears in syrup) are less cariogenic when combined with a particular noncariogenic food (e.g., cheese)

5. Importance of carbohydrates in periodontal health
   a. Energy source for the growth and repair of periodontal tissues
   b. Protein-sparing nutrient
   c. Firm texture of complex carbohydrates can promote circulation in gingival tissue
   d. Dietary monosaccharides and disaccharides enhance supragingival bacterial growth and plaque formation; these bacteria set the stage for the growth and development of subgingival bacteria and plaque, which are responsible for the destructive effects of periodontitis

J. Requirements
   1. 130 g/day of digestible carbohydrate is the recommended daily allowance (RDA) for adults and children. Minimum adult intake (50 to 100 g of digestible carbohydrate) prevents use of body protein as an energy source; pregnant and lactating women need additional carbohydrates to prevent ketosis
   2. Recommendations
      a. The Food and Nutrition Board recommends that 45% to 65% of calories should come from carbohydrates[2]
      b. Calories from simple carbohydrates (monosaccharides and disaccharides)—10% or less of the total caloric intake
      c. The majority of calories should come from complex carbohydrates (including fiber)

K. Dietary modifications for persons with disease conditions
   1. Obesity—reduce total calories and percentage of simple carbohydrates (concentrated sweets) to increase the nutrient density of a lower-calorie diet
   2. Genetic defects
      a. Lactose intolerance (inability to hydrolyze lactose)—eat fewer milk products, use fermented products, or add a commercial lactose enzyme (lactase) to milk
         (1) Yogurt with active-bacteria culture is recommended because the lactose is digested by the yogurt
         (2) The main concern for oral and systemic health is an inadequate intake of calcium and vitamin D; a hydrogen breath test can be used for diagnosis
         (3) Types of lactose intolerance
             (a) Primary—congenital absence of lactase (a brush-border enzyme)
             (b) Secondary—temporary or permanent loss of lactase activity resulting from intestinal injury, disease such as Crohn's disease, or infections which cause injury to the GI mucosa
      b. Galactosemia—congenital inability to metabolize galactose; lactose and milk products should be removed from the diet
      c. Fructose intolerance—congenital inability to metabolize fructose; fructose and sucrose should be removed from the diet; individuals with fructose intolerance have significantly fewer dental caries
   3. Dental caries and periodontal disease—a protective diet should be implemented
      a. A diet that is low in retentive carbohydrates
      b. Avoidance of cariogenic snacks
      c. A diet that is adequate in all nutrients (Table 12-3)
      d. Inclusion of foods of firm or hard texture

TABLE 12-3 Dietary Reference Intake, Adequate Intake, and Tolerable Upper Limits of Nutrients Specific to Bone Health

Nutrient	Dietary Reference Intake (DRI)/ Recommended Dietary Allowance (RDA)*	Therapeutic Range[†] (Adequate Intake)	Tolerable Upper Limit
Calcium (mg/d)	—	[‡]210–1300	2.5 for children and adults
Phosphorus (g/d)	460–1250 for most healthy children and adults	[‡]100–275 for infants	[§]3–4 for healthy individuals
Magnesium (mg/d)	80–420 for most healthy children and adults	[‡]30–75 for infants	[§]65–350 for healthy individuals
Vitamin D (μg/d)	—	[‡]5–15	[§]25–50 for healthy individuals
Fluoride (mg/d)	—	[‡*]0.01–4	[§]0.7–10 for healthy individuals

*Adequate intake (AI), also known as a therapeutic range, is the mean intake for healthy individuals that is used when an RDA value cannot be determined.
[†]Recommended dietary allowance values meet the needs of 97% of individuals in a group. Daily reference intake values are groups of values that provide quantitative estimates of nutrient intake for planning and assessing diets for all healthy individuals.
[‡]The lower number represents the adequate intake for infants and children, and the higher range of numbers will vary depending on life stage and gender group. Refer to the National Academy Press Web site (http://nap.edu/) for more in-depth information. The therapeutic range, also referred to as adequate intake, is the dose at which physiologic benefits for healthy individuals and decreased risk for toxicity may exist.
[§]The lower number represents the upper limits for infants and children, and the higher number represents upper limits for males and females (pregnant and lactating). The tolerable upper limit is the highest level of daily nutrient intake that is likely to pose no risk of adverse health effects.

4. Diabetes (inability to regulate glucose because of insufficiency or relative ineffectiveness of insulin)—dietary treatment (see the section on "Diabetes Mellitus" in Chapter 19)
   a. Two major forms
      (1) Type 1 diabetes—persons with type 1 diabetes require:
         (a) Daily injections of insulin
         (b) Routine blood testing to monitor blood sugar levels
         (c) Routine urine testing to monitor ketone levels
      (2) Type 2 diabetes—persons with type 2 diabetes require:
         (a) Medication to facilitate glucose metabolism
         (b) Specialized diet to help control the disease
         (c) Routine blood testing to monitor blood sugar levels
   b. Signs and symptoms of diabetes mellitus
      (1) Frequent urination (polyuria)
      (2) Excessive thirst (polydipsia)
      (3) Recurring gingival infections
      (4) Extreme hunger (polyphagia)
   c. Dietary recommendations
      (1) Type 1 diabetes
         (a) Is managed primarily with insulin therapy
         (b) A regular pattern of three meals per day, with one or more snacks between meals
         (c) A diet that is rich in complex carbohydrates and dietary fiber
         (d) A diet high in carbohydrates replaced with unsaturated fat and dietary fiber, if elevated triglycerides are present
      (2) Type 2 diabetes
         (a) Regular meal patterns
         (b) Regular physical activity
         (c) Monitoring carbohydrate intake and increasing the consumption of unsaturated fat and dietary fiber, if elevated triglycerides are present
5. Reactive hypoglycemia—rare; symptoms of dizziness, hunger, and heart palpitations are lessened with a low-carbohydrate diet
6. Dumping syndrome—occurs after gastric surgery; postprandial symptoms of nausea, dizziness, cramping, and diarrhea are lessened by a low-monosaccharide, low-disaccharide diet
7. Alcoholism—overconsumption of alcohol may cause malnutrition (see the section on "Chronic Alcohol Abuse and Dependence" in Chapter 19)
   a. Depresses the appetite
   b. Empty-calorie food—provides energy but few other nutrients (e.g., concentrated sweets, alcohol, and fats)
   c. Causes vitamin B depletion because the liver needs niacin and thiamine to metabolize alcohol
   d. Causes folate and iron deficiency
   e. Depresses antidiuretic hormone, causing loss of magnesium, potassium, and zinc in urine
8. Alcohol consumption during pregnancy—has a direct teratogenic effect on the developing fetus: fetal alcohol syndrome (see the section on "Fetal Alcohol Spectrum Disorders" in Chapter 19)

9. Carbohydrate regulation in some hyperlipoproteinemias—total carbohydrate and alcohol intake is controlled; concentrated sweets are restricted

Proteins

A. Definition—complex biologic compounds of high molecular weight that contain nitrogen, hydrogen, oxygen, carbon, and small amounts of sulfur; each protein has a specific size and is made up of amino acid building blocks linked through peptide bonds in a specific arrangement

B. Classifications
  1. Chemical
    a. Simple proteins—contain amino acids only
    b. Compound (conjugated) proteins—contain simple proteins and a nonprotein group
      (1) Nucleoproteins
      (2) Metalloproteins
      (3) Phosphoproteins
      (4) Lipoproteins
    c. Derived proteins—fragments produced during digestion or hydrolysis (e.g., peptides, peptones, and proteases)
  2. Biologic
    a. Complete proteins contain sufficient amounts of the essential amino acids for normal metabolic reactions; found in foods of animal origin
      (1) A total of 20 essential amino acids that cannot be synthesized by humans and must be provided in the diet in sufficient amounts to meet the body's needs
        (a) Adult—histidine, isoleucine, leucine, lysine, methionine, phenylalanine, threonine, tryptophan, and valine
        (b) Infant—all of the above plus histidine and probably taurine
        (c) Premature infant—all of the above plus cysteine
      (2) Nonessential amino acids can be synthesized by the body and need not be provided by the diet but are necessary for normal metabolic reactions; include alanine, arginine, aparagine, aspartic acid, cysteine, glutamic acid, glutamine, glycine, proline, serine, and tyrosine
    b. Incomplete proteins have insufficient quantities of one or more essential amino acids to support protein synthesis in humans; plant proteins are often incomplete (e.g., corn protein is low in lysine; legume protein is low in methionine)
    c. Complementary proteins are proteins that are incomplete when ingested singly but, when combined, provide sufficient essential amino acids
      (1) In a "vegan" (or strict vegetarian) diet, the complementing of plant proteins can be accomplished by combining appropriate incomplete proteins; the amino acids in different foods can complement one another, even when eaten at different meals; persons on a strict vegetarian diet are at the greatest risk for developing deficiencies in calcium, iron, zinc, and vitamin B_{12} because the major food sources of these nutrients come from animal products
      (2) In an "ovo-lacto" vegetarian diet, milk and egg proteins can provide the essential amino acids that are inadequate in incomplete plant proteins; however, this diet still may be deficient in iron
    d. Protein quality is a measure of a protein's ability to support protein synthesis; it is measured by comparing the test protein with a reference protein, usually egg protein
      (1) Amino acid or protein chemical score (CS)—compares the essential amino acid content in a dietary protein to that of a reference protein
      (2) Protein efficiency ratio (PER)—measures a protein's ability to support growth
      (3) Biologic value (BV)—expression of the percentage of nitrogen retained for maintenance and growth compared with the amount absorbed
      (4) Net protein utilization (NPU)—expression of the percentage of retained nitrogen compared with the amount ingested; differs from BV because it takes into account the protein's digestibility
      (5) Protein-digestibility-corrected amino acid score (PDCAAS)—compares the amino acid balance of a food protein with the amino acid requirements of preschool-aged children and then corrects for digestibility; used by the FDA for labeling

C. Structure
  1. Primary—linear sequence of the component amino acids
  2. Secondary—steric interaction of amino acids that are close to one another in the linear sequence (e.g., the α-helix and β-sheet)
  3. Tertiary—steric interaction between amino acids that are far apart in the linear sequence, which causes folding and the ultimate functional structure of the protein (e.g., disulfide bonds)

4. Quaternary—steric interaction between subunits of proteins with more than one polypeptide chain (e.g., hemoglobin)

D. Digestion, absorption, and transport (see Table 12-1 and Figure 12-1)

1. Mouth—mechanical breakdown and moistening

2. Stomach

   a. Hydrochloric acid from parietal cells denatures or unfolds proteins and activates pepsinogen to give pepsin

   b. Pepsin begins the hydrolysis of the peptide bonds of proteins to form peptides and proteoses

3. Small intestine

   a. The pancreas secretes bicarbonate into the duodenum to neutralize the acidic products from the stomach and proteolytic enzymes into an inactive form; enzymes activated by trypsin through a hormonal feedback mechanism are chymotrypsin, aminopeptidase, and carboxypeptidase; each hydrolyzes peptide bonds formed by different classes of amino acids

   b. Enzymes of the brush border are dipeptidases that hydrolyze dipeptides to amino acids

4. Absorption—at the brush border of the microvilli of the small intestine, absorption occurs both by simple diffusion along a concentration gradient and by active transport at specific amino acid sites involving carrier enzymes, a sodium–ATP pump, and vitamin B_6

5. Transport—absorbed amino acids collected by the portal blood system and transported to the liver

E. Metabolism (see Figure 12-2)

1. Amino acid pool—a collection of amino acids in a dynamic equilibrium in the liver, blood, and other cells that provides the raw material for the body's protein and amino acid needs

   a. Input into the pool comes from proteins in the diet, breakdown of body proteins, and synthesis of nonessential amino acids

   b. Output from the pool is for synthesizing body structures, specialized substances (e.g., melanin from tyrosine), and energy, as needed

2. Anabolism

   a. De novo synthesis—requires deoxyribonucleic acid (DNA), messenger ribonucleic acid (mRNA), and ribosomal ribonucleic acid (rRNA)

     (1) In the nucleus, DNA carries the genetic information in groups of three bases that provide the code for the individual amino acids comprising a specific protein

     (2) mRNA transports a copy of the code from DNA into the cytoplasm

     (3) mRNA attaches to a ribosome and acts as a template for the alignment of amino acids that are attached to transfer RNA (tRNA)

     (4) If the proper amino acids are in the correct proportions and the synthetic enzymes and energy are available, the polypeptide chain is synthesized

   b. Transamination

     (1) Nonessential amino acids can be synthesized from the corresponding α-keto acids, an α-amino acid (as the NH_3^+ donor), a specific transaminase enzyme, and the coenzyme pyridoxal phosphate (vitamin B_6)

     (2) The intermediate complex formed in this reaction is called a *Schiff base*

3. Catabolism—amino acids in excess of those needed for the synthesis of proteins and other biomolecules cannot be stored or excreted; they may, however, be deaminated and the α-keto acid used as a metabolic fuel for immediate energy needs or for long-term energy storage as fat

   a. Amino group

     (1) Deamination—loss of the α-amino group, usually in the liver, through transfer to α-ketoglutarate to form glutamate; glutamate is then oxidatively deaminated to yield ammonia (NH_3)

     (2) Urea cycle—series of steps whereby the ammonia produced during deamination is converted to urea for excretion

   b. α-Keto acid

     (1) Ketogenic amino acids are those whose carbon skeleton, after deamination, yields acetyl-CoA or acetoacetyl-CoA, which then yields ketone bodies; high concentrations of ketone bodies lead to some of the undesirable side effects of high-protein, low-carbohydrate diets, for example, ketoacidosis

     (2) Glucogenic amino acids are those that yield pyruvate, α-ketoglutarate, and other intermediates of the citric acid cycle that can, if needed, be converted to glucose

4. Nitrogen balance—comparison measurement of the amount of nitrogen ingested with the amount excreted (e.g., urinary nitrogen plus approximately 1 g/day for nail, hair, skin, and perspiration losses) made to determine whether net protein catabolism, anabolism, or equilibrium exists

a. Positive balance—intake is greater than output; indicates net protein synthesis and is the normal situation for anyone building protein-containing tissue, such as during childhood, pregnancy, and recovery from undernutrition, surgery, or illness

b. Negative balance—intake is less than output; indicates net protein breakdown, when the body must break down its own protein to meet energy or metabolic needs; can result from insufficient protein (or essential amino acids) or energy intake or from fever, infection, anxiety, or prolonged stress

F. Metabolic regulation

  1. Hormones

    a. Anabolic—growth hormone, insulin, normal thyroid hormone, and sex hormones

    b. Catabolic—adrenocortical hormones and large amounts of thyroid hormone

  2. Vitamins—pyridoxine and riboflavin are necessary for protein synthesis; when they are deficient in the diet, synthesis may be limited

G. Functions

  1. Structural—formation of:

    a. Collagen and elastin

    b. Bone and tooth matrix

    c. Myosin fibrils

    d. Keratin

  2. Dynamic

    a. Transport of nutrients by:

      (1) Lipid-soluble and fat-soluble vitamins

      (2) Iron—transferrin

      (3) Hemoglobin and myoglobin—oxygen

      (4) Protein-bound molecules

      (5) Membrane transport

    b. Regulation and control by:

      (1) Immunoglobulins

      (2) Buffers

      (3) Hormones

      (4) Enzymes

      (5) Blood coagulation—fibrin

      (6) Muscle contraction—actin and myosin

  3. Energy source (4 kilocalories [kcal]/g)

  4. Role of proteins in oral biology

    a. Pre-eruptive effects on teeth—essential for all cells and therefore necessary for normal tooth bud and pulp formation and synthesis of protein matrix for enamel and dentin

    b. Post-eruptive effects on teeth

      (1) Essential for maintaining the integrity of pulpal tissue throughout life

      (2) Chemical nature of protein foods can neutralize acids produced by oral bacteria

    c. Periodontal health and disease

      (1) Essential for all cells in the growth, development, and maintenance of the periodontium

      (2) Essential for the normal function of cellular defenses against subgingival bacteria and toxins

      (3) Necessary in the healing and repair of injured tissues from periodontitis or periodontal surgery

H. Requirements

  1. Determination and estimates of protein requirements

    a. Studies of nitrogen balance are used to determine the lowest protein intake that will support homeostasis or equilibrium

    b. Average requirement for reference proteins of 0.8 g/kg/day for young adult males; other groups by extrapolation or interpolation

    c. Estimates for growth needs in infants are based on the amount of protein provided by that quantity of human milk that ensures a satisfactory growth rate

  2. Recommended dietary allowances—developed by the National Research Council; based on 1985 World Health Organization recommendations, which use nitrogen balance data; these allowances assume ingestion of good-quality protein in a mixed diet; adjustments are made for growth, pregnancy, and lactation

  3. Food sources—protein needs of an average adult can be met by choosing two or more servings per day of meats, poultry, fish, eggs, dried beans, and nuts

I. Dietary modifications for disease

  1. Genetic disorders

    a. Phenylketonuria (PKU)—inherited enzyme defect in which individuals cannot metabolize the phenylalanine found in nearly all proteins; the prescribed diet provides only enough phenylalanine to meet growth and maintenance needs; dietary protein is restricted, but amino acids are provided by a synthetic formula from which the phenylalanine has been removed

    b. Other genetic disorders—maple syrup urine disease, homocystinuria, tyrosinemia, methylmalonic aciduria, propionic acidemia, and isovaleric acidemia are genetic disorders in which amino acid metabolism is altered; treated with low-protein diets and synthetic amino acid formulas

    c. Gout—characterized by excessive uric acid production leading to the formation of urate crystals deposited in the joints; treatment often includes restriction of protein to limit purine and uric acid production

2. Protein needs are increased during fever, after severe injury and surgery, and by intestinal malabsorption, increased protein loss from the kidneys, or diminished protein synthesis by the liver
3. Dietary protein must be restricted when the kidneys can no longer remove nitrogenous wastes from the body or in severe liver disease when the nitrogenous byproducts of protein catabolism can no longer be synthesized
4. Protein-energy (calorie) malnutrition (PEM or PCM)
   a. Kwashiorkor (classic)—failure of the young child to grow because of insufficient protein intake (usually following weaning from mother's milk); edema often masks muscle wasting
   b. Marasmus (classic)—failure of the infant or young child to grow because of partial starvation; total caloric and protein intakes are insufficient
   c. Adult PEM or PCM—seen even in the developed countries among alcoholics and long-term hospitalized patients with acquired immune deficiency syndrome (AIDS), tuberculosis, and anorexia nervosa

Lipids (Fats)

A. Definition—biochemical compounds composed of carbon, hydrogen, oxygen, and small amounts of phosphorus; insoluble in water and soluble in fatty substances and organic solvents
B. Classification
   1. Simple lipids
      a. True fats—contain fatty acids attached to glycerol (a trihydroxy alcohol) through an ester linkage; these may be monoglycerides, diglycerides, or triglycerides, depending on the number of glycerol–hydroxyl groups esterified; chemical and biochemical characteristics of glycerides depend on the number, order, and kinds of fatty acids attached
         (1) Saturated fatty acids—contain no double bonds and are found in lipids from animal sources; are solids at room temperature (high melting point)
         (2) Unsaturated fatty acids—contain one or more double bonds and come from plant sources; are usually liquids at room temperature (low melting point)
         (3) Hydrogenation—addition of hydrogen to some or all of the double bonds; used in the manufacture of margarine or butter

substitutes from vegetable oils; in partial hydrogenation, some *trans* bonds are formed and may present a health risk
         (4) Rancidity—addition of oxygen to some of the double bonds of fatty acids that contributes to spoilage; occurs spontaneously in foods and can be reduced by the addition of antioxidants, such as butylated hydroxytoluene (BHT)
         (5) Iodine number—chemical indication of the degree of unsaturation of a fatty acid; the more molecules of iodine bound by the fatty acid, the more unsaturated and the higher is the iodine number
      b. Waxes—esters of a fatty acid and an alcohol other than glycerol; the body is unable to use waxes because digestive enzymes do not hydrolyze their ester linkage
   2. Compound lipids contain compounds added to the glycerol and fatty acids
      a. Phospholipids (glycerol + 2 fatty acids + phosphate group = R group)
         (1) Water-soluble emulsifiers (e.g., lecithin, with choline as the R group)
         (2) Membrane constituents (e.g., sphingomyelin)
         (3) Active intermediates in metabolism of lipid compound (e.g., CoA)
      b. Glycolipids—contain a carbohydrate component and are found in the brain and nervous tissue (e.g., cerebrosides)
      c. Lipoproteins—are water soluble and responsible for carrying lipids throughout the body
         (1) Chylomicrons—approximately 2% protein; carry exogenous (absorbed from the diet) triglycerides around the body
         (2) Very-low-density lipoproteins (VLDLs)—9% protein; carry endogenous triglycerides around the body
         (3) Low-density lipoproteins (LDLs)—21% protein; carry mostly cholesterol from the liver to peripheral sites
         (4) High-density lipoproteins (HDLs)—50% protein; carry cholesterol back to the liver; can be elevated by exercise
   3. Derived lipids are compounds whose synthesis begins like fatty acid synthesis, with acetyl groups added on one at a time
      a. Sterols—all have a polycyclic nucleus
      b. Cholesterol is a precursor for the synthesis of many steroid compounds and a constituent of cell membranes
         (1) Sources
            (a) Exogenous—average dietary intake is 400 to 600 milligrams (mg) from foods of animal origin

(b) Endogenous—average synthesis in the body is 1 to 2 g/day

(2) Regulation of cholesterol—dietary cholesterol, percentage of fat, ratio of polysaturated to monosaturated to unsaturated fat, and amount of certain fibers in the diet

c. Steroids—similar to sterols but with side-chain modification (e.g., bile acids, sex hormones, adrenocortical hormones, and vitamin D)

4. Artificial fats—substances developed for use in foods; have the flavor, appearance, and feel of dietary fats without their physiologic effects

a. Olestra—a zero-kilocalorie (0-kcal) artificial fat made from an indigestible combination of sucrose and fatty acids; may help serum cholesterol levels by directly interfering with cholesterol absorption; may increase the requirement for vitamin E; approved for use in snack foods

b. Simplesse—has approximately 15% of the kilocalorie of the fat it replaces; made by microparticulation of protein; the small protein particles have the feel of fat; not suitable for use in cooking but used in fat-free dairy products and salad dressings

c. Oatrim and maltodextrim—carbohydrate-based fat replacements; mimic the texture and feel of fat by forming gels; are digestible and contribute some calories

C. Digestion, absorption, and transportation (see Table 12-1 and Figure 12-1)

1. Digestion

a. Mouth—no enzymatic action; mechanical and moistening action only

b. Stomach—gastric lipase hydrolyzes some short-chain and medium-chain fatty acids from triglycerides

c. Small intestine

(1) Gallbladder—bile salts emulsify fats before digestion

(2) Pancreas—pancreatic lipase hydrolyzes fatty acids from triglycerides to form diglycerides and monoglycerides

(3) Intestinal mucosa—lecithinase converts lecithin to fatty acids, monoglyceride, phosphate, and choline

2. Absorption and transport

a. Short-chain fatty acids can be absorbed into the portal system

b. Medium-chain and long-chain fatty acids are water insoluble, require bile as a carrier (emulsifier), and are absorbed in stages

(1) Bile separated out at the intestinal wall and recirculated

(2) Complete breakdown of triglycerides within the mucosal cells by mucosal lipase

(3) Resynthesis of new triglycerides that combine with protein carriers to form chylomicrons

(4) Passage into the lymph system (lacteals) and blood through the thoracic duct

(5) At its destination, lipoprotein lipase hydrolyzes the triglycerides, clearing chylomicrons from blood

(6) Lipoprotein carriers (VLDLs, LDLs, and HDLs) carry endogenous lipids and cholesterol

D. Metabolism (see Figure 12-2)

1. Anabolism

a. Lipogenesis—synthesis of triglycerides for long-term storage of energy; starting material is acetyl-CoA, which can come from glucogenic amino acids, carbohydrates, or breakdown of dietary lipids; lipogenesis takes place in nearly all cells but is most active in adipose cells

b. Synthesis of steroids occurs in all cells

c. Synthesis of lipoproteins occurs mainly in the liver

2. Catabolism

a. β-Oxidation—fatty acids are broken down in a stepwise manner to yield one molecule of acetyl-CoA for every two carbon atoms; acetyl-CoA can be catabolized further by means of the TCA and oxidative phosphorylation

b. Ketone production—when the body's supply of carbohydrates is low, the TCA is depressed and acetyl-CoA from β-oxidation accumulates; alternative route for acetyl-CoA is ketone production; acetoacetone, acetone, and β-hydroxybutyrate are the ketone bodies; excess ketone production can cause ketosis, ketonuria, and ketoacidosis (which is sometimes fatal)

E. Metabolic regulators

1. Vitamins as coenzyme precursors

a. Anabolism—biotin, riboflavin (in flavin adenine dinucleotide [FAD]), niacin (in nicotinamide–adenine dinucleotide [NAD]), and pantothenic acid (in CoA) (see Figure 12-2)

b. Catabolism—riboflavin, niacin, and pantothenic acid

2. Hormones

a. Anabolism—insulin

b. Catabolism—ACTH, thyroid-stimulating hormone (TSH), epinephrine, and glucagon

3. Enzymes necessary for the metabolism of lipids are synthesized or inhibited in response to the relative amounts of substrates and products available

F. Biologic role and functions of lipids
  1. Structural components of cell membrane
  2. Energy source
    a. Provide 9 kcal/g (compared with 4 kcal/g for protein or carbohydrates)
    b. Long-term storage of energy
  3. Carrier medium of fat-soluble vitamins
  4. Protective padding for body organs
  5. Insulation for the maintenance of body temperature
  6. Role of lipids in oral biology
    a. Cariostatic properties
      (1) Lipids provide a coating on the tooth's surface and form a protective pellicle on the tooth.
      (2) Lipids act by neutralizing the acids produced by bacterial metabolism of the plaque biofilm; they raise the pH and decrease risk of the demineralization of enamel.
    b. No relationship between dietary fat and periodontal disease

G. Nutritional requirements
  1. Essential fatty acids (EFAs)—cannot be synthesized in sufficient amounts to meet the body's needs; must be supplied in the diet; for humans the only EFAs are linoleic (ω-6) and linolenic (ω-3); requirement is approximately 3% of total kilocalories
    a. Function—necessary for the synthesis of membranes and prostaglandins (local hormone)
    b. Deficiency symptoms—seen in infants on low polyunsaturated fatty acid (PUFA) diets and in adults receiving total parenteral nutrition feedings without lipids; the deficiency is characterized by slow growth, reproductive failure, and skin lesions
  2. Recommendations (dietary goals as recommended by the AHA)
    a. Total fats—≤30% of total kilocalories; majority of calories should come from monounsaturated and polyunsaturated fatty acids
    b. Cholesterol—≤300 mg/day; 200 mg/day for high-risk individuals
    c. Saturated fats—avoid saturated and trans fatty acids (found in processed foods); less than 10% of total kilocuries should come from saturdated fatty acids
    d. Two weekly servings of fatty fish such as tuna or salmon
  3. The seventh edition of *Dietary Guidelines for Americans* makes similar recommendations for healthy persons ages 2 years and older

H. Dietary modifications for disease
  1. Cardiovascular disease (CVD)—blood vessel lumens become narrower and sometimes completely blocked because of the plaques caused by the accumulation of fatty substances, cellular debris, and calcium; blood pressure and the work required of the heart increase; formation of clots increase, and the result may be a heart attack (myocardial infarction) or stroke
    a. Hyperlipoproteinemias—for diagnosis, elevation of serum VLDL, LDL, and chylomicron levels indicates that a client is at risk for CVD; a genetic predisposition for certain hyperlipoproteinemias exists; elevated HDL levels may exert a protective effect against CVD; routine exercise elevates HDL levels in most people
    b. Dietary factors that may increase serum lipids—high intake of cholesterol, saturated fats, total fats, sucrose, fructose, and ethanol (alcohol)
    c. Dietary factors that may decrease serum lipids—monounsaturated and polyunsaturated fatty acids, omega fatty acids (fish oils), and pectin; ethanol in moderate amounts may have a protective effect by increasing HDL levels; unidentified substances in garlic, yeast, onions, and some wines may also have a protective effect
  2. Obesity—because fats are a concentrated source of calories (9 kcal/g), most reducing diets recommend a decrease in fat intake; fat should not be too severely restricted because it adds to the palatability and satiety of the diet
  3. Gallbladder disease and chronic pancreatitis—often cause pain after lipid ingestion; diet may have to be restricted in fats until the conditions are corrected
  4. Cystic fibrosis and malabsorption disorders—often treated with synthetic medium-chain triglyceride formulas that are more easily absorbed
  5. Dumping syndrome and gastric ulcers—often treatment involves increasing fat in the diet to delay gastric emptying
  6. Epilepsy—children with some types of epilepsy may be effectively treated with a ketogenic diet that is high in fats, is low in carbohydrates, and causes a ketotic condition

Vitamins

A. Definition—organic substances that are essential to life and are needed in very small amounts; serve in regulatory functions and often act as coenzymes or precursors of coenzymes; some vitamins can be produced in precursor form or activated in the body

B. Classification
  1. Water-soluble vitamins
    a. Vitamin C
    b. B-complex vitamins
  2. Fat-soluble vitamins
    a. Vitamin A
    b. Vitamin D
    c. Vitamin E
    d. Vitamin K
C. Chemistry and general properties
  1. Water-soluble vitamins
    a. Soluble in water
    b. Sensitive to heat, light, and oxygen
    c. Contain the elements carbon, hydrogen, oxygen, and nitrogen, and, in some cases, other elements such as cobalt or sulfur
    d. Absorbed into blood by both active and passive transport from the upper portion of the digestive tract (see Figure 12-1); vitamin B_{12} requires the intrinsic factor for absorption
    e. Transported free and unbound to cells by blood
    f. Minimal storage of excess dietary vitamins except for:
      (1) Vitamin C—stores may last 30 to 90 days
      (2) Vitamin B_{12}—stores may last many years in those without pernicious anemia
      (3) Folic acid—stores may last 4 to 5 months
    g. Are excreted in urine
    h. Should be supplied in the diet nearly every day
    i. Deficiency symptoms often develop rapidly
    j. Are relatively nontoxic with excessive dietary intake, although the increased use of over-the-counter "megavitamin" preparations has caused the appearance of toxic symptoms
  2. Fat-soluble vitamins
    a. Soluble in fat and fat solvents (some water-soluble derivatives are available)
    b. More stable than water-soluble vitamins in light, heat, and oxygen
    c. Contain only elements of carbon, hydrogen, and oxygen
    d. Must be emulsified and carried across the membranes of the intestinal cells in the presence of fat and bile (see Figure 12-1); any conditions that decrease the digestion, absorption, or transport of lipids will lower the usable amount of fat-soluble vitamins
    e. Absorbed into the lymphatic system and transported by attachment to protein carriers
    f. Not readily excreted
    g. Not absolutely necessary in the diet every day
    h. Amount ingested in excess of the daily need is stored in the liver and fatty tissues
    i. Deficiency symptoms slow to develop
    j. Toxic with chronic excessive intake
D. General functions
  1. Water-soluble vitamins
    a. Form coenzymes for energy metabolism
    b. Synthesis of red blood cells and DNA
  2. Fat-soluble vitamins—play a role in:
    a. Vision
    b. Maintenance of the body's mucosal linings and epithelial cells
    c. Integrity of mineralized tissues of bone and teeth by regulating the calcium and phosphorus levels in the body
    d. Cellular antioxidant
    e. Normal blood clotting
E. Nutritional requirements—dietary reference intake (DRIs) and RDA are based on vitamin and mineral intake from food, not supplements; for an elaboration of DRI and RDA, see the section on "Methods for Assessment of Dietary Intake" later in this chapter. Refer to "Food and Nutrition" at the National Academy Press Web site of the National Academy of Science, available at http://nap.edu/; also see Web Site Information and Resources table at the end of this chapter
F. Dietary sources, specific body functions, and symptoms of deficiencies and toxicities (Table 12-4)
G. Role of vitamins in oral biology
  1. Functions
    a. Tooth formation (Table 12-5)
    b. Periodontium (see Table 12-5)
  2. Oral manifestations of deficiencies and toxicities (see Table 12-4)

Minerals

A. Definition—inorganic elements that are essential to life; serve both structural and regulatory functions
B. Classification (see Table 12-4)
  1. Macrominerals—present in relatively high amounts in body tissues
  2. Trace elements—present at less than 0.005% of body weight
C. Chemistry and general functions
  1. Exist as inorganic ions
  2. Chemical identity not altered in the body or in food
  3. Indestructible
  4. Soluble in water and tend to form acidic or basic solutions
  5. Vary in amounts absorbed and in pathways of excretion (see Figure 12-1)
  6. Some readily absorbed into blood and transported freely

TABLE 12-4 Nutrients and Their Related Effects on the Oral Cavity

Nutrient	Dietary Sources	Major Body Functions	Oral Manifestations of Nutrient Deficiency	Oral Manifestations of Nutrient Excess
Vitamins Vitamin A	Provitamin A, orange, yellow, and green vegetables and fruit Retinol: milk, cheese, butter, fortified margarine, egg yolk	Antioxidant, Constituent of rhodopsin Maintains epithelial tissue involved in bone growth and remodeling	Ameloblast atrophy Faulty bone and tooth formation Enamel hypoplasia Xerostomia Cleft lip Increased risk of candidiasis Decreased taste sensitivity	Hypertrophy of bone Cracking and bleeding lips Cheilosis Erythemic gingivae
Vitamin D	Sunlight, oily fish, eggs, dairy, fortified milk, margarine	Promotes growth and mineralization of bones and teeth Increases absorption of calcium at intestine	Loss of alveolar and mandibular bone Delayed dentition Increased caries rate Loss of lamina dura around roots of tooth Failure of bones to heal	Pulp calcification Enamel hypoplasia
Vitamin E	Vegetable oils, seeds, green leafy vegetables, margarine and whole grain or fortified cereals, wheat germ, nuts	Antioxidant Involved in cellular respiration and synthesis of body compounds, prevents hemolysis of red blood cells (RBCs)	Loss of resistance to inflammation in peridontium	No effect noted
Vitamin K	Green and yellow vegetables, meats, microflora in the gut	Important in blood clotting Involved in the formation of active prothrombin	Gingival hemorrhage Increased risk of candidiasis	No effect noted
Vitamin C	Citrus fruits, tomatoes, green peppers, broccoli, strawberries, melons	Important in collagen synthesis Important in the body's use of iron, B_{12}, and folic acid	Odontoblast atrophy Porotic dentin formation Gingival inflammation Cyanotic gingival tissues Ulceration and necrosis Slow wound healing Defects in collagen formation	No effect noted
Thiamin	Pork, whole grains, nuts, legumes	Coenzyme in reactions involving removal of carbon dioxide in carbohydrate metabolism Synthesized by intestinal bacteria in large intestine	Increased sensitivity and burning sensation of oral mucosa Loss of taste and appetite	No effect noted
Riboflavin	Dairy products, grains	Functions as a coenzyme in the metabolism of carbohydrate, protein, and fat Synthesized by intestinal bacteria in the large intestine	Angular cheilosis Atrophy of filiform papillae Enlarged fungiform papillae Shiny, red lips Painful tongue Glossitis	No effect noted
Niacin	Liver, meat, fish, poultry, cereals, legumes, peanuts,	Coenzyme in energy (ATP) production	Loss of filiform and fungiform papillae Mucositis Stomatitis Glossitis Ulcerative gingivitis Glossodynia	No effect noted

Continued

TABLE 12-4 Nutrients and Their Related Effects on the Oral Cavity—cont'd

Nutrient	Dietary Sources	Major Body Functions	Oral Manifestations of Nutrient Deficiency	Oral Manifestations of Nutrient Excess
Pyridoxine	Meat, poultry, fish, vegetables, whole-grain cereals, egg yolk	Coenzyme involved in amino acid metabolism Converts tryptophan to niacin Role in hemoglobin synthesis	Angular cheilosis Sore, burning mouth Glossitis Glossodynia Stomatitis Deficiency usually occurs in combination with other B vitamins	No effect noted
Pantothenic acid	Organ meats, whole-grain cereals, broccoli, avocados	Constituent of coenzyme A, which plays a central role in energy metabolism	No effect noted	No effect noted
Cobalamin	Meat, poultry, eggs, fish, shellfish, dairy products	Coenzyme involved in synthesis of single carbon units in nucleic acid metabolism Important in RBC formation and myelin synthesis	Stomatitis Hemorrhagic gingiva Pale to yellow mucosa Glossopyrosis Glossitis Atrophy and burning tongue Altered taste Halitosis Oral paresthesia Detachment of periodontal fibers Bone loss Xerostomia Aphthous ulcers	No effect noted
Folate	Fortified grain products, liver, kidney, yeast, mushrooms, leafy green vegetables, legumes	Coenzyme involved in ribonucleic acid (RNA) and deoxyribonucleic acid (DNA) synthesis Important in the proper formation of neural tubes during fetal development	Glossitis Enlargement of fungiform papillae Ulcerations along edge of tongue Gingivitis Neural tube defects: cleft palate and lip	Excess can mask cobalamin deficiency Pale mucosa Angular cheilosis
Biotin	Liver, kidney, milk, egg yolk, cereals	Coenzyme required for the synthesis and oxidation of fats and carbohydrates and for the deamination of proteins	Glossitis Gray mucosa Atrophy of lingual papillae	No effect noted
Minerals Calcium	Milk, cheese, dark green vegetables, fortified breads, juices and cereals, canned salmon	Bone and tooth formation Blood clotting Nerve transmission Muscle contraction	Incomplete calcification of teeth Risk of hemorrhage Increased susceptibility to caries and periodontal disease	No effect noted
Phosphorus	Milk, cheese, meat, poultry, grains, eggs	Bone and tooth formation Acid–base balance Release of energy (adenosine triphosphate [ATP]/adenosine diphosphate [ADP])	Incomplete calcification of teeth Failure of dentin formation Increased susceptibility to caries during tooth development Increased susceptibility to periodontal disease	No effect noted

TABLE 12-4 Nutrients and Their Related Effects on the Oral Cavity—cont'd

Nutrient	Dietary Sources	Major Body Functions	Oral Manifestations of Nutrient Deficiency	Oral Manifestations of Nutrient Excess
Sulfur	Meat, fish, poultry, legumes	Important in oxidation reduction reactions Body water balance	No effect noted	No effect noted
Potassium	Meats, milk, many fruits, fish, eggs	Acid–base balance Body water balance Nerve function Affects heart muscle contraction	No effect noted	No effect noted
Chlorine	Table salt, cured and pickled foods, water	Formation of gastric juice Body water balance Acid–base balance	No effect noted	No effect noted
Sodium	Table salt; cured, processed, canned, and pickled foods; broth	Acid–base balance Body water balance Nerve function	Decrease in salivary flow	Dry, sticky tongue and oral mucous membranes
Magnesium	Whole grains, green leafy vegetables, nuts, beans, bananas	Activates enzymes involved in energy metabolism Maintains calcium homeostasis	Alveolar bone fragility Gingival hyperplasia Enamel hypoplasia Widening of periodontal ligament	No effect noted
Iron	Egg yolk, meats, liver, whole grains, dark green vegetables, dried fruits	Constituent of hemoglobin and enzymes involved in energy metabolism	Angular cheilosis Pallor of lips or oral mucosa Atrophy of filiform papillae Decreased resistance to infection Glossitis Increased risk of candidiasis	No effect noted
Fluoride	Drinking water, tea, seafood	Important in the maintenance of bone structure Forms strong apatite crystals during tooth formation	Decreased resistance to dental caries	Enamel fluorosis
Zinc	Lamb, beef, oysters, eggs, peanuts, whole grains	Required for synthesis of DNA, RNA, and protein Bone growth and metabolism	Impaired taste Loss of tongue sensation Delayed wound healing Impaired keratinization of epithelial cells Increased susceptibility to periodontal disease Flattened filiform papillae	No effect noted
Copper	Shellfish, oysters, crabs, liver, nuts, soy products, legumes	Important catalyst in hemoglobin synthesis	Decreased trabecular pattern Decreased tissue vascularity Fragility of tissue	No effect noted
Selenium	Seafood, kidney, liver, dairy products, whole grains, nuts	Antioxidant	No effect noted	Associated with increased dental caries

Continued

TABLE 12-4 Nutrients and Their Related Effects on the Oral Cavity—cont'd

Nutrient	Dietary Sources	Major Body Functions	Oral Manifestations of Nutrient Deficiency	Oral Manifestations of Nutrient Excess
Manganese	Whole grains, legumes, nuts, tea, green leafy vegetables	Normal skeletal development Involved in fat synthesis, urea formation, and energy release	No effect noted	Associated with increased dental caries
Iodine	Marine fish and shellfish, table salt, eggs	Constituent of thyroid hormones Regulates energy metabolism	No effect noted	No effect noted
Molybdenum	Legumes, whole grain cereals, organ meats	Constituent of enzymes involved in uric acid formation and oxidation of aldehydes	No effect noted	No effect noted
Chromium	Vegetables, whole grains, wheat germ, nuts, mushrooms, beer and wine	Involved in carbohydrate and lipid metabolism	No effect noted	No effect noted
Cobalt	Liver, kidney, fish, poultry eggs, tempeh	Important in RBC formation as a component of B_{12}	No effect noted	No effect noted
Other Nutrients Carbohydrates	Breads, cereals and grains, starchy vegetables, fruits	Source of energy	Decrease in caries rate as carbohydrate intake decreases in population and individuals	Cariogenic; causative risk factor for dental caries Form, frequency, and total contact time influence cariogenicity
Fats	Cooking oils, butter, fats found in meat, fish, poultry with skin, dairy products, etc.	Source of energy Cariostatic; antimicrobial action that produces an oily film on enamel and protects against cariogenic challenges	Difficult to develop a deficiency	Cariostatic; antimicrobial action that produces an oily film on enamel and protects against cariogenic challenges
Protein	Meat, lean meat, fish, poultry, eggs, legumes, tofu, dairy products, peanut butter	Source of energy Cariostatic	Defects in composition, eruption pattern, and resistance to decay during periods of tooth development Increased susceptibility to soft tissue infection, poor healing, and tissue regeneration	No effect noted
Water	Tap water, bottled water, water used in coffee and tea; some fruits and vegetables contain water	Source of hydration	Dehydration Fragility of epithelial tissues Decreased muscle strength for chewing Xerostomia Fissured tongue	No effect noted

Data from DePaola DP, Touger-Decker R, Rigassio-Radler D, and Faine MP: Nutrition and dental medicine. In Shils ME, et al, editors: Modern nutrition in health and disease, *ed 10, Baltimore, 2005, Williams & Wilkins, p 1171; and from Davis JR, Stegeman CA:* The dental hygienist's guide to nutritional care, *ed 3, Philadelphia, 2010, Saunders; Palmer C:* Diet and nutrition in oral health, *ed 2, Upper Saddle River, 2007, Pearson Prentice Hall, pp 169–173.*

TABLE 12-5 Effects of Nutrients on Oral Tissues and Their Role in Tooth Formation

Nutrients	Effects on Oral Soft and Hard Tissue	Role in Tooth Formation
Vitamin A	Synthesis and function of epithelial cells Maintenance of the integrity of the sulcus Normal growth and function of salivary glands Essential for activity of epiphyseal cartilage cells and normal endochondral bone growth	Normal growth of dentin and enamel Normal growth of periodontal tissues and maintenance of epithelium
Vitamin D	No effects noted	Controls calcification of dentin and enamel by regulating calcium absorption in the intestines
Vitamin C	Synthesis of connective tissue Essential for integrity of capillaries and oral mucosa Needed for normal bone matrix formation Needed for normal phagocytic function and antibody synthesis in host defense system	Integrity of blood vessels in gingival and pulpal tissues Hydroxylation of proline and lysine in collagen synthesis Normal formation of dentin
B-complex vitamins		
Niacin	Integrity of oral tissues	No effects noted
Folacin	Normal synthesis of protein compounds in oral tissues (e.g., hemoglobin and enzymes)	No effects noted
Thiamin	Normal energy metabolism during development and maintenance of oral tissue	No effects noted
Riboflavin	Energy metabolism of oral tissues	No effects noted
Pyridoxine	Normal carbohydrate metabolism and hemoglobin synthesis in oral tissues	No effects noted
Cobalamin	Integrity of nerve tissue and normal red blood cell formation in oral tissues	No effects noted
Calcium–phosphorus ratio	No effects noted	Normal tooth and bone mineralization
Fluoride	No effects noted	Forms dentin and enamel
Iron	Normal hemoglobin formation and carbon dioxide transport to tissue	No effects noted
Fiber	Stimulates salivary flow and integrity of periodontal tissues	No effects noted
Protein	Synthesis of antibodies and leukocytes Synthesis of epithelial and connective tissues in the healing process Maintains integrity of periodontal tissues	Formation of matrix of dentin and enamel Collagen formation

Data from DePaola DP, Touger-Decker R, Rigassio-Radler D, and Faine M: Nutrition and dental medicine. In Shils ME, et al, editors: Modern nutrition in health and disease, ed 10, Baltimore, 2005, Williams & Wilkins, p 1171.

7. Some require carriers for absorption and transportation
8. Excessive intake can be toxic
D. General functions
   1. Maintenance of acid–base balance
   2. Coenzymes or catalysts for biologic reactions
   3. Components of essential body compounds
   4. Maintenance of water balance
   5. Transmission of nerve impulses
   6. Regulation of muscle contraction
   7. Growth of oral and other body tissues

E. Nutritional requirements (see information on the National Academy Press Web site)
F. Dietary sources, specific body functions, and symptoms of deficiencies and toxicities (see Table 12-4)
G. Role of minerals in oral biology
   1. Function
      a. Tooth formation (see Table 12-5)
      b. Periodontium (see Table 12-5)
   2. Oral manifestations of deficiencies and toxicities (see Table 12-4)

Water

A. Definition—essential nutrient abundantly found in foods and beverages; makes up 50% to 60% of total body weight; survival without water is possible only up to 2 or 3 days

B. Total body water
1. Body water, as a percentage of body weight, decreases with age, ranging from 69% in newborn infants to 49% in women
2. Distribution—majority is intracellular, with the remainder being extracellular in serum, cerebrospinal fluid, tissue spaces, and saliva
   a. Intracellular
      (1) Enclosed within the cell membrane
      (2) Accounts for two thirds of the total
      (3) Increases with increased body cell mass
   b. Extracellular compartment
      (1) Intravascular
         (a) Approximately 3 liters (L)
         (b) Includes water in blood vessels
      (2) Intercellular (interstitial)
         (a) Approximately 12 L
         (b) Fluids that leave blood vessels
         (c) Fluids present in spaces between and surrounding each cell

C. Biologic role and functions
1. Is the medium in which most of the body's reactions take place
2. Is the means for transporting vital materials to cells and waste products away from cells
3. Regulates a constant body temperature
4. Maintains a constant composition of elements in body fluids (e.g., calcium, sodium, and fluoride)
5. Is part of the chemical structure of compounds that form cells (e.g., proteins)
6. Is active in many chemical reactions (e.g., digestion of a disaccharide)
7. Serves as a solvent (e.g., amino acids dissolve in water); this permits their transport to body cells
8. Lubricates and protects sensitive tissue around joints and mucosal linings

D. Water balance
1. Intake—controlled by thirst sensations; total daily intake need ranges from 1 to 3 L at a minimum to replace daily water losses; sources of water intake are:
   a. Ingested liquids and foods—1200 to 2000 milliliters (mL) per day
   b. Metabolic water from the oxidation of foods—250 to 350 mL per day
2. Elimination—total water output is 1500 to 3000 mL daily
   a. Sensible or measurable losses—occur through the kidneys as urine and through the bowel

as feces; constant daily losses amount to 650 to 1800 mL
   b. Insensible or unmeasurable losses—occur through the lungs with expired air and through the skin as perspiration; daily losses vary considerably, with an average of 850 to 1200 mL

E. Regulation
1. Potassium and sodium concentrations are responsible for maintaining water balance; when extracellular sodium equals intracellular potassium, water will not move into or out of the cell
2. Mechanisms of regulation
   a. Thirst response—when sodium increases, it stimulates the hypothalamus and heightens the the urge to drink
   b. Excretion regulation
      (1) Increased sodium stimulates the hypothalamus to signal the pituitary to release antidiuretic hormone (ADH), and water is resorbed in the kidney tubules
      (2) Decreased sodium causes the release of aldosterone, which causes resorption of sodium at the kidney tubules

F. Requirements—include water from liquids and food
1. For men, the adequate intake (AI) is 15 cups (3.7 L) per day
2. For women, the adequate intake (AI) is 11 cups (2.7 L) per day

G. Causes of water deficiency and conditions of toxicity
1. Dehydration
   a. Malfunction of kidneys
   b. Blood loss
   c. Vomiting
   d. Diarrhea
   e. Inadequate fluid intake
2. Water intoxication
   a. Edema
   b. Hypertension
   c. Sodium retention

SPECIALIZED CELLS OF ORAL TISSUES—EFFECTS OF NUTRIENTS

A. Epithelial cells
1. Important in tooth formation during the embryonic period
2. Make up the outer layers of tissue in the oral mucosa
   a. Rapid cell renewal, especially in the sulcular area
   b. Cell renewal more frequent with increasing age

3. Important in the normal development of salivary glands

4. Vitamin A and protein are essential for the normal proliferation of epithelial cells

B. Fibroblasts

1. Synthesize collagen fibrils in connective tissues of the gingiva, periodontal ligament, and pulp

2. Throughout life, fibroblasts maintain a rate of collagen synthesis equal to that of collagen breakdown; nutrient deficiencies can interfere with this equilibrium and cause a net loss of collagen tissue

3. Vitamin C, zinc, copper, and protein are important in collagen formation

C. Cementoblasts and cementocytes

1. Synthesize the protein matrix for cementum; vitamin C, zinc, copper, and protein are essential

2. Calcify the protein matrix; protein, calcium, phosphorus, and vitamin D are essential

3. Cementum is avascular and part acellular

4. Cellular cementum consists of cementocytes that depend on diffusion from the periodontal ligament for their nutrient supply

D. Ameloblasts

1. Synthesize the protein matrix for enamel; vitamins A and C, zinc, copper, and protein are essential

2. Calcify the protein matrix; protein, calcium, phosphorus, and vitamin D are essential; fluoride improves the quality of the apatite crystals formed

3. Once enamel is formed, no metabolic cells are present

E. Odontoblasts

1. Synthesize the protein matrix for dentin; vitamins A and C, zinc, copper, and protein are essential

2. Calcify the protein matrix; protein, calcium, phosphorus, and vitamin D are essential; fluoride improves the quality of the apatite crystals formed

3. Once dentin is formed, no metabolic cells are present, except in reaction to trauma; with trauma, new odontoblasts can form (possibly from pulpal tissue), and secondary dentin can be laid down

F. Osteocytes—osteoblasts and osteoclasts

1. Function in the synthesis of the alveolus

2. Function in the lifelong process of bone apposition (osteoblasts) and resorption (osteoclasts) in the alveolus

3. Nutrients important in the formation and maintenance of the alveolus are protein; vitamins A, C, and D; zinc; copper; calcium; and phosphorus

ENERGY BALANCES AND WEIGHT CONTROL

A. Definition—energy balance is a dynamic state in which the calories from food are equal to the caloric needs of the body; changes in energy balance result in a relative gain or loss in body weight

1. Lean body mass is highly metabolically active; basal metabolism is generally higher in people with greater amounts of lean body mass

2. In older adults, increases in body weight and body fat are not attributed to increased intake but are related to decrease in energy expenditure from loss of lean body mass

B. Measurement of energy

1. By calorimetry—food sample is burned in oxygen in an enclosed vessel surrounded by water; 1 kcal is the amount of heat produced sufficient to raise the temperature of 1 kg of water to $1^\circ C$; (the commonly used term *calorie* has the same definition)

2. In the body—carbon, hydrogen, and oxygen (from protein, carbohydrates, alcohol, or fats) are converted to carbon dioxide, water, and energy; energy is produced in the form of ATP; when needed, each ATP molecule loses a high-energy phosphate bond and becomes adenosine diphosphate (ADP) with a release of approximately 7.3 kcal/mole

C. Energy-producing systems

1. Blood glucose—immediate and preferred source of energy for cellular metabolism; glycogen stores provide glucose through glycogenolysis during the short periods of fasting between meals and in response to hormonal signals during sudden movement or intense exercise

a. Protein—can be used as an energy source when the blood glucose level falls; glucogenic amino acids are converted to glucose after deamination by gluconeogenesis; in a starvation state, body proteins are used for energy, which may cause irreversible damage if the essential protein components of the body are catabolized

b. Fat—mobilized from adipose tissue; triglycerides are broken down into glycerol and fatty acids in the liver; fatty acids are catabolized by β-oxidation to acetyl-CoA

c. Ethanol (alcohol)—can be oxidized to acetaldehyde, which is then converted into acetyl-CoA

2. Acetyl-CoA—enters the TCA from many sources

3. ATP—made during the process of oxidative phosphorylation in the mitochondria; proteins, carbohydrates, and fats do not yield the same number of ATP molecules per molecule of starting material because of their difference in molecular structure; to estimate the stored energy of foods, use these approximations: protein, 4 kcal/g; carbohydrate, 4 kcal/g; fat, 9 kcal/g; and ethanol, 7 kcal/g

D. Energy-using systems—ATP produced during catabolism is used by the body for biosynthetic activities, muscle contraction, ion transport, nerve conduction, and maintenance of body temperature
  1. Energy for basal metabolism—basal metabolic rate (BMR) is a measure of the energy required to maintain a living state while at rest and without food; includes respiration, circulation, maintenance of body temperature, muscle tone, glandular activities, and cellular metabolism
     a. Conditions for BMR measurement—postabsorptive state; muscles totally relaxed; awake; environmental temperature between 20°C and 25°C (68°F and 77°F); free of emotional stress; not during ovulation
     b. Factors influencing the BMR—age, genetics, gender, body size, nutritional state, muscular training, pathologic conditions, thyroid gland activity, climate, and altitude
  2. Energy for activity—the activity component of the energy requirement is for voluntary physical activity and varies from 20% of the BMR for sedentary activity to 50% or more of the BMR for heavy activity; factors influencing energy needs for the activity component include the size of the individual and the intensity and duration of the activity
  3. Thermic effect of food (TEF)—energy required to digest, absorb, and metabolize food; also called *nonshivering thermogenesis* because a slight elevation in body temperature occurs after a meal; not a clearly defined phenomenon; believed to include the energy needed to increase muscular contractions of the digestive tract, increases the synthesis of digestive enzymes and transports molecules; amounts to about 5% to 10% of the BMR and activity energy components

E. Nutritional requirements: determined by intake of food energy that allows the maintenance of ideal weight; data have been gathered from animal studies, balance studies, and intake surveys
  1. Recommendations represent the average needs of people in each age group and within a given activity category
  2. Recommendations are influenced by body size, gender, climate, age, and activity level

F. Weight management and control
  1. Calculating caloric intake needs—body mass index (BMI) and ideal body weight (IBW); see

TABLE 12-6 Body Mass Index Classification Chart

	Obesity Class	Body Mass Index (BMI) (1 kg/m²)
Underweight	—	<18.5
Normal	—	18.5–24.9
Overweight	—	25.0–25.9
Obesity	I	30.0–34.9
	II	35.0–39.9
Extreme obesity	III	>40

Adapted from National Institutes of Health: Clinical guidelines on the identification, evaluation, and treatment of overweight and obesity in adults: Obesity initiative. *Washington, DC, 1998, NIH.*

the section on "Complete Nutritional Assessment" later in this chapter
     a. BMI—approximate positive correlation of height and weight with body fat (r = +0.7–0.8); used to assess obesity and as an indicator of optimal weight for health (Table 12-6); for example, overweight adults with a BMI > 25 are at risk for comorbid diseases
        (1) Calculate BMI by dividing body weight in kilograms (kg) by the height in square meters (m²); for example, a man weighing 270 pounds (122.7 kg) who is 6 feet (3.34 m²) tall has a BMI of approximately 37
        (2) BMI does not differentiate between lean body mass and fat mass; so could inaccurately label an individual as obese
     b. Waist circumference is a more accurate method of determining central obesity, also known as abdominal obesity in an individual. Abdominal obesity puts an individual at greater risk of cardiovascular disease.
        (1) Women with waist measurements >35 inches are at risk for comorbid conditions
        (2) Men with waist measurements >40 inches are at risk for comorbid conditions
        (3) Waist circumference standards used for the general population may not apply to individuals under 5 feet in height or with a BMI of 35 or above
     c. Determining IBW
        (1) Males' IBW = 106 + (6 × inches over 5 feet tall)
        (2) Females' IBW = 100 + (5 × inches over 5 feet tall)
        (3) For individuals under 5 feet, subtract 2 pounds (lb) for each inch below 5 feet

d. Alternative method—decreasing usual caloric intake by 500 kcal/day usually allows a weight loss of 1 lb per week; this loss may reach a plateau as the body adjusts to a new BMR. Refer to www.choosemyplate.gov to determine individual caloric needs

2. Types of diet modifications
a. Balanced, low-calorie— the safest and healthiest reducing diet (e.g., Weight Watchers diet), if calories are approximately 1200 kcal/day and the intake is balanced and varied
b. Low-carbohydrate, high protein—risk of development of ketosis (e.g., Atkins diet, the Zone diet, South Beach diet) exists
c. Low-fat—may deprive the individual of essential fatty acids and fat-soluble vitamins; causes rapid emptying of the stomach (low satiety) and may make food seem flavorless; most individuals can decrease their usual fat intake without any harmful effects
d. High-fiber—increases fiber and bulk in the diet and allows a more rapid transit time for food in the GI tract; fiber also binds other nutrients, so they are not completely absorbed; moderate increases in the fiber content of the diet (e.g., in well-designed vegetarian diets) appear to be helpful in treating diabetes, diverticulosis, and hypercholesterolemia as well as in decreasing the total caloric intake of reducing diets; very-high-fiber diets cause GI discomfort and may induce mineral deficiencies
e. Single food (monotonous) diet—no one food by itself can provide a balance of nutrients; diets that promote a single food with unrealistic claims are not recommended (e.g., the grapefruit diet, the cabbage soup diet)
f. Liquid formulas (protein)—very low-calorie diets; have been successfully used in treating morbidly obese persons in carefully monitored hospital settings but are not recommended for the individual (e.g., Optifast)

3. Prescription drugs used for weight loss are recommended for individuals with a BMI ≥30 with no obesity-related risk factors or for those with a BMI of 27 to 29.9 with obesity-related risk factors; adverse side effects have been observed in long-term use of such drugs; prescription drugs include:
a. Noradrenergic drugs for short-term weight loss
(1) Diethylpropion
(2) Phentermine (e.g., Zantry, Adipex-P, Fastin)
(3) Mazindol

b. Serotonergic drugs
(1) Fenfluramine (also phentermine plus fenfluramine, or Phen-Fen) and dexfenfluramine (Redux) were removed from the U.S. market because of reports of primary pulmonary hypertension, heart valve abnormalities, and death associated with their use
(2) Fluoxetine (not FDA approved for treating obesity)
c. Sibutramine (Meridia) is an approved combination of serotonin and adrenergic drugs; centrally acting agent that increases satiety but has little effect on hunger
d. Orlistat (Xenical prescription or Alli over the counter) is a lipase inhibitor; interferes with fat digestion; taking the drugs with meals inhibits fat absorption by 30%

4. Activity in weight management—even moderate activity such as walking will increase caloric expenditure and should be considered in every weight-loss program; moderate exercise also improves muscle tone, stimulates circulation, increases BMR, and often creates a sense of well-being

5. Behavior modification—eating habits and attitudes often must be changed to prevent weight regain; many successful diet programs combine decreased food intake and increased activity with an analysis and modification of eating behaviors; group programs such as Weight Watchers help make behavioral changes

6. Dietary aids—represent a multimillion-dollar business, and although they may help cause an initial rapid weight loss, they are no more effective than mere calorie cutting in long-term weight maintenance; moreover, most diet drugs have the potential for serious side effects if used habitually over a long period or by persons with certain medical conditions; types most often used are appetite suppressants, stimulants, laxatives, diuretics, and bulk-producing agents

7. Surgical therapy: gastric bypass surgery may be recommended to individuals with BMI >40 or those with BMI >35 and comorbid conditions. This surgical approach is used to reduce the size of the stomach to decrease its reserve capacity. Bloating, nausea, vomiting, dumping syndrome, anemia, and nutrient deficiencies may result if diet instructions are not followed after surgery
a. Fluids are consumed separately from meals; more frequent small meals throughout the day are recommended
b. Increased risk of caries because of alterations in eating habits

G. Eating disorders
1. Treatment
    a. Correction of any underlying physiologic causes of weight loss
    b. Increased caloric intake with foods that are concentrated sources of energy; several small meals per day
    c. Limiting weight-gain goals to 1 to 2 lb per week
    d. Team approach; physician, registered dietitian, psychotherapist, or all should be involved in the treatment
2. Signs and symptoms of disordered eating
    a. Erosion of tooth enamel (perimylolysis)
    b. Halitosis
    c. Severe weight loss
    d. Dental caries
    e. Lanugo
    f. Enlarged tongue
    g. Angular cheilosis
    h. Enlarged parotid glands
    i. Xerostomia
    j. Goose bumps on skin
    k. Glossitis
3. Anorexia nervosa—state of PEM brought on by voluntary starvation (and often with the use of diet aids, intense exercise, and self-induced vomiting); seen most often in middle-income and upper-income adolescent females, who are typically described as perfectionists, overachievers, and models of good behavior; they begin dieting because they have a distorted perception of body shape and weight; death may occur from failure of multiple organ systems; treatment usually includes specially tailored counseling and hospitalization before voluntary weight gain is possible; treatment encourages regular mealtimes, varied and moderate intake, and gradual introduction of feared foods; the client should be referred to a physician, a registered dietitian, or a psychologist for treatment
4. Bulimia—condition of alternate food gorging and purging by vomiting; occasional use of laxatives to maintain weight; most often found in adolescent females who appear to be of normal weight; is more prevalent than anorexia nervosa; treatment involves counseling; self-induced vomiting can cause swelling of the salivary glands and esophagus and the destruction of tooth enamel by acid that results in sensitive teeth; the client should be referred to a physician, a registered dietitian, or a psychologist for treatment
5. Eating Disorders Not Otherwise Specified (EDNOS)—a broad category in which individuals do not meet the strict criteria for anorexia nervosa or anorexia bulimia; binge eating disorder falls into this category

NUTRITIONAL ASSESSMENT AND COUNSELING

Malnutrition

A. Overconsumption of nutrients such as:
1. Fat—can result in excess weight gain; associated with coronary heart disease (CHD), obesity, and certain types of cancers
2. Sugar—can result in excess weight gain; associated with obesity, dental caries, and plaque-induced gingivitis
3. Salt or sodium—can result in retention of excess body fluid; associated with high blood pressure; increased sodium may also decrease calcium levels
4. Excess calories—can result in obesity; associated with CHD, hypertension, and diabetes mellitus type 2
5. Vitamin and mineral supplements—"megadoses" may result in toxicity of one or many nutrients and inhibition of others
B. Nutrient deficiencies—the health of a person is at risk because of the unavailability of nutrients for cellular activities; end result of deficiencies is the same, but the multiple causes can be classified as primary or secondary
1. Primary deficiency is a result of an inadequate food intake and can result from the following conditions:
    a. Fad diets—low-calorie or imbalanced diet plans
    b. Economics—inadequate resources to obtain a healthy diet
    c. Illness—loss of appetite
    d. Improper food preparation—destruction of nutrients because of delayed storage and overcooking of foods
    e. Accessibility to food—nutritious foods unavailable because of problems with transportation or market supplies encountered by individuals
    f. Ignorance—lack of nutritional knowledge
    g. Flavor preferences—palatability of sweets and fats can lead to a diet high in empty-calorie foods
    h. Time constraints—inadequate time for food preparation can lead to the use of highly processed convenience foods, which tend to have low nutrient density
    i. Poor oral health—inability to masticate food because of edentulism or oral disease;

altered taste perceptions result from oral disease

2. Secondary deficiency is the result of inability to digest, absorb, and use foods consumed; an individual may eat a balanced diet, but other factors interfere with the body's use of nutrients in foods; examples of these conditioning factors include:
   a. Disease—any GI or metabolic disease can interfere with the digestion and use of foods and nutrients (e.g., ulcers, lactase deficiency, partial obstruction of the GI tract, and inborn errors of metabolism)
   b. Drug–nutrient interactions—certain drugs can interfere with and reduce the absorption, transportation, and metabolism of nutrients (e.g., grapefruit juice with high blood pressure medication)
   c. Nutrient–nutrient interactions—excess or deficiency of certain nutrients can affect the absorption of other nutrients (e.g., vitamin C and iron)
   d. Allergies—sensitivity to certain foods or chemicals in foods can lead to malabsorption syndromes (e.g., gluten sensitivity as in celiac disease)

3. Manifestations of primary and secondary deficiencies
   a. Gradual decreases in the tissue level of nutrients
      (1) Earliest sign of malnutrition
      (2) Determined by blood and urine analyses for each nutrient
   b. Biochemical disturbances
      (1) Occur if duration of deficiency is long enough to deplete the body's stores and interfere with cellular metabolism
      (2) Determined by blood and urine analysis for alterations in cellular levels of enzymes and metabolites
   c. Anatomic lesions
      (1) Signs of chronic and severe malnutrition, leading to destruction of body tissues
      (2) Determined by clinical examination of body tissues

Complete Nutritional Assessment

A. Health and pharmacologic history
   1. Factors that influence food intake
      a. Socioeconomic conditions—food purchasing power
      b. Home environment—culture, family values, and eating practices
      c. Client motivation and education—interest and awareness of the principles of a nutritious diet

   d. Prescriptive drugs that may suppress appetite, alter taste perception, or negatively interact with foods
   2. Factors that influence food use
      a. Oral health—ability to masticate, saliva production, and presence of oral disease
      b. Systemic health—ability to digest, absorb, and metabolize nutrients in food; therapeutic diets for disease control
      c. Mental health—desire to eat
      d. Drug use—alcohol abuse and illegal drugs

B. Assessment of dietary intake
   1. Collection of objective data on what a person eats
      a. Assessment tools—screening questionnaire for food intake frequency, 24-hour recall method, and food record or diary
         (1) Food-frequency questionnaires—ask how often food items are consumed; elicit specific details; work better with large groups in the community setting
         (2) 24-hour recall method—mental recall of everything eaten in the previous 24 hours; useful for individual counseling in a clinical setting; does not represent "usual" diet
         (3) Food record diary—exact record of everything eaten in a specific period; more accurate account
         (4) Combining 3- to 7-day food record with a 24-hour recall method presents a more accurate measure of intake
      b. Specific amounts or quantities of foods eaten must be recorded to use assessment tools effectively
   2. Analysis and evaluation of food intake
      a. Methods of analysis—the USDA MyPlate (Figure 12-3)
      b. Methods of evaluation—comparing results of diet analysis with standards of adequacy
   3. Diet modifications
      a. Adding foods to the diet to correct for nutrient deficiencies
      b. Eliminating or reducing excessive nutrient intake for disease control and prevention (e.g., sugar, fat, oils, or sodium)
      c. Collaborate with a registered dietitian for in-depth analysis and modification of dietary intake

C. Biochemical analysis and immune function
   1. Blood and urine analyses
      a. Most objective and precise assessment data
      b. Determine marginal nutritional deficiencies before overt clinical signs appear by measuring either the concentration of a nutrient or the functional activity of the nutrient

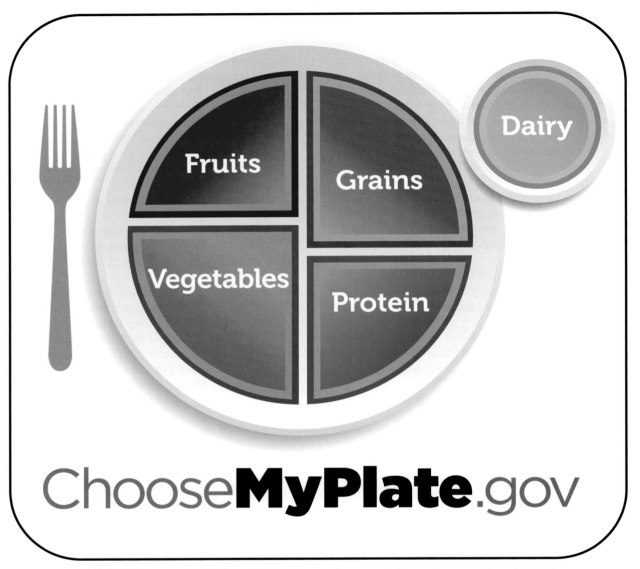

FIGURE 12-3 Anatomy of MyPyramid. *(From www.choosemyplate.gov: Accessed June 2, 2011)*

2. Delayed cutaneous hypersensitivity skin tests
   a. Assessment of host defense mechanisms by evaluating the client's reaction to common skin test antigens as a nonspecific indicator of malnutrition
   b. Most useful for evaluating the critically ill client's ability to withstand the stresses of surgery
D. Clinical examination of body tissues—indicator of systemic health and nutritional status (see Table 12-4)
   1. Oral tissues
      a. Dental caries—excessive sugar or acid exposure (supports *S. mutans* and *Lactobacillus acidophilus*)
      b. Gingivitis and periodontal disease—excessive sugar intake (supports growth of plaque biofilm and nutritional deficiencies)
      c. Glossitis—nutritional deficiencies affecting the papillae and color of the tongue
      d. Stomatitis—nutritional deficiencies affecting oral soft tissues
      e. Cheilosis—nutritional deficiencies affecting the lips and the corners of the mouth
      f. Necrotizing ulcerative gingivitis (NUG)—excessive sugar and caffeine intake, smoking, stress, and poor oral hygiene combined with nutritional deficiencies result in lowered host resistance to bacterial plaque biofilm and bacterial challenges
   2. Anthropometric analysis—determines the body structure, form, and composition (e.g., content of lean body mass and fat tissue); the following tools are useful, but each has its limitations:

a. BMI, IBW, and waist circumference (see the section on "Energy Balances and Weight Control" in this chapter)
b. Skinfold thickness measurements
  (1) Obtained by using skinfold calipers to measure subcutaneous fat in millimeters in selected areas (e.g., triceps and subscapular regions)
  (2) Measurements are compared with standards to estimate total body fat composition
c. Arm muscle circumference
  (1) Sensitive indicator of the muscle mass that reflects protein stores
  (2) Determined by measuring the arm circumference at the midpoint of the upper arm and by measuring triceps skinfold
d. Bioelectrical impedance and ultrasound methods
  (1) Potential predictors of total body fat
  (2) Lean body mass conducts electricity better than fat mass
e. Underwater weighing
  (1) Measures body weight when the person is under water
  (2) One of the most accurate methods used to determine body volume
f. Dual-energy x-ray absorptiometry (DEXA)—can distinguish fat mass, fat-free mass, and bone mineral loss; most accurate method to determine body fat

Methods for Assessment of Dietary Intake

A. Dietary intake standards
  1. *Dietary Reference Intake (DRI)* and *Recommended Dietary Allowance (RDA)*
    a. Published by the Panel on Micronutrients of the Food and Nutrition Board, Institute of Medicine, National Academy of Sciences; principally used as measurement tools by nutrition professionals who plan and evaluate food supplies for groups; to establish guidelines for new food products; used as the basis for regulatory standards in determining nutritional quality; and used to set standards for nutritional labeling (e.g., percentage of daily value)
    b. DRI is the updated version of the RDA established by the National Academy of Science, Food and Nutrition Board; DRI values are based on the observed average or experimentally set intake by individuals that appear to sustain a defined nutritional status

    (1) Unlike RDA values, DRI values aim to prevent nutrient deficiency as well as reduce the likelihood of chronic disease
    (2) DRI includes five sets of standards:
      (a) RDA—intake level sufficient to meet nutrient requirements of nearly all healthy individuals
      (b) AI (adequate intake)—value based on approximation of nutrient intake by a group of healthy people, used when an RDA value cannot be determined
      (c) UL (upper limit)—highest level of daily nutrient intake that is likely to pose no risk of adverse health effects to almost all individuals in the general population; risk of adverse effects increases as intake increases above the UL
      (d) EAR (estimated average requirement)—nutrient intake value that is estimated to meet the requirements of half the healthy individuals in a group
      (e) EER (estimated energy requirement)—average calorie need estimates for various life stage groups and genders

  2. *Dietary Guidelines for Americans* are issued by the U.S Department of Agriculture (USDA) and the U.S. Department of Health and Human Services (USDHHS). The guidelines are revised every 5 years. The 7th edition of the *Dietary Guidelines for Americans* (2010) includes 23 key recommendations for the general population and 6 additional key recommendations for special populations.[3] Special populations include children and adolescents, women capable of becoming pregnant, pregnant women, women who are breastfeeding, older adults and adults at high risk of chronic disease. The updated guidelines are intended for Americans ages 2 years and older, including those with chronic disease. Two common themes are weaved throughout the updated guidelines: encouragement of balanced caloric intake to manage body weight and the consumption of nutrient-dense foods and beverages.[3]

  The recommendations for the general public are grouped into five general chapters:
  a. Balancing Calories to Manage Weight
  b. Foods and Food Components to Reduce
  c. Foods and Nutrients to Increase
  d. Building Healthy Eating Patterns
  e. Helping Americans Make Healthy Choices

  The key recommendations within these chapters include the following:[3]

a. Men ages 19 and older should eat between 2000 and 3000 calories a day depending on degree of activity; women should limit themselves to 1600 and 2400. Individuals should aim for the lower caloric levels if inactive

b. SoFAS (solid fats and added sugars) should make up no more than 13% of your daily caloric intake based on a 2000-calorie diet

c. Reduce consumption of refined grains. Half of grain consumption should come from whole grains. Based on a minimum consumption of 6 ounces—3 ounces should come from whole grain foods

d. Limit sodium intake to 2300 mg a day. African Americans and individuals 51 and older or who have hypertension, diabetes, or chronic kidney disease should decrease their intake to 1500 mg

e. Increase intake of fruits and vegetables. Consume 2 cups of fruit and 2.5 cups of vegetables (including beans and peas) each day

f. Aim for 3 cups of low fat or fat free dairy foods each day

g. Consume at least 8 ounces of seafood a week.

h. Limit protein foods; consume no more than 5.5 ounces daily.

i. Consume a variety of food sources to ensure optimum intake of potassium, calcium, and vitamin D. Choose whole food sources of nutrients—limit use of supplements

3. Dietary guidelines for oral health

a. Eat a balanced diet representing moderation and variety as shown by MyPlate, and follow the recommendations of the *Dietary Guidelines for Americans* (2010)[3]

b. Combine and eat foods in sequence to enhance mastication, saliva production, and oral clearance; for example, combine dairy foods with sweet or starchy foods, or combine protein-rich foods with cooked or processed starches

c. Plan eating intervals that allow time for the pH of the plaque to return to neutral; for example, up to 120 minutes may be needed for the plaque pH to return to neutral after exposure to a fermentable carbohydrate

d. Take care not to replace other foods needed to maintain optimum health with sweets and soft drinks; obtain most calories from whole grains, fruits and vegetables, low-fat or nonfat dairy products, and lean meats or meat alternatives

e. Drink water often; consume sweetened and acidic beverages *with* meals to allow for a

buffering action, rather than consuming soft drinks *between* meals

f. Limit the consumption of sugar-free beverages and sports drinks; demineralization of tooth structure can still occur as a result of the low pH of these beverages; consume these with meals

4. The Food and Nutrition Board's recommendations for healthy adult Americans

a. Maintain a healthy weight by balancing energy intake and energy expenditure

b. If the requirement for energy is low (e.g., weight-reducing diet), reduce the consumption of foods such as alcohol, sugars, fats, and oils that provide calories but few other essential nutrients

c. Use salt in moderation; recommended intake is no more than 2300 mg (1 teaspoon) per day; 1500 mg/day for those with hypertension

d. Select a nutritionally adequate diet from the foods available by each day consuming appropriate servings of low-fat dairy products, lean meats or legumes, vegetables, fruits, cereals, grains, and breads (Table 12-7)

e. Select as wide a variety of foods in each of the major food groups as is practical to ensure a high probability of adequate quantities of all essential nutrients

5. The USDA MyPlate (see Figure 12-3)

a. Graphic design is similar to a pie chart; organizes foods into four colorful sections with a side portion for dairy.

(1) Red represents fruits; green is for vegetables; orange is for grains; purple is for protein. There is a separate blue section for dairy on the side of the plate.

(2) Encourages healthier eating habits and the consumption of a more plant-based diet

(3) Promotes balanced proportions of each food group to be consumed at meals

(a) Half of your plate should be fruits and vegetables

(b) At least half of your grains should be whole grains

(c) Make the switch to fat free or low fat milk

(d) Balance calories

(e) Avoid oversized portions

(4) Recommends reduced intake of those foods high in sodium; read labels to compare

(5) Supports the consumption of water over sugary drinks

TABLE 12-7 Daily Guide to Food Choices

Food Group	Source of	DAILY RECOMMENDED SERVINGS		
		1600 kilocalories (kcal)	2200 kcal	2800 kcal
Water	Fluids to maintain water balance and hydration	64 ounces (oz)	64 oz	64 oz
Breads, cereals, grains	Riboflavin, thiamin, niacin, iron, protein, fiber, magnesium	5 oz	7 oz	10 oz
Vegetables	Vitamins A and C, folate, potassium, magnesium, iron, fiber, phytochemicals	2 cups	3 cups	3.5 cups
Fruits	Vitamins A and C, potassium, iron phytochemicals, fiber	1.5 cups	2 cups	2.5 cups
Milk, yogurt, cheese	Calcium, protein, riboflavin, vitamins A and D, phosphorus	3 cups	3 cups	3 cups
Meat and meat alternatives	Protein, zinc, iron, vitamin B_{12}, niacin, thiamin, vitamin A, folacin, pyroxidine, magnesium, phosphorus, vitamin B_6	5 oz	6 oz	7 oz
Fats and oils	Essential fatty acids, energy	5 teaspoon (tsp)	6 tsp	8 tsp
Sugars	Energy	Women: 6 tsp Men: 9 tsp	Women: 6 tsp Men: 9 tsp	Women: 6 tsp Men: 9 tsp
Alcohol	Energy	—	—	—

Courtesy of Connie Mobley, RD, PhD, The University of Texas Health Science Center, Department of Community Dentistry, San Antonio, TX. My Pyramid Food Intake Patterns. U.S. Department of Agriculture, Center for Nutrition Policy and Promotion, MyPyramid Food Guidance System, April 2005: Available at http://www.pyramid.gov/downloads/MyPyramid_Food_Intake_Patterns.pdf: Accessed May 27, 2010. Johnson RK, Appel LJ, Brands M, et al: Dietary sugars intake and cardiovascular health: A scientific statement from the American Heart Association, Circulation 120:1011–1020, 2009.

B. Methods for collecting data on food intakes
  1. Nutritional Screening and Assessment of Dietary Intake Questionnaire (Figure 12-4)
   a. Description—interviewer collects data from the client about all food consumed in the previous 24-hour period; additional questions help determine frequency of sugar and food group intake
   b. Nutrition tools used to guide recommendations
    (1) USDA MyPlate
    (2) *Dietary Guidelines*
    (3) *Dietary Reference Intake (DRI)* based on life stage
   c. Advantages
    (1) Can be filled out by the client while waiting in the oral health care setting
    (2) Requires only 15 to 20 minutes to complete
    (3) Allows analysis of food group consumption
    (4) Allows evaluation of sugar intake
   d. Limitations
    (1) No nutrient analysis
    (2) Relies on the client's memory

  2. Twenty-four-hour dietary recall
   a. Description—interviewer collects data from the client about all food consumed in the previous 24-hour period
   b. Advantages
    (1) Requires 20 minutes or less for the interview
    (2) Allows nutrient analysis
    (3) Allows analysis of food group consumption
    (4) Allows evaluation of sugar intake
   c. Limitations
    (1) Requires a trained interviewer
    (2) Relies on the client's memory
    (3) Represents only 1 day of food consumption
    (4) Requires a nutrient data file on foods to analyze nutrients
  3. 3- to 7-day food record or diary
   a. Description—client keeps a record of food and eating times for 3 to 7 days
   b. Advantages
    (1) No interviewer required except to give directions on how to fill out the record

Nutritional Screening and Assessment of Dietary Intake Questionnaire

Client's Name _____ Gender: M F Age: _____

Height _____ Weight _____ # IBW _____ Occupation/Activity Level _____

FOR THE EDENTULOUS CLIENT, COMPLETE ONLY THOSE ITEMS WITH AN ASTERISK (*).

*_____ Complete Oral Health Evaluation   CRA Score†: low moderate high very high

*Review client chart and Oral Health Evaluation Form for the following:

____ Does client have a chronic disease (diabetes, hypertension, etc.)?
____ Is client taking medication or a dietary supplement with nutritional implications?
____ Does client have periodontal disease or xerostomia?
____ Does client have a dietary screening score greater than 3?

*Obtain typical dietary intake information: (record 24-hour recall of dietary intake)
*Use nutritional tools as a guide to making recommendations (USDA MyPlate, Dietary Guidelines, DRIs/RDIs)

Determine if diet is caries promoting, using the following criteria:	If YES, circle:
a.	Do the total number of servings from the combined sugars and sweet beverages group exceed the number of servings from the grains group?	**4 points**
b.	Are food and beverage sources of sugars consumed alone?	**2 points**
c.	Are foods from the grains group consumed alone? Are foods from the grains group consumed in combination with foods that are sources of sugars? Are these combined foods eaten alone?	**2 points**
d.	Is diet lacking foods and/or adequate servings of foods from 1 or more food groups? Do number of servings for food groups exceed recommendations?	**2 points**

e.	Does the client have an unusual meal pattern?
	  –Eating snacks or drinking beverages in place of meals
	  –Spacing meals/snacks more than 6 hours apart
	  –Eating or drinking every 1–2 hours
		1 point

f.	Does the client eat or drink late in the evening or immediately prior to bedtime?	**1 point**
g.	Does the client report chewing gum that is not sugar free?	**1 point**
Total Score (6=caries promoting diet)	

*Chart findings using SOAP format.

*Educate client, using appropriate nutrition education handouts and models. Refer client to other healthcare professionals, as appropriate.

FIGURE 12-4 Nutritional Screening and Assessment of Dietary Intake Questionnaire. *CRA, caries risk assessment; the CRA score is determined from an oral health evaluation tool that is used to determine the level of caries risk on an individual basis. *(Modified from Connie Mobley, RD, PhD, University of Nevada Las Vegas, School of Dental Medicine, Las Vegas, Nevada.)*

(2) Allows for analyses of both nutrients and food groups

(3) Allows for evaluation of sugar intake

(4) An average intake of several days may be more representative of client's food intake than that of just 1 day

c. Limitations

(1) Represents the food consumption of only the days included in the record

(2) Relies on the cooperation and ability of the client to keep the record

(3) Requires a nutrient data file for nutrient analysis

C. Methods for evaluating food intake

1. MyPlate

a. Nutrient contributions (see Table 12-7)

(1) Role in general health

(2) Role in oral health

b. Advantages for use in counseling

(1) Client participation

(2) Simple

(3) Inexpensive

(4) Fairly accurate

(5) Detailed nutrient analysis

c. Limitations

(1) No provisions made for combination foods (e.g., pizza or casseroles); need to break down into ingredients that correspond to the six groups

(2) Web site can be difficult to navigate

2. Computerized analysis of diet

a. Definition—food nutrient data are individually entered into a computer program, and the specific amounts of each nutrient for each food consumed are calculated

b. Nutrient data file (software)—lists foods and their nutrients;[4,5] the USDA has a nutrient database Web site: http://fnic.nal.usda.gov/. MyPlate has an online dietary assessment tool MyPyramid Tracker that can be accessed at http://www.mypyramidtracker.gov (see the Web Site Information and Resources table at the end of this chapter)

c. DRI and RDA values—used as a standard for comparison with the client's daily nutrient intake

d. Advantages

(1) Accurate

(2) Specific

(3) Cost-efficient when technology is available

(a) Computers in oral healthcare settings with internet access

(b) Services available for a fee outside the oral healthcare setting

e. Limitations

(1) Limited client participation and home use

(2) Hardware and software availability

(3) Expense

(4) Requires training for accurate interpretation of output

3. Sugar analysis and evaluation

a. Dental caries and periodontal disease are multifactorial infectious diseases that result from the interaction of the resistance of oral tissues (host factor) with the destructive effects of bacterial plaque and acids (agent factor) produced from the metabolism of dietary sugars (diet or environment factor); dental disease occurs when all three factors exist simultaneously; often called the "triad" of dental disease; nutritional assessment of exposure to sugar is an essential part of nutritional counseling in disease prevention programs and can be conducted by using precise or simplified methods

(1) Precise analysis—computer analysis of the diet for carbohydrate content: total carbohydrate in grams, monosaccharides and disaccharides in grams (e.g., grams of sucrose), and fiber in grams; percentage of the total daily calorie intake from simple and complex carbohydrates can be calculated and compared with the recommendations: Added sugars should contain no more than 25% of total calories consumed; fiber needs range from 21 to 38 g, depending on age and gender[2]

(2) Simplified analysis—dietary sugars (sweets and foods processed with sugars; see Table 12-3) are circled on the food record or recall; cariogenicity of the diet is assessed on the basis of frequency and form of sugar exposure; frequent exposure to retentive solid sugars, especially between meals, is harmful; acid production potential of the diet can be calculated by using the following formula:

Total daily *solid* sugar exposures × 40 min

+

Total daily *liquid* sugar exposures × 20 min

= Total min acid exposure to oral tissues from *all* dietary sugars

Total should not exceed 100 min of exposure

The formula is based on research that shows glucose-rich food products (either liquid or sugar) result in a decrease of oral pH below the critical level (pH 5.5, the point at which acids decalcify enamel) and that it takes 20 minutes after consumption of liquid sugars for healthy saliva to neutralize acids and raise the pH to a safe level; solid sugars adhere to teeth and have approximately double the potential for acid production

b. Caries activity tests—often involve counting the number of acidogenic bacteria or measuring the acids produced by these bacteria; provide information about the current oral environment and help to detect dental caries risk; are valuable adjuncts in plaque-control programs and can be used to monitor a client's progress in oral home care and diet modifications.

Nutritional Counseling Techniques

A. Direct approach—counseling technique that focuses on the dietary problem
   1. Role of the client—the client provides information about his or her diet; is passive and listens to the counselor
   2. Role of the counselor—the counselor controls the session; analyzes and evaluates the client's diet and makes recommendations for improvement
   3. Advantages—easier for the counselor and often requires less time than a more client-oriented approach
   4. Limitations—fosters client dependence; little chance of success if the client is not committed to dietary changes; client is not involved in decision making
B. Nondirect or behavior-modification approach—counseling technique that focuses on the client
   1. Role of the client—the client actively participates in the diet analysis, evaluation, and modification program
   2. Role of the counselor—the counselor provides information on the causes of dental disease, the role of the diet, and the use of dietary assessment tools
   3. Method
      a. Assumption—dietary habits are learned behaviors and can be "unlearned" and replaced with new behaviors
      b. Collection of baseline data
      c. Client takes ownership of his or her dietary problems and is committed to change
      d. Client determines his or her behavioral changes and goals; develops own reward system to use when goals are met

e. Changes are gradually made in small steps; appropriate changes are rewarded and failures ignored
      f. Close monitoring of progress until new behaviors become self-reinforcing
   4. Advantages—fosters client independence; success is more likely because the client is in control of the change process
   5. Limitations—more time and effort needed to arrive at appropriate solutions to dietary problems and rewards for behavior modification
C. Factors that influence the client's food intake—any combination of the following influences affects food choices and needs to be addressed in a modification program:
   1. Environmental influences—economics, lifestyle, geography, seasons, markets
   2. Social influences—family, culture, religion, social pressures, marketing strategies
   3. Psychological influences—self-image, emotions, stresses, values, priorities
D. Determinants for dental client selection
   1. High-risk clients—those with conditions that would benefit most from nutritional counseling
      a. Pregnancy—nutrient needs are high; hormonal changes may lead to exaggerated responses to plaque and bacterial toxins; maternal diet affects the formation of fetal oral tissues
      b. Adolescence—nutrient needs are high; vulnerable to nutritional problems from fad diets for weight loss and muscle building; frequent snacking on empty-calorie foods; problems of anorexia and bulimia can lead to enamel erosion, irritation of oral mucosa, and infected or enlarged salivary glands, with possible xerostomia
      c. Rampant caries—high bacterial plaque and calculus and a positive caries-activity test may indicate a problem of frequent exposure to sugar
      d. Periodontal disease or NUG—frequent exposure to sugar and nutritional deficiencies can contribute to the development and progression of these conditions
      e. Oral and maxillofacial surgery—nutritional counseling before and after surgery is important for optimal surgical recovery; postsurgical nutrient needs are high because of blood loss, tissue repair, and host defense activities; modifications in food texture (e.g., soft foods) are made according to the client's ability to masticate
      f. Edentulism—inability to masticate can result in nutrient deficiencies because of the limited nutrient content in soft and liquid foods

(1) Food choices are altered because of difficulties with chewing or fear of choking; reduced intake of meats, fresh fruits, and vegetables; softer foods are usually eaten

(2) Lowered intake of magnesium, folic acid, fluoride, zinc, and calcium

   g. Oral cancer—nutrient needs are high because of host defense activities and tissue repair from cancer and its treatment; cancer or treatment may result in inadequate food intake because of decreased appetite, altered taste perceptions, irritated oral tissues, and xerostomia

2. Dental office resources—availability of trained personnel, time, and facilities to conduct nutrition counseling services

3. Client factors—level of client motivation to use and benefit from nutritional counseling and financial and intellectual capabilities for using nutritional counseling services

Dietary Modifications for Specific Dental Conditions

A. Dental caries (see Tables 12-4 and 12-5)
   1. Role of nutrients in tooth formation
      a. Pre-eruptive effects—nutrients are used systemically for enamel, dentin, and pulp formation; tooth bud formation begins at 6 weeks in utero, and calcification is completed at 13 years
      b. Post-eruptive effects—fluoride aids in the remineralization of small enamel lesions; evidence indicates that specific minerals or combinations of minerals and fats have local cariostatic properties
   2. Local effect of dietary carbohydrates on bacteria growth and plaque formation
   3. Role of diet and nutrients in salivary gland function
      a. Nutrients are used systemically for the normal development and secretory function of salivary glands
      b. Foods of firm texture (e.g., raw vegetables) enhance mastication, stimulate the salivary flow rate, and modify the concentration of constituents in saliva, possibly improving antibacterial properties and the buffering capacity to neutralize decalcifying acids
B. Periodontal disease (see Table 12-5)
   1. Role of nutrients in the formation of periodontal tissues

   a. Nutrients are used systemically for the normal development of the gingiva, periodontal ligament, cementum, and alveolus
   b. Periodontal tissues are metabolically active throughout a person's life, and nutrients are constantly needed for maintenance (e.g., the cell population of the sulcal epithelium completely renews itself within 3 to 6 days)
   2. Local effect of dietary carbohydrates on bacteria growth and plaque formation
   3. Role of nutrients in the host defense system
      a. During the initial stages of periodontitis, the nutritional status of the client is important in cellular immunocompetence for combating bacterial insults to the periodontium
      b. After periodontal surgery, cellular immunocompetence is important for optimal healing and preventing infection
C. Oral and maxillofacial surgery
   1. Presurgical nutritional counseling
      a. Adequate nutrient intake is needed to build up nutrient reserves in tissues to cope with postsurgical nutrient demands and complications
      b. Counseling is helpful for advising the client to plan and purchase appropriate foods before surgery in anticipation of convalescence
      c. Need for referral to registered dietitian prior to surgery should be evaluated
   2. Postsurgical nutritional counseling
      a. Nutrient requirements are high because of blood loss, increased catabolism, tissue repair, and host defense activities
      b. Dietary intake is influenced by surgical complications of anorexia, dysphagia, and oral discomfort; a liquid diet should be used initially for the first few days, followed by a soft diet until the client can eat normally; during convalescence, high-protein liquid products fortified with vitamins and minerals (e.g., Ensure, Sustacal, and Instant Breakfast) are helpful but contain cariogenic sweeteners; safe levels of vitamin and mineral supplements (100% to 200% of DRI or RDA values) may be recommended
D. Prosthodontics
   1. Nutritional counseling in the preparation of the mouth for a prosthesis
      a. Nutrients—systemically important for the health of oral soft tissues and the alveolar ridge
         (1) Surgery—if surgery is necessary, nutrient requirements will be higher for postsurgical healing

(2) Tissue state—if any inflamed or soft tissue injuries and bone resorption conditions exist, nutrient requirements will be higher for repair and host defense activities

b. Dietary sugars—condition of the remaining dentition is important for maintaining the use of a new prosthesis; cariogenic sugars need to be restricted to control bacterial growth, acid production, and bacterial plaque formation

c. Texture of foods—partial or fully edentulous clients will often need to eat chopped, soft foods; if nutrient intake is compromised, fortified liquid products or nutrient supplements are helpful

2. Nutritional counseling after prosthesis insertion

a. Food texture—liquid foods for the first 24 hours, followed by soft foods and chopped or cut-up foods; this minimizes biting and chewing and allows time for the muscles and tongue to adjust to the new prosthesis

b. Counter-dislodgement forces—for every bite of food, food should be evenly divided in the right and left sides of the mouth before chewing to equalize occlusal forces

c. Nutrients—adequate intake for the integrity of the oral mucosa and alveolar ridge

d. Dietary sugars—should be restricted to prevent bacterial growth, acid production, and bacterial plaque formation on the remaining dentition and prosthesis

e. Food flavors—initially, flavors of foods will be altered because of the new prosthesis, but this side effect will eventually disappear with continued denture use

E. Orthodontics

1. Role of nutrients—systemically important for the integrity of periodontal tissues; requirements are higher as stresses of tooth movement result in more bone apposition and the synthesis of a new periodontal ligament; nutrients are needed for the healing and repair of gingival injuries and irritations from orthodontic bands

2. Role of sugars—to prevent enamel erosion and decay, dietary sugars (especially retentive sweets) must be restricted during the wearing of appliances

3. Role of food textures—when appliances or bands are tightened, chewing hard-textured foods may be painful, and liquid and soft foods should be eaten temporarily; retentive and sticky foods should be avoided because they become trapped in the appliance and are difficult to remove

Dietary Considerations for the Immunocompromised and Clients with Special Needs

A. Oral cancer

1. Nutritional support for healing and cellular immunocompetence

a. Compromised nutritional status—weight loss and nutrient deficiencies increase the risk of not withstanding the physiologic stresses of cancer and anticancer therapies

b. Surgical treatment—primary method in treating cancer; nutrient requirements are higher as a result of the increased catabolic activities, tissue repair, and host defense activities

c. Chemotherapy and radiation treatment—nutrient needs are higher because of the destruction of healthy cells and tissues that occurs during these types of treatments

d. Possible need for referral to registered dietitian to monitor client's dietary intake during the compromised state

2. Diet modifications useful in treating complications from cancer or cancer treatments

a. Client unable to ingest or digest food

(1) Home enteral feedings can provide nutrients (e.g., nasogastric tube feedings)

(2) Home parenteral feedings can provide nutrients (e.g., intravenous feedings)

b. Eating problems arising from complications or side effects of anticancer therapies

(1) Nausea and vomiting—client should suck on ice chips; eat frequently; eat dry, bland foods; eat and drink slowly; avoid highly spiced and fatty foods; new antinausea medications are effective

(2) Loss of appetite—client should eat foods that are appealing; make up nutrient requirements at times when the appetite is good; eat foods with a high nutrient density

(3) Food aversions and alterations in taste and smell—client should eliminate offending foods; include highly spiced and distinctive textures to improve taste perceptions; cook and serve food in plastic utensils rather than in metal utensils

(4) Dry mouth (xerostomia)—client should use xylitol-containing gum, mints, and sprays; suck on ice chips or use synthetic saliva; drink liquids with meals; eat cold-temperature foods rather than hot-temperature foods; concentrate on highly nutritious liquids

    (5) Radiation-induced caries—client should restrict cariogenic foods; because of changes in both the quality and quantity of saliva following cancer treatment, rapid demineralization of the tooth surface can occur

    (6) Glossitis and stomatitis—client should eat a variety of soft, easy-to-chew foods; eat stewed foods rather than broiled and fried foods; avoid highly spiced or acidic foods; eat moderate-temperature foods; use straws if swallowing is difficult

B. HIV (human immunodeficiency virus)

  1. Causes of malnutrition in HIV-infected persons

    a. Reduced food intake

      (1) Drug treatments cause vomiting, nausea, and food aversions

      (2) Fatigue, depression, and fear cause anorexia

      (3) Oral infections alter taste, cause pain, and reduce saliva flow

      (4) Esophageal infections and respiratory complications hamper swallowing

    b. Increased nutrient loss

      (1) Cancers of the GI tract cause malabsorption

      (2) Drugs cause diarrhea and malabsorption

      (3) PEM leads to malabsorption

    c. Altered metabolism

      (1) Cancer, infections, and fevers increase BMR

      (2) Drug therapy alters nutrient utilization

  2. Nutrient support

    a. Any subclinical nutrient deficiencies and weight loss should be corrected at the time of positive HIV test

    b. At least 100% of the DRI or RDA values of all vitamins and minerals must be provided

    c. Client must avoid all foodborne illnesses

    d. The nutrition plan should be designed on the basis of individual complications, with emphasis on controlling weight loss by eating nutrient-dense foods throughout the day

    e. Dietary recommendations should only be regulated by an MD, an RD, or both.

C. Clients with special needs (see Chapter 19)

  1. Dental problems—unmet oral health care needs in this population significantly exceed those in the general population

    a. The oral caries rate may be higher than that of the general population because of poor oral hygiene and cariogenic food habits

    b. Increased periodontal disease as compared with the general population because of the following:

      (1) Poor oral hygiene; limited self-care

      (2) Diets consisting of soft-textured foods

      (3) Frequent exposures to fermentable carbohydrates

      (4) Metabolic disturbances affecting disease resistance and the reparative process

      (5) Nutritional deficiencies associated with diet or metabolic disturbance

      (6) Malocclusion and developmental defects

    c. Barriers to health care

  2. Nutritional problems—slow growth, excessive weight loss or gain, and nutrient deficiencies can occur in the following situations:

    a. Inability to consume an adequate diet

      (1) Absence or weak sucking response (e.g., cleft lip and palate)

      (2) Poor control of arm and head (e.g., cerebral palsy)

      (3) Inadequate control of jaw, lip, and tongue (e.g., tongue thrust and tonic bite)

      (4) Attention deficit (e.g., intellectual disability and hyperactivity)

    b. Impaired nutrient use

      (1) Malabsorption conditions (e.g., cystic fibrosis)

      (2) Inborn errors of metabolism (e.g., phenylketonuria)

      (3) Drug-nutrient interactions (e.g., anticonvulsant medications can interfere with calcium and phosphorus use)

      (4) Poor muscle control (e.g., constipation)

    c. Excessive intake of foods, calories, and sweets

      (1) Food, especially sweets, often used to reinforce good behavior

      (2) Overfeeding because of parental guilt

      (3) Overemphasis on feeding because mealtime is perceived as the most important time for parent–child interaction

      (4) Excessive calorie intake resulting from inactivity and the pleasurable aspects of eating

@ WEB SITE INFORMATION AND RESOURCES

SOURCE	WEB SITE ADDRESS	DESCRIPTION
Food and Nutrition Center: U.S. Department of Agriculture National Agricultural Library	http://fnic.nal.usda.gov/	Resource for *Dietary Nutrient* database, *Dietary Guidelines*, and the *Food Guide Pyramid*
Healthy People 2010 and 2020	http://www.healthypeople.gov	*Information on Healthy People 2010 and 2020*; includes tips for speakers; valuable resource for community-based activities
American Dental Association	http://ada.org/public/topics/diet.asp	*Information about Your Diet and Dental Health*
The National Academy of Science	http://www.nap.edu	Information about dietary values and standards (RDA, DRI)
Choose My Plate	http://www.choosemyplate.gov	Provides guidance on balance, moderation and adequate consumption of essential food groups; interactive resource for individual groups. Provides specific dietary requirement based on age, gender, and level of physical activity.

REFERENCES

1. Johnson RD, Lawrence LJ, Brands M, et al: Dietary sugars intake and cardiovascular health scientific statement from the American Heart Association, *Circulation* 120: 1011–1020, 2009.
2. Institute of Medicine (IOM), National Academy of Sciences, Food and Nutrition Board: *Dietary Reference Intakes for energy, carbohydrates, fiber, fat, fatty acids, cholesterol, protein, and amino acids*, Washington, DC, 2010, The National Academy Press: Available at http://www.nap.edu/openbook.php?record_id=10490: Accessed May 27, 2010.
3. U.S. Department of Agriculture and U.S. Department of Health and Human Services: *Dietary guidelines for Americans, 2010*, ed 7, Washington, DC: U.S. Government Printing Office, December 2010.
4. Axxya Systems: Nutritionist Pronutrition analysis software, 4800 Sugar Grove Blvd, Suite 602, Stafford, TX 77477: Available at http://www.axxya.com: Accessed May 27, 2010.
5. ESHA Research: Food processor nutrition and fitness analysis software, P.O. Box 13028, Salem, Oregon 97309-1028: Available at: http://www.esha.com: Accessed May 27, 2010.

SUGGESTED READINGS

American Dietetic Association: Position of the American Dietetic Association (ADA): Oral health and nutrition, *J Am Diet Assoc* 107:1418–1428, 2007: Available at http://www.eatright.org/public/files/oral_health.pdf; Accessed May 27, 2010.

Harper Mallonee LF: Nutrition counseling. In Darby M: *Dental hygiene: theory and practice*, ed 3, St Louis, 2010, Saunders.

Palmer CA: *Diet and nutrition in oral health*, ed 2, New Jersey, 2006, Pearson Prentice Hall.

Romito LM: *Nutrition and oral health, The Dental Clinics of North America*, Philadelphia, 2003, Saunders.

Stegeman CA, Davis JR: *The dental hygienist's guide to nutritional care*, ed 3, St Louis, 2010, Saunders.

Touger DR, Sirois DA, Mobley CC: *Nutrition and oral medicine*, ed 1, New Jersey, 2005, Humana Press.

CHAPTER 12 REVIEW QUESTIONS

Answers and Rationales to the Review Questions are available on this text's accompanying Evolve site. See inside front cover for details.

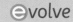

1. **Which one of the following monosaccharides is the most important physiologically?**
   a. Hexoses
   b. Trioses
   c. Pentoses
   d. Tetroses

2. **Which one of the following is an example of a simple carbohydrate composed of two monosaccharide units?**
   a. Glucose
   b. Sucrose
   c. Fructose
   d. Amylose

3. _____is the synthesis of blood glucose from noncarbohydrate sources.
   a. Glycogenolysis
   b. Gluconeogenesis
   c. Glyconeogenesis
   d. Glycolysis

4. **Anabolic hormones are metabolic regulators that raise the blood glucose level. Catabolic hormones lower the blood glucose level.**
   a. The first statement is TRUE; the second statement is FALSE
   b. The first statement is FALSE; the second statement is TRUE
   c. Both statements are TRUE
   d. Both statements are FALSE

5. **Soluble fibers regulate the use of sugars and slow down gastric emptying. All of the following are examples of soluble fibers EXCEPT one. Which one is the EXCEPTION?**
   a. Pectin
   b. Oat bran
   c. Lignin
   d. Mucilages

6. **What is the recommended fiber intake for adults?**
   a. 50 g per day
   b. 35–40 g per day
   c. 20–30 g per day
   d. 15 g per day

7. **All of the following are biologic roles and functions of carbohydrates EXCEPT one. Which one is the EXCEPTION?**
   a. Provide precursors of structural and functional molecules
   b. Provide 9 kcal/g
   c. Provide bulk and palatability to the diet
   d. Spare protein

8. **Nutritive sweeteners are used by the body as an energy source. Which of the following is an example of a nutritive sweetener?**
   a. Aspartame
   b. Xylitol
   c. Saccharin
   d. Sucralose

9. **Which of the following dietary habits is MOST likely to contribute to caries risk?**
   a. Form of simple sugar consumed
   b. Timing of ingestion of simple sugars
   c. Frequency of simple sugar consumption
   d. Total intake of simple sugars

10. **The RDA for digestible carbohydrate is 130 g/day. The minimum adult intake is 50 to 100 g to prevent use of body protein as an energy source.**
    a. The first statement is TRUE; the second statement is FALSE
    b. The first statement is FALSE; the second statement is TRUE
    c. Both statements are TRUE
    d. Both statements are FALSE

11. **Secondary lactose intolerance can occur as a result of all the following EXCEPT one. Which one is the EXCEPTION?**
    a. Congenital absence of lactase
    b. Certain disease conditions that affect the gastrointestinal mucosa
    c. Intestinal injury
    d. Infections that cause injury to the gastrointestinal mucosa

12. **Which of the following is only required by persons with type 2 diabetes?**
    a. Routine blood testing
    b. Daily injections of insulin
    c. Specialized diet to help control the disease
    d. Routine urine testing to monitor ketone levels

13. **Which one of the following terms refers to excessive thirst, a common symptom of diabetes?**
    a. Polyuria
    b. Polyol
    c. Polyphagia
    d. Polydipsia

14. **Which of the following is considered a non-essential amino acid?**
    a. Histidine
    b. Methionine
    c. Phenylalanine
    d. Tyrosine

15. De novo synthesis is an anabolic process that requires all of the following EXCEPT one. Which one is the EXCEPTION?
   a. Deoxyribonucleic acid (DNA)
   b. Messenger ribonucleic acid (mRNA)
   c. Ribosomal ribonucleic acid (rRNA)
   d. α-Keto acid

16. Negative nitrogen balance indicates net protein breakdown. It occurs during childhood, pregnancy, and recovery from undernutrition, surgery, or illness.
   a. The first statement is TRUE; the second statement is FALSE
   b. The first statement is FALSE; the second statement is TRUE
   c. Both statements are TRUE
   d. Both statements are FALSE

17. The following are examples of proteins' various roles in oral biology EXCEPT one. Which one is the EXCEPTION?
   a. Maintain the integrity of pulpal tissue throughout life
   b. Essential for all cells in growth, development, and maintenance of the periodontium
   c. Provide a coating on the tooth's surface and prevent retention of food particles
   d. Essential for the normal function of cellular defenses against subgingival bacteria and toxins.

18. Which of the following conditions is characterized by excessive uric acid production?
   a. Phenylketonuria
   b. Gout
   c. Homocystinuria
   d. Maple syrup urine disease

19. All of the following hormones are anabolic EXCEPT one. Which one is the EXCEPTION?
   a. Insulin
   b. Adrenocortical hormones
   c. Growth hormone
   d. Sex hormones

20. Lipoproteins are responsible for carrying lipids throughout the body. Which of the following lipoproteins primarily carry cholesterol from the liver to peripheral sites?
   a. Very-low-density lipoproteins (VLDL)
   b. Chylomicrons
   c. Low-density lipoproteins (LDL)
   d. High-density lipoproteins (HDL)

21. Cholesterol is a precursor of many steroid compounds and a constituent of cell membranes. Cholesterol comes from all of the following sources EXCEPT one. Which one is the EXCEPTION?
   a. Exogenous sources
   b. Endogenous sources
   c. Plant-based foods
   d. Foods of animal origin

22. All of the following are important post-eruptive effects of carbohydrate on the teeth EXCEPT one. Which one is the EXCEPTION?
   a. Streptococcus mutans synthesize polysaccharides from sucrose which enhances bacterial plaque formation
   b. Carbohydrates provide an energy source for oral bacteria
   c. Lactic acid, pyruvate acid, or acetyl-coenzyme A are the end products of glycolysis for acidogenic bacteria
   d. Carbohydrates contribute to enamel remineralization

23. All of the following describe water-soluble vitamins EXCEPT one. Which one is the EXCEPTION?
   a. They are sensitive to heat, light, and oxygen
   b. They are absorbed by active transport
   c. They contain elements of carbon, hydrogen, oxygen, nitrogen; can also contain cobalt and sulfur
   d. They are absorbed by passive transport
   e. Can be toxic with chronic excessive intake

24. All of the following statements are true about fat, soluble vitamins EXCEPT one. Which one is the EXCEPTION?
   a. Fat-soluble vitamins are not absolutely necessary in the diet every day
   b. Fat-soluble vitamins must be emulsified and carried across the membranes of the intestinal cells in the presence of fat and bile
   c. Fat-soluble vitamins are not readily excreted in urine
   d. Fat-soluble vitamin intake in excess of the daily need is stored in the body

25. Increased caries rate is attributed to a deficiency of vitamin D. Pulp calcification can occur if an excess of vitamin D exists.
   a. The first statement is TRUE; the second statement is FALSE
   b. The first statement is FALSE; the second statement is TRUE
   c. Both statements are TRUE
   d. Both statements are FALSE

26. What role does vitamin C have in tooth formation?
   a. Is involved in the formation of the matrix of dentin and enamel
   b. Is important to the normal growth of dentin and enamel
   c. Controls calcification of dentin and enamel
   d. Is involved in the hydroxylation of proline and lysine in collagen synthesis

27. **Body water, as a percentage of body weight, increases with age. The majority of body water is intracellular.**
    a. The first statement is TRUE; the second statement is FALSE
    b. The first statement is FALSE; the second statement is TRUE
    c. Both statements are TRUE
    d. Both statements are FALSE

28. **Each of the following is associated with dehydration EXCEPT one. Which one is the EXCEPTION?**
    a. Sodium retention
    b. Diarrhea
    c. Malfunction of kidneys
    d. Blood loss

29. **Osteocytes function in the synthesis of the alveolus. They function in the process of bone apposition and resorption. All of the following vitamins are important in the synthesis of the alveolus EXCEPT one. Which one is the EXCEPTION?**
    a. Vitamin C
    b. Vitamin A
    c. Vitamin D
    d. Calcium

30. **In a healthy individual, if the amount of glucose in the blood exceeds the body's immediate energy needs, all of the following can occur EXCEPT one. Which one is the EXCEPTION?**
    a. Glucose will be converted to fat and stored in adipose tissue
    b. Glucose will be stored as glycogen in liver and muscle
    c. Excess glucose will be excreted in urine
    d. Excess glucose can be converted to keto acids to be used in protein synthesis

31. **What is the immediate and preferred source of energy for cellular metabolism?**
    a. Protein
    b. Glucose
    c. Fat
    d. Ethanol

32. **Which of the following is TRUE about the basal metabolic rate (BMR)?**
    a. The BMR should be measured while a person sleeps
    b. The BMR is influenced by climate and altitude
    c. The BMR includes the energy necessary for normal muscle activity
    d. The BMR should be measured at an environmental temperature of 98.6°F

33. **A person with a body mass index (BMI) of _____ is considered overweight.**
    a. 18.5–24.9
    b. 25.0–25.9
    c. 30.0–34.9
    d. >40

34. **Which of the following is not a sign or symptom of disordered eating?**
    a. Periodontitis
    b. Perimylosis
    c. Severe weight loss
    d. Lanugo

35. **Anorexia bulimia is a condition of binging and purging most commonly seen in adolescent females who appear normal in weight. Anorexia nervosa occurs more commonly in females from lower socioeconomic groups who are typically underachievers.**
    a. The first statement is TRUE; the second statement is FALSE
    b. The first statement is FALSE; the second statement is TRUE
    c. Both statements are TRUE
    d. Both statements are FALSE

36. **Thermic effect of food (TEF) is the energy needed to digest, absorb, and metabolize food. Age, gender, and body size are among a few of the factors that influence TEF.**
    a. The first statement is TRUE and the second statement is FALSE
    b. The first statement is FALSE and the second statement is TRUE
    c. Both statements are TRUE
    d. Both statements are FALSE

37. **Vitamins are inorganic substances that are essential to life. Megadoses of vitamins may result in toxicity of one or many nutrients and inhibition of others.**
    a. The first statement is TRUE; the second statement is FALSE
    b. The first statement is FALSE; the second statement is TRUE
    c. Both statements are TRUE
    d. Both statements are FALSE

38. **From which of the following conditions can primary nutrient deficiency result?**
    a. Accessibility to food
    b. Drug–nutrient interactions
    c. Allergies
    d. Metabolic disease

39. **Biochemical disturbances occur as a manifestation of primary and secondary deficiencies. Which of the following statements is TRUE about biochemical disturbances?**
    a. They are the earliest sign of malnutrition
    b. They are determined by clinical examination of body tissues
    c. They occur if duration of deficiency is long enough to deplete the body's stores
    d. They present as signs of chronic and severe malnutrition

40. **Which of the following methods of dietary assessment presents a TRUE measure of intake and is (are) suitable to use with individuals in the clinical setting?**
    a. Food frequency record and 24-hour recall
    b. 24-hour recall and food record diary
    c. Food record diary and food frequency questionnaire
    d. Multiple 24-hour recalls

41. **All of the following are limitations of the direct approach to nutritional counseling EXCEPT one. Which is the EXCEPTION?**
    a. It fosters client dependence
    b. With the indirect approach (also known as the behavior modification approach) more time and effort are required to arrive at solutions to dietary problems
    c. The client is not involved in decision making
    d. Little chance of success exists if the client is not committed

42. **Of the following methods of anthropometric analysis, which one is the MOST accurate measurement for body volume?**
    a. Dual energy x-ray absorptiometry (DEXA)
    b. Skinfold thickness measurement
    c. Bioelectrical impedance
    d. Underwater weighing

43. **Which of the following statements BEST describes the dietary reference intake (DRI)?**
    a. The intake level sufficient to meet nutrient requirements of nearly all healthy individuals
    b. Value based on the observed average or experimentally set intake by individuals that appear to sustain a defined nutritional status
    c. Nutrient intake value estimated to meet the requirements of half the healthy individuals in a group
    d. Value based on approximation of nutrient intake by a group of healthy people

Answer questions 44 to 46 based on Case A.

Case A

Charlie is an 80-year-old male patient, who presents to the dental clinic for routine prophylaxis. His wife passed away about a year ago. Charlie has had several missing teeth on both his maxillary and mandibular arch. He lives on a limited income, so he does not want to have any type of prosthetic dental work done. He says, "I'm old, and I don't need to spend the money on fake teeth—I eat just fine." After reviewing Charlie's health and pharmacologic history, the dental hygienist notes that he has lost a considerable amount of weight in the past 6 months. In addition, four new areas of decay are identified during the oral examination. The hygienist questions Charlie about his dietary habits. Charlie reports that he eats about two meals a day and that he buys a lot of convenience foods because they are much easier to prepare. He adds that he drinks black coffee with two tablespoons of sugar in a day.

44. **The new dental caries activity in Charlie's mouth is most likely caused by all of the following EXCEPT one. Which one is the EXCEPTION?**
    a. Sugar added to coffee
    b. Timing of the foods consumed
    c. Forms of foods consumed
    d. Consumption of only two meals a day

45. **Which of the following statements is TRUE regarding the diet of individuals who are edentulous or who have limited mastication because of loss of teeth?**
    a. Intake of dairy products is reduced
    b. Intake of grains is reduced
    c. Intake of meats is reduced
    d. More fruits and vegetables are consumed

46. **All of the following nutrients are typically lower in those individuals who are edentulous or who have limited mastication because of loss of teeth EXCEPT one. Which one is the EXCEPTION?**
    a. Magnesium
    b. Folic acid
    c. Zinc
    d. Vitamin B_{12}

Answer questions 47 to 49 based on Case B.

Case B

Maria, an 8-year-old girl with cerebral palsy, presents to the dental clinic for her 6-month continued care appointment. The dental hygienist performs an oral examination and updates her dental charting. Maria has severe malocclusion, which makes it difficult for her to clean her teeth adequately. Her gingiva is inflamed. The dental hygienist finds several incipient caries. A periodontal assessment reveals probing depths of 4 to 5 mm isolated to the posterior teeth. Maria's plaque score is 64%. The dental hygienist questions Maria about her daily oral hygiene habits. Maria's mother, who is also attending the appointment, states that her daughter is very diligent about brushing her teeth after meals. However, Maria's limited dexterity affects her oral self-care ability. Maria's diet consists of three balanced meals per day and snacks. Her mother is very diligent about preparing vegetables for Maria, slightly overcooking the vegetables so that they are easy for Maria to eat. Maria consumes three or four glasses of 100% fruit juice daily. Her mother offers juice with meals and also during snack time. Sugar-containing foods are not kept at home, so Maria only consumes them on special occasions.

47. **Individuals with special needs often have more periodontal disease compared with the general population. Which of the following is the MOST LIKELY reason for Maria's increasing pocket depths?**
    a. Poor oral hygiene and malocclusion
    b. Diet
    c. Fruit juice consumption
    d. Nutritional deficiencies

48. **Maria has several areas of incipient decay. All of the following are potential factors to Maria's new areas of decay EXCEPT one. Which one is the EXCEPTION?**
    a. Form of foods consumed
    b. Frequency of foods consumed
    c. Timing of foods consumed
    d. Amount of food consumed

49. **The dental hygienist asks Maria to fill out a dietary intake questionnaire with the assistance of her mother. This type of assessment tool has many advantages. On the basis of the scenario presented above, which of the following would be the best rationale for Maria to use the questionnaire?**
    a. Can be filled out by the client in the oral health care setting
    b. Takes only 15 to 20 minutes to complete
    c. Allows analysis of food group consumption
    d. Allows evaluation of sugar intake

50. **All of the following types of dietary fiber play a role in lowering blood cholesterol EXCEPT one. Which one is the EXCEPTION?**
    a. Pectin
    b. Oat bran
    c. Lignin
    d. Mucilages

CHAPTER 13 Biomaterials

Stephen C. Bayne, John M. Powers, Edward J. Swift, Jr., and Jeffrey Y. Thompson

Biomaterials, restorative materials, and tissue engineering are fundamental to the dental hygiene process of care and are used in a variety of dental hygiene roles and practices. This chapter reviews the general considerations of specific biomaterials as well as preventive and restorative materials, including applications, terminology, and classifications for each; the structures of materials in terms of the starting components, reactions involved in their use, and manipulation procedures; and the properties of materials, including physical, chemical, mechanical, and biologic characteristics.

Direct applications of these materials include dental amalgams; dental composites; pit-and-fissure sealants; infiltrants for lesions; bonding agents; cement liners, cement bases, and other cements; fluoride-releasing restorative materials, topical fluorides, and fluoride varnishes; dentifrices and prophylactic pastes; and bleaching agents. Indirect applications include impression materials, provisional materials, models, casts, dies, waxes, investment materials, casting alloys, dental solders, chromium alloys for partial dentures, porcelain-fused-to-metal (PFM) alloys, dental ceramics, crown-and-bridge cements, acrylic appliances, acrylic denture bases, denture teeth, denture liners, denture cleansers, mouth protectors, veneers, computer-assisted design and computer-assisted machining (CAD/CAM) and copy-milled restorations, and dental implants.

INTRODUCTION

General Considerations

A. Applications for dental biomaterials
  1. Direct preventive and restorative dental procedures
  2. Indirect preventive and restorative dental procedures

B. Definitions and terminology
  1. Materials science terminology
  2. Biomaterials terminology for classification
C. Classification of materials for applications by:
  1. Key parts of composition-influencing properties
  2. Extent of cavity preparation

Structure

A. Composition
  1. Generally two components in a specific ratio
    a. Powder and liquid (P/L)
    b. Powder and powder (P/P)
    c. Water and powder (W/P)
    d. Paste and paste (p/p)
    e. Paste and light
  2. Generally, the liquid part is the major reactant
B. Reaction during use
  1. Physical reaction—solidification by drying or cooling with no chemical reaction
  2. Chemical reaction—solidification by creating new primary bonds within the composition
C. Manipulation
  1. Proportioning variables
    a. Ratio of parts
    b. Temperature
    c. Relative humidity
  2. Mixing variables
    a. Manual mixing
      (1) Method of combining components, for example, stirring and stropping
      (2) Rate of mixing, for example, fast and slow
    b. Auto-mixing
  3. Stages of manipulation
    a. Definitions of times
      (1) Mixing time—time elapsed from onset to completion of mixing
      (2) Working time—time elapsed from onset of mixing to onset of initial setting time

(3) Initial setting time—time at which sufficient reaction has occurred to cause the materials to be resistant to further manipulation

(4) Final setting time—time at which the material is practically set, as defined by its resistance to indentation

b. Definitions of intervals
  (1) Mixing interval—length of time of mixing stage
  (2) Working interval—length of time of working stage
  (3) Setting interval—length of time of setting stage

c. All water-based materials lose their gloss at the time of setting

Properties

A. Physical properties—events that do not involve changes in composition or primary bonds
  1. Descriptive properties
    a. Weight—gravitational force that attracts a body
    b. Mass—resistance of a body to acceleration (or being moved)
    c. Volume—a defined region in three-dimensional space
    d. Density—a body's weight per unit of volume
  2. Thermal properties
    a. Linear coefficient of thermal expansion (LCTE, α)
      (1) Rate of expansion or contraction of one dimension of a material with temperature change (Figure 13-1)
      (2) LCTE = $[(L_2 - L_1)/(L_1)]/(T_2 - T_1)$ where
        (a) L_1 = original length
        (b) L_2 = new length
        (c) T_1 = original temperature
        (d) T_2 = new temperature
      (3) Values reported as: in/in/°F (inch per inch per degree F), $10^{-6}/°F$; cm/cm/°C, (centimeter per centimeter per degree C), 10–6/°C; ppm/°C (parts per million per degree C)
      (4) LCTE values—tooth, 9 to 11 ppm/°C; amalgam, 25 ppm/°C; composite, 35 to 45 ppm/°C; inlay wax, 300 ppm/°C
      (5) When the thermal expansion of restorative material does not match the tooth structure, percolation of fluids occurs at the margins during cyclic heating and cooling
    b. Thermal conductivity
      (1) Insulators transmit heat poorly, for example, dental enamel, dental cements, acrylic polymers, dental porcelain, and ceramic restorations
      (2) Conductors transmit heat easily, for example, dental amalgam and cast gold alloys
      (3) Teeth with metal restorations may be sensitive to hot and cold foods because of their good thermal conduction
      (4) Individuals wearing dentures may not sense normal temperature differences attributable to the thermal insulation of the acrylic denture base
      (5) To be an effective insulator, the material must be at least 0.5 mm thick
  3. Electrical properties—electrical conductivity
    a. Conductors transmit electrons easily, for example, metals
    b. Semiconductors transmit electrons sometimes, for example, ceramics and often composites
    c. Insulators transmit electrons poorly, for example, ceramics and polymers
  4. Surface properties
    a. Contact angle—internal angle of liquid droplet with solid surface
      (1) Good wetting (angle = 0 degrees)
      (2) Spreading (angle < 90 degrees)
      (3) Poor wetting (angle ≥ 90 degrees)
    b. Reflection—degree of surface back-scattering
  5. Color properties
    a. Perception—physiologic response to physical stimulus by the eye, which can distinguish three parameters
      (1) Dominant wavelength—blue, green, yellow, orange, and red
      (2) Luminance—lightness of color from black to white
      (3) Excitation purity—saturation of light

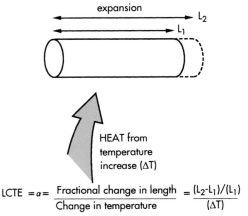

$$LCTE = \alpha = \frac{\text{Fractional change in length}}{\text{Change in temperature}} = \frac{(L_2\text{-}L_1)/(L_1)}{(\Delta T)}$$

FIGURE 13-1 Linear coefficient of thermal expansion.

b. Measurement
(1) Munsell Color System (e.g., 5R 6/4)
(a) Hue—color family (R, YR, Y, GY, G, BG, B, PB, P, RP)
(b) Value—lightness from black to white (0/ to 10/)
(c) Chroma—saturation from gray upward (/0 to /18)
(2) Instrumentation techniques—record the spectral reflectance versus wavelength curves (405 to 700 nm)
(3) L*a*b* color system
(a) L* is value
(b) a* is red, −a* is green
(c) b* is yellow, −b* is blue
(4) Dental manufacturer shade guides
(a) Custom product shades guides
(b) VITA shade guide
(c) VITA Linearguide 3D Master
c. Definitions
(1) Metamerism—colors with different spectral energy distributions that look the same under certain lighting conditions but look different with different light sources
(2) Fluorescence—emission of light by a material when a beam of light is shined on it
(3) Opacity—degree of light absorption by a material
(4) Translucency—degree of internal light reflection
(5) Transparency—degree of light transmission through a material

B. Chemical properties
1. Primary chemical bonding types
a. Types
(1) Metallic, for example, metals
(2) Ionic, for example, ceramics
(3) Covalent, for example, ceramics and polymers
b. Events related to changes in primary chemical bonding
(1) Contraction attributable to chemical reaction
(a) Rate of contraction of size of material during chemical reaction or phase change at constant temperature
(b) Linear change (percent) = $[(L_1 - L_0)/(L_0)] \times 100\%$
where
L_0 = original length
L_1 = final length (after 24 hours)
(c) Values reported as percentage changes
(2) Corrosion of surfaces

2. Secondary chemical bonds
a. Types
(1) Hydrogen bonding—where hydrogen is attracted to an electronegative element; found in most water-based liquids
(2) Van der Waals forces—dispersion forces caused by fluctuating dipoles; found in dental composites and acrylics
b. Events related to changes in secondary chemical bonding
(1) Adsorption—uptake "onto" the surface of the solid
(2) Absorption—uptake "into" the solid
(a) Example—water absorbed by denture
(b) Example—moisture absorbed by alginate (imbibition)
(3) Desorption—fluid lost from the solid; for example, water lost from alginate (syneresis)
(4) Solubility—material loss by dissolution of surface
(5) Disintegration—material loss by disruption of solid, usually by absorbed water

3. Corrosion
a. Chemical corrosion—chemical reaction at surface
(1) Products may be soluble
(2) Products may be insoluble and form layers (tarnish)
b. Electrochemical corrosion—chemical reaction that requires an anode (e.g., dental amalgam), a cathode (e.g., gold crown), an electrolyte (e.g., saliva), and an electrical circuit (e.g., contact) for electron flow (Figure 13-2)
(1) Galvanic corrosion—dissimilar metals in contact (examples above)
(2) Local galvanic corrosion (structure selective corrosion)—dissimilar phases in the same metal in contact
(3) Crevice corrosion—corrosion in the crack under plaque, between a restoration and the tooth structure, or in the scratch on the surface of a restoration, where the metals may be the same but the electrolytes are different locally
c. Corrosion potential
(1) Immune—does not corrode (i.e., cathodic)
(2) Active—corrodes readily (i.e., anodic)
(3) Passive—corrosion produces protective film, for example, chromium oxide film on stainless steel

C. Mechanical properties
1. Resolution of forces (Figure 13-3)
a. Uniaxial (one-dimensional) forces—compression, tension, and shear

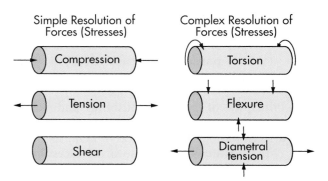

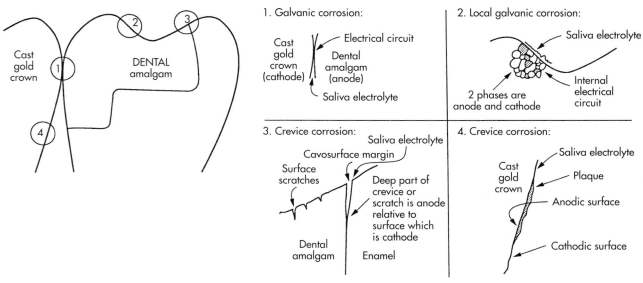

FIGURE 13-2 Electrochemical corrosion.

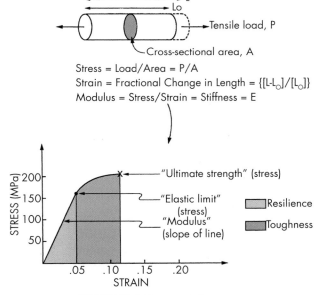

FIGURE 13-3 Resolution of forces.

FIGURE 13-4 Stress–strain curve.

b. Complex forces—torsion, flexure, and diametral tension or compression
2. Normalization of forces and deformations
   a. Stress
      (1) Applied force (or material's resistance to force) per unit area
      (2) Stress = force/area
          Lb/in^2 (pounds per square inch, psi)
          Kg/cm^2 (kilogram per square centimeter)
          MN/m^2 (megapascals, MPa
   b. Strain (Figure 13-4)
      (1) Change in length per unit of length because of force
      (2) Strain = $(L - l_0)/(l_0)$; dimensionless units
3. Stress-strain diagrams
   a. Plot of stress (vertical) versus strain (horizontal)
      (1) Allows convenient comparison of materials

      (2) Different curves for compression, tension, and shear
      (3) Curves depend on rate of testing and temperature
   b. Analysis of curves (see Figure 13-4)
      (1) Elastic behavior
         (a) Elastic strain—initial response to stress (elastic—when the stress is removed, the strain returns to zero and the material returns to its original length)

(b) Elastic modulus—slope of first part of curve; represents the stiffness of the material, or the resistance to deformation under force

(c) Elastic limit (proportional limit)—stress above which the material no longer behaves totally elastically

(d) Yield strength—stress that is an estimate of the elastic limit at 0.002 permanent strain

(e) Hardness—value on a relative scale that estimates the elastic limit in terms of a material's resistance to indentation, for example, Knoop hardness scale, Diamond pyramid hardness scale, Brinnell hardness scale, Rockwell hardness scale, Barcol scale, Shore A hardness scale, and Mohs' hardness scale (Table 13-1); hardness values are used to determine the ability of abrasives to alter the substrates they contact

(f) Resilience—area under the stress–strain curve up to the elastic limit; estimates the total elastic energy that can be absorbed before the onset of plastic deformation

(2) Elastic and plastic behavior

(a) Beyond the stress level of the elastic limit, a combination of both elastic and plastic strain exists

(b) Ultimate strength—highest stress reached before fracture; the ultimate compressive strength is greater than the ultimate shear strength and the ultimate tensile strength

(c) Elongation (percent elongation)—percent change in length up to the point of fracture = strain × 100%

(d) Brittle materials—<10% elongation at fracture

(e) Ductile materials—>10% elongation at fracture

(f) Toughness—area under the stress–strain curve up to the point of fracture (it estimates the total energy absorbed up to fracture)

(3) Time-dependent behavior

(a) Strain rate sensitivity—the faster a stress is applied, the more likely a material is to store the energy elastically and not plastically

(b) Creep (i.e., strain relaxation with time in response to a constant stress, such as dental wax deforming because of built-in stresses created during cooling)

(c) Stress relaxation (with time in response to a constant strain)

(d) Fatigue—failure caused by cyclic loading

4. Principles of cutting, polishing, and surface cleaning

a. Terminology

(1) Cutting—gross removal of excess material from the surfaces of restorations or teeth

(2) Finishing—fine removal of surface material in an effort to produce finer surface scratches

(3) Polishing—smoothing of surfaces by removal of fine scratches

(4) Debriding—removal of unwanted material attached to surfaces

(5) Air abrasion (air-polishing)—removal or polishing of hard tissue by the kinetic energy from particles sprayed against the surface

(6) Microabrasion—removal of stains by a mixture of an abrasive and hydrochloric acid

b. Surface mechanics for materials (Table 13-2)

(1) Cutting—requires materials with the highest possible hardness to produce the cuts

(2) Finishing—requires materials with the highest possible hardness for the best effect, except at the margins of restorations, where the tooth structure may be inadvertently affected

TABLE 13-1 Mohs' Scale for Hardness*

Number	Hardness
10	Diamond
9	Corundum
8	Topaz
7	Quartz
6	Orthoclase
5	Apatite
4	Fluorite
3	Calcite
2	Gypsum
1	Talc

*Standard for checking hardness of abrasives and substrates.

TABLE 13-2 Hardness Values for Dental Substrates*

Hardness Value	Number
CAD/CAM ceramic	6–7
Porcelain	6–7
Composite	5–7
Glass	5–6
Dental enamel	5–6
Dental amalgam	4–5
Dentin	3–4
Hard gold alloys	3–4
Pure gold	2–3
Acrylic	2–3
Cementum	2–3

*Based on Mohs' scale: diamond = 10; talc = 1 (see Table 13-1).

(3) Polishing—requires materials with a Mohs' hardness that is only 1 to 2 units above that of the substrate
(4) Debriding—requires materials with a Mohs' hardness that is less than or equal to that of the substrate to prevent scratching
c. Factors affecting cutting, polishing, and surface cleaning
(1) Applied pressure
(2) Particle size of abrasive
(3) Hardness of abrasive
(4) Hardness of substrate
(5) Speed of rotary instrument
d. Factors affecting air abrasion
(1) Abrasive particle size—27 μm or 50 μm aluminum oxide
(2) Air pressure—higher air pressure cuts faster but may cause discomfort
e. Precautions
(1) During cutting, heat will build up and change the mechanical behavior of the substrate from brittle to ductile and encourage smearing
(2) Instruments may transfer debris onto the cut surface from their own surfaces during cutting, polishing, or cleaning operations (this has important implications in cleaning dental implant surfaces)
D. Biologic properties
1. Definitions of biohazards
a. Toxicity—cell or tissue death attributable to material concentration

b. Sensitivity—systemic reaction to a substance
(1) Allergy—reaction to relatively small amounts of a material
(2) Hypersensitivity—reaction to minute amounts of a material
2. Definitions of local tissue interactions with biomaterials
a. Fibrous tissue capsule formation (tissue encapsulation)
b. Integration at the interface (osseo-integration)
(1) Bone ingrowth
(2) Bone ongrowth
c. Biodegradation (desorption or resorption)
3. Classification of biologic materials—tissue interfaces
a. Intraoral and supragingival—in enamel or dentin
b. Intraoral, pulpal, or periapical
c. Transcutaneous
d. Subcutaneous
e. Intraosseous
4. Clinical analysis of biocompatibility
a. Risk versus benefits
b. Safety and efficacy
5. Agencies that oversee materials, devices, and therapeutics
a. Regulatory agencies—U.S. Food and Drug Administration (FDA)
b. Standards development for manufacturing practices (for physical, chemical, mechanical, and biologic properties and for clinical testing)
(1) American Dental Association (ADA)—Council on Scientific Affairs
(2) American National Standards Institute (ANSI)
(3) Federation Dentaire Internationale (FDI)
(4) International Standards Organization (ISO)

DIRECT PREVENTIVE AND RESTORATIVE MATERIALS

Dental Amalgam

A. General considerations
1. Applications
a. Load-bearing restorations for posterior teeth (class I, class II)
b. Pin-retained restorations
c. Buildups (foundations) or cores for cast restorations
d. Retrograde root canal filling material

2. Terminology
   a. Amalgam alloy—powder particles of Ag-Sn-Cu-(Zn) (*Note*: Minor elements are indicated in parentheses)
   b. Amalgam—reaction product of any material with mercury
   c. Dental amalgam—reaction product of amalgam alloy (Ag-Sn or Ag-Sn-Cu) with mercury
3. Classification of dental amalgam by:
   a. Powder particle shape
      (1) Irregular (comminuted, filing, or lathe-cut)
      (2) Spherical (spherodized)
      (3) Blends, for example, irregular–irregular, irregular–spherical, or spherical–spherical
   b. Total amount of copper
      (1) Low-copper alloys (conventional, traditional); <5% copper (Ag-Sn-Cu)
      (2) High-copper alloys (corrosion-resistant); 12% to 28% copper (Ag-Sn-Cu)
   c. Presence of zinc
   d. Other modifications
4. Examples
   a. Low-copper, irregular-particle alloy, for example, 70Ag-26Sn-4Cu
   b. High-copper, blended-particle alloy with irregular particles, for example, 70Ag-26Ag-4Cu and spherical particles, for example, 72Ag-28Cu
   c. High-copper, spherical-particle alloy, for example, 60Ag-27Sn-13Cu

B. Structure
1. Components
   a. Mercury mixed with amalgam alloy
   b. Mercury reacts with periphery of alloy particle to produce crystalline silver–mercury, tin–mercury, and copper–tin phases
2. Reaction (Figure 13-5)
   a. Setting reactions
      (1) Low-copper dental amalgam
         Hg + Ag-Sn → Ag-Sn + Ag-Hg + Sn-Hg
      (2) High-copper dental amalgam
         Hg + Ag-Sn-Cu → Ag-Sn-Cu + Ag-Hg + Cu-Sn
         and

Hg + Ag-Sn + Ag-Cu → Ag-Sn + Ag-Cu + Ag-Hg + Cu-Sn
   b. Phases in set amalgams
      (1) Residual alloy (Ag-Sn, Ag-Sn-Cu, or Ag-Cu)—strongest; most corrosion-resistant
      (2) Ag-Hg (=γ_1) = major matrix phase in low-copper or high-copper dental amalgams
      (3) Sn-Hg (=γ_2) = second matrix phase in low-copper dental amalgams
      (4) Cu-Sn (η or ε) = second matrix phase in high-copper dental amalgams
3. Manipulation
   a. Selection—based on clinical requirements for strength
   b. Packaging
      (1) Powder or pressed tablets; mercury
      (2) Precapsulated powder and mercury
   c. Mixing
      (1) Mercury-alloy—specific to each product but generally less than 1:1 so that amalgam contains 41% to 50% mercury
      (2) Mechanical amalgamators—variable time, speed (frequency and amplitude), and amalgamator motion for different equipment; variables affect the mixing process
      (3) Each amalgamator has specific settings for each different amalgam alloy (e.g., high-copper amalgams require 5 to 10 seconds)
      (4) Amalgamator capsules are disposable
      (5) Pestle may be included in the capsule for mixing efficiency
      (6) Overmixed mass is difficult to remove from capsule
      (7) Undermixed mass is crumbly
   d. Condensation
      (1) Adaptation of amalgam to cavity walls
      (2) Removal of excess mercury-rich matrix produces a stronger and more corrosion-resistant amalgam because it minimizes the formation of the matrix phases of amalgam, which are the least desirable parts of the set material
      (3) Amalgams with spherical alloys are more fluid and require larger-tipped condensers
      (4) It is important to condense in small increments, overpack restoration, avoid delays, and avoid saliva contamination
   e. Finishing
      (1) The anatomy shouldbe carved within a few minutes after condensing
      (2) The surface should be burnished or the final finish performed at least 24 hours later

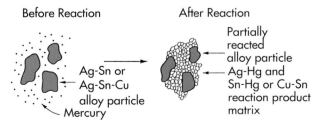

FIGURE 13-5 Amalgam reaction.

C. Properties
  1. Physical
    a. Coefficient of thermal expansion = 25 ppm/°C
    b. Thermal conductivity—high (therefore, the amalgam may need an insulating liner or base in very deep cavity preparations)
  2. Chemical
    a. Dimensional change on setting, should be less than ±20 μm (excessive expansion can produce postoperative pain)
    b. The cavity varnish or the bonding agent electrically insulates a dental amalgam restoration, but it does not prevent corrosion
    c. Chemical corrosion produces a black or green tarnish on the surface that is aesthetically unacceptable but is not detrimental to oral health
    d. Electrochemical corrosion produces penetrating corrosion of low-copper amalgams but produces only superficial corrosion of high-copper amalgams
  3. Mechanical
    a. Compressive strength—ranges from 310 to 480 MPa, comparable with enamel (410 MPa) but is not significant in preventing marginal fracture
    b. Because of low tensile strength, enamel support is needed at the margins
    c. Spherical high-copper alloys develop high tensile strength quickly and can be polished sooner than enamel
    d. Excessive creep occurs during the Ag-Hg phase of incorrectly mixed amalgams and contributes to early marginal fracture
    e. Marginal fracture is correlated with creep and electrochemical corrosion in low-copper amalgams (Figure 13-6)
    f. Bulk fracture (isthmus fracture) occurs across the thinnest portions of amalgam restorations because of high stresses during traumatic occlusion, the accumulated effects of fatigue, or both
    g. Dental amalgam is relatively resistant to abrasion, that is, wear
  4. Biologic
    a. Mercury hygiene
      (1) All personnel must be trained; all personnel must be made aware of mercury sources in the oral care setting
      (2) A proper work-area design is important; personnel must work in well-ventilated spaces; the treatment area atmosphere must be periodically checked for mercury vapor
      (3) Pre-encapsulated products should be stored in tight containers
      (4) Mercury should not come into contact with the skin.
      (5) Spills should be cleaned up immediately to minimize mercury vaporization
      (6) Amalgamators should be used with covers enclosing the mixing arm
      (7) High-vacuum suction should be used during amalgam alloy placement, setting, polishing, or removal when mercury may be vaporized
      (8) All scrap amalgam should be salvaged and stored in tightly closed containers and recycled in accordance with applicable laws
      (9) Mercury-contaminated items must be disposed of in sealed bags and not in medical waste containers
      (10) The dental office personnel must be aware of aerosols created by vacuuming mercury spilled on the floor or the carpet
      (11) Floor coverings should be replaced every 5 years to eliminate accumulated spilled mercury that might have accumulated in carpet pores
      (12) Professional clothing must be removed before leaving the workplace
    b. Mercury bioactivity
      (1) Depends on whether the form is metallic, inorganic, or organic mercury
      (2) Metallic mercury is the least toxic form and is absorbed primarily through the lungs rather than through the gastrointestinal (GI) tract or skin
      (3) Mercury accumulated in the body may come from air, water, food, dental sources (a low amount), or medical sources
      (4) Average half-life for mercury elimination from the body is 55 days
      (5) Occupational Safety and Health Administration (OSHA) has set the average level

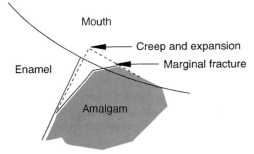

FIGURE 13-6 Marginal ditching in an amalgam restoration is produced by creep and expansion, which elevate the margins of the amalgam, and functional stresses produce marginal fracture.

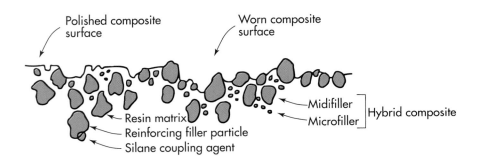

FIGURE 13-7 Hybrid dental composite.

for mercury toxicity by exposure as <50 μg/m³ per 40-hour workweek

(6) Incidence of mercury hypersensitivity is estimated to be <1 per 100 million persons

c. Environment issues-important to:
(1) Use best management practices (BMPs)
(2) Use precapsulated alloys
(3) Manage mercury through recycling—recycle used disposable amalgam capsules; salvage, store, and recycle noncontact amalgam; salvage amalgam pieces from restorations after removal, and recycle amalgam waste; use chairside traps to retain amalgam and recycle contents; recycle contents retained by vacuum pump filter or other amalgam-collection devices; disinfect extracted teeth that contain amalgam restorations using bleach, and recycle them with chairside trap wastes.

D. Amalgam alternatives
1. Indium-containing amalgam can have lower mercury vapor pressures than conventional dental amalgam
2. Esthetic filling materials (composites, all-ceramic restorations, compomers)
3. Cast-gold, PFM, or all-ceramic restorations

Dental Composites

A. General considerations
1. Applications
a. Anterior restorations created for aesthetic purposes (class III, IV, and V cervical erosion, or abrasion lesions)
b. Low-stress posterior restorations (small class I and II)
c. High-stress posterior restorations with certain formulations
d. Veneers
e. Cores for cast restorations
f. Cements for ceramic restorations
g. Cements for resin-bonded bridges

h. Repair systems for composites or ceramic restorations

2. Terminology (Figure 13-7)
a. Composite—physical mixture of materials to average the properties of the materials involved
b. Dental composite—restoration material resulting from the mixture of ceramic reinforcing filler particles in a monomer matrix that is converted to polymer on setting
c. Polymerization—reaction of small molecules (monomers) into very large molecules (polymers)
d. Cross-linking—tying together of polymer molecules by chemical reaction between the molecules to produce a continuous three-dimensional network

3. Classification by:
a. Amount of filler—25% to 75% by volume, 45% to 85% by weight
(1) Very high—packable
(2) High—hybrid or all-purpose composite
(3) Moderate—flowable composite
(4) Low—microfill
b. Filler particle size
(1) Average sizes—minifill = 0.1 to 1.0 μm; microfill = 0.01 to 0.1 μm; nanofill = 0.001 to 0.01 μm
(2) Mixture of sizes—hybrid (micro-hybrid = mini + micro)
(3) Presence of precured composite (heterogeneous)
c. Polymerization method
(1) Auto-cured (also self-cured, SC)
(2) Visible light-cured (VLC)
(3) Dual-cured (VLC + SC)
d. Matrix chemistry
(1) Bisphenol A–glycidylmethacrylate Bis-GMA or Bis-GMA–like monomers
(2) Urethane dimethacrylate (UDM or UDMA) monomers
(3) TEGDMA (tetraethyleneglycol dimethacrylate)—diluent monomer to reduce viscosity

(4) Oxirane (or oxetane) expanding monomers—to control overall polymerization shrinkage

B. Structure
  1. Components
  a. Filler particles—colloidal silica, crystalline silica (quartz), or silicate glasses (noncrystalline) of various particle sizes (containing Ba, Li, Al, Zn, Yr, and others)
  b. Matrix—Bis-GMA (or UDMA) with lower-molecular-weight diluents (e.g., TEGDMA) that co-react during polymerization; ring-opening monomers
  c. Coupling agent—silane, which chemically bonds the surfaces of the filler particles to the polymer matrix
  2. Reaction
  a. Free-radical polymerization—monomers + initiator + accelerators → polymer molecules
  b. Initiators—start polymerization by decomposing and reacting with monomer
  (1) Benzoyl peroxide typically used in SC systems
  (2) Camphorquinone typically used in VLC systems
  c. Accelerators—speed up initiator decomposition; different amines used for accelerating initiators in SC and VLC systems
  d. Retarders or inhibitors—prevent premature polymerization
  3. Manipulation
  a. Selection
  (1) Microfill composites or micro-hybrids for anterior class III, IV, and V restorations
  (2) Micro-hybrids for class I, II, III, IV, and V restorations
  b. Conditioning of enamel and dentin (see bonding agents)
  (1) Total-etch technique:
    (a) Acid-etch with 15% to 38% phosphoric acid
    (b) Have the client rinse for 5 to 10 seconds with water
    (c) Air-dry enamel for 5 to 10 seconds, but do not desiccate or dehydrate
    (d) Apply bonding agent and polymerize
  (2) Self-etch technique (apply bonding system)
  c. Mixing (if required)—two pastes are mixed for 20 to 30 seconds
  (1) Self-cured composite—working time is 60 to 120 seconds after mixing
  (2) Light-cured composite—working time is nearly unlimited; used for most anterior and some posterior composite restorations; natural light and dental chair lights may slowly start the reaction
  (3) Dual-cured composite—working time is 5 to 8 minutes
  d. Placement—a plastic instrument or syringe or a unidose compule should be used
  e. Light curing—it is important to:
  (1) Check the output of the light-curing unit
  (2) Use high-intensity QTH (quartz-tungsten-halogen) or LED (light-emitting-diode)
  (3) Cure incrementally in ≤1.5-mm–thick layers; use a matrix strip, where possible, to produce a smooth surface and to contour the composite
  f. Finishing and polishing—it is important to:
  (1) Remove the oxygen-inhibited layer
  (2) Use stones, carbide burrs, or diamonds for gross reduction
  (3) Use multi-fluted carbide burrs or special diamonds for fine reduction
  (4) Use aluminum oxide strips or discs for finishing or rubber points, cups, and discs
  (5) Use fine aluminum oxide or diamond finishing pastes
  (6) Microfill and nanofill composites develop smoothest finish because of small size of filler particles
  (7) Keep in mind that liquid polishes provide short-term smooth surface coatings

C. Properties—generally improve with filler content
  1. Physical
  a. Radiopacity depends on the ions in silicate glass
  b. The coefficient of thermal expansion is 35 to 45 ppm/°C and decreases with increasing filler content
  c. Thermal and electrical insulators
  2. Chemical
  a. Water absorption is 0.5% to 2.5% and increases with polymer content
  b. Acidulated topical fluorides (e.g., acidulated phosphate fluoride [APF]) tend to dissolve glass particles, and thus composites should be protected with a non-petroleum based jelly during these procedures, or a different topical fluoride such as neutral sodium fluoride should be used
  c. Major color changes have occurred in resin matrix with time because of oxidation, which produces colored byproducts, but the newer products are highly color stable
  3. Mechanical
  a. The compressive strength is 310 to 410 MPa, which is adequate

b. Wear resistance—improves with higher filler content, higher percentage of conversion in curing, use of microfiller, and closer interparticle spacing of fillers

c. Surfaces that are rough from wear retain plaque biofilm and stain more readily

4. Biologic—the components may be cytotoxic, but the cured composite is biocompatible as restorative filling material

Pit-and-Fissure Sealants

A. General considerations—see the section on "Dental Sealants" in Chapter 16
  1. Applications
     a. Occlusal surfaces of newly erupted posterior teeth
     b. Lingual surfaces of anterior teeth with fissures
     c. Occlusal surfaces of teeth in older persons with reduced flow of saliva (because low levels of saliva increase susceptibility to dental caries)
  2. Classification by:
     a. Polymerization method
        (1) Self-curing
        (2) Light-curing—90% of current products
     b. Filler content
        (1) Unfilled—many systems are unfilled because filler tends to interfere with and wear away from self-cleaning occlusal areas; sealants are designed to wear away, except where no self-cleaning action occurs; a common misconception is that sealants should be wear resistant
        (2) Lightly filled—10% to 30% by weight
B. Structure
  1. Components
     a. Monomer—Bis-GMA–like or UDMA monomers with TEGDMA, a diluent monomer, to facilitate flow into pits and fissures before cure
     b. Initiator—benzoyl peroxide (in self-cured) and camphorquinone (in light-cured)
     c. Accelerator—amine
     d. Opaque filler—1% titanium dioxide or other colorant to make the material detectable on tooth surfaces
     e. Reinforcing filler—silicate glass (generally not added because wear resistance is not required within pits and fissures)
     f. Fluoride—may be added for slow release
  2. Reaction—free radical reaction (see the section on "Dental Composites")

3. Manipulation
   a. Preparation—this involves:
      (1) Cleaning the pits and fissures of organic debris
      (2) Etching the occlusal surfaces, pits, and fissures with 37% phosphoric acid
      (3) Washing the occlusal surfaces for 5 to 10 seconds
      (4) Drying the etched area for 5 to 10 seconds with clean air spray
      (5) Applying the sealant and polymerizing
   b. Mixing or dispensing
      (1) Self-cured—equal amounts of liquids are mixed in a Dappen dish for 5 seconds with a brush applicator
      (2) Light-cured—syringes or unidose tips are used for dispensing
   c. Placement—pits, fissures, and occlusal surfaces; this involves:
      (1) 60 seconds for self-cured materials to set
      (2) Light-curing according to manufacturer's instructions
   d. Finishing
      (1) Unpolymerized (air-inhibited layer) and excess materials should be removed
      (2) The hardness and marginal adaptation of the sealant should be examined
      (3) Occlusal adjustments should be made, where necessary, in the sealant; most unfilled sealant materials are self-adjusting
C. Properties
  1. Physical—wetting: low-viscosity sealants wet acid-etched tooth structure the best
  2. Mechanical
     a. Wear resistance should not be too great because the sealant should be able to wear off the self-cleaning areas of tooth
     b. To prevent loss, sealants should be protected during polishing procedures with air-abrading units
  3. Biologic—no apparent biologic problems
  4. Clinical efficacy
     a. Effectiveness is 100% if retained in pits and fissures
     b. Requires routine clinical evaluation (every $1\frac{1}{2}$ to 2 years) to check the integrity and resealing of defective areas if sealant loss is attributable to poor retention
     c. Sealants resist attack from topical fluorides (also applied for prevention of dental caries)

Infiltrants

A. General considerations
  1. Applications—approximal and smooth-surface uncavitated lesions where sealing would not be

a permanent solution to stop lesion growth and create good aesthetics

2. Definition—a resin system capable of penetrating through slightly porous enamel, embedding into an existing decalcified region of dentin, stopping lesion activity by preventing the diffusion of organic acids below plaque and restoring the aesthetics of the tooth structure

3. Classification—this is a new and novel approach to minimally invasive dentistry for interproximal uncavitated lesion repair; currently, only one system is available on the market
  a. Approximal application kit
  b. Smooth surface application kit

B. Structure
  1. Components—acrylic monomer infiltrant after use of a hydrochloric (HCl) acid etchant to create micropores in the enamel overlying the lesion and to allow resin penetration
  2. Reaction—the resin is light-cured
  3. Manipulation (approximal repair)
    a. Wedging of teeth to separate interproximate contacts
    b. Application of acid etchant (>90s with 15% aqueous HCl) to create micropores through the overlying enamel by using a unique holder and a film packet to deliver materials
    c. VLC materials

C. Properties
  1. Physical—the tooth structure appears to have normal color and opacity after infiltration
  2. Chemical—no evidence of dentin decalcification after infiltration
  3. Mechanical—previously decalcified dentin is restored to approximately the same hardness
  4. Biologic—no evidence of any threat to the pulp before setting

Bonding Agents

A. General considerations
  1. Applications—composites, resin-modified glass ionomers, compomers, bonded ceramic restorations, veneers, orthodontic brackets, desensitizing dentin by covering exposed tubules, resin-bonded bridges, composite-repair and ceramic-repair systems, and amalgams
  2. Definitions
    a. Smear layer—thin layer of compacted debris on enamel and dentin resulting from the cavity-preparation process (Figure 13-8) that is weakly held to the surface (5 to 6 MPa) and that limits bonding agent strength if not removed
    b. Etching (or conditioning)—smear layer removal and production of microspaces for

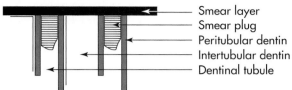

[Cavity preparation]

— Smear layer
— Smear plug
— Peritubular dentin
— Intertubular dentin
— Dentinal tubule

FIGURE 13-8 The surface of cut dentin, with a smear layer and smear plugs occluding the dentinal tubules.

micromechanical bonding by dissolving minor amounts of surface hydroxyapatite crystals
      (1) Total-etch (or etch-and-rinse)—phosphoric acid should be used
      (2) Self-etch—reliance on acidic monomer to dissolve smear layer, etch surface of intertubular dentin, and embed collagen fibers
    c. Priming—micromechanical (and possibly chemical) bonding to the microspaces created by the conditioning step
    d. Conditioning and priming agent (self-etching primer)—agent that accomplishes both actions
    e. Bonding—formation of resin layer that connects the primed surface to the overlying restoration, for example, composite

  3. Classification
    a. Major substrate
      (1) Enamel and dentin bonding system—for bonding to enamel and dentin composite or other restorative materials
      (2) Amalgam bonding system—for bonding amalgam to enamel and dentin to amalgam
      (3) Universal bonding system—for bonding an appliance to enamel, dentin, amalgam, porcelain, or any other substrate that may be necessary for a restorative procedure using the same set of procedures and materials
    b. Number of components and type of etching (Figure 13-9)
      (1) Three-component total-etch system—etching + priming + bonding (E + P + B) (also called *fourth-generation*; involves two layers of material)
      (2) Two-component total-etch system—etching + priming/bonding (E + PB) (also called *fifth-generation*; involves one layer of material)
      (3) Two-component self-etch system—etching/priming + bonding (EP + B) (also called *sixth-generation type-1*; involves two layers of material)

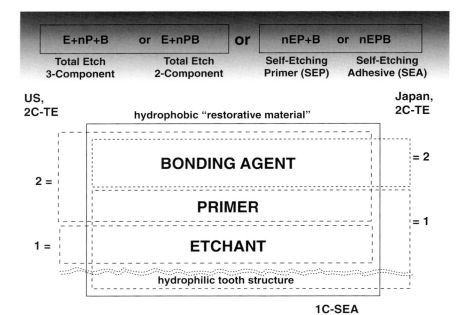

FIGURE 13-9 Evolution of bonding system types with fewer components.

(4) One-component self-etch system—etching/priming/bonding) (EPB)—materials are mixed (if necessary) and scrubbed onto the surface to be bonded using the applicator tip (also called *sixth-generation type-2*; involves 1 layer of material)

B. Structure

1. Components of bonding systems

a. Conditioning agent—mineral (e.g., 10% to 40% phosphoric acid), organic acid (e.g., polyacrylic acid), or acrylic monomer acid (e.g., phosphonate)

b. Priming agent—resin and monomer in alcohol, acetone, or water

c. Bonding agent—Bis-GMA or UDMA monomers

2. Reaction

a. Bonding occurs primarily by intimate micromechanical retention, with the relief created by the conditioning step

b. Chemical bonding is possible but is not recognized as contributing significantly to the overall bond strength

3. Manipulation (manufacturer's instructions should be followed)

a. Conditioning

(1) Total-etch technique—this involves:

(a) Applying phosphoric acid solution or equivalent

(b) Rinsing and drying without desiccation (dentin should be kept moist with "glistening" appearance)

(c) In case of overdried dentin, remoistening surface with water or a rewetting solution for 10 to 15 seconds

(2) Self-etch technique—this involves applying an acidic primer or a bonding agent

b. Priming—this involves:

(1) Applying a priming agent, and gently drying to remove excess solvent (but airthinning must not be done unless recommended by manufacturer)

(2) Applying several layers until dentin is fully impregnated to surface

c. Bonding—this involves:

(1) Applying one to two coats of bonding agent when bonding composites

(2) Applying multiple coats of the bonding agent or mixing it with a thickening agent in preparation for bonding with amalgam restorations

C. Properties

1. Physical—thermal expansion and contraction may create fatigue stresses that debond the interface and permit microleakage

2. Chemical—water absorption into the bonding agent may chemically alter the bonding

3. Mechanical—mechanical stresses may produce fatigue that can debond the interface and permit microleakage

a. Enamel bonding—adhesion occurs by macrotags (between enamel prisms) and microtags (into enamel prisms) to produce micromechanical retention

b. Dentin bonding—adhesion occurs by removal of smear layer and formation of microtags within intertubular dentin to produce a hybrid zone (interpenetration or diffusion zone) that microscopically intertwines collagen bundles and bonding agent polymer. Macrotags within tubules do not add much to retention because they are poorly polymerized and poorly adapted

4. Biologic

   a. Conditioning agents may be locally irritating if they come into contact with soft tissue

   b. Uncured priming agents, particularly those based on hydroxyethyl methacrylate (HEMA), may become skin sensitizers for dental personnel after several contacts

   (1) Hands and face must be protected from inadvertent contact with unset materials and their vapors

   (2) HEMA and other priming monomers may penetrate through rubber gloves in relatively short times (60 to 90 seconds)

Cement Liners (Calcium Hydroxide; Zinc Oxide–Eugenol)

A. General considerations—applications (if remaining dentin thickness is <0.5 mm)

   1. Thermal insulation where the cavity preparation is close to the pulp

   2. Delivering medications to the pulp

   a. Calcium hydroxide (CH) liners—in self-cured and light-cured versions that stimulate reparative dentin

   b. Zinc oxide–eugenol relieves pain by desensitizing nerves

B. CH structure (for zinc oxide–eugenol types; see the section on "Dental Sealants")

   1. Components

   a. Paste of CH reactant powder, ethyl toluene sulfonamide dispersant, zinc oxide filler, and zinc stearate radiopacifier

   b. Paste of glycol salicylate reactant liquid, titanium dioxide filler powder, and calcium tungstenate radiopacifier

   2. Reaction

   a. Chemical reaction of calcium ions with salicylate to form methylsalicylate salts

   b. Moisture absorbed to allow CH to dissociate into ions to react with salicylate

   c. Mixture sets from outside surface to inside as water diffuses

   3. Manipulation

   a. Dentin should not be dehydrated, or material will not set

b. A drop each of the pastes should be mixed together for 5 seconds

c. The material should be applied to dentin; 1 to 2 minutes should be allowed for the material to set

C. CH properties

   1. Physical—good thermal and electrical insulator

   2. Chemical—poor resistance to water solubility, so may dissolve

   3. Mechanical—low compressive strength (0.7 to 3.4 MPa)

   4. Biologic—releases constituents, which diffuse toward the pulp and stimulate reparative dentin formation

Cement Bases

A. General considerations (limited use)

   1. Applications

   a. Thermal insulation below a restoration (Figure 13-10)

   b. Mechanical protection where dentin is inadequate to support amalgam condensation pressures

   2. Classification (many materials have been used in the past)

   a. Glass ionomer (GI) cement bases

   b. Resin-modified glass ionomer (RMGI)—light-curing compositions

B. Structure (see the section on "Luting cements")

   1. Components

   a. Self-curing cements (ZP, PC, GI)—reactive powder (chemically basic) and reactive liquid (chemically acidic)

   b. Light-curing cements (RMGI)—paste

   2. Reaction

   a. Self-curing cement—acid–base reaction that forms salts or cross-linked matrix; reaction may be exothermic

   b. Light-curing cements—monomer polymerization is exothermic

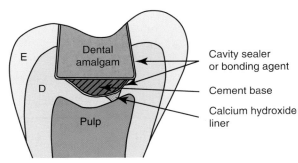

FIGURE 13-10 Sealer, liner, and base applications for use with dental amalgam. *E*, Enamel; *D*, dentin.

3. Manipulation—consistency for basing includes more powder, which improves all of the cement properties
C. Properties
  1. Physical—excellent thermal and electrical insulation
  2. Chemical—much more resistant to dissolution than cement liners
    a. PC and GI cements are chemically adhesive to tooth structure
    b. Solubility of all cement bases is lower than that of cement liners if they are mixed at higher powder-to-liquid ratios
  3. Mechanical—much higher compressive strengths (80 to 210 MPa) than those of luting cements
    a. Light-cured RMGI cements are the strongest
    b. Zinc oxide–eugenol cements are the weakest
  4. Biologic (see the section on "Luting cements" for details)—PC, GI, and RMGI cements, properly handled, provide good biocompatibility with pulp

Other Cement Applications

A. Root canal sealers
  1. Applications
    a. Cementing of silver cone or gutta-percha point
    b. Paste filling material
  2. Classification
    a. Zinc oxide–eugenol cement types
    b. Noneugenol cement types
    c. Therapeutic cement types
    d. Flowable composite types
  3. Important properties
    a. Physical—radiopacity
    b. Chemical—insolubility
    c. Mechanical—flow; tensile strength
    d. Biologic—inert
B. Gingival tissue packs
  1. Application—provide temporary displacement of gingival tissues
  2. Composition—slow-setting zinc oxide–eugenol cement mixed with cotton twills for texture and strength

C. Surgical dressings
  1. Application—gingival covering after periodontal surgery
  2. Composition—modified zinc oxide–eugenol cement (containing tannic acid, rosin, and various oils)
D. Orthodontic cements
  1. Application—cementing of orthodontic bands
  2. Composition—composite (see the sections on "Luting Cements" or "Bonding Agents")
  3. Manipulation
    a. Resin (composite) cements use total etch or self-etch bonding systems for improved bonding
    b. Band, bracket, or cement removal requires special care

Fluoride-Releasing Restorative Materials

A. General considerations
  1. Applications for glass ionomers, resin-modified glass ionomers, compomers, and atraumatic restorative technique (ART) materials
    a. Class V restorations—glass ionomers and resin-modified glass ionomers for geriatric dentistry
    b. Class I and II restorations—resin-modified glass ionomers and compomers in pediatric dentistry; and ART temporary restorations in people living in the underserved regions of the world
    c. Class III restorations—resin-modified glass ionomers and compomers
  2. Classification by composition
    a. Conventional glass ionomers—limited use
    b. Metal-modified glass ionomers—limited use
    c. Resin-modified glass ionomers (hybrid ionomers)—popular use
    d. Compomers—limited use (Figure 13-11)
    e. Giomers—limited use
    f. Resin-reinforced glass ionomers (ART materials)—extremely popular use for temporaries, ART, and permanent restorations in pediatric dentistry applications (representing

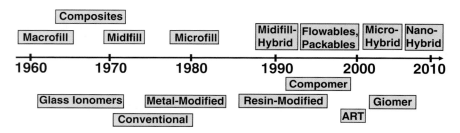

FIGURE 13-11 Evolution of glass ionomer composites over 35 years, leading toward composites.

the largest use of glass ionomer restorative material)

B. Structure

1. Components

a. Conventional glass ionomers—aluminosilicate glass powder and liquid water solution of co-polymers (or acrylic acid with maleic, tartaric, or itaconic acids)

b. Metal-modified glass ionomers—used for cores

c. Resin-modified glass ionomers—aluminosilicate glass powder and liquid with water solution of co-polymers (or acrylic acid with maleic, tartaric, or itaconic acids) and water-soluble monomers, for example, HEMA

d. Compomers—hybrid of resin-modified glass ionomer and composite

e. Giomers—compomers with precured glass ionomer particles blended into a mixture

f. Resin-reinforced (ART materials)—high F-releasing conventional glass ionomer that may have small amounts of resin added for increased tackiness

2. Reactions (may involve several reactions and stages of setting)

a. Glass ionomer reaction (acid–base reaction of polyacid and ions released from aluminosilicate glass particles)

(1) Calcium, aluminum, fluoride, and other ions released by the outside of the powder particle dissolving in acidic liquid

(2) Calcium ions initially cross-link acid-functional co-polymer molecules

(3) Calcium cross-links are replaced in 24 to 48 hours by aluminum ion cross-links, with increased hardening of system

(4) If no other reactants are present in the cement (e.g., resin modification), then protection from saliva is required during the first 24 hours, unless otherwise indicated by manufacturer's instructions

b. Polymerization reaction (polymerization of double bonds from water-soluble monomers or pendant groups on the co-polymer to form cross-linked matrix)

(1) Polymerization reaction can be initiated with chemical (self-curing) or light-curing steps

(2) Cross-linked polymer matrix ultimately interpenetrates the glass ionomer matrix

(3) Occurs in resin-modified glass ionomer materials and compomers

3. Manipulation

a. Self-curing materials—powder and liquid components may be manually mixed or may be pre-encapsulated for mechanical mixing; light-curing materials—directly placed from a syringe or a unidose tip

b. Placement—mixture is normally placed by using a syringe

c. Finishing—can be immediate if the system is resin modified or is a compomer system (but otherwise must be delayed 24 to 72 hours until aluminum ion replacement reaction is complete)

d. Sealing—the resin sealer is applied to smooth the surface (and to protect against moisture affecting the glass ionomer reaction)

C. Properties

1. Physical

a. Good thermal and electrical insulation

b. Better radiopacity than with most composites

c. Linear coefficient of thermal expansion and contraction is closer to that of the tooth structure than that of composites (but is less well matched for resin-modified and compomer systems)

d. The aesthetics of resin-modified and compomer systems are not quite as good as those of most composites

2. Chemical

a. Reactive acid side groups of co-polymer molecules produce chemical bonding to the tooth structure

b. Fluoride ions are released

(1) Rapid release at first because of excess fluoride ions in the matrix

(2) Slow release after 7 to 30 days because of slow diffusion of fluoride ions out of aluminosilicate particles (Figure 13-12)

(3) Presence of fluoride in topical fluorides and fluoride-containing toothpastes may recharge the fluoride content in the cement matrix temporarily for 2 to 3 days

c. The solubility resistance of resin-modified systems is close to that of composites

3. Mechanical

a. Compressive strength of resin-modified systems and compomers is much better than that of conventional glass ionomers but not quite as strong as that of composites

b. Glass ionomers are more brittle than are composites

4. Biologic

a. Ingredients are biologically compatible with pulp

b. Fluoride ion release may reduce the incidence and severity of secondary caries (see Figure 13-12), but no definitive clinical research studies exist

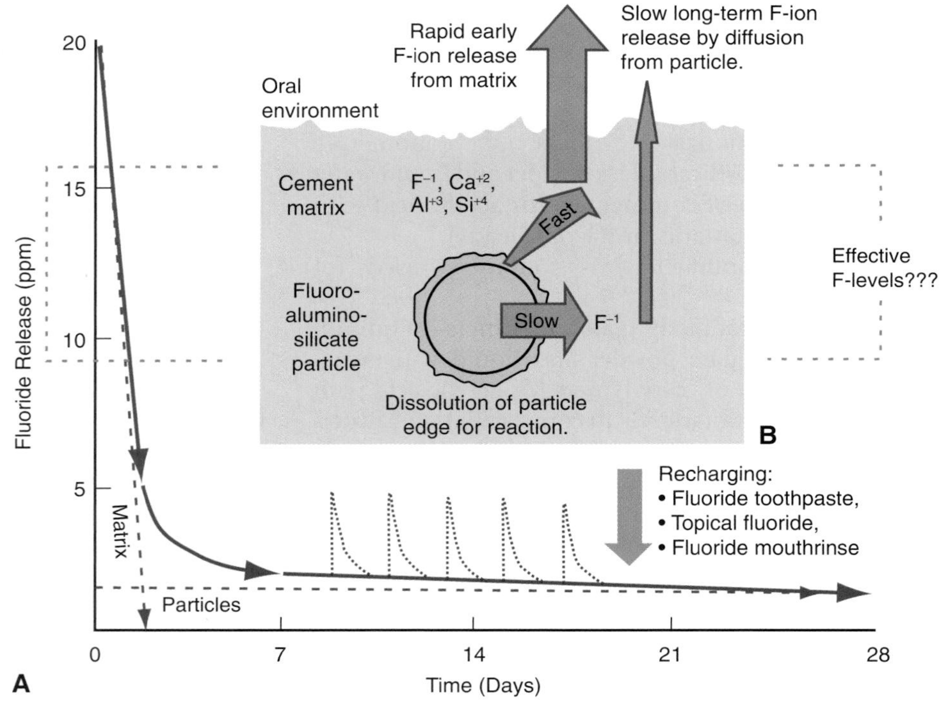

FIGURE 13-12 A, Fluoride ion release from glass ionomer. Diffusion from cement. **B,** Fluoride concentration released over time. *(From Bayne SC, Thompson JY: Biomaterials. In Roberson TM, Heymann HO, Swift EJ, editors: Sturdevant's art and science of operative dentistry, ed 5, St Louis, 2006, Mosby.)*

Topical Fluorides and Fluoride Varnishes

A. General considerations (see the section on "Fluoride Agents for Professional Application" in Chapter 16)
   1. Applications—used to prevent smooth-surface caries
   2. Classification
      a. Acidulated phosphate fluoride (APF) gels (acid pH)
      b. Neutral fluoride gels (sodium fluoride at neutral pH)
      c. Fluoride varnishes (5% sodium fluoride, 2.26% fluoride, 22,600 ppm fluoride)
B. Structure for APF
   1. Composition
      a. APF
         (1) Fluoride ion concentration ranges from 1.22% to 1.32%
         (2) Ingredients—2% sodium fluoride, 0.34% hydrogen fluoride, 0.98% orthophosphoric acid, thickening agent, flavoring agent, coloring agent, and aqueous gel
         (3) pH ranges from 3 to 4; may dissolve glass in restorations, thus those surfaces must be protected
      b. Neutral fluoride gels

   c. Fluoride varnishes—fluoride source mixed with urethane or other resin and dissolved in solvent
   2. Reactions
      a. APF—acid demineralization of the outer layer of enamel; fluoride accelerates the remineralization of demineralized enamel; fluoride ions are incorporated to produce fluoride-substituted hydroxyapatite
      b. Neutral fluoride gels—form fluoride salts on surfaces of teeth
      c. Fluoride varnishes—provide temporary film to allow longer-term fluoride diffusion from varnish into enamel
   3. Manipulation
      a. Gels are applied in a soft, spongy tray after extrinsic stain removal; teeth should be free from saliva; maxillary and mandibular trays are loaded, placed in position, and squeezed to mold the trays tightly around teeth; the tray is held in position for 4 minutes (shorter applications are not effective); the client is told not to eat, smoke, or drink for 30 minutes
      b. Varnishes are painted onto all tooth surfaces; wear away after several hours
C. Properties
   1. Chemical—enamel solubility is decreased by fluoride ion incorporation

2. Biologic—enamel is more resistant to carious dissolution

Dentifrices and Prophylactic Pastes

A. General considerations
1. Cleansing—removal of exogenous stains, pellicle, materia alba, and other oral debris without causing undue abrasion to tooth structure
2. Polishing—smoothing surfaces (without significant abrasion) of amalgam, composites, glass ionomers, ceramic, and other restorative materials
3. Factors influencing cleaning and polishing
    a. Hardness of abrasive particles versus that of the substrate (see Tables 13-1 and 13-2)
    b. Particle size of abrasive particles
    c. Pressure applied during procedure
    d. Temperature of abrasive materials
    e. Speed of the rotating instrument used (easiest factor to control)

B. Structure
1. Composition—contain abrasives, such as kaolinite, silicon dioxide, calcined magnesium silicate, diatomaceous silicon dioxide, pumice, sodium–potassium–aluminum silicate, or zirconium silicate; some pastes also may contain sodium fluoride or stannous fluoride, but they have not been shown to produce therapeutic effects
2. Reactions—abrasion for cleansing and polishing
3. Manipulation (see the section on "Principles of Cutting, Polishing, and Surface Cleaning")

C. Properties
1. Mechanical
    a. Products with pumice and quartz enable more efficient cleansing but also generate greater abrasion of enamel and dentin
    b. Coarse pumice is the most abrasive
    c. Dentin is abraded five to six times faster than enamel, regardless of the product used, and cementum is abraded even more quickly than is dentin
    d. Polymeric restorative materials such as denture bases, denture teeth, composites, and composite veneers can easily be scratched during polishing
    e. Ceramic restorations that are externally characterized should not be polished, or the surface color will be lost
2. Biologic—no known problems

Whitening Agents

A. General considerations
1. Lighten discolored teeth

2. Classification by:
    a. Site of application
        (1) External—applied to the tooth surface
        (2) Internal—applied inside the pulpless (endodontically treated) tooth
    b. Method of application
        (1) In-office—applied professionally
        (2) At-home—dispensed by the dentist or obtained over the counter (OTC) and applied by the client

B. Structure
1. In-office systems use light, heat, or both to "activate" a high concentration (up to 30% to 39%) hydrogen peroxide gel or paste, but little evidence that light or heat provides any benefit exists
2. At-home systems typically use a 10% carbamide peroxide (equivalent to 3.4% hydrogen peroxide) or higher (15% to 20% carbamide peroxide) concentration that is applied in a custom-fitted, mouthguard-type soft plastic tray
3. New systems use thin polyethylene strips impregnated with 5.3% hydrogen peroxide (OTC) and 14% hydrogen peroxide (office dispensed)

C. Properties
1. The effectiveness of whitening depends on application time and dose
2. In-office whitening can provide faster results but is more expensive than at-home bleaching
3. Yellow-colored teeth bleach more rapidly than do gray-colored teeth
4. Tetracycline-stained teeth whiten very slowly (several months of daily at-home treatment needed) or not at all
5. Most common side effects are tooth sensitivity and gingival irritation; both are transient

INDIRECT PREVENTIVE AND RESTORATIVE MATERIALS

Impression Materials

A. General considerations
1. Applications
    a. Dentulous impressions for casts for prosthodontics
    b. Dentulous impressions for pediatric and orthodontic appliances
    c. Dentulous impressions for study models for orthodontics
    d. Edentulous impressions for casts for denture construction
2. Terminology
    a. Rigid—inflexible and cannot be removed from undercut area

TABLE 13-3 Impression Materials

Materials	Type	Reaction	Composition	Manipulation	Initial Setting Time
Plaster (Limited use)	Rigid	Chemical	Calcium sulfate hemihydrate, water	Mix powder and liquid (P/L) in bowl	3–5 min
Compound (Limited use)	Rigid	Physical	Resins, wax, stearic acid, and fillers	Soften by heating	Variable (sets on cooling)
Zinc oxide–eugenol [Limited use]	Rigid	Chemical	Zinc oxide powder, oils, eugenol, and resin	Mix pastes on pad	3–5 min
Agar-agar (Limited use)	Flexible	Physical	12%–15% agar, borax, potassium sulfate, and 85% water	Conditioned in heated bath	Variable (sets on cooling)
Alginate	Flexible	Chemical	Sodium alginate, calcium sulfate, retarders, and 85% water	Mix P/L in bowl	4–5 min
Polysulfide (Limited use)	Flexible	Chemical	Low-molecular-weight (Low MW) mercaptan polymer, fillers, lead dioxide, copper hydroxide, or peroxides	Mix pastes on pad	5–7 min
Silicone (Limited use)	Flexible	Chemical	Hydroxyl functional dimethyl siloxane, fillers, tin octoate, and orthoethyl silicate	Mix pastes on pad	4–5 min
Polyether	Flexible	Chemical	Aromatic sulfonic acid ester and polyether with ethylene imine groups	Mixing gun or mixing machine	4–6 min
Polyvinyl siloxane (Addition silicone)	Flexible	Chemical	Vinyl silicone, filler, chloroplatinic acid, Low MW silicone, and filler	Mixing gun or mixing machine	4–5 min

b. Flexible—can be removed from undercut area
c. Hydrocolloid—gel produced by interconnection of small particles (colloid, <1 µm) dispersed in water
d. Elastomeric—based on flexible polymeric material

3. Classification
   a. Rigid impression materials (very limited use)
      (1) Plaster
      (2) Compound
      (3) Zinc oxide–eugenol
   b. Flexible hydrocolloid impression materials
      (1) Agar-agar (reversible hydrocolloid)
      (2) Alginate (irreversible hydrocolloid)
   c. Flexible, elastomeric, general-purpose impression materials
      (1) Polysulfide elastomer (mercaptan rubber [limited use])
      (2) Silicone elastomer (condensation silicone [laboratory use])
      (3) Polyether (PE) elastomer
      (4) Polyvinyl siloxane (PVS) (addition silicone)
      (5) PE–VPS hybrid

d. Precision impression materials used for prosthodontics
   (1) Addition silicones—contain surfactants to make surface wetting easier
   (2) Polyethers—more hydrophilic

B. Structure
   1. Components (Table 13-3)
      a. Most contain fillers to control shrinkage
      b. Matrix
   2. Reaction (see Table 13-3)
      a. Physical reaction—cooling causes reversible hardening
      b. Chemical reaction—irreversible reaction during setting
   3. Manipulation
      a. Mixing
         (1) P/L types mixed in bowl (plaster and alginate)
         (2) Thermoplastic materials not mixed (compound and agar-agar)
         (3) Hand-mix—paste–paste types are hand mixed on a pad (zinc oxide–eugenol, polysulfide rubber, silicone rubber, polyether rubber, and polyvinyl siloxane)

(4) Auto-mix—paste–paste types are mixed through a disposable nozzle on an auto-mixing gun (polyvinyl siloxane, polyether)

(5) Machine-mix—components mixed and extruded through a disposable nozzle using small machine, for example, Penta-mix 2

b. Placement

(1) Mixed material—carried in a tray to the mouth (full arch, quadrant, or triple tray)

(2) The material sets in the mouth more quickly because of higher temperature

c. Removal—rapid removal of the impression encourages deformation to take place elastically rather than permanently (elastic recovery requires approximately 20 minutes)

d. Cleaning and disinfection of impressions (see the section on "Maintaining the Treatment Area During Client Care" in Chapter 10)

e. Problems—polyvinyl siloxane may be inhibited from bonding at the surface of the preparation wall by the dentin-bonding agent and also may be dissolved by subsequent infection-control solutions; components from latex gloves can contaminate the impression

Provisional Materials

A. General considerations

1. Applications

a. While waiting for laboratory fabrication of cast restoration

b. While observing the reaction of pulp tissue

2. Terminology

a. Temporary—provisional or nonpermanent; range of use is 2 to 52 weeks

b. Short-term use—2 to 6 weeks

c. Longer-term use—6 to 52 weeks

d. Provisional materials—usually include both provisional restoration and provisional cement

e. Direct—set intraorally (in situ)

f. Indirect—set out of the mouth

3. Objectives

a. Physiologic objectives—protection of hard and soft tissues, pulpal protection, delivery of medication, stabilization of tooth, provision of function for chewing, and provision of patient comfort

b. Aesthetic objectives—short-term resistance to staining

c. Clinical objectives—ease of use, low cost, ease of repair, low polymerization exotherm, minimal surface reactions on curing, absence of sensitivity reactions

d. Material performance objectives—fracture resistance, wear resistance

4. Classification

a. Provisional resins

b. Temporary or provisional cements

B. Structure

1. Components

a. Provisional restorations

(1) Zinc oxide–eugenol cement, with cotton fibers

(2) Acrylic P/L products

(3) Bis-acryl and bis-methacryl resin products

b. Provisional cements

(1) Zinc oxide–eugenol-based cements

(2) Calcium hydroxide cements

(3) Admix cements (cements mixed with petroleum jelly)

(4) Composite cements (without bonding systems)

2. Reaction (see the sections on "Dental Composites" and "Cement Liners")

3. Manipulation (see the sections on "Dental Composites" and "Cement Liners")

C. Properties

1. Physical

a. Excellent thermal and electrical insulation

b. Percolation resistance is good for cements but poor for resins

2. Chemical—generally good resistance to dissolution

3. Mechanical

a. Good short-term resistance to fracture

b. Poor resistance to abrasion

c. Limited color stability and stain resistance

4. Biologic—cements are biocompatible, but resins with low-molecular-weight monomers may cause pulpal inflammation if cured in situ without caution

Model, Cast, and Die Materials

A. General considerations

1. Applications

a. Gold casting, ceramic, and porcelain-fused-to-metal veneer fabrication procedures

b. Orthodontic and pediatric appliance construction

c. Study models for occlusal records

2. Terminology

a. Models—replicas of hard and soft tissues for study of dental symmetry

b. Casts—working replicas of hard and soft tissues for use in the fabrication of appliances or restorations

TABLE 13-4 Gypsum Products

Characteristics	Plaster	Stone	Diestone
Chemical name	β-Calcium sulfate hemihydrates	α-Calcium sulfate hemihydrate	α-Calcium sulfate hemihydrate
Formula	$CaSO_4 \cdot \frac{1}{2}H_2O$	$CaSO_4 \cdot \frac{1}{2}H_2O$	$CaSO_4 \cdot \frac{1}{2}H_2O$
Uses	Plaster models, impression plaster	Cast stone, investments	Improved stone, diestone
Water (W)			
Reaction water	18 mL	18 mL	18 mL
Extra water	32 mL	12 mL	6 mL
Total water	50 mL	30 mL	24 mL
Powder (P)	100 g	100 g	100 g
W/P ratio	0.50	0.30	0.24

c. Dies—working replicas of one tooth (or a few teeth) used for the fabrication of a restoration

d. Duplicates—second casts prepared from original casts

3. Classification by materials
   a. Models (model plaster or orthodontic stone)
   b. Casts (regular stone)
   c. Dies—may be electroplated (very limited use)
      (1) Diestone—gypsum product
      (2) Epoxy dies—epoxy polymer; abrasion-resistant dies

B. Structure of gypsum products
   1. Components (Table 13-4)
      a. Powder (calcium sulfate hemihydrate = β-$CaSO_4 \cdot \frac{1}{2} H_2O$)
      b. Water (for mixing and reacting with powder)
   2. Reaction
      a. Calcium sulfate hemihydrate (one-half mole of water) crystals dissolve and react with water
      b. Calcium sulfate dihydrate (two moles of water) form and precipitate new crystals
      c. Unreacted (excess) water is left between crystals and slowly evaporates
   3. Manipulation
      a. Selection—based on strength for models, casts, or dies
      b. Mixing
         (1) Appropriate proportions of water and powder are dispensed (see Table 13-4)
         (2) The powder is sifted into the water in a rubber mixing bowl
         (3) A stiff-blade spatula is used to mix the mass on the side of the bowl
         (4) The mixing is completed in 60 seconds

   c. Placement
      (1) Vibration is used to remove air bubbles created through mixing
      (2) Vibration is used to keep the mixture wet and help it flow into the impression

C. Properties
   1. Physical
      a. Excellent thermal and electrical insulator
      b. Dense
      c. Excellent dimensional accuracy (setting expansion)
         (1) Plaster: 0.20%
         (2) Stone: 0.10%
         (3) Diestone: 0.05%
         (4) High-expansion diestone: 0.20% (for all-ceramic restoration fabrication)
      d. Good reproduction of fine detail of hard and soft tissues
   2. Chemical
      a. Heating will reverse the reaction, that is, decompose the material into calcium sulfate hemihydrate, the original dry component
      b. Models, casts, and dies should be wet during the grinding or cutting to prevent heating
   3. Mechanical
      a. Better powder packing and lower water content at mixing lead to higher compressive strengths (plaster < stone < diestone)
      b. Poor resistance to abrasion (polymer added to improve resistance)
   4. Biologic
      a. Materials are safe for contact with external epithelial tissues
      b. Masks should be worn during grinding or polishing operations, which are likely to produce gypsum dust

Waxes

A. General considerations
 1. Applications
  a. Making impressions
  b. Registering of tooth or soft tissue position
  c. Creating restorative patterns for laboratory fabrication
  d. Aiding in laboratory procedures
 2. Terminology
  a. Inlay wax—used to create a pattern for inlay, onlay, or crown for subsequent investing and casting in a metal alloy
  b. Casting wax—used to create a pattern for metallic framework for removable partial dentures
  c. Baseplate wax—used to establish the vertical dimension, plane of occlusion, and initial arch form of a complete denture
  d. Corrective impression wax—used to form a registration pattern of soft tissues on an impression
  e. Bite registration wax—used to form a registration pattern for the occlusion of opposing models or casts
  f. Boxing wax—used to form a box around an impression before pouring a model or cast
  g. Utility wax—soft, pliable adhesive wax for modifying appliances, such as alginate impression trays
  h. Sticky wax—sticky when melted and used to temporarily adhere pieces of metal or resin in laboratory procedures
 3. Classification
  a. Pattern waxes—inlay, casting, and baseplate waxes
  b. Impression waxes—corrective and bite registration waxes
  c. Processing waxes—boxing, utility, and sticky waxes
B. Structure
 1. Components
  a. Base waxes—hydrocarbon (paraffin) or ester waxes
  b. Modifier waxes—carnauba, ceresin, beeswax, rosin, gum dammar, or microcrystalline waxes
  c. Additives—colorants
 2. Reaction—waxes are thermoplastic (soften on heating, harden on cooling)
C. Properties
 1. Physical
  a. High coefficients of thermal expansion and contraction
  b. Insulators (cool unevenly); should be placed in increments to allow heat dissipation
 2. Chemical
  a. Degrade prematurely if overheated
  b. Designed to degrade into CO_2 and H_2O during burnout for inlay waxes
 3. Mechanical—stiffness, hardness, and strength depend on modifier waxes used and on temperature

Investment Materials

A. General considerations
 1. Applications
  a. Mold-making materials for casting alloys or castable ceramics to facilitate the creation of oversize mold space to compensate for shrinkage during cooling of casting alloy
  b. Mold-making materials for denture production
 2. Terminology—*investment* refers to the mold-making material
 3. Classification
  a. Gypsum-bonded investments (GBI)—based on gypsum products for matrix
  b. Phosphate-bonded investments (PBI)
  c. Silicate-bonded investments (SBI)
  d. Specialty investments—for glass ceramics, titanium alloys, and other specialized fabrication procedures
B. Structure—66% filler, 33% binder (matrix forms on setting), 1% modifiers
 1. Components
  a. Liquid—water or other reactant starts the formation of the matrix binder by reacting with the powder
  b. Powder—reactant powder, filler, or modifiers
 2. Reactions and mold expansion
  a. Setting expansion while material reacts, forming crystals that push on each other
  b. Hygroscopic expansion while setting mold placed under water
  c. Thermal expansion during heating of mold to casting temperature
  d. Filler expansion caused by the inversion of crystalline lattice during heating
 3. Manipulation
  a. P/L is mixed and placed in a container around the wax pattern
  b. After setting, the investment is heated to eliminate the wax pattern in preparation for casting

Casting Alloys

A. General considerations
 1. Applications—inlays, onlays, crowns, and bridges

2. Terminology
   a. Precious (metals)—based primarily on valuable elements (Au, Pt, Pd, Ag, Ir, Rh, Rd)
   b. Noble or immune—corrosion-resistant element or alloy
   c. Base or active—corrosion-prone alloy
   d. Passive—corrosion-resistant because of surface oxide film (*passivation* is the prevention of corrosion by the formation of a thin, adherent oxide film on the metal surface, which acts as a barrier to further oxidation)
   e. Purity by weight (99.99% = 4 nines pure)
   f. Karat (24 karat is 100% gold; 18 karat is 75% gold)
   g. Fineness (1000 fineness is 100% gold; 500 fineness is 50% gold)

3. Classification
   a. High-gold alloys are >75% wt gold or other noble metals (= 50% atoms that are immune)
      (1) ADA type I—83% wt noble metals, for example, in simple inlays
      (2) ADA type II—≥78% wt noble metals, for example, in inlays and onlays
      (3) ADA type III—≥75% wt noble metals, for example, in crowns and bridges
      (4) ADA type IV—≥75% wt noble metals, for example, in partial dentures
   b. Medium-gold alloys are 25% wt to 75% wt gold or other noble metals
   c. Low-gold alloys are <25% wt gold or other noble metals
   d. Gold-substitute alloys do not contain gold
      (1) Palladium-silver alloys—passive because of mixed oxide film
      (2) Cobalt–chromium or nickel–chromium alloys—passive because of Cr_2O_3 oxide film
   e. Titanium alloys are based on 90% to 100% titanium; passive because of TiO_2 oxide film

B. Structure
   1. Components of gold alloys
      a. Gold contributes to corrosion resistance
      b. Copper contributes to hardness and strength
      c. Silver counteracts orange color of copper
      d. Palladium increases melting point and hardness
      e. Platinum increases melting point
      f. Zinc acts as oxygen scavenger during casting
   2. Manipulation
      a. Heated to just beyond melting temperature for casting
      b. Cooling shrinkage causes substantial contraction

C. Properties
   1. Physical
      a. Electrical and thermal conductors
      b. Relatively low coefficient of thermal expansion
   2. Chemical
      a. Silver content affects susceptibility to tarnish
      b. Corrosion resistance is attributed to high noble metal content or passivation
   3. Mechanical
      a. High tensile and compressive strengths but relatively weak in thin sections such as margins; can be deformed relatively easily
      b. Good wear resistance except in contact with ceramic

Dental Solders

A. General considerations
   1. Applications—fabrication of cast bridges and metallic orthodontic appliances
   2. Terminology
      a. Soldering—joining using filler metal that melts below 500°C
      b. Brazing—joining using filler metal that melts above 500°C
      c. Welding—melting and alloying of pieces to be joined
      d. Fluxing
         (1) Oxidative cleaning of area to be soldered
         (2) Oxygen scavenging to prevent oxidation of alloy being soldered
      e. Numeric terminology: 16 to 650 = 650 fineness solder to be used with 16-karat alloys; fineness refers to the gold or other precious metal content
   3. Classification
      a. Gold solders—bridges
      b. Silver solders—gold-substitute bridges and orthodontic alloys

B. Structure of gold solders
   1. Composition—lower gold content than of alloys being soldered
   2. Manipulation—solder must melt below melting temperature of alloy

C. Properties
   1. Physical—similar to alloys being joined
   2. Chemical—more prone to chemical and electro-chemical corrosion
   3. Mechanical—similar to alloys being joined but weaker
   4. Biologic—similar to alloys being joined

Chromium Alloys for Partial Dentures

A. General considerations
   1. Applications—casting partial denture metal frameworks

2. Classification
   a. Cobalt–chromium
   b. Nickel–chromium
B. Structure
   1. Composition
      a. Chromium—produces a passivating oxide film for corrosion resistance
      b. Cobalt—increases the rigidity of the alloy
      c. Other elements—increase strength and castability
   2. Manipulation
      a. Require higher temperature investment materials (PBI or SBI)
      b. More difficult to cast because less dense than gold alloys; usually require special casting equipment
      c. Much more difficult to finish and polish because of higher strength and hardness
C. Properties
   1. Physical—less dense than gold alloys
   2. Chemical—passivating corrosion behavior
   3. Mechanical—stronger, stiffer, and harder than gold alloys
   4. Biologic
      a. Nickel may cause sensitivity in some individuals (approximately 6% of men, and 11% to 24% of women)
      b. Beryllium in some alloys forms oxide that is toxic, which is a significant problem for dental laboratory technicians if grinding dust is inhaled

Porcelain-Fused-to-Metal Alloys

A. General considerations
   1. Applications—substructures for porcelain-fused-to-metal (PFM) crowns and bridges
   2. Classification
      a. High-gold alloys
      b. Palladium–silver alloys
      c. Cobalt–chromium alloys
B. Structure
   1. Composition
      a. High-gold alloys are 98% gold, platinum, palladium, or both
      b. Palladium–silver alloys are 50% to 60% palladium and 30% to 40% silver
      c. Chromium–cobalt alloys are 60% to 65% chromium and 25% to 30% cobalt, with other metals
   2. Manipulation
      a. Must have melting temperatures above that of porcelains (low-fusing porcelains) that will be fabricated onto their surfaces
      b. More difficult to cast (see the section on "Chromium Alloys for Partial Dentures")

C. Properties
   1. Physical
      a. Except for high-gold alloys; others are less dense alloys
      b. Alloys are designed to have low thermal expansion coefficients that must be matched to the veneering porcelain
   2. Chemical—high-gold alloys are immune to corrosion; others passivate
   3. Mechanical—high modulus and hardness
   4. Biologic—biologically acceptable if they do not corrode

Dental Ceramics

A. General considerations
   1. Applications
      a. Veneering material for PFM crowns and bridges
      b. All-ceramic, high-strength inlays, onlays, crowns, and bridges
      c. Denture teeth
   2. Terminology
      a. Ceramic—any inorganic material containing metallic and nonmetallic elements, generally formed at a high temperature
      b. Porcelain—ceramic composition based primarily on silica, alumina, and potassium oxide; created by mixing clay, feldspar, and quartz, and then heating
      c. PFM restoration—metal-based coping (substructure) coated with a porcelain veneer
      d. All-ceramic—inlay, onlay, crown, bridge, or veneer made entirely of ceramic
      e. Fusing—coalescence of packed layer of particles into a single porcelain mass
      f. High-strength ceramics—ceramics that include one or more phases or strengthening mechanisms to make the composition mechanically more crack-resistant than conventional porcelains
      g. Glass-ceramics—initially noncrystalline (glassy) ceramics from which some crystalline phase is precipitated for strengthening
      h. Glass-infiltrated ceramic—partially sintered ceramic particles that are infused with a glassy matrix, for example, InCeram
   3. Classification
      a. Feldspathic porcelains—produced by traditional laboratory fabrication with porcelain particles painted into position as a water slurry (condensed) and then heated for particle coalescence (sintered)
         (1) High-fusing porcelains—for denture teeth
         (2) Medium-fusing porcelains—for jacket crowns; not commonly used

(3) Low-fusing porcelains—veneering material for PFM restorations

b. High-strength ceramics—produced by specialized laboratory fabrication technique

(1) Lucite-reinforced porcelains—pressure molded

(2) Alumina-reinforced porcelains

(3) High-density alumina core materials

(4) Glass-infiltrated core materials, for example, spinel, alumina, and zirconia

(5) Hydroxyapatite-based materials

c. Glass-ceramics

(1) Mica-based glass-ceramics—used as starting blanks for CAD/CAM or copy-milled restorations

(2) High-strength glass-ceramic core materials, for example, lithia disilicate glass-ceramics

d. High-strength crystalline single-phase materials

(1) Alumina

(2) Zirconia (yttria-stabilized tetragonal zirconia)

B. Porcelain structure

1. Components

a. Large number of oxides—principally silicon oxide (silica), aluminum oxide (alumina), and potassium oxide, created by combining clay, feldspar, and quartz raw materials

b. Minor oxides contribute properties of opacity, translucency, and color

2. Manipulation

a. Traditional porcelain fabrication

(1) Porcelain powder mixed with water, padded onto substrate, compacted, and heated to produce coalescence with shrinkage

(2) Shrinkage is approximately 30% on firing (sintering), thus porcelain layer must be made oversized and built up by several stages of application

b. Special ceramic laboratory fabrication procedures—require specialized equipment and furnaces

c. Milling—requires specialized equipment

C. Properties

1. Physical

a. Excellent electrical and thermal insulation

b. Low coefficient of thermal expansion and contraction

c. Good color and translucency; excellent aesthetics (superior to all other materials)

2. Chemical

a. Not resistant to fluorine-containing acids and can be dissolved by contact with APF topical fluoride treatments

b. Can be acid etched with hydrofluoric acid or other strong acids for providing micromechanical retention for cements

3. Mechanical

a. Harder than tooth structure and will cause opponent wear, although some glass-ceramics are comparable in hardness to enamel

b. Can be polished with diamond pastes

c. Poor fatigue behavior when compared with metal alloys

4. Biologic—relatively inert

Crown-and-Bridge Cements

A. General considerations (Table 13-5)

1. Applications

a. Luting inlays, onlays, crowns, and bridges

b. Luting orthodontic bands and brackets

2. Terminology—luting: attachment by gross mechanical interdigitation with crown and tooth surfaces

3. Classification

a. Traditional cements (typically P + L) (Rarely used)—zinc oxide–eugenol (ZOE) and zinc phosphate (ZP)

b. Polymeric cements (typically precapsulated or paste–paste)—polycarboxylate (PC), glass ionomer (GI), resin-modified glass ionomer (RMGI), resin or composite (CC), and universal cement (UC)

B. Structure

1. Components (see Table 13-5)

a. Traditional cements—powder (reactant; chemically basic); liquid (reactant; chemically acidic)

b. Polymeric cements—polymer cross-linking reaction (PC, GI), polymerization reaction (RMGI, CC, UC), or both

2. Reaction

a. Traditional cements—acid–base reaction that forms salt; great excess of powder leaves residual powder as filler

b. Polymeric cements—setting produced by cross-linking reactions similar to glass ionomer or composite setting reactions

3. Manipulation

a. Traditional cements—all reactions are exothermic; reaction controlled by chilling components, chilling mixing slab, or incrementally adding powder to the liquid

b. Polymeric cements—powder is added to liquid as quickly as possible to complete mixing in 30 seconds or mixed in triturators and used quickly; may include preplacement of bonding system as well

TABLE 13-5 Luting Cements

Cement	Abbreviation	Powder or Filler Components	Liquid or Matrix Components
Traditional (or conventional) types Zinc oxide–eugenol (ZOE), unmodified (Limited use)	ZOE	Zinc oxide	Eugenol
Zinc phosphate (ZP) (Limited use)	ZP	Zinc oxide	Phosphoric acid in water
Polymeric (or Resin) Types Polycarboxylate	PC	Zinc oxide	Polyacrylic acid in water
Glass ionomer, conventional	GI*	Fluoro-aluminosilicate glass	Polyacrylic acid in water
Resin-modified glass ionomer	RMGI*	Fluoro-aluminosilicate glass	Copolymer acid in water; water-soluble monomers
Compomer	CM*	Fluoro-aluminosilicate glass; silicate glass	Bis-GMA–like monomers
Universal cement† (Esthetic resin cement, RC)	UC of RC*	Fluoro-aluminosilicate glass	Bis-GMA–like monomers
Composite	CP*	Colloidal silica	Bis-GMA–like monomers

*Principal cements in use today.
†Self-adhesive resin cement and adhesive resin cement versions.

C. Properties
   1. Physical properties
      a. All luting cements are electrical and thermal insulators
      b. All luting cements have low coefficients of thermal expansion and contraction
   2. Chemical properties
      a. In acidic environments, cements tend to disintegrate
      b. Polycarboxylate and glass ionomer cements will adhere chemically to calcium ions on the surface of tooth structure and to oxides contained within the set cements
      c. Polycarboxylate and glass ionomer are most resistant to microleakage
      d. Glass ionomer cements release fluoride ions (and most polycarboxylate cements initially release fluoride because of small CaF_2 contents included as mixing aids)
   3. Mechanical properties—compressive strength; composite has the highest compressive strength, and ZOE has the lowest
   4. Biologic properties
      a. Eugenol-based cements produce obtundent (pain-soothing) effects
      b. Polycarboxylate and glass ionomer cements are most gentle to the dental pulp (when manipulated correctly)

Acrylic Appliances

A. General considerations
   1. Application—space maintenance and tooth movement for orthodontics and pediatric dentistry
   2. Classification—none
B. Structure
   1. Components
      a. Powder—PMMA (polymethylmethacrylate) powder, peroxide initiator, and pigments
      b. Liquid—MMA (methylmethacrylate) monomer, hydroquinone inhibitor, cross-linking agents, and chemical accelerators (N, N-dimethyl-p-toluidine)
   2. Reaction
      a. The PMMA powder makes mixture viscous for manipulation before curing
      b. Chemical accelerators cause the decomposition of benzoyl peroxide into free radicals that initiate the polymerization of the monomer
      c. New PMMA is formed as a matrix that surrounds the PMMA powder
      d. Linear shrinkage of 5% to 7% during setting, but dimensions of appliances are not critical

3. Manipulation
   a. The mixture of powder and liquid is painted onto the working cast to create the shape for the acrylic appliance
   b. Orthodontic wires may be part of the appliance
   c. After curing the mixture, the shape and fit are adjusted by grinding with burrs and stones, with a slow-speed handpiece
      (1) Caution—acrylic dust is irritating to epithelial tissues of nasopharynx and skin and may produce allergic dermatitis or other reactions
      (2) Grinding may heat the polymer to temperatures that depolymerize and release monomer vapor, which may be an irritant
C. Properties (see the section on "Acrylic Denture Bases")
   1. Physical
   2. Chemical—may contain 2% to 3% unreacted monomer that can cause soft tissue irritation in approximately 4% of the population
   3. Mechanical
   4. Biologic

Acrylic Denture Bases

A. General considerations
   1. Application—used to support artificial teeth
   2. Classification
      a. PMMA/MMA dough systems
      b. PMMA/MMA injected resin systems
      c. PMMA/MMA pour resins
      d. UDMA VLC resins
B. Structure of PMMA/MMA types
   1. Components
      a. Powder—PMMA polymer, peroxide initiator, and pigments
      b. Liquid—MMA monomer, hydroquinone inhibitor, and cross-linking agents
   2. Reaction
      a. Heat (or chemicals) used as an accelerator to decompose peroxide into free radicals
      b. Free radicals initiate polymerization of MMA into PMMA
      c. New PMMA is formed as a matrix around residual PMMA powder particles
      d. Linear shrinkage—5% to 7% of monomer on polymerization; reduced by processing procedures
   3. Manipulation
      a. P/L mixed to form dough or fluid resin to fill mold
      b. Mold heated to start and control reaction

C. Properties
   1. Physical
      a. Thermal insulator—prevents the patient's sensations of food temperature
      b. High coefficient of thermal expansion and contraction
      c. Poor distortion resistance at higher temperatures; therefore, dentures should not be cleaned in hot water
      d. Good resistance to color change
   2. Chemical
      a. Stored in water before delivery to reach equilibrium absorption level
      b. Absorbs water and must be kept hydrated
      c. Not resistant to strong oxidizing agents
   3. Mechanical
      a. Low strength, but flexible; good fatigue resistance
      b. Poor scratch resistance; clean tissue-bearing surfaces of denture with soft brush and do not use abrasive cleaners
   4. Biologic—occasional allergic reactions to minute residual monomer have been reported in newly processed dentures

Denture Teeth

A. General considerations
   1. Applications—complete or partial dentures
   2. Classification
      a. Porcelain teeth
      b. Acrylic resin teeth—95% of all denture teeth
      c. Abrasion-resistant teeth—composite veneered and interpenetrating network (IPN) teeth
B. Structure and properties
   1. Porcelain teeth (high-fusing porcelain)
      a. Bonded into denture base mechanically
      b. Harder than natural teeth or other restorations and are capable of abrading those surfaces
      c. Good aesthetic appearance
      d. Used when clients have good ridge support and sufficient room between the arches
   2. Acrylic resin teeth—PMMA
      a. Bonded pseudochemically into the denture base; teeth are wetted with monomer before forming denture base
      b. Soft and easily worn by abrasive foods
      c. Good initial aesthetics
      d. Used for clients with poor ridges and those who are opposed to natural teeth
   3. Abrasion-resistant teeth (composite veneered)
      a. Bonded pseudochemically into the denture base
      b. Much better abrasion resistance than acrylic resin teeth but poorer bonding

Denture Soft Liners

A. General considerations
    1. Applications—for clients with soft tissue irritation
    2. Classification
        a. Long-term liners (soft liners)—used over a period of months for patients with severe undercuts or continually sore residual ridges
        b. Short-term liners (tissue conditioners)—used to facilitate tissue healing over several days
B. Structure
    1. Soft liners—plasticized acrylic co-polymers or silicone rubber
    2. Tissue conditioners—PEMA (polyethylmethacrylate) plasticized with ethanol and aromatic esters
C. Properties
    1. Liners flow under low pressure, allowing adaptation to soft tissues, but are elastic during chewing forces
    2. Low initial hardness, but the liner becomes harder as plasticizers are leached out during intraoral use
    3. Some silicone rubber liners support the growth of yeasts

Denture Cleansers

A. General considerations
    1. Applications—for removal of soft debris by light brushing and then rinsing of denture; hard deposits require professional repolishing
    2. Classification
        a. Alkaline perborates—do not remove bad stains; may harm liners
        b. Alkaline hypochlorites—may cause bleaching, corrode base-metal alloys, and leave residual taste on appliance
        c. Dilute acids—may corrode base-metal alloys
        d. Abrasive powders and creams—can abrade denture surfaces
    3. Techniques recommended for denture cleaning
        a. Full dentures without soft liners—immerse denture in solution of one part 5% sodium hypochlorite (Clorox) and three parts water
        b. Full or partial dentures without soft liners—immerse denture in solution of 1 teaspoon of sodium hypochlorite (Clorox) and 2 teaspoons of glassy phosphate (Calgon) in a half glass of water
        c. Lined dentures—clean any soft liner with a cotton swab and cold water; clean the denture with a soft brush

B. Properties
    1. Chemical—cleansers can swell plastic surfaces or corrode metal frameworks
    2. Mechanical—cleansers can scratch the surfaces of denture bases or denture teeth

Mouth Protectors (Athletic Mouthguards)

A. General considerations
    1. Applications—to protect against blows to the chin, the top of the head, and the face or to prevent grinding of teeth; typically used by football, basketball, soccer, and hockey players (contact sports)
    2. Terminology—mouth protectors, teeth protectors, or athletic mouthguards
    3. Classification
        a. Stock protectors—least desirable because of poor fit
        b. Mouth-formed protectors ("boil-and-bite")—made by client; improved fit compared with stock type
        c. Custom-made protectors—fabrication by dentist is preferred because of durability, low levels of speech impairment, and comfort
B. Structure
    1. Components
        a. Stock protectors—thermoplastic co-polymer of polyvinyl acetate–polyethylene (PVA-PE)
        b. Mouth-formed protectors—thermoplastic co-polymer
        c. Custom-made protectors—thermoplastic co-polymer or polyurethane
    2. Reaction—hardening during cooling
    3. Fabrication
        a. Alginate impression made of maxillary arch
        b. High-strength stone cast poured immediately
        c. Thermoplastic material is heated in hot water and vacuum-molded to cast
        d. Mouth protector trimmed to within 2 mm of labial fold, clearance provided at the buccal and labial frena, and edges smoothed by flaming
        e. Gagging, taste, irritation, and impairment of speech are minimized with properly fabricated mouth protector
    4. Instructions for use—client must:
        a. Rinse before and after use with cold water
        b. Clean protector occasionally with soap and cool water
        c. Store the protector in a rigid container
        d. Protect the protector from heat and pressure during storage
        e. Evaluate the protector routinely for evidence of deterioration

C. Properties
   1. Physical—thermal insulators
   2. Chemical—absorbs water and stains during use
   3. Mechanical—tensile strength, modulus, and hardness decrease after water absorption, but elongation, tear strength, and resilience increase
   4. Biologic—nontoxic as long as no bacterial, fungal, or viral growth occurs on surfaces between uses

Veneers

A. General considerations
   1. Applications—generally anterior maxillary teeth
   2. Terminology
      a. Extracoronal—bonded over existing enamel, that is, no tooth preparation
      b. Intracoronal—bonded into an intraenamel cavity preparation
   3. Classification by materials
      a. Direct composite veneer
      b. Indirect composite veneer (laboratory processed)
      c. Ceramic veneer (stacked or pressed ceramic)
      d. CAD/CAM ceramic veneer
B. Structure
   1. Components—composite, porcelain, or ceramic
   2. Manipulation
      a. Bonding—enamel etching and bonding
      b. Finishing and polishing must be done with care to avoid scratching the surfaces
   3. Maintenance
      a. Polishing with abrasive materials or scaling with metal instruments must be avoided
      b. The protector must be protected with petroleum jelly during topical APF fluoride treatments, or neutral sodium fluoride must be used
C. Properties
   1. Physical—good aesthetic appearance; but some coloring may occur because of the composite resin cement used for bonding the veneer
   2. Chemical
      a. Composite veneers have good acid resistance
      b. Ceramic and CAD/CAM veneers should be protected from APF or other acids
   3. Mechanical
      a. Composite veneers are subject to scratching
      b. Ceramic and CAD/CAM veneers have good abrasion resistance
   4. Biologic—no known problems

CAD/CAM and Copy-Milled Restorations

A. General considerations
   1. Applications—inlays, onlays, veneers, crowns, bridges, implants, and implant prostheses
   2. Stages of fabrication of CAD/CAM restorations
      a. CSD—computerized surface digitization; acquisition of surface contours and geometry
      b. CAD—computer-aided (assisted) design; digital design of restoration
      c. CAM—computer-aided (assisted) machining; fabrication of restoration from block of material
   3. Stages of fabrication for copy milling
      a. Fabrication of wax or composite dies that duplicate the contours and geometry of the restoration to be fabricated
      b. Dies and ceramic or composite blocks mounted in tandem for copy-milling operation
   4. Classification
      a. Chairside or in-office CAD/CAM systems
      b. Laboratory CAD/CAM systems
      c. Laboratory copy-milling systems
      d. Examples of CAD/CAM and copy-milling systems in dentistry:
         (1) Automill (Alldent, Liechtenstein)
         (2) Avanza 100 (Ceramatic Dental, Sweden)
         (3) Bego Medifacturing (Bego Medical, Germany)
         (4) Cad-esthetics (Decim Norden, Sweden)
         (5) Cadim (Advance, Japan)
         (6) Celay (Mikrona Technology, Switzerland)
         (7) Ce.novation (Inocermic, Germany)
         (8) Cercon (Dentsply/Degudent, USA/Germany)
         (9) Cerec AC/InLab (Sirona, Germany)
         (10) Cicero (Elephant Dental, Netherlands)
         (11) DCS Precident (DCS Dental, Switzerland)
         (12) DECSY (Digital Process, Japan)
         (13) Dental CAD/CAM GN1 (GC, Japan)
         (14) Digident (Girrbach Dental, Germany)
         (15) E4D Dentist (D4D Technologies, USA)
         (16) Etkon (Etkon, Germany)
         (17) iTero (Cadent, USA)
         (18) Kavo-Everest (Kavo, Germany)
         (19) Lava (3M ESPE, USA/Germany)
         (20) Premium Dental System (I-mes, Germany)
         (21) Pro 50 (Cynovad, Canada)
         (22) Procera (Nobel Biocare, Sweden)
         (23) Wol-ceram (Woldent, Germany)
         (24) XAWEX Production System (I-mes, Germany)

B. Structure
  1. Materials
     a. Feldspathic porcelains (Vita Mark II, ProCAD)
     b. Machinable leucite-reinforced ceramic (IPS Empress CAD)
     c. Machinable lithium disilicate (IPS e.Max CAD)
     d. Machinable high-strength ceramics (Inceram spinel, Inceram alumina, Inceram zirconia, Procera alumina, Procera zirconia, Lava zirconia, Cercon zirconia, Crystal zirconia, IPS e.Max ZirCAD zirconia)
     e. Metal alloys (limited use)
     f. Composites—newer use
  2. Cementing
     a. Etching enamel and dentin for micro-mechanical retention
     b. Bonding agent for retention to etched surface
     c. Composite as a luting cement for reacting chemically with bonding agent and with silanated surfaces of restoration
     d. Silane for wetting and chemical bonding to etched ceramic (or metal) restorations and for co-reaction with luting composite cement
     e. Hydrofluoric acid for gel etching or sandblasting to create spaces for micro-mechanical retention on surface of restoration
     f. Ceramic primer for alumina or zirconia
C. Properties
  1. Physical properties
     a. Thermal expansion coefficient well-matched to tooth structure
     b. Good resistance to plaque biofilm adsorption or retention
     c. Good aesthetics (for shade matching)
  2. Chemical properties—not resistant to hydrofluoric acid and should be protected from APF
  3. Mechanical properties
     a. Excellent wear resistance (but may abrade opposing teeth)
     b. Some wear of luting cements but self-limiting
     c. Excellent toothbrush abrasion resistance
     d. Limited fatigue resistance caused by brittleness (low-fracture toughness) and initiation and propagation of cracks
  4. Biologic properties—excellent compatibility with natural tissues

Dental Implants

See the sections on "Dental Implants" in Chapter 14 and "Advanced Instrumentation Techniques" in Chapter 17.

A. General considerations
  1. Applications
     a. Single-tooth implants
     b. Abutments for bridges (freestanding, attached to natural teeth)
     c. Abutments for overdentures
  2. Terminology
     a. Endosseous—into the bone; represents >90% of all current types
     b. Subperiosteal—below the periosteum but above the bone; second most frequently used type
     c. Transosteal—through the bone
     d. Endodontic—through the root canal space and into the periapical bone
     e. Intramucosal—within the mucosa
  3. Classification by geometric form
     a. Endosteal root forms
        (1) Screws
        (2) Cylinders
     b. Other endosteal forms
        (1) Blades
        (2) Staples
     c. Circumferential
  4. Classification by materials type
     a. Metallic—titanium (majority of types; uncoated and coated), stainless steel, and chromium/cobalt
     b. Polymeric—PMMA
     c. Ceramic—hydroxyapatite, carbon, and sapphire
  5. Classification by attachment design
     a. Bioactive surface retention by osseo-integration—integration of bone with implant; most favored type of attachment
     b. Nonactive porous surfaces for micro-mechanical retention by osseo-integration
     c. Nonactive, nonporous surface for ankylosis by osseo-integration
     d. Gross mechanical retention designs (e.g., threads, screws, channels, or transverse holes)
     e. Fibro-integration by formation of fibrous tissue capsule
     f. Combinations of the above designs
B. Structure
  1. Components
     a. Root (for osseo-integration)
     b. Neck (for epithelial attachment and percutaneous sealing)
     c. Intramobile elements (for shock absorption)
     d. Prosthesis (for dental form and function)
  2. Manipulation
     a. Selection—based on remaining bone architecture and dimensions
     b. Sterilization—RF glow discharge leaves the biomaterial surface uncontaminated and sterile; autoclaving or chemical sterilization contraindicated for some designs

c. Handling—must be handled with an instrument of like composition, that is, titanium instruments used to handle titanium implants to avoid metallic contamination and localized electrochemical corrosion

C. Properties
   1. Physical—should have low thermal and electrical conductivity
   2. Chemical
      a. Should be resistant to electrochemical corrosion
      b. Do not expose surfaces to acids, for example, APF fluorides
      c. The effects of adjunctive therapies, for example, 0.12% chlorhexidine gluconate mouthrinse must be kept in mind
   3. Mechanical
      a. Should be abrasion resistant and have a high modulus
      b. During scaling operations, care must be taken to avoid abrading (e.g., with metal scalers or air-abrasive systems); see the sections on "Advanced Instrumentation Techniques," "Instrumentation of Dental Implants," and "Selective Stain Removal" in Chapter 17.
   4. Biologic—depend on osseo-integration and epithelial attachment

Tissue Engineering

See the section on "Genetics" in Chapter 7.
A. General considerations
   1. Applications—replacement of any oro-facial tissues, particularly intraoral tissues
   2. Terminology
      a. Tissue engineering—attempt to regenerate tissue for the body, either in the laboratory or in the patient, through manipulation of cellular material, biologic mediators, and natural or synthetic matrices
      b. Cells (in tissue engineering)—living cells that are either precursors of more differentiated cells or disorganized collections of cells that grow, divide, and organize into physiologically functioning tissue
      c. Signals—any physical, chemical, or biologic mediators (extracellular or intracellular) that initiate, propagate, or otherwise stimulate cellular development into fully organized tissue
      d. Scaffolds—any extracellular matrix structure (natural or synthetic, temporary or permanent, hard or soft) that provides a foundation for cells to become attached, organized, and proliferate to generate the tissue of interest

3. Classification by materials by tissue-replacement therapies
   a. Autografts—from one's own body
      (1) Best chance of clinical success
      (2) Genetic match (no immunity problems)
   b. Allografts (or homografts)—from same species (usually from cadavers)
      (1) Can be antigenic (sensitize the patient)
      (2) Concerns about transmitted diseases
   c. Xenografts—from different species
      (1) Limited range of use, for example, porcine heart valve
      (2) Heavily treated prior to use
   d. Synthetics—entirely manmade
      (1) Can be metals, ceramics, polymers, or composites
      (2) Prone to long-term mechanical breakdown
      (3) Can produce a toxic response
   e. Tissue-engineered replacement—rebuilding tissues in the laboratory to be implanted, or causing the body to artificially "rebuild the tissue" in situ
      (1) Use of mixture of natural and synthetic materials
      (2) Offers the possibility of a "near-perfect" replacement
      (3) Can potentially solve transplant availability problems
B. Structure
   1. Components
      a. Cells (cellular material)
         (1) Stem cells (undifferentiated)
         (2) Specific cells, for example, osteoblasts, fibroblasts
      b. Signals (biologic mediators)
         (1) Growth factors, for example, bone morphogenic proteins (BMPs)
         (2) Genetic material
      c. Scaffolds (matrices)
         (1) Polymers—native, for example, collagen; or synthetic, for example, PLA/PGA
         (2) Ceramics—native, for example, bone chips; or synthetic, for example, Bioglass
         (3) Composites—combination of native and synthetic, for example, hydroxyapatite-coated collagen fibers
   2. Manipulation
      a. Design and grown human tissues outside of the body for later implantation to repair or replace diseased tissues
         (1) Not necessarily patient specific
         (2) Ideal for large-volume need, for example, skin grafts
      b. Implantation of cell-containing or cell-free devices (with appropriate signal molecules)

that induce the regeneration of functional human tissues; guided tissue regeneration, for example, use of Perioglass combined with appropriate growth factors in treatment of severe periodontal disease

c. Development of external or internal devices containing human tissues designed to replace the function of diseased internal tissues

(1) Involve use of stem cells or specific differentiated cells from the patient

(2) Ideal for load-bearing tissues, for example, bone, tendon

C. Properties—physical, chemical, and mechanical properties should be similar to those of natural tissues

@ WEB SITE INFORMATION AND RESOURCES

SOURCE	WEB SITE ADDRESS	DESCRIPTION
Academy of General Dentistry	http://www.agd.org	Abstracts on dental and related topics
American College of Prosthodontists	http://www.prosthodontics.org/	General information about prosthodontics
American Dental Association (ADA)	http://www.ada.org/	Information about all approved dental materials and ADA standards for dental materials
American Dental Education Association	http://www.adea.org/	Extensive series of links to dental schools and to biomaterials teaching activities
Clinicians Reports	http://www.cliniciansreport.org	Updates on dental materials and devices
International Association for Dental Research (IADR) Dental Materials Group	http://www.dentalresearch.org/DMG/	List of all dental materials sites and dental materials manufacturer Web sites
MEDLINE/PubMed	http://www.ncbi.nlm.nih.gov/sites/entrez?db=pubmed	Public access to National Library of Medicine (NLM) abstract index that includes all dental research abstracts for published articles in dental journals
The Dental Advisor	http://www.dentaladvisor.com/	Evaluation of current dental products
University of Michigan Biomaterials Properties Database	http://www.lib.umich.edu/health-sciences-libraries/introduction-biomaterials-properties-database	List of all physical and mechanical properties of dental materials
Dental Evaluation and Consultation Service	http://www.airforcemedicine.afms.mil/decs	List of current reviews and analyses of dental materials, instruments, and devices; evaluation of current dental products

SUGGESTED READINGS

Anusavice KJ, Phillips RW: *Phillip's science of dental materials,* ed 11, Philadelphia, 2003, Saunders.

Bayne SC, Thomson JY: *Biomaterials science [digital only],* Chapel Hill, NC, 2004, Brightstar.

Hatrick CD, Eakle WS, Bird WF: *Dental materials, clinical applications for dental assistants and dental hygienists,* ed 2, St Louis, 2011, Saunders.

Powers JM, Wataha JC: *Dental materials: Properties and manipulation,* ed 9, St Louis, 2008, Mosby.

O'Brien WJ: *Dental materials and their selection,* ed 4, Philadelphia, 2009, Quintessence.

Powers JM, Sakaguchi RL: *Craig's restorative dental materials,* ed 13, St Louis, 2012, Mosby.

CHAPTER 13 REVIEW QUESTIONS

1. **Which of the following mixing methods is NOT used for dental materials?**
   a. Two liquids mixed through a mixing nozzle
   b. Powder and liquid precapsulated and mixed in a triturator
   c. Powder and liquid mixed on a mixing pad
   d. Two liquids agitated together using a vibrating stirrer
   e. Powder and water mixed together with a spatula in a mixing bowl

2. **What is *mixing time*?**
   a. Time elapsed from the start of mixing until the end of mixing
   b. Time elapsed from the beginning of mixing until the beginning of setting
   c. Time elapsed from the beginning of the working interval until the end of the setting interval
   d. The working interval
   e. The time required by the operator to handle and place a dental material

3. **Which one of the following materials does NOT set by polymerization?**
   a. Flowable dental composite
   b. Hybrid glass ionomer cement
   c. Dental plaster
   d. Polyvinyl siloxane impression material
   e. Polysulfide impression material

4. **Why is the linear coefficient of thermal expansion important for restorative materials?**
   a. It predicts the mismatch in expansion and contraction at the interface of restorative materials
   b. It predicts the loss in strength of a restorative material as the temperature increases
   c. It indicates the insulating characteristics of a restorative material
   d. It indicates the resistance to thermal degradation of a material
   e. It indicates the amount of expansion and contraction on polymerization

5. **Which of the following materials undergoes problematic imbibition?**
   a. Gold restorations
   b. Dental sealant
   c. Dental composite
   d. Dental cement
   e. Alginate impression material

6. **Which one of the following is a rapid thermal conductor?**
   a. Dental enamel
   b. Dentin
   c. Dental amalgam
   d. Dental composite
   e. Zirconia all-ceramic inlays

7. **Which one of the following is BEST for pulpal insulation?**
   a. 1 mm of calcium hydroxide liner
   b. 1 mm of remaining dentin thickness
   c. 3 mm of composite restoration
   d. 5 mm of dental amalgam restoration
   e. Surface sealant over restoration

8. **Which one of the following terms is NOT important for color matching?**
   a. Hue, Chroma, Value
   b. Ambient lighting conditions
   c. Surface gloss
   d. Translucency
   e. Imbibition

9. **Which one of the following is NOT associated with electrochemical corrosion events?**
   a. Plaque
   b. Crevices
   c. Stress
   d. Passivation
   e. Translucency

10. **Engineering stress is computed as:**
    a. Applied load divided by original cross-sectional area of the object
    b. Deformation divided by the volume of the object
    c. Modulus multiplied by the plastic deformation
    d. Difference between the total strain and plastic strain
    e. Deformation divided by the original length

11. **Engineering strain is computed as:**
    a. Change between the initial and final strain divided by the time
    b. Area under the stress–strain curve
    c. Load at yield divided by elastic deformation
    d. Applied load divided by the total elastic deformation
    e. Deformation divided by the original length of the object

12. **What is another name for a material's modulus?**
    a. Stiffness
    b. Elastic limit
    c. Toughness
    d. Fatigue resistance
    e. Brittleness

13. **Loading of a restoration beyond the material's elastic limit produces:**
    a. Only plastic deformation
    b. Only elastic deformation
    c. Fatigue fracture
    d. Elastic and plastic deformation
    e. Stress relaxation

14. **What is the point at which loading begins to produce both plastic and elastic strain at the same time?**
    a. Fracture
    b. Toughness
    c. Fatigue
    d. Modulus
    e. Elastic limit

15. **What is the Mohs' hardness value for enamel?**
    a. 10
    b. 7
    c. 5–6
    d. 3–4
    e. 1

16. **Which phase in dental amalgam restorations is MOST likely to corrode?**
    a. Ag-Hg
    b. Ag-Sn
    c. Ag-Sn-Cu
    d. Sn-Hg
    e. Cu-Sn

17. **Which phase of the dental amalgam is the strongest?**
    a. Sn-Hg
    b. Ag-Cu
    c. Cu-Sn
    d. Ag-Hg
    e. Ag-Sn

18. **Which method is recommended to minimize the escape of mercury vapor during amalgam mixing?**
    a. Mortar and pestle
    b. Friction-fit capsule
    c. Precapsulated alloy and mercury
    d. Covered mixing arm on the triturator
    e. None of the above

19. **What range of copper is involved in the composition of high-copper dental amalgam alloys?**
    a. 0.1% to 0.5%
    b. 0.5% to 1%
    c. 1% to 5%
    d. 6% to 12%
    e. 12% to 30%

20. **What is the major advantage of high-copper dental amalgam restorations over low-copper dental amalgam restorations?**
    a. Better mechanical properties
    b. Lower coefficient of thermal expansion
    c. Greater polishability
    d. Lower corrosion tendency
    e. Lower thermal conductivity

21. **What is the Occupational Safety and Health Administration (OSHA) limit for exposure to mercury vapor in air during a 40-hour workweek?**
    a. 10 $\mu g/m^3$
    b. 20 $\mu g/m^3$
    c. 30 $\mu g/m^3$
    d. 40 $\mu g/m^3$
    e. 50 $\mu g/m^3$

22. **What is the melting temperature of the Ag-Hg matrix phase in a set dental amalgam restoration?**
    a. 87°C
    b. 107°C
    c. 127°C
    d. 147°C
    e. 167°C

23. **What is the major problem associated with polishing a dental amalgam?**
    a. Creation of marginal ditching
    b. Burnishing of surface corrosion products into the amalgam
    c. Production of a grayish color
    d. Localized melting of the amalgam with mercury smearing
    e. Smearing amalgam onto enamel to cause staining

24. **What is the incidence of hypersensitivity to mercury from dental amalgam restorations in the general population?**
    a. 1 per 1000 patients
    b. 1 per 50,000 patients
    c. 1 per 1 million patients
    d. 1 per 5 million patients
    e. 1 per 100 million patients

25. **What is the principal reason for the shift away from dental amalgam use?**
    a. Toxicity of mercury to office personnel
    b. Environmental concerns about ineffective mercury recycling from dental offices
    c. Much improved mechanical properties of other esthetic materials such as composites
    d. Patient hypersensitivity problems to mercury released from amalgams
    e. Lower cost of procedures for alternative restorative materials

26. **Which one of the following is the main criterion for failure of a high-copper dental amalgam restoration?**
    a. Accumulation of black or green tarnish on exposed surfaces
    b. Marginal ditching along occlusal margins
    c. Creep of the restoration out of the cavity preparation in proximal areas
    d. Wear facets along the occlusal contact areas
    e. None of the above

27. **Which restorative material is most often substituted for dental amalgam in posterior restoration applications?**
    a. All-ceramic
    b. Dental composite
    c. Hybrid glass ionomer
    d. Direct gold
    e. Atraumatic restorative technique (ART) material

28. **Which one of the following is TRUE about pit-and-fissure sealants?**
    a. Uncured sealant along air-exposed surfaces will finish curing in 24 hours
    b. Sealants should be filled to improve their mechanical properties
    c. Tinted sealants are more useful than colorless ones
    d. Sealant inspection is unnecessary after 2 years
    e. Partial sealing of pits and fissures is better than no sealing at all

29. **Which event does not alter the aesthetics of existing composite restorations?**
    a. Whitening techniques
    b. Extensive tea exposure
    c. Acidulated phosphate fluoride (APF) application
    d. Tobacco use
    e. Gum chewing

30. **What is the MOST appropriate way to manage long-term wear or discoloration of posterior dental composite restoration surfaces?**
    a. Replace the composite with a dental amalgam
    b. Repair the worn areas with resin-modified glass ionomer
    c. Resurface the old composite with new composite
    d. Replace the restoration with a new high-strength ceramic
    e. Adjust the occlusion of the opponent tooth

31. **Which one of the following procedures does NOT require etching with phosphoric acid solution?**
    a. Dental sealant
    b. Ceramic orthodontic bracket attachment
    c. Total-etch dentin bonding procedure
    d. Self-etch dentin bonding procedure
    e. Amalgam bonding procedure

32. **What is TRUE about the dentin smear layer?**
    a. 50- to 100-micron-thick debris layer
    b. Composed mostly of collagen and water
    c. Dissolved by acid etching during bonding procedures
    d. Easily removed with air-water spray
    e. Effectively seals dentin

33. **What is required to produce good bond strength to dentin?**
    a. Long conditioning (etching) times
    b. Drying of dentin
    c. Preapplication of chlorhexidine
    d. Postcuring materials with visible light
    e. Hybrid layer formation

34. **How do self-etching bonding systems work?**
    a. Acidic monomers replace need for phosphoric acid etching
    b. New monomers chemically adhere to hydroxyapatite
    c. Phosphoric acid is mixed with other components of the bonding system
    d. Chemical bonding to collagen replaces need for micromechanical bonding
    e. Wetting agent helps adaptation and replaces need for micromechanical bonding

35. **Where are water-miscible acrylic monomers MOST likely to be found?**
    a. Polishing pastes
    b. APF
    c. Pit-and-fissure sealants
    d. Dentin primers
    e. Resin surface sealers

36. **Which component of the dentin bonding system is MOST likely to cause skin sensitization in dental personnel?**
    a. Phosphoric acid
    b. Hydroxyethyl methacrylate (HEMA)
    c. Ethanol
    d. Urethane dimethacrylate (UDMA)
    e. Bisphenol A–glycidylmethacrylate (Bis-GMA)

37. **What is the shorthand representation for a self-etching primer adhesive?**
    a. E + P + B
    b. E + PB
    c. EP + B
    d. EPB
    e. E

38. **Which of the following restorations requires surface protection with non-petroleum based jelly during APF applications?**
    a. Porcelain ceramics
    b. Amalgams
    c. Dental sealants
    d. Cast gold
    e. Orthodontic wire

39. **Which one of the following constituents may have a palliative action on the dental pulp?**
    a. HEMA
    b. Calcium hydroxide
    c. Bis-GMA
    d. 4-Methacryloxyethyl trimellitate anhydride (4-META)
    e. Eugenol

40. **What is the primary filler component composite cement?**
    a. Aluminum oxide
    b. Polymethylmethacrylate (PMMA)
    c. Silica
    d. Zinc oxide
    e. Calcium oxide

41. **Which one of the following dental cements does NOT include polymer as part of the matrix?**
    a. Zinc oxide–eugenol cement
    b. Polycarboxylate cement
    c. Glass ionomer cement
    d. Resin-modified glass ionomer cement
    e. Composite cement

42. **What ions on tooth structure permit glass ionomer chemical adhesion?**
    a. Aluminum ions
    b. Calcium ions
    c. Fluoride ions
    d. Carboxylic acid ions
    e. Hydrogen ions

43. **Which one of the following materials does NOT release fluoride?**
    a. Traditional glass ionomer
    b. Resin-modified glass ionomer
    c. ART restorations
    d. Provisional restorations
    e. Compomer

44. **Which of the following choices is MOST similar to a compomer?**
    a. Polycarboxylate
    b. Glass ionomer
    c. Zinc phosphate cement
    d. Composite
    e. Giomer

45. **What pattern does the fluoride-release from glass ionomers follow?**
    a. Rapid decrease to a low level after 24 hours
    b. Rapid decrease over 7 to 14 days
    c. Decrease after 30 days
    d. Increase after many months
    e. No release after 1 year

46. **Which of the following applications is MOST typical for an ART material?**
    a. Class III aesthetic restorations
    b. Class II restorations
    c. Class IV restorations in permanent teeth
    d. Liner under composite restorations
    e. Temporary restoration

47. **Which impression material is a hydrogel?**
    a. Alginate
    b. Zinc oxide–eugenol (ZOE)
    c. Polysulfide
    d. Polyether
    e. Polyvinyl siloxane

48. **Which one of the following impression materials is typically mixed by extrusion through a disposable nozzle?**
    a. Alginate
    b. ZOE
    c. Polyvinyl siloxane
    d. Silicone
    e. None of the above

49. **Which application typically requires the strongest gypsum material?**
    a. Orthodontic model
    b. Master cast
    c. Repairing casts
    d. Removable die
    e. Denture fabrication

50. **What is the chemical composition of set gypsum products?**
    a. Calcium sulfate trihydrate
    b. Calcium sulfate dihydrate
    c. Calcium sulfate monohydrate
    d. Calcium sulfate unhydrated
    e. Calcium sulfate hemihydrate

51. **What is the chemical composition of gypsum powder that is to be mixed with water to form models?**
    a. Calcium phosphate
    b. Calcium chloride
    c. Calcium sulfate hemihydrate
    d. Calcium carbonate
    e. Calcium fluoride

52. **How much "water of reaction" is required for the actual setting of 100 g of calcium sulfate hemihydrate powder?**
    a. 12 mL
    b. 18 mL
    c. 24 mL
    d. 32 mL
    e. 50 mL

53. **What is the major difference between plaster and stone powders?**
    a. Hydration state
    b. Color
    c. Crystal structure
    d. Powder particle packing
    e. Sterilization techniques

54. **Why does die stone require less water for mixing than plaster?**
    a. Die stone powder particles pack more efficiently
    b. Die stone undergoes a different reaction from that of stone
    c. Die stone powder particles are less porous and imbibe less water
    d. Die stone chemical reaction generates less heat and requires less cooling
    e. Die stone contaminants are minimized by adding less water

55. **Why should molten wax application onto dies be accomplished slowly and in thin layers when creating a casting pattern?**
    a. Careful use minimizes porosity
    b. This promotes wetting of the wax on the dies
    c. This avoids distortion from thermal contraction during wax cooling
    d. This has a tendency to sag because of low modulus
    e. This has susceptibility to water absorption

56. **What is the role of paraffin in MOST dental waxes?**
    a. Increases tackiness
    b. Increases hardness
    c. Increases thermal stability
    d. Acts as main low-melting component
    e. Reduces thermal expansion

57. **What is the goal for the design of MOST dental inlay waxes?**
    a. High hardness
    b. Low cost
    c. Low melting temperature
    d. Complete pyrolysis on heating to carbon dioxide (CO_2) and (H_2O)
    e. Low coefficient of thermal expansion

58. **What are the primary components of an investment material?**
    a. Matrix, binder, and accelerators
    b. Water and two powders
    c. Two liquid reactants and powder
    d. Matrix, filler, and modifier
    e. Two pastes

59. **What is the principal advantage of phosphate bonded investment (PBI) over gypsum bonded investment (GBI)?**
    a. More stability at higher temperatures
    b. Stronger
    c. Less setting expansion
    d. Faster reacting
    e. Lower cost

60. **What is the karatage of an alloy that is 80% gold (Au) by weight?**
    a. 8 karat
    b. 12 karat
    c. 16 karat
    d. 19 karat
    e. 22 karat

61. **In high-gold casting alloys, which element produces a protective oxide on the surface of the molten alloy during the casting process?**
    a. Au
    b. Zn
    c. Ag
    d. Cu
    e. Pd

62. **In high-gold casting alloys, which element is primarily responsible for hardness?**
    a. Ag
    b. Cu
    c. Zn
    d. Au
    e. Pd

63. **What element is responsible for producing the corrosion resistance of stainless steel instruments?**
    a. Cr
    b. Fe
    c. C
    d. Co
    e. Ni

64. **What level of chromium is required in steel alloys to produce effective passivation?**
    a. 10–14%
    b. 14–18%
    c. 18–28%
    d. 28–40%
    e. >40%

65. **Which one of the following terms is NOT specifically related to soldering?**
    a. Filler metal
    b. Brazing
    c. Joining
    d. 600 to 650 fine
    e. Precious metal content

66. **Which application does NOT use gold alloys?**
    a. Cast alloy crown
    b. Cast alloy bridge
    c. Partial denture framework
    d. Cast post and core
    e. Implant

67. **Which of the following dental materials CANNOT cause nickel sensitivity?**
    a. Dental amalgam
    b. Stainless steel crowns
    c. Some PFM alloys
    d. Some partial denture framework alloys
    e. Some orthodontic wires

68. **What is the general incidence of nickel sensitivity in men?**
    a. 30%
    b. 25%
    c. 20%
    d. 10%
    e. Lower than in women

69. **What events contribute to a relatively high nickel sensitivity level in women?**
    a. Greater contact with metal coinage
    b. Contact dermatitis from nickel-based jewelry
    c. Greater contact with stainless steel
    d. Genetic differences
    e. Less protective skin and hair during contact

70. **What are the three principal components of dental porcelains?**
    a. Silica, calcium oxide, and alumina
    b. Alumina, zinc oxide, and calcium fluoride
    c. Alumina, potassium oxide, and calcium oxide
    d. Calcium oxide, magnesium oxide, and chromium oxide
    e. Silica, alumina, and potassium oxide

71. **What component of dental porcelain contributes primarily to aesthetics?**
    a. Alumina
    b. Silica
    c. Potassium oxide
    d. Chromium oxide
    e. Titanium oxide

72. **What component is involved with very-high-strength dental ceramics?**
    a. Silica
    b. Silicon carbide
    c. Potassium oxide
    d. Chromium oxide
    e. Zirconia

73. **What is NOT TRUE for feldspathic porcelain?**
    a. Excellent translucency
    b. Relatively low coefficient of thermal expansion
    c. Ductile
    d. Used to veneer most dental porcelains
    e. High hardness

74. **Which is TRUE of all traditional dental cements?**
    a. Precapsulated
    b. Endothermic reactions
    c. Acid–base reactions
    d. Good esthetics
    e. High strength

75. **Which one of the following dental cement compositions requires staged additions of powder to the liquid during mixing on a chilled glass slab to control the reaction?**
    a. Compomer cement
    b. Polycarboxylate cement
    c. Resin-modified glass ionomer cement
    d. Zinc phosphate cement
    e. Universal cement

76. **What is the primary monomer involved in denture base fabrication?**
    a. HEMA
    b. EMA
    c. Bis-GMA
    d. MMA
    e. UDM

77. **Why are acrylic resin teeth popular for denture fabrication?**
    a. Light weight
    b. Excellent wear resistance
    c. Ease of cleaning
    d. Easily bonded to denture base
    e. Best esthetics

78. **What is the major problem for tissue conditioners over the first few days?**
    a. Increased hardness
    b. Discoloration
    c. Bad taste
    d. Loss of bonding
    e. Fungal growth

79. **Mouth protectors should be cleaned with:**
    a. Dilute chlorhexidine solutions
    b. Ultrasonic agitation in baking soda solutions
    c. Dilute chlorine bleach in water
    d. Denture-cleaning solutions
    e. Cool soap-and-water solutions

80. **Which one of the following materials practically CANNOT be fabricated using CAD/CAM procedures?**
    a. Dental composite
    b. Dental porcelain
    c. Gold alloys
    d. Zirconia
    e. Alumina

81. **What does NOT harm the protective titanium dioxide surface on dental implants?**
    a. APF application
    b. Scaling with metal instruments
    c. Use of polishing agents
    d. Abrasive dentifrices
    e. Dental floss

82. **What are the major requirements for tissue engineering?**
    a. Cells, signals, scaffolds
    b. Cells and bone
    c. Cells and collagen
    d. Collagen, hydroxyapatite, and signals
    e. Cells and scaffolds

83. **Which of the following biomaterials uses tissue from a cadaver?**
    a. Autograft
    b. Allograft
    c. Xenograft
    d. Synthetic tissue
    e. Engineered tissue

84. **Which of the following is NOT a scaffold material for tissue engineering?**
    a. Bone chips
    b. Gold mesh
    c. Polylactic acid (PLA)
    d. Bioglass
    e. Collagen

Periodontics

Denise M. Bowen

The vast majority of periodontal needs are related to the treatment of gingivitis and early periodontitis, the prevention of periodontal disease, and the maintenance of periodontal health after therapy. These services are provided by dental hygienists; the demand for these services and the dental hygienists who provide them continues to grow. Understanding of periodontics is critical to the process of dental hygiene care.

BASIC FEATURES OF THE PERIODONTIUM

A. The periodontium (Figure 14-1) is composed of gingiva, periodontal ligament, cementum, and alveolar bone
B. The function of the periodontium is to attach the teeth to the alveolar bone tissues of the mandible and the maxilla

Gingiva

Definition
A. Part of the oral masticatory mucosa that surrounds the cervical portion of the teeth and covers the alveolar process of the jaws
B. Components
  1. Marginal gingiva (unattached or free gingiva)
    a. Unattached cuff-like tissue that surrounds teeth facially, lingually, and interproximally
    b. Parts of marginal gingiva
      (1) Gingival margin—most coronal portion; surrounds the teeth in a scalloped outline; located at or approximately 0.5 millimeters (mm) coronal to the cemento-enamel junction (CEJ)
      (2) Gingival groove—present in only 50% of gingival surfaces; when present, it is located 1 to 1.5 mm apical to the gingival margin at the base of the gingival sulcus
      (3) Gingival sulcus—space formed by the tooth and the sulcular epithelium laterally and by the coronal end of the junctional epithelium (base of the sulcus) apically; in periodontal health, almost no gingival sulcus exists; a sulcular measurement of 1 to 2 mm facially and lingually and 1 to 3 mm interproximally is considered normal
      (4) Interdental gingiva—occupies the interdental space coronal to the alveolar crest (clinically, it fills the embrasure space beneath the area of tooth contact)
        (a) Interdental gingiva—consists of two interdental papillae (one facial and one lingual) that are connected by the concave interdental col
        (b) Col is absent when teeth are not in contact
        (c) Interdental gingiva, like facial and lingual gingivae, is attached to the tooth by the junctional epithelium and connective tissue fibers
  2. Attached gingiva
    a. Portion of the gingiva that is attached to the underlying periosteum of the alveolar bone and to the cementum by connective tissue fibers and the epithelial attachment
    b. Boundaries
      (1) Apically demarcated from the alveolar mucosa by the mucogingival junction
      (2) Coronally demarcated by the base of the gingival sulcus
    c. Width varies from 1.8 to 4.5 mm
      (1) Generally widest in the facial anterior maxillary areas and narrowest in the mandibular premolar facial areas

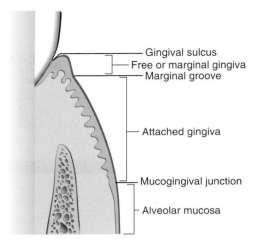

FIGURE 14-1 Anatomy of the periodontium.

(2) The width is not measured on the palate as the palate cannot be clinically distinguished from the palatal mucosa
   3. Changes in the width of attached gingiva result from changes at the coronal end

Histologic Features[1,2]

See the sections on "Oral histology," "Oral mucosa," and "Dento-gingival junction," in Chapter 2.
A. Epithelium
   1. Sulcular (crevicular) epithelium—stratified squamous, nonkeratinized epithelium that is continuous with the oral epithelium; lines the peripheral surface of the sulcus extending to the coronal border of the junctional epithelium
   2. Junctional epithelium—part of the dento-gingival junction; stratified squamous, nonkeratinized epithelium that surrounds and attaches to the tooth on one side and attaches on the other side to the gingival connective tissue; new cells originate from the cells in the apical portion adjacent to the tooth and from the cells in contact with the connective tissue; epithelial cells are shed (desquamation) at the coronal end of the junctional epithelium, which forms the base of the gingival sulcus
      a. The junctional epithelium is more permeable to cells and fluids than is the oral epithelium
      b. The junctional epithelium serves as the route for the passage of fluid and cells from the connective tissue into the sulcus and for the passage of bacteria and bacterial products from the sulcus into the connective tissue
      c. The junctional epithelium is easily penetrated by the periodontal probe; penetration is increased in inflamed gingiva

   d. The length of the junctional epithelium ranges from 0.25 to 1.35 mm; most coronal portion of the anchoring periodontium in health
   3. Epithelial attachment—basal lamina, hemidesmosomes, adhesion proteins (laminins), and anchoring fibrils that connect the junctional epithelium to the tooth surface at or slightly coronal to the CEJ
B. Connective tissue (or lamina propria)—composed of gingival fibers (connective tissue fibers), intercellular ground substance, cells, and vessels and nerves (see Chapter 2, Figures 2-20 and 2-27)
   1. Gingival fibers—composed of collagen fibers (60% of connective tissue volume) and an elastic fiber system composed of oxytalan, elaunin, and elastin fibers; fiber bundle groups provide support for marginal gingiva, including the interdental papilla (see also Chapter 2, Figure 2-28, B, and the section on "Oral histology, periodontal ligament for gingival fiber groups")
   2. Intercellular ground substance (or matrix)–similar to connective tissue in periodontal ligament
   3. Cells
      a. Fibroblasts (predominant cells)
         (1) Produce various types of fibers found in connective tissue
         (2) Instrumental in synthesis of intercellular ground substance
         (3) Wound healing or healing after therapy is regulated by fibroblasts (see the section on "Regeneration and wound healing" in Chapter 7)
      b. Other connective tissue cellular components—host defense cells
   4. Vessels and nerves (see the section on "Blood supply to the periodontium")

Normal Clinical Features

See Figure 14-2.
A. Color—in light-skinned individuals, pale or coral pink; in dark-skinned individuals, coral pink to brown; color varies, depending on the degree of vascularity, amount of melanin, epithelial keratinization, and thickness of epithelium
B. Texture
   1. Gingival margin—dull, smooth surface
   2. Attached—stippled, "orange peel" surface present on facial surfaces; may not always be present in health
C. Consistency
   1. Gingival margin—firm and resilient; resists displacement
   2. Attached gingiva—firmly bound to the underlying alveolar bone and cementum

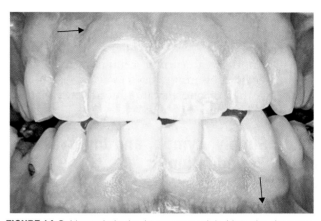

FIGURE 14-2 Normal gingiva in a young adult. Note the demarcation, referred to as the *mucogingival line* (*arrows*), between the attached gingival and the darker alveolar mucosa. *(From Newman MG, Takei H, Klokkevold PR, Carranza FA:* Carranza's clinical periodontology, *ed 11, St Louis, 2012, Saunders.)*

D. Contour and shape
  1. Papillary contour—pointed; papilla fills proximal embrasure space to the contact point
  2. Marginal contour—most coronal edge should form a knife-like edge with a scalloped configuration mesiodistally (follows the CEJ)
  3. The contour varies with the shape and alignment of teeth and with the size and position of contacts

Periodontal Ligament

See the section on "Periodontal ligament" and Figure 2-27 in Chapter 2.

Functions

A. Physical—attachment of the tooth to the bone, transmission of occlusal forces to the bone, absorption of the impact of occlusal forces, and maintenance of the proper relationship of gingival tissues to teeth
B. Formative—participation in formation of cementum and bone and remodeling of the periodontal ligament by activities of connective tissue cells (cementoblasts, fibroblasts, osteoblasts)
C. Resorptive—by the activity of connective tissue cells (primarily osteoclasts)
D. Nutritive—nutrients carried through blood vessels to cementum, bone, and gingiva
E. Sensory—proprioceptive and tactile sensitivity provided by innervation to the ligament

Clinical Considerations

A. Thickness varies from 0.05 to 0.25 mm (mean, 0.2 mm), depending on the stage of eruption, the person's age, and the function of a tooth; the ligament is thickest in the apical area and is thicker in functioning than in nonfunctioning teeth and in areas of tension than in areas of compression
B. Periodontal ligament cells that form collagen in ligament bundles can also remodel the ligament through secretion of new collagen (fibroblasts) and resorption of older collagen (fibroclasts), as well as lateral resorption of adjacent bone (osteoclasts) when altered forces are applied (e.g., orthodontics)
C. Accidentally exfoliated teeth can be reimplanted if handling of torn ligament is minimized before reimplantation

Cementum

See the section on "Cementum" in Chapter 2.

Clinical Considerations

A. Compensates for occlusal wear and continuous eruption by apical deposition of cementum throughout life
B. Protects the root surface from resorption during tooth movement
C. Has a reparative function, which permits re-establishment of new connective tissue attachment after certain types of periodontal therapies
D. When enamel and cementum do not meet, cervical hypersensitivity and caries are more likely

Alveolar Process

See the section on "Alveolar bone" and Figure 2-26 in Chapter 2.

Shape, Thickness, and Location

A. The contour of the alveolar bone follows the contour of the CEJ and the arrangement of the dentition
B. The shape of the alveolar crest is generally parallel to the CEJ of adjacent teeth; is approximately 1.5 to 2 mm apical to the CEJ
C. Cortical plates generally are thicker in the mandible than in the maxilla
D. Posterior areas—bone generally is thick, and cancellous bone separates the cortical plate from the alveolar bone proper
E. Anterior areas—bone is thin, with little or no cancellous bone separating the cortical plate from the alveolar bone proper
F. Dehiscence—situation in which the marginal alveolar bone is denuded, forming a defect extending apical to the normal level, exposing an abnormal amount of root surface
G. Fenestration—situation in which the margin of alveolar bone is intact; an isolated lack of alveolar

bone on the root surface leaves it covered only by the periosteum and overlying gingiva

Radiographic Features of the Normal Periodontium

See Figure 14-3.

A. Alveolar crest—thin, radiopaque line continuous with the lamina dura; the shape is dependent on the following:
  1. Proximity of adjacent teeth and roots
  2. Level of adjacent CEJs
B. Interdental septum—proximal alveolar bone bordered by the alveolar crest
C. Lamina dura—radiographic image of the alveolar bone proper; may or may not be present as a thin radiopaque line surrounding the bone adjacent to the periodontal ligament
D. Periodontal ligament space—thin radiolucent line surrounding each tooth between the root and adjacent alveolar bone
E. Supporting bone—radiopacity of the trabecular pattern varies, depending on the amount, pattern, and presence of cancellous and cortical bone
F. Limitations of radiographs—radiographs:
  1. Do not show the relationships between soft and hard tissues
  2. Do not show the initial signs of early bone loss
  3. May not accurately show interproximal bony changes

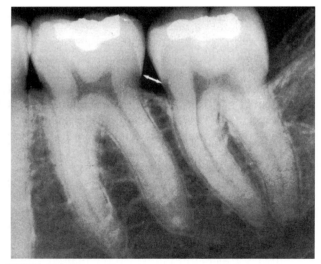

FIGURE 14-3 Crest of interdental septum, which is normally parallel to a line drawn between the cemento-enamel junction of adjacent teeth (*arrow*). Note the radiopaque lamina dura around the roots. *(From Newman MG, Takei H, Klokkevold PR, Carranza FA: Carranza's clinical periodontology, ed 11, St Louis, 2012, Saunders.)*

4. Do not show bone changes on facial or lingual surfaces; these bony plates are obscured by teeth roots
5. Do not reveal current cellular activity; only reflect past events
6. Have their diagnostic value affected by variations in technique

Blood Supply, Lymph, and Innervation of the Periodontium[1,2]

See the section on "Blood and lymph" and "Nerve tissue" in Chapter 2.

A. Blood supply originates from the inferior and superior alveolar arteries
B. Lymph drains into larger lymph nodes and veins
C. The nerve supply is derived from the branches of the trigeminal nerve and thus is sensory in nature; nerve branches terminate in the periodontal ligament, on the surface of alveolar bone, and within gingival connective tissue; receives stimuli for pain (nociceptors) and for position and pressure (mechanoreceptors and proprioceptors)

▌ DISEASES OF THE PERIODONTIUM

Classification of Periodontal Diseases[1-3]

See the section on "Periodontal diseases" in Chapter 9.

A. Importance of disease classification
  1. Useful for dental hygiene diagnosis, prognosis, care plans, and legal documentation
  2. Classifications of periodontal diseases are changing as new information about causes, pathogenicity, and host factors continues to evolve
B. Current classifications of periodontal diseases[3]
  1. Gingival diseases
    a. Dental plaque–induced gingival diseases—can occur on a periodontium with no attachment loss that is not progressing; include plaque-associated gingivitis and gingival diseases modified by systemic factors such as disorders of the endocrine system (hormonal), blood dyscrasias, medications, and malnutrition
    b. Non–plaque-induced gingival lesions—include gingival diseases of specific bacterial, viral, fungal, or genetic origin; gingival manifestations of systemic conditions such as mucocutaneous disorders and allergic reactions; and traumatic lesions, foreign body reactions, and otherwise nonspecified gingival lesions

2. Chronic periodontitis—localized or generalized

3. Aggressive periodontitis—localized or generalized

4. Periodontitis as a manifestation of systemic diseases (i.e., hematologic or genetic)

5. Necrotizing periodontal diseases

6. Abscesses of the periodontium

7. Periodontitis associated with endodontic lesions

8. Developmental or acquired deformities and conditions

Gingival Diseases[1,3]

A. Common characteristics
  1. Signs and symptoms confined to the gingiva
  2. Presence of bacterial plaque, which initiates or exacerbates the lesion
  3. Clinical signs of inflammation
  4. No loss of attachment or stable attachment levels; possible precursor to attachment loss

B. Dental plaque–induced gingivitis
  1. Inflammation of the gingiva resulting from bacterial plaque biofilm at the gingival margin
  2. Most common form of periodontal disease; prevalent in all age groups
  3. Change in gingival color and contour (redness, swelling, enlargement); increased sulcular temperature and gingival exudate; bleeding on provocation; reversible with plaque removal
  4. Sensitivity or tenderness can occur, although not necessarily present in all clients
  5. Absence of attachment loss and bone loss is characteristic; after active periodontal treatment and resolution of inflammation in periodontitis, tissue becomes healthy, but attachment loss remains; dental plaque–induced gingivitis on a reduced periodontium can occur in these cases if gingival inflammation arises without evidence of progressive attachment loss

C. Gingival diseases associated with endocrine changes or endogenous sex hormones
  1. Periodontal tissues are modulated by androgens, estrogens, and progestin
  2. Most information exists about sex hormone–induced effects in women: menstruation, pregnancy, and puberty
  3. Gingival response requires bacterial plaque in conjunction with steroid hormones
    a. Puberty-associated gingivitis—occurs in adolescents during puberty in both genders when the dramatic rise in hormone levels has a transient effect on gingival inflammation; signs of gingivitis exist in the presence of relatively sparse deposits
    b. Menstrual cycle–associated gingivitis—significant and observable inflammatory changes occur most frequently during ovulation
    c. Pregnancy-associated gingivitis—some of the most remarkable endocrine changes occur during pregnancy owing to increased plasma hormone levels; features are similar to plaque-induced gingivitis, but relatively little bacterial plaque may be present
    d. Pregnancy-associated pyogenic granuloma (pregnancy tumor)—pronounced response of gingiva to bacterial plaque at gingival margin in the form of a sessile or pedunculated protuberant mass; more common interproximally; regresses after parturition

D. Gingival diseases associated with medications (drug-influenced gingival diseases)[2-4]
  1. Drug-influenced gingival enlargement—overgrowth of the gingiva most commonly associated with the following:
    a. Anticonvulsant agents (e.g., phenytoin)—occurs in about 50% of users
    b. Immunosuppressant agents (e.g., cyclosporin A)—occurs in about 30% of users
    c. Calcium channel blockers (e.g., nifedipine, verapamil, diltiazem, sodium valproate)—occurs in 6% to 20% of users
  2. Occurs most frequently in the anterior gingiva, especially in children; onset within 3 months of drug regimen
  3. Changes in gingival contour, size, and color all because of enlargement; increased gingival exudate and bleeding on provocation can coexist; first occurs interproximally
  4. Found in the gingiva, with or without bone loss; not associated with attachment loss
  5. Plaque control can limit the severity of the pronounced inflammatory response of the gingiva
  6. Oral contraceptive–associated gingivitis—also can occur in the presence of marginal plaque because of the pronounced inflammatory response of the gingiva in women using certain oral contraceptive agents; inflammation and enlargement are reversible when the drug is discontinued

E. Gingival diseases associated with systemic diseases
  1. Diabetes mellitus–associated gingivitis—found in children with poorly controlled type 1 diabetes mellitus
  2. Leukemia-associated gingivitis (hematologic gingival disease)—primarily found in persons with acute leukemia
  3. Both diseases manifest with pronounced inflammatory response to bacterial plaque; changes in gingival color and contour; increased bleeding on provocation
  4. Plaque biofilm control can limit severity

F. Gingival diseases associated with malnutrition
  1. Malnutrition leads to compromised host response and defense mechanisms
  2. Increased susceptibility to infection may exacerbate gingival response to bacterial plaque
  3. Scurvy can also result from ascorbic acid (vitamin C) deficiency; the resultant gingival lesions are described as erythematous, bulbous, hemorrhagic, swollen, and spongy
G. Non–plaque-induced gingival lesions[3]
  1. Infectious gingivitis—includes specific bacteria (e.g., *Neisseria gonorrhoeae*, *Treponema pallidum*, streptococci), viruses (e.g., herpes simplex types 1 and 2, varicella zoster, and papillomavirus), fungi (e.g., *Candida* species), or genetic conditions (e.g., hereditary gingival fibromatosis) (see the section on "Periodontal diseases" in Chapter 9); linear gingival erythema occurs in individuals who have acquired immune deficiency syndrome (AIDS) or other immunocompromising diseases
    a. Clinical changes—distinct band of severe erythema on marginal gingiva; can be localized or generalized; sometimes punctuated red dots are also present on attached gingiva; no ulceration or loss of attachment occurs
    b. Radiographic changes—none; normal findings
    c. Cause—immunosuppressed host response to bacterial plaque
    d. Treatment—scaling and debridement with povidone–iodine irrigation for antimicrobial and topical anesthetic effect; prescription of antifungal agents if candidiasis is also present; critical importance of thorough self-care practices, including mechanical removal of bacterial plaque and twice-daily 0.12% chlorhexidine rinses, 1-month re-evaluation, and continued care, must be stressed to the client
  2. Dermatologic diseases, including lichen planus, pemphigoid, pemphigus vulgaris, erythema multiforme, psoriasis, and lupus erythematosus, also may present with gingival manifestations; the diagnosis depends on clinical findings and biopsy specimens (see the sections on "Major aphthous ulcers," "Skin diseases," and "White lesions" in Chapter 8)
  3. Allergic reactions in the oral mucosa are uncommon but can be caused by dental restorations, dentifrices, mouthwashes, and food allergens; signs and symptoms do not resolve when oral hygiene is instituted
  4. Foreign body reactions occur when ulceration of the gingival epithelium allows entry of a substance into the gingival connective tissue; most commonly is an amalgam tattoo

  5. Mechanical trauma can be accidental, iatrogenic, or factitious; results in gingival or tooth abrasion, recession, ulceration, inflammation, or laceration

Chronic Periodontitis[2,3]

A. Slowly progressive; most common in adults; can also occur in children and adolescents
B. The disease results from the inflammatory process originating in the gingiva (gingivitis) and extending into the supporting periodontal structures; may have periods of activity and remission; has slow to moderate progression; may have periods of rapid progression
  1. Can be further classified on the basis of extent and severity
    a. Extent—number of sites involved
      (1) Localized—30% of sites or less
      (2) Generalized—more than 30% of sites
    b. Severity—clinical attachment loss (CAL)
      (1) Early—progression of gingival inflammation into the deeper periodontal structures and alveolar bone crest, with slight bone loss; with normal gingival contour, usual periodontal probing depth is 2 to 3 mm, with slight loss of connective tissue attachment and alveolar bone; average 1 to 2 mm attachment loss
      (2) Moderate—a more advanced state of the above condition, with increased destruction of periodontal structures and noticeable loss of bone support, possibly accompanied by an increase in tooth mobility; average probing depth of 4 to 5 mm, with normal gingival contour; average 3 to 4 mm attachment loss
      (3) Advanced—further progression of periodontitis, with major loss of alveolar bone support >30%;[5] usually accompanied by increased tooth mobility; furcation involvement in multiple-rooted teeth is likely; recession is common; average probing depth 6 mm or more, with normal gingival contour; average ≥5 mm attachment loss
  2. Radiographic features (see the section on "Changes in the periodontium associated with disease")
  3. Cause—host response to bacterial plaque biofilm; the amount of destruction is consistent with the presence of local factors; subgingival calculus is frequently seen; is associated with various microbial patterns; can be associated with local predisposing factors; may be modified by systemic diseases and other risk factors

4. Treatment—nonsurgical or surgical periodontal therapy, or both, depending on extent and severity, followed by periodontal maintenance procedures

C. Chronic periodontitis can be recurrent and refractory (nonresponsive); not all cases of periodontitis have successful treatment outcomes

Aggressive Periodontitis[1–3,6]

A. Can occur at any age; may be localized or generalized

B. Common features

1. Occurs in persons otherwise healthy
2. Rapid attachment loss and bone loss, which may or may not be self-arresting
3. Familial aggregation
4. Secondary features that are less universal include the following:
   a. Bacterial plaque inconsistent with the severity of periodontal destruction
   b. Elevated proportions of *Aggregatibacter actinomycetemcomitans* and sometimes *Porphyromonas gingivalis*
   c. Phagocyte abnormalities and poor antibody response
   d. Progression of attachment loss and bone loss can be self-arresting

C. Localized aggressive periodontitis

1. Circumpubertal onset most common
2. Localized incisor and first-molar onset with interproximal attachment loss on at least two teeth (one first molar) and involving no more than two teeth other than incisors and first molars

D. Generalized aggressive periodontitis

1. Most common before age 30, but may also occur in older persons
2. Pronounced episodic nature of bone loss and attachment loss
3. Generalized interproximal attachment loss affecting at least three permanent teeth other than incisors and first molars

E. Treatment—same as for chronic periodontitis; systemic antibiotic (tetracycline derivative or metronidazole and amoxicillin therapy) and diligent periodontal maintenance procedures

Periodontitis as a Manifestation of Systemic Diseases[2,3]

A. Systemic factors modify all forms of periodontal disease, but some systemic diseases cause periodontitis; the listing is categorized under broad headings; other diseases may be added to the list in the future

B. Hematologic disorders—see the section on "Blood dyscrasias" in Chapter 8

1. Neutrophil deficiencies cause severe destruction of periodontal tissues; leukocyte activities such as chemotaxis, phagocytosis, and killing or neutralization of ingested organisms or substances must be integrated for adequate protection
2. Quantitative leukocyte disorders
   a. Neutropenia—the malignant form involves necrosis and ulceration of marginal gingiva and bleeding; more cyclic or chronic forms involve deep periodontal pockets with extensive, generalized bone loss
   b. Leukemia—most common in the acute form; symptoms include generalized gingival enlargement, swelling caused by cellular infiltrate, and bleeding related to associated thrombocytopenia

C. Genetic disorders[1,6] (see the section on "Genetics" in Chapter 7)

1. Genetic disorders usually manifest early in life and have similar signs and symptoms as those of aggressive forms of periodontitis; host genetic factors are believed to be important determinants in a person's susceptibility to periodontitis
2. Disorders associated with periodontitis include familial and cyclic neutropenia, Down syndrome, leukocytic deficiency syndrome, Papillon-Lefèvre syndrome, Chédiak-Higashi syndrome, histiocytosis syndrome, glycogen storage disease, infantile genetic agranulocytosis, Cohen syndrome, Ehlers-Danlos syndrome (types IV and VIII), and hypophosphatasia; rare conditions such as Papillon-Lefèvre syndrome, Chédiak-Higashi syndrome, and Ehlers-Danlos syndrome have the strongest evidence linking genetic mutations with periodontitis[6]

Necrotizing Periodontal Diseases[2,3]

A. Necrotizing ulcerative gingivitis (NUG)—inflammatory destructive disease of the gingiva that has a sudden onset with periods of remission and exacerbation; predisposing conditions may be preexisting (e.g., gingivitis, smoking, period of severe stress, deficient diet or sleep)

1. Clinical findings are characterized by crater-like depressions at the crest of the interdental papilla that progress into the marginal gingiva
   a. Surface of the lesion(s) is covered by a gray, necrotized slough surrounded by an obvious erythematous (red) zone; interproximal necrosis
   b. Bleeding may be spontaneous and will occur even when necrotic tissue is removed gently

c. Initially, moderate pain increases as the disease advances

d. Strong fetid odor and increased salivation

e. Swelling and tenderness of regional lymph nodes (especially submandibular nodes)

f. Fever and malaise may be present

2. Radiographic findings—normal, unless the disease has not been treated and has led to the destruction of supporting structures (necrotizing ulcerative periodontitis)

3. Causes—predisposing factors are present, with intermediate-sized spirochetes (*Treponema* and *Selemonas*), *Fusobacterium*, and *Prevotella intermedia* found within the tissue; the primary causative factor is uncertain; has been associated with immunosuppression

4. Treatment

a. Debridement for plaque biofilm and debris removal—initially by the clinician and then daily by the client (who may find it difficult to do because of pain); ultrasonic debridement may be beneficial

b. Reappoint in 24 to 48 hours to evaluate healing; after removal of bacterial challenge, rapid response in individuals with normal immune function; no response in the immunocompromised; complete and thorough scaling, root planing, and periodontal debridement performed at this appointment; pain is markedly reduced if healing has begun

c. The recurrent nature of NUG and the critical role of self-care practices and frequent continued-care visits must be stressed

d. Antibiotics may be prescribed for the treatment of systemic symptoms (lymphadenopathy, fever)

e. Soft nutritious diet and the avoidance of spicy foods, alcohol, and tobacco use are important

B. Necrotizing ulcerative periodontitis

1. Occurs in persons who have human immunodeficiency virus (HIV) infection or AIDS, other immunocompromising diseases, or severe malnutrition

2. Characterized by severe soft tissue necrosis and rapid destruction of periodontal attachment and bone; may lead to the exposure of alveolar bone and sequestration

3. Chief complaint may be "jaw pain" or "deep aching pain"

4. Can be localized or generalized

5. Treatment requires medical consultation and conventional periodontal therapy with povidone–iodine irrigation and pain control; rigorous self-care practices for mechanical plaque biofilm removal in conjunction with twice daily 0.12% chlorhexidine mouthrinsing, judicious use of systemic antibiotics, or both; adjunctive antifungal therapy, if indicated; more frequent maintenance therapy than indicated for persons with adult periodontitis

Abscesses of the Periodontium[2,3]

See Table 14-1.

A. Microbiology—*Streptococcus viridans* is the most common isolate; similar to microbiota found in deep periodontal pockets

B. Factors associated with abscess formation

1. Occlusion of pocket orifices or incomplete calculus removal during treatment of a periodontal pocket

TABLE 14-1 Characteristics of Periodontal and Endodontic Abscesses

Characteristic	Periodontal Abscess	Endodontic Abscess
Pain	Less severe than with periapical abscess	Usually severe
Discharge	Through pocket	Usually over apex, but possibly at gingival margin
Swelling	More gingivally	Over apex
Area of maximum tenderness	More gingivally	Over apex
Timing	Usually swelling before pain	Usually pain before swelling
Tender to percussion	Not usually, or mild	Usually very tender
Pocket formation	Yes	Not always, but can occur
History of trauma or previous restoration	Not necessarily	Usually
Previous symptoms of pulpitis	Not necessarily	Frequently
Vitality of tooth	Usually vital	Nonvital (but partial vitality may exist with multiple-rooted teeth)
Radiographic appearance	Marginal bone loss evident	May be apical rarefaction

Adapted from Chapple ILC, Lumley PJ: The periodontal-endodontic interface, Dent Update 26(8):338–341, 1999; and Guerenlian JR: The periodontal enigma, Access 15(3):28–32, 2001.

2. Furcation involvement

3. Systemic antibiotic treatment

4. Diabetes mellitus

C. Classification of abscesses of the periodontium

　1. Gingival abscess—a localized purulent infection involving the marginal gingiva or interdental papilla; may have bluish hue; does not involve the underlying periodontium

　2. Periodontal (or lateral) abscess—localized, purulent area of inflammation within periodontal tissue

　　a. Clinical findings—the abscess may:

　　　(1) Be in the supporting periodontal tissues on the lateral aspect of the root, which results in a sinus (fistula) opening through the bone extending out to the external surface

　　　(2) Develop in the soft tissue wall of a deep periodontal pocket, adjacent to a periapical lesion, or after deep scaling or periodontal debridement

　　　(3) Be acute or chronic

　　　　(a) Acute—extreme pain, sensitivity, mobility, enlarged lymph nodes; the gingival area is edematous, red, and smooth with a shiny surface; exudate may be expressed from the gingival margin on pressure

　　　　(b) Chronic—usually asymptomatic or episodes of dull pain; elevation of the tooth; desire to grind on the tooth (may have acute episodes); usually has a sinus opening onto the gingival mucosa along the root

　　b. Radiographic findings (many variations according to the location, stage, and extent of the lesion)—typical appearance is that of a discrete radiolucent area along the lateral aspect of the root

　　c. Treatment—debridement with 0.12% chlorhexidine or povidone–iodine irrigation; antibiotics if fever, swelling, or lymph node involvement is present; combined periodontal–endodontic therapy if related to periapical abscess

　3. Pericoronal abscess—inflammation of the tissue flap (operculum) surrounding the crown of a partially erupted tooth; also called *pericoronitis*; most common in third-molar areas; may be acute, subacute, or chronic

　　a. Clinical findings if acute

　　　(1) An extremely red, swollen lesion with exudate is present

　　　(2) The area is extremely tender; pain radiates to the ear, throat, and floor of the mouth

　　　(3) A foul taste is present in the mouth

　　　(4) Inflammation may progress so that swelling, inability to close the jaw, fever, and malaise occur; the symptoms are less obvious when chronic

　　b. Cause—accumulation of food debris and bacterial growth between the soft tissue flap and the tooth; tissue inflammation may be compounded by trauma from the opposing tooth

　　c. Treatment

　　　(1) Antibiotics if fever, swelling, or lymphadenopathy is present

　　　(2) Cleansing of the area (lavage, débridement) and creation of access for the drainage of the exudate

　　　(3) Frequent rinsing with warm water by the client and return for continued care after 24 hours

　　　(4) Extraction of the involved tooth or removal (excision) of the soft tissue flap after the pain subsides and the infection is controlled

Periodontitis Associated with Endodontic Lesions[3]

See Table 14-1. Combined periodontal–endodontic lesions—either a deep periodontal pocket or an endodontic infection may be the cause or the result of the other, or both may develop independently; require combined endodontic and periodontic treatment

Developmental or Acquired Deformities and Conditions[1,3]

A. Localized tooth-related factors that modify or predispose to dental plaque–induced gingival diseases and periodontitis

　1. Tooth anatomic factors—enamel pearls, furcation, tooth position, root proximity, open contacts, root abnormalities

　2. Dental restorations and appliances—marginal discrepancies, overhangs

　3. Root fractures—periodontal lesions commonly accompany vertical root fractures

　4. Cervical root resorption and cemental tears—if the lesion is located coronally on the root, communication with the oral environment allows bacterial invasion

B. Mucogingival deformities and conditions around teeth; gingival recession (or gingival atrophy)—exposure of the root surface caused by an apical shift in the position of the gingiva

　1. The severity of the recession is determined by the actual position of the gingiva

2. The recession may be partially clinically visible and partially hidden (covered by inflamed pocket wall)

3. The term *recession* refers only to the location of the gingiva, not to the condition of the gingiva; recession of gingiva may be inflamed or noninflamed

4. Causes—the following factors have been implicated as possible causative factors:
   a. Gingival inflammation
   b. Faulty toothbrushing (gingival abrasion)
   c. Tooth position
   d. Location and amount of pull on the margin of the frenum attachment
   e. Dehiscence
   f. Advancing age

5. Clinical significance
   a. Exposed roots are susceptible to dental caries and abrasion
   b. Wearing away of cementum on the exposed surface exposes dentin, which may be sensitive to mechanical, chemical, or thermal stimuli
   c. Interproximal recession creates space for the accumulation of bacterial plaque biofilm and other debris

6. Treatment—nonsurgical or surgical
   a. Removal of causative or risk factors
   b. Daily thorough oral self-care practices and periodontal maintenance
   c. Root desensitization, if needed
   d. Gingival graft, regenerative or periodontal flap surgery may be performed

C. Mucogingival deformities or conditions on edentulous ridges—similar to dentulous areas, as well as the following factors:
   1. Vertical or horizontal ridge deficiency, or both
   2. Decreased vestibular depth

Epidemiology of Periodontal Diseases and Related Risks[1,2,7]

A. Basic terminology
   1. Incidence—number of new cases in an identified population during a specific period
   2. Prevalence—percentage of affected people in an identified population
   3. Extent—number or percentage of teeth or sites affected by a disease or condition
   4. Severity—degree of severity or advancement of a given disease or condition
   5. Risk factor—environmental, behavioral, or systemic characteristics or exposures that are associated strongly with a disease, without causality established; usually confirmed through longitudinal studies
   6. Risk indicator—a probable or putative risk factor that has been associated with a given condition or disease through cross-sectional studies; not always confirmed in longitudinal studies
   7. Risk predictor or marker—a factor that has been associated with future development of a given disease or condition; considered potentially predictive without established causality
   8. Odds ratio—odds represent the ratio of the probability that an event will occur to the probability that the event will not occur; an odds ratio of 1.0 means that people exposed to a particular event or factor are no more likely than a normal, healthy individual to develop that disease or condition; greater than 1.0 is more likely

B. Natural history of periodontal disease[8-10]
   1. Classic studies of the natural history of periodontal disease have established important features of the disease
      a. Severe disease tends to cluster in a small percentage of the population
      b. Pronounced differences in susceptibility to periodontal destruction can be independent of the environment
   2. Landmark longitudinal studies in which Löe and coworkers examined the course of periodontal disease during a 20-year period in two cohorts: Sri Lankan tea workers who were generally healthy but had never received dental care and did not know of toothbrushing, and students and academicians from Norway who had lifelong dental care and oral self-care education[8-10]
   3. Plaque, calculus, and gingivitis, which were common conditions in both groups, led to a slow loss of periodontal attachment with increasing age
   4. Periodontal attachment loss progressed at a rate of 0.3 mm per year in Sri Lanka and 0.1 mm per year in Norway; professional and self-care prevented or slowed the progression of disease
   5. In the Sri Lankan group with no periodontal therapy, the disease patterns identified were:
      a. No progression beyond gingivitis (11%)
      b. Moderate progression of 4-mm attachment loss (81%)
      c. Rapid progression of 9-mm attachment loss (8%)
   6. Periodontal diseases are most often slowly progressive; however, while some individuals show no progression even without care, others show rapid progression
   7. Because plaque, calculus, and gingival inflammation were present in both cohorts in the study by Löe and coworkers, other risk factors must play a role in progression of periodontal disease

C. Current model of pathogenicity
   1. All individuals are not equally susceptible to periodontal disease
   2. Only a low percentage of sites with gingivitis will develop into periodontitis
   3. Periodontal disease is a highly complex disease, and variations in its epidemiology can be attributed to both local (environmental) factors and host susceptibility
   4. From a health-maintenance perspective, a person with multiple strong risk factors is not of greater concern than one with few risk factors; even one risk factor may significantly augment a person's expression of disease
D. Epidemiology of periodontal diseases[1,2,11,12]
   See also the section on "Epidemiology of oral diseases and conditions" in Chapter 20
   1. Gingivitis
      a. Prevalence—large-scale national studies in the United States have estimated that 50% of adults have gingivitis; this is an underestimation because of study designs; gingival bleeding in at least one site was seen in 63% of adults; this is more prevalent, severe, and extensive in groups of subjects with extensive dental deposits, low socioeconomic status, limited access to health education and dental care, less education, and low health literacy and in adolescents, underserved minorities, and cognitively and developmentally challenged persons
      b. Risk factors—may be environmental or systemic
         (1) Systemic conditions that produce vascular changes, for example, acute leukemia, hemophilia, Sturge-Weber syndrome, and Wegener's granulomatosis
         (2) Systemic conditions that affect host response, for example, diabetes mellitus, Addison's disease, thrombocytopenia, combined immunodeficiency diseases, and HIV infection
         (3) Systemic conditions related to hormonal changes, for example, pregnancy, puberty, steroid therapy, and birth-control medications
         (4) Environmental factors or local factors such as plaque-retentive factors (calculus, ill-fitting restorations), tooth malalignment or crowding, and smoking, which decrease normal inflammatory response and have a greater effect on the risk of periodontitis than of gingivitis
      c. Causative factors—cause and effect studied
         (1) Bacterial plaque biofilm is causative in gingivitis—it is both necessary and sufficient to cause gingivitis; plaque-retentive factors such as calculus, incorrect restorative margins, prostheses, and orthodontics increase risk of gingival inflammation; gingivitis is preventable in most people with frequent and effective personal and professional plaque control measures
         (2) Prescription drugs can cause drug-influenced gingival enlargement, resulting, in whole or in part, from systemic drug use; these drugs can cause drug-influenced gingival enlargement, or their effects can be exacerbated by bacterial plaque
      d. Possible influence of diet and nutrition
         (1) No direct link has been established between nutrition and periodontal disease except in the case of scurvy and severe ascorbic acid (vitamin C) deficiency
         (2) The relationship of diet and nutrition to disease susceptibility, tissue integrity, and defense mechanisms cannot be ignored
   2. Chronic periodontitis[1,2,11]
      a. Prevalence—varies significantly, depending on the population being treated or untreated; greatest increases in mean CAL found in untreated groups; most recent U.S. surveys indicate 35% of adults over 30 years of age have periodontitis, including 22% mild and 13% moderate-to-severe forms; severity highest in older age groups
      b. Risk factors with positive association
         (1) Tobacco use—strongest environmental risk factor, predictor of future disease, and modifier of periodontal treatment outcomes; smokers are more likely to have periodontitis than nonsmokers; dose-related—development of severe disease increases with number of cigarettes smoked per day and with years of smoking; all forms of tobacco implicated; most likely related to effects on host immune response; smoking has been found to depress the number of helper lymphocytes, impair vascularization, inhibit collagen production, increase collagenase activity, and inhibit healing after periodontal therapy; although the past effects of smoking on the periodontium are not reversed, smoking cessation is beneficial to periodontal health[13]
         (2) Diabetes mellitus—especially in persons with poor metabolic control and type 1 diabetes; associated with more severe and

rapid disease progression and with poor treatment outcomes; effects appear to be cumulative and related to host immune response

(3) HIV infection—especially when HIV converts to AIDS with CD4 counts below 200/µL and in those who are severely immunocompromised, including those with HIV infection and AIDS, immunosuppression, leukemia, hemophilia, neutropenias, uncontrolled diabetes mellitus, agranulocytosis, Wegener's granulomatosis, Addison's disease, Sjögren's syndrome, Crohn's disease, Sturge-Weber syndrome, Down syndrome, and others; necrotizing periodontal diseases have been associated with immunocompromised status

(4) Osteoporosis—especially in conjunction with higher calculus scores; most likely caused by common pathways shared in the pathogenesis of periodontitis and that of osteoporosis

(5) Psychological stress—weakly associated; believed to be related to behavioral changes and immune system effects, especially in those who have poor coping skills; it also is likely that systemic diseases associated with periodontal disease share psychosocial stress as a common risk factor

c. Risk indicators
(1) Age—positive association; rate of progression is not related to age; however, prevalence, severity, and extent are greater in older groups of people perhaps because of the cumulative nature of the disease
(2) Gender—in the developed nations, males tend to have a higher prevalence of periodontal disease than do females who have access to dental care
(3) Socioeconomic status (SES), education, and access to dental care—negative association; lower SES, education, and number of dental visits are related to more periodontal destruction
(4) Bacterial plaque biofilm alone is not a sufficient causative factor for periodontitis; however, untreated populations and those with poor oral hygiene and higher calculus scores are at risk for greater disease progression and attachment loss; poor plaque control also has been associated with poor treatment outcomes
(5) Dental factors—sites previously affected by periodontitis; increased probing depth

and loss of clinical attachment or multiple residual periodontal pockets after active treatment increase the risk for continued attachment loss

(6) Local predisposing factors can be associated with periodontal disease; tooth-related or iatrogenic factors, missing teeth, mobile teeth, mouthbreathing, and areas of food impaction increase the risk of periodontal disease

3. Aggressive periodontitis
a. Prevalence—true prevalence and incidence are difficult to determine because of few longitudinal, prospective, and even careful retrospective studies as well as variations in diagnostic criteria and protocols in larger studies; frequency of affected individuals increases between puberty and 25 years of age
b. Risk indicators
(1) Race—aggressive periodontitis seems to be more prevalent among African Americans (10%) and Mexican Americans (5%) than in Caucasian Americans (1.3%); however, it is difficult to isolate racial differences from access to care and socioeconomic factors
(2) Genetics—studies in twins have shown that heredity accounts for the significant variance in measures of adult periodontitis, possibly related to the encoding of interleukin 1 (IL-1) affecting a person's susceptibility to the disease; leukocyte chemotaxis and phagocytosis defects and prevalence rates increase in parents, siblings, and offspring of those who have aggressive periodontitis; the disease is consistently present in several genetic or inherited disorders such as leukocyte adhesion deficiency, acatalasia, Chédiak-Higashi syndrome, Ehler-Danlos syndrome, Papillion-Lefèvre syndrome, hypophosphatasia, and prepubertal periodontitis (see the section on "Genetics" in Chapter 7)

CHANGES IN THE PERIODONTIUM ASSOCIATED WITH DISEASE

See the section on "Inflammation" in Chapter 7.
A. Pathogenesis and stages of the periodontal lesion[1-2,14]
1. Pathogenesis—mode of origin or development of a disease; bacterial virulence factors, constituents, or metabolites that are capable of disrupting protective host mechanisms or causing

disease initiation, progression, or both are required for the occurrence of periodontal disease

2. Stage I gingivitis, or initial lesion—2 to 4 days after bacterial plaque biofilm accumulation
   a. Changes are not clinically visible; subclinical lesion
   b. Histologic changes
      (1) Brief vasoconstriction followed by "widening" of small capillaries (vasodilation), margination, emigration, and migration of polymorphonuclear neutrophils (PMNs)
      (2) Increase in leukocytes, particularly PMNs (neutrophils) and macrophages, in the connective tissue, junctional epithelium, and gingival sulcus; neutrophils are the earliest responders, or the first line of defense, in inflammation
      (3) Host systems (e.g., complement and kinin systems and arachidonic pathways)
      (4) Increase in the flow of gingival crevicular fluid into the sulcus
      (5) Inflammatory infiltrate occupies 5% to 10% of the gingival connective tissue where collagen has been lost

3. Stage II gingivitis or early lesion—begins 4 to 7 days after bacterial plaque accumulation; may persist for 21 days or longer
   a. Clinical signs of gingivitis appear (erythema, edema, and bleeding on stimulation)
   b. Histologic changes
      (1) Persistence of inflammation from initial lesion
      (2) Inflammatory infiltrate in the connective tissue dominated by lymphocytes (75%); primarily T cells, with some macrophages, plasma cells, and mast cells
      (3) The junctional epithelium becomes densely infiltrated with inflammatory cells and begins to proliferate into connective tissue
      (4) Destruction of collagen fibers (especially circular and dento-gingival) in the infiltrated area; fibroblasts are altered
      (5) Migration of leukocytes, macrophages, and lymphocytes into the junctional epithelium and the gingival sulcus
      (6) The gingival crevicular fluid peaks at 6 to 12 days after clinical signs of gingivitis
      (7) The sulcular lining is ulcerated (allowing bleeding)

4. Stage III gingivitis or established (chronic) lesion—the period varies; may persist for months or years without progressing to stage IV (periodontitis)

   a. Clinical changes
      (1) Erythema (redness) of the gingiva as a result of proliferation of capillaries (begins in the papillary area) or a bluish hue superimposed over the reddened gingiva as a result of congested blood vessels, sluggish blood flow, or both
      (2) Bleeding may occur on probing as a result of thinning of the sulcular epithelium, ulceration of the sulcular epithelium, or both
      (3) Color changes begin in the papillary area and the gingival margin and then spread to the attached gingiva
      (4) Consistency may be either soft and spongy or firm and leathery; depends on whether destructive changes or reparative changes within the gingiva are dominant
      (5) Texture may be either of the following:
         (a) Smooth and shiny (destructive, exudative factors dominant)
         (b) Stippled and nodular (reparative, fibrotic proliferation dominant)
      (6) Increase in size of gingiva (enlargement)
      (7) Increase in depth of the gingival sulcus—may be caused by enlargement of the gingival tissue only; creates a gingival or pseudopocket (Figure 14-4)
         (a) Begins with papillary enlargement
         (b) Extends into margins, producing rounded and bulbous gingival margins

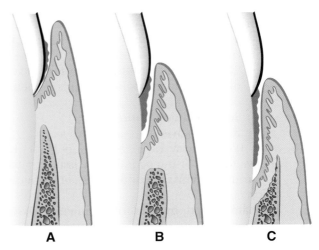

| A | B | C |

FIGURE 14-4 Different types of periodontal pockets. **A,** Gingival pocket. No destruction of the supporting periodontal tissues is seen. **B,** Suprabony pocket. The base of the pocket is coronal to the level of the underlying bone. Bone loss occurs horizontally. **C,** Infrabony pocket. The base of the pocket is apical to the level of the adjacent bone. Bone loss occurs vertically. *(From Newman MG, Takei H, Klokkevold PR, Carranza FA:* Carranza's clinical periodontology, *ed 11, St Louis, 2012, Saunders.)*

(8) Progression of inflammation orchestrated by the progression of cytokines
  (a) May remain only within gingival tissue (gingivitis)
  (b) May extend into supporting periodontal tissue in stage IV (periodontitis)
  Note: Periodontitis must be preceded by gingivitis, but gingivitis does not always progress to periodontitis

b. Histologic changes
  (1) Vascular proliferation and increase in number and predominance of B cells and plasma cells (produced by B lymphocytes) invade deep into the connective tissue; blood vessels are congested and blood flow is impaired
  (2) Widened intercellular spaces in the junctional epithelium contain lysosomes, lymphocytes, and monocytes; pathogens such as *A. actinomycetemcomitans* and *P. gingivalis* invade host tissues
  (3) Periodontal pathogens found in plaque biofilm such as *A. actinomycetemcomitans*, *P. gingivalis*, and *Tannerella forsythensis* produce collagenase and elastinase, enzymes that destroy connective tissue; *A. actinomycetemcomitan*, *P. gingivalis*, and *Treponema denticola* also produce a trypsin enzyme that kills lymphocytes; *Prevotella intermedia*, *Capnocytophaga*, and *P. gingivalis* degrade antibodies
  (4) The junctional epithelium continues to protrude into the connective tissue
  (5) Collagenase and other enzymes actively break down connective tissue, resulting in continued loss of collagen
  (6) Simultaneous proliferation of collagen fibers and epithelium (enlargement) occurs
  (7) Sulcular lining is ulcerated
  (8) Bone loss has not occurred

5. Stage IV—pathway of inflammation from the gingiva to supporting periodontal tissue (transition from gingivitis to periodontitis), or advanced lesion
  a. Characterized by loss of connective tissue attachment to teeth, including gingival and periodontal ligament fibers and their attachment to cementum, concurrent gingival inflammation, resorption of alveolar bone, and apical migration of the epithelial attachment along the root surface(i.e., CAL)
  b. Generally follows the course of blood vessels through soft tissues and into alveolar bone;

the pattern of inflammatory pathway affects the pattern of bone destruction
  c. Initially, the inflammation penetrates and destroys gingival fibers near the gingival fiber attachment to cementum and then spreads
    (1) Interproximally—into bone and the periodontal ligament
    (2) Facially and lingually—from bone to the periodontal ligament, from the gingiva to the outer periosteum and periodontal ligament, and from the periosteum into bone

B. Formation of the periodontal pocket[2]
  1. Persistent, chronic gingivitis may progress to periodontitis, which results in loss of connective tissue attachment, bone destruction, and periodontal pocket formation (see Figure 14-4)
  2. Periodontal pocket—pathologic deepening of the gingival sulcus produced by the destruction of supporting tissue and apical migration of the junctional epithelium
  3. Classification
    a. Suprabony pocket—base of the pocket is coronal to the alveolar crest; also called *supracrestal* or *supra-alveolar pocket*
    b. Infrabony pocket—base of the pocket is apical to the alveolar crest; also called *intrabony*, *intra-alveolar*, or *subcrestal pocket*
  4. Histopathology
    a. The gingival epithelium may show evidence of inflammatory changes
    b. Connective tissue changes
      (1) Inflammatory cells infiltrate the connective tissue and proceed through it
      (2) Degeneration of gingival connective tissue fibers; gingival cells release mediators or chemicals that destroy bone
      (3) Tissue invasion by periodontal pathogens
    c. Changes within supporting bone as inflammatory process progresses
      (1) Cytokines and effector molecules (e.g., interleukins, prostaglandin E_2 [PGE_2], MMP [matrix metalloproteinase]) have proinflammatory effects and stimulate osteoclastic cells that degenerate mineral content of bone; PMN, macrophage, and mononuclear cells degenerate organic matrix of bone by producing collagenase
      (2) Bone marrow component (fatty tissue) is replaced by inflammatory cell infiltrate, fibroblastic proliferation, and deposition of collagen fibers
      (3) The cortical plate of the interdental septum (crestal area) is the first area to be involved

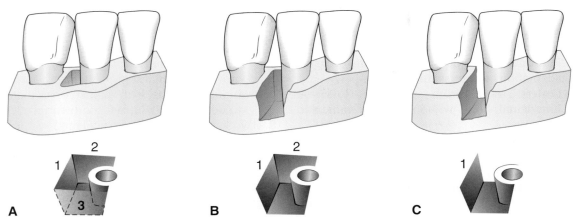

FIGURE 14-5 One-, two-, and three-wall vertical defects on the right lateral incisor. **A,** Three bony walls: distal (*1*), lingual (*2*), and facial (*3*). **B,** Two-wall defect: distal (*1*) and lingual (*2*). **C,** One-wall defect: distal only (*1*). *(From Newman MG, Takei H, Klokkevold PR, Carranza FA:* Carranza's clinical periodontology, *ed 11, St Louis, 2012, Saunders.)*

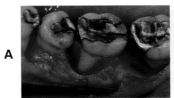 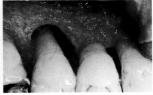

FIGURE 14-6 Angular defects. Circumferential vertical defect in relation to the maxillary canine and premolars, **A.,** Infrabony pockets around the molars, **B.** *(From Newman MG, Takei HH, Klokkevold PR, Carranza FA:* Carranza's clinical periodontiology, *ed 10, St Louis, 2006, Saunders.)*

(4) Once this central breakthrough has occurred, supporting bone is destroyed in a lateral direction; bone loss is accompanied by both resorption and formation

(5) Periodontal pockets are constantly undergoing repair

C. Common clinical changes associated with periodontitis

1. Similar changes in the gingiva as seen in gingivitis, but usually more chronic

2. Areas of gingival recession

3. Bleeding on probing

4. Periodontal attachment loss

5. True periodontal pockets

6. Loose, extruded, or migrated teeth; diastemas may develop

7. Exudate from the gingival margin in response to pressure; suppuration (pus) is a sign of secondary infection

8. Symptoms—generally painless; client may complain of itching gums, loose teeth, food impaction, and bad taste; relief is felt with pressure applied to the gums

9. Furcation involvement

D. Radiographic changes associated with periodontitis (usually follow this sequence)

1. Fuzziness and discontinuity of the lamina dura at the proximal aspects of the crest of the interdental septum

2. Wedge-shaped radiolucent area formed between the mesial or distal aspects of the alveolar crest and the root surface of the involved tooth; also called *triangulation*

3. Center of the crestal portion of the interdental septum also becomes fuzzy, and faint cup-shaped areas of alveolar crest bone loss appear; bony crater

4. Bone destruction patterns in periodontitis (Figures 14-5 and 14-6)

a. Horizontal bone loss is most common; bone is reduced in height but remains parallel to the tooth surface

b. Osseous defects or bone deformities

(1) Vertical or angular defects occur in an oblique direction; most commonly, infrabony pockets accompany vertical defects

(2) Classified by number of walls; may have one, two, or three walls

c. Osseous craters are concavities in the crest of interdental bone, common in posterior segments

d. Bulbous bone or bony enlargements occur as adaptations to excess function

e. Craters result from complete loss of interdental bone without loss of radicular bone

5. Limitations of radiographs in the diagnosis of periodontitis

a. The radiograph does not reveal minor destructive changes in bone

b. The involvement of facial and lingual surfaces cannot be seen

c. Angulation errors can affect radiographic image of alveolar bone

d. The internal morphology of infrabony craters or defects cannot be seen

e. As a general rule, bone loss is always greater than that revealed by the radiograph

E. Periodontal disease activity

1. Refers to the stage(s) of periodontal disease characterized by loss of alveolar bone and connective tissue attachment

2. Implies that the natural history of periodontal disease has periods of active destruction and periods of relative inactivity, although chronic inflammation persists

BACTERIAL PLAQUE BIOFILM[1,2]

See the sections on "Microbiology of the oral cavity" and "Bacterial plaque" in Chapter 9.

A. Definition—complex community of bacteria that forms on any surface that is exposed to the fluids in the mouth; communication of bacteria within the biofilm allows for production of byproducts; dense, noncalcified, highly organized; firmly adherent to teeth or other hard materials within the mouth; cannot be washed off by salivary or water flow

1. Biofilms protect bacteria housed within them (sessile), offering greater potential than freestanding (planktonic) bacteria

2. Microorganisms produce a matrix called *glycocalyx* and extracellular proteins that encase and coat bacteria in the biofilm, providing protection from the oral environment, retentive qualities essential to being adherent to the tooth surfaces, and pathogenic byproducts (e.g., dextrans and levans, uronic acid, and others); referred to as the *slime layer*

3. The matrix, or slime layer, of a biofilm provides a barrier from antimicrobial and antibiotic agents, making the biofilm resistant to chemotherapy

4. The matrix or slime layer provides structure for the biofilm, nutritional advantages required for growth and maturation of bacteria within the biofilm, and strength against forces that attempt to detach bacteria from tooth surfaces

B. Two categories of bacterial plaque—supragingival and subgingival

C. Stages in plaque formation

1. Acquired pellicle

2. Bacterial plaque biofilm

a. Complex microbial community forms, allowing for communication of bacteria within the biofilm and providing firm adherence to the tooth, restoration, or other such surfaces

b. Rate of formation varies from person to person and from tooth to tooth, and varies even between areas on the same tooth; seen on teeth after 24 to 48 hours without oral hygiene

c. Growth of microcolonies within the matrix and co-aggregation and adhesion of bacteria allow for increased thickness of plaque biofilm; shifts in the types of microorganisms occur as plaque ages; bacteria deep within the biofilm are more metabolically active and better protected than those on the surface that can be more easily dislodged

D. Supragingival versus subgingival plaque biofilms

1. Supragingival plaque

a. As plaque ages, the percentage of gram-positive organisms decreases

b. As plaque ages, aerobic bacteria decrease and anaerobic bacteria increase

2. Subgingival plaque[15]

a. Inflammatory changes in the gingival sulcus or periodontal pocket resulting from supragingival plaque modify the relationship between the gingival margin and the tooth surface, creating a protected subgingival area that is bathed by gingival crevicular fluid

b. This environment allows subgingival bacteria to colonize and adhere to other bacteria, the tooth, or the epithelial tissue surrounding the sulcus or the pocket

c. Pathogenic anaerobic bacteria and spirochetes become well established in the subgingival plaque biofilm

d. Subgingival plaque may be attached or loosely adherent (epithelium-associated)

(1) Attached subgingival plaque (also called *tooth-associated subgingival plaque*)

(a) Similar to supragingival bacterial plaque, inner layers are dominated by gram-positive rods and cocci, such as *Streptococcus sanguis, Actinomyces viscosus,* and *Actinomyces naeslundii;* gram-negative rods and cocci also are found

(b) Apical portions are dominated by gram-negative rods, with some filaments present; secondary colonizers such as *P. intermedia, Capnocytophaga* species, *F. nucleatum,* and *P. gingivalis* co-aggregate

(c) Associated with calculus formation and root caries[16]

(2) Loosely adherent subgingival plaque (also called *epithelium-associated* or *unattached plaque*)

(a) Extends from the gingival margin apical to the junctional epithelium, adjacent to the gingival epithelium or the pocket lumen

(b) Primarily gram-negative rods as well as motile organisms, filaments, and spirochetes that are not highly organized; predominance of species such as *P. gingivalis, A. actinomycetemcomitans, T. denticola, P. intermedia, T. forsythensis* (formerly *Bacteroides forsythus*) (pathogenic), and *Capnocytophaga ochracea* (beneficial)

(c) Associated with different forms of periodontitis[16]

e. Bacterial invasion of periodontal tissues

(1) Bacteria have been found within diseased periodontal tissue in disease

(2) Widened intercellular spaces in the gingival epithelium or the pocket lining may allow for the penetration of organisms from subgingival bacterial plaque

(3) Bacterial invasion may occur, or the presence of bacteria within the tissue may be a result of displacement or manipulation rather than actual invasion

(4) *A. actinomycetemcomitans* and *P. gingivalis* are believed to be tissue-invading organisms

E. Bacterial specificity

1. Specific plaque hypothesis—suggests that specific combinations of bacteria cause various forms of periodontal disease; only certain plaque microorganisms are pathogenic

2. Research is further defining the bacterial causes and host response effects of destructive periodontal disease

F. Dental calculus—bacterial plaque that has mineralized

1. Calculus plays a secondary role in the etiology of periodontal diseases by serving as a plaque-retentive factor; not all plaque necessarily calcifies; all calculus in humans is covered by bacterial plaque

2. Earliest mineralization occurs along the inner surface of the plaque or in attached subgingival plaque; calcium and phosphorus come from the saliva for the mineralization of supragingival calculus and from the gingival crevicular fluid (GCF) for the mineralization of subgingival calculus

3. Its porosity serves as a reservoir for bacteria and endotoxins that are destructive to the periodontium; impossible for the client to remove

4. Modes of attachment to teeth

a. By acquired pellicle

b. By direct attachment of the calculus matrix to the tooth surface; penetration into cementum

c. By mechanically locking into tooth surface irregularities

5. Effect on the periodontium—because bacterial plaque always covers calculus, it is primarily a bacterial irritant (not mechanical); calculus plays a significant role as a secondary, contributing factor in the pathogenesis of periodontal disease; a plaque-retentive factor

G. Pathogenic effect on periodontium (see discussions on acute and chronic inflammation in the section on "Inflammation" in Chapter 7)

1. Bacterial plaque biofilm contributes to periodontal breakdown by direct injury to tissue and by stimulating host-mediated responses that result in tissue injury

2. Direct injury is caused by toxins and enzymes produced by bacteria and proinflammatory metabolic byproducts of bacterial metabolism; most significant pathologic effects during the early stages of disease

a. Exotoxins are proteins and other metabolic byproducts such as hydrogen sulfide, uric acid, and fatty acids released by organisms that cause direct injury to tissue

b. Endotoxins called *lipopolysaccharides* or cytotoxic agents are cellular components of gram-negative bacteria that are toxic to surrounding cells, contribute to the inflammatory process, and induce bone resorption; endotoxins are released from the cell wall on the death of gram-negative bacteria, initiating inflammation and tissue destruction

c. Enzymes—mainly proteases, collagenase, hyaluronidase, chondroitin sulfatase, fibrinolysin, and phospholipase A—directly degrade surrounding tissue and penetrate by breaking down structural barriers

3. Indirect toxicity results when subgingival bacteria act as antigens and a resultant local immune reaction occurs; the host response attempts to control the bacterial attack, and some destruction of tissue results by a variety of immunopathologic reactions

H. Host response—protective (see Figures 7-1 to 7-4 in Chapter 7); host-mediated destructive processes play a role in the cause of inflammatory periodontal infections once the protective elements of the periodontium are overwhelmed

I. Host response—destructive
1. Cytokines, including ILs and PGE_2, participate in periodontal pathologic changes; they are low-molecular-weight (LMW) proteins produced by fibroblasts and inflammatory cells (e.g., monocytes and lymphocytes); lipo-polysaccharide (LPS) stimulates cytokines
2. Collagenase and lysosomal enzymes destroy connective tissue
3. Aspartate aminotransferase—an intracellular enzyme that indicates cell death or tissue destruction when present extracellularly
4. Elevated levels of host-derived enzymes (e.g., collagenase, aspartate aminotransferase, β-glucuronidase, elastase) in GCF can be used as markers for periodontitis
5. Tumor necrosis factor alpha (TNF-α)—an inflammatory mediator that contributes to bone resorption; shares properties with ILs
6. MMP—produces collagenase contributing to loss of attachment

CLINICAL ASSESSMENT OF THE PERIODONTIUM[15,16]

A. Indices—system for documenting clinical observations to help clients become aware of their current status, to demonstrate changes in the client's health over a certain period, and to survey large populations for current status and trends in health (see Table 20-6 in Chapter 20)
B. Periodontal documentation
1. Used to document existing periodontal status; baseline for future reference
2. Updated periodically to determine changes in periodontal health or disease progression
3. Necessary for care planning
4. Serves as a guide for the clinician during treatment and evaluation
5. Serves as a legal document
6. Serves as a technique for managing risks associated with failure to diagnose and treat periodontal disease

C. Periodontal assessment—complete periodontal documentation should be based on a thorough periodontal assessment, which includes the following:[15-17]
1. A description of gingival tissue—includes visual signs of inflammation
2. Findings from examination of the periodontium with a periodontal probe (see the section on "Instrumentation for assessment" in Chapter 17), which include the following:[1,15,16]
   a. Presence of bleeding—widely accepted as an indicator of gingival inflammation; more sensitive than visual signs; however, inflamed sites do not always bleed, and bleeding is a poor predictor of attachment loss (only 30%), unless multiple sites are found in conjunction with deep pockets, attachment loss, or both; these combined conditions help make important risk prediction for attachment loss; some suggest prediction increases by 70% to 75%; results when sulcular lining is ulcerated as a result of infection; may also result with repeated probing of a given site because of trauma
   b. Probing depth (also called *sulcus* or *pocket depth*)—gives a historical record of past periodontal disease activity; useful in monitoring the success of periodontal therapy; important in determining client's ability to maintain health through plaque biofilm control; the periodontal probe remains the best diagnostic aid for detecting periodontal pockets and CAL; multiple sites of deep pockets help better predict attachment loss; absence of deep pockets is a good predictor of periodontal stability
   c. Clinical attachment level—measures from the CEJ to the attachment; determines the amount of apical migration of the junctional epithelium or the amount of lost periodontal connective tissue attachment to the tooth; most accurate measure of severity of periodontal disease because the measurement is not influenced by the position of the gingival margin influenced by inflammation and recession and because CEJ is a static reference point when measuring CAL
      (1) Because the gingival attachment is located slightly apical to the CEJ in a fully erupted tooth and the gingival margin is slightly coronal to the CEJ in normal gingival contour, probing depth will be slightly greater than CAL
      (2) When gingival recession is present and the gingival margin is apical to the CEJ,

the probing depth will be less than CAL; therefore, a normal sulcus depth can be present in an area of connective tissue and bone loss

   (3) If the gingival margin meets the CEJ, the probing depth and CAL are equal

  d. Recession—measured from the CEJ to the gingival margin; indicates apical migration of the gingiva

  e. Presence of purulent exudate (suppuration)—in response to lateral digital pressure on the gingival margin or probing; suggests advanced lesion of periodontitis and secondary infection at site

  f. Adequacy of width of attached gingiva—measured from attachment to mucogingival junction; the amount varies, depending on location; adequate zone necessary to withstand stresses from mastication; if none is present, the gingival margin will move with alveolar mucosa; if inadequate, a mucogingival problem or defect exists

3. Alternatives to use of standard periodontal probe for periodontal examination (see the section on "Periodontal assessment" in Chapter 15)[1,2]

  a. Periodontal screening and recording system (PSR)—designed to provide thorough screening and recording for all clients while saving time in recording aspect of initial examination[1,2]

  b. Electronic periodontal probes[1,2,17]

   (1) Increase accuracy by reducing the margin of error, standardizing pressure, or both; the latter type is also called *controlled-force probes*

   (2) Reduce time required for probing and recording; some are voice activated; some provide printouts of probing depths, attachment loss, or both, for example, Florida probe, Toronto probe, Foster-Miller probe, pressure probe, pressure-sensitive probe (PSP), Hunter probe, Interprobe

   (3) The advantages of computer-linked probes include automatic probe recordings and enhanced infection control due to elimination of mouth-to-paper chart recordings; computerized client records integrate all client data

   (4) The disadvantages of controlled-force probes include decreased tactile sensitivity and increased client discomfort

  c. Dental remote access terminal (e.g., Dental RAT)—a foot-controlled mouse that enables hands-free periodontal charting, thereby offering benefits of infection control and electronic printouts

4. Presence and distribution of bacterial plaque and calculus (may use indices)

5. Condition of tooth proximal contacts—loose or open contacts permit food impaction

6. Degree of pathologic tooth mobility (see the section on "Periodontal assessment" in Chapter 15 for a specific classification system)

  a. Pathologic tooth mobility is caused by loss of periodontal support (bone loss), trauma from occlusion, inflammation extending into the periodontal ligament from the gingiva or the apex (abscesses), periodontal surgery (temporarily), hormonal changes associated with pregnancy and sometimes menstruation or use of hormonal contraceptives, pathologic processes of the jaws that destroy the bone or roots of teeth (e.g., osteomyelitis or tumors)[16]

  b. Tooth mobility is most commonly assessed by using the blunt ends of the handles of two dental instruments (single-ended); can be measured electronically for objective data (e.g., Periotest)

7. Presence of furcation involvement (see the section on "Periodontal assessment" in Chapter 15 for a specific classification system)

8. Presence of malocclusion or malposition of teeth

9. Presence and condition of dental restorations and prosthetic appliances; missing teeth; dental implants

10. Presence of overhanging restorations (overhangs)—contributing causative factor in periodontal disease from accumulation of bacterial plaque and food impaction

11. Assessment of disease progression by longitudinal comparison of probing depths, attachment levels, and interproximal bone height (radiographic)

12. Interpretation of a satisfactory number of bitewing and periapical radiographs of diagnostic quality (see the section on "Radiographic image interpretation" in Chapter 6)

  a. Level of alveolar crest in relation to the CEJ and interdental bone

  b. Furcation areas

  c. Width of periodontal ligament space

  d. Existing dental restorations and caries

  e. Periapical disease

  f. Length, shape, and position of roots

13. Alternative to traditional radiography (see the section on "Supplemental techniques and specialized imaging modalities" in Chapter 6)

D. Documentation of oral habits
1. Bruxing (grinding) or clenching of teeth
2. Chewing on fingernails or foreign objects
3. Smoking or drinking (alcohol) habits
4. Temporomandibular joint (TMJ) trauma (evidenced by crepitus, tenderness, or deviations)

E. Assessment of occlusion—includes:
1. Classification and anterior relationships
2. Excessive wear patterns (facets)
3. Defective prematurities—isolated occlusal contacts that cause deflection in the pathway of physiologic mandibular movement
4. Teeth, restorations, or prosthetic appliances that may interfere with the normal movements of the mandible
5. TMJ discomfort
6. Fremitus—vibration of root surfaces as the client "taps" teeth together
7. Tooth sensitivity to pressure and to hot and cold substances

F. Classification of occlusal trauma[2]
1. Primary occlusal trauma—trauma results from excessive occlusal forces when periodontal support is normal; result could be mobility, excessive wear of a tooth or teeth, sensitivity of involved teeth, or fremitus
2. Secondary occlusal trauma—the supporting periodontium is not normal (some loss of supporting structures because of periodontitis); one or more teeth are not able to withstand even normal occlusal forces, and particularly excessive occlusal forces; could result in mobility or sensitivity

G. Additional information obtained through client interview
1. Complete documentation of the client's past and current health status, including pharmacologic history and risk factors
2. Complete documentation of the client's dental, fluoride, social, and cultural histories
3. Client's daily oral hygiene routine
4. Client's knowledge level and attitude toward oral health

H. Supplemental diagnostic tests[1,2,17]
1. Traditional approach to periodontal diagnosis measures only the results of periodontal inflammation and destruction; the goals for developing newer diagnostic approaches include the ability to detect the presence of disease early to predict destruction before it occurs; prognostic devices or tests also would be able to assess the risk of disease in the future
2. Validity of a diagnostic test is determined by calculating its sensitivity and specificity
   a. Sensitivity—the probability of a test being positive when a disease truly is present
   b. Specificity—the probability of a test being negative when a disease truly is not present
   c. Predictive value—refers to the probability that a disease will be present when the test is positive or not present when the test is negative; influenced by the prevalence of disease in a particular population
3. Prognostic device or test—predicts the likelihood that a disease will occur in the future
4. Supplemental diagnostic tests can be used for screening (to separate the diseased from healthy individuals) or to detect sites or individuals at high risk for progressive disease
5. General categories of supplemental diagnostic tests
   a. Detection of substances associated with periodontal pathogens (microbiologic monitoring)
      (1) DNA (deoxyribonucleic acid) probes—paper points are inserted into specific site(s) and sent to a laboratory for analysis; the laboratory report returned in 2 days specifies levels of eight known periodontal pathogens; provide general information on antibiotic selection; have high degree of sensitivity and specificity
      (2) Culturing—plaque samples from specific sites are placed in a vial containing transport medium and sent to a laboratory for analysis; specific percentages of various bacterial species are identified, and specific recommendations for antibiotic sensitivity can be obtained; a highly detailed technique is required
      (3) Enzyme-linked immunosorbent assay (ELISA)—matches plaque sample DNA and bacterial antigens to periodontal pathogens; used in research rather than in clinical practice in the United States; a rapid chairside test may be available in the future
      (4) Enzymatic tests—immunoassay technology matches the fingerprint of the bacterial antigen to those of selected periodontal pathogens; limited to only three key microorganisms, but all have been linked to periodontal destruction; ease of use and immediate chairside results are advantages, for example, GCF enzyme assays; highly sensitive and moderately specific
   b. Local measures of host response;[1,14] host-derived enzymes in GCF, which are produced by inflamed pocket wall and primarily composed of inflammatory cells and serum proteins as well as inflammatory mediators

and tissue breakdown and bacterial bypro-ducts (e.g., collagenase, PGE_2, aspartate aminotransferase)
  c. Genetic testing[6]—determines genotype status through an in-office test for periodontal disease susceptibility (e.g., Periodontal Susceptibility Test) (see the section on "Genetics" in Chapter 7)
  d. Automatic calculus detection systems
    (1) Fiberoptic probe—lights up and sounds when subgingival calculus is detected (e.g., DetecTar®)
    (2) Periodontal endoscope—a specific type of endoscopy developed to explore and visualize the periodontal pocket, including the root surface, furcation areas, root fractures, and root caries (e.g., Perios-copyTM System)
  e. Risk assessment tool—Web-based Periodon-tal Risk Calculator (Previser Oral Health Information Suite™) that assesses a person's risk for periodontal disease on the basis of nine weighted risk factors
  f. Bacterial risk assessment test (BANA)—tests three anaerobes commonly associated with periodontal disease risk; based on chairside incubation and testing of samples of sub-gingival plaque

PERIODONTAL MEDICINE[1,2,18]

A. The traditional view that systemic diseases modify the effects of bacterial plaque biofilm on the initia-tion and progression of periodontal disease remains true; systemic diseases play an important role in predisposing an individual to periodontal infection by affecting host response to bacterial plaque
B. Some classifications of periodontal disease include a group of periodontal diseases that actually are caused by systemic diseases (see previous section on classification of periodontal diseases)
C. Periodontal medicine—a discipline that studies the relationship of periodontal disease as a risk factor for systemic diseases
D. Periodontal disease is a chronic, sustained inflam-matory response to a given stimulus (virulent bac-teria in the plaque biofilm) similar to other conditions such as coronary heart disease, athero-sclerosis, rheumatoid arthritis, type 2 diabetes, obesity, and osteoporosis. A relationship between periodontal disease and these diseases has been documented, and periodontal disease is a known risk factor for these systemic diseases, although a cause-and-effect connection has not been established

1. Periodontal infection presents a chronic inflam-matory burden at the systemic level
2. Bacterial pathogens can enter tissues; recurrent transient bacteremias occur
3. Systemic exposures to gram-negative pathogens and LPS trigger inflammatory mediator expres-sion related to other organisms
4. Client-based clinical outcomes such as disease morbidity and mortality and surrogate markers (e.g., serum inflammatory markers such as cross-reactive protein) are used instead of traditional markers or outcomes (bleeding, pocket depth, etc.)
E. Research into the associations between oral infec-tions, notably periodontal diseases, and the occur-rence and severity of the following systemic diseases and conditions is still ongoing.

TREATMENT[1,2,19,20–22]

Initial Care Plan

See the section on "Planning" in Chapter 15.
A. Collection of data to assess the status of the peri-odontium (see the section on "Clinical assessment of the periodontium")
B. Formulation of initial care plan based on data col-lection and assessment
  1. Determination of all causative and contributing factors (risk factors and risk indicators)
  2. Removal or control of etiologic and risk factors in an organized, logical sequence
    a. Plaque removal and control and removal of any plaque-retentive factors
    b. Reduction, control, or elimination of risk factors
    c. Elimination of inflammation; pocket reduc-tion or elimination
  3. Order of treatment will depend on:
    a. The severity of the client's periodontal condi-tion and prognosis
    b. The general health status of the client
    c. The client's motivation, cooperation, needs, and desires
C. Contributing factors influencing the prognosis
  1. Local factors
    a. Degree of periodontal destruction (amount of attachment loss)
    b. Rate of periodontal destruction (amount of attachment loss per unit of time)
    c. Presence of contributing local factors (e.g., malocclusion, parafunctional habits, position of teeth in alveoli, malalignment, root prox-imity, missing teeth)
    d. Quality of restorations present

2. Risk factors—related to the client's general health (presence or absence of systemic disease), factors affecting host response, and environmental factors (stress, smoking)

Nonsurgical Periodontal Therapy (Initial Therapy or Phase I Therapy)[1,16,19,20–22]

A. Principles of nonsurgical periodontal therapy (NSPT) (see the section on "Debridement concepts" in Chapter 17)
  1. Elimination or suppression of pathogenic microorganisms through the removal and control of bacterial plaque and plaque-retentive factors
  2. Control of the source of infection and prevention of reinfection
  3. Resolution or elimination of inflammation
  4. Consideration and, if possible, control of behavioral, systemic, and environmental host risk factors; the aim is to:

  a. Address all risk factors; increase protective factors
  b. Minimize potential impact of systemic factors
5. Restoration or maintenance of comfort, function, and aesthetics
6. Decreasing the likelihood of disease progression
B. Elimination of inflammation by reducing and controlling pathogenic microorganisms
  1. Directly removing and controlling bacterial plaque
    a. Oral hygiene self-care, including plaque biofilm removal and control
    b. Periodontal instrumentation—scaling, root planing, and periodontal debridement
    c. Adjunctive use of antiplaque and antigingival agents, as indicated (Table 14-2)
  2. Elimination of factors that favor bacterial accumulation to indirectly decrease number of

TABLE 14-2 Commercially Available Antiplaque and Antigingivitis Agents

Active Ingredients (Example Products)	Alcohol (%)	Mechanism of Action	Efficacy	Directions for Use	Adverse Effects
Chlorhexidine 0.12% (Peridex*† and PerioGard†)	11.6	Cell wall destruction	45–61% plaque and gingivitis reduction	Rinse with 15 mL for 30 seconds, twice a day	Tooth staining, altered taste, increase in supragingival calculus
Stannous fluoride gels (Gel-Kam® 0.4%) or dentifrice (Crest® ProHealth™*‡)	0	Interferes with bacterial metabolism	15–25% gingivitis reduction	Brush twice daily	Tooth staining in some patients
Stannous fluoride rinse (prescription 0.64%) PerioMed™, ProDentRx™ Periocheck™)	0	Interferes with bacterial metabolism	20–25% gingivitis reduction	Rinse daily	Tooth staining
Thymol 0.06%, eucalyptol 0.09%, methyl salicylate 0.06%, menthol 0.04% (Listerine® Antiseptic‡)	21.6–26.9	Inhibits plaque formation and bacterial adherence	30–35% reduction	Rinse with 2/3 oz or 4 tsp for 30 seconds	Burning or sloughing of oral mucosa
Cetylpyridinium chloride 0.045–0.5% (Crest® ProHealth™*‡, Scope®)	0 to 18%	Disrupts cell wall integrity	14%–24%	Rinse as directed	Soft-tissue irritation
Chlorine dioxide (Oxyfresh, Clo-Syst II Retardent)	0	Inactivates volatile sulfur compounds	Further research needed; benefit is reduction in halitosis	Rinse after brushing	Mucosal irritation
Triclosan (Colgate Total®*‡)		Broad-spectrum antimicrobial activity	25% plaque reduction 20% gingivitis reduction, calculus reduction	Brush twice daily	None known

*Approved by the U.S. Food and Drug Administration (FDA).).
†Demonstrated substantivity.
‡Accepted by the Council on Dental Therapeutics of the American Dental Association (ADA); note that the Seal of Acceptance is no longer given by the ADA to prescription products

pathogens (e.g., calculus, overhangs, food impaction, improper contacts, mouthbreathing)
C. Client as co-therapist–self-care, goal setting, long-term commitment
D. Components of NSPT
  1. Plaque biofilm control—involves both clinician and client in eliminating and controlling bacterial plaque; customized oral hygiene instruction, correction of plaque-retentive factors, and supragingival and subgingival débridement are key elements; antimicrobial or antigingival agents or devices may be used as adjuncts to mechanical oral self-care methods; long-term success of NSPT depends on adequate bacterial plaque control
  2. Oral prophylaxis versus NSPT
    a. The objective of oral prophylaxis is to prevent the initiation of gingivitis and, failing that, to prevent the conversion of gingivitis to periodontitis
    b. Oral prophylaxis is performed for clients with healthy periodontium and to clients with plaque-induced gingivitis; NSPT is performed for clients with slight to moderate loss of periodontal support
    c. Oral prophylaxis includes supragingival and subgingival debridement to remove deposits; removal or correction of plaque-retentive factors (e.g., overhanging margins, open contacts, defective restorations); and, finally, selective coronal polishing, if necessary, for plaque and stain removal or for client satisfaction
    d. The term *scaling* refers to supragingival or subgingival calculus removal without intentional removal of tooth surface
    e. The therapeutic goal of prophylaxis is to establish gingival health through the elimination of causative factors; the goals of NSPT are to alter or eliminate periodontal pathogens, address contributing risk factors, arrest progression of periodontitis, and preserve the health, comfort, and function of the dentition
  3. Nonsurgical periodontal therapy
    a. Objective—to treat and manage established periodontal disease and to create conditions conducive to health; contributing risk factors must be addressed because they affect treatment outcomes
    b. Rationale—periodontal instrumentation and plaque control result in a significant reduction of gram-negative periodontal pathogens and encourage repopulation with the gram-positive cocci and rods that are associated with health; a reduction in inflammatory cytokines that are responsible for tissue damage occurs after the bacterial composition is altered; calculus, overhanging restorations, and other plaque-retentive factors that harbor bacterial plaque also are removed; all of these components of NSPT reduce inflammation, promote tissue regeneration, and create a biologically acceptable root surface; control, alteration, or elimination of risk factors (e.g., diabetes, smoking, stress, medications, substance abuse, medications, etc.) alters the host response to bacterial plaque and has the potential to slow periodontal disease progression
    c. Supragingival and subgingival scaling, periodontal debridement, root planing, or a combination of all is performed; all these procedures are technically demanding; definitive treatment procedures are designed to remove cementum or surface dentin that is diseased, embedded with calculus, toxins, or microorganisms; treatment often requires local anesthesia; when performed thoroughly, some soft tissue removal, termed *incidental curettage*, is unavoidable; in the case of root planing, the need for extensive cementum removal to obtain a glassy, smooth surface is still being debated because of a lack of clarity about its absolute necessity, the possibility of overtreatment, and resultant hypersensitivity
      (1) Complete removal of calculus from root surfaces is unlikely, especially as pocket depth and inaccessibility increase; complete removal of detectible calculus remains the initial clinical endpoint because thorough instrumentation remains paramount to the success of therapy, whether nonsurgical or surgical
      (2) The areas most susceptible to residual deposits after treatment include furcations, line angles, root concavities, and the CEJ.
    d. NSPT most often requires multiple appointments after assessment for treatment (e.g., four appointments 1 week apart for a quadrant therapy approach) to remove or correct all detectible deposits and plaque-retentive factors; some evidence suggests longer appointments within 24-hour and 48-hour periods for complete mouth debridement, termed *full-mouth disinfection*, are necessary to reduce cross-contamination from untreated areas to treated areas
    e. Hand activated or mechanized instruments may be effectively used for root planing and periodontal debridement; ultrasonic instruments are advocated for debridement

f. NSPT has been shown to be successful in treating early to moderate periodontitis, especially for initial pocket depths of 4 to 6 mm; results are less predictable in periodontal pockets more than 6 mm in depth, if tooth movement occurs, or when furcation involvement is present

   (1) Pocket reduction in 4-mm to 6-mm areas occurs

   (2) NSPT is the definitive treatment for early to moderate periodontitis and an initial therapy for those expected to require surgical therapy

g. Root planing in healthy sulcus areas or shallow crevices is contraindicated; has been shown to cause a loss of attachment in crevices <3 mm

h. Use of lasers in periodontics requires further long-term study to determine safety and effectiveness[23]

i. Initial evaluation of NSPT—occurs during and on completion of instrumentation by careful tactile exploration of tooth and root surfaces; a clear field, adequate illumination, and use of air facilitate assessment are required

   (1) The term *periodontal debridement* refers to treatment of periodontal disease through mechanical removal of tooth and root surface irregularities (including bacterial plaque, clinically detectable calculus, and all plaque-retentive factors) depending on the health of adjacent soft tissue; removal of calculus is only considered important from the perspective of its plaque-retentive nature

   (2) The difference between periodontal debridement and root planing is in the desired initial endpoint and its effect on the extent of instrumentation; root planing is performed until root smoothness is obtained with reasonable time and effort, whereas débridement attempts to preserve tooth surface by removing only enough deposits and plaque-retentive factors to achieve periodontal health

   (3) Ultimate evaluation of NSPT—tissue response

4. Thorough re-evaluation 4 to 6 weeks after scaling, root planing, or periodontal debridement to determine the need for additional therapy (e.g., surgery, physician referrals, antimicrobials, antibiotics); initial evaluation is followed by the evaluation of the outcomes of NSPT or initial therapy, or by the re-evaluation of NSPT, after an appropriate time following initial therapy by means of a periodontal examination; it is critical to determine if clinical judgment regarding the extent of root planing and periodontal debridement was adequate to achieve periodontal health; if unsuccessful, retreatment is indicated; a period of 4 to 6 weeks is considered appropriate for the resolution of inflammation and periodontal tissue healing; relevant findings of the re-evaluation are documented in the patient's legal treatment record

5. Re-evaluation includes:

a. Evaluation and reinforcement of the client's self-care

b. Updated periodontal assessment, including bleeding points, probing depths, and attachment levels

c. Reassessment of the clinical health of tissues; if areas still show signs of inflammation, the cause should be determined

   (1) Bacterial plaque and calculus self-care should be reviewed; it is then necessary to deplaque, scale, debride, or root plane if the condition is localized; the need for rescheduling and retreatment with active therapy should be determined if the condition is generalized

   (2) If no plaque, calculus, and inflammation are noted, the client's success should be reinforced and the importance of continued care for periodontal maintenance should be stressed

   (3) If the pocket depth is still moderate to severe, controlled drug delivery and surgical procedures might be warranted; the client must be referred for evaluation by periodontist[24]

   (4) If inflammation, and bleeding are still severe, unexplained, or generalized, physical examination by a physician, including differential blood counts and complete physical examination for a possible previously undetected systemic host risk factors, should be considered

E. Use of topical antimicrobial agents as adjuncts; also referred to as *local chemotherapy* (see the section on "Mouthrinses" in Chapter 16)

1. Can be employed in initial or nonsurgical therapy, during the healing stage following periodontal surgery, or during continuing care for periodontal health maintenance

2. Indicated for control of supragingival plaque and gingivitis; effectiveness in periodontitis has not been documented; used to augment oral self-care efforts of clients that are only partially effective; also recommended for extensive restorative cases and dental implants; aids healing after periodontal surgery (see the sections on

"Oral irrigation" and "Dental implant maintenance" in Chapter 16)

3. Antiplaque and anti-gingivitis agents (see Table 14-2)
   a. Chlorhexidine gluconate
      (1) Most effective antimicrobial agent for reducing plaque and gingivitis in the long term (45% to 61%); the "gold standard" for topical antimicrobial mouthrinses; 0.12% concentration in the United States and 0.2% outside the United States
      (2) High substantivity—ability to adhere to soft and hard tissues for a long duration while releasing active ingredient; a cationic bisbiguanide that ruptures bacterial cell membranes
      (3) Adverse effects—staining, reversible desquamation, poor taste or alteration of taste, increase in supragingival calculus deposits; especially with long-term use
      (4) Examples-Peridex® or PerioGard® by prescription (the American Dental Association [ADA] no longer gives the Seal of Acceptance to prescription drugs)
      (5) Alcohol content 11.6%, or alcohol free
      (6) Twice-daily use promotes compliance; client should be instructed to use 15 mL of rinse for 30 seconds; rinse should be separate from dentifrice by 30 minutes for full effectiveness
      (7) Also recommended for wound healing after surgery or as pre-rinse to reduce salivary bacterial load and aerosols during periodontal therapy and mechanized instrumentation
   b. Phenolic compounds (essential oils)
      (1) Antiseptic form approved by the ADA as a safe and effective antimicrobial and anti-gingivitis agent (e.g., Listerine®Antiseptic); carries the ADA Seal of Acceptance
      (2) Long-term studies indicate approximately 30% to 35% reduction in plaque and gingivitis, although results have varied from 15% to 37%
      (3) Available antiseptic products have variable alcohol content (21.6% to 26.9% alcohol); thymol, menthol, eucalyptol, and methyl salicylate are active ingredients; act by bacterial cell wall disruption and inhibition of bacterial enzymes
      (4) Adverse effects—burning sensation and bitter taste; some report soft tissue irritation; caution with xerostomia and recovering alcoholics; some formulations have high alcohol content; some are now alcohol free

      (5) Twice-daily use promotes compliance; client should be instructed to use 15 mL of rinse for 30 seconds after brushing
      (6) Also recommended as pre-procedural rinse to reduce salivary bacterial load and aerosols during periodontal therapy and mechanized instrumentation
   c. Triclosan
      (1) Approved by the ADA as a safe and effective antimicrobial and antigingivitis agent (e.g., Colgate Total®); carries the ADA Seal of Acceptance
      (2) A bisphenol that has broad-spectrum antimicrobial activity, especially when combined with zinc citrate for additional antiplaque effects; also used alone or in combination with a co-polymer of polyvinylmethyl and maleic acid to increase substantivity and to provide some anticalculus properties
      (3) Dentifrice formulation promotes compliance; shown to reduce plaque formation by 25% and gingivitis by 20%; can be combined with fluoride, unlike other antimicrobial agents, which often are not compatible or synergistic
4. Other agents used in periodontal therapy
   a. Povidone iodine
      (1) An iodophor with polyvinyl-pyrrolidone added to iodine; effective against many organisms, including bacteria, viruses, and fungi
      (2) Primarily used as a pre-procedural rinse or during mechanized instrumentation for antiseptic lavage or irrigation; often recommended for use during treatment of immunocompromised clients who might have multiple organisms affecting their oral health; can be effective antimicrobial and antigingivitis agent, but only with short-term use
      (3) Adverse effects—concern for iodine toxicity with prolonged use; contraindicated in those with iodine sensitivity or allergy, and thyroid dysfunction and pregnant or lactating women; temporary extrinsic tooth staining can be removed by tooth polishing
   b. Stannous fluoride
      (1) Antimicrobial mechanism of action appears to be related to the stannous (tin) ion rather than fluoride
      (2) Long-term studies have shown significant reductions in gingivitis without concurrent significant reductions in plaque

scores and concurrent reductions; further long-term study is warranted

(3) Available in dentifrice (e.g., Crest® Pro-Health™); in gel form (e.g., Stop®, Gel-Kam®, Omni Gel™) 0.4% concentration; or in rinses containing 0.63% concentrations (e.g., PerioMed™, ProDenRx™, Periocheck™)

(4) Stannous fluoride has low to moderate substantivity; twice-daily use promotes compliance

(5) Adverse effects may include unpleasant taste in the mouth and tooth staining after prolonged use (2–3 months) in some individuals

(6) Has the ADA's Seal of Acceptance for their ability to deliver fluoride for anti-caries activity; the dentifrice formulation has been approved for bacterial plaque-reducing and gingivitis-reducing properties; dentifrice and some gels also approved for dentinal hypersensitivity reduction; the product label should be checked for the ADA Seal of Acceptance

c. Quaternary ammonium compounds (cetyl-pyridinium chloride)

(1) The most common formulation is cetyl-pyridinium chloride used alone or with domiphen bromide; cationic surface active agents rupture bacterial cell walls; the compound binds to oral tissues but releases rapidly, which limits its substantivity and, therefore, effectiveness in the oral cavity

(2) Six-month studies show 14% to 24% reduction in bacterial plaque and gingivitis; the therapeutic value of the product is questionable

(3) May have some benefit in reducing halitosis; clients purchase the product for mouth-freshening benefits

(4) Adverse reactions are minimal; may include possible slight staining and burning sensation

(5) Well-known representatives of this group are Pro Health™ Rinse, Scope®, Cepacol®, Oral B® Rembrandt, and Clear Choice; several of these are alcohol free

d. Oxygenating agents—hydrogen peroxide: anti-inflammatory properties decrease the clinical signs of inflammation, but bacterial pathogens may not be reduced; studies do not support long-term use of 100% hydrogen peroxide as oral rinse; safety issues such as tissue injury and co-carcinogenicity, have

been raised with long-term use of hydrogen peroxide. Some oxygenating agents available on the market include Amosan and Gly-Oxide

e. Oxidizing agents (chlorine dioxide)—have no therapeutic value but are recommended for breath freshening; also have been shown to effectively reduce halitosis; reduce volatile sulfur compounds (VSC) that are believed to be responsible for halitosis; well-known representatives of this group are Oxyfresh, Enfresh, Therafresh, Profresh, and Clo-Syst II

5. Methods for topical delivery of antimicrobial agents

a. Most common methods of delivery for anti-microbials are dentifrices, mouthrinsing, and oral irrigation

b. Mouthrinses, dentifrices, and gels deliver agents supragingivally; subgingival penetration is 0 to 1 mm

c. Oral irrigation can deliver agent subgingivally; complete plaque removal is not achieved, but periodontal pathogens found in loosely adherent plaque can be removed; must be used as an adjunct to mechanical plaque biofilm control; often used during the maintenance of periodontal health after completion of active periodontal therapy (e.g., Water Pik®, Hydrofloss®)

d. Oral irrigation can be accomplished with water or antimicrobial agents; both reduce bleeding and gingivitis, but antimicrobials are more effective in removing bacterial plaque and making it less pathogenic; effect on periodontitis is not well documented

e. Depth of penetration with oral irrigation is related to type of tip used[25]

(1) Standard jet tip—shallow penetration of 1.8 mm (3-mm to 6-mm pockets only 44% depth)

(2) Subgingival tip—90% coverage in pockets of 6 mm or less; decreasing coverage as pocket becomes deeper

(3) Cannula—75% to 100% coverage if the tip reaches the base of the pocket; safety is a concern with home use

f. Oral irrigation can have value in conjunction with daily self-care regimen for mechanical plaque biofilm removal in the treatment of gingivitis or in periodontal maintenance therapy

g. Professionally administered oral irrigation, with and without root planing and periodontal debridement, has been studied; the main benefit is from mechanical debridement; a single application of an antimicrobial irrigant has little value because of low substantivity in the periodontal pocket

F. Sustained-release, local drug delivery systems (also called *controlled drug delivery*)[1,2,26]

1. Systems are available for site-specific, sustained, local delivery of antibiotics or antimicrobials to specific subgingival sites (e.g., gels, chips, collagen film, bioabsorbable materials); the objective is to eliminate periodontal pathogens; these methods of local delivery provide for the benefits of antibiotic or antimicrobial therapy with greater safety and compliance; delivery mechanisms allow the antibiotic or antimicrobial agent to be delivered for up to 14 days (varies by product) after placement; controlled delivery releases the material's active ingredient over time, maintaining a constant and sufficient release of the active ingredient

2. Controlled delivery offers the advantage of sustained release of a high concentration of the active ingredient to the site of periodontal infection without systemic involvement; can be used in conjunction with scaling, debridement, and root planing during initial periodontal therapy in pockets >5 mm with bleeding on probing, at re-evaluation for recalcitrant sites, or during continuing care for localized sites needing adjunctive therapy for the maintenance of periodontal health; few use these systems as a monotherapy

3. Contraindicated in the presence of allergy to the active ingredient or to any component of the delivery system and during pregnancy or lactation; not useful for treatment of generalized diseased sites

4. Studies have shown that these controlled delivery systems cause an improvement in clinical attachment levels or probing depths of ≥2 mm at 30% to 40% of sites treated in multiple-center, randomized clinical trials, a level considered both statistically and clinically significant

5. Currently available sustained-release systems for subgingival application
   a. Chlorhexidine chip—2.5-mg chlorhexidine gluconate in a hydrolyzed gelatin biodegradable film; self-retentive on contact with moisture, placed using cotton pliers immediately following scaling and root planing in pockets >5 mm for retention; statistically significant improvement in probing depths and attachment levels, compared with scaling and root planing alone, with minimal clinical change in probing depth; use limited to eight sites; can use a total of three applications at intervals of 3 months (PerioChip)
   b. Minocycline hydrochloride microspheres (2%)—consist of antibiotic minocycline hydrochloride in a bioabsorbable polymer of poly-D, L-lactide-CO-glycolide; are designed for use as adjunctive therapy with scaling and root planing; microspheres are dispensed subgingivally from a capsule placed in a syringe; the tip is inserted into the base of the pocket and then withdrawn after the drug has been applied; shown to be clinically superior to scaling and root planing alone at initial therapy; the client is instructed not to brush for 12 hours or floss for 10 days (Arestin); minocycline is also available as a gel and ointment outside of the United States
   c. Doxycycline hyclate gel (10%)—solidifying liquid, biodegradable polymer that hardens after exposure to fluid in the periodontal pocket; delivered via injection from a syringe with a blunt cannula inserted into the pocket; studied and approved by the U.S. Food and Drug Administration (FDA) as monotherapy, although not often used as such; studies also show clinically significant reductions in probing depths and gains in attachment levels with scaling and root planing; the client is instructed not to brush or floss sites for 7 days (Atridox)

G. Use of systemic antibiotics[25]—drugs that target the bacterial load

1. Sometimes used in conjunction with periodontal therapy (surgical or nonsurgical); however, no evidence that antibiotics alone arrest periodontal disease exist; may be prescribed for clients who are nonresponsive to periodontal therapy, acute periodontal infections with systemic manifestations, for prophylaxis in medically compromised clients, and in conjunction with surgical or nonsurgical therapy when systemic health or classification of periodontal disease warrants use after consideration of risks and benefits
   a. Generalized recurrent or refractory periodontal disease despite appropriate treatment—often related to impaired host resistance or persistent, superinfecting microorganisms[27]
   b. Aggressive forms of periodontitis—related to neutrophil defects and tissue-invasive microorganisms (*A. actinomycetemcomitans* and *P. gingivalis*)
   c. Acute, severe infections (e.g., periodontal abscess, NUG)—especially with fever, malaise, lymphadenopathy, or other systemic signs and symptoms

d. Immunocompromised status—used with extreme caution to avoid development of resistant strains

2. Not recommended for the routine treatment of gingivitis or chronic periodontitis; problems such as adverse drug reactions, drug hypersensitivity, development of antibiotic-resistant strains, interactions with other prescribed medications taken by the client, and client nonadherence limit widespread use; the Centers for Disease Control and Prevention (CDC) recommends judicious use of antibiotics because of growing concerns about overuse and consequently the development of drug-resistant strains of bacteria, which has led to a resurgence of diseases previously well controlled by antibiotics (e.g., tuberculosis, staphylococcal infections, diphtheria); particular concerns about use in pregnant or lactating women do exist, and a higher risk of drug interactions is present with long-term use of cardiovascular disease, asthma, seizures, and diabetes medications

   a. Common side effects include nausea, vomiting, diarrhea, rashes, changes in vaginal or intestinal flora, and allergy; prolonged use can be associated with bleeding problems

   b. Specific reactions include the Antabuse effect of metronidazole taken with alcohol, discoloration or deformed teeth with tetracycline use in children under 8 years of age, and increased risk of pseudomembranous colitis with clindamycin

3. Restricted use and careful selection are indicated on the basis of response to mechanical therapy, medical history analysis, possible drug interactions, and risks; indiscriminate use is prohibited; microbial analysis, antimicrobial sensitivity testing, or a combination of both before prescribing systemic antibiotics for periodontal therapy is recommended[25,27]

4. Common agents include tetracylcines (doxycycline), nitromadazoles (metronidazole), lincomycins (clindamycin), quinalones (ciprofloxacin), macrolide (azithromycin but not erythromyacin); combination therapy includes metronidazole and amoxicillin or metronidazole and ciprofloxacin; the combination is synergistic and increases the spectrum of drug activity; penicillins and cephlosporins are not considered drugs of choice

H. Use of host-modulating drugs;[1,2] host response is the target

1. Subantimicrobial dose doxycycline (SDD)[28]— used systemically in subantimicrobial doses to inhibit proteases and periodontal disease progression; downregulates the activity of matrix metalloproteinases (MMPs) that are active during periods of periodontal tissue breakdown and thus play a major role in inflammation and the destruction of collagen and bone

   a. Has not been shown to substitute for meticulous home care and periodontal maintenance

   b. Administered 20 mg twice per day (instead of the 50-mg or 100-mg dosage used as antibiotic) for a period of 6 to 9 months or up to 12 months concurrent with periodontal therapy; a low dose eliminates most side effects, although SDD is contraindicated when known allergy to tetracylines is present

   c. Research has shown slight but statistically significant gains in clinical attachment and reductions in probing depths

2. Nonsteroidal anti-inflammatory drugs (NSAIDs) have been shown to inhibit PGE_2 and arachidonic acid metabolites that are proinflammatory mediators in bone loss, inflammation, and pocket depth in periodontitis (e.g., ibuprofen, flurbiprofen, naproxen, meclofenamate, ketorolac); are not approved in the United States for the treatment of periodontal disease; generally used for short-term treatment of postoperative pain; long-term use has been shown to have adverse affects on the gastrointestinal tract and on cardiovascular health

3. Bisphosphonates—have been used experimentally in animals to inhibit bone resorption and bone mineral content and to interfere with the breakdown of collagen in periodontium; are under investigation as host modulators in the management of periodontal disease

   a. Used to treat Paget's disease and osteoporosis

   b. Examples include risedronate (Actonel), alendronate sodium (Fosamax), ibandronate (Boniva)

Additional Clinical Interventions

A. Gingival curettage[29]—a procedure to remove the ulcerated, chronically inflamed tissue lining a periodontal pocket; evidence fails to support the efficacy of this procedure

B. Historical overview

1. In the past, gingival curettage was a recommended procedure for the treatment of areas of gingival inflammation or to reduce inflammation and probing depths through shrinkage of tissues and healing by a long junctional epithelium

2. Studies of gingival curettage have almost always combined this technique with root planing

3. Research indicates that gingival curettage is ineffective and that root planing alone can, in most cases, reduce inflammation, shrink tissue, and promote healing
4. In some states, gingival curettage is a legally permissible procedure that can be performed by dental hygienists
5. On the basis of research findings, gingival curettage has limited, if any, current application in the treatment of chronic periodontitis
6. If new connective tissue attachment is the goal of a particular periodontal treatment plan, curettage has no justifiable application; healing occurs by means of a longer junctional epithelium and tissue shrinkage as it does with root planing or periodontal debridement; surgical intervention is the therapy of choice when new attachment is the desired endpoint

C. Treatment of occlusal trauma[1,30]
1. Definitions
   a. Occlusal trauma—injury to the periodontal attachment apparatus resulting from occlusal forces when those forces exceed the reparative and adaptive capacity of the attachment apparatus
   b. Primary occlusal trauma—injury to the periodontium as a result of excessive occlusal forces when the periodontal attachment apparatus and the attachment level are normal
   c. Secondary occlusal trauma—injury to a compromised periodontium with loss of attachment or bone loss resulting from normal or excessive occlusal force
2. Clinical features and diagnosis
   a. When injury to the periodontal ligament occurs, collagen is destroyed, vascular elements are affected, and osteoclasts are increased on the pressure side; all of this results in a widening of the periodontal ligament space because of the lateral resorption of the bony socket wall, especially in the crestal area when the force is great enough to cause necrosis of the ligament; when a back-and-forth motion, or "jiggling," of the tooth in the socket (fremitus) occurs from occlusal trauma, changes are seen on both the tension and the pressure side, resulting in a funnel-shaped widening of the periodontal ligament and loss of bone; as such, mobility is the hallmark of occlusal trauma, and radiographic findings reveal widening of the ligament space, infrabony defects, or both; parafunctional habits such as bruxism and clenching or iatrogenic factors causing premature contacts (e.g., "high" restorations) most frequently result in occlusal trauma; tissues can regenerate on removal of the occlusal force that is causing destruction; therefore, constant evaluation and re-evaluation are indicated
   b. Although necrosis of the ligament and loss of bone can occur from occlusal trauma, it is important to note that attachment loss characterized by apical migration of the periodontal attachment such as that caused by periodontitis does not occur solely from occlusal trauma; occlusal trauma can contribute to advancing loss of attachment once attachment loss or bone loss from periodontitis has weakened tooth support
   c. Positive diagnosis is made on the basis of signs and symptoms of injury (e.g., tooth mobility or migration; pain on percussion or chewing; radiographic changes such as widened periodontal ligament, crestal infrabony [angular] defects, and condensing osteitis, or root resorption; TMJ dysfunction, severe wear facets; crown or root fractures; or *fremitus* (a term used when tooth movement or vibration occurs with the teeth occluded and grinded in all functional positions); clinicians correlate clinical findings with radiographic findings; pathologic occlusion shows evidence of disease interfering with comfort, function, or aesthetics that can be attributed to occlusal forces
   d. Pulp vitality testing, evaluation of parafunctional habits, clinical assessment of occlusal discrepancies and bone, fremitus and mobility, radiographic assessment of the periodontal ligament and bone, and other adjunctive diagnostic procedures generally are required for differential diagnosis
3. Once diagnosed, occlusal traumatism may be treated; however, plaque-induced inflammation also must be eliminated
   a. Occlusal adjustment—selective grinding of teeth to equalize the distribution of occlusal forces
   b. Construction of occlusal appliances (e.g., night mouthguard, removable orthodontic appliance, clenching suppression appliance) to manage parafunctional habits, to minimize the effect of destructive forces, and for minor tooth movement to improve tooth alignment
   c. Splinting of teeth for temporary or permanent stabilization
   d. Restorative dentistry to improve the occlusal plane and replace missing teeth or occlusal reconstruction
   e. Orthodontics to correct malocclusion
   f. Extraction of selected teeth

Surgical Interventions[2,5,31]

A. Principles of periodontal surgery
   1. Rationale
      a. Eliminate active infection
      b. Render the periodontium more cleansable by the client and maintainable by the professional
         (1) Improvement in the contours of hard and soft tissues
         (2) Pocket elimination or reduction
      c. Replace damaged or destroyed periodontium
         (1) Soft tissue replacement (gingival grafts)
         (2) Hard tissue replacement (osseous grafts)
      d. Surgery is rarely performed solely to remove inflammation or infection but, rather, in an attempt to:
         (1) Eliminate both hard and soft defects created by disease
         (2) Restore normal architecture and physiologic function
         (3) Gain regeneration or new attachment of the supporting structures
   2. Case preparation (see the sections on "Implementation" and "Evaluation" in Chapter 15)
      a. Clients need to complete the initial therapy before entering the surgical phase; initial care aims to remove the causative factors, control active disease, and educate the client in the role as a co-therapist
      b. Completion of initial therapy prepares tissue for surgery by reducing marginal inflammation and improving tissue tone, which allows more predictable incisions and suturing and reduces surgical bleeding
      c. The prognosis is improved overall after initial preparation or therapy
      d. The client's response to NSPT is assessed in relation to healing response; motivation and supplemental self-care devices may be needed for adequate healing
      e. Completion of initial therapy can reduce the number of sites requiring surgery or even eliminate the need for surgery in a given sextant or quadrant
B. Types of surgical intervention
   1. Resective periodontal surgery
      a. Gingivectomy—surgical procedure for pocket reduction by excision of the soft tissue pocket wall
         (1) Indications—gingival pockets composed of enlarged fibrotic tissue, pockets of generally universal shape with horizontal bone loss, correction of gingival form aesthetic problems such as gingival craters, gingival overgrowth, increase in clinical crown length, when ostectomy is not required; involves only the gingiva
         (2) Contraindications—reduction of infrabony pockets or osseous craters or when the base of the pocket extends apical to the mucogingival junction, presence of mucogingival problems such as inadequate keratinized gingiva, inadequate self care, acutely inflamed gingiva, and presence of large exostoses or osseous ledges
      b. Gingivoplasty—reshaping of the gingiva to obtain a physiologic form similar to that characteristic of healthy tissue by using a rotary instrument; frequently combined with gingivectomy
      c. Periodontal flap procedures—may be used as a method of surgical curettage (e.g., modified Widman flap) or for pocket elimination by apically repositioning the soft tissue; most common form of surgery
         (1) Advantages (depending on the type of flap)
            (a) Better access to achieve thorough scaling and root planing when clear access and visibility are not possible through nonsurgical procedures
            (b) Thorough removal of the pocket lining from deep pockets, furcations, or other areas of complex anatomy
            (c) Elimination or reduction of pockets in areas of minimal gingival width that render gingivectomy or gingivoplasty procedures difficult
            (d) Means to obtain access to alveolar bone to correct osseous defects
         (2) Indications
            (a) Probing depths in the presence of infrabony defects; probing depths >5 mm after initial therapy; furcation involvement; presence of root anomalies or irregularities not accessible through nonsurgical procedures
            (b) To enhance the cleansability of areas inaccessible to home care for long-term maintenance of periodontal health
            (c) To provide access for grafting, ridge augmentation, and regenerative periodontal procedures
         (3) Contraindications
            (a) Possibility to treat and control periodontal disease by a more conservative approach (NSPT)
            (b) In the presence of excessive mobility

(c) Advanced attachment loss; poor prognosis

(d) Inadequate gingiva, poor crown–root ratios, or anatomic preclusions

(e) Systemic disorders that are contraindications for surgery

(f) Noncompliant client

d. Excisional new attachment procedure (ENAP)—uses internally beveled incision to remove the crevicular lining and the junctional epithelium, allowing for root preparation

e. Tuberosity reductions—common with flap procedures in maxillary tuberosity or retromolar areas to reduce pockets distal to the last tooth in the arch

f. Osseous resective surgery or osseous resection
   (1) Objectives—removal of alveolar bone to produce a more physiologic architecture or contour; ultimately, pocket reduction in one-walled infrabony or vertical defects; also for lengthening the clinical crown for root restoration; the goal is to remove a minimal amount of bone; may include ostectomy, osteoplasty, or both
   (2) Indications—vertical alveolar defects or exostoses requiring reshaping (osteoplasty) or surgical crown lengthening (ostectomy) for access to deep root caries lesions or fractures

g. Root resection or hemisection—the objective is removal of the crown, root, or both to eliminate the involved furcation when osseous resection or regenerative surgery is not feasible; *resection* is removal of one molar root when two roots are involved to include class II or III furcations; also requires endodontics and restorative dentistry; *hemisection* is converting a two-rooted tooth into a single-rooted tooth by removing both one root and a portion of the crown

2. Regenerative and reconstructive surgery
   a. Bone grafts and regenerative surgery
      (1) Objective—to promote regeneration of connective tissue, periodontal ligament, cementum, and alveolar bone
      (2) Indications—two-walled and three-walled vertical defects, class II furcation defects, circumferential defects (see Figures 14-5 and 14-6)
   b. Options available
      (1) Guided tissue regeneration (GTR) and guided bone regeneration (GBR)—involve using a semi-permeable membrane between the epithelium and the underlying ligament and bone to prevent rapid downgrowth of the epithelium or connective tissue, which would interfere with connective tissue regrowth after surgical débridement of the defect; non-resorbable (e.g., expanded polytetrafluoroethylene [e-PTFE] or Teflon, Gore-Tex, rubber dam) or resorbable (e.g., Guidor or Resolute) membranes are used; the former must be removed approximately 6 weeks after surgery, so the latter is most commonly employed

      (2) Bone grafts—involve placing bone-grafting material into a debrided defect to the level of the uninvolved crest to promote bone healing and regeneration (osseo-induction); the graft stimulates new bone formation and thus new attachment; autografts are obtained from the same client, allografts are transferred from genetically dissimilar individuals within the same species, for example, processed human cadaver bone that is freeze-dried or demineralized; alloplastic grafts use biologic fillers (e.g., bioactive glass ionomers, biocompatible composite polymers) or organic materials such as coral and bone; xenografts are obtained from another species

      (3) Biologic and biomimicry mediators—biologic agents such as enamel matrix derivative or synthetic biomimicry agents such as platelet-derived growth factors, platelet-rich plasma, and bone morphogenetic proteins are being studied for their potential to enhance periodontal regeneration

3. Periodontal plastic and reconstructive surgery
   a. Periodontal plastic and reconstructive surgery includes mucogingival surgery to correct defects or deficiencies in the shape, position, or amount of keratinized, attached gingiva surrounding teeth; mucogingival therapy to correct these types of defects in soft tissue and underlying bone; periodontal plastic surgery to create morphology and appearance that is acceptable to the client and the clinician, including root coverage, crown lengthening, ridge preservation, and augmentation; aesthetic surgery around implants; and exposure of teeth for orthodontics

   b. Includes gingival augmentation to increase the width of the attached gingiva, establish vestibular depth, arrest progressive gingival recession, and facilitate self-care; frenectomy for the elimination of abnormal frenum often in conjunction with a soft tissue graft;

alveolar ridge augmentation occurring as a result of tooth loss; aesthetic crown lengthening when anterior teeth are shorter than normal; papillary retention and reconstruction to correct deficient interproximal height of papillary gingiva; or surgical movement of impacted teeth for orthodontics (e.g., closed orthodontic eruption)

    c. The numerous procedures include, but are not limited to, the previously discussed flap procedures and osseous resection; however, grafts (most commonly autografts and occasionally allografts) also are employed to cover exposed root surfaces, including free soft tissue grafts obtained from a donor site that is distant from the recipient site and thus maintains none of its own blood supply; soft tissue–only grafts for ridge augmentation; subepithelial connective tissue grafts for either of these purposes; a tunnel technique can be employed for single-tooth autografts or ridge augmentation, thus precluding the need for reflecting a flap

Healing Following Periodontal Therapy

See the section on "Regeneration and wound healing" in Chapter 7.

A. In health, periodontal tissue constantly undergoes renewal; the oral epithelium maintains thickness by the mitotic activity of epithelial cells, fibroblasts generate and regenerate connective tissue, and cementoblasts form new cementum; periodontal ligament cells and bone are continually remodeled by fibroblasts and osteoblasts

B. Basic healing processes after all forms of periodontal therapy are the same

    1. Regeneration—growth and differentiation of new cells and intercellular substances to form or re-form tissues or parts of the same type as the precursor; primary means of healing following NSPT, creating a longer junctional epithelium

    2. Repair—also referred to as *healing by scar tissue* or *fibrosis*; does not necessarily restore the original architecture or function of the tissue or part

    3. Epithelial adaptation—close adaptation of the marginal gingival epithelium without complete pocket elimination; occurs with shrinkage of the gingiva following therapy; often occurs in conjunction with the regeneration of a longer junctional epithelium

    4. New attachment—embedding of new periodontal ligament fibers into new cementum and formation of a new gingival attachment in an area previously degenerated by disease rather than

repair of the periodontal attachment apparatus after an injury (reattachment)

    a. Goal of periodontal surgery—the rapid downgrowth of the epithelium must be prevented to allow the formation of connective tissue and bone; this is the basis of using a barrier in regenerative surgery

    b. Requires adequate removal of local etiologic factors via débridement; immobilization of mobile teeth and elimination of occlusal stress in a weakened periodontium are necessary

Sutures

A. Objectives

    1. Used to hold soft tissue in place until the healing process has progressed to the point at which tissue placement can be self-maintained

    2. Stabilization of the soft tissue helps:

        a. Maintain blood clotting around the wound

        b. Protect the wound area during the healing process

B. Types of suture materials

    1. Absorbable—surgical gut (from intestines of sheep); polyglactin (coated Vicryl and Vicryl Rapide) and polyglecaprone (Monocryl); absorb through proteolysis by enzymes in saliva in 7 to 10 days, thus eliminating the need for removal

    2. Nonabsorbable—surgical silk most common; expanded polytetrafluoroethylene (or Teflon, Gore-Tex) in GTR; must be professionally removed after 7 to 10 days

C. Procedure for suture removal

    1. Grasp the knotted end of suture with cotton pliers, and gently pull it away from the tissue

    2. Insert the tip of scissors under the suture, and cut the suture material that had been in the tissue

    3. Gently pull the knotted end so that only the suture material that had previously been incorporated within the tissue will pass through the tissue during the removal process

    4. Count and record the number of sutures removed, and compare this number with the suture placement record

    5. Gently cleanse the wound sites, and check for bleeding; control the bleeding, as needed

Periodontal Dressings

A. The rationale for the use of periodontal dressing is to protect the tissues after surgery; have no curative properties; wound healing progresses at the same rate with or without dressings; sometimes used for client comfort or for protection of the wound area

B. Types—dressings using metallic oxide and fatty acids (noneugenol) are most common (e.g., Coe-Pak, Periocare); clear, translucent light-cured dressings (e.g., Barricaid™) are preferred by some clinicians for aesthetics

C. Procedure for dressing placement

   1. Explain the process to the client; ensure that the bleeding has stopped

   2. Mix the dressing material according to the manufacturer's instructions; most materials come in two tubes, and equal lengths are mixed for a rubbery consistency

   3. Gently place the dressing, and establish retention in the embrasure spaces

   4. Ensure that the dressing does not cover more than the cervical third of the tooth, does not overextend into the mucobuccal fold and is not forced between the flap and the root surface; does not interfere with frenum attachments or with the client's occlusion; and the surface of the dressing is smooth and well contoured

   5. Provide postsurgical instructions to the client (see the section on "Client instructions and education")

D. Removal of the periodontal dressing

   1. Remove the dressing within 5 to 7 days; tease the edges of the dressing away from teeth with a curet or cotton pliers; be sure that sutures are not embedded in the dressing

   2. After the pack has been removed, gently cleanse the area with warm water or dampened cotton tips; remove sutures; assess tissue healing, but do not probe sulcular areas

POSTOPERATIVE CARE

Client Instructions and Education

A. Discomfort—the client should:

   1. Expect some discomfort after the local anesthesia wears off; use the prescribed pain medication

   2. Rest and limit physical activities during the first few days to prevent excessive bleeding and promote healing

   3. Use an ice pack to prevent swelling

   4. Eliminate spicy, hot, cold, hard, or sticky foods and liquids and tobacco use to limit tissue irritants and protect the dressing

B. Home-care recommendations—provide the following instructions to the client:

   1. Do not rinse the mouth on the first day because this may disturb the process of blood clotting that is necessary for wound healing

   2. After the first day, rinse gently with lukewarm water or a small amount of an antimicrobial rinse (e.g., chlorhexidine gluconate) to help control bacterial plaque biofilm; brush and floss nonsurgical areas as usual but gently

   3. Using a soft brush and water, very gently clean the surface of the dressing

   4. Slight seepage of blood during the first few hours is normal; any unusual, persistent bleeding should be reported to the periodontist

Follow-Up Care

A. Client returns approximately 7 days after surgery

B. Dressing and sutures are removed; new dressing may or may not be applied

C. Dentinal hypersensitivity may be experienced; desensitization is indicated for dentinal hypersensitivity; desensitization methods may be prescribed (see the section on "Control of dentinal hypersensitivity" in Chapter 16)

D. Home-care instructions are provided for plaque biofilm control

E. Long-term postoperative care requires periodic evaluation (also known as *periodontal maintenance care, continued care,* or *recare*)

Periodontal Maintenance[2,32,33]

A. An extension of periodontal therapy; also called *periodontal maintenance care, continued care,* or *recare* (no longer called *supportive periodontal therapy*)

   1. Initiated after completion of active periodontal treatment and continued at various intervals for the life of the dentition or its implant replacements

   2. Periodontal maintenance is an extension of active therapy, whether nonsurgical or surgical

B. The objectives of periodontal maintenance care is to:

   1. Minimize any recurrence and progression of periodontal disease in previously treated clients

   2. Reduce tooth loss incidence by monitoring the client's periodontal status at regular intervals

   3. Re-evaluate results after active periodontal therapy (nonsurgical or surgical) over the long term

   4. Reinforce self-care instructions and encourage client's long-term protective oral health behaviors

   5. Determine the need for additional treatment in a timely manner

C. Components of periodontal maintenance care

   1. Need for the cooperation of client, dental hygienist, dentist, and periodontist

   2. Emphasis on scaling, root planing, and periodontal debridement; extrinsic stain removal; and re-instruction of client in self-care to maintain attachment levels

3. Optimization of protective factors; minimization and elimination of risk factors
D. Periodic re-evaluation and assessment
  1. Review and update of client's health, pharmacologic, and dental histories; review and control of associated risk factors
  2. Radiographic review
  3. Examination of extraoral and intraoral soft tissues
  4. Dental charting of caries, tooth mobility and fremitus, and other tooth-related problems
  5. Periodontal assessment and charting of gingival recession, probing depths, bleeding on probing; levels of plaque and calculus, furcation involvement, exudation, occlusal trauma, tooth mobility; and other signs or symptoms of periodontal disease
  6. Evaluation of client's oral self-care behavior, attitude, values, and skill
  7. Examination of dental implants and peri-implant tissues
E. Treatment—based on assessment
  1. Always encourage the client; provide oral self-care re-instruction, and reinforce client's compliance with recommended maintenance intervals
  2. Healthy periodontium—removal of supragingival deposits; no root planing indicated
  3. Presence of bleeding or inflammation of the gingiva—treatment depends on the cause and pocket depths; removal of deposits and contributing factors, as necessary; possible use of an antimicrobial rinse (e.g., 0.12% chlorhexidine) or sustained-release, locally delivered antibiotic or antimicrobial agent
  4. Presence of periodontal pockets—scaling, periodontal debridement, and root planing followed by re-evaluation in 4 to 6 weeks to determine the need for adjunctive therapy or possible periodontal surgery
  5. Determination of frequency of periodontal maintenance must be individualized
    a. The frequency increases when clients have less than optimal oral self-care practices
    b. Longer intervals are acceptable if clients can control bacterial plaque biofilm, unless systemic disease or advanced periodontitis exists
    c. The goal is to control the clinical signs of inflammation and to stabilize attachment levels
    d. Frequent intervals (≤3 months) are generally necessary for subgingival and supragingival plaque and calculus removal in the presence of periodontitis
    e. Generally, the shorter the interval, the greater is the long-term success, particularly during the healing phase (1 year) after surgery

F. Indications for re-treatment
  1. Increase in probing depth or attachment loss of ≥2 mm
  2. Bleeding on probing that does not respond to periodontal maintenance procedures
  3. Severity—to be considered in determining treatment regimens (nonsurgical or surgical); retaining questionable teeth is not recommended
  4. Generalized deterioration—systemic complication might be suspected.
  5. Dental implants with bone loss or mobility

DENTAL IMPLANTS[1,2,34,35]

See the sections on "Dental implants" in Chapter 13 and "Advanced instrumentation techniques" in Chapter 17.
A. Definition—artificial replacements of teeth that are permanently affixed into alveolar bone by a biomedical device and usually composed of an inert metal or a metallic alloy
  1. Implants offer an alternative to removable dentures to edentulous or partially edentulous persons; single or multiple teeth can be replaced
  2. Implants provide a permanent anchor for artificial teeth by serving as an abutment for fixed or removable prostheses
    a. Implant—portion surgically placed within the bone
    b. Abutment—metallic post attached to the implant so that a restoration can be placed over it
    c. Superstructure—prosthetic replacement (e.g., crown, bridge, or denture) that is affixed to the abutment or a removable replacement tooth that the client can remove and clean
    d. Implant-assisted prosthesis—removable tissue dentures (overdentures) supported in the arch by endosseous dental implants
B. Limiting factors
  1. Systemic—age is a consideration only if the client's jaws are still growing because implants are contraindicated until full growth is attained; any condition or disease that affects an individual's ability to fight infection should be carefully considered because implant failure is commonly caused by infection; greater failure also occurs in poor quality and density of bone, so conditions such as osteoporosis also require careful consideration; cigarette smoking is a documented risk factor for implant failure, so tobacco use cessation is essential before implant placement; factors affecting the client's ability to withstand surgery also are paramount (e.g., malnutrition, recent cardiac arrest, bleeding problems)

2. Local—unfavorable ridge morphology or other bone quality and density changes caused by resorption; sufficient bone and soft tissue for implant positioning must be similar to that of a natural tooth within the tissue and the alveolar ridge—orthodontics and surgical augmentation or correction may be possible; severe malocclusion or parafunctional habits that would cause excessive trauma would contraindicate implants; uncontrolled periodontal disease is also a contraindication; an immobile implant generally is not attached to a natural tooth with periodontal ligament mobility

C. Implant design

  1. Systems—either two-stage (submerged) or one-stage (nonsubmerged)

    a. Submerged—designed to protect the implant from occlusal stress and bacterial exposure during the healing phase; the implant is placed in two steps, allowing osseo-integration for 3 to 6 months before exposing the implant to the oral cavity for abutment placement; a prosthetic device is later connected to the implant

    b. Nonsubmerged—the implant has a collar that extends through tissue and attaches the prosthesis supragingivally or slightly subgingivally at the time of placement; only one surgery is involved for client comfort and convenience

    c. Shape and size vary in either system; most common are screw-shaped, root-shaped, or cylinder-shaped implants

  2. Materials commonly used for dental implants—must be biocompatible

    a. Titanium—a metallic element; pure, plasma sprayed, or titanium alloy

    b. Hydroxyapatite—plasma sprayed

D. Two major types of implants

  1. Subperiosteal—custom-fabricated framework of metal that is supra-alveolar (on top of the bone) but beneath oral tissue; rests on bone for support

    a. Posts protrude through tissue to provide anchor for the final bridge or denture

    b. Two-step surgery required—initial surgery to deflect soft tissue and make an impression of alveolar bone; followed by placement of fabricated implant framework

    c. Subperiosteal implants are not used frequently; used if bone mass is inadequate for root-type implants

  2. Endosteal or endosseous (inside bone)

    a. The implant is placed directly into a socket, which has been prepared through a process called *trephining*; uses a series of specially prepared drills and burs

      (1) Osseo-integration refers to the implant being in direct contact with bone without intervening connective tissue (i.e., no periodontal ligament or connective tissue attachment); the implant is, in effect, "ankylosed" within bone

      (2) After initial loss of 1-mm to 2-mm alveolar bone during the first year, crestal bone should be stable with no more than 0.1 to 0.2 mm per year thereafter

    b. After bone and soft tissue heal, the final bridge or denture is placed

  3. Transosteal implants—means "through the bone"; mandibular denture anchors are placed all the way through the mandible from under the border into the oral cavity

  4. Endodontic implants—placed inside the tooth through to pulpal canal to stabilize the tooth; used infrequently

E. Implant–tissue interface

  1. Controversy exists regarding the implant–tissue interface, although it is agreed that this is the basis of implant success

  2. The epithelial attachment to the implant may be similar to the attachment to a natural tooth (i.e., basal lamina and hemidesmosomes); no periodontal ligament; called *perimucosal seal*

  3. Perimucosal seal, or biologic seal, is defined as the adaptation of keretinized or nonkeretinized epithelium to the abutment cylinder of an implant; critical to implant retention

  4. Osseo-integration—contact established between normal and remodeled bone and the implant surface without the interposition of connective tissue

F. Criteria for successful treatment outcomes

  1. Immobility of the implant

  2. No peri-implant radiolucency on the radiograph

  3. Absence of signs and symptoms such as pain, bleeding, infections, paresthesia, or mandibular canal involvement

  4. Minimum success rate of 85% at 5 years and 80% percent at 10 years of observation

G. Implant management

  1. Periodic evaluation of implants, surrounding tissue, and oral hygiene essential to long-term success; considerations in periodic evaluation include:

    a. Extent of plaque biofilm and dental calculus

    b. Clinical appearance of peri-implant soft tissue

    c. Radiographic appearance—no periodontal ligament space or bone loss; no peri-implant radiolucency

    d. Absence of occlusal interference or trauma; stability of implant and prostheses—no mobility

e. Probing depths (if other signs of disease present)—gentle, careful technique must be used
f. Absence of bleeding or exudate
g. Adequacy of maintenance interval
h. Client comfort and function
2. Goals
   a. Maintenance of the health of the implant and supporting tissue
   b. Prevention of loss of perimucosal seal
   c. Prevention of gingivitis and, failing that, prevention of conversion of gingivitis to peri-implantitis, a periodontitis-like disease process that can affect dental implants

(1) Infectious failure—failing implants with a primarily infectious cause
(2) Traumatic failure—failing implants with a primarily traumatic cause
d. Provision of preventive and maintenance therapies with minimal damage, or surface scratching, to implants
e. Control of bacterial plaque biofilm
H. Preventive instrumentation (see the sections on "Dental implant maintenance" in Chapter 16 and "Instrumentation of dental implants" in Chapter 17)

@ WEB SITE INFORMATION AND RESOURCES

SOURCE	WEB SITE ADDRESS	DESCRIPTION
American Academy of Periodontology	www.perio.org	Position papers, parameters of care, scientific information, and related links in periodontics as well as related information for consumers
Cochrane Collaboration	www.cochrane.org	Evidence-based health care databases; site search for "periodontal" provides excellent related systematic reviews
International Centre for Evidence-Based Oral Health, Eastman Dental Institute	www.eastman.ucl.ac.uk	Systematic reviews as part of an overall mission for the synthesis of periodontal research
National Center for Dental Hygiene Research	www.usc.edu/hsc/dental/dhnet	Current topics in dental hygiene and periodontics with links to related government sites, product companies, and professional associations
University of Minnesota School of Dentistry, Division of Periodontology	www1.umn.edu/perio/tobacco/	Information on tobacco use cessation and related links
University of California Los Angeles (UCLA) Periodontal Information Center	www.dent.ucla.edu/pic	Free courses for dental professionals on current topics in periodontics; can earn continuing education units with annual fee

REFERENCES

1. Weinberg MA, Westphal C, Froum SJ, Palat M, Schoor RS: *Comprehensive periodontics for the dental hygienist*, ed 3, Upper Saddle River, New Jersey, 2010, Pearson.
2. Newman MG, Takei HH, Carranza FA: *Carranza's clinical periodontology*, ed 11, St Louis, 2012, Saunders.
3. Armitage GC: Development of a classification system for periodontal diseases and conditions, *Ann Periodontol* 4(1):1–6, 1999: Available at http://www.perio.org/resources-products/classification.pdf: Accessed September 1 2010.
4. American Academy of Periodontology Research, Science, and Therapy Committee: Drug-associated gingival enlargement, *J Periodontol* 75:1424–1431, 2004: Available at http://www.perio.org/resources-products/posppr3-3.html: Accessed September 1 2010.
5. Ad Hoc Committee on Parameters of Care, American Academy of Periodontology: Parameter on chronic periodontitis with advanced loss of periodontal support,

J Periodontol 71(Suppl 5):856–858, 2000: Available at http://www.perio.org/resources-products/posppr3-2.html: Accessed September 1 2010.
6. American Academy of Periodontology Research, Science, and Therapy Committee: Periodontal diseases in children and adolescents, *J Periodontol* 74:1696–1704, 2003: Available at http://www.perio.org/resources-products/posppr3-3.html: Accessed September 1 2010.
7. American Academy of Periodontology: Statement on risk assessment, *J Periodontol* 79:202, 2008: Available at http://www.perio.org/resources-products/posppr3-4.html: Accessed September 1 2010.
8. Löe H, Anerud A, Boysen H: Natural history of periodontal disease in man: Prevalence, severity, and extent of gingival recession, *J Periodontol* 63:489–495, 1992.
9. Löe H, Anerud A, Boysen H, Morrison E: Natural history of periodontal disease in man: Rapid, moderate and no loss of attachment in Sri Lankan laborers 14 to 46 years of age, *J Clin Periodontol* 13:431–445, 1986.

10. Löe H, Anerud A, Boysen H, et al.: Natural history of periodontal disease in man: The rate of periodontal destruction after 40 years of age, *J Periodontol* 49:607–620, 1978.

11. Brown LJ, Brunelle JA, Kingman A: Periodontal status in the United States, 1988–1991: Prevalence, extent, and demographic variation, *J Dent Res* 75(Spec Iss): 672–683, 1996.

12. Dye BA, Nowjack-Raymer R, Barker LK, et al.: Overview sand quality assurance for the oral health component of the National Health and Nutrition Examination Survey (NHANES) 2003–04, *J Public Health Dent* 68(4): 218–226, 2008.

13. Heasman L, Stacey F, Preshaw PM, McCracken GI, Hepburn S, Heasman PA: The effect of smoking on periodontal treatment response: A review of clinical evidence, *J Clin Periodontol* 33(4):241–253, 2006.

14. American Academy of Periodontology Research, Science, and Therapy Committee: The pathogenesis of periodontal diseases, *J Periodontol* 70:457–470, 1999: Available at http://www.perio.org/resources-products/posppr3-3. html: Accessed September 1, 2010.

15. American Academy of Periodontology Research, Science and Therapy Committee: Guidelines for periodontal therapy, *J Periodontol* 72:1624–1628, 2001: Available at http://www.perio.org/resources-products/posppr3-3. html: Accessed September 1, 2010.

16. American Academy of Periodontology: Parameters of care, *J Periodontol* 71(5 Suppl):847–883, 2000: Available at http://www.perio.org/resources-products/pos/ppr3-2. html: Accessed September 1, 2010.

17. American Academy of Periodontology Research, Science, and Therapy Committee: Diagnosis of periodontal diseases, *J Periodontol* 74:1237–1247, 2004: Available at http://www.perio.org/resourcesproducts/posppr3-3. html: Accessed September 1, 2010.

18. American Academy of Periodontology: The mouth body connection: Available at http://www.perio.org/ consumer/mbc.top2.htm: Accessed June 1, 2010.

19. Darby ML, Walsh MM: *Dental hygiene theory and practice*, ed 3, St Louis, 2010, Saunders.

20. American Academy of Periodontology Research, Science and Therapy Committee: Treatment of plaque-induced gingivitis, chronic periodontitis and other clinical conditions, *J Periodontol* 72:1790–1800, 2001: Available at http://www.perio.org/resourcesproducts/posppr3-3. html: Accessed September 1, 2010.

21. Ad Hoc Committee on Parameters of Care, American Academy of Periodontology: Parameter on plaque-induced gingivitis, *J Periodontol* 71(Suppl 5):851–852, 2000: Available at http://www.perio.org/resources-products/posppr3-2.html: Accessed September 1, 2010.

22. Ad Hoc Committee on Parameters of Care, American Academy of Periodontology: Parameter on chronic periodontitis with slight to moderate loss of periodontal support, *J Periodontol* 71(Suppl 5):853–855, 2000: Available at http://www.perio.org/resources-products/ posppr3-2.html: Accessed September 1, 2010.

23. American Academy of Periodontology: Statement on use of lasers for excisional new attachment procedure (ENAP): Available at http://www.perio.org/resources products/posppr3-4.html: Accessed September 1, 2010.

24. American Academy of Periodontology: Guidelines for the management of patients with periodontal diseases, *J Periodontol* 77:1607–1161, 2006: Available at http:// www.perio.org/resources-products/pdf/management. pdf: Accessed September 1, 2010.

25. American Academy of Periodontology Research, Science and Therapy Committee: Systemic antibiotics in periodontics, *J Periodontol* 75:1553–1565, 2004: Availble at http://www.perio.org/resourcesproducts/posppr3-3. html: Accessed September 1, 2010.

26. American Academy of Periodontology: Statement on local delivery or controlled release antimicrobials as adjunctive therapy in the treatment of periodontitis, *J Periodontol* 77:1458–14, 2006: Available at http:// www.perio.org/resourcesproducts/posppr3-3.html: Accessed September 1, 2010.

27. Ad Hoc Committee on Parameters of Care, American Academy of Periodontology: Parameter on "refractory" periodontitis, *J Periodontol* 71(Suppl 5):859–860, 2000: Available at http://www.perio.org/resources-products/ posppr3-2.html: Accessed September 1, 2010.

28. American Academy of Periodontology: Statement on Periostat® as an adjunct to scaling and root planing for the treatment of adult periodontitis, 2000: Available at http://www.perio.org/resourcesproducts/posppr3-4. html: Accessed September 1, 2010.

29. American Academy of Periodontology: Statement on gingival curettage, *J Periodontol* 73(10):1229–1230, 2002: Available at http://www.perio.org/resourcesproducts/ posppr3-4.html: Accessed September 1, 2010.

30. Ad Hoc Committee on Parameters of Care, American Academy of Periodontology: Parameter on occlusal traumatism in patients with chronic periodontitis, *J Periodontol* 71 (Suppl 5):873–875, 2000: Available at http://www.perio.org/resources-products/posppr3-2. html: Accessed September 1, 2010.

31. Torosian J: Surgical intervention. In Hodges KD, editor: *Concepts in nonsurgical periodontal therapy*, New York, 1997, Delmar.

32. American Academy of Periodontology Research, Science and Therapy Committee: Periodontal maintenance, *J Periodontol* 74:1395–1401, 2003: Available at http:// www.perio.org/resources-products/posppr3-3.html: Accessed September 1, 2010.

33. Ad Hoc Committee on Parameters of Care, American Academy of Periodontology: Parameter on periodontal maintenance, *J Periodontol* 71(Suppl 5):849–850, 2000: Available at http://www.perio.org/resources-products/posppr3-2.html: Accessed September 1, 2010.

34. American Academy of Periodontology: Position paper. Dental implants in periodontal therapy, *J Periodontol* 71:1934–1942, 2000: Available at http://www.perio.org/ resources-products/posppr3-3.html: Accessed September 1, 2010.

35. Ad Hoc Committee on Parameters of Care, American Academy of Periodontology: Parameter on placement and management of the dental implant, *J Periodontol* 71(Suppl 5):870–872, 2000: Available at http:// www.perio.org/resources-products/posppr3-2.html: Accessed September 1, 2010.

CHAPTER 14 REVIEW QUESTIONS

Answers and Rationales to Chapter Review Questions are available on this text's accompanying Evolve site. See inside front cover for details.
Use Case A to answer questions 1 to 12.

evolve

| Synopsis
Client
History | Age: _56_
Sex: _M_
Height: _5' 11"_
Weight: _180 lb_ | **VITAL SIGNS**
Blood pressure: _142/94 mm Hg_
Pulse rate: _65 bpm_
Respiration: _18 rpm_ |

Case A

1. Under the care of a physician   ✔ YES   ___NO
         Condition: _Diabetes_
2. Hospitalization within the last five years   ✔ YES   ___NO
3. Has or had the following conditions:

Rheumatic fever or rheumatic heart disease   ___YES   ✔_NO

Congenital heart disease (bicuspid aortic valve)   ___YES   ✔_NO

Heart attack   ___YES   ✔_NO

Angina pectoris   ___YES   ✔_NO

Hypertension   ___YES   ✔_NO

Diabetes mellitus type 1   ✔_YES   ___NO

Hepatitis   ___YES   ✔_NO

Bleeding disorder   ___YES   ✔_NO

Fainting spells, seizures, or epilepsy   ___YES   ✔_NO

Asthma   ___YES   ✔_NO

Allergies (medication, food)   ✔_YES   ___NO

         Allergic to: _penicillin_   Other:_____

4. Current medications:

Anticoagulants	___YES	✔_NO	Nitroglycerin	___YES	✔_NO
Insulin	✔_YES	___NO	High blood pressure medication	___YES	✔_NO
Antibiotics	___YES	✔_NO	Corticosteroids	___YES	✔_NO
Aspirin	___YES	✔_NO	Oral contraceptives	___YES	✔_NO

Other: _____

5. Smokes or uses tobacco products   ✔_YES   ___NO

MEDICAL HISTORY: The client reports that he last had a physical examination to monitor his diabetes about a year ago. His HbA1c was 7.5. The physician stated that his condition was under control, but that he must monitor his diet, blood glucose, and insulin levels more carefully. He is allergic to penicillin.

DENTAL HISTORY: The client states that he has trouble controlling his diabetes. From his dental record, he was treated nonsurgically for periodontal disease a year ago. He did not return for his periodontal maintenance therapy visits since that time, even though he is on a three-month continued-care interval. The client reports toothbrushing one to two times daily and no flossing.

SOCIAL HISTORY: The client works 60 hours per week, travels, and supports a family of five.

CHIEF COMPLAINT: "My gums bleed when brushing and I am concerned about bad breath."

SUPPLEMENTAL
ORAL EXAMINATION
FINDINGS: The client has no third molars and is missing teeth #15 and #30. Extrinsic stain is generalized on crowns of teeth.

Gingival bleeding is present upon probing around all teeth. All areas have proximal and marginal bacterial plaque and moderate calculus.

Recession and inadequate zones of attached gingiva are present around the facial gingiva of teeth #23 to #26.

Client has slight to moderate bone loss, and 4-mm to 6-mm pocket depths are generalized throughout the mouth. These findings are similar to the last appointment with 1-mm increase in probe readings in the molar areas.

1. Which of the following statements is MOST accurate regarding this client's health history assessment?
   a. His general health requires no treatment modification, precautionary measure, or referral
   b. Signs and symptoms of a possible uncontrolled condition exist, and physician referral is warranted
   c. The client's poorly controlled diabetes is the cause of his periodontal disease
   d. Prophylactic antibiotic premedication for prevention of infective endocarditis is indicated before any invasive procedures

2. On the basis of the assessment findings reported, what is the MOST accurate preliminary diagnosis for this client?
   a. Dental plaque–induced gingivitis
   b. Aggressive periodontitis
   c. Chronic periodontitis
   d. Periodontitis as a manifestation of systemic disease
   e. Refractory periodontitis

3. The recession noted in the mandibular anterior region requires evaluation by a dentist or periodontist. If periodontal surgery is indicated, a gingivectomy would be performed to correct this condition.
   a. Both statements are TRUE
   b. Both statements are FALSE
   c. The first statement is TRUE, and the second statement is FALSE
   d. The first statement is FALSE, and the second statement is TRUE

4. Smoking is the primary cause of this client's periodontal disease. Infrequent professional oral health care is an additional environmental risk factors contributing to his periodontitis also should be addressed in the dental hygiene care plan.
   a. Both statements are TRUE
   b. Both statements are FALSE
   c. The first statement is TRUE, and the second statement is FALSE
   d. The first statement is FALSE, and the second statement is TRUE

5. Which of the following devices would be MOST effective for plaque biofilm removal in the mandibular anterior region?
   a. Dental floss
   b. Dental tape
   c. Oral irrigation
   d. Interproximal brush

6. Controlled drug delivery (sustained-release drug delivery) of antibiotics should be considered in the care plan because the patient's systemic health warrants use of antibiotics for control of advancing periodontitis.
   a. Both the statement and the reason are correct and related
   b. Both the statement and the reason are correct but NOT related
   c. The statement is correct, but the reason is NOT correct
   d. The statement is NOT correct, but the reason is correct
   e. NEITHER the statement NOR the reason is correct

7. An oxygenating mouthrinse would be beneficial for this client because he has inadequate oral hygiene and a weakened host response.
   a. Both the statement and the reason are correct and related.
   b. Both the statement and the reason are correct but NOT related.
   c. The statement is correct, but the reason is NOT correct.
   d. The statement is NOT correct, but the reason is correct.
   e. NEITHER the statement NOR the reason is correct.

8. In addition to professional dental hygiene care and proper oral hygiene measures, which of the following procedures or agents would address the client's chief concerns?
   a. Selective stain removal
   b. Chlorine dioxide mouthrinse
   c. Tooth whitening
   d. Daily fluoride mouthrinse

9. Which of the following periodontal therapies would be BEST recommended for this case?
   a. Regenerative periodontal surgery
   b. Gingival curettage
   c. Nonsurgical periodontal therapy
   d. Oral prophylaxis
   e. Periodontal maintenance therapy

10. All of the following are concerns related to potential outcomes of dental hygiene care in this case EXCEPT one. Which one is the EXCEPTION?
    a. Lack of client motivation and adherence to recommendations
    b. Delayed healing following treatment
    c. Poorly controlled diabetes mellitus
    d. Genetic predisposition

11. **Which of the following would be the BEST indicator of treatment success at the re-evaluation appointment 4 to 6 weeks following initial periodontal therapy?**
   a. Relatively free of plaque biofilm
   b. Stable periodontal probing depths
   c. Absence of gingival inflammation and bleeding
   d. No re-formed dental calculus deposits

12. **What is the maximum continuing-care interval recommended for periodontal maintenance therapy for this client?**
   a. 3 months
   b. 4 months
   c. 6 months
   d. 1 year

13. **What change in alveolar bone on a dental radiograph indicates early loss of bone?**
   a. Fuzziness in the crest of the bone
   b. Faint cup-shaped areas interproximally
   c. Vertical or angular defects
   d. Furcation involvement

14. **After bacterial virulence is established and the periodontal lesion is initiated, which is the first inflammatory cell to respond?**
   a. B lymphocytes
   b. Plasma cells
   c. Neutrophils
   d. T lymphocytes
   e. Macrophages

15. **All of the following tissue changes result in true periodontal pocket formation EXCEPT one. Which one is the EXCEPTION?**
   a. Apical migration of the junctional epithelium
   b. Apical migration of the gingival margin
   c. Destruction of the connective tissue attachment
   d. Resorption of the alveolar bone

16. **Which of the following diagnostic procedures is MOST accurate for determining severity of periodontal attachment loss?**
   a. Full-mouth digital radiographic survey
   b. Microbial testing of plaque biofilm
   c. Detection of pathologic tooth mobility or furcations
   d. Periodontal probing of all sulcular areas
   e. Determining presence or absence of bleeding on probing

17. **Which of the following are characteristic of aggressive periodontitis?**
   a. A long-standing inflammatory disease with periods of remission and exacerbation
   b. A slowly progressive disease that usually manifests itself around puberty
   c. A degenerative disease of the periodontium initially characterized by bone loss in anterior teeth and first molars
   d. A rapidly progressive inflammatory disease that most often affects the entire dentition equally
   e. A disease that most commonly affects children and adolescents with medically compromising conditions

18. **In cases of periodontitis, what is the first area to be involved in bone resorption?**
   a. Facial and lingual aspects of supporting bone
   b. Cribriform plate or lamina dura
   c. Cancellous portion of supporting bone
   d. Cortical plate of the interdental septum
   e. Bone surrounding the apical area of the tooth

19. **Which one of the following differentiates subgingival plaque biofilm from supragingival plaque?**
   a. Chromogenic bacteria influence the color
   b. Gram-negative anaerobes predominate
   c. Aerobic bacteria predominate in the slime layer
   d. The biofilm becomes calcified over time

20. **Which of the following types of cells are responsible for resorption of cementum and bone in orthodontic tooth movement ?**
   a. Cementoblasts
   b. Fibroblasts
   c. Osteoblasts
   d. Cementoclasts
   e. Osteoclasts

21. **Which of the following histologic changes in inflamed gingiva results in bleeding?**
   a. Vasodilation within the gingival connective tissue
   b. Ulceration of the sulcular lining
   c. Lymphoid cell accumulation
   d. Collagenase destroying the lamina propria
   e. Alteration of fibroblasts in the connective tissue

22. **Tooth mobility and fremitus are hallmarks of occlusal trauma because trauma is the primary cause of clinical attachment loss when occlusal trauma is present.**
   a. Both the statement and the reason are correct and related
   b. Both the statement and the reason are correct but NOT related
   c. The statement is correct, but the reason is NOT correct
   d. The statement is NOT correct, but the reason is correct
   e. NEITHER the statement NOR the reason is correct

23. All of the following conditions can be determined by radiographic examination EXCEPT one. Which one is the EXCEPTION?
    a. Extent and severity of bone loss
    b. Height of crestal bone
    c. Widening of the periodontal ligament space
    d. Presence of periodontal pockets
    e. Presence of dental calculus

24. Which radiographic findings will MOST likely be seen in dental plaque–induced gingivitis?
    a. Widened periodontal ligament space and triangulation
    b. Slight changes in the lamina dura
    c. Condensing osteitis
    d. Normal lamina dura and crestal bone

25. Oral examination findings for a 16-year-old female with good general health status include localized 4-mm and 5-mm periodontal probing depths, with radiographic bone loss visible on teeth #3, #14, #24, and #25; slight gingival inflammation in the mandibular anterior region; fair oral hygiene with minimal deposits is present; and no active caries are visible. On the basis of these findings, which of the following would be the MOST accurate preliminary diagnosis?
    a. Necrotizing ulcerative gingivitis
    b. Chronic periodontitis
    c. Dental plaque–induced gingivitis
    d. Localized aggressive periodontitis
    e. Hormone-associated gingivitis

26. A 35-year-old client with early chronic periodontitis who smokes and has challenges with self-care is new to your health care facility. All of the following initial or nonsurgical periodontal therapies are appropriate to recommend for this client EXCEPT one. Which one is the EXCEPTION?
    a. Topical antimicrobial mouthrinse
    b. Gingival curettage
    c. Scaling and periodontal débridement
    d. Selective stain removal
    e. Periodontal maintenance and supportive periodontal therapy

27. Which of the following antimicrobial and antigingivitis agent is the MOST effective because it is highly substantive?
    a. Essential oils
    b. Chlorhexidine gluconate
    c. Povidone iodine
    d. Cetylperidium chloride
    e. Stannous fluoride

28. Which of the following structures demarcates the attached gingiva from the alveolar mucosa?
    a. Gingival groove
    b. Junctional epithelium
    c. Gingival margin
    d. Base of the sulcus
    e. Mucogingival junction

29. All of the following tissues comprise nonkeratinized epithelium EXCEPT one. Which one is the EXCEPTION?
    a. Crevicular epithelium
    b. Attached gingiva
    c. Interdental papilla
    d. Junctional epithelium
    e. Marginal gingiva

30. Which of the following bacteria are tissue invading and thus associated with destruction of collagen and resorption of bone in periodontitis?
    a. *Actinomyces viscosus*
    b. *Porphyromonas gingivalis*
    c. *Streptococcus sanguis*
    d. *Treponema pallidum*
    e. *Capnocytophaga ochracea*

31. Which of the following types of drugs have been associated with gingival overgrowth?
    a. Oral contraceptives
    b. Antidepressants
    c. Calcium channel blockers
    d. Antihistamines
    e. Quinolones

32. All of the following conditions can cause periodontitis as a manifestation of systemic disease EXCEPT one. Which one is the EXCEPTION?
    a. Diabetes mellitus
    b. Chédiak-Higashi syndrome
    c. Papillion-Lefèvre syndrome
    d. Ehler-Danlos syndrome
    e. Leukemia

33. Which of the following BEST describes the junctional epithelium?
    a. Keratinized epithelium
    b. Basal cell epithelium
    c. Squamous cell epithelium
    d. Orthokeratinized epithelium
    e. Parakeratinized epithelium

34. Which type of periodontal disease is characterized by gray, sloughing tissue, pain, and spontaneous bleeding?
    a. Pericoronitis
    b. Pregnancy-related gingivitis
    c. Necrotizing ulcerative gingivitis
    d. Gingival abscess
    e. Aggressive periodontitis

35. Which of the following indicates that gingivitis has progressed to periodontitis?
    a. Widened periodontal ligament space on radiographs
    b. Periodontal probing depth ≥4 mm
    c. Clinical attachment loss
    d. Gingival recession
    e. Bleeding on probing

36. Which condition should be suspected when a radiolucent area occurs at the apex of the root of a tooth on a radiograph?
    a. Periodontal abscess
    b. Pyogenic granuloma
    c. Occlusal traumatism
    d. Periapical abscess
    e. Mucogingival problem

37. Which area within the periodontium is LEAST susceptible to tissue breakdown in periodontal disease?
    a. Gingival crevice
    b. Dentogingival junction
    c. Interdental col
    d. Junctional epithelium
    e. Attached gingiva

38. All of the following are possible causes of gingival recession EXCEPT one. Which one is the EXCEPTION?
    a. Faulty toothbrushing
    b. Bacterial plaque biofilm
    c. Dehiscence
    d. Dental caries
    e. Tooth position in the arch

39. All of the following are environmental risk factors associated with periodontal disease EXCEPT one. Which one is the EXCEPTION?
    a. Smoking
    b. Rough restorative margins
    c. Mouthbreathing
    d. Age
    e. Dental calculus

40. At a re-evaluation appointment with a client 6 weeks after completion of nonsurgical periodontal therapy, the hygienist notes generalized gingival inflammation and bleeding. Periodontal probing depths remain unchanged. Plaque control is acceptable, although re-instruction is indicated on the lingual of the mandibular molars. What is the MOST probable explanation for these findings?
    a. Residual dental calculus deposits are present
    b. Plaque removal was absent for the past 24 hours
    c. Systemic disease influencing host response is present
    d. Plaque removal was enhanced immediately before appointment

41. All of the following risk factors have been associated with the prevalence of gingivitis EXCEPT one. Which one is the EXCEPTION?
    a. Socioeconomic status
    b. Level of education
    c. Dietary habits
    d. Tooth alignment
    e. Sites previously affected by periodontitis

42. Which of the following situations would be an indication for regenerative periodontal surgery?
    a. An edematous 5-mm pseudopocket
    b. Severe drug-influenced gingival enlargement
    c. An infrabony pocket of 6 mm on the distal aspect of tooth #30
    d. Gingival recession that extends into the alveolar mucosa
    e. A periodontal abscess

43. Which of the following is an objective of periodontal regenerative surgery?
    a. Improve the aesthetics of the client's face
    b. Create gingival contour and appearance acceptable to the client
    c. Remove alveolar bone to improve contour and correct defects
    d. Remove enlarged tissue to assist the client in daily plaque control
    e. Promote regeneration of connective tissue, periodontal ligament, cementum and alveolar bone

44. All of the following are substances produced by the host response to bacterial plaque biofilm EXCEPT one. Which one is the EXCEPTION?
    a. Lipo-polysaccharide
    b. Matrix metalloproteinase (MMP)
    c. Cytokines
    d. Interleukin 1 (IL-1)
    e. Prostaglandin E_2 (PGE_2)

45. Which type of periodontal surgery is used to reduce probing depths and arrest periodontal disease by promoting new attachment of periodontal tissues?
    a. Gingivoplasty
    b. Guided tissue regeneration
    c. Osseous resection
    d. Bone grafting
    e. Mucogingival surgery

46. What has the discipline of periodontal medicine shown about the relationship between periodontal diseases and systemic diseases?
    a. Periodontitis causes systemic diseases such as heart disease and cerebrovascular disease
    b. Persons with weakened host response have increased susceptibility to periodontitis
    c. Periodontal disease is treated with systemic antibiotics
    d. Periodontitis has been associated with systemic diseases as a possible risk factor
    e. Genetic mutations affecting susceptibility and progression of systemic diseases also affect periodontitis

47. All of the following are necessary for new attachment after periodontal surgery EXCEPT one. Which one is the EXCEPTION?
    a. Thorough removal of bacterial irritants
    b. Immobilization of mobile teeth
    c. Regeneration or generation of new tissues or parts
    d. Adequate number of fibroblasts and osteoblasts
    e. Rapid apical growth of epithelium

48. All of the following are advantages of controlled drug delivery (sustained-release drug delivery) over systemic drug administration in periodontal therapy EXCEPT one. Which one is the EXCEPTION?
    a. Less concern about client adherence throughout indicated time frame
    b. Site-specific antimicrobial action in periodontal pocket
    c. High concentration delivered to the site of infection
    d. Can be used when periodontal infection is generalized or severe

49. What is the advantage of synthetic absorbable sutures?
    a. Do not require the client to return for removal
    b. Have antibacterial properties
    c. Cause less tissue reaction than silk or gut sutures
    d. Are not treated by the surrounding tissue as a foreign body

50. Periodontal dressings improves the rate of wound healing following periodontal surgery. These materials also minimize client discomfort.
    a. Both statements are TRUE
    b. Both statements are FALSE
    c. The first statement is TRUE, and the second statement is FALSE
    d. The first statement is FALSE, and the second statement is TRUE

51. Joe Smith, age 50, returns for periodontal maintenance therapy every 3 months for 1 year after nonsurgical periodontal treatment for chronic periodontitis. The inflammation has been resolved, and periodontal probing depths have decreased from 5 mm or 6 mm to 4 mm or less in most treated areas, with the exception of the distal surface of #2, where the probing depth has increased from 4 mm to 6 mm. Radiographs reveal no change on #2 distal. Which of the following explains this finding?
    a. Continuing clinical attachment loss
    b. Error in periodontal probing technique
    c. Calculus deposits affecting accuracy of initial reading
    d. Inaccessibility and poor visibility in pocket areas
    e. Healing of periodontal tissues

52. Which of the following factors could limit a recommendation for dental implants?
    a. Complete edentulism
    b. Age over 65 years
    c. Minimal bone density
    d. Single missing tooth

53. What is the most common material used for dental implants?
    a. Stainless steel
    b. Porcelain
    c. Gold
    d. Titanium

54. Which of the following findings would indicate a failed dental implant?
    a. Peri-implant inflammation
    b. Bleeding on provocation
    c. Alveolar bone loss
    d. Loosening of the prosthetic crown
    e. Mobility

55. A client with dental implants returns for continuing care 6 months after dental implant placement. Which of the following factors assessed during oral examination and re-evaluation would be MOST effective for assessing success of previous dental hygiene care delivered?
    a. Amount and distribution of bacterial plaque deposits
    b. Condition of gingival tissue
    c. Radiographic examination of alveolar bone
    d. Presence or absence of dental calculus deposits
    e. Efficacy of oral hygiene techniques demonstrated

CHAPTER 15 Dental Hygiene Process of Care

Kristin H. Calley

The dental hygiene process—a systematic, problem-solving approach to quality oral health care—provides a framework for dental hygienists to individualize care and ensure that clients' needs are met. This approach provides a framework for evidence-based decision making and sound clinical judgment while identifying and resolving client needs within the dental hygiene practice.[1]

The process is a standard of practice recognized by the American Dental Hygienists' Association (ADHA), and an educational standard of the American Dental Association (ADA) Commission on Dental Accreditation.[2,3] This chapter addresses the major components of the dental hygiene process of care: assessment, diagnosis, planning, implementation, evaluation that includes prognosis, legal–ethical considerations, and documentation.

DENTAL HYGIENE PARADIGM[1]

Basic Concepts

A. A paradigm is composed of major concepts selected for study by a discipline
B. The paradigm for the discipline of dental hygiene includes four concepts[4]
   1. Clients—recipients of dental hygiene care; include persons, families, groups, and communities from all age, cultural, gender, and economic groups
   2. Environment—external factors that affect the client's optimal oral health; includes economic, psychological, cultural, physical, legal, educational, ethical, and geographic dimensions
   3. Health and oral health—status of the overall health and the oral wellness or illness of the client
   4. Dental hygiene actions—interventions that a dental hygienist initiates to promote wellness,

prevent and control oral disease, and encourage active client participation and collaboration
C. Dental hygiene practice—based on a systematic process of care that involves assessment, diagnosis, planning, implementation, and evaluation (Figure 15-1)
D. The dental hygiene process of care provides a logical system for determining the health and disease status of the client and for selecting appropriate interventions and measuring treatment outcomes
E. The dental hygiene process of care is integrated with the client's comprehensive dental hygiene diagnosis and care plan

HUMAN NEEDS THEORY AND ASSESSMENT[1,5-7]

See the section on "Human behavior principles" in Chapter 16.

Basic Concepts

A. Most widely known model in the discipline of dental hygiene—human needs conceptual model; requires assessment of each client's human needs as the framework for providing care
B. Based on the theory that human activity is dominated by behaviors aimed at need fulfillment; an internal drive exists in all humans to satisfy unmet needs; unmet needs motivate specific behaviors to eliminate the perceived deficit; the model encourages establishing an environment that is more client oriented than task oriented
C. The human needs model uses eight needs relevant to oral health that should be considered in the implementation of the dental hygiene process of care[8] (Figure 15-2)

Assessment
- Health, pharmacologic, cultural and dental history and vital signs
- Extraoral and intraoral clinical assessment
- Dentition assessment
- Periodontal and oral hygiene assessment
- Risk assessment

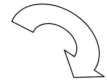

Evaluation

- Measure outcomes in terms of the client's goals and record an evaluative statement for each goal

- Modify plan and continue the dental hygiene process

Diagnosis
- Synthesizing, analyzing, and interpreting client data
- Identifying unmet human need related to dental hygiene
- Formulating and validating the dental hygiene diagnosis
- Prioritizing the dental hygiene diagnosis

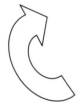

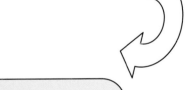

Implementation

- Educational interventions for personal dental biofilm control, diet, preventive agents, tobacco/alcohol and other risk factors related to both oral and systemic diseases and conditions
- Professional preventive and therapeutic services for management of periodontal diseases, caries, etc.

Planning
- Establish priorities for care
- Set goals and evaluation measures related to existing dental hygiene problems
- Identify interventions appropriate for client needs
- Develop a written care plan for use during dental hygiene therapy

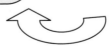

FIGURE 15-1 Dental hygiene process-of-care algorithm.

D. During baseline assessment, deficits in eight human needs are identified, and the dental hygiene diagnosis is made; planning, implementation, and evaluation of dental hygiene care are carried out to address the client's unmet needs

E. Human needs assessment form—an instrument to assist in the summarization and organization of gathered assessment data; used to provide a written record of unmet needs, dental hygiene diagnoses, client goals, care plans, and outcome evaluations of dental hygiene care (see Figure 15-3)

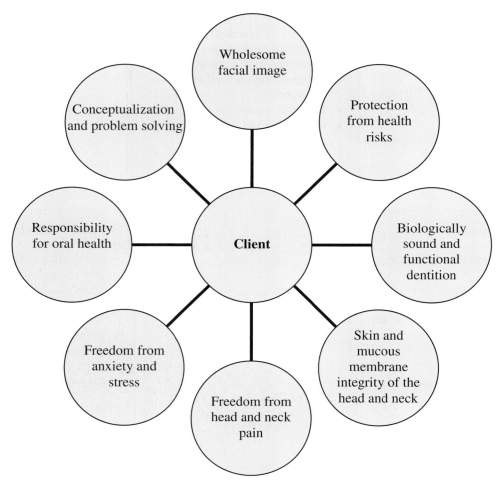

FIGURE 15-2 Eight human needs related to oral health and disease. *(Adapted from Walsh MM, Darby ML: Human needs theory and dental hygiene care. In Darby ML, Walsh MM, eds: Dental hygiene theory and practice, ed 3, St Louis, 2010, Saunders.)*

ASSESSMENT

Basic Concepts

A. Definition—comprehensive and systematic collection, analysis, and permanent documentation of data to identify the client's needs and oral health problems

B. Assessment—first phase of dental hygiene process of care

C. Data collection—continuous process of collection, documentation, and analysis of objective and subjective data needed to provide comprehensive care

D. Data are continuously updated and documented during the dental hygiene process of care

E. Data are collected by interview, questionnaire, observation, measurement, and examination

F. Data recordings are discussed with the client and other health care professionals responsible for client care

G. Data collection and documentation—includes comprehensive personal, health, and dental histories; pharmacologic history; identification of the client's chief concerns and human needs; clinical examination; periodontal examination; analysis of appropriately updated diagnostic radiographs; microbiologic or other tests for assessing the periodontal status of selected patients or sites also may be indicated[9]

HEALTH HISTORY EVALUATION

A. Health history—taken to identify and evaluate predisposing conditions and risk factors that may affect dental hygiene care, client management, potential for an emergency, and treatment outcomes[9]

1. Such conditions and factors include, but are not limited to, allergies, diabetes mellitus, hypertension, osteoporosis, cardiac and pulmonary diseases, pregnancy, tobacco use, substance abuse, medications

2. In the presence of a condition that, in the judgment of the dental hygienist, requires further

ASSESSMENT (circle signs and symptoms present)

1) WHOLESOME FACIAL IMAGE
   *expresses dissatisfaction with appearance
   –teeth –gingiva –facial profile –breath *other _____

2) FREEDOM FROM ANXIETY/STRESS
   *reports or displays:
   –anxiety about proximity of clinician, confidentiality, or
    previous dental experience
   –oral habits   –substance abuse

   *concern about:
   –infection control, fluoride therapy, fluoridation, mercury
    toxicity

3) SKIN & MUCOUS MEMBRANE INTEGRITY OF HEAD
   AND NECK
   –extra-/intra-oral lesion   –pockets ≥4 mm
   –swelling   –attachment loss ≥4 mm
   –gingival inflammation   –xerostomia
   –bleeding on probing   –other _____

4) PROTECTION FROM HEALTH RISKS
   *BP outside of normal limits   *need for prophylactic
   *potential for injury   antibiotics
                                  *risk factors
   *other _____

5) FREEDOM FROM HEAD AND NECK PAIN
   *extra-/intra-oral pain or sensitivity
   *other _____

6) BIOLOGICALLY SOUND & FUNCTIONAL DENTITION
   *reports difficulty in chewing
   *presents with:
   –defective restorations   –ill-fitting dentures, appliances
   –teeth with signs of disease –abrasion erosion
   –missing teeth   –rampant caries
   *other _____

7) RESPONSIBILITY FOR ORAL HEALTH
   *plaque & calculus present
   *inadequate parental supervision of oral health care
   *no dental exam within the last 2 years
   *other _____

8) CONCEPTUALIZATION & UNDERSTANDING
   *has questions about DH care and/or oral disease
   *other _____

DENTAL HYGIENE DIAGNOSIS (List the human need not met, then be specific about the etiology and signs & symptoms evidencing a deficit)

(Unmet Human Need)   (Etiology)   (Signs & Symptoms)
                       DUE TO   EVIDENCED BY

CLIENT GOALS	INTERVENTIONS (Target etiologies)	EVALUATION (goal met, partially met, or unmet)

Appointment Schedule: _____

Continued-care recommendations:

FIGURE 15-3 American Dental Association (ADA) health history form. *(Copyright 2011 American Dental Association. All rights reserved. Reprinted with permission.)*

evaluation, consultation with an appropriate health care provider should be obtained

B. Health history form—legal document that provides past and present information about the client's health to meet the client's human need for safety[10]

1. Provides baseline information about the client's health status and assists in medical and dental diagnoses

2. Information used to assess the overall physical and emotional health of the client

   a. Conditions that necessitate precautions to ensure the client's need for safety is met during health care procedures and that medical emergencies are prevented

   b. Conditions that require the client to be referred to a physician

   c. Diseases, conditions, or medications that contraindicate dental or dental hygiene care

   d. Previous history of reactions to medications or drugs

   e. Infectious diseases that could endanger other individuals

   f. Physiologic state of the client, including pregnancy, puberty, menopause, and use of hormones

3. Health history questionnaire should be completed in ink, and comprehensive information should be recorded on a questionnaire form or a summary sheet; this may also be a component of the electronic client record

4. The health history should be reviewed by the client and the dental hygienist and updated at each subsequent visit

5. The client should sign the written health history form at each appointment to confirm its accuracy; if the client is a minor, a parent or legal guardian should sign and date the health history form; electronic signatures are used in the electronic client record

6. The dental hygienist should sign the health history form at each appointment to indicate that medical and pharmacologic updates were obtained and verified; electronic signatures are used in the electronic client record

7. The health history form should be thorough but not contain redundant information and should use simple language to facilitate understanding

8. The health history form questions may include those shown in Figure 15-4.

   a. Personal, social, and cultural histories related to health and disease

   b. Dental history information should include:

      (1) Main concern—why the client is seeking dental or dental hygiene care

      (2) In the case of new clients, the date of the last dental or dental hygiene care received to determine responsibility for oral health

      (3) Areas of pain or discomfort identified during interviewing, but not associated with client's main concern

      (4) Nervousness or anxiety about treatment; history of an upsetting experience; the client's need for freedom from anxiety and stress should be addressed

      (5) Pain, swelling, or bleeding in gums

      (6) The client's satisfaction with his or her teeth and oral health

      (7) Past or current orthodontics, periodontal surgery, extractions, temporomandibular joint (TMJ) problems, occlusal equilibration, fixed and removable dentures

      (8) Oral habits such as clenching or grinding, biting lips or cheeks, mouthbreathing, and holding foreign objects between teeth

   e. Radiographic history information (see the section on "Ethical considerations regarding the use of ionizing radiation" in Chapter 6)

      (1) Purpose—the radiation exposure history of the client should be obtained to make safe decisions for radiographic prescriptions

      (2) Information should include:

         (a) Whether the client is regularly exposed to radiation in his or her work environment

         (b) The dates and total number of dental and medical films exposed during a 5-year period

   f. Health history information (see Chapters 7, 8 and 19 for more detailed discussions of conditions) should include:

      (1) Screening questions designed to assess risk factors or undiagnosed diseases and to enable the clinician to determine the need for a physician consultation or referral before dental hygiene care (Table 15-1)

      (2) Detailed questions designed to identify diseases or conditions that a client previously had or currently has and to determine the need for precautionary measures, physician consultation before dental hygiene care, or need for antibiotic prophylaxis (Table 15-2)

         (a) When practitioner questions the client regarding his or her disease status, specific information should include:

            [1] Type and onset of disease

            [2] Treatment received in the past

            [3] Severity of disease or extent of damage

            [4] Type of current medical care

REQUEST FOR MEDICAL CONSULTATION

Date: _____

TO: **CLIENT INFORMATION**

_____   RE: _____
Physician's Name   Client's name

_____   _____
Address   Address

_____   Gender:_____ Birthdate:_____
Address

Request: It is anticipated that dental hygiene treatment will extend for (# of appointments) over (time period) (weekly/monthly) for (appointment length) hour durations. Your Client reported (or we observed) the following:

_____Cardiac arrhythmia, diagnosed _____   _____Diabetes, Type 1, glucose level _____
_____High blood pressure (readings(s)/date) _____   _____Diabetes, Type 2, glucose level_____
_____Congential heart disease (CHD)_____   _____Total joint replacement (type & date replaced)
_____ Anticoagulant therapy, (medication dose/name)   _____Other:_____

The treatment planned for _____ includes:
_____Deep scaling and root planing/debridement (hemorrhage will occur)
_____Use of local anesthesic agent
_____Use of nitrous oxide-oxygen analgesia
_____Other:_____

Our concerns for _____ include the need for:
_____Antibiotic prophylactic according to the AHA guidelines (2007)
_____Evaluation of high blood pressure prior to dental hygiene care
_____Evaluation of prothrombin time prior to dental hygiene care; INR score___
_____ Evaluation of glucose level of control. Please provide most recent diabetes laboratory test results _____ H1A$_{1c}$
_____Other:_____._____

_____   _____
Dentist   Registered Dental Hygienist

RECOMMENDATIONS: Please indicate the definitive diagnosis and/or level of control. Also provide applicable laboratory test results in the space provided:

_____   _____
Physician Signature   Date

Adapted with permission from Idaho State University, Department of Dental Hygiene

FIGURE 15-4 Request for medical consultation.

TABLE 15-1 Health History Screening Questions

Risk Factor Category	Sample Questions	Significance of Finding
Overall health	How do you rate your general health? Has there been any change in your general health within the past year? Have you been under the care of a medical doctor during the past 2 years? What is the date of your last physical examination? Have you ever been hospitalized or had a serious illness?	Hospitalization history can provide a good record of past serious illnesses that may be significant to dental hygiene care Knowledge of why a client was hospitalized is used to evaluate the client's ability to tolerate stress involved during treatment Knowledge of any problems for which the client required medical intervention can increase the ability to evaluate the patient's condition before treatment
Weight fluctuation history	Have you unintentionally lost or gained more than 10 pounds in the past year? Are you on a medically recommended diet?	Unexpected weight changes may indicate heart failure, hypothyroidism, hyperthyroidism, or uncontrolled diabetes Information may identify an underlying systemic problem such as diabetes, hyperthyroidism, or cancer
Cardiovascular disease	When you walk up stairs or take a walk, do you ever have to stop because of pain in your chest or shortness of breath or because you are very tired? Do your ankles swell during the day? Do you require more than two pillows to sleep, or do you have an elevated bed?	Clients with cardiovascular disease are more susceptible to physical or emotional challenges during dental hygiene care These signs may indicate possible valvular disease, arrhythmia, or congestive heart failure
Diabetes	Are you on a medically recommended diet? Do you have to urinate more than six times a day? Are you frequently thirsty? Does your mouth frequently become dry? If yes, what is the probable cause?	Determine family history or potential for diabetes; consultation with a physician may be indicated Complications of diabetes include blindness, hypertension, kidney failure, and delayed healing
Tuberculosis or other respiratory diseases	Do you have a nonproductive persistent cough? Do you have a productive persistent cough? Do you have night sweats? Do you have difficulty breathing?	May indicate current or past history of tuberculosis History of the disease must be defined, and medical consultation may be indicated
Hematologic disorder	Do you bruise easily? Do you have a tendency to bleed longer than normal? Have you ever had a blood transfusion?	Need to determine whether a blood disorder is present; medical consultation may be indicated; Concerns about delayed healing, prolonged bleeding, and infection
Latex allergy	Have you experienced a skin reaction (redness, rash, hives, or itching) to adhesive tape, adhesive strips, kitchen gloves, or rubber or latex products? Have you experienced swelling of the lips, tongue, or skin after dental treatment, after blowing up a balloon, or after contact with rubber or latex products? Have you experienced a runny nose, itchy eyes, scratchy throat, or difficulty breathing after contact with rubber or latex products? Do you have an allergy to bananas, kiwis, potatoes, tomatoes, avocados, chestnuts, or other foods?	Need to assess risk for reaction May need medical consultation to determine risk of anaphylaxis Provide a latex-reduced environment

TABLE 15-2 American Heart Association (AHA) and American Association of Orthopedic Surgeons (AAOS) Antibiotic Premedication Guidelines for Professional Oral Health Care

Dental Procedures That Require Premedication in Highest Risk Clients*	2007 AHA Recommendations for Cardiac Conditions	2009 AAOS Recommendations for Orthopedic Conditions	Other Conditions That May Necessitate Antibiotic Premedication Based on Physician Consultation
All dental procedures that involve manipulation of gingival tissues or the periapical region of teeth, or perforation of the oral mucosa †NOTE: Clients can receive antibiotic coverage within a 2-hour period if unexpected bleeding occurs, if during treatment the client discloses additional health history information that would indicate need for premedication, or both	Highest Risk Category: Only people at the greatest risk of bad outcomes from infective endocarditis (IE) should receive short-term preventive antibiotics before identified dental (and medical) procedures. Patients at the greatest danger of adverse outcomes from IE and for whom preventive antibiotics are worth the risks include those with: —artificial heart valves —a history of having had IE —certain specific, serious congenital heart conditions, including: —unrepaired or incompletely repaired cyanotic congenital heart disease, including those with palliative shunts and conduits —a completely repaired congenital heart defect with prosthetic material or device, whether placed by surgery or by catheter interventions, during the first 6 months after the procedure —any repaired congenital heart defect with residual defect at the site or adjacent to the site of a prosthetic patch or prosthetic device —a cardiac transplant that develops a problem in a heart valve	Antibiotic premedication recommended for all persons who have undergone total joint replacement All patients with prosthetic joint replacement Immunocompromised or immunosuppressed patients Inflammatory arthropathies (e.g., rheumatoid arthritis, systemic lupus erythematosus) Drug-induced immunosuppression Radiation-induced immunosuppression Patients with comorbidities (e.g., diabetes, obesity, human immunodeficiency virus [HIV], smoking) Previous prosthetic joint infections Malnourishment Hemophilia HIV infection Insulin-dependent (type 1) diabetes Malignancy Megaprostheses	Prophylaxis consultation recommended Renal transplants or dialysis Immunosuppressive therapy (e.g., cyclosporine) Uncontrolled diabetes Sickle cell anemia Spina bifida (ventriculoatrial shunt)

*Every attempt should be made to complete procedures and services in as few appointments as possible; follow-up appointments should be scheduled at least 9 days apart if client is premedicated.
†Clinical judgment may indicate antibiotic use in selected circumstances that may cause significant bleeding.
Adapted from Committee on Rheumatic Fever, Endocarditis, and Kawasaki Disease: Prevention of infective endocarditis: Guidelines from the American Heart Association, by the, Circulation, e-published April 19, 2007: Available at www.americanheart.org/presenter.jhtml?identifier=3004539: Accessed March 15, 2011; and from American Academy of Orthopedic Surgeons American Association of Orthopedic Surgeons: Antibiotic prophylaxis for bacteremia in patients with joint replacements, Available at http://www.aaos.org/about/papers/advistmt/1033.asp: Accessed March 15, 2011.

[5] Results of follow-up testing
[6] Classification of the client's risk for a medical emergency using the American Society of Anesthesiologists (ASA) Physical Status Classification System (Table 15-3)

(b) Questions regarding cardiovascular disease (CVD) are significant because clients with various forms of CVD are especially vulnerable to physical or emotional challenges that may be encountered during dental hygiene care; for most CVDs, the

TABLE 15-3 American Society of Anesthesiologists (ASA) Physical Status Classification System and Stress-Reduction Protocols

ASA Classification	Client Risk Description	Examples of Medical Conditions	Precautionary Measures for Stress Reduction
Physical status 1	Normal healthy client without systemic disease Little or no anxiety Elective dental hygiene care can be implemented	Physiologically and psychologically sound	Determine client's level of anxiety Schedule morning appointment Minimize waiting time Consider shorter appointments for anxious clients Optimize adequate pain control during therapy
Physical status 2	Client with mild systemic disease Healthy client with extreme anxiety Elective dental hygiene care can be implemented with minimal risk, but measures for stress reduction should be taken	Well-controlled disease of one body system: asthma, diabetes, epilepsy, cigarette smoking without chronic obstructive pulmonary disease (COPD), thyroid disease, hypertension (blood pressure between 140–159 systolic and 90–94 diastolic mm Hg)	Identify the client's medical risk potential Complete a physician consultation before starting dental hygiene care, as indicated Schedule a morning appointment time Take and record vital signs at each appointment
Physical status 3	Client with severe systemic disease that limits activity but is not incapacitating Elective dental hygiene care is not contraindicated, but risk is increased and precautionary measures for stress reduction should be taken	Stable angina pectoris, myocardial infarction or cerebrovascular accident (CVA) more than 6 months earlier, well-controlled diabetes, congestive heart failure (CHF), COPD, exercise-induced asthma, epilepsy not well controlled, symptomatic thyroid disorders, blood pressure between 160 and 199 mm Hg systolic or 95 and 114 mm Hg diastolic	Optimize adequate pain control during therapy Shorter appointments, not to exceed 90 minutes Arrange appointments during the beginning of the week (Monday through Wednesday)
Physical status 4	Client with incapacitating systemic disease that is a constant threat to life Elective dental hygiene care is contraindicated until the medical condition has improved to at least ASA class III status	Unstable angina pectoris, myocardial infarction and CVA within past 6 months, severe CHF or COPD; uncontrolled epilepsy, diabetes, thyroid disease; blood pressure of 200 mm Hg or higher systolic or 115 mm Hg or higher diastolic	Immediate medical consultation

Adapted from American Society of Anesthesiologists: ASA physical status classification system: Available at www.asahq.org/clinical/physicalstatus.htm:. Accessed May 30, 2011; Malamed SF: Knowing your patients, J Am Dent Assoc 141:3S–7S, 2010. Note: Physical statuses 5 and 6 are used primarily in medical practice.

stress-reduction protocol, based on the ASA system, is necessary (see the sections on "Vasoconstrictors" in Chapter 18; "Congenital heart disease," "Cardiac arrhythmias/dysrhythmias," "Hypertensive disease," "Ischemic heart disease," "Cerebrovascular disease," and "Congestive heart failure" in Chapter 19; and "Vital signs," in Chapter 21)

[1] Hypertension can result in myocardial infarction (MI) and stroke and contribute to arteriosclerosis, impaired kidney function, and cardiac enlargement; hypertension guidelines must be followed during professional care to reduce the risk of a medical emergency (Table 15-4)

[2] When CVD is identified, it is important for the clinician to conduct a thorough interview to assess the severity and level of control of disease and to determine alterations in care (e.g.,

TABLE 15-4 Classification of Adult Blood Pressure and Precautionary Measures

Category	Systolic (mm Hg)		Diastolic (mm Hg)	Dental Management Considerations
Normal	<120	and	<80	Routine dental management Recheck at continued-care (recare) visit
Prehypertension	120–139	or	80–89	Routine dental management Advise client of status; and recommend lifestyle management Recheck at recare visit
Stage I Hypertension	140–159	or	90–99	Monitor blood pressure at consecutive appointments If all exceed these guidelines, seek medical consultation Stress-reduction protocol Recheck at recare visit
Stage II Hypertension	≥160–170	or	≥100–110	Recheck blood pressure in 5 minutes If still elevated within this range, seek and receive medical consultation before dental hygiene therapy Noninvasive care only Definitive emergency care only if blood pressure is <180/110 Stress-reduction protocol Continue to monitor blood pressure at consecutive appointments Recheck at each visit
Hypertensive Crisis	>180	or	>110	Recheck blood pressure in 5 minutes If still elevated, immediate medical consultation is indicated No dental or dental hygiene care, elective or emergent, until blood pressure is decreased Noninvasive emergency care with drugs: analgesics or antibiotics are indicated Refer to hospital for immediate invasive dental care

From Chobanian AV, Bakris GL, Black HR, Cushman WC, Green LA, Izzo JL, Jr., et al: Seventh Report of the Joint National Commission on Prevention, Detection, Evaluation, and Treatment of High Blood Pressure, Hypertension, 42:1206–1252, 2003; Little JW, Miller C, Rhodus NL, Falace D: Dental management of the medically compromised patient, St Louis, 2008, Mosby; Adapted from U.S. Department of Health and Human Services; National Institutes of Health; National Heart, Lung, and Blood Institute; National High Blood Pressure Education Program: JNC 7 Express. The seventh report of the Joint National Committee on Prevention, Detection, Evaluation, and Treatment of High Blood Pressure. National Institutes of Health/National Heart, Lung, and Blood Institute, Bethesda, MD, NIH publication 03-5233, 2004: Available at http://www.nhlbi.nih.gov/guidelines/hypertension/jnc7full.htm; Accessed March 15, 2011; and Malamed SF: Handbook of local anesthesia, ed 5, St Louis, 2004, Mosby.

physician consultation, antibiotic prophylaxis, stress reduction protocol)

[a] Clients undergoing corrective surgery for congenital heart disease and have prosthetic material or device are susceptible to transient bacteremias for up to 6 months and must receive antibiotic prophylaxis; at 6 months after surgery, antibiotic prophylaxis is not usually recommended (see Table 15-2)

[b] When antibiotic prophylaxis is necessary, 9 to 10 days should be scheduled between appointments to allow oral bacteria to return to the original state; clients currently on an antibiotic regimen must use an alternative regimen of antibiotic therapy; if antibiotic medication is inadvertently missed, administer within 2 hours after the procedure

(c) Questions regarding diseases of the immune system and blood disorders assess the client's potential risk for infection in dental hygiene care and his or her ability to handle stress through the appointment; primary concerns include prolonged bleeding, delayed healing, and secondary infections; physician consultation may be required for more chronic or involved conditions

[1] In the case of clients with diabetes, concerns about a hypoglycemic incident, susceptibility to oral infections (abscesses and periodontal diseases), impaired wound healing, and impaired glycemic control because of the presence of periodontal disease exist; consultation with a physician is indicated in most cases and referral is based on health history, dialogue, and oral conditions

[2] Oral assessment should be initiated to determine the presence of infections and the extent of periodontal disease before consultation with the appropriate physician; glycated hemoglobin values (A_{1c}) and blood glucose levels are requested from physician; the client should be asked to bring his or her glucometer, or a glucometer should be available in the oral care facility (Box 15-1)

[3] In clients with well-controlled diabetes, no alteration of the care plan is indicated unless complications of diabetes such as hypertension, congestive heart failure (CHF), MI, angina, or renal failure are present

[4] Clients with controlled diabetes should eat before appointments; appointments should be scheduled no later than midmorning, and a sugar source must be available in the oral care facility in case of any incidence of hypoglycemia or hyperinsulinism

(d) Metabolic syndrome (MetS) is closely associated with insulin resistance, in which the body cannot use insulin efficiently; patients with MetS are at increased risk of coronary heart disease, stroke, peripheral vascular disease, and type 2 diabetes

---

BOX 15-1 Glycemic Management for Adults (without pregnancy) with Diabetes

Blood Glucose Level (mg/dL)

<70	Tendency toward hypoglycemia. Give 15 g*of carbohydrate, and wait 15 minutes; monitor again to assess whether the treatment should continue; notify client's physician
70–130 (Preprandial)	Acceptable
<180 (Peak postprandial)†	
180–239	Risk for infection
>240	Unacceptable for treatment. Refer to a physician, and reschedule or postpone treatment until the client reports control and acceptability of treatment
Glycosylated hemoglobin	Level periodically determined to assess plasma glucose control during the preceding 1 to 3 months
Hemoglobin A_{1c} (HbA$_{1c}$)	Normal range <6.5%

*15 g = 3 glucose tablets, a tube of glucose gel, or 4 ounces of fruit juice.
†Postprandial glucose measurements should be made 1 to 2 hours after the beginning of the meal.
Adapted from: American Diabetes Association: Standards of medical care in diabetes, Diabetes Care 33(Suppl 1):S11S61.

---

[1] MetS is identified by the presence of three or more components: obesity measured by waist circumference (men >40 inches and women >35 inches), fasting blood triglycerides (>150 mg/dL), blood high-density lipoprotein (HDL) cholesterol (men <40 mg/dL and women <50 mg/dL), blood pressure (>130/85 mm Hg), and fasting glucose (>100 mg/dL)

[2] Physician referral, medical consultation, or both may be required for clients who do not have regular medical care to determine the presence of associated conditions or the level of control of existing conditions

(e) Questions regarding respiratory disease or chronic obstructive pulmonary disease (COPD) assess the level of compromised respiratory function; clinicians should use precautionary measures to avoid further depression of respiration (see the section on "Chronic obstructive pulmonary disease" in Chapter 19)

(f) Musculoskeletal system disorders may be associated with chronic use of salicylates or nonsteroidal anti-inflammatory drugs (NSAIDs), which can alter blood clotting and corticosteroid therapy and increase the risk of acute adrenal insufficiency

(g) Neurologic and psychological disorders must to be identified and the degree of control determined; medications used to control seizures can cause drug-influenced gingival enlargement, and psychiatric drugs have the potential to interact adversely with the vasoconstrictors in local anesthetic agents

(h) Other disorders such as glaucoma, sexually transmitted infections (STIs), herpes, chemical dependency, and tobacco use have significant implications for treatment: in glaucoma, anticholinergics are contraindicated because they increase intraocular pressure; chemical dependency and tobacco use are risk factors for infectious diseases, malignancies, CVD, pulmonary diseases, and periodontal diseases; dental hygiene care for clients with active herpes or STIs should be postponed until the disease is no longer active

(i) The physiologic state of women identifies their status related to pregnancy and endocrine changes

(j) The identification of the risk of latex allergy is essential to reduce the chances of an allergic reaction; types of reactions include irritant contact dermatitis, allergic contact dermatitis (delayed hypersensitivity), and latex allergy

[1] Irritant contact dermatitis,—the most common reaction; causes dry, itchy areas of irritation on the skin

[2] Allergic contact dermatitis (type IV hypersensitivity reaction) —results from exposure to chemicals added to latex during harvesting of rubber, processing, or manufacturing

[3] Latex allergy, or immediate allergic urticaria (type I hypersensitivity reaction)—results from certain proteins in latex rubber; symptoms range from skin redness, rash, hives, or itching to runny nose, itchy eyes, asthma, and anaphylaxis

[4] Clients at risk for latex reaction should be treated in a latex-reduced environment; physician consultation is indicated for clients with risk of an anaphylactic reaction

(k) Listing of current medications—used to determine medications taken by the client and possible interactions with other medications; these medications may be the only clue to the client's existing condition (*Physicians' Desk Reference* or *Mosby's Dental Drug Reference* can help with the identification of adverse reactions, precautions, contraindications, and dental considerations)

(l) Identification of medication allergies informs health care professionals of the client's previous adverse reactions to medications

(m) Vital signs (see the section on "Vital signs" in Chapter 21)

[1] Vital signs are values given to measurements of blood pressure, respiration, pulse, and temperature; are important as they serve as a baseline in a medical emergency

[2] Abnormal or elevated blood pressure values should be brought to the client's immediate attention; on the basis of the blood pressure values, monitoring of pressure at every appointment or a physician consultation may be required before initiation of dental hygiene care (see Table 15-4)

[3] Blood pressure, respirations, and pulse are measured and recorded before the administration of local anesthetic agents or nitrous oxide–oxygen analgesia

(3) Conditions being treated with medications—may influence or contraindicate certain procedures; for example, anticoagulant therapy may require a lower dose; antihypertensive drugs may alter the choice of local anesthetic; antipsychotic medications may alter the choice of nitrous oxide–oxygen analgesia (see the sections on "Anticoagulants" in Chapter 11; "Toxicity," "Vasoconstrictors," and "Nitrous oxide–oxygen conscious sedation" in Chapter 18; and Chapter 21)

(4) Physician consultations—may be necessary, depending on the information obtained from health history or physical examination; written documentation from the physician is necessary (Figure 15-1)

   (a) Written informed consent is obtained from the client before submitting the request for physician consultation

   (b) Medical consultation can be faxed or mailed to the concerned physician's office

9. Health history information is gathered through interviews, written questionnaires, or a combination of both

  a. The interview method allows the dental hygienist to develop client rapport and ensures that the client understands the questions

  b. The self-administered written questionnaire is the most common format used to gather information pertaining to the client's health status

  c. Use of both the interview and the written questionnaire is the best approach to collect accurate and comprehensive health information

EXTRAORAL AND INTRAORAL ASSESSMENT

A. Purpose—to assess and recognize deviations from normal conditions significant to the client's health

B. Establishment of an assessment sequence that is followed systematically

  1. Skills used in performing extraoral and intraoral examination include direct observation, palpation, auscultation, and olfaction

    a. Direct observation—visual inspection techniques used to examine the client's movement, body symmetry, color, texture, contour, consistency, and form of skin and mucous membrane

    b. Palpation—sense of touch used to examine for tenderness, texture, masses, and variations in structure and temperature within the head and neck region. Forms of palpation include:

     (1) Digital palpation—use of single (index) finger to move or press against the tissue of the floor of the mouth or hard palate

     (2) Bi-digital palpation—use of one or more fingers and thumb to move or compress the tissue of lips, tongue, cheeks, and vestibule

     (3) Bimanual palpation—simultaneous use of the index finger of one hand and the fingers and thumb of the other hand to move or compress the tissue of the floor of the mouth

     (4) Manual palpation—use of all the fingers of one hand to move and compress tissue to assess cervical lymph nodes

     (5) Bilateral palpation—use of both hands simultaneously to move or press the tissue on the contralateral sides of the head to assess the submandibular nodes, TMJ, inferior border of mandible, and temporalis and masseter muscles

     (6) Circular compression—use of fingers that move in a rotating, circular motion while slight pressure is applied

    c. Auscultation—listening to and detecting sounds made by the body, for example, clicking (crepitation) of the TMJ; speech disorders; and vocal hoarseness

    d. Olfaction—use of the olfactory sense to detect variations in breath odors such as alcohol breath, fruity ketosis (diabetic acidosis), and halitosis associated with dental caries, periodontitis, and necrotizing ulcerative gingivitis

  2. Extraoral examination procedure (see Chapter 4)

    a. Head, neck, and face

     (1) The overall appearance of client should be assessed via visual inspection

     (2) The symmetry of skin, eyes, nose, and ears should be observed; areas of unusual discoloration should be inspected

      (a) Skin (see the section on "Skin diseases" in Chapter 8)

       [1] Normal texture is continuous, firm, and pigmented in relation to normal variations associated with race and ethnicity

       [2] Abnormal textures or pigmentations should be recorded (e.g., scarring, swelling, moles, freckles, pallor, redness, severe acne, tumors, jaundice)

[3] Abnormal lesions should be measured and documented in writing, with details about color, size, shape, and surface texture

(b) Face

[1] Face and head should be symmetrical and have normal function

[2] Asymmetry or lack of function may be associated with injury, Bell's palsy, tumor, abnormal growth and development, difficulty swallowing, Parkinson's disease, Tourette's syndrome, and abuse

[3] Facial expression can indicate the client's general frame of mind (e.g., anxious, happy, sad, angry)

(c) Eyes (see the section on "Visual impairment" in Chapter 19)

(d) Nose

[1] Breathing should be assessed; flared nostrils or ragged breath could indicate difficulty breathing

[2] An enlarged, bulbous, and red nose may be associated with an overgrowth of sebaceous and sweat glands from alcohol abuse (rhinophyma)

(e) Ears (see the section on "Hearing impairment" in Chapter 19)

(3) The symmetry of bones, muscles, lymph nodes, and salivary glands should be observed

(a) The inferior border of the mandible should be assessed for asymmetry by using bimanual palpation from the midline to the posterior angle

(b) The TMJ and the muscles of mastication should be inspected

[1] The TMJ should be assessed for deviation, pain, crepitus, grinding, and reduced range in opening or closing; evaluated via client interview and bilateral palpation with index fingers anterior to outer meatus; client is asked to open and close the mouth slowly several times; any deviation or symptomatology is recorded

[2] Masseter and temporalis muscles are assessed for overdevelopment, pain, swelling, and unusual hardness by using bilateral circular compression; the client is asked to clench the teeth together while the muscles are palpated

(c) The mentalis muscle is assessed for overdevelopment and smoothness of contraction during the swallowing movement; evaluated by digital palpation; tissue is moved over the mandible and he client is asked to swallow

(d) The larynx is assessed for unrestricted movement by bimanual palpation; the larynx is gently moved from side to side to check movement

(e) Lymph node chains are assessed (Figure 4-7, Chapter 4)

[1] Occipital lymph nodes are assessed for pain, swelling, enlargement, unusual hardness, or fixed position by using bilateral palpation

[2] Auricular and parotid lymph nodes are examined for pain, swelling, enlargement, unusual hardness, or fixed position by using bilateral palpation

[3] Superficial cervical lymph nodes are assessed for pain, enlargement, unusual hardness, and fixed position by placing the client's head to one side with the chin slightly lowered and by palpating with fingers along the sternocleidomastoid muscle

[4] Deep cervical lymph nodes are examined for pain, enlargement, unusual hardness, and fixed position by placing the client's head upright and by palpating the deep tissues along the sternocleidomastoid muscles with the thumb and fingers

[5] Submental and submandibular glands are examined for asymmetry, noncontinuous borders, pain, tenderness, swelling, enlargement, unusual hardness, or difficulty in swallowing by bilateral digital palpation

(f) The thyroid gland is assessed for asymmetry and enlargement by a combination of bi-digital palpation and circular compression; the client is asked to sit upright and to swallow (see Figure 4-8, Chapter 4)

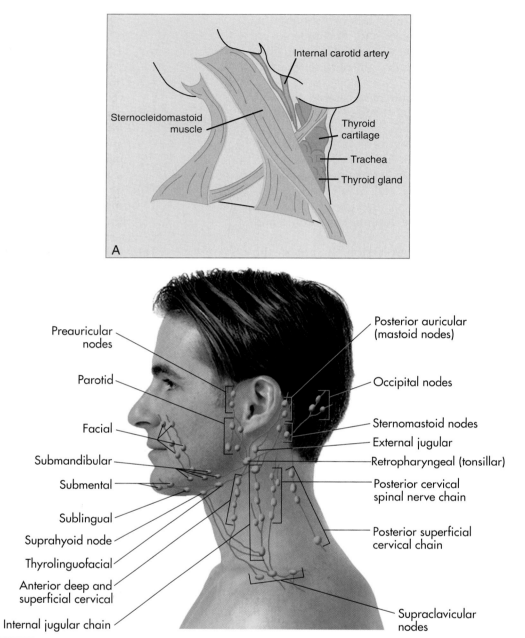

FIGURE 15-5 A, Location of the thyroid gland and major muscle groups. **B,** Lymph nodes of the head and neck region. *(Adapted from Seidel HM, Ball JW, Flynn,JA, et al: Mosby's guide to physical examination, ed 7, St Louis, 2011, Mosby.)*

(g) Parotid glands are examined for pain, swelling, enlargement, and hardness by using bilateral circular compression; salivary flow can be observed at the opening of Stensen's duct when the gland is compressed

3. Intraoral examination procedure

   a. Screen the client to detect lesions that may be pathologic, particularly lesions that may be cancerous

   b. Prevent the development of advanced, irreversible, or untreatable oral disease through early recognition of initial lesions

   c. Oral piercing is a popular form of body art

     (1) Inspect the tongue, lips, cheeks, frenum, and uvula for piercings

     (2) Barbells and rings are the most common types of jewelry

     (3) Complications from piercing include excessive hemorrhage; transmission of

communicable diseases; nerve damage; infection; bacteremia; Ludwig's angina; cracked, fractured, or abraded teeth; recession; dehiscence; aspiration or ingestion of jewelry[11]

(4) Jewelry should be removed during the radiography procedure

d. The oral mucosa, lips, floor of the mouth, tongue, salivary ducts, hard and soft palates, and oropharynx should be examined and evaluated (see Table 5-1 and Figures 5-1 to 5-8 in Chapter 5)

(1) The lips are examined by visual inspection and palpation for:

   (a) Changes in size—may be caused by swelling or allergic reaction

   (b) Chapping—may be caused by mouth breathing or nutritional deficiency

   (c) Blistering—may be associated with herpetic lesions

   (d) Cracking—may be associated with angular cheilosis, candidiasis, or vitamin B deficiency (see the section on "Vitamins" and Table 12-4 in Chapter 12)

   (e) Scar tissue or irritations—may be associated with habitual lip biting or trauma; bruising at commissures may indicate binding or gagging associated with physical abuse

   (f) Abnormal texture, lack of moistness or firmness—may be associated with dehydration and excessive sun exposure

   (g) Limitations of opening; muscle elasticity, and muscle tone—may be associated with stroke or TMJ dysfunction

(2) Labial and alveolar mucosa and the gingiva are examined by using bilateral and bi-digital palpation

   (a) Signs of tissue trauma from biting, toothbrush abrasion, burns, or physical abuse; lacerated or torn frenum (tissue tags) may indicate binding, gagging, or forced feeding

   (b) Ulcerated lesions such as herpetic lesions or aphthous ulcers

   (c) Tight or low frenum attachments, which can cause gingival defects such as recession and loss of attached gingiva

   (d) Spit tobacco lesion (leukoplakia), hyperkeratinized tissue; white, sometimes corrugated, in appearance;

the client should be taught self-assessment techniques

   (e) Amalgam tattoo, blue-and-black coloration, size variations—can be found on any area of soft tissue (see section on "Abnormalities of oral soft tissues" in Chapter 8)

   (f) Fordyce granules—ectopic sebaceous glands

(3) The buccal mucosa is assessed by using bi-digital palpation; the mouth mirror is used to reflect light and to inspect the buccal mucosa

   (a) The buccal mucosa is examined for color and texture

   (b) The parotid papilla and duct (Stensen's duct) are evaluated; the duct is palpated to assess salivary function

   (c) Atypical findings include traumatic lesions related to cheek biting, linea alba adjacent to occlusal plane, ectopic sebaceous glands (Fordyce granules)

(4) Hard and soft palates and alveolar ridges are examined by visual inspection; the mouth mirror is used to reflect light; digital palpation is used on the hard palate and alveolar ridges; palpation is not recommended for soft palate to avoid triggering the gag reflex

   (a) The hard palate, including the incisive papilla, rugae, and palatine fovea, is examined and assessed for:

      [1] Shape of the palate—low, high, narrow vault; alterations in shape may require alteration in oral radiographic techniques

      [2] Petechiae, torus palatinus, trauma (food burns, denture irritation), stomatitis (nicotine, ulcerative, necrotizing, and denture), fistulas from draining abscesses, denture-related candidiasis (see Chapter 8)

   (b) The soft palate is assessed for inflammation, petechiae, trauma, stomatitis, and bifid uvula

   (c) Alveolar ridges are assessed for impacted third molars, scarring from third molar extractions, opercula, and exostosis

(5) The oropharynx is assessed by visual inspection with a mouth mirror

   (a) The client is asked to say "Ah" to relax and lower the posterior portion of the tongue

(b) The anterior and posterior pillars are assessed for inflammation, petechiae, trauma, stomatitis, and enlarged tonsillar tissues

(6) The floor of the mouth is examined by visual inspection and bimanual palpation

(a) The function of the submandibular gland is tested by wiping each Wharton's duct with gauze and compressing it with a gloved finger to observe salivary flow

(b) The entire floor of the mouth is palpated; the finger of one hand and the finger and thumb of the other hand are placed under the client's chin to palpate

(c) Enlargement or masses, Wharton's duct, sublingual caruncle, and lingual frenum are assessed

(d) Varicosities, tight frenum attachment (ankyloglossia), and blocked salivary duct are inspected

(e) Exostosis along lingual surface of mandible and mandibular tori—significant if interfering with prosthetic appliances

(7) The tongue is examined by visual inspection and digital palpation

(a) The dorsal surface is inspected; the entire tongue is palpated and the lateral borders of the tongue are examined by using gauze to gently hold the tongue

(b) The ventral surface is examined by having the client touch the palate with the tongue

(c) The tongue is assessed for:

[1] Coating on the dorsal surface and the condition of papillae; the extent is assessed

[2] Size; macroglossia associated with Down syndrome or cretinism (see the section on "Down syndrome" in Chapter 19)

[3] Lingual frenum; tight frenum restricting movement (ankyloglossia)

[4] Fissured tongue; deep grooves and crevices along the lateral borders and the dorsal surface; the lateral borders are common sites of oral cancer

[5] Geographic tongue—benign condition in which a sporadic migration of dorsal papilla occurs; tenderness is assessed

[6] Nutritional deficiencies; burning or glossy tongue (see the section on "Abnormalities affecting the tongue" in Chapter 8)

[7] Black hairy tongue related to proliferation of filiform papillae; caused by irritants such as smoking and alcohol (see the section on "Abnormalities affecting the tongue" in Chapter 8)

[8] Hairy leukoplakia caused by extensions of keratin on the lateral borders of the tongue; associated with human immunodeficiency virus (HIV) infection

[9] Atypical lesions, including aphthous ulcerations, trauma-associated fibroma, hemangiomas, and white plaque

ASSESSMENT OF DENTITION

A. Purpose—to assess and document the exact location and condition of teeth, restorations, and dental caries, noting normal and abnormal findings on detailed dentition chart; used for care planning, communication with the client, legal documentation, forensic use, and financial audits; composed of study models, occlusion assessment, dentition charting, pulpal vitality testing, and stain determination, (see Chapter 5)

B. Components of dentition assessment include:

1. Study models—impressions for study models taken to obtain visual reproduction of teeth, gingiva, and adjacent intraoral structures and to assist with dentition and periodontal charting

2. Occlusion assessment—presence of malocclusion or tooth position determined; signs of parafunctional habits resulting in occlusal traumatism noted (see the sections on "Intra-arch and interarch relationships" in Chapter 5 and "Clinical assessment of the periodontium" in Chapter 14)

3. Dentition charting—graphic representation of the client's teeth at assessment; includes developmental anomalies and defects, condition of teeth, dental caries activity, restorative history, and other problems; a combination of radiographs and direct visual inspection is used to assist with accurate recording of tooth assessment (Box 15-2); office guides and professional organizations' dentition charting symbols may be adopted for use; the ADA's National Board Dental Examination (NBDE) provides a dental charting symbol key in each client case used.

BOX 15-2 Systematic Approach for Dentition Charting

Sequence

Complete a general appraisal of teeth, and note developmental anomalies and defects affecting tooth shape, number of teeth, tooth size, and presence of partial or complete dentures (e.g., generalized moderate fluorosis, amelogenesis imperfecta, peg laterals, number of teeth present, mandibular partial denture)

Chart all missing or erupted supernumerary teeth before recording specific tooth-by-tooth information

Using radiographs, chart all unerupted or impacted teeth

Chart teeth indicated for extraction

Chart existing restorations (amalgam, tooth-colored, and temporary restorations; inlays, onlays, and gold foils; crowns, veneers, and bridges)

Chart signs of tooth damage (dental caries, risk areas, attrition)

Chart areas of plaque-retentive factors and defective restorations needing replacement (overhangs, deficient margins, unpolished amalgam restorations, fractured restorations, improper anatomic contour, occlusal surfaces indicated for pit-and-fissure sealants)

When treatment has been completed on teeth indicated for restorative or supportive care, update the chart using a different color to quickly identify teeth that were restored after original baseline charting

Update the dentition charting at each recare visit, and record any areas of change

---

a. Universal Numbering System—most widely used notation system; permanent teeth numbered from 1 to 32 and primary teeth lettered from A to T; 1 to 16 or A to J are located on the maxillary arch, moving right to left; 17 to 32 or K to T are located on the mandibular arch, moving left to right (from the client's perspective)

b. Developmental anomalies that affect enamel and dentin, developmental defects that affect tooth shape, number of teeth, and tooth size are noted (see the section on "Abnormalities of teeth" in Chapter 8)

c. Tooth positions, eruption patterns, and missing teeth are recorded (see the sections on "Eruption" and "Intra-arch and interarch relationships" in Chapter 5)

d. Tooth damage that results in loss of integrity of tooth surface is recorded; common forms of damage include attrition, abrasion, erosion, fracture, and dental caries (see the section on "Abnormalities of teeth" in Chapter 8)

e. Dental caries is an infectious, transmittable, and mulifactorial disease of bacterial origin; carious lesions are classified by the type and location of the lesion by using visual inspection with magnification, laser fluorescence, light fluorescence, digital imaging, fiberoptic transillumination, gentle probing, and radiographic examination with standard bitewing or digitized view[12]

(1) Classification for carious lesions includes rate, direction, and type of disease progression; used to determine level of priority for restorative therapy

(a) Rampant caries—a rapidly progressive decay process that affects the smooth surfaces of numerous teeth and requires urgent intervention; commonly found with early childhood caries (formerly called *nursing bottle syndrome*)

(b) Chronic caries—slowly progressive decay process

(c) Arrested caries—carious lesion that has been reversed because of the remineralization process

(d) Backward caries—lateral spread of decay at the dentino-enamel junction through an undermining process; the surface lesion appears small, but destruction is extensive underneath[13]

(e) Recurrent or secondary caries—new decay located around existing restorations

(2) Carious lesions described by specific location on tooth surface (see the section on "Dental caries" in Chapter 9)

(a) Pit-and-fissure caries—develop in the pits and grooves of the occlusal surfaces of premolars and molars, lingual pits of maxillary incisors, buccal grooves of mandibular molars, and lingual grooves of maxillary molars; pit-and-fissure sealants are an effective preventive strategy to protect tooth surfaces (see the sections on "Pit-and-fissure sealants" in Chapter 13 and "Dental sealants" in Chapter 16)

(b) Smooth surface caries—found on the facial, lingual, mesial, and distal surfaces of teeth

(c) Root caries—found on exposed root surfaces

(3) G.V. Black's classification of dental caries and restorations provides a precise description of the types and location of caries and restorations

(a) Class I—pits and fissures on the occlusal, buccal, and lingual surfaces of posterior teeth and the lingual surfaces of anterior teeth

(b) Class II—proximal surface of posterior teeth, usually involving the occlusal surfaces

(c) Class III—proximal surfaces of incisors and canines, not including the incisal edge

(d) Class IV—proximal surfaces of incisors and canines, including the incisal edge

(e) Class V—gingival third of facial or lingual surfaces of any tooth

(f) Class VI—cusp tips of posterior teeth and the incisal edge of anterior teeth

f. Charting of existing restorations, treatment procedures (endodontics, apicoectomy), and tooth-replacement methods (implants, crown, bridge) completed by using commonly accepted dental symbols

(1) Restorations should be charted with G.V. Black's classification system and should reflect the actual restoration

(2) The restoration morphology, margin quality and location, and biocompatibility of restorative material with soft tissue are evaluated[14]

(a) The restoration and the surrounding tooth structure are assessed for new or recurrent dental caries

(b) The marginal and structural integrity assessed for open margins or signs of restorative material fatigue or fractures; the appropriate margin is smooth to tactile evaluation and does not show any overhang

(c) The interproximal and occlusal contours and the proximal contact are assessed; the appropriateness of faciolingual and occlusocervical dimensions are determined; indication for amalgam polishing or recontouring to improve restoration is assessed

(d) Surface finish is assessed to determine whether it meets the functional and aesthetic requirements of the client; indication for amalgam polishing or finishing is assessed

(3) Faulty restorations are usually in need of replacement because of the presence of recurrent dental caries, fractures, or factors that encourage microbial plaque biofilm retention and may contribute to the development of secondary caries, periodontal disease, and dentinal hypersensitivity

(4) Overhangs on class II restorations should be assessed for removal (margination procedures) to correct defective margins and to provide a smooth surface that will not harbor bacterial plaque biofilm[14,15]

(a) Type I overhang—less than one third of the interproximal space; treated with margination procedure and repolishing of restoration; may be detected radiographically

(b) Type II overhang—one third to one half of the interproximal embrasure space; treated with margination procedure if the predicted final result is good (the prognosis for the tooth, complexity, and cost of replacement are considered); usually radiographically and clinically detectable

(c) Type III overhang—more than one half of the interproximal embrasure space; treated with replacement of restoration; clinically and radiographically detectable

g. Implant identification (see the sections on "Dental implants" in Chapters 13 and 14)—to assess for peri-implantitis and the stability of the implant

h. Prosthetic appliances—assessed for stability and functionality

4. Pulpal vitality testing, when applicable (see the section on "Pulpal vitality and testing devices" in Chapter 16)

5. Stain assessment (see the section on "Selective stain removal" in Chapter 17) to determine the extent and type of stain present

a. Stains are primarily factors related to aesthetics; result from deposits of chromogenic bacteria, foods, and chemicals

b. Heavy tobacco stains encourage bacterial plaque biofilm retention

PERIODONTAL ASSESSMENT

See the section on "Clinical assessment of the periodontium" in Chapter 14.

A. Recognition of oral health, gingivitis, or periodontitis must occur through systematic and comprehensive periodontal examination to determine whether oral prophylaxis, nonsurgical periodontal therapy (NSPT), periodontal maintenance (PM), or other periodontal therapy is indicated and to what extent[9,16] (Table 15-5)

TABLE 15-5 Periodontal Assessment Symbols

Term	Procedure	Symbol
Gingiva Blunted papilla	Indicate by placing a straight horizontal line in the affected interproximal space	
Cratered papilla	Indicate by drawing the shape of the crater in the affected interproximal space from the buccal or lingual space	
Inadequate amount of attached gingiva	Indicate when <1 mm of attached gingiva is present; calculate by measuring from the margin of free gingiva to the mucogingival junction, and subtract from the pocket depth measurement	NAG | IAG NAG = no attached gingiva IAG = inadequate attached gingiva
Recession	Measure the amount of recession in millimeters from the margin of the free gingiva to the cemento-enamel junction; draw the gingival margin	
Loss of attachment	Measure the amount of recession in millimeters from the margin of the free gingiva to the cemento-enamel junction; add to the depth of the pocket	PD 222 212 LOA 4 3
Frenum pull	Indicate any abnormal muscle pull on the gingiva, attachment of the free gingiva, or tight frenums by placing a symbol in the area where it occurs	
Exudate	Indicate by placing an X above the affected tooth	X DATE 1/6/02 PD 645 434 423 PD LOA AG
Probing depth	Measure from the margin of the free gingiva to the junctional epithelium; record all readings and all areas of hemorrhage	

Continued

TABLE 15-5 Periodontal Assessment Symbols—cont'd

Term	Procedure	Symbol
Pathology Furcation involvement (class I, II, III, or IV)	Use Roman numerals on the affected area to depict the extent of the furcation from the buccal or lingual bifurcation or trifurcation or use a triangle in the furcation area showing class I (partial triangle), class II (complete triangle unfilled), or class III (triangle completely filled in)	
Mobility (class 1, 2, or 3 or I, II, or III)	Record on the basis of degree of tooth movement	
Periodontal pathology	Outline the affected area, approximating the size and location of the radiolucency observed on the radiograph	
Other Factors Marginal ridge discrepancy	Place an N in the area of the occlusal contact when adjacent marginal ridges are not equal in height	
Food impaction	Indicate by placing a zigzag arrow in the interproximal space	
Deficient contacts	Indicate a loose contact by drawing a single vertical line in the interproximal space. Indicate an open contact by drawing two vertical lines in the interproximal space	

B. During general periodontal examination, anatomic features such as position, size, and shape of gingiva and interdental papillae and position of frena must be recorded

1. The presence, location, and severity of gingival inflammation are assessed—soft-tissue description (color, texture, consistency, and marginal and papillary shape)
2. Mucogingival relationships are evaluated to identify the deficiencies of keratinized tissue, abnormal frenulum insertions, and other tissue abnormalities such as clinically significant gingival recession (e.g., recession, loss of attachment/clinical attachment level, and attached gingiva)

C. Periodontal probing is done to assess the periodontal probing depth and to provide information on the health of subgingival areas and the presence of bleeding on probing (see the section on "Assessments with periodontal probes" in Chapter 17)

1. Probing depths are measured on six tooth sites (distofacial, facial, mesiofacial, distolingual, lingual, mesiolingual) and recorded on the periodontal chart
2. Using diagnostic radiographs and probing depths, the presence of pseudopockets (false or gingival pockets) or periodontal pockets is determined

D. Periodontal soft tissues, including peri-implant tissues, should be examined

E. The presence and types of purulent exudates and gingival crevicular fluid analysis should be determined; increased gingival crevicular fluid and purulent exudate indicate inflammatory changes within the pocket wall; these are considered risk factors for disease progression and require further assessment to determine cause and to plan interventions

F. The presence and distribution of bacterial plaque biofilm and calculus—location, extent, and tenacity of deposits are identified to assist with appropriate care planning and instrument selection (see the section on "Assessments with dental explorers" in Chapter 17)

G. Degree of mobility of teeth and dental implants

1. Mobility—risk factor for periodontal disease progression; should be measured when moderate to advanced disease is present
2. Measured by bi-digital evaluation when teeth are not occluded and via direct observation (fremitus) when teeth are occluded; classified by degree of movement
   a. Class 1 or I—slight mobility, greater than normal
   b. Class 2 or II—moderate mobility, greater than 1 mm
   c. Class 3 or III—severe mobility, tooth can move in all directions and can be depressed into the socket
3. Contributing factors—trauma from occlusion, inflammation in periodontal ligament, periodontal surgery, physiochemical changes (pregnancy or hormonal changes) in periodontal tissues, and pathologic conditions (tumors)[17]

H. The presence, location, and degree of clinical furcation involvements are determined

1. Occurs when loss of attachment extends into bifurcation or trifurcation of multiple-rooted teeth; classified by degree of involvement
   a. Class I—exposure of furcation; but bone remains between roots
   b. Class II—loss of some bone between roots; but not complete communication from one surface to another
   c. Class III—through-and-through involvement with complete loss of bone between roots; opening covered by gingiva
   d. Class IV—through-and-through involvement with complete loss of bone between roots; entrance clearly visible
2. Furcation involvement—risk factor in predicting periodontal breakdown; compromises the prognosis of a tooth; detection and thorough periodontal debridement essential at the earliest point

I. Bacterial culturing, genetic testing, deoxyribonucleic acid (DNA) or ribonucleic acid (RNA) probes, and antibody and enzyme markers should be implemented, when indicated (see the section on "Clinical assessment of the periodontium" in Chapter 14)

1. Microbial assessments are not recommended routinely because tests fail to identify specific diseases or predict disease progression
2. Commercially available genetic tests assess susceptibility to chronic periodontitis; assist in risk assessment; are still being studied for use as a diagnostic test[16]
3. Microbiologic monitoring may be used in clients who continue to experience disease progression in spite of regular NSPT, surgical intervention, and effective oral self-care; those who are at high risk for disease progression or medically compromised clients with aggressive periodontitis may benefit from microbiologic monitoring

RADIOGRAPHIC EVALUATION

See the sections on "Oral radiographic procedures" and "Radiographic image interpretation" in Chapter 6.

A. A satisfactory number of diagnostic-quality periapical and bitewing radiographs are exposed and interpreted during the assessment phase of therapy

B. Depending on the diagnostic needs of the client, current radiographs are used for the proper evaluation and interpretation of the status of the dentition, periodontium, and dental implants

C. Any radiographic abnormalities are noted in the client's chart, and appropriate follow-up or referral is done

D. Digital subtraction radiology is used to detect and measure small changes in living bone (progressive bone loss or bone fill) that would otherwise go unnoticed with traditional technology

ORAL HYGIENE ASSESSMENT

A. Oral hygiene assessment—review of current home care practices, adherence levels, oral health and hygiene knowledge and skill levels, and psychosocial factors that might influence behaviors and oral habits; assists in the development of effective self-care educational sessions during the implementation phase of care (see the section on "Oral health education" in Chapter 16)

B. Indices—tools to measure and score periodontal assessment factors such as plaque biofilm, calculus, and bleeding for the benefit of both the clinician and the client (see the section on "Clinical assessment of the periodontium" in Chapter 14 and Table 20-6 in Chapter 20)

C. Oral self-care methods—used by the client to remove or reduce bacterial biofilm both supragingivally and subgingivally (1 to 3 mm); oral hygiene measures, oral home care, plaque biofilm control, and mechanical plaque biofilm removal are synonymous with oral self-care methods (see the sections on "Dental plaque biofilm detection," "Mechanical plaque biofilm control on facial, lingual, and occlusal tooth surfaces," "Interdental biofilm control," "Specialized plaque biofilm control devices," and "Care of fixed and removable prostheses" in Chapter 16)

    1. Determination of the use, frequency, and methods of plaque biofilm removal devices, dentifrices, mouthrinses, and fluorides

    2. Determination of the frequency of tobacco use, oral habits, and sugar intake

    3. Assessment of the client's skill level for oral self-care methods to determine whether the responsibility for oral health need is being met

      a. Skill deficiency—present if the client does not have the knowledge and the psychomotor ability to perform mechanical plaque biofilm removal

      b. Management deficiency—present if the client possesses the ability but does not perform plaque biofilm removal effectively on a daily basis

    4. Assessment of the motivation and readiness of the client to learn to determine whether the need for conceptualization and problem solving is being met; the Learning Ladder Continuum concept, a common approach to assessing the client's readiness to learn; describes learning that occurs in a progressive series of steps or intervals (see the section on "Stages in making a commitment to a new behavior" in Chapter 16)

D. Evaluation of dietary risk factors for dental caries; recommendations offered to reduce total sugar clearance time per day (see the section on "Nutritional assessment and counseling" in Chapter 12)

RISK-FACTOR ASSESSMENTS

A. Risk factors—factors that significantly increase the risk for the onset or progression of a specific disease; include systemic health, oral and pharyngeal cancers, caries, and periodontal disease risk factors

B. Systemic disease—risk factor for periodontal disease; systemic conditions include CVD, diabetes mellitus, respiratory disease, osteoporosis, preterm low birth weight, and behavioral and psychosocial status of client (see Chapter 14); when these conditions are present, consider the following American Academy of Periodontology recommendations[18,19]

    1. Diagnose the periodontal condition, and inform the client of his or her risk for systemic disease[17]

    2. Consultation with client's physician may be indicated to advise the physician about the client's periodontal status and the proposed care plan

    3. Determine the level of control or the status of disease such as gestational period, medications used, and glycemic control

    4. Provide self-care education regarding the relationship of periodontal infection to systemic health and of systemic health to periodontal disease

    5. Provide adequate NSPT, and encourage the client to commit to periodontal maintenance care

C. Oral and pharyngeal cancer risk—determined by evaluating risk factors such as socioeconomic status, tobacco use, race, alcohol use, sun exposure, gender, and age to formulate appropriate care plan and intervention to reduce risk

1. Assessment of tobacco use
2. Use the three A's (the ADHA's tobacco cessation initiative includes ASK, ADVISE, REFER)
   ASK the client about tobacco use
   ADVISE the client who wants to quit
   ASSIST the client in stopping
   ARRANGE for follow-up services
3. Teach the client oral cancer self-evaluation examination (see the section on "Oral cancer self-examination" in Chapter 16)
4. Have the client apply tobacco-cessation strategies
5. Refer the client to community-based resources or online resources such as Smokefree.gov

D. Caries risk—determined by assessing causative factors (e.g., frequency of sugar intake, high cariogenic bacteria count, biofilm removal ability, salivary dysfunction, socioeconomic status, biofilm-retentive factors, and fluoride history) to formulate appropriate care plan to reduce the client's risk (Table 15-6)
   1. Sugar intake assessment includes determining the form and frequency of exposure and offering appropriate recommendations to reduce exposure
   2. Bacterial plaque biofilm is a key factor in caries development; therefore, self-care education should focus on assisting the client with developing effective plaque biofilm removal methods
   3. Plaque-retentive factors (restoration overhangs, defective and ill-fitting crown margins, dental caries, exposed root surfaces, excess cement, and xerostomia) should be identified and eliminated or minimized
   4. Use of topical fluoride or chemotherapeutic agents (e.g., antimicrobial mouthrinses and dentifrices, products with xylitol) should be assessed and prescribed if not already being used by the client
   5. Recare regularity is evaluated and adjusted on the basis of the level of caries risk

E. Periodontal risk—assessed by determining dental and host–environmental risk factors and risk indicators (e.g., history of previous aggressive disease, increased pocket probing depth, loss of clinical attachment, infrequent dental visits, stress, poor oral hygiene, specific bacterial pathogens, tobacco use, diabetes mellitus with poor glycemic control, inherited risk), and by determining signs and symptoms of disease to assist with the formulation of accurate diagnosis and plan of care (see the section on "Changes in the periodontium associated with disease" in Chapter 14)

EVIDENCE-BASED DECISION MAKING[20,21]

A. Health care professionals must be able to assess the value of the information available in scientific literature and to use current best evidence when providing dental hygiene care
B. Evidence-based decision making integrates clinical expertise, client values, and best evidence into the decision-making process to achieve successful therapeutic outcomes
C. Evidence-based decision making begins during the process of care when the client presents with a specific clinical question or when a question arises during dental hygiene care; the four elements of an evidence-based question ("PICO") are:
   1. Patient, or problem
   2. Intervention, cause, or prognosis
   3. Comparison, or control
   4. Outcome, or outcomes
D. The hygienist develops a well-defined clinical question (PICO) related to the diagnosis, therapy, prognosis, cause, or harm to answer the client-related question (Table 15-7)
E. A computerized literature search is conducted to answer the PICO question—randomized controlled clinical trials, systematic reviews, or meta-analysis studies provide the best evidence for answering the question
F. Evidence obtained from literature search is critically evaluated to determine validity and clinical applicability—studies are reviewed to identify the results and determine whether they are valid and whether they apply to the client
G. Evidence gathered from literature appraisal is applied to clinical practice by discussing the findings with client and offering recommendations for treatment
H. The process and the clinician's performance are evaluated

ASSESSMENT AND DOCUMENTATION

A. Accurate documentation of all assessment findings is the legal responsibility of all clinicians (Table 15-8)
B. Assessment findings should be clearly recorded and dated using ink on appropriate data-collection forms (health history forms, extraoral and intraoral examination forms, dentition and periodontal charting forms, and radiographic interpretation forms)
   1. Documentation and monitoring of abnormal lesions must be followed; if after 1 week to

TABLE 15-6 Classification of Caries Risk

Risk Level	Children (0 to 5 years)	Children (6 years and older) and Adults
Low	No evidence of: —carious or incipient lesions, restorations or tooth loss caused by caries in past 2 years —caries activity in the mother or other siblings in the past 2 years —dental or orthodontic appliances —plaque biofilm present —inadequate salivary flow —special care health needs —not eligible for government programs Evidence of: —optimal fluoride exposure —regular recare intervals —eating sugar or starchy foods/drinks with meals or having infrequent exposure	No evidence of: —carious or incipient lesions, restorations or tooth loss caused by caries in past 3 years —caries activity in the mother or other siblings in the past 2 years —interproximal restorations or restorations with plaque-retentive factors or open contacts) —dental or orthodontic appliances —exposed root surfaces —plaque biofilm present special care health needs chemotherapy or radiation therapy —smokeless tobacco use —eating disorders —drug/alcohol abuse Evidence of: —adequate salivary flow —optimal fluoride exposure —regular recare intervals —eating sugar or starchy foods or drinks with meals or infrequent exposure —low count of cariogenic bacteria —well-coalesced pits and fissures
Moderate	No evidence of: —fluoride exposure —regular recare or dental home Evidence of: —caries activity in the mother or other siblings in the past 7–23 months —frequent or prolonged exposure to sugar or starchy foods or drinks between meals —dental or orthodontic appliances —visible plaque biofilm	No evidence of: —fluoride exposure —regular recare or dental home Evidence of: —1 or 2 new carious or incipient lesions, restorations or tooth loss caused by caries in the past 3 years —caries activity in the mother or other siblings in the past 7–23 months —interproximal restorations or restorations with plaque-retentive factors or open contacts) —dental or orthodontic appliances —exposed root surfaces —visible plaque biofilm —special care health needs —smokeless tobacco use —eating disorders —drug or alcohol abuse —deep pits and fissures or developmental defects
High	No evidence of: —fluoride exposure —regular recare or dental home Evidence of: —caries activity in the mother or other siblings in the past 6 months —carious or incipient lesions —restorations or tooth loss caused by caries in the past 2 years —bottle or sippy cup at bedtime with juice or sugar (cariogenic agent) —eligibility for government program —special care health needs —inadequate saliva flow related to hyposalivary medications, cancer treatment, or genetic factors	No evidence of: —fluoride exposure —regular recare or dental home Evidence of: —3 or more carious or incipient lesions, restorations or tooth loss caused by caries in the past 3 years —caries activity in the mother or other siblings in the past 6 months —high levels of cariogenic bacteria *Streptococcus mutans* (105 colony—forming units [cfu]/mL) lactobacilli (103 cfu/mL) —frequent or prolonged exposure to sugar or starchy foods or drinks between meals —special care health needs —chemotherapy or radiation therapy —inadequate saliva flow related to hyposalivary medications, cancer treatment, or genetic factors

Adapted from Jenson L, Budenz AW, Featherstone J, Ramos-Gomez F, Spolsky VW, Young DA: Clinical protocols for caries management by risk assessment, J Calif Dent Assoc, 35(10):714–723, 2007; and American Dental Association, Councils on Dental Practice and Scientific Affairs: Caries risk assessment form: Available at http://gsa.ada.org/search?as_sitesearch=www.ada.org/sections/professionalResources/docs&q=caries+risk&searchButton.x=0&searchButton.y=0&site=ADAorg_Collecti on&client=ADAFrontEnd&proxystylesheet=ADAFrontEnd&output=xml_no_dtd&ie=UTF-8&ip=24.117.153.112&access=p&sort=date%3AD%3AL%3Ad1&entqr=3&oe= UTF-8&ud=1: Accessed April 13, 2010.

TABLE 15-7 Asking the Clinical Question: PICO Mnemonic

Element (PICO)	Descriptive Question(s) to Ask	Example
Patient, or problem	How would I describe a group of clients similar to mine? What are the most important characteristics for this client?	A client with generalized marginal biofilm and inflammation
Intervention, cause, or prognosis	Which main intervention or prognostic factor am I considering for this client?	A powered toothbrush
Comparison, or control	What is the main alternative to compare with the intervention?	Compared with a manual toothbrush
Outcome, or outcomes	What can I hope to accomplish, measure, or improve?	Decrease marginal biofilm and inflammation

Adapted from Forest JL, Miller SA: Translating evidence-based decision making into practice: EBDM concepts and finding the evidence, J Evid Based Dent Pract 9:(2), 59–72, 2009.

10 days the lesion or abnormality remains, procedures should be implemented to diagnose the condition (e.g., excisional or incisional biopsy, brush biopsy) (see the section on "Diagnostic tools for oral cancer detection" in Chapter 16)
2. Active disease or any deviations from normal should be documented and monitored
C. Additional information that was assessed (e.g., risk factors) and discussed with client, but not charted, should be recorded on a record of services form

DIAGNOSIS

A. Definition—clinical diagnosis by licensed dental hygienist that identifies actual or potential unmet human needs (deficits) related to oral health or disease that dental hygienist is educated and licensed to treat or refer for care;[7] the second phase in the dental hygiene process of care (see Figure 15-1)
B. Dental diagnosis identifies a specific oral disease, whereas dental hygiene diagnosis identifies human needs deficits related to dental hygiene care
C. Interpretation of collected data during assessment phase of care is necessary to identify significant findings, recognize deviations from normal, describe abnormalities, and analyze significance of the abnormalities

TABLE 15-8 Components of Dental Hygiene Care

General assessment	Medical and dental history Chief concern Clinical examination Radiographic analysis Microbiologic, genetic, biochemical diagnostic tests Extraoral and intraoral examinations
Periodontal and restorative assessment	Risk assessment Plaque or biofilm, calculus Dental restorations Caries assessment Dental implants Probing depth (bleeding and suppuration) Clinical attachment level and gingival recession Furcation status Prosthetic appliances Occlusion (mobility, occlusal discrepancy, fremitus) Proximal contact relationships Periodontal–systemic inter-relationships
Self-care education	Risk factors Disease theory education Skill enhancement Behavior interventions (nutrition counseling, tobacco cessation, medical referral)
Instrumentation and supportive therapy	Pain and anxiety control methods Plaque biofilm and calculus removal Restoration overhang removal Desensitization for dentinal hypersensitivity Fluoride therapy Sealant application Local or systemic chemotherapeutic agents Implant maintenance Mouthguard fabrication
Selecting polishing procedures	Selective stain removal (polishing) Restoration enhancement (finishing, polishing)
Referrals	Medical consultation Restorative therapy Periodontal surgery Orthodontics Endodontics Oral surgery Oral pathology diagnosis

Adapted from American Academy of Periodontology: Statement on comprehensive periodontal therapy, 2010: Available at http://www.perio.org/resources-products/posppr3-4.html: Accessed May 30, 2011.

1. Analysis of assessment data used to identify deviations from normal values and to identify patterns or relationships within data
2. Synthesis combines elements from data to develop explanations for symptoms

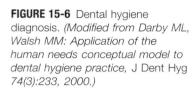

FIGURE 15-6 Dental hygiene diagnosis. *(Modified from Darby ML, Walsh MM: Application of the human needs conceptual model to dental hygiene practice,* J Dent Hyg *74(3):233, 2000.)*

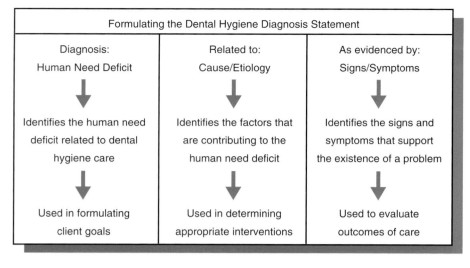

Formulating the Dental Hygiene Diagnosis Statement		
Diagnosis: Human Need Deficit	Related to: Cause/Etiology	As evidenced by: Signs/Symptoms
↓	↓	↓
Identifies the human need deficit related to dental hygiene care	Identifies the factors that are contributing to the human need deficit	Identifies the signs and symptoms that support the existence of a problem
↓	↓	↓
Used in formulating client goals	Used in determining appropriate interventions	Used to evaluate outcomes of care

a. Inductive reasoning finds possible patterns in observations to predict new information

b. Deductive reasoning begins with generalizations and proceeds to discover specific facts

D. Identification of unmet human needs related to oral health or systemic problems provides a unique focus for the provision of dental hygiene care

E. Validation allows for the recognition of errors and discrepancies, the need for additional information from the client or from other health care professionals, or the reinterpretation of documented evidence

F. Diagnostic statements are formulated after data analysis and validation; become framework for planning, implementation, and evaluation phases of care; three major components of written diagnostic statements are shown in Figure 15-6

1. Condition or problem, or potential problem, as identified by unmet human needs (diagnosis) related to dental hygiene care; used to formulate client goals

2. Identification of contributing or causative factors related to unmet human needs; used to determine appropriate dental hygiene interventions

3. Signs and symptoms (evidence) of unmet human needs that support existence of problem; used to evaluate outcomes of dental hygiene care

PLANNING

A. Definition—identification and prioritization of current and potential dental and dental hygiene care needs, establishment of client goals, and determination of interventions and outcomes to meet these needs

B. Clients are more likely to express their wants, needs, and desires and to commit to a care plan if they are actively involved in the development of goals, priorities, interventions, and appointment planning

C. Assessment data and diagnosis should be used to develop a logical plan of therapy to eliminate disease, slow disease progression, and maintain and promote health[22]

D. Four components to consider when completing written care plan:

1. Establish priorities for care that require a collaborative approach among the client, the dental hygienist, and the dentist; address the following:

a. Needs of the client based on conditions that pose the greatest threat to comfort, life, health, and safety

b. Main concerns or preferences of the client (chief complaint)

c. Motivational level of the client

2. Set client-oriented goals and evaluation measures that reflect the expected and desired outcomes of dental hygiene care

a. For each dental hygiene diagnosis, at least one goal and intervention should be established; some diagnoses may require multiple interventions

b. Goals should focus on cognitive, affective, or psychomotor domains and contain a subject, verb, measurement criteria, and specific time element

(1) Cognitive goals focus on increasing knowledge level

(2) Affective goals focus on changes in beliefs, attitudes, and values

(3) Psychomotor goals focus on skill development when skill deficiencies are present

c. Expected outcomes and evaluation measures are used to determine whether goals are being met during care or after completion of therapy; when indicated, modify the diagnosis or care plan if goals are not being met; two forms of evaluation should be considered when planning care:
   (1) Evaluation that occurs throughout the implementation phase of care
   (2) Evaluation or re-evaluation that occurs after the completion of initial therapy

3. Identify interventions as part of care planning that specifically address the dental hygiene diagnosis (see Table 15-8).
   a. Traditional phases of dental care planning include[23]
      (1) Preliminary phase—focuses on treating periodontal or dental emergency needs
      (2) Phase I therapy—focuses on controlling the risk factors responsible for disease; includes self-care education, diet control, removal or correction of biofilm-retentive factors, antimicrobial therapy, and dental caries management
      (3) Phase II therapy—focuses on surgical care; includes periodontal surgery, placement of implants, and endodontic therapy
      (4) Phase III therapy—focuses on prosthetic treatment and final management of dental caries along with periodontal examination to re-evaluate response to restorative procedures
      (5) Phase IV therapy—focuses on long-term periodontal maintenance therapy; includes assessment, self-care education, deposit removal, and evaluation of continued-care (recare) interval
   b. Common system of periodontal disease classification; includes overall disease extent (localized and generalized), severity (case type), and activity (chronic, aggressive, or necrotizing) (see the section on "Diseases of the periodontium" in Chapter 14)
      (1) Case type I—gingivitis
      (2) Case type II—mild periodontitis
      (3) Case type III—moderate periodontitis
      (4) Case type IV—advanced periodontitis
      (5) Case type V—refractory periodontitis
   c. Some interventions for common forms of periodontal disease are as follows:
      (1) Therapy for gingivitis (case type I)—includes oral self-care education, supragingival and subgingival debridement, antimicrobial agents, and correction of plaque biofilm–retentive factors

completed during a 1-hour appointment; may include re-evaluation at another appointment if extensive bleeding occurs on probing or pseudopockets are present
      (2) Therapy for mild periodontitis (case type II)—includes elimination, modification, or control of systemic diseases and other risk factors; oral self-care education; and supragingival and subgingival debridement, including scaling and root planing with a quadrant approach, during four 60- to 90-minute appointments and re-evaluation
      (3) Therapy for moderate periodontitis (case type III)—includes elimination, alteration, or control of systemic diseases and other risk factors; oral self-care education; and supragingival and subgingival debridement, including scaling and root planing with a sextant or quadrant approach, during four to six 60- to 90-minute appointments and re-evaluation for surgery
      (4) Therapy for advanced periodontitis (case type IV)—includes elimination, modification, or control of systemic diseases and risk factors; oral self-care education; débridement, including scaling and root planing; subgingival microbial sampling; and extraction of teeth that have a poor prognosis with a sextant approach during six 60- to 90-minute appointments and re-evaluation for surgery
      (5) Therapy for refractory periodontitis (case type V)—includes self-care education, debridement, scaling and root planing, control of risk factors, systemic antibiotics, locally delivered antibiotics, microbial diagnostic testing, and antimicrobial therapy, with a sextant or quadrant approach, based on number of sites involved; re-evaluation for surgery; and periodontal maintenance therapy

4. Writing care plan provides permanent documentation that becomes a contract between the dental hygienist and the client; elements of care plan include:
   a. Procedure—course of action or procedures to be rendered
   b. Appointment sequence order in which therapy will be given
   c. Approximate time for each procedure and total time for each appointment
   d. Expected outcomes and limitations of care

CASE PRESENTATION

A. Definition—presentation of assessment data to include dental and dental hygiene diagnosis and proposed care plan

B. Purpose—to satisfy legal and ethical responsibilities for care, reach agreement for therapy, and obtain informed consent

C. A collaborative approach between client and clinician should be encouraged

D. Case presentation should be accurate, direct, and concise; should describe:

1. Existing oral conditions and related causative and contributing factors presented in terms that are understandable to the client
2. Treatment procedures and how therapy may differ from previous appointments (e.g., number of appointments, length, purpose of each appointment, services to be incorporated, and description of services)
3. Desired outcomes of treatment and provisional prognosis
4. Risks and benefits of all treatment options involved
5. Consequences of rejecting treatment or not proceeding with all components of care
6. Alternative approaches to care, if any exist (e.g., mechanized versus hand-activated instrumentation, NSPT versus surgery when advanced disease is present)
7. Client's responsibility as a co-therapist (e.g., commitment to self-care and continued-care recommendations)
8. Client's right to decline care by providing an opportunity to initially consent for care and to withdraw from treatment at any time
9. Time and cost involved in professional care

INFORMED CONSENT

A. Definition—process by which a client agrees to a proposed treatment after a complete case presentation (see Chapter 22)

B. Includes use of a written informed consent form, signed by the client or the guardian, the clinician, and a witness, stating that all treatment descriptions, risk, benefits, outcomes of treatment, alternative treatments, and an opportunity for questions and answers were provided; should be completed before implementation of care plan

C. An informed refusal form is completed when the client declines some or all of the care plan; includes:

1. Proposed dental and dental hygiene care planned
2. Risks involved without treatment
3. List of procedures being refused
4. Date the informed refusal form was signed
5. Signature of the client, the dental hygienist or the dentist, and a witness

CLIENT MANAGEMENT WITH EFFECTIVE COMMUNICATION

A. Communication—giving or exchanging information, signals, or messages through facial expression, behavior, talking, gestures, and writing; effective communication is essential in creating an environment conducive to modifying a client's psychomotor skills, level of knowledge, values, attitudes, and lifestyles

B. Intrapersonal communication—processing a message within oneself; often affected by one's personal life experiences, culture, beliefs, and values

C. Interpersonal communication—messages between two or more people; focuses on the interaction and interpretation of a conversation with nonverbal behaviors and spoken words; effective interpersonal communication may reduce the incidence of miscommunication and client management problems and increase the client's commitment to care

1. Nonverbal behaviors—nonspoken messages, including body orientation, posture, facial expressions, gestures, touch, distance, voice tone, and hesitation in speech
2. Verbal behaviors—spoken messages, including language, active listening, paraphrasing, and reflective responding
   a. The language used in communication should be carefully selected based on the client's characteristics and presented in a straightforward and nonthreatening manner
   b. Active listening requires maintaining eye contact and concentration and focusing on what the client is communicating
   c. Paraphrasing is restatement or summarization of what the client said; provides the opportunity to correct any misunderstandings
   d. Reflective responding addresses the actual feelings of the client; response is presented in manner that restates, rewords, or reflects what the client said

D. Enhancement of client–dental hygienist relationship through confidence and trust requires:

1. Acceptance—accepting the client without judgment
2. Comfort—ability to deal with embarrassing or emotionally painful topics related to an individual's health
3. Concreteness—communicating in a clear and precise manner with terms understandable to a client

4. Empathy—listening and understanding the emotions and feelings of an individual
5. Genuineness—communicating in an open and honest manner
6. Respect—ability to convey honor and esteem for an individual
7. Responsiveness—ability to reply to messages at the very moment they are sent
8. Self-disclosure—sharing personal experiences with a client
9. Warmth—displaying personal feelings and empathy

IMPLEMENTATION

See the section on "Nonsurgical periodontal therapy" in Chapter 14.
A. Definition—delivery of preventive and therapeutic procedures identified in an individualized care plan to meet a client's human needs (see Table 15-8)
   1. Activities—reduction or elimination of risk factors for disease, health promotion, self-care education, mechanical and mechanized instrumentation, pharmocotherapeutic interventions, pain control strategies, selective polishing; supporting interventions, including overhang removal, desensitization, dietary assessment and counseling, dental caries management, and occlusal therapy
   2. Modifications to the initial care plan are made as new assessment criteria become available during the implementation of care (i.e., improved self-care, increase in healing response time)
B. Self-care education—teaching disease control, health maintenance, and health promotion strategies to target the client's diagnosed problems; should occur at each appointment before instrumentation procedures; strategies are those implemented by the client at home (see the section on "Oral health education" in Chapter 16)
C. Pain and anxiety control should be used when indicated to prevent or manage apprehension and pain and promote the client's cooperation and compliance; includes local anesthetic agents, nitrous oxide–oxygen analgesia, topical anesthetic agents, and psychosomatic methods (see Chapter 18)
D. Instrument selection—based on intraoral conditions discovered in the assessment phase of care: periodontal pocket depth, furcation involvement, root concavities, deposit size, configuration, mode of attachment, and location (see Chapter 17)
   1. Hand-activated instrumentation—use of sharp curets and files, with fundamental instrumentation principles during scaling and debridement

2. Mechanized instrumentation—ultrasonic and sonic scaling equipment and techniques for scaling and debridement
E. Polishing procedures—use of abrasive agents, prophy angle, low-speed handpiece or toothbrush, and air abrasion unit to remove bacterial plaque biofilm and stain and to produce a smooth, lustrous tooth surface
   1. Selective polishing—aesthetic procedure accomplished with a rubber cup and paste or air-polishing unit (airbrasion) to remove extrinsic stain remaining after periodontal instrumentation (see the section on "Selective stain removal" in Chapter 17)
   2. Polishing and finishing restorations prevent recurrent caries and deterioration of restorations, maintain periodontal health, and prevent occlusal problems
F. Maintenance therapy (formerly known as *supportive therapy*)—a term used for interventions directed at sustaining oral health and controlling disease progression (e.g., débridement for the control of periodontal diseases and the maintenance of periodontal health, fluoride therapy, sealant application, occlusal appliance fabrication, oral irrigation, desensitization, local or systemic antibiotics, and implant maintenance) (see the sections on "Nonsurgical periodontal therapy" and "Periodontal maintenance" in Chapter 14; "Oral irrigation," "Fluorides," "Mouthrinses," "Dental sealants," "Care of fixed and removable prostheses," "Dental implant maintenance," "Tobacco use interventions," and "Control of dentinal hypersensitivity" in Chapter 16.
G. Ergonomics focuses on the prevention of exposure to injury within the work environment; involves clinician and client positioning, tasks and procedures performed, equipment design and use, and impact of these actions on musculoskeletal health
   1. Cumulative trauma disorders (also known as *repetitive strain disorders*)—musculoskeletal and nerve impairments caused by repetitive work activities, especially when performed aggressively, in awkward positions, or both
   2. Prevention of ergonomic hazards—involves daily application of ergonomic principles while providing dental hygiene care (e.g., posture, grasp, properly fitted gloves, instrument and equipment design, exercise for hand and body, positioning of equipment and materials in the environment)

EVALUATION

See the sections on "Treatment" and "Periodontal maintenance" in Chapter 14.

A. Definition—measurement of extent to which client has achieved specified goals in care plan and determination of success of interventions; ensures that high-quality care has been provided

B. The quality of dental hygiene care is assessed by certain criteria and standards
1. Criteria—qualities or characteristics by which the knowledge, skill, or oral health status of the client is measured through descriptions of acceptable levels of performance of client or dental hygienist (e.g., probing attachment levels are reduced by 1 to 2 mm and no sites with bleeding on probing)
2. Standards—acceptable and expected levels of performance by the dental hygienist or other health care professionals, which have been established through national consensus[2]

C. Measurement of outcomes of dental hygiene interventions involves collecting evaluation data to determine whether the client's goals established during the planning phase of care have been met, partially met, or not met

D. *Supervised neglect* occurs when the client needs further professional care to achieve higher levels of oral wellness or to prevent or control oral disease process but has been discharged from care, under the false assumption that a healthy state was achieved

E. Two forms of evaluation
1. Evaluation—occurs continually throughout implementation phase of care; provides the mechanism for modifying the care plan as new assessment criteria become available during treatment (e.g., improved client self-care, increase in healing response time)
2. Re-evaluation—occurs 4 to 6 weeks after therapy is completed to evaluate response to initial care and to recommend additional therapy as needed (e.g., decrease in probing depths, elimination of bleeding points)

F. Elements of re-evaluation appointment include components of the dental hygiene process of care: assessment, diagnosis, planning, and implementation
1. Assessment
   a. Reassessment of initial assessment data and periodontal status to evaluate improvement such as effective self-care methods, reduction by 1 to 2 mm in probing measurements, no bleeding on probing, and healthy-appearing gingival tissue
   b. Determination of the presence of residual deposits, newly accumulated deposits, or unresponsive areas indicated by bleeding on probing or gingival inflammation
   c. Re-evaluation of the client's self-care practices
2. Diagnosis—re-evaluation of dental or dental hygiene diagnosis, if indicated, based on assessment data
3. Planning—care plan developed on the basis of assessment findings; includes, when indicated, modification to self-care practices, localized debridement, chemotherapy, appropriate referrals, and the establishment of continued-care schedule or periodontal maintenance therapy
4. Implementation—provision of self-care education; removal of residual deposits and plaque biofilm–retentive factors; debridement of nonresponsive areas; provision of indicated therapy and reassessment of continued-care schedule

G. The continued-care (recare) schedule is determined on the basis of individual client needs, degree of risk for oral disease, and disease progression; the client is informed of the rationale for and the importance of continued care[24]
1. Continued-care schedules with intervals of 1 to 3 months are recommended to clients who display poor results after therapy, have significant risk factors, have advanced or aggressive disease, have poor self-care, have furcation involvement, or have complicated prostheses
2. Intervals of 3 months are recommended to clients who complete routine NSPT with uneventful healing and demonstrate moderate to high risk for oral diseases and disease progression
3. Intervals of 3 to 4 months are recommended to clients who have maintained generally good results for 1 year or longer after therapy but display significant risk factors (e.g., inconsistent or poor oral hygiene, heavy calculus formation, systemic disease or condition, tobacco use, localized pockets, occlusal problems, complicated prostheses, ongoing orthodontic therapy, dental caries activity, and localized teeth with less than 50% of alveolar bone support)
4. Intervals of 6 months to 1 year are recommended to clients who maintain excellent results for 1 year or longer and have been able to eliminate or control risk factors for oral disease (e.g., good oral hygiene, minimal calculus, no occlusal problems, no complicated prosthesis, no remaining pockets, no teeth with less than 50% of alveolar bone remaining, and low risk for dental caries)

H. Documenting the outcomes of dental hygiene care aids in preventing possible legal charges related to inadequate documentation and the client feeling inadequately informed about his or her oral health status; should include:

1. Status and prognosis for the case, sites at risk for disease progression, and sites with disease progression
2. Sites with plaque biofilm and calculus, bleeding, and areas of inflammation
3. Need for restorative and periodontal treatment and for referral to a specialist
4. Discussion that took place with the client regarding his or her health or disease status
5. Past commitment of the client and recommendations suggested by the clinician
6. Time interval required for the next appointment (continued-care interval)
7. Acceptance or rejection of any further needed therapy

PROGNOSIS

A. Definition—prediction of duration, course, and termination of disease and response to treatment; usually determined after diagnosis and before care is planned
B. Overall prognosis considers both oral and systemic health and the significance of factors present (e.g., type of periodontal disease, age, socioeconomic status, systemic conditions, malocclusion, periodontal status, complicated prosthesis, tobacco use, and cooperation of the client)
C. Prognosis for individual teeth made after overall prognosis is determined and relates to mobility, periodontal pockets, adequacy of attached gingiva, mucogingival involvement, furcation involvement, tooth morphology, status of teeth serving as abutments, bone level surrounding tooth, and extensive caries
D. Level of prognosis established through collaboration of the dental hygienist and the dentist after comprehensive assessment[25]
   1. Excellent prognosis—no bone loss, excellent gingival conditions, and adequate client commitment to care
   2. Good prognosis—adequate remaining bone support, adequate possibilities to control causative and risk factors, and adequate client commitment to care
   3. Fair prognosis—less than adequate remaining bone support, some tooth mobility, grade I furcation involvement, adequate maintenance possible, and acceptable client commitment to care
   4. Poor prognosis—moderate to advanced bone loss, tooth mobility, grade I and II furcation involvement, difficult areas to maintain, and doubtful client commitment to care

5. Questionable prognosis—advanced bone loss, grade II and III furcation involvement, tooth mobility, and inaccessible areas
6. Hopeless prognosis—advanced bone loss, areas not maintainable, and extraction or extractions indicated

ETHICAL, LEGAL, AND SAFETY ISSUES

See Chapter 22. Provision of comprehensive, quality care by licensed dental hygienists includes legal, ethical, and safety issues that must be kept in mind.
A. Ethical issues that place hygienist at risk are:
   1. Failure to refer to a medical professional or other dental specialist when indicated
   2. Failure to maintain client confidentiality
   3. Failure to perform thorough case presentation so that the client can make an informed decision about the dental hygiene care
   4. Failure to perform comprehensive assessment to detect oral diseases and abnormalities and degree of client risk for disease or disease progression
B. Legal issues that place hygienist at risk are:
   1. Failure to comply with HIPAA (The Health Insurance Portability and Accountability Act); the clinician must verify that clients have read the HIPAA policy and obtain a written Acknowledgment of Receipt of the Notice from the client
   2. Failure to assess, diagnose, treat, or refer for disease; even when under the supervision of a dentist, a licensed dental hygienist is accountable and responsible for client care
   3. Failure to obtain written informed consent before initiating care
   4. Failure to provide necessary care on the basis of assessment findings; constitutes supervised neglect
   5. Failure to provide evidence-based care
   6. Failure to document assessment, care plan, informed consent, services rendered, and client response to care
C. Safety issues that place the dental hygienist and the client at risk are:
   1. Failure to protect the client from harm during care
   2. Failure to accurately assess the client's health and pharmacologic history and to make necessary physician referrals
   3. Failure to allow time during appointment for the provision of adequate care
   4. Failure to evaluate therapy after completion of care or to recommend an appropriate continued-care interval

5. Failure to follow established protocol that protects the clinician and the client during therapy (e.g., standard precautions; see Chapter 10)
6. Failure to use instrumentation in effective and responsible manner (e.g., not using sharp instruments, not selecting appropriate instruments based on conditions present, and causing tissue trauma)
7. Failure to follow the manufacturer's instructions in the use of equipment, devices, and dental materials

@ WEB SITE INFORMATION AND RESOURCES

SOURCE	WEB SITE ADDRESS	DESCRIPTION
Medline and PubMed	www.ncbi.nlm.nih.gov/pubmed/	Used for evidence-based decision making
Medline Plus	www.nlm.nih.gov/medlineplus/	Patient information on health topics and medication; medical encyclopedia
National Center for Dental Hygiene Research	www.usc.edu/hsc/dental/dhnet/	Focus for many dental hygiene research-related topics and links
Healthfinder	www.healthfinder.gov	Patient information on health topics, special population topics, health care, directory
Dimensions of Dental Hygiene	www.dimensionsofdentalhygiene.com/	Online journal with dental and dental hygiene–related topics
National Institutes of Health	www.nih.gov	Health topics, funding, news and events
American Academy of Periodontology	www.perio.org	Association Web site; parameters of practice and position papers related to the treatment of periodontal diseases
National Institute of Dental and Craniofacial Research	www.nidcr.nih.gov	Oral health information, educational resources and research
National Guideline Clearinghouse	www.guideline.gov	Evidence-based clinical practice guidelines
Centers for Disease Control and Prevention	www.cdc.gov	Health and safety topics, publications, data and statistics
Occupational Safety and Health Administration	www.osha.gov	Information on the health and safety of employees
RxList	www.rxlist.com/script/main/hp.asp	Information related to prescription medications
Merck Manual	www.merck.com	Information related to medical conditions
MyMedicineListTM	www.safemedication.com	Database containing important medication information
Aetna InteliHealth® (Harvard Medical School-Intelihealth Partnership)	www.intelihealth.com	Consumer information related to health and medicine
U.S. Department of Health & Human Services	www.hhs.gov/ocr/privacy/	Health information privacy

REFERENCES

1. Darby ML, Walsh MM: *Dental hygiene theory and practice,* ed 3, St. Louis, 2010, Saunders.
2. American Dental Hygienists' Association (ADHA): *Standards for clinical dental hygiene practice,* Chicago, 2008, ADHA.
3. Commission on Dental Accreditation: *Accreditation standards for dental hygiene education programs,* Chicago, 2010, American Dental Association.
4. American Dental Hygienists' Association: *Policy manual: ADHA framework for theory development—1,* Chicago, 2005, ADHA.
5. Darby ML, Walsh MM: A proposed human needs conceptual model for dental hygiene: Part I, *J Dent Hyg* 67(6):326–334, 1993.
6. Darby ML, Walsh MM: Application of the human needs conceptual model of dental hygiene to the role of the clinician: Part II, *J Dent Hyg* 67(6):335–346, 1993.

7. Darby ML, Walsh MM: Application of the human needs conceptual model to dental hygiene practice, *J Dent Hyg* 74(3):230–237, 2000.

8. Yamamoto J, Hannebrink R, Finta L, et al: Development of an instrument to measure outcomes of dental hygiene care. Paper presented at the Annual Session of the American Dental Hygienists' Association, Chicago, 1995.

9. American Academy of Periodontology: Statement on comprehensive periodontal therapy, (2010): Available at http://www.perio.org/resources-products/posppr3-4.html: Accessed October 1, 2010.

10. Pickett AF: Personal, dental and health histories. In Darby ML, Walsh MM, editors: *Dental hygiene theory and practice*, ed 3, St Louis, 2010, Saunders.

11. WebMD Oral Health Guide: Available at www.webmd.com/oral-health/guide/oral-piercing: Accessed November 5, 2010.

12. Fontana M, Young DA, Wolff MS, Pitts NB, Longbottom C: Defining dental caries for 2010 and beyond, *Dent Clin North Am* 54(3):423–440, 2010.

13. Pimlott JF, Leakey JD: Assessment of the dentition. In Darby ML, Walsh MM, editors: *Dental hygiene theory and practice*, ed 3, St Louis, 2010, Saunders.

14. Hinrichs JE: The role of dental calculus and other predisposing factors. In Newman MG, Takei HH, Klokkevold PR, Carranza FA, editors: *Clinical periodontology*, ed 10, St Louis, 2006, Saunders.

15. Chan DCN, Chung AKH: Management of idiopathic subgingival amalgam hypertrophy—the common amalgam overhang, *Operat Dent* 34(6):753–758, 2009.

16. American Academy of Periodontology: Implications of Genetic Technology for the Management of Periodontal Diseases, *J Periodontol* 76:850–857, 2005.

17. American Academy of Periodontology: Parameter on occlusal traumatism in patients with chronic periodontitis, *J Periodontol* 71:873–875, 2000.

18. Friedewald VE, Kornman KS, Beck JD, et al: The American Journal of Cardiology and Journal of Periodontology Editors' Consensus: Periodontitis and Atherosclerotic Cardiovascular Disease, *J Periodontol* 80:1021–1032, 2009.

19. American Academy of Periodontology: Parameter on systemic conditions affected by periodontal diseases, *J Periodontol* 71:880–883, 2000.

20. Forrest JL: Introduction to the basics of evidence-based dentistry: Concepts and skills, *J Evid Based Dent Pract* 9(3):108–112, 2009.

21. Forrest JL, Miller SA: Translating evidence-based decision making into practice: EBDM concepts and finding the evidence, *J Evid Based Dent Pract* 9(2):59–72, 2009.

22. American Academy of Periodontology: Guidelines for periodontal therapy, *J Periodontol* 72:1624–1628, 2001.

23. Newman MG, Takei HH, Klokkevold PR, Carranza FA: *Clinical periodontology*, ed 11, St Louis, 2012, Saunders.

24. Merin RL: Supportive periodontal treatment. In Newman MG, Takei HH, Klokkevold PR, Carranza FA, editors: *Clinical periodontology*, ed 11, St Louis, 2012, Saunders.

25. Novak KF, Goodman SF, Takei HH: Determination of prognosis. In Newman MG, Takei HH, Klokkevold PR, Carranza FA, editors: *Clinical periodontology*, ed 10, St Louis, 2006, Saunders.

SUGGESTED READINGS

American Academy of Periodontology: Guidelines for the management of patients with periodontal diseases, *J Periodontol* 77(9):1607–1611, 2006.

Beemsterboer PL: *Ethics and law in dental hygiene*, ed 3, Philadelphia, 2010, Saunders.

Friedewald VE, Kornman KS, Beck JD, et al: The American Journal of Cardiology and Journal of Periodontology Editors' Consensus: Periodontitis and atherosclerotic cardiovascular disease, *J Periodontol* 80:1021–1032, 2009.

Featherstone J, Roth JR: Curing the silent epidemic: Caries management in the 21st century and beyond, *J Calif Dent Assoc* 35(10):681–685, 2007.

Featherstone J, Young DA, Domejean-Orliaguet S: Caries risk assessment in practice for age 6 though adult, *J Calif Dent Assoc* 35(10):703–713, 2007.

Forrest JL: Introduction to the basics of evidence-based dentistry: Concepts and skills, *J Evid Based Dent Pract* 9(3):108–112, 2009.

Forrest JL, Miller SA: Translating evidence-based decision making into practice: EBDM concepts and finding the evidence, *J Evid Based Dent Pract* 9(2):59–72, 2009.

Little JW, Miller C, Rhodus NL, Falace D: *Dental management of the medically compromised patient*, ed 7, St Louis, 2008, Mosby.

Malamed SF: *Medical emergencies in the dental office*, ed 6, St Louis, 2007, Mosby.

Mealey BL, Oates TW: Diabetes mellitus and periodontal diseases, *J Periodontol* 77:1289–1303, 2006.

Miller SA, Forrest JL: Translating evidence-based decision making into practice: Appraising and applying the evidence, *J Evid Based Dent Pract* 9(4):164–182, 2009.

Ramos-Gomez F, Crall J, Gansky S, et al: Caries risk assessment appropriate for the age 1 visit (infants and toddlers), *J Calif Dent Assoc* 35(10):687–702, 2007.

Wartenberg D, Thompson WD: Privacy versus public health: The impact of current confidentiality rules, *Am J Public Health* 100(3):407–412, 2010.

Wun E, Dym H: How to implement a HIPAA compliance plan into a practice, *Dent Clin North Am* 52(3):669–682, 2008.

CHAPTER 15 REVIEW QUESTIONS

Answers and Rationales to Chapter Review Questions are available on this text's accompanying Evolve site. See inside front cover for details.
Use Case A to answer questions 1 to 4.

e volve

CASE A

A 44-year old man presents as a new client for dental hygiene care. His medical history reveals type 2 diabetes, high blood pressure controlled with medication and a hip replacement. He reports no blood glucose monitoring and controls diabetes with diet and exercise. His last physical examination was last year. However, he is not sure of the examination results. He assumes everything is fine. You record his blood pressure reading at 150/102 mm Hg.

1. **Which of the following should be considered before implementing invasive dental hygiene care for this client?**
   a. Dental hygiene care can be implemented immediately without any considerations
   b. Dental hygiene care can be started immediately as long as the client consents to treatment
   c. Consult with client's physician to establish a definitive diagnosis of diabetes and level of control for diabetes and hypertension before initiating invasive dental hygiene care
   d. Appointments should be longer than normal to reduce the number of appointments needed and to reduce stress

2. **What is this client's ASA physical status classification?**
   a. PS1
   b. PS2
   c. PS3
   d. PS4

3. **What is the BEST course of action for the dental hygienist related to the blood pressure reading?**
   a. Recheck blood pressure in five minutes; if it is still elevated within that range, dismiss the client and seek immediate consultation with physician
   b. Recheck blood pressure at each appointment; if it is still within range for three consecutive appointments, refer to physician
   c. Recheck blood pressure in five minutes; if it is still elevated within that range, continue with noninvasive care only and consult with physician before dental hygiene therapy
   d. Recheck blood pressure in five minutes, and continue with dental hygiene care

4. **Which human need should be considered during the dental hygiene process of care?**
   a. Freedom from head and neck pain
   b. Protection from health risks
   c. Skin and mucous membrane integrity of head and neck
   d. Wholesome facial image

Use Case B to answer questions 5 to 11.

CASE B

A 25-year old female presents for dental hygiene care. Her records indicated that 10 months have lapsed since receiving dental hygiene care and she scheduled the appointment because her teeth are sensitive when she eats candy and her "gums" hurt when she brushes her teeth. She reports an arrhythmia but is not sure of the type or cause and irregularly takes the prescribed medication for its treatment. Her vital signs are within normal limits.

During the dental and periodontal assessment, you record generalized marginal gingival inflammation, generalized moderate interproximal subgingival calculus deposits, generalized bleeding on probing, with 2-4 mm probing depths. Existing restorations include teeth #14-MO, #4-MOD, #13-MO, #18-MO, and #19-B. Radiographs reveal no evidence of bone loss, proximal carious lesions on 29D, 30M, and 19M and restoration overhangs on #14M and #4D. She brushes once a day and does not use an interproximal cleaning aid.

5. **Which of the following conditions represents the MOST accurate periodontal disease classification?**
   a. Case type I - gingivitis
   b. Case type II – mild periodontitis
   c. Case type III – moderate periodontitis
   d. Case type IV – advanced periodontitis

6. **All of the following human need categories relates to the client's current conditions EXCEPT one. Which one is the EXCEPTION?**
   a. Protection from health risks
   b. Freedom from anxiety and stress
   c. Skin and mucous membrane integrity of head and neck
   d. Biologically sound and functional dentition

7. All of the following are related to the overhanging restorations EXCEPT one. Which one is the EXCEPTION?
   a. Increase bacterial plaque biofilm retention
   b. Restorations should be replaced
   c. Restorations are risk factors for periodontal disease
   d. Restorations are treated using margination procedures

8. Based on the oral assessment findings, what is the classification of caries risk for this client?
   a. Low risk
   b. Moderate risk
   c. High risk
   d. Not enough data to determine

9. The restoration on tooth #14 would be BEST classified as a:

a. Class I restoration
b. Class II restoration
c. Class III restoration
d. Class IV restoration

10. Based on the periodontal assessment, what is the BEST re-evaluation interval for this client?
    a. One to two weeks
    b. Four to six weeks
    c. Three to four months
    d. Six months to one year

11. What is the overall prognosis for this client after phase I therapy?
    a. Excellent
    b. Good
    c. Fair
    d. Poor

Use Case C to answer questions 12 and 13.

CASE C

A heavy tea drinker just purchased over-the-counter whitening strips to see if her discolored teeth could be whitened. She wants to know if using whitening strips is better than using the professional custom bleaching tray system at home. You want to provide an evidence-based answer (based on a search of the research literature).

12. Which of the following would be an example of a well-developed question to help narrow your research literature search?
    a. For clients with discolored teeth, are whitening strips the best method to increase whitening?
    b. Are whitening strips the best method to increase whitening?
    c. Are whitening strips more effective than custom tray bleaching systems?
    d. For clients with tooth discoloration from tea stain, are whitening strips more effective in increasing teeth whitening when compared with professional at-home custom tray bleaching?

13. Which type of study will provide the BEST evidence to answer the client's question?
    a. Case-control studies
    b. Randomized controlled clinical trials
    c. In vitro research
    d. Case reports

14. A dental hygienist records a client's blood pressure as 152/85 mm Hg. What blood pressure category is represented?
    a. Prehypertension
    b. Stage I hypertension
    c. Stage II hypertension
    d. Stage III hypertension

15. What phase of dental care focuses on periodontal surgery?
    a. Preliminary phase
    b. Phase I
    c. Phase II
    d. Phase III

16. The written care plan includes all of the following components EXCEPT one. Which one is the EXCEPTION?
    a. Appointment sequence for therapy to be provided
    b. Approximate time for each appointment
    c. Cost of each presented procedure
    d. Expected outcomes and limitations of care

17. All of following procedures, EXCEPT *one*, are required when localized bleeding on probing is noted during a four to six week re-evaluation appointment. Which one is the EXCEPTION?
    a. Determining presence of residual or new deposits
    b. Establishment of continued-care (recare) interval
    c. Evaluation of self-care practices
    d. Referral to physician

18. **Which is a correct statement regarding the assessment phase of care?**
    a. Includes the comprehensive collection, analysis, and permanent documentation of client data.
    b. Involves the collection of only subjective information
    c. Assessment data should be updated only during continued-care (recare) appointments
    d. Data should not be discussed with the client or appropriate health care providers

19. **When reviewing a health history, the client has indicated that he has allergies to kiwis, avocados, and bananas. To what condition is this client at risk?**
    a. Acute adrenal insufficiency
    b. Asthma
    c. Diabetes
    d. Latex allergy

20. **The American Academy of Periodontology (AAP) classification for advanced periodontitis is:**
    a. Case type I
    b. Case type II
    c. Case type III
    d. Case type IV

21. **Each of the following factors is considered when providing dental hygiene care for diabetic clients EXCEPT one. Which one is the EXCEPTION?**
    a. Cardiovascular conditions
    b. Continued-care (recare) interval
    c. Susceptibility to oral infection
    d. Rapid healing

22. **Individuals with stable angina pectoris, COPD and/or mild congestive heart failure are in which ASA physical status classification category?**
    a. PS1
    b. PS2
    c. PS3
    d. PS4

23. **What phase of the dental hygiene process of care immediately follows diagnosis?**
    a. Assessment
    b. Evaluation
    c. Implementation
    d. Planning

24. **All of the following are components of assessment, EXCEPT one. Which one is the EXCEPTION?**
    a. Health history
    b. Intraoral photographs
    c. Periodontal probing
    d. Self-care education

25. **After a comprehensive assessment, findings show chronic periodontitis with moderate bone loss, generalized pocket depths of 4 to 6 mm with bleeding, light subgingival biofilm and calculus on the maxillary arch and moderate to heavy subgingival biofilm and tenacious calculus on the mandibular arch. Based on these findings, what would be a realistic approach to NSPT for this client?**
    a. A 60-minute appointment consisting of oral self-care education and supragingival and subgingival debridement
    b. Two 60-minute appointments consisting of oral self-care education, debridement, and scaling and root planing
    c. Five 60- to 90-minute appointments consisting of oral self-care education, debridement, scaling and root planing, and re-evaluation
    d. Six 60- to 90-minute appointments consisting of oral self-care education, debridement, scaling and root planing, and re-evaluation

26. **When client-oriented goals are developed during the planning phase of care, to what do affective goals relate?**
    a. Increasing client's knowledge level about bacterial biofilm
    b. Influencing changes in beliefs and attitudes
    c. Providing information related to bacterial biofilm
    d. Modifying a toothbrushing method

27. **When reviewing a health history, the client has indicated that she urinates more than six times a day, is frequently thirsty, and her mouth is always dry. What condition manifests these characteristics?**
    a. Asthma
    b. Diabetes mellitus
    c. Hypertension
    d. Thyroid disease

28. **Which of the following conditions is indicated by yellow sclera of the eye?**
    a. Difficulty breathing
    b. Drug abuse
    c. Jaundice
    d. Medical emergency status

29. **What is the G.V. Black classification of dental caries and restorations located on the gingival buccal third of #18?**
    a. Class II
    b. Class III
    c. Class IV
    d. Class V

30. **A client presents with a type III overhang on an amalgam restoration. Which of the following statements related to this overhang is correct?**
    a. Covers less than one third of interproximal space
    b. Restoration indicated for replacement
    c. Indicated for a margination procedure
    d. Clinically not detectable

31. Each of the following represents standard client assessment information that is necessary for planning comprehensive dental hygiene care EXCEPT one. Which one is the EXCEPTION?
    a. Extraoral assessment
    b. Current self-care practices
    c. Dentition evaluation
    d. Fluoride varnish application

32. A 53-year-old client presents for a periodontal maintenance appointment. When developing a dental hygiene care plan, which of the following should be addressed first?
    a. Chlorhexidine stain on teeth
    b. Localized light plaque
    c. Pain on tooth #28
    d. Smoking habit

33. What is the BEST method for examining the mentalis muscle?
    a. Circular compression
    b. Digital palpation
    c. Indirect vision
    d. Auscultation

34. Which of the following is LEAST significant when determining the continued-care (recare) interval for periodontal maintenance therapy?
    a. Presence of light plaque, biofilm
    b. Elimination of pocket depths
    c. Bleeding on probing
    d. Cost of care

35. Assessment findings reveal that an 11-year-old client has deep pits and fissures, generalized areas of heavy plaque, marginal gingival inflammation, incipient carious lesions on teeth #3 and #14, #19 and #30. Given these findings, what would be the degree of caries risk?
    a. Low
    b. Moderate
    c. High
    d. No risk

36. The client is *not* able to correctly demonstrate the use of the floss threader with floss. The discrepancy in performance is MOST likely the result of which of the following?
    a. Management deficiency
    b. Motivation
    c. Readiness to learn
    d. Skills deficiency

37. To engage in effective verbal behaviors, which one of the following skills is necessary?
    a. Appropriate voice tone
    b. Gestures
    c. Paraphrasing
    d. Posture

38. All of the following are included in the case presentation, EXCEPT one. Which one is the EXCEPTION?
    a. Desired outcomes of treatment
    b. Alternative approaches to care
    c. Risks of all proposed therapeutic options
    d. Treatment outcome guarantee

39. Which of the following BEST identifies the procedure that is immediately followed after a client declines a component of the dental hygiene care plan?
    a. Alternative approaches to care are suggested
    b. Outcomes of therapy are explained
    c. Informed refusal form is completed
    d. Client's right to decline care is clarified

40. What would be a reasonable prognosis for a client with chronic periodontitis and moderate bone loss with localized areas of grade II furcation involvements, improvable oral self-care methods, and irregular continued-care (recare) intervals?
    a. Excellent
    b. Good
    c. Fair
    d. Poor

41. Failure to refer a client to a medical professional when indicated constitutes which one of the following issues?
    a. Ethical
    b. Legal
    c. Safety
    d. Breach of contract

42. When implementing a tobacco cessation program into practice, the second step is which of the following?
    a. Ask
    b. Advise
    c. Assist
    d. Arrange

43. When providing dental hygiene care, all of the following relate to safe practice issues EXCEPT one. Which one is the EXCEPTION?
    a. Failure to obtain written informed consent
    b. Failure to provide comprehensive care
    c. Failure to follow infection-control protocol
    d. Failure to use proper instrumentation during the provision of dental hygiene care

44. What is a grade III furcation involvement?
a. Exposure of furcation with bone remaining between roots
b. Complete loss of bone between roots
c. Loss of some bone between roots
d. Severe bone loss and furcation are clearly visible

45. To determine a care plan that is BEST for a client, which one of the following actions should be addressed first?
a. Periodontal debridement for the entire mouth
b. Consultation and treatment for areas of pain
c. Tobacco cessation counseling
d. Consultation for periodontal surgery

46. When reviewing the health history, the client indicates that he has a persistent cough that is nonproductive, difficulty breathing, and night sweats. What condition is manifested by these characteristics?
a. Acute adrenal insufficiency
b. Asthma
c. Tuberculosis
d. Common cold

47. Which of the following conditions is commonly related to a nutritional deficiency?
a. Black hairy tongue
b. Burning tongue
c. Geographic tongue
d. Macroglossia

48. The term *prognosis* refers specifically to which factor?
a. Diagnosis
b. Care planning
c. Evaluation
d. Prediction

49. What recare interval is recommended for a client who has maintained good results for the first year following routine nonsurgical periodontal therapy, but displays localized pockets?
a. One to two months
b. Three to four months
c. Four to six months
d. Six months

50. The submental glands are BEST examined using which type of palpation?
a. Bilateral digital
b. Circular compression
c. Digital palpation
d. Auscultation

51. Which of the following conditions require prophylactic antibiotic premedication for dental hygiene care?
a. Rheumatic heart disease
b. Functional heart murmur
c. Prosthetic heart valve
d. Mitral valve prolapse with regurgitation

Strategies for Oral Health Promotion and Disease Prevention and Control

M. Anjum Shah

The promotion of oral health and the prevention of oral diseases and disease progression are the focus of dental hygiene practice. As an educator and provider of preventive and therapeutic services, the dental hygienist must use evidence-based strategies and interventions that support prevention-oriented health care. Because the success of preventive oral health programs depends on the client's self-care behaviors, the dental hygienist must ensure client adherence to appropriate self-care regimens. This chapter focuses on the dental hygienist's role as a facilitator of client oral health behaviors and as a provider of educational services for health promotion and oral disease prevention and control.

GENERAL CONSIDERATIONS

Dental Hygiene Process of Care[1,2]

See Chapter 15.
- **A.** Dental hygiene practice is based on a process of care that involves the steps of assessment, diagnosis, planning, implementation, and evaluation
- **B.** Inherent in the process model is a continuum of care that supports a logical system of determining a client's health and disease status and selecting appropriate interventions
- **C.** The dental hygiene process is integrated into the client's comprehensive dental diagnosis and oral health care plan

ORAL HEALTH EDUCATION

Basic Concepts

- **A.** Initiation and progression of dental diseases depend on the interaction of host, agent, and environmental factors; thus, prevention and control of these diseases require attention to all primary and modifying factors in each category
- **B.** Dental caries and the inflammatory periodontal diseases are complex disease states that require the colonization by specific pathogenic bacteria in dental plaque biofilm; none will occur in the absence of pathogenic bacteria in biofilm; thus, the control of plaque biofilm is essential in any oral disease prevention program
- **C.** In dentistry, the emphasis is to prevent disease, maintain oral health, and halt disease progression
- **D.** Effective preventive programs identify active disease and assess disease risk; clients at high risk for dental caries, periodontal disease, and oral lesions require multiple preventive strategies applied frequently and aggressively (see the sections on "Periodontal disease risk factors" in Chapter 14 and "Caries risk factors" in Chapter 15; see also Table 15-6)
- **E.** The prevention of oral diseases requires the participation of clients with adequate knowledge of the disease process and personal level of risk, sufficiently developed skills in implementing oral care procedures, and the motivation to practice preventive behaviors over time to decrease the level of risk
- **F.** Many strategies can facilitate changes in the health behaviors of clients; a grasp of the basic concepts underlying educational, motivational, and behavioral theory is necessary to understand the variables influencing a person's oral health beliefs, attitudes, values, and behaviors
- **G.** Educating clients in effective oral care practices follows the process-of-care model

Appointment Sequencing

A. Instructions for the control of dental plaque biofilm are given to the client before any treatment is instituted
  1. Clients will see positive changes from their actions (limited soft tissue changes may occur before debridement of tooth surfaces)
  2. Improved gingival health can result from improved toothbrushing even in the presence of calculus
  3. Clients will recognize the primary importance of self-care
B. Biofilm control instructions should be given to the client throughout dental and dental hygiene care
  1. Clients need time to practice dental hygiene
  2. Clients need time to progress through the stages involved in learning and habituation
  3. Evaluation and modifications can occur over time
  4. Tissue changes can be demonstrated effectively when treatment and dental plaque biofilm control are integrated

Stages in Making a Commitment to a New Behavior

Learning-Ladder or Decision-Making Continuum
A. One approach to mastering the behavior of dental plaque biofilm control is based on the concept that humans learn in a series of sequential steps, referred to as the *learning-ladder continuum* or the *decision-making continuum*[2]
B. The dental hygienist first determines the client's entry level on the ladder and then plans for the client's moving up the steps in sequence
C. Steps in the process
  1. Unawareness or ignorance—client lacks information or has incorrect information about the problem; unmet human need (deficit) in conceptualization and problem solving
  2. Awareness—the client knows a problem exists or may occur but does not act on this knowledge; unmet human need (deficit) in responsibility for oral health
  3. Self-interest—the client recognizes the problem and indicates a tentative inclination toward action
  4. Involvement—the client's attitudes and feelings are affected, and the desire for additional knowledge increases
  5. Action—new behaviors directed toward solving problem are instituted by the client

6. Habit or commitment—new behaviors are practiced over a period and eventually become a lifestyle change

Trans-theoretical Model[3]

A. Conceptualizes behavior change through a series of steps; progression through the steps is dependent on the balance of the advantages and disadvantages of the decision
B. Provides a framework to determine and select appropriate interventions to assist clients in improving their health behaviors
C. Stages of change include:
  1. Precontemplation—the client has no intention of making a change within the next 6 months
  2. Contemplation—the client intends to make a change within the next 6 months
  3. Preparation—the client intends to make a change within the next 30 days and has taken some behavioral steps in this direction
  4. Action—the client has practiced changed behaviors for less than 6 months
  5. Maintenance—the client has practiced changed behaviors for more than 6 months

Learning Domains

A. To be considered successful, disease-control education must result in behavioral changes; once a client's learning needs have been assessed, a plan for teaching and learning can be designed
B. Three domains of learning have been classified in a hierarchy and are used to specify the learning objectives:
  1. Cognitive domain—concerned with knowledge outcomes and the client's intellectual abilities and skills; the major hierarchical steps are knowledge, comprehension, application, analysis, synthesis, and evaluation
  2. Affective domain—concerned with the client's attitudes, interests, appreciation, and modes of interest; the major hierarchical steps are receiving, responding, valuing, organizing, and characterizing
  3. Psychomotor domain—concerned with the client's technical or motor skills; the major hierarchical steps are perception set, guided response, mechanism, complex overt response, adaptation, and organization

Instructional Principles

See Table 19-14 for dental management considerations with clients who have special needs.

A. Effective teaching involves the direction and facilitation of learning to help make positive changes in a person's behaviors

B. To maximize learning, the following principles apply to the design of an educational plan:

1. Small step size—present only what person can assimilate in one session; provide conceptual or factual information when the "need to know" is evident
2. Active participation—provide time and opportunity for the person to ask questions; offer suggestions and monitor the practicing of new skills to enhance learning and retention
3. Immediate feedback—provide the learner with early and frequent information regarding progress; make suggestions for improvement, and use positive reinforcement to support and encourage learning
4. Self-pacing—recognize that each person will progress at a different pace; recognize the learner's needs, and establish an instructional pace tailored to each client

C. Visual aids enhance verbal instructions

1. Use of visual aids available in print, video, internet, or DVD can enhance client comprehension of oral hygiene instructions
2. Demonstration of dental plaque biofilm control techniques on models before intraoral demonstration may be helpful
3. Written instructions and illustrated pamphlets reinforce in-office instructions
4. Clients can access consumer health information from the Internet
5. Use of an intraoral camera that projects images on a monitor enables the client to see the conditions in his or her own mouth

Human Behavior Principles

A. Values

1. Values form the basis for behaviors
2. Clients come to the dental hygienist with existing values
3. Conflicts between clients' existing values and those values that support and enable preventive oral health care practices must be recognized and resolved
4. Clients who have value systems that support preventive health behaviors will adopt new behaviors that fit readily into their existing value system

B. Motivation

1. Defined as a desire to fulfill an unmet human need (deficit); an inner force that causes a person to act
2. May be internally or externally generated
   a. Internally generated motivation focuses on one's own perceived needs; generally longer lasting
   b. Externally generated motivation is based on offers of reward or punishment; generally of shorter duration

C. Motivation theories—locus of control

1. Internal locus of control—clients feel that they have control over their own outcomes and that their behavior will make a difference; they are most likely to adopt preventive health behaviors
2. External locus of control—clients feel that the outcomes are out of their control and that whatever they do will not affect the outcomes; they are less likely to change behaviors and rely more on the dental professional to take care of their problems

D. Attribution

1. Involves explanations given for performance; influences client's feelings about himself or herself
2. The success or failure at performing a behavior is influenced by the client's thoughts[1]
3. Self-efficacy—the client's level of self-confidence affects his or her belief in the success of performing a behavior

PREVENTION-ORIENTED HEALTH MODELS

Health Belief Model

A. Based on the concept that one's beliefs direct behavior; the model is used to explain and predict health behaviors and acceptance of health recommendations; the emphasis is on the perceived world of a client, which may differ from objective reality

B. Components

1. Susceptibility—clients must believe that they are susceptible to a particular disease or condition
2. Severity—clients must believe that if they get the particular disease or condition, the consequences will be serious
3. Asymptomatic nature of disease—clients must believe that a disease may be present without their being fully aware of it
4. Benefit of behavior change—clients must believe that effective means of preventing or controlling

the potential or current problem exist and that action on their part will produce positive results

C. Cues to action—once these beliefs have been accepted, the client will act on them, when necessary; the stronger the beliefs, the greater is the potential that appropriate action will occur

Agent–Host–Environment Theory

A. Theory that disease is result of an imbalance in one or all three factors, that is, agent, host, environment

B. Factors
1. Primary—aimed at preventing disease or injury; health promotion activities (such as biofilm control) and specific protection (such as dental sealants and mouth protectors)
2. Secondary—involves early detection and treatment of disease; interventions—such as oral cancer screening programs and regular self-examinations—are designed to stop or minimize the progression of disease in the early stages
3. Tertiary—interventions that prevent disability, restore function, or prevent further destruction of tissues (hard or soft), for example, periodontal or restorative therapies

Maslow's Hierarchy of Needs

A. Theory about human nature that is used to explain the motivational process; Maslow suggested that inner forces (needs) drive a person to action; he classified needs in a pyramid according to their importance to the client, his or her ability to motivate self, and the importance placed on the needs being satisfied; only when a client's lower needs are met will the client become concerned about higher-level needs; once the needs have been met, they no longer function as motivators (Figure 16-1)

B. Hierarchy of needs
1. Physiologic—survival needs are the most powerful and must be met before any others; include the components necessary for body homeostasis, such as food, water, oxygen, sleep, temperature regulation, and sex
2. Security and safety—these needs are required for protection against physical or psychological damage and are more cognitive than physiologic in nature; include shelter, a job for economic self-sufficiency, and a well-organized and stable environment
3. Social—once the physiologic and security needs have been met, then the needs for love and social belonging become prime motivators; include belonging to a group and having the chance to give and receive friendship and love

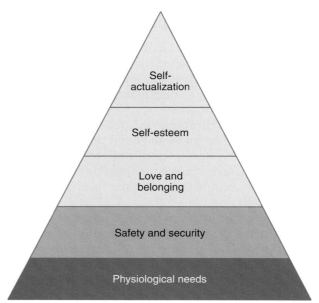

FIGURE 16-1 Maslow's hierarchy of needs. *(From Darby ML, Walsh MM:* Dental hygiene theory and practice, *ed 3, St Philadelphia, 2010, Saunders. Modified from Potter PA, Perry AG:* Fundamentals of nursing, *ed 7, St Louis, 2009, Mosby.)*

4. Esteem or ego—of the two categories of needs that exist at this level, one involves feelings of worth, such as competence, achievement, mastery, and independence; the other involves gaining the esteem of others and triggers learning and the desire to acquire status, power, and higher-level skills
5. Self-actualization or self-realization—these needs drive the client to reach the very top of his or her field; based on positive actions toward development, growth, and self-enhancement

C. Application—assessment of a client's level of needs may aid in the identification of motivational factors that can be targeted for enhancing behavior change

Factors Influencing Client Adherence to Preventive Regimen

A. Client–clinician interaction
1. The quality of communication between the client and the hygienist is critical to achieving client adherence
2. Clients must be encouraged to share the responsibility for their oral health
3. Authoritarian or autocratic verbal and nonverbal messages from the dental hygienist will be less effective than messages that allow for genuine client involvement and assumption of responsibility

4. The dental hygienist must recognize that established behaviors are hard to change because they generally satisfy needs; new behaviors are adopted slowly

B. Client's support systems

 1. Client's lifestyle and significant others influence his or her willingness and ability to carry out self-care regimens

 2. Support systems are important, especially with children and clients with disabilities, who must depend on caregivers to carry out home-care practices

C. Complexity of therapy

 1. Clients must agree that time and effort required to practice preventive behaviors are reasonable

 2. Changes in basic lifestyle are harder to achieve than modest modifications to existing behaviors

 3. Product cost and availability affect adherence to oral self-care regimens

Prevention Principles for Children

A. Proactive counseling of parents about anticipated developmental changes in their children

B. Information provided to parents or caregivers in appropriate-sized "bites" on the basis of the developmental milestone anticipated in their children

C. Guidance is based on the rationale that people are ready to apply information that is most relevant to them and their children

D. Box 16-1 provides suggestions for obtaining compliance from pediatric clients

DENTAL PLAQUE BIOFILM DETECTION

General Considerations

A. Because dental plaque biofilm is relatively invisible and tooth surfaces are not easily accessed, teaching

---

BOX 16-1 Tips for Dental Hygienists Working with Children

When a child visits your practice, your priority is to create a positive dental experience. The child is more important than his or her teeth. Incorporating the ideas from this fact sheet as you interact with children will help them become both comfortable and compliant.

Make the reception area a friendly, colorful place. Include toys, games, and videos. Books about visiting a dental office and a doll dressed as an oral health care provider will help children discuss any fears they may have

Each staff member should greet the child by name in a friendly and welcoming manner. Bend down or squat so that you are at the level of the child's head, and listen to what he or she has to say

The treatment room should be decorated in a way that is visually assessable and appealing to children. Show the child the instruments you will be using and explain how they are used. Make everything that looks unfamiliar look friendly. For example, you might draw friendly faces on the masks used for demonstration; or, as some practitioners like to, call the suction instrument "Mr. Thirsty." Demonstrate the buttons on the chair and how the chair moves up and down, but do not put the chair back if doing so makes the child nervous

Allow the parent into the treatment area if the child so desires, especially for the first visit. Both you and the room will look less frightening with a familiar person present

Explain exactly what you are going to do during the appointment. Use age-appropriate terms to explain why it is important that teeth be kept healthy

Turn the appointment into a game. For example, count eyes, ears, and fingers before moving on to counting teeth. Always give the child a choice of flavors. Write down preferences so that you will have all of the child's favorites ready for the next visit. If the light shines in the child's eyes, produce a pair of sunglasses and say how "cool" he or she looks.

Use a new toothbrush during the brushing lesson. Apply fluoride varnish. Let the child know that you are in control with a fast solution to every problem.

Praise the good, but do not criticize the bad. A child may take "these teeth don't look so good" very personally and feel that he or she has done something wrong. Concentrate on teaching the right way to take care of teeth

Do not use tricks or lies; keep your promises. If you say "Just let me do one more thing," do just one more thing and then let the child go. If the child will not cooperate, try again another day

When the visit is over, let the child pick a treat from a "treasure box." Praise good behavior, and let the child give the parent(s) the "good news" about his or her teeth

Snap a picture of the child's sparkling smile and create a gallery of photos in the office. Seeing his or her own picture is something a child looks forward to at the next appointment

Modified from American Dental Hygienists' Association: Tips for dental hygienists working with kids *[members only section, requires registration and password].*

clients dental disease-control skills can be challenging

B. Agents that make biofilm visible supragingivally can enhance the teaching–learning process by:

1. Demonstrating a relationship between the presence of plaque biofilm and the clinical signs of disease

2. Guiding the development of skills that are applied before biofilm removal

3. Allowing evaluation of the effectiveness of skills that are applied after biofilm removal

4. Promoting self-evaluation of skills that are applied by the client at home

C. The presence of subgingival plaque biofilm cannot be demonstrated by using disclosing agents

D. The plan for disease-control education should include establishing the associations among the presence of plaque, clinical signs of disease such as bleeding, the presence of risk factors, and possible links to systemic disease

E. Subgingival biofilm detection by the client is best managed when the client has an understanding of the gingival sulcus (or pocket) and of the clinical changes that occur with ineffective plaque biofilm removal

Disclosing Agents

A. Erythrosin (FD&C Red No. 3 or No. 28)

1. A red dye available in tablet or solution form; most widely used agent

2. Can be dissolved into a solution or chewed to dissolve in mouth

3. Tends to stain soft tissues, making post-application evaluation of gingiva difficult

B. Fluorescein dye (FD&C Yellow No. 8)

1. Plaque biofilm stained with sodium fluorescein; visible only with use of an ultraviolet light source

2. More expensive to use but has the advantage of not interfering with gingival assessment or leaving a visible stain on oral tissues

C. Two-tone dyes (FD&C Red No. 3 and Green No. 3)

1. Combination solution; has the advantage of differentiating mature plaque biofilm (stains blue) from new plaque biofilm (stains red)

2. Discloses plaque biofilm but not gingival tissues

Application Methods for Disclosing Agents

A. Solutions are applied with a cotton swab; the tablets are chewed and swished; the client is instructed to rinse and expectorate; single-unit doses are available

B. The agents do not stain biofilm-free tooth surfaces unless roughness (i.e., decalcification, pitting) is present

C. Precautions

1. Avoid staining restorative materials that may be susceptible to permanent discoloration

2. Dispense the solution into a disposable cup; do not contaminate the solution by introducing applicators into the storage container bottle

3. Erythrosin solutions contain alcohol, which can evaporate over time and alter the concentration of the solution (verify that the client is not an alcoholic, recovering alcoholic, or on Antabuse)

4. To avoid staining the lips, apply a light coat of nonpetroleum or water-based lubricant (e.g., K-Y jelly)

5. Avoid using the agent before application of a dental sealant

6. Avoid any risk of staining clothing, that is, provide appropriate protective drapes to the client, and use small amounts of the solution

Plaque and Gingival Indices

Recording a plaque score at consecutive appointments enables the client to see progress (see Table 20-6 for information on indices and computing indices).

MECHANICAL PLAQUE BIOFILM CONTROL ON FACIAL, LINGUAL, AND OCCLUSAL TOOTH SURFACES

Basic Concepts

A. Microbial population of dental plaque biofilm contributes to the initiation of dental caries and periodontal diseases

B. Mechanical disruption of organized plaque biofilm colonies, both supragingivally and subgingivally, is effective and widely used to prevent and control dental diseases

C. Toothbrushing—most widely used and effective means of controlling plaque biofilm on the facial, lingual, and occlusal surfaces of teeth

D. Toothbrushes are available in many shapes, sizes, and textures; new designs based on in vivo and in vitro studies, manufacturers' claims of superior biofilm control, and consumer appeal are being marketed

E. The selection of the type of toothbrush should be based on the client's needs, oral characteristics, and preferences

F. Special attention to subgingival plaque biofilm control in areas >3 mm is essential; toothbrushes are generally ineffective in depths >3 mm and in furca; additional tools must be selected

G. Toothbrushes should be replaced after 2 to 3 months of use and when filaments become bent or splayed

H. Clients who are immunosuppressed, debilitated, or diagnosed with a known infection and those about to undergo surgery should disinfect their toothbrushes or use disposable ones

Manual Toothbrushes

A. Description
   1. Parts include the handle, head, and shank; the head, or the working end, holds clusters of bristles (tufts) in a pattern
   2. Design variables
      a. Handle can be in the same plane with the head or offset at an angle
      b. The length varies, with adult brushes being longer than those recommended for children
      c. Tuft placement can be in 2 to 4 rows, with 5 to 12 tufts per row; bristles may be of varying lengths
      d. The brushing planes can be even, flat, or uneven
      e. Many brushes have contoured or thick handles, angled shanks, and flexible heads
   3. Bristle characteristics
      a. Natural bristles come from hog or boar hairs and are hollow and nonuniform in diameter, texture, or durability; hollow bristles may harbor bacteria and absorb water, making them soft and soggy with repeated use; these are seldom used today because of their disadvantages
      b. Nylon bristles, or filaments, are manufactured for uniformity in texture, shape, and size; nonabsorbent nylon bristles are easily cleaned, dry quickly, and are more durable than natural bristles
      c. Relative stiffness—the diameter and length of filaments determine whether the brush will be ranked hard, medium, soft, or extra-soft; variations exist among products from different manufacturers
      d. The filament ends (tips) can be cut flat or polished to be rounded
B. Desirable characteristics of toothbrushes
   1. Conform to individual requirements in size, shape, and texture
   2. Easily and efficiently manipulated
   3. Readily cleaned and aerated
   4. Impervious to moisture
   5. Durable and inexpensive
   6. Flexible and soft
   7. Contain rounded-end filaments
C. Factors in toothbrush selection and recommendations
   1. Oral health status
   2. Recommended method of brushing
   3. Periodontal status
   4. Client's age, dexterity, and ability to use the brush in an effective, nontraumatic manner
   5. Client's preference and motivation
   6. Unique, special needs of the client (e.g., those with arthritis, Parkinson's disease; see Chapter 19)
D. Soft, multiple-tufted brushes are generally recommended on the basis of their usefulness in both supragingival and subgingival plaque disruption with minimal likelihood of trauma to soft and hard tissues; many toothbrushes have received the American Dental Association (ADA) Seal of Acceptance, the Canadian Dental Association (CDA) Seal of Recognition, or both[4]

Manual Toothbrushing Methods

Although the Bass (sulcular) method is widely recognized as being the most effective and most often recommended, it is helpful to know all the major methods. The method selected should disrupt both supragingival and subgingival plaque biofilm to the extent possible. The issue of gingival stimulation is of less importance than plaque control. Although a horizontal scrub technique is often used, it is not recommended because of potential trauma to hard and soft tissues.

In all of the following methods, the handle is placed parallel to the occlusal plane for posterior (facial and lingual) and anterior facial surfaces and parallel to the long axis of the tooth (using the toe of the brush) for anterior lingual surfaces. Occlusal surfaces are cleaned with a scrubbing motion.

A. Bass or sulcular brushing method
   1. Technique—direct the bristles into the sulcus at a 45-degree angle to the long axis of the tooth; vibrate the bristles in a short back-and-forth motion
   2. Indications—plaque biofilm disruption at and under the gingival margin; good gingival stimulation; widely recognized as an effective control technique
B. Stillman's method
   1. Technique—position the bristles on the attached gingiva and direct them apically at a 45-degree angle to the long axis of the tooth; use firm, gentle vibration holding the bristles stationary
   2. Indication—gingival stimulation

C. Roll method
1. Technique—place the sides of the bristles on the attached gingiva and direct them apically; turn the wrist to roll or sweep the bristles over the gingiva and the tooth
2. Indications—facial and lingual tooth surfaces; often combined with the Bass, Charters', or Stillman's method
D. Charters' method
1. Technique—position the bristle tips toward the occlusal surfaces at a 45-degree angle to the long axis of the tooth; move the bristles in a short back-and-forth motion
2. Indications—cleaning orthodontic appliances, fixed appliances; following periodontal surgery when sulcular brushing must be avoided to allow wound healing
E. Fones (circular) method
1. Technique—with upper and lower teeth together, place the bristles perpendicular to the buccal tooth surfaces; use a wide circular motion to cover the gingiva and tooth surfaces of both arches; on the lingual surfaces, use smaller circles to brush each arch separately
2. Indications—when technique must be easy to learn and execute; can be mastered by children
F. Combination methods
1. Modified-Bass method—combination of Bass and roll methods
2. Modified-Stillman's method—combination of Stillman's and roll methods
G. Leonard (vertical) method
1. Technique—with teeth in the edge-to-edge position, place the toothbrush bristles perpendicular to teeth; apply a vigorous up-and-down stroke with gentle pressure, followed by a slight circular motion or rotation as the toothbrush strikes the gingival margin; in the embrasure space, apply pressure that is sufficient to force the bristles into the space without damaging the gingiva
2. Indication—not recommended

Power Toothbrushes

A. General description
1. Brush heads contain bundles of bristles arranged on a variety of brush head shapes; toothbrushes with different brush head shapes are available on the market
2. The bristles can have flat, bi-level, or multi-level trims; designed for occlusal and smooth surfaces or interdental proximal surface cleaning
3. The handles are larger than those of manual brushes

4. Several power toothbrushes have the ADA Seal of Acceptance or the CDA Seal of Recognition for reduction of plaque biofilm and gingivitis[4]
5. Power toothbrushes move in directions and at speeds unattainable by manual toothbrushes
6. Power toothbrushes have timers to ensure adequate brushing duration and a pressure sensor to monitor the force applied on the toothbrushes
B. Power source—electric rechargeable handle-base; replaceable, rechargeable, and nonreplaceable batteries
C. Motion—distinctly different stroke movement from the motion of manual toothbrushes; motions occur in one of the following directions:
1. Side-to-side, arcuate, or back-and-forth
2. Oscillating or rotating
3. Rotating or counter-rotating
4. High-frequency pulsating, combined with an oscillating or rotating movement
5. Sonic vibratory motion from low-frequency acoustic energy
D. Indications for use—recommended for all clients because of the effectiveness of power toothbrushes in removing plaque biofilm and reducing gingivitis; especially valuable to those who:
1. Lack the manual dexterity, discipline, or motivation to master an effective manual toothbrushing technique, especially children and adolescents who are physically and mentally challenged (recommended to the caregivers who may be doing the toothbrushing for these children and adolescents)
2. Have orthodontic appliances or implants
3. Prefer a power toothbrush
4. Have extrinsic dental stain or are prone to dental stain
5. Are aggressive brushers, or exhibit abrasion, erosion, abfraction, or gingival recession
6. Have periodontal disease or are undergoing periodontal maintenance therapy

Power Toothbrushing Methods

A. Client variables and manufacturer instructions guide the need for individualized modifications
B. General principles
1. Follow the manufacturer's instructions for use and care
2. Select a low-abrasive dentifrice to avoid tooth abrasion
3. Apply a small amount of dentifrice over teeth to minimize spatter

4. Position the bristles on teeth before activating the power toothbrush; vary positions and brush head, as needed, to access tooth surfaces
5. Monitor the pressure applied to avoid trauma to soft and hard tissues
6. Replace the brush head, as necessary

Comparison of Power Toothbrushes and Manual Toothbrushes: Reported Effectiveness[2,4–7]

A. Power toothbrushes consistently remove more plaque biofilm than do manual brushes
B. Several brands carry the ADA Seal of Acceptance or the CDA Seal of Recognition for biofilm removal and reduction in gingivitis
C. Power toothbrushes reduce plaque biofilm and gingivitis better than the manual toothbrush can, with or without floss[7]

Single-Tufted Brushes

A. Design—flat or tapered
B. Suggested use—to remove plaque biofilm from surfaces not accessible with larger brushes, including areas of crowded or malpositioned teeth, distal surfaces of terminal molars, around pontics, in furcations, and on lingual surfaces of molars; also used on type II or III embrasure (depending on design) and fixed dental prosthesis[1]
C. Technique—tufts are positioned at or just under the gingival margin, and a sulcular brushing stroke is used; placement of the tapered angled side against teeth allows for the insertion of the bristles several millimeters subgingivally

Factors in Toothbrushing Effectiveness

A. Sequence
   1. A methodical, systematic approach enhances effectiveness
   2. Suggested sequence: begin systematic, overlapping strokes at the facial aspect of the maxillary right or left terminal tooth; continue around the arch to the terminal tooth on the opposite side; switch to the lingual aspect, and begin working back toward the starting side; use the same pattern for the mandible, and then brush the occlusal surfaces
B. Duration
   1. Monitor the brushing time in an area by counting strokes or seconds after each time the brush is moved

2. The total manual brushing time of 2 minutes is often recommended; the average brushing time is ≤1 minute; some power toothbrushes have built-in 2-minute timers to encourage clients to brush for longer duration[1]
C. Frequency
   1. Thorough removal of plaque biofilm every day is the goal of client self-care and for maintenance of oral health
   2. Toothbrushing should be performed twice daily; however, the frequency should be increased when gingival or periodontal conditions warrant it or when caries risk is high
   3. Thoroughness in daily brushing is more important than frequency
   4. Emphasis should be placed on effective oral cleaning, not just toothbrushing
D. Skill level
   1. Careful attention should be given to evaluating skill development in all components of toothbrush manipulation, including grasp, placement, activation, wrist movement, and amount of pressure applied
   2. Control of toothbrush placement and motion is essential for effectiveness

Improper Toothbrushing

A. Need to assess
   1. Improper toothbrushing—may result from lack of education in proper technique, incorrect application following instruction, or long-established habits
   2. The dental hygienist should evaluate the client's toothbrushing technique and monitor the conditions of hard and soft tissues at each continued-care visit
   3. Faulty placement, overly vigorous motion or pressure, and use of a brush with frayed, splayed, or broken bristles can lead to unwanted consequences
B. Acute consequences—soft tissue injuries such as denuded attached gingiva, lesions that appear "punched out" and red, and clusters of small ulcerations at the gingival margin
C. Chronic consequences
   1. Soft tissue—loss of gingival tissue or change in contour; malpositioned or prominent teeth and an inadequate band of attached gingiva are predisposing factors
   2. Hard tissue—loss of tooth structure and creation of a wedge-shaped defect at the cervical third of tooth (noncarious cervical lesion); malpositioned or prominent teeth may contribute to the problem; brushing without toothpaste is recommended in cervical abraded

areas to avoid additional loss of tooth structure (fluoride should be applied by other means)[1]

Toothbrush Maintenance

A. Toothbrushes should be rinsed clean after each use and then allowed to air-dry in the upright position

B. Toothbrushes should be replaced when the bristles splay or lose resiliency; generally, should not be used longer than 2 to 3 months

C. Some toothbrushes have color-indicator bristles to alert the user about replacement time

D. After an acute illness and an oral infection, toothbrushes should be replaced or disinfected with 0.12% chlorhexidine gluconate; power toothbrushes with a built-in sanitizer unit help control toothbrush contamination[1]

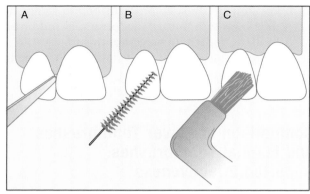

FIGURE 16-2 Interproximal embrasure types and corresponding interdental cleansers. **A,** Type I—no gingival recession: dental floss. **B,** Type II—moderate papillary recession: interdental brush. **C,** Type III—complete loss of papillae: uni-tufted brush. *(From Darby ML, Walsh MM: Dental hygiene theory and practice, ed 3, St Louis, 2010, Saunders. Modified from Newman MG, Takei H, Klokkevold PR, Carranza FA: Carranza's Clinical Periodontology, ed 11, St Louis, 2012, Saunders.)*

INTERDENTAL PLAQUE BIOFILM CONTROL

Basic Concepts

A. Toothbrushes—effective in removing plaque biofilm from facial, lingual, and occlusal surfaces of teeth; relatively ineffective on proximal surfaces

B. Interdental cleaning devices—designed for access to interproximal surfaces; essential for effective control of plaque biofilm

C. Interdental col area—protected area that harbors microorganisms that can initiate disease

D. Anatomy of the interdental area—significant factor in both disease initiation and control

Factors to Consider When Selecting Interdental Cleaning Methods

A. Soft-tissue variables include the level of health or disease and the position and architecture of the gingiva and attachment (Figure 16-2); three types of embrasures[1]
1. Type I embrasures are occupied by interdental papillae
2. Type II embrasures have slight to moderate recession of interdental papillae
3. Type III embrasures have extensive recession or complete loss of interdental papillae

B. Hard tissue variables include tooth position, root anatomy, and status of restorations or prostheses

C. Client variables include level of manual dexterity, adherence, skill development, and personal preferences

Flosses

A. Dental floss—most frequently recommended device for interdental cleaning of type I embrasures[1] (Figure 16-3)

B. Flossing may precede or follow brushing in a home-care regimen

C. As gingival recession increases, as in type II and type III embrasures, the effectiveness of flossing decreases; other interdental plaque-control aids should be selected

D. Agents to enhance color, taste, and therapeutic value have been incorporated into the dental floss; evidence to confirm the effectiveness of the addition of fluoride and whitening agents is limited

E. Floss type
1. Unwaxed—unbound filaments are spread on the tooth and have more friction for cleaning; filaments hold plaque and debris for easier removal; the floss slips through contacts more easily
2. Waxed—resists tearing and shredding on faulty restorations or when moved through very tight contacts; limited research is available on the efficacy of the waxed floss in biofilm removal compared with the unwaxed floss[8]
3. Polytetrafluoroethylene (PTFE) floss—slides through contacts easily; does not fray
4. Tape or ribbon—wider, flatter type of floss that covers a broad surface
5. Variable diameter—a tufted segment combined with the floss acts like a brush against the proximal surfaces; accesses concavities and irregular surfaces; recommended for type II or III embrasures

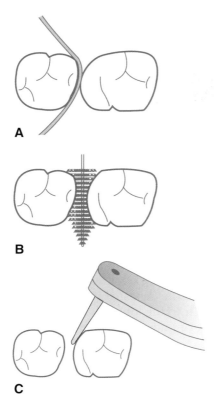

FIGURE 16-3 Use of interdental plaque biofilm control devices. **A,** Dental floss. **B,** Interdental brush. **C,** Toothpick in holder. *(From Darby ML, Walsh MM: Dental hygiene theory and practice, ed 3, St Louis, 2010, Saunders.)*

6. Braided nylon—for use with dental implants; has a stiff nylon end for threading under implant prostheses

Flossing Technique

A. Floss length—varies with holding technique; 10 to 15 inches when forming a loop; 12 to 24 inches when wrapping around fingers
B. Holding technique
  1. Ends may be tied together to form a loop, wrapped around middle fingers, or tucked into the palm of the hand
  2. With equal tension in both hands, grasp with both thumbs or with the thumb and the forefinger for use on the maxilla or with both forefingers for use on the mandible; leave one-inch to two-inch length between fingers
C. Insertion
  1. Approach the embrasure space obliquely, and ease the floss past the contact with a back-and-forth motion
  2. Snapping through contact can cause tissue injury

D. Adaptation and stroke
  1. Position fingers such that the floss wraps securely against the proximal surface and forms a "C" shape against the tooth
  2. Slide beneath the gingival margin, and move in an apico-coronal direction several times

Improper Flossing

A. Acute consequences—snapping through contacts, failure to curve the floss against the proximal surfaces, and application of excessive pressure can result in floss cuts of interdental papillae
B. Chronic consequences
  1. Soft tissue—excessive pressure applied submarginally can be destructive to attachment fibers
  2. Hard tissue—repeated heavy sawing movements in a facio-lingual direction can abrade proximal tooth structure

Flossing Aids

A. Types of aids
  1. Floss holders
    a. General description—the floss is threaded through and held on a double-pronged plastic device, forming a span between the prongs
    b. Technique—the prepared holder is positioned for insertion, then adapted and activated in much the same manner as the handheld floss; special care should be taken not to snap the floss through the contacts
    c. Indications for use—client's lack of dexterity to floss properly and client preference
  2. Floss threaders
    a. General description—firm, flexible, blunt-ended devices for moving the floss through closed contacts or under pontics or orthodontic wires; a variety of designs are available
    b. Technique—position the floss in the threader with even lengths on each side; pass the threader through the embrasure from the buccal aspect to the lingual aspect, leaving sufficient length on the buccal aspect; remove the threader and use the floss in the normal manner; slide through the space to remove it

Supplementary Devices for Plaque Biofilm Removal

Interdental Brushes
A. General description
  1. Soft nylon filaments are twisted onto a stainless steel wire to form a tapered or a nontapered small brush; the wire may be plastic coated for

use around dental implants and for client comfort

2. Interdental brushes must be used with a special handle; some have small handles, and some have contra-angled handles

3. Interdental brushes provide excellent access to root concavities, furcation areas, and proximal surfaces where papillae do not fill the interdental spaces, as in type II and type III embrasures (see Figure 16-3)

4. Most recently, interdental brushes have come in a variety of sizes, with thin wires and a tapered brush to remove interproximal plaque biofilm from all types of embrasures; for example, Butler Go-Betweens Cleaners® which the manufacturer claims can fit into 0.8-mm interproximal spaces

B. Technique

1. Choose a brush of appropriate size, insert interproximally, and use an in-and-out motion from the buccal aspect to the lingual aspect, and vice versa

2. Brushes may be used in furcation areas in a similar manner

3. The filaments get compressed when the brush moves through constricted areas and flare out to adapt to larger spaces

4. Access into the interproximal pockets may be achieved with careful vertical placement and movement

C. Precautions

1. Avoid forcing through tight, tissue-filled areas to prevent trauma

2. Do not aim the wire into tissue

3. Discard the tip when the filaments lose their original shape

4. Do not use a brush with a stainless-steel wire on an implant; the brush must have a plastic-coated wire to prevent damage to the implant

D. Indications for use—in types II and III embrasure spaces, when access permits; for disrupting plaque biofilm from root concavities, proximal surfaces, and furcation areas; for delivery of antimicrobial agents

Toothpicks[1]

A. Suggested use—for proximal surfaces and concavities and in exposed furcation areas

B. Technique—round toothpicks can be used alone or inserted into special holders; moisten the tip with saliva, and adapt it to the surface to be cleaned; subgingivally, use a 45-degree angle to the tooth; move the toothpick in and out several times for cleaning the interproximal surfaces, and follow the tooth contour on the facial or lingual surfaces

C. Precautions—rigid pointed tips can cause injury if forced into tight tissue areas; over time, papillae will abrade if toothpicks are used improperly

Interdental Wedges[1]

A. Suggested use—for cleaning the proximal surfaces or just under the gingival margin; triangular in cross-sections; should be used interproximally only when adequate space for insertion is available (e.g., type II and III embrasures)

B. Technique—moisten the tip, position the flat base of the triangle at the gingival border, insert with the tip angled slightly toward the occlusal surface, and move the wedge in and out, with moderate pressure against the surface

C. Precautions—discard tips as soon as splaying occurs; using a fulcrum position increases control and reduces the risk of inserting the wedge with too much pressure; repeated insertion with the tip perpendicular to the long axis of the tooth may cause blunting of interdental papillae

Interdental Tip

A. Suggested uses—for proximal surfaces, in exposed furcations, and under gingival margins; conical or pyramidal flexible rubber or plastic tip; may be used to maintain interproximal gingival contours or to recontour papillae following periodontal surgery; rubber tips are also used for massaging the gingiva to improve blood circulation, increase keratinization, and provide epithelial thickening[1]

B. Technique

1. Dental plaque biofilm removal—trace the gingival margin with the tip aimed into the sulcus; move the tip in and out in a bucco-lingual direction along the proximal tooth surface apical to contact areas

2. Contouring gingiva—place the tip, without forcing it, into the interdental contour, being careful to follow the gingival form; press the side of the tip against the gingiva, and use a firm rotary motion to apply intermittent pressure

C. Precaution—avoid flattening interdental papillae; use of interdental tips made from rubber should be avoided on clients with latex sensitivity

Power Interdental Cleaning Devices[1]

A. Power flossing devices are available to make interdental cleaning easier; include flossers, interdental brushes, and dental water jets

B. Technique—usually the unit comes with an attachment (similar to a floss holder, interdental brush, or single-tufted or end-tufted brush); the brush is activated by turning it on after attaching the brush handle; requires only one hand to operate; the tip is aimed into the interproximal space

C. Suggested use—alternative to the handheld floss; client preference

Dental Water Jet[1]

A. General description—motor-driven pulsating device with a reservoir and specially designed tips to deliver the irrigant to the gingival pocket; depending on the size of the tip selected, this device has the ability to reach deep periodontal pockets; dental water jets that produce a steady stream of fluid, including those that can be attached to a faucet, are available but have not been tested clinically for their efficacy

B. Technique—the reservoir is filled with water or an antimicrobial agent; after inserting the appropriate tip into the handle, the pressure gauge is adjusted to the client's comfort setting; starting with posterior teeth, the tip is placed at a 90-degree angle to the long axis of the tooth, following each tooth along the gingival margin

C. Indications for use—clients with fixed orthodontics, dental implants, crowns, and bridges; those with gingivitis; and persons in periodontal maintenance program; research suggests that the use of oral irrigation does not reduce plaque biofilm; however, it does improve gingival health compared with regular oral hygiene[9]

D. Precaution—each manufacturer's product differs; follow each model's instructions for use; some units may only require diluted solution to operate effectively

▌ DENTIFRICES

Basic Concepts

A. Definition—substance used with a toothbrush on accessible tooth surfaces; currently available in gel and paste forms

B. Purposes
   1. Cosmetic—tooth surfaces are cleaned and polished; breath is freshened
   2. Cosmetic and therapeutic—certain nontherapeutic substances augment the efficiency of brushing in the removal of plaque biofilm, debris, and stain
   3. Therapeutic—vehicle for transporting biologically active ingredients such as fluoride, which inhibits tooth demineralization and promotes remineralization, to the tooth and its environment

C. Basic ingredients[1]
   1. Detergents—lower surface tension to loosen debris and stain; provide foaming characteristic;

sodium lauryl sulfate, a commonly used foaming agent, has been implicated in causing aphthous ulcers in susceptible clients

2. Cleaning and polishing agents—abrasives that help remove stain, plaque biofilm, and debris from tooth surfaces and give a luster to the tooth surface; should provide maximal cleaning benefit with minimal abrasion; examples include calcium carbonate, silica, calcium pyrophosphate, aluminum oxide, insoluble calcium metaphosphate, magnesium carbonate, and bicarbonate

3. Humectants—retain moisture to ensure a chemically and physically stable product; for example, glycerin, mannitol, sorbitol, synthetic cellulose, vegetable oils, and propylene glycol

4. Binding agents—prevent separation by increasing the consistency of a mixture of liquid and solid ingredients; for example, mineral colloids, natural gums, and seaweed colloids

5. Flavoring and sweetening agents—provide a pleasant and refreshing flavor and aftertaste, and cover unpleasant flavors; for example, peppermint, cinnamon, wintergreen, noncariogenic artificial sweeteners such as glycerin, sorbitol, menthol, and xylitol

6. Coloring agents—contribute to the product's attractiveness and desirability; vegetable dyes and titanium dioxide

7. Preservatives—prevent bacterial growth and prolong shelf life of the product; for example, alcohol, benzoates, and dichlorinated phenols

Therapeutic and Active Ingredients

A. Definition—biologically active ingredients that produce a beneficial effect on hard or soft tissue; dentifrices claiming therapeutic effects are eligible for acceptance by the ADA Council on Scientific Affairs or the CDA; updated lists from the ADA and the CDA should be consulted at least annually[4]

B. Remineralizing agents
   1. Fluoride—substantial data exist to show that approved fluoride dentifrices reduce the incidence of dental caries; fluorides currently used in dentifrices are sodium fluoride (NaF), stannous fluoride (SnF_2), SnF_2–sodium hexametaphosphate, and sodium monofluorophosphate ($Na_2\text{-}PO_3F$)[1]

   2. Dentifrices containing fluoride may carry the ADA Seal of Acceptance or the CDA Seal of Recognition for their effectiveness in preventing dental caries

   3. Amorphous calcium phosphate—calcium and phosphate were traditionally added to dentifrices as abrasives and lubricants and now for caries control; peer-reviewed research on the efficacy of amorphous calcium phosphate as an anticaries agent is limited

4. Xylitol—a sugar substitute, which has anticaries and anti-plaque properties; *Streptococcus mutans* cannot metabolize xylitol, which allows a less acidic environment for tooth demineralization[1]

C. Antimicrobial agents—triclosan is the primary agent used in the United States; its antigingivitis and anti-plaque efficacy has been demonstrated

D. Desensitizing agents— desensitization agents work in one of two ways; they either block dentinal tubules (high concentration of fluoride, calcium phosphates, and oxalate salts) or block nerve repolarization (potassium salts including potassium nitrate or potassium citrate); potassium nitrate is the primary agent used in desensitizing dentifrices[10]

E. Anticalculus agents—function by interfering with the calcium phosphate bond in the calculus matrix; effective only against the formation of supragingival calculus on enamel surfaces
1. Pyrophosphate system—pyrophosphate has a negative charge, attracts positively charged calcium ions, and interferes with calculus formation
2. Zinc system—zinc has a positive charge, attracts negatively charged phosphate ions, and interferes with calculus formation

F. Whitening agents—several dentifrices are marketed for their ability to remove or bleach stains; several whitening dentifrices have low abrasive levels; may be effective for the maintenance of cosmetic restorations; some whitening agents include papain (Citroxain), silica, hydrogen peroxide, and carbamide peroxide; dentifrices may carry the ADA Seal of Acceptance for their effectiveness in stain removal[4]

G. Baking soda—manufacturers claim benefits from the addition of baking soda to neutralize acids in the mouth and prevent the demineralization of tooth surfaces; it is also added in combination with peroxide for whitening purposes; use caution when recommending dentifrices containing baking soda to clients with hypertension

Guidelines for Dentifrice Selection

A. Products selected should carry the ADA Seal of Acceptance or the CDA Seal of Recognition; this ensures that adequate evidence of safety and efficacy has been demonstrated in controlled clinical trials, that advertising claims comply with ADA and CDA standards for accuracy and truthfulness, and that the therapeutic ingredient will be bioavailable when the dentifrice is used

B. All ADA-accepted and CDA-recognized dentifrices have safe levels of abrasiveness

C. Dentifrices containing fluoride are granted acceptance on the basis of their caries-reduction properties

D. Anticalculus dentifrices contain fluoride; those that carry the ADA Seal of Acceptance or the CDA Seal of Recognition have gained acceptance for the proven efficacy of their fluoride mechanism, not for their anticalculus properties because calculus does not cause disease

E. Desensitizing dentifrices that carry ADA and CDA Seals have gained acceptance for their proven efficacy in the control of dentinal hypersensitivity

Guidelines for Dentifrice Use[11]

A. Daily use of fluoride dentifrice should be recommended to all clients, regardless of caries risk, because these products promote tooth remineralization

B. Young children (under age 6) should be supervised when using a fluoride dentifrice—use of a small, pea-sized amount of a toothpaste or gel containing no more than 1100 ppm (parts per million) fluoride is recommended because children under 6 will most likely swallow the dentifrice

CONTROLLING ORAL MALODOR

A. Identifying malodor
1. Oral malodor (bad breath, or halitosis)—common problem that originates approximately 90% of the time from the mouth and from the oropharynx region (tongue coating, gingivitis, periodontitis, pharyngitis, and tonsillitis); systemic causes account for 10% of oral malodor[12]
2. Malodors are produced by microorganisms on the tongue and teeth; proteolytic activity results in foul-smelling compounds or volatile sulfur compounds (VSCs)[13]
3. Oral dryness (xerostomia) exacerbates malodor; smoking, medications, alcohol, and caffeine increase oral dehydration
4. As in adults, malodor in children is related primarily to oral factors and is associated with postnasal drip and nasal odor[14]
5. Bad breath caused by high levels of VSCs is often associated with periodontal infections and overnight denture wearing[15-17]
6. Malodor can be measured by sensory or organolectic (smell) instruments such as gas chromatography (GC) that monitor VCSs (hydrogen sulfide, methyl mercaptan, andimethyl sulfide)[18]

B. Controlling malodor
1. Improve oral hygiene by including tongue cleaning in the process

2. Abstain from tobacco and alcohol use
3. Avoid caffeine
4. Stimulate salivary flow by chewing sugarless gum with xylitol
5. Use ADA-accepted or CDA-recognized antimicrobial mouthrinses
6. Use saline nasal sprays and humidifiers to control dryness of throat and nasal passages
7. Use sugar-free (with xylitol) breath sprays, breath fresheners, or drops

C. Technique for tongue cleaning
1. Brushing
    a. With the tongue extended, place the toothbrush on the dorsum of the tongue with the tips directed toward the throat; place the toothbrush as far posterior as can be tolerated
    b. Apply light pressure, and move the toothbrush forward and out; repeat to cover the entire surface; avoid vigorous scrubbing
2. Tongue-cleaning devices
    a. Tongue-cleaning devices are available in various designs, but all have some sort of flexible or rigid scraping surface or strip; tongue cleaning can be achieved by either a power toothbrush or a manual toothbrush
    b. The device is placed toward the back of the tongue on the dorsal surface and then pulled forward while light pressure is applied; this method is repeated until a coating-free tongue is achieved
    c. The same technique is applied with a toothbrush as with other tongue-cleaning devices to achieve a coat-free tongue

ORAL IRRIGATION

Basic Concepts

Oral irrigation can be a valuable adjunct to maintaining oral cleanliness and health; oral irrigating devices force a steady or pulsating stream of water over gingival tissue and teeth, with the goals of removing unattached debris and reducing the concentration of microorganisms and cellular end products that may be present; irrigators also are used to deliver antimicrobial agents supragingivally and subgingivally

Home Irrigation

A. Home uses
1. Before toothbrushing and flossing to remove debris or retained food particles, or after toothbrushing to deliver antimicrobial agents

2. Debridement of recessed areas of fixed prosthetic or orthodontic appliances; around dental implants
3. Flushing of periodontal pockets with a controlled, low-intensity, pulsating stream of water

B. Types of irrigators
1. Hand syringes—blunt tip, side-port cannula; requires high level of dexterity and motivation; not recommended for most clients
2. Power-driven device—unit with a water reservoir; plugs into an electrical outlet to create a pulsating jet of water; water pressure is regulated by an adjustable dial or sliding switch
3. Water pressure–driven device—attaches directly to a faucet to deliver a constant stream of water; pressure is controlled by regulating water flow from the faucet
4. Tips—standard jet tip or flexible subgingival tip; tips with a side-port design or an end-port design show similar effectiveness

C. Client technique for use of power irrigators
1. Adjust the water stream to a low-pressure setting
2. Lean over the washbasin
3. Direct the tip at right angle (90 degrees) to tooth surfaces; the stream should move in a horizontal direction through the gingival embrasure and around teeth
4. Soft tips designed for subgingival access may be angled into the sulcus

D. Use with antimicrobial agents[1,19]
1. Some studies have documented greater benefits with the addition of antimicrobial agents
2. Since standard irrigation tips are unable to access periodontal pockets completely, no significant benefits in treating periodontitis is found; demonstrated benefits are limited to parameters such as plaque and bleeding indices, gingivitis, and reduction of bleeding on probing
3. The use of water alone is as effective as the use of chemotherapeutic agents

E. Precautions—contraindications to use
1. Clients should be trained in the proper use of irrigating devices and be monitored for adverse effects
2. Transient bacteremias may occur following oral irrigation, particularly when untreated disease is present; persons at highest risk for infective endocarditis can use irrigation as part of their oral self care
3. Contraindicated in persons with periodontal abscess or ulcerative lesions and in clients with dexterity problems

In-Office Irrigation[4,20]

A. In-office uses
   1. As an adjunct to mechanical debridement
   2. Benefits of in-office irrigation not supported by research; controlled-release agents such as chlorhexidine chip, minocycline microspheres, and 10% doxycycline hyclate gel are more effective
B. Types of office irrigators
   1. Hand syringe—blunt tip, side-port cannula
   2. Part of an ultrasonic scaling unit
   3. Air-driven handpiece attachment
C. Technique for use
   1. Techniques for hand syringe and power irrigators are essentially the same; pressure must be controlled for both
   2. Use adequate suction throughout the procedure
   3. Fill the reservoir or the syringe with full-strength or diluted antimicrobial solution; power irrigators usually use a solution diluted with equal parts water
   4. Bend the cannula by using a protective sheath
   5. Adjust the flow rate of the power unit to a low setting; settings vary with the viscosity of the solution selected
   6. Insert the cannula to the base of the pocket, or sulcus, and retract 1 mm
   7. Release the irrigant into all areas to be irrigated
   8. Consult the manufacturer's instructions for the cleaning and maintenance of the unit; dispose of the cannula in a biohazard container for sharp objects
D. Antimicrobial agents
   1. Stannous fluoride—1.64% SnF_2; dispense equal parts of 3.28% SnF_2 concentrated gel and distilled water; use a fresh mixture for each client
   2. Chlorhexidine digluconate—0.12% in the United States and 2% in Europe; may be diluted to 0.06% concentration; may become less effective in the presence of sodium laurel sulfate, fluoride, blood, and protein
   3. Essential oils mouthrinse; may be diluted with equal parts water for use in a power irrigator, but most studies use it at full strength
   4. Povidone–iodine, metronidazole, and tetracycline have been used with varying results
E. Precautions
   1. Use of low pressure prevents gingival tissue trauma and allows better access to the base of the pocket
   2. Some patients may require a physician consult

CARE OF FIXED AND REMOVABLE PROSTHESES

Dental prostheses are replacements for one or more teeth or other oral structures, ranging from a single tooth to a complete denture. Clients wearing fixed or removable dental prostheses have unique needs that require specific procedures for maintaining the prosthesis as well as retained natural teeth; relevant terminology follows:[20]

A. Appliance—in dentistry, a general term referring to a device used to provide a functional or therapeutic effect
B. Abutment—tooth, root, or dental implant used for the support and retention of a fixed or removable dental prosthesis
C. Clasp—retains and stabilizes the denture by attaching it to the abutment teeth
D. Denture—artificial substitute for missing natural teeth and adjacent tissues
E. Pontic—artificial tooth on a fixed, partial denture or isolated tooth on a removable, partial denture that replaces lost natural tooth, restores its function, and usually occupies space previously occupied by a natural crown
F. Fixed prosthesis—dental prosthesis firmly attached to natural teeth, roots, or dental implants usually by a cementing agent; cannot be removed by client
G. Obturator—maxillofacial prosthesis that includes an intraoral structure that replaces all or part of the palate or the maxilla; it may also have a palatal lift that aids in speech or swallowing
H. Overdentures—dentures with retained natural teeth or dental implants
I. Removable prosthesis—dental prosthesis that can readily be placed in the mouth and removed by the wearer
J. Orthodontic bracket—a small metal attachment fixed to a band that serves as a means of fastening the archwire to the band
K. Orthodontic band—a thin metal ring that secures orthodontic attachments to a tooth
L. Orthodontic wire—a slender, pliable rod or thread of metal used as a source of force to direct teeth to move in desired directions
M. Implant, or dental implant—a device surgically inserted into the jawbone to be used as a prosthodontic abutment; may be used to support complete dentures
N. Grills "Grillz/fronts"—a decorative, jewel-encrusted encasement for teeth; often used by persons in some cultures and sub-cultures; usually made of precious metals such as gold, platinum, or other metals[21]

Fixed Prosthesis Maintenance

A. Fixed prostheses such as fixed bridges and orthodontic bands and wires increase the potential for plaque biofilm and debris retention and make access to the proximal surfaces more difficult

B. Home care armamentarium

1. Floss threaders—allow the floss to move beneath pontics and between pontics and abutments

2. Interdental brushes—access interdental spaces apical to closed contacts

3. Special brushes and toothpicks

a. Orthodontic bi-level toothbrushes—three rows wide, with shorter middle row; moves into and around orthodontic appliances; adapts to areas between the orthodontic appliance and the gingival margin

b. Two-row brushes—for cleaning of sulci; adapt to narrow areas between brackets and gingivae

c. Toothpick holders—for cleaning type II embrasures, furca, and margins of appliances, brackets, and sulci

d. Single-tuft or end-tuft brushes—for use in type III embrasure areas, furca, margins of appliances and brackets, and single-teeth abutments

e. Oral irrigators—flushing action removes loose debris and food material; dental hygienists should instruct clients in proper use

Removable Prosthesis Maintenance

A. Clients with removable appliances, including orthodontic appliances, must be taught about the importance of conscientious home care

B. Debris, stain, plaque biofilm, and calculus will collect on removable appliances, if the appliances are not cleaned regularly

C. Inadequate cleaning may contribute to the development of soft tissue lesions underlying the appliance or of carious lesions on abutting tooth surfaces; chronic *Candida albicans* infection also may result

D. Removable prostheses can be maintained by:

1. Brushing with water and a mild oral detergent or dentifrice after each meal and before retiring to bed at night

a. Special denture brushes have two different arrangements of filaments to access both the inner curved surface and the outer and occlusal surfaces

b. Special clasp brushes have a narrow, tapered cylindrical design that can adapt to the inner clasp surface, a prime site for plaque biofilm formation and retention

2. Immersion in a solvent or a detergent solution that chemically loosens or removes stains and deposits is recommended; the appliance should be brushed after soaking it to remove residual debris and chemicals; commonly used soaking agents include dilute sodium hypochlorite (bleach), alkaline peroxide, vinegar, and various enzyme solutions that render proteins less adherent; bleach causes corrosion and is not recommended on metal appliances

3. Antifungal denture solutions help prevent candidiasis

E. Removable appliances should be taken out at night and stored in a covered container with one of the solvents or denture solutions listed above

F. Cleansing procedures

1. Hold the appliance securely to avoid dropping it and breaking it

2. When brushing, hold the appliance over a sink partly filled with water or lined with a cushioning material

3. Avoid overzealous brushing and use of strong abrasives; the plastic resin material can be scratched or abraded to the extent of compromising denture fit

4. If any denture adhesive material is used, it should be removed from the appliance and the underlying mucosa several times a day

5. Brush the underlying mucosa at least once a day with a soft toothbrush

6. Solutions used for cleansing or soaking a denture should be renewed for each use

G. All removable appliances and prostheses, including fluoride carriers, night guards, mouth guards, and bleaching trays should be cleaned and appropriately stored after use[20]

H. Clients with "grills" may need to be educated on the importance of oral hygiene; these clients should be well informed on the importance of cleaning the appliance on a regular basis; the significance of oral hygiene and the use of fluoride products should be emphasized at each continued care appointment; a 3-month continued-care interval with fluoride therapy may be recommended to prevent tooth demineralization[21]

Dental Implant Maintenance

See the sections on "Dental implants" in Chapters 13 and 14 and "Instrumentation of dental implants" in Chapter 17.

A. Osteo-integrated implants and superstructures require special home maintenance, products, and techniques; clients must learn the techniques for plaque biofilm control that prevent damage to the implant material and superstructure

B. The home-care armamentarium may include:
1. Soft-bristled, multiple-tufted nylon tooth-brushes
2. Interdental brushes with nylon coating over metal wire cores; coating prevents scratching of the implant material (usually titanium)
3. Flat and tapered end-tuft brushes
4. Dental floss
5. Implant flossing aids—braided nylon filaments with a hook leader for insertion is recommended; flat cotton floss; or floss containing a soft filament brush component
6. Rubber tip stimulator; wood sticks
7. Disclosing tablets or liquid; may be most useful during initial education on plaque biofilm control
8. Antimicrobial mouthrinse; chlorhexidine used twice a day is the rinse of choice after treatment; other antimicrobial mouthrinses may be used for long-term treatment
9. Small amount of ADA-approved or CDA-recognized gel or fine-abrasive, fluoridated toothpaste; abrasive toothpastes must be avoided; anticalculus formulas are acceptable
10. Oral irrigators may be used on the lowest setting, with the tip directed perpendicular to the long axis of the tooth or implant; water, chlorhexidine 0.12%, phenol-based, or plant alkaloid mouthrinses may be used

C. Plaque biofilm control skill development
1. Clients must be shown how to control plaque biofilm on all areas of the implant and the superstructure
2. Sufficient supervised practice will ensure adequate skill development
3. Plaque biofilm control must be monitored at each continued-care appointment and techniques modified, as indicated
4. Research indicates that tobacco use increases implant failure[22]

CARIES MANAGEMENT

Fluorides[23]

See the sections on "Topical fluorides and fluoride varnishes" in Chapter 13 and "Preventing and controlling oral disease" in Chapter 20.

General Considerations
A. Most effective agent for the prevention and control of dental caries, especially on smooth surfaces
B. A multi-therapeutic approach is most effective; three categories of administration:

1. Systemic—community water supplies, institutional water supplies, and dietary supplementation
2. Professional application—gels and varnishes
3. Self-applied—dentifrices, rinses, and gels
C. Safe when used in recommended amounts and concentrations; dental hygienists must be alert to the potential for acute and chronic adverse effects
1. Large quantities of fluoride products should not be stored in the home
2. Institutions that have fluoride programs must handle and store fluoride products safely
3. Parents and caregivers must be educated about supervising home use of products containing fluoride by young children to prevent acute toxic reactions or long-term effects (e.g., dental fluorosis)
4. Products intended for topical application should not be swallowed
5. If excessive amounts have been ingested, vomiting should be induced immediately with ipecac or manually; calcium solution or milk should be administered to slow the absorption rate; emergency medical care should be obtained (see the section on "Drug-related emergencies and poisoning" in Chapter 21)
6. Fluoride therapy is used based upon the client's risk assessment

Ingested Fluorides
A. Drinking optimally fluoridated water (0.7 ppm) during tooth formation and then later as a topical from drinking the water provides a significant decrease in the overall percentage of dental caries in both children and adults
B. Maximum benefits are obtained when fluoride is provided from the onset of tooth development until tooth eruption is complete and then used continuously for drinking
C. Fluoride works primarily and most effectively via topical (surface) mechanisms (whether delivered in the drinking water, foods, beverages, or products) to inhibit demineralization, enhance remineralization, and inhibit plaque bacteria
D. Dietary supplementation is not recommended for pregnant and lactating women who drink water that is less than optimally fluoridated
E. The dental hygienist has a key role in educating parents, caregivers, and children about the value of fluoride and its topical benefits

Fluoride Agents for Professional Application
A. Neutral sodium fluoride (NaF)
1. Characteristics—first fluoride used for topical application; commonly available in 2% concentration foam or gel and 5% concentration varnish

2. Application
   a. A 2% NaF solution is administered in a series of four applications at 1-week intervals that coincide with the eruption of primary and permanent teeth; suggested ages for application are 3, 7, 10, and 13 years; old method
   b. Applications of 2% NaF at 6-month intervals as a substitute for acidulated phosphate fluoride (APF) when porcelain or certain types of composite restorations are present have not been substantiated in the literature; 4-minute application
   c. Fluoride varnish—contains a 5% NaF concentration, approved by the FDA for use as a desensitizing agent and cavity liner; the varnish is used as a topical fluoride treatment; painted on teeth; the varnish is retained on the tooth surface for 3 to 4 hours, which maintains fluoride reaction with the underlying enamel[24]
   3. Advantages—stable solution in plastic containers; relative absence of taste; does not stain teeth or irritate soft tissues; safe for use in dentition with porcelain crowns and composite restorations; varnish is easily applied on the teeth of young children; research highly supports the efficacy of fluoride varnish for caries prevention compared with other professional fluoride methods[24,25]
B. Acidulated phosphate fluoride (APF)
   1. Characteristics—available as foam, gels, and thixotropic gels; 1.23% NaF with 1 molar (M) orthophosphoric acid concentration
   2. Application intervals—every 6 months, or more frequently when caries risk is high; 4-minute application
   3. Advantages—stable when stored in plastic container; high level of client acceptance; nonirritating to soft tissues; does not discolor tooth structure; highest documented efficacy; most commonly used in-office treatment; 1-minute application not supported by the research literature
   4. Disadvantages and precautions—low pH of 3.5 for enhanced fluoride uptake may cause etching of dental sealants and porcelain and some composite restorations; sealants, porcelains, and composites should be protected with a water-based lubricant, or use NaF as an alternative
C. APF and SnF_2 combination solutions
   1. Characteristics—available as 0.32% APF and 1.64% SnF_2; to be mixed together as a rinse application; fluoride products in these concentrations have not received the ADA Council on Scientific Affairs Seal of Acceptance

2. Application intervals—single application at 6-month continued-care intervals; more frequently if indicated
3. Advantages—ease of application, good client acceptance
4. Disadvantages and precautions—lack of ADA approval and lack of CDA recognition indicates insufficient clinical evidence to support efficacy; not recommended for use

Indications for Professional Application
A. Topical fluoride therapy is an accepted part of the prevention-oriented care plan
B. Assessment of client's risk for dental caries will determine a client's fluoride therapy plan
C. Therapy regimen may include both professionally applied and self-applied agents
D. Inclusion of topical fluoride in client's care plan should be based on the following criteria:[23]
   1. For children and adults at moderate, high or highest risk for dental caries—fluoride varnish or fluoride gel is the treatment of choice at continued-care intervals[25]
   2. Less than optimally fluoridated drinking water
   3. Fair or poor oral hygiene
   4. Decalcification, white spots, or incipient lesions are present; secondary or recurrent caries; active caries
   5. Following root instrumentation, dentin can be exposed and dentinal tubules opened; hypersensitive root surfaces that often result can be controlled by fluoride application
   6. Fluoride application reduces incidence of root caries and dentinal hypersensitivity associated with exposed root surfaces resulting from gingival recession
   7. Irregular professional dental visits
   8. Inappropriate dietary practices (e.g., frequent sugar intake)
   9. When xerostomia is present as a result of irradiation to the head and neck, certain medications, and salivary gland dysfunction resulting in changes in quality and quantity of saliva; caries destruction occurs rapidly and is generalized when salivary production is minimal; multiple fluoride treatments are used to control high risk for dental caries associated with xerostomia
   10. Clients wearing orthodontic or prosthodontic appliances

Application Principles—General Guidelines for Client Preparation
A. Explain the indication(s), the steps involved, and the time required for the procedure, the need to control salivary flow and to avoid ingestion, and

post-application restriction of ingesting anything by mouth for 30 minutes after application

B. Position the client to facilitate salivary control and reduce potential for gagging

C. Calculus, extrinsic stains, materia alba, and heavy plaque biofilm should be removed before the application of fluoride

Application Methods

Tray Systems

A. Designed for use with fluoride gels; trays cover all teeth in an arch, come in a variety of materials, shapes, and sizes; tray systems are not appropriate for solutions because they cannot be adequately retained within tray boundaries

B. Tray examples—most commonly used
  1. Disposable styrofoam—available in a variety of sizes and shapes; soft, pliable, and comfortable; good retention of gel, also available with foam liner; used for professional fluoride application; the ADA and the CDA do not recommend the use of fluoride foam because of lack of sufficient scientific evidence for its efficacy in caries prevention; the ADA and the CDA recommend only 4-minute fluoride gel application[25]
  2. Custom-fitted polyvinyl—used by the client for self-application of fluoride gel; provides excellent coverage; must be remade as the dentition matures; relatively expensive

C. Factors in tray selection—appropriate tray selection critical to the success of the procedure; criteria used to evaluate tray suitability are as follows:
  1. Adapts to facial and lingual surfaces without extreme gapping
  2. Achieves complete coverage; the depth is sufficient to reach the exposed root surfaces
  3. Minimizes any loss of the agent into the mouth
  4. Comfortable for the client
  5. Reasonable cost

D. Application procedure
  1. Assemble the armamentarium—trays, fluoride, a saliva ejection device, gauze squares, and a timer or a clock
  2. Protect the dental sealants and the porcelain or composite restorations with a water-based lubricant for APF application, or, preferably, use neutral NaF
  3. Place a thin ribbon of gel in the tray and spread it
  4. Thoroughly dry each arch; this prevents dilution of the material and controls for a potential salivary barrier
  5. Insert the tray(s); one or two trays can be inserted at once; tray type, client variables, and clinician preference will influence the method selected
  6. Insert the saliva ejection device, which reduces the potential for ingestion, nausea, and vomiting
  7. Adapt the tray(s); the dental hygienist or the client can gently press on the trays to close any small anterior gaps
  8. Have the client apply gentle biting pressure to force the gel interproximally
  9. Begin timing; trays are left in position for 4 minutes; the efficacy of 1-minute applications recommended by some manufacturers is not supported by clinical studies
  10. Remove the tray(s); if only one tray was inserted initially, insert the second tray at this point; do not allow the client to rinse between insertions
  11. Clear any excess agent from the mouth; instruct the client to expectorate and swab the tongue, teeth, and soft tissues with gauze squares
  12. Provide post-treatment instructions; clients are instructed not to eat, rinse, or drink for at least 30 minutes; this increases the total contact time of fluoride exposure

Paint-On System When clients have a limited number of teeth or have root exposure that a tray fails to cover, fluoride agents must be applied with a technique that allows for small amounts to be continuously applied to properly prepared tooth surfaces; gels and varnishes may also be applied with this technique

A. Components of the application procedure for gels (varnishes are painted on even in a wet environment and the varnish remains until worn off)
  1. Assemble the armamentarium—long and short cotton rolls and cotton roll holders, fluoride solution or gel and container, saliva ejection device, applicator (cotton pellets and cotton pliers, or cotton-tipped applicator), gauze squares, a timer or a clock
  2. Protect the dental sealants and the porcelain or composite restorations with a water-based lubricant (e.g., K-Y jelly) for APF application; or, preferably, use neutral NaF
  3. Isolate teeth using cotton rolls and a suitable holder (optional); a long curved cotton roll can be placed on the buccal aspect and a short one placed on the lingual aspect until full mouth isolation is achieved; depending on client variables and clinician experience, it may be advisable to treat only one half of the mouth at a time
  4. Insert the saliva ejection device
  5. Dry the isolated teeth using a systematic approach

6. Begin timing (no timing is required with fluoride varnish)
7. Apply the prepared fluoride by using a thoroughly moistened applicator; when using a solution, swab teeth continuously for 4 minutes
8. Remove the cotton rolls and holders
9. Clear any excess agent; use optimal evacuation methods, and ask the client to expectorate
10. Do not allow the client to rinse
11. Provide post-treatment instructions

B. Advantages
1. Allows for selective omission of an area or tooth; the agent can be kept from surfaces where fluoride use is contraindicated
2. Allows for direct observation of gel, or varnish during application; dental hygienist can control the placement of gel or varnish and evaluate the status of salivary control, thus reducing potential for ingestion

C. Disadvantages—a dry field must be maintained for the gel; salivary contamination does not affect the effectiveness of the varnish

Self-Applied Fluorides

A. Frequent, low doses of fluoride exposure to tooth surfaces are important for enamel remineralization and prevention of demineralization
B. Rinses—available by prescription, except as noted
1. Daily use—low potency, high frequency
   a. 0.044% APF rinse supplement
   b. 0.05% NaF (available over the counter [OTC])
   c. 0.1% SnF_2 rinse (0.63% plus water)
2. Weekly use—high potency, low frequency
   a. 0.2% NaF
   b. Most commonly used concentration for school-based fluoride rinse programs
3. Many commercially prepared fluoride rinses contain alcohol and should not be recommended for persons with a history of alcoholism or xerostomia; use alcohol-free rinses with children and clients who need to avoid exposure to alcohol
4. Fluoride rinses are not recommended for children under 6 years old; swallowing small doses of fluoride over a period may lead to dental fluorosis

C. Gels—available OTC and by prescription
1. 0.4% SnF_2 (brush-on or tray application)
2. 1.1% NaF (brush-on or tray application, also available in paste)
3. 0.05% APF (tray application)

D. Some studies indicate that SnF_2 may have antiplaque, antihypersensitivity, and anticaries effects

Amorphous Calcium Phosphate[1,26]

A. Amorphous calcium phosphate (ACP) contains the same minerals as the hydroxyapatite crystals of tooth enamel; research on the efficacy of ACP in tooth remineralization is limited
B. Casein phosphopeptide–amorphous calcium phosphate (CPP-ACP), a milk protein peptide, is usually added to stabilize and localize the calcium and phosphate ions on the tooth surface, promoting remineralization of enamel
C. Products that contain ACP should not be substituted for fluoride therapy; ACP should be used in conjunction with fluoride to enhance fluoride uptake[27]
D. Several professionally applied and OTC self-applied products, including dentifrices, tooth whitening agents, prophylaxis paste, and fluoride varnish, contain ACP
E. At this point, a body of scientific evidence to substantiate the validity of ACP-containing products is not available

Xylitol for Dental Caries Prevention[1,28]

A. Xylitol is a noncariogenic artificial sweetener; S. mutans cannot metabolize xylitol, which causes a decrease in S. mutans infections
B. Evidence shows that xylitol inhibits the attachment and transmission of S. mutans, reduces plaque biofilm formation, and stimulates salivary secretion
C. Xylitol-containing salivary stimulants can be beneficial for people with xerostomia and diabetes
D. Several products contain xylitol, for example, chewing gum, lozenges, and mints; when used for therapeutic purposes, products must contain 1.55 g xylitol and must be used minimum of four to five times throughout the day

Caries Management by Risk Assessment[1,29,30] See Table 15-6 "Classification of Caries Risk" in Chapter 15.

Caries Management by Risk Assessment (CAMBRA), an evidence-based approach to dental caries prevention, in which the clinician assesses the client for caries risk factors and protective factors and determines whether the client is at low, medium, or high caries risk. Based on the identified level of risk, a client-specific care plan is developed to manage the individual's caries risk.

A. Present and past caries assessment—risk identified through clinical examination; the presence of each of the following will place the client in the high-risk category:
1. Teeth with frank lesions that radiographically show penetration into dentin
2. Evidence of radiographic caries limited to enamel in interproximal surfaces
3. White spots on surfaces
4. Teeth restored within the past 3 years

B. Biologic factors contributing to caries—factors that assist clinician understand why an individual has an ongoing caries problem
  1. Medium or high level of streptococci and lactobacilli counts
  2. Presence of heavy biofilm on teeth
  3. Frequent snacking between meals
  4. Deep pits and fissures
  5. Recreational drug use
  6. Inadequate salivary flow caused by medication, radiation, or systemic diseases
  7. Exposed roots
  8. Orthodontic appliance
C. Caries management behaviors—biologic or therapeutic factors related to the client's practice of oral hygiene that can counterbalance the challenge presented by caries risk factors; also referred to as *protective factors*
  1. Drinks fluoridated water on a regular basis
  2. Uses a fluoride toothpaste at least once or more daily
  3. Uses fluoride-containing mouthrinse daily
  4. Has had fluoride varnish applied in the past 6 months
  5. Has received an in-office topical fluoride treatment in the past 6 months
  6. Has used prescription chlorhexidine daily for a week in each of the past 6 months
  7. Has used xylitol gum or lozenges four to five times daily in the past 6 months
  8. Has used calcium and phosphate supplement during the past 6 months
  9. Has adequate salivary flow

MOUTHRINSES OR CHEMOTHERAPEUTICS[4]

A. May have cosmetic and therapeutic value
B. Effectiveness of many mouthrinses is limited to dislodging gross debris, temporarily reducing microorganisms, and providing a feeling of freshness
C. One category of commercial mouthrinses is approved by the ADA Council on Scientific Affairs: phenol-related essential oil compounds gained acceptance for control of both plaque biofilm and gingivitis and carry the ADA Seal of Acceptance; the ADA no longer gives the Seal to prescription agents
  1. Chlorhexidine gluconate (Peridex®, PerioGard®, Pro Dentx®, PerioRx®)
    a. Available by prescription only
    b. 0.12% concentration in an aqueous solution containing 11.6% alcohol, pH 5.5; also made without alcohol for persons who cannot use alcohol (ask the pharmacist)

c. Clinical effects are comparable with 0.2% percent mouthrinse used for many years outside the United States; extensive clinical research has documented its efficacy
    d. Review of numerous studies has established chlorhexidine's safety, stability, and substantivity, which make it effective in preventing and controlling plaque biofilm and reducing and inhibiting gingivitis
    e. May cause brownish-yellow stain and supragingival calculus
    f. Unpleasant taste may hinder client acceptance
    g. Recommended for short-term use only; one 2-ounce, 30-second rinse, twice daily for 6 months
    h. Available in alcohol-free formulation
  2. Phenol-related essential oils (Listerine® and many equivalent generic store brands)
    a. Available without a prescription
    b. Contains thymol, menthol, eucalyptol, and methylsalicylate in a hydroalcohol solution, 21.6% to 26.9% alcohol, pH 5.0
    c. Low substantivity
    d. Listerine®'s efficacy in inhibiting bacterial plaque biofilm and gingivitis has been documented and has facilitated its acceptance by the ADA Council on Scientific Affairs[4]
    e. Various flavors available to enhance client acceptance and adherence to manufacturer's recommendation for a 30-second rinse twice daily
    f. Essential-oil mouthrinses, using basically the same formula as Listerine®, are marketed under many store brand names and are also accepted by the ADA Council on Scientific Affairs as having anti-plaque and antigingivitis effects
    g. Can be used as pre-procedural mouthrinses before aerosol-producing procedures; or as a pre-procedural subgingival irrigant
    h. Used to decrease S. *mutans*[31]
    i. Anticalculus formulation of Listerine® containing zinc chloride; inhibits supragingival calculus accumulation; has the ADA Seal of Acceptance
    j. Available in alcohol-free formulation; efficacy under investigation
D. Mouthrinses are recommended as adjuncts to, not replacements for, mechanical plaque biofilm control
E. Effective on supragingival biofilm only, unless delivered subgingivally with irrigators
F. Approved mouthrinses should be considered for clients with the following conditions:
  1. Inability to achieve acceptable mechanical plaque biofilm control

2. Fixed splinting, prostheses, dental implants, and overdentures

3. Orthodontic appliances

4. Postperiodontal or other oral surgery

5. Clients at high risk for dental caries

6. Medication-induced gingival enlargement

7. Immunosuppression

8. Pre-procedural application to minimize bacteremia and disease transmission

G. Commercially prepared mouthrinses may contain alcohol or be alcohol-free; other ingredients are water, flavoring, coloring, sweetening agents, and a variety of active ingredients such as:

1. Antimicrobials to reduce or inhibit biofilm activity (cetylpyridinium chloride, chlorhexidine, sanguinarine, phenolic compounds, triclosan); the ADA states that most people can benefit from using an ADA-accepted mouthrinse

2. Oxygenating agents to debride and release oxygen (hydrogen peroxide)

3. Astringents to shrink tissue (citric acid, zinc chloride)

4. Anodynes to alleviate pain

5. Buffering agents to reduce acidity, dissolve mucinous films, and relieve soft tissue pain

6. Deodorizing (sodium bicarbonate) and oxidizing (chlorine dioxide) agents to neutralize odors and eliminate volatile sulfur compounds

7. Fluorides to decrease dental caries risk (see the section on "Self-applied fluorides")

8. Whitening agent such as hydrogen peroxide to reduce intrinsic stains

H. Inexpensive mouthrinses may be prepared by the client (not recommended for clients on a low-salt or sodium-free diet) and used following thorough periodontal debridement

1. Isotonic (normal) saline solution: ½ teaspoon salt in 8 ounces of water

2. Hypertonic saline solution: ½ teaspoon salt in 4 ounces of water

3. Sodium bicarbonate solution: ½ teaspoon sodium bicarbonate (baking soda) in 8 ounces of warm water

I. Mouthrinse use should be monitored by both the client and the dental hygienist; any adverse effects indicate that use should be evaluated and possibly discontinued

J. Mouthrinses containing quaternary ammonium compounds, zinc and copper salts, cetylpyridinium, octenidine, and stannous fluoride have been effective in short-term studies and may warrant further evaluation

K. Mouthrinses, sprays, or swab sticks contain moisteners and possibly fluoride; recommended to relieve oral symptoms of xerostomia

L. Detergent prebrushing mouthrinses (e.g., Plax®) containing sodium benzoate have failed to document efficacy[4]

M. The dental hygienist should teach clients how to be wise consumers of mouthrinses, helping clients to recognize the benefits, limitations, and appropriate therapeutic regimens for mouthrinses

DENTAL SEALANTS

General Considerations

See the section on "Pit-and-fissure sealants" in Chapter 13.

A. Although systemic and topical fluorides provide increased resistance to carious destruction, the pit-and-fissure surfaces do not benefit from fluoride use to the same degree as do smooth surfaces

B. Sealants are a thin resin or glass ionomer coating placed in the pits and fissures of teeth to act as a physical barrier to oral bacteria

1. Preventive sealant—placed in caries-free pits and fissures

2. Therapeutic sealant—placed in pits and fissures with incipient carious lesions to halt caries process

C. Pits and fissures allow for the accumulation and stagnation of fermentable substrates and serve as accumulation sites for acidogenic microorganisms capable of demineralizing tooth tissue

D. The effectiveness of dental sealants in the prevention of pit-and-fissure caries has been clearly demonstrated in research settings

E. Protection from caries approaches 100% when pits and fissures remain completely sealed; numerous clinical trials have documented the efficacy of sealants

F. Comprehensive prevention programs incorporate the complementary use of sealants and fluorides

G. Sealants classified by method of polymerization

1. Auto-polymerizing—chemically cured or self-curing

2. Photo-polymerizing—cured by visible light

H. Sealants classified by filler content

1. Filled sealant—composite resin sealant containing particles of glass and quartz

2. Unfilled sealants—composite resin sealant without particles; less resistant to long-term wear

3. Glass ionomer—salivary control not a critical factor; ideal for teeth when moisture control is an issue

4. Fluoride releasing—promotes remineralization

5. Calcium phosphate—promotes remineralization

I. Sealants classified by color—available in clear, tinted, and opaque color; the color aids in detection and in monitoring retention

Indications for Application

A. Factors to consider
1. Dental caries activity, risk, and pattern
2. Depth of pits and fissures
3. Dietary patterns
4. Current and past fluoride exposure
5. Eruption status
6. Frequency of preventive services

B. Procedure for sealant placement[1]
1. Clients or guardians should be informed about sealants as a primary preventive measure
2. Clients who can benefit from sealant application are:
   a. Children with newly erupted teeth with pits and fissures
   b. Persons whose lifestyle, behavior patterns, physical or emotional development, or lack of fluoride exposure put them at high risk for dental caries
   c. Children and adults whose teeth have deep pits and fissures
   d. People with xerostomia or persons with orthodontic appliances
   e. Other persons who desire sealants as a preventive measure to protect pits and fissures

C. Teeth with questionable or incipient carious lesions should be sealed; incipient lesions are arrested after sealant placement[1,32]

Contraindications to Sealant Application

A. Client behavior does not allow for maintenance of dry field necessary for successful application

B. Presence of frank carious lesion on occlusal surface

C. Presence of carious lesion on proximal surface that necessitates preparation of occlusal surface

D. Previously restored tooth, except as noted in item C above

E. Life expectancy of the primary tooth predicted to be short

Application Guidelines[1]

A. Mechanical cleansing of enamel
1. Debride the pit-and-fissure surface of plaque biofilm and surface debris
2. Cleansing agents include:
   a. Watery slurry of flour or pumice
   b. Toothbrush

c. Air polishing
d. Dental explorer

B. Isolating
1. Salivary contamination of etched enamel surfaces is a major reason for resin sealant failure
2. Isolation—using either a rubber dam or cotton rolls and bibulous (absorbent) pads—is essential for consistent success

C. Drying
1. Dry isolated tooth thoroughly in preparation for the application of conditioner or etchant
2. Avoid water contamination if using air-water syringe

D. Conditioning or etching
1. Acid conditioning etches enamel surface before the application of resin or glass ionomer (sealant) material; etching removes a layer of enamel and increases the total surface area by rendering the deeper enamel regions porous; the sealant's resin material fills the enamel micropores, producing a mechanical "lock" when polymerized
2. Acid conditioning agents (30% to 50% phosphoric acid)—available in either solution or gel form
   a. Apply the solution by gently dabbing the enamel surface with a saturated cotton pellet, sponge, or brush; avoid rubbing the surface because it causes a breakdown of lattice-like micropores
   b. Gels are applied with a special applicator, brush, cotton tip, or cotton pellet
   c. Whether using gel or solution, cover all susceptible surfaces and cuspal inclines with the etchant
   d. Contact between the etching agent and soft tissues should be avoided
   e. Etch the tooth surface for 10 to 20 seconds; check the manufacturer's instructions for etching time

E. Rinsing the conditioned tooth
1. Thoroughly rinse the etched enamel surfaces by using a water syringe and a high-speed evacuation system; do not allow the client to swish; rinsing time may need to be increased to ensure complete removal
2. Salivary contamination at this point results in substantial reduction in resin sealant bond strength
   a. Do not allow client to close the mouth, rinse, or touch the conditioned surface with the tongue
   b. When using cotton rolls or bibulous (absorbent) pads, change them as needed, being careful to avoid salivary contamination

F. Drying the conditioned tooth
1. Prepare the tooth for resin sealant application by drying it thoroughly with compressed air for at least 10 seconds; a completely dry tooth surface is essential for effective application of the resin sealant; it is not as critical when using glass ionomer sealants
2. Examine the conditioned surface; properly etched surfaces will appear dull and chalky; re-etch the tooth surface when these changes are not seen or salivary contamination occurs

G. Applying the sealant material—all susceptible pits and fissures, including the buccal pits of mandibular molars and the lingual grooves of maxillary molars, should be sealed, when possible
1. Visible light-cured sealants—the resin sealant is applied to the etched surface; the tip of the light source is placed 2 mm from the sealant (see the manufacturer's instructions)
   a. Light must be delivered for polymerization to occur and for the prevention of sealant failure
   b. Once polymerization is complete, the sealant should be wiped with a wet cotton roll or pellet to remove any air-inhibited layer of nonpolymerized resin; failure to remove this layer will result in an unpleasant taste
   c. The sealant material is delivered in a variety of ways; unit dose dispensers contain enough sealant for one quadrant; this method reduces the risk of cross-contamination, when used properly
2. Chemical or self-curing sealants—the catalyst and the sealant are mixed and then placed immediately onto the prepared tooth surface with a brush or a custom dispenser; working time from mixing to setting is 1 to 3 minutes; it is important not to disturb the layer of applied sealant during polymerization
3. The sealant material should be allowed to flow into all areas to minimize entrapment of air bubbles
4. Applying excess sealant to the occlusal surface should be avoided, as this could alter the client's occlusion

H. Evaluating the results
1. Examine the sealant to determine the adequacy of bond strength and the absence of voids, underextensions, overextensions, or undercuring
2. The sealed surface should feel completely smooth
3. Floss teeth to ensure that the sealant has not flowed into interproximal spaces

4. For the filled-type sealant material, occlusion should be checked with articulating paper; frank high spots should be reduced with a finishing bur or fine stone; in the case of unfilled-type sealant materials, high spots self-adjust after a few days
5. Evaluate sealant retention at each appointment; replace the material, as needed
6. Most sealant failures result from "operator error," for example, oil, debris, or moisture contamination, or from not following manufacturer's instructions

I. Document on client's chart the type of sealant used and the teeth sealed

TOBACCO USE INTERVENTIONS

General Considerations

A. Although the overall percentage of smokers is declining in the United States, a significant number of adolescents continue to initiate tobacco use. The two types of tobacco are smoked tobacco and unsmoked tobacco. Examples of smoked tobacco include *bidis*, cigars, pipes, cigarettes, water pipe (*hookah*), and clove cigarettes. Unsmoked tobacco is also known as *spit tobacco*, *snuff*, or *smokeless tobacco*.[33] Tobacco cessation is considered to have occurred when an individual permanently discontinues the use of tobacco.[1]

B. Smoking is a primary risk factor for:
1. Lung cancer
2. Chronic obstructive lung disease
3. Heart disease
4. Head and neck, oropharyngeal, and other cancers
5. Periodontal disease[34,35]

C. Oral effects of tobacco use: oral and pharyngeal cancer, failure of periodontal therapy, failure of dental implants, dental caries, tobacco abrasion, extrinsic stain, halitosis, attrition, delayed wound healing, nicotine stomatitis, oral leukoplakia, and tooth loss[1,36]

D. From a host-response perspective, smoking has been found to interfere with the normal function of helper lymphocytes critical to antibody production, impair revascularization in both soft and hard tissues, inhibit collagen production, and increase collagenase activity[37]

E. Spit tobacco use is associated with oral, laryngeal, and pharyngeal cancers; oral mucosal lesions and gingival recession are mostly observed in individuals using spit tobacco. Oral mucosal lesions often disappear after spit tobacco use is discontinued[1]

F. Dental hygienists must assume the responsibility for helping clients abstain from tobacco use and to encourage and appreciate nonusers[33,38]

G. Nicotine itself is not a carcinogen, but it is physiologically addictive; clients trying to quit may experience withdrawal symptoms (e.g., insomnia, irritability, weight gain); embedded social and psychological factors also contribute to the challenge

H. Dental hygienists should take an active role in the community and in legislative efforts to reduce all tobacco use

Tobacco Cessation Interventions[33,38,39]

A. Oral and all health care facilities should be tobacco free

B. Oral health care professionals should strive to quit all tobacco-related habits and serve as positive role models

C. Tobacco use by all clients should be addressed, assessed, and documented in the clients' permanent records

D. The Agency for Healthcare Research and Quality's Clinical Practice Guideline on Treating Tobacco Use and Dependence recommends five components for successful client-provider interaction:[38]

  1. Ask—at every visit of every client, identify and document tobacco use status

  2. Advise—a clear, strong, personalized message to refrain from all tobacco use should be communicated to each client who uses tobacco

  3. Assess—determine if the client is willing to make an attempt to quit

  4. Assist—if client is willing to make an attempt to quit, counseling and pharmacotherapeutic agents should be used; FDA-approved pharmacotherapeutic agents include:

    a. Nicotine reduction therapy—nicotine transdermal patch, gum, lozenge, nasal spray, and oral inhaler

    b. Non-nicotine agents for managing nicotine addiction—sustained-release bupropion hydrochloric acid (HCl) (Zyban) tablets and varenicline (Chantix)

  5. Arrange—a follow-up contact should be scheduled within the first week following the quit date

E. The American Dental Hygienists' Association Smoking Cessation Initiative (SCI) recommends the following steps:

  1. Ask—ask every client about his or her tobacco use at every visit; ask if the client is a current, former, or never tobacco user

  2. Advise—advise every tobacco user to quit; advise those who have tried and not succeeded to try again; employ the teachable moment by linking clinical findings with advice

  3. Refer—refer the client to QUITLINES, Web sites, and local cessation programs; find programs and assistance at www.smokefree.gov, www.askadviserefer.org, or call 1-800-QUIT NOW (1-800-784-8669); these Web sites provide resources to use at the chairside

F. Teenagers, preteens, and children should be considered potential users of smoked and spit tobacco products; interventions include:

  1. Questioning them about tobacco use (e.g., cigarettes, cigars, pipes, water pipes [*hookahs*], chewing tobacco, snuff)

  2. Educating them about the health risks of tobacco use

  3. Educating them about the negative effects of tobacco on their physical appearance and athletic prowess

  4. Encouraging them to resist peer pressure and media messages to start using tobacco

G. Tobacco-use assessment should be part of history taking; assessment should include:

  1. Form of tobacco used

  2. Amount used

  3. Duration of habit

  4. Previous quit attempts

  5. Reasons for quitting or abstaining from tobacco use

H. Client readiness for cessation—clients should be asked if they are ready to quit; the transtheoretical model can be used to assess stages of readiness to quit; clients should set their own quit date[1,40] (see Table 20-9 in Chapter 20)

I. Approximately 70% of adult smokers would like to quit

J. Typically, smokers try to stop multiple times before they succeed

ORAL CANCER

Self-Examination and Basic Concepts

A. Many oral cancers are, unfortunately, not detected until they have invaded deep tissues and require radical surgery, extensive chemotherapy, irradiation, or all three interventions

B. Assessment and reduction of risk factors—early detection and early treatment are the best ways to manage oral cancer; self-examination can supplement a thorough in-office head and neck, extraoral, and intraoral examination

C. Whereas all clients can potentially benefit from self-examination skills, it is especially important to educate high-risk persons

D. Clients need to be taught about mutable and nonmutable risk factors for oral cancer

1. Mutable risk factor—can be changed or eliminated (e.g., smoking, sun exposure, or drinking behavior)

2. Nonmutable risk factor—cannot be changed or eliminated (e.g., genetic makeup or gender)

E. Strategies for reducing risk factors should be part of the dental hygiene care plan

High-Risk Factors

A. Tobacco use
   1. Clients who smoke are estimated to be at greater risk than nonsmokers
   2. Clients who use snuff and spit tobacco are prone to squamous cell carcinomas at or near the site where the tobacco is held

B. Alcohol use—the combination of smoking and alcohol use is responsible for 80% to 90% of all head and neck cancers[1]

C. Virus—certain viruses, for instance, hepatitis B virus (HBV), human immunodeficiency virus (HIV), and human papillomavirus (HPV), and *Helicobacter pylori* are linked to the development of cancers such as cancer of the liver, nasopharynx, cervix, and lymphatic system[1,41]

D. Sun exposure—clients who work outdoors, especially those with fair complexions, are at higher risk for basal cell tumors of the skin (predominating about the face and lips)

Examination Technique

Materials Needed

A. Large mirror and adequate light source are essential for self-examination procedures

B. A flashlight, a mouth-sized mirror, and gauze or tissue squares help better access to and visualization of intraoral structures

Systematic Approach

A. Face and neck
   1. Symmetry—one-sided irregularities should be further investigated; both right and left sides should have the same outline and shape; lesions that fail to heal within 2 weeks should be suspect
   2. Skin—have the client remove eyeglasses; check for sores, bumps, and discolorations
   3. Neck—palpate lymph chains for lumps or tender areas

B. Lips and gums
   1. Have the client remove full or partial dentures
   2. Retract the lips; look for sores or color changes (Figure 16-4)
   3. Palpate the lips; run a finger over the gingiva to feel for irregularities, tenderness, or roughened areas

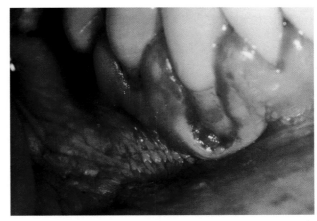

FIGURE 16-4 Keratotic and dysplastic tissue present on the attached and marginal gingiva of the mandibular canine at the site of tobacco placement. *(Photo courtesy of University of Maryland Dental School.)*

C. Cheek
   1. Retract the right side and then the left side to visualize the inner surface; look for red, white, brown, or speckled patches
   2. Palpate for lumps or tenderness
   3. Run a finger over the inside surface to check for rough or raised places

D. Roof of mouth
   1. Tilt the head back and use a flashlight for better visualization
   2. Use a mouth-sized mirror to reflect the image in a larger mirror
   3. Look for sores or color changes; feel for lumps or areas of tenderness

E. Tongue
   1. Have the client extend the tongue, and look at the dorsum
   2. Grasp the tongue with a gauze square; pull and roll the tongue to the right side and then to the left side
   3. Look for sores, color changes, and irregularities (Figure 16-5)
   4. Feel for lumps, areas of tenderness, or roughened surfaces

F. Floor of mouth
   1. Have the client place the tip of the tongue against the roof of the mouth
   2. Look for any asymmetry, sores, or color changes
   3. Place the fingers of one hand under the client's jaw, and use the index finger of the other hand to compress structures
   4. Check for lumps, tenderness, or irregularities

Teaching Factors

A. Provide the client with an assessment of his or her mutable and nonmutable risk factors; help the client to reduce the risks for oral cancer

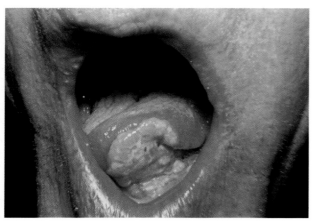

FIGURE 16-5 Tongue and floor of the mouth of a client with epidermoid squamous cell carcinoma. *(Photo courtesy of University of Maryland Dental School.)*

B. Several demonstrations of the self-assessment procedure will probably be necessary for mastery; pamphlets and Web sites that demonstrate techniques are extremely helpful

C. Introduce the concept of "normal range," and familiarize the client with what is normal in his or her mouth

D. Provide the criteria for determining significant deviations from normal
   1. Sores that fail to heal within 2 weeks
   2. Appearance of white, red, or dark-colored patches
   3. Presence of swellings, lumps, bumps, or growths

E. Reinforce need for a systematic approach to ensure thoroughness

F. Define the oral health professional's role in interpreting findings; the client should report unusual findings, but not self-diagnose him/herself

G. Establish the concept that self-examination is not meant to be a substitute for periodic regular professional evaluation

H. Free publications can be ordered from the National Cancer Institute at 1-800-4-CANCER

DIAGNOSTIC TOOLS FOR ORAL CANCER DETECTION

General Consideration

A. The combination of visual examination and palpation is the main approach to detecting epithelial changes in the oral mucosa[42-45]

B. Routine examination for the detection of oral cancer should be completed for each client (see the section on "Extraoral and intraoral assessment" in Chapter 15)

C. Routine oral cancer screenings can reduce oral cancer incidence and mortality rate[45,46]

D. The diagnosis of a suspicious lesion is established by traditional biopsy[45]

Exfoliative Cytology

Definition
Exfoliative cytology—a nonsurgical technique for collecting surface cells from a suspicious oral lesion for microscopic evaluation; not recommended

Advantages
A. Nonsurgical, noninvasive procedure requiring minimal client preparation and no postoperative care

B. Easily and efficiently implemented in any setting, making it ideal for mass screening or use in remote areas

C. Clinical laboratory and professional personnel costs are relatively low

Disadvantages
A. Lacks precision
   1. Only surface lesions can be evaluated because only surface (not basal) cells are collected
   2. Heavily keratinized lesions will not yield adequate cells for examination

B. May delay definitive treatment
   1. Definitive treatment cannot be decided on the basis of the sample smear results alone; valuable time may be lost obtaining and analyzing a smear specimen
   2. When clinical evidence suggests a malignant lesion, biopsy, which is more precise, is the procedure of choice

C. Yields a high number of false negatives

D. No longer a recommended technique in dentistry and dental hygiene

Procedure
A. Fix the sample—to prevent cell dehydration, quickly cover sample surface with layer of 70% alcohol, or apply a spray fixative; allow the sample to air-dry in an area protected from airborne contamination

B. Prepare for transfer to laboratory for analysis and interpretation

Brush Biopsy

Definition
A. Trans-epithelial oral biopsy—samples the superficial, intermediate, and basal epithelial layers to detect oral cancer at its earliest stages (Figure 16-6); indicated for small, innocuous-appearing lesions that have no apparent cause and that are observed

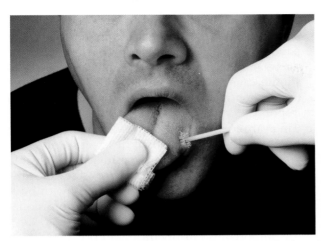

FIGURE 16-6 Brush biopsy technique being used in evaluation of a suspect intraoral lesion. *(Photo courtesy of Oral CDx, Suffern, New York.)*

on a routine basis on thorough oral examination; it should be noted that larger, typically less innocuous–appearing lesions should be referred to a dentist or physician for scalpel biopsy
B. Accurate detection of precancerous or cancerous areas requiring scalpel biopsy
C. The dental hygienist's role is to identify red, white, or mixed lesions as well as ulcerated, thickened, traumatized, or irritated oral epithelium to be evaluated using brush biopsy
D. Dental hygienists should consult their state regulatory board or state statutes to determine whether they are legally permitted to perform brush biopsies

Advantages
A. Easy, chairside test to evaluate epithelial changes and lesions that may have received only a clinical follow-up before this test became available
B. Rapid results, generally within 3 days to detect dysplasia or carcinoma
C. Minimally invasive; does not require topical or local anesthesia to obtain a sample[47]
D. Each specimen is evaluated by both computer-assisted analysis and a pathologist

Disadvantages
A. Costs for both obtaining and analyzing the specimen are incurred by the client; may be covered by some insurance plans
B. As with any biopsy method, false negatives are possible; selecting the correct location(s) to brush on a lesion may be difficult, sometimes resulting in false negatives[47,48]
C. Brush biopsies with negative results require careful follow-up

Procedure
A. Armamentarium (see www.oralcdx.com)
  1. Sterile brush instrument for biopsy
  2. Microscope specimen slide
  3. Fixative
  4. Laboratory forms
B. Obtaining and preparing the sample
  1. Using the client's saliva, moisten the biopsy brush
  2. Firmly press the biopsy brush against the lesion
  3. While pressing, rotate the brush over the surface of the lesion until pink tissue or pinpoint areas of bleeding occur; number of rotations will vary, depending on the thickness of the lesion
  4. Use of topical anesthesia is contraindicated because it may distort the sample
  5. To prepare the glass slide, transfer as much of the cellular sample as possible by rotating and dragging brush lengthwise on the slide
  6. Apply the fixative to thoroughly cover the slide; allow drying for 15 minutes
  7. Package the sample and send it to the laboratory for evaluation

Laboratory Findings for Exfoliative Cytology or Brush Biopsy

A. Classification categories
  1. Unsatisfactory—specimen is not adequate for diagnosis
  2. Class I: Normal—only normal cells are present
  3. Class II: Atypical—some cellular changes may be present; no suggestion of malignancy is present
  4. Class III: Intermediate—changes may suggest malignancy, but findings are not clear; biopsy is recommended
  5. Class IV: Suggestive of cancer—cells with malignant characteristics are present; biopsy is mandatory
  6. Class V: Positive for cancer—cells are obviously malignant; scalpel biopsy is mandatory
B. Follow-up needs
  1. Unsatisfactory—the client should be scheduled for another smear or brush biopsy
  2. Class I or II findings—the client should be monitored for healing of lesion or re-evaluated if the lesion fails to resolve; as with all biopsy methods, false-negative reports are possible; a healed lesion is the best reassurance for reports in categories I and II
  3. Class III, IV, or V findings—the client should be referred for scalpel biopsy

ViziLite®

A. Definition—an FDA-approved technology that screens for oral abnormalities, potentially indicative of oral cancer; this tool helps oral health care professionals identify lesions before they appear on oral tissue surfaces. ViziLite® illumination cannot distinguish keratotic, inflammatory, malignant, or possibly malignant lesions; clinical judgment, and scalpel biopsy are essential for proper patient care[43]

B. Procedure

1. The client rinses with a solution that penetrates 22-cell layers
2. The oral health care professional activates a patented light stick intraorally
3. The light stick illuminates any suboral lesions during the oral cancer screening examination (www.vizilite.com)

C. Studies have shown inconsistent results with the use of ViziLite®; further controlled clinical studies are needed to determine the usefulness of this device[45,46,49]

VELscope®

A. Definition—an FDA-approved handheld device that uses oral fluorescence technology to identify precancerous and cancerous lesions in the oral cavity; the fluorescence technology shows healthy tissue as green and potentially cancerous lesions as dark magenta, brown, or black; changes in tissue can be detected while the change is still subepithelial and otherwise not visualized during conventional oral examination; surgical margins can be determined, which will help guide complete removal of oral cancers in the operatory[50]

B. Procedure

1. Shine the VELscope® light intraorally by maintaining a distance of at least 2 inches
2. Abnormal oral tissue appears irregular and dark, whereas normal areas appear green

C. This device should be used as an adjunct to clinical screening; clinical judgment and scalpel biopsy are essential for the diagnosis of oral cancer lesions[45,51,52]

D. Because of the higher risk of false-positive results with this test, further testing in controlled clinical settings are needed to determine the usefulness of VELscope®[45]

CONTROL OF DENTINAL HYPERSENSITIVITY

General Considerations

A. Dentinal hypersensitivity—abnormal condition that occurs when vital dentin is exposed to the environment of the oral cavity; the result is painful stimuli that can reach the pulp and cause pain

B. Thermal, evaporative, tactile, osmotic, or chemical stimuli cause fluid movement within the dentinal tubule, exciting the nerve and signaling the pulp to respond

C. Gingival recession and loss of enamel should be minimized to avoid dentinal hypersensitivity

D. Treatment of dentinal hypersensitivity is a valuable client service; symptoms cause considerable discomfort to the client and may interfere with both control of plaque biofilm and professional treatment

E. It is important to distinguish pain reaction caused by dentinal hypersensitivity (items 1 to 4 below) from pain attributable to other causes

1. Rapid onset
2. Sharp pain
3. Short duration
4. Response to stimuli

Etiology

A. Primary causes of hypersensitivity are exposed dentin and open dentinal tubules

B. Dentin exposure occurs:

1. In 10% of all teeth; during development, enamel and cementum do not join
2. When enamel or cementum is lost through abrasion, erosion, abfraction, dental caries, or overinstrumentation
3. When soft tissue is lost because of gingival recession, periodontal surgery, or an aggressive toothbrushing technique
4. Diet exposing the exposed dentin to foods and beverages with a low pH; soft drinks, sport drinks, coffee, fruit juices, and fruit drinks; citrus fruits; yogurt; and some alcoholic beverages; plaque biofilm acids
5. Loss of hard and soft tissues is believed to be accelerated from the combination use of mechanical brushing and a dentifrice applied immediately following exposure to acidic food or drink

Pain Mechanism

A. Hydrodynamic theory—the most widely accepted

B. Explains the following:

1. Dentinal tubules are exposed
2. Pain-producing stimuli are present
3. Pain-producing stimuli initiate the flow of lymphatic fluid within dental tubules
4. Odontoblasts and their processes act as receptors and transmitters of sensory stimuli

5. The movement of tubular fluids causes nerve endings at the pulpal wall to be stimulated and produce pain

Pain Stimuli

A. Thermal or evaporative stimuli—foods and liquids at extreme temperatures, cold air, and too-rapid drying of a tooth surface; cause a concurrent rapid drop in tooth temperature; are more problematic than hot air changes
B. Mechanical stimuli—instrumentation, home-care devices, eating utensils, and friction from removable prosthetic or orthodontic devices
C. Chemical stimuli—foods high in acid or sugars; some topical medications; plaque acids

Desensitizing Agents

A. Modes of action—desensitizing agents:
  1. Seal dentinal tubules by surface precipitation of ions, subsurface incorporation of ions, or stimulation of secondary dentin
  2. Decrease the excitability of sensory nerves, thereby making the nerve less sensitive to stimuli
B. Optimal characteristics—professionally applied desensitizing agents should act rapidly and should be nontoxic, easy to apply, and have consistent outcomes and long-term effects

Types of Desensitizing Treatments

A. No single agent or form of treatment is effective for all persons
B. Numerous agents have varying degrees of success; they include:
  1. Solutions, gels, or pastes of fluoride in varying compounds and percentages, stannous fluoride, calcium hydroxide, strontium chloride, potassium nitrate, sodium citrate, formaldehyde, glutaraldehyde, arginine and insoluble calcium, casein phosphopeptide–amorphous calcium phosphate complex, or potassium or ferric oxalate
  2. Adhesive, varnish, or bonding materials
  3. Polymerizing agents[1]
    a. Glass ionomer cements (GIC)—used in cervical abrasion and abfraction; the sensitive area is etched with 50% citric acid, rinsed with water, and dried before application of the glass ionomer cement
    b. Adhesive resin primers—reduces dentin permeability by occluding open tubules; the material is rubbed on the sensitive area for approximately 30 seconds and air-dried

4. Iontophoretic devices—iontophoresis is the application of an electrical current to impregnate tissues with ions from dissolved salts; fluoride iontophoresis is thought to result in the increased uptake and penetration of fluoride ions into dentin; devices are technique sensitive
5. Laser therapy—one-time treatment that reduces or eliminates dentin sensitivity by sealing dentinal tubules; sensitive dentin treated with laser is found to be harder compared with untreated dentin[1]
6. Restorations—restoration may be placed on the surface where dentin is exposed to help reduce sensitivity

Desensitization Methods

A. Self-care regimens
  1. Effective plaque biofilm control strategies are important in gaining and maintaining control of hypersensitivity; modifications to minimize aggressive brushing are critical
  2. Specially formulated toothpastes containing 5% potassium nitrate to desensitize the nerve are often combined with fluoride, which promotes remineralization
  3. Daily use of a fluoride gel or rinse is advisable when the problem is generalized or recurrent; 0.4% SnF_2 gels carry the ADA Seal of Acceptance for desensitization
B. Professionally delivered regimens should support and make possible self-care regimens
  1. General guidelines
    a. Remove all deposits; involved surfaces must be free of barriers to the agent
    b. Local anesthesia is appropriate when instrumentation procedures or the application of the agent are too painful
    c. Isolate the sensitive tooth and control saliva
    d. Dry the affected tooth with cotton pellets or gauze; avoid using an air syringe
    e. Apply the agent according to the manufacturer's instructions for method and time required; pastes are usually burnished in with a wooden point, whereas solutions, gels, or varnishes are painted or bathed on; some clients may experience an acute pain reaction to the agent; immediately remove the agent, wait a few minutes, and then attempt re-application
    f. Remove any excess agent to avoid ingestion by the client
    g. Test for change in pain reaction; this will not be possible with anesthetized areas
    h. Plan for future re-application if desensitization has not occurred

2. Precaution—some agents have very high concentrations of fluoride; to prevent nausea, use proper application and salivary flow–control techniques

PULPAL VITALITY AND TESTING DEVICES

Basic Concepts

A. Teeth may become nonvital from bacterial invasion of the pulp associated with caries or periodontal disease or from injuries such as mechanical or thermal trauma

B. Any tooth suspected of being nonvital should be tested for pulpal vitality

C. The preferred method of testing is that which provides a qualitative assessment

D. Tests should correlate with or mimic the client's chief complaint

E. Palpation, percussion, and radiographic findings (e.g., widened periodontal ligament [PDL]) are other sources of data for pulpal assessment

Types of Pulp Vitality Testing Methods

Laser Doppler Flowmetry[53,54]

A. Noninvasive, painless, semi-quantitative method; measures pulpal blood flow through assessment of the vascular supply by the passage of light through a tooth; monitors blood flow in response to pressure changes and administration of local anesthesia

B. This device is useful in young children whose responses are usually unreliable

C. Studies have shown that blood circulation is the most accurate determinant in assessing pulp vitality[55]

D. Laser doppler flowmetry is more reliable at identifying vital and nonvital teeth earlier compared with other pulp vitality tests

Pulse Oximetry[53,56,57,58]

A. Definition—Noninvasive oxygen monitoring instrument used in medical practice to measure pulse rate as well as oxygen saturation of blood during administration of anesthesia

B. This objective test requires no response from the client; used in dentistry to evaluate vascular supply to teeth

C. The instrument consists of two light-emitting diodes (LEDs) and a photodetector; normal arterial blood flow is required for accurate assessment

Traditional Electrical Testing Devices

A. The electrical pulp tester (also known as a *vitalometer*) and the digital pulp tester use gradations of electrical current to excite a response in pulpal tissue and thus assess response to stimulus; pulp testers have either a portable battery or a plug-in electrical power source; all testers have rheostats, with a scale (e.g., 1–10 or 1–50) that indicates the relative amount of current being applied; digital pulp testers provide a digital reading; electrical pulp testers can be used safely on clients with implanted cardiac devices

B. Procedure

1. Armamentarium

a. Testing device

b. Cotton rolls

c. Toothpaste or other conducting medium

2. Client preparation

a. Explain the procedure to the client; use the minimal stimulation necessary to evoke a response

b. Instruct the client to raise a hand when the slightest warmth or tingling sensation is felt

c. To acquaint the client with the type of sensation created and to determine a normal response pattern, first test the teeth adjacent and contralateral to the tooth being tested

3. Obtaining a reading

a. Isolate and dry the teeth to be tested; this prevents the conduction of current into the soft tissue

b. Apply a small amount of toothpaste, or an alternative conductor, to the tester tip

c. Place the tip on sound tooth structure within the middle third of the crown for a single-rooted tooth and within the middle third of each cusp for a multiple-rooted tooth; a clip resting on the client's lip and attached to the handpiece is necessary to create a closed electric circuit and to activate the tester

d. Avoid any contact with restorations and soft tissue

e. Slowly advance the rheostat from zero to increasingly higher numbers until a sensation is felt by the client; the rheostat should not be moved above that point for that tooth

4. Documentation

a. Two readings should be taken for each tooth tested and the readings averaged

b. For all teeth tested, record the lowest average reading, the type of testing device and conductor used, and any client actions or reactions that may have affected the results

C. Variables affecting results

1. Pulpal conditions may vary from early inflammation to complete necrosis; client responses vary with each condition; the pulp of the tooth that is tested is considered to be degenerating when, compared with a control, much more current is required to gain a response
2. Metallic restorations conduct electrical charges more rapidly than tooth structure and can produce false readings
3. Teeth with splints, bridges, or proximal restorations may produce false-positive reactions because the circuit can be transferred from adjacent vital teeth
4. Multiple-rooted teeth may have some combination of vital and nonvital canals and give false-positive results
5. Pain reactions are influenced by the client's attitude, age, gender, anxiety, emotions, fatigue, culture, and medications

Thermal Testing

This type of testing employs a hot or cold thermal stimulus to test for pulpal response. The cold test is used most often; the heat test is useful when an unidentified tooth is heat sensitive.

ETHICAL, LEGAL, AND SAFETY ISSUES

A. Dental hygienists must have knowledge of evidence-based preventive products and strategies

B. A combination of frequent review of the literature; focus on information from controlled clinical trials and systematic review articles; the practitioner's knowledge, clinical experience, and judgment; and client preferences leads to appropriate evidence-based decision making and best practices

C. Thorough, accurate, and confidential chart documentation is essential; adherence to the regulations of the Health Insurance Portability and Accountability Act (HIPAA) is mandatory

D. The client's progress with regard to self-care should be documented in the client record and should include the client's response, knowledge, adherence, involvement, skills, and measurable oral changes

E. The dental hygienist should discuss all the procedures with clients on an appropriate level for comprehension, obtain informed consent, and encourage client participation in the dental hygiene care plan

F. Dental hygiene interventions are offered within the scope of dental hygiene practice and within the legal jurisdiction of the employment setting

G. Clients have the right to accept or reject the dental care plan and still retain the respect of the dental hygienist

H. Clients have the right to receive individualized, cutting edge, evidence-based recommendations and care

@ WEB SITE INFORMATION AND RESOURCES

SOURCE	WEB SITE ADDRESS	DESCRIPTION
National Center for Dental Hygiene Research	http://www.usc.edu/hsc/dental/dhnet/	Resources and links for dental hygienists
American Academy of Periodontology	http://www.perio.org	Periodontics resources and position papers
Campaign for Tobacco Free Kids	http://www.tobaccofreekids.org/index.php	Information and initiatives to keep children tobacco free
ADHA Ask. Advise. Refer. Campaign	http://www.askadviserefer.org	Information about smoking cessation
American Lung Association—Freedom from Smoking	http://www.lungusa.org/	Information about lung diseases and tobacco use cessation

REFERENCES

1. Darby ML, Walsh MM: *Dental hygiene theory and practice,* ed 3, Philadelphia, 2010, Saunders.

2. Walsh MM: Improving health and saving lives, *Dimensions Dent Hyg* 1(7):20, 2003.

3. Tillis TS, Stach DJ, Cross-Poline GN, Annan SD, Astroth DB, Wolfe P: The transtheoretical model applied to an oral self-care behavior change: development and testing of instruments for stages of change and decisional balance, *J Dent Hyg* 77(1):16–25, 2003.

4. Ciancio SG: *ADA guide to dental therapeutics,* ed 5, Chicago, 2009, American Dental Association.

5. Moritis K, Jenkins W, Hefti A, Schmitt P, McGrady M: A randomized, parallel design study to evaluate the effects of a Sonicare and manual toothbrush on plaque and gingivitis, *J Clin Dent* 19(2):64–68, 2008.

6. Biesbrock AR, Bartizek RD, Gerlach RW, Terézhalmy GT: Oral hygiene regimens, plaque control, and gingival health: a two-month clinical trial with antimicrobial agents, *J Clin Dent* 18(4):101–105, 2007.

7. Rosema NA, Timmerman MF, Versteeg PA, van Palenstein Helderman WH, Van der Velden U, Van der Weijden GA: Comparison of the use of different modes of mechanical oral hygiene in prevention of plaque and gingivitis, *J Periodontol* 79(8):1386–1394, 2008.

8. Salvi GE, Della Chiesa A, Kianpur P, et al: Clinical effects of interdental cleansing on supragingival biofilm formation and development of experimental gingivitis, *Oral Health Prev Dent* 7(4):383–391, 2009.

9. Husseini A, Slot DE, Van der Weijden GA: The efficacy of oral irrigation in addition to a toothbrush on plaque and the clinical parameters of periodontal inflammation: a systematic review, *Int J Dent Hygiene* 6(4): 304–314, 2008.

10. Wilkins EM: *Clinical practice of the dental hygienist,* ed 10, Baltimore, 2009, Lippincott Williams & Wilkins.

11. ADA Council on Access, Prevention and Interprofessional Relations, Caries Diagnosis & Risk Assessment: A review of preventive strategies and management, *J Am Dent Assoc* 126(Suppl):15, 1995.

12. Awano S, Koshimune S, Kurihara E, et al: The assessment of methyl mercaptan, an important clinical marker for the diagnosis of oral malodor, *J Dent* 32:555–559, 2004.

13. Bosy A: Oral malodor: philosophical and practical aspects, *J Can Dent Assoc* 63(3):196–201, 1997.

14. Amir E, Shimonov R, Rosenberg M: Halitosis in children, *J Pediatr* 134(3):338–343, 1999.

15. Figueirido LC, Rosetti EP, Marcantonio E Jr, Marcantonio RA, Salvador SL: The relationship of oral malodor in patients with and without periodontal disease, *J Periodontol* 73:1338–1342, 2002.

16. Lee C, Kho HS, Chung SC, Lee SW, Kim YK: The relationship between volatile sulfur compounds and major halitosis-inducing factors, *J Periodontol* 74:32–37, 2004.

17. Nalcad R, Baran I: Oral malodor and removable complete dentures in the elderly, *Oral Surg Oral Med Oral Pathol Oral Radiol Endod* 105(6):5–9, 2008.

18. Amano A, Yoshida Y, Oho T, Koga T: Monitoring ammonia to assess halitosis, *Oral Surg Oral Med Oral Pathol Oral Radiol Endod* 94(6):692–696, 2002.

19. Greenstein G, Research, Science and Therapy Committee, American Academy of Periodontology: Position paper. The role of supra-and subgingival irrigation in the treatment of periodontal disease, *J Periodontol* 76:2015–2027, 2005.

20. Daniel SJ, Harfst SA, Wilder R: *Mosby's dental hygiene: concepts, cases and competencies,* St Louis, 2007, Mosby.

21. Hollowell WH, Childers NK: A new threat to adolescent oral health: the grill, *Pediatr Dent* 29(4):320–322, 2007.

22. Strietzel FP, Reichart PA, Kale A, Kulkarni M, Wegner B, Küchler I: Smoking interferes with the prognosis of dental implant treatment: a systematic review and meta-analysis, *J Clin Periodontol* 34:523–544, 2007.

23. Centers for Disease Control and Prevention: Recommendations for using fluoride to prevent and control dental caries in the United States, *MMWR* 50(RR14):1, 2001.

24. Azarpazhooh A, Main PA: Fluoride varnish in the prevention of dental caries in children and adolescents: a systematic review, *J Can Dent Assoc* 74(1):73–79, 2008.

25. American Dental Association Council on Scientific Affairs: Professionally applied topical fluoride evidence-based clinical recommendations, *J Am Dent Assoc* 137(8):1151–1159, 2006.

26. Reynolds EC: Remineralization of enamel subsurface lesions by casein phosphopeptide-stabilized calcium phosphate solution, *J Dent Res* 76:1587–1595, 1997.

27. Reynolds EC, Cai F, Cochrane NJ, et al: Fluoride and casein phosphopeptide-amorphous calcium phosphate, *J Dent Res* 87(4):344–348, 2008.

28. Ashley D, Barbieri S: The use of xylitol in caries prevention, *Access* 19(10):24–27, 2005.

29. Featherstone JD, Domejean-Orliaguet S, Jenson L, et al: Caries risk assessment in practice for age 6 through adult, *J Calif Dent Assoc* 35:703–707, 710–713, 2007.

30. Jenson L, Brideny AW, Featherstone JDB, et al: Clinical protocols for caries management by risk assessment, *J Calif Dent Assoc* 35:714–723, 2007.

31. Fine DH, Furgang D, Barnett ML, et al: Effect of an essential oil-containing antiseptic mouthrinse on plaque and salivary *Streptococcus mutans* levels, *J Clin Periodontol* 27:157–161, 2000.

32. Mertz-Fairhurst EJ, Curtis JW Jr., Ergle JW, et al: Ultraconservative and cariostatic sealed restorations: results at year 10, *J Am Dent Assoc* 129(1):55–66, 1998.

33. Walsh MM, Ellison JA: Treatment of tobacco use dependence: the role of the dental professional, *J Dent Educ* 69(5):521–537, 2005.

34. Position paper: Tobacco use and the periodontal patient. Research, Science and Therapy Committee of the American Academy of Periodontology, *J Periodontol* 70(11): 1419–1427, 1999.

35. Johnson GK, Hill M: Cigarette smoking and the periodontal patient, *J Periodontol* 75:196–209, 2004.

36. U.S. Department of Health and Human Services: *The health consequences of smoking: what it means to you,* Bethesda, MD, 2004, U.S. Department of Health and Human Services, Centers for Disease Control and

Prevention, National Center for Chronic Disease Prevention and Health Promotion, Office of Smoking and Health.

37. Loos BG, Roos MT, Schellekens PT, van der Velden U, Miedema F: Lymphocyte numbers and function in relation to periodontitis and smoking, *J Periodontol* 75: 557–564, 2004.

38. Fiore MC, Anderson JE, Jorenby DE, Scott WJ: *Treating tobacco use and dependence: clinical practice guidelines*, Rockville, MD, 2000, U.S. Department of Health and Human Services.

39. Walsh MM: Treating tobacco dependency, *Dimension Dent Hyg* 2(1):2, 2004.

40. Prochaska JO, DiClemente CC: Stages of change in the modification of behavior problems, *Prog Behav Modif* 28:184, 1992.

41. American Cancer Society: Cancer facts and figures 2008: Available at: http://www.cancer.org/downloads/STT/2008CAFFfinalsecured.pdf: Accessed March 28, 2010.

42. Ram S, Siar CH: Chemiluminescence as a diagnostic aid in the detection of oral cancer and potentially malignant epithelial lesions, *Int J Oral Maxillofac Surg* 34: 521–527, 2005.

43. Farah CS, McCullough MJ: A pilot case control study on the efficacy of acetic acid wash and chemiluminescent illumination (ViziLite) in the visualization of oral mucosal white lesions, *Oral Oncol* 43:820–824, 2007.

44. Epstein JB, Silverman S Jr, Epstein JD, Lonky SA, Bride MA: Analysis of oral lesion biopsies identified and evaluated by visual examination, chemiluminescence and toluidine blue, *Oral Oncol* 44:538–544, 2008.

45. Trullenque-Eriksson A, Muñoz-Corcuera M, Campo-Trapero J, Cano-Sánchez J, Bascones-Martínez A: Analysis of new diagnostic methods in suspicious lesions of the oral mucosa, *Med Oral Patol Oral Cir Bucal* 14(5):E210–E216, 2009.

46. Kujan O, Glenny AM, Oliver RJ, Thakker N, Sloan P: Screening programmes for the early detection and prevention of oral cancer, *Cochrane Database Syst Rev* 3:CD004150, 2006.

47. Svirsky JA, Burns JC, Carpenter WM, et al: Comparison of computer-assisted brush biopsy results with follow up scalpel biopsy and histology, *General Dent* 50: 500–503, 2002.

48. Christian DC: Computer-assisted analysis of oral brush biopsies at an oral cancer screening program, *J Am Dent Assoc* 133:357–362, 2002.

49. Mehrotra R, Singh M, Thomas S, Nair P, Pandya S, Nigam NS, Shukla P: A cross-sectional study evaluating chemiluminescence and autofluorescence in the detection of clinically innocuous precancerous and cancerous oral lesions, *J Am Dent Assoc* 141(2):151–156, 2010.

50. Poh CF, Zhang L, Anderson DW, et al: Fluorescence visualization detection of field alterations in tumor margins of oral cancer patients, *Clin Cancer Res* 12:6716–6722, 2006.

51. VELscope, the Oral Cancer Screening System. LED Dental Inc.: Available at http://www.velscope.com: Accessed April 16, 2010.

52. Paulis M: The influence of patient education by the dental hygienist: acceptance of the fluorescence oral cancer exam, *J Dent Hyg* 83(3):134–140, 2009.

53. Samraj RV, Indira R, Srinivasan MR Kumar A: Recent advances in pulp vitality testing, *Endodontology* 15: 14–19, 2003.

54. Jafarzadeh H: Laser Doppler flowmetry in endodontics: a review, *Int Endod J* 42(6):476–490, 2009.

55. Evans D, Reid J, Strang R, Stirrups D: A comparison of laser Doppler flowmetry with other methods of assessing the vitality of traumatized anterior teeth, *Endod Dent Traumatol* 15:284–290, 1999.

56. Gopikrishna V, Pradeep G, Venkateshbabu N: Assessment of pulp vitality: a review, *Int J Paediatr Dent* 19(1):3–15, 2009.

57. Gopikrishna V, Kandaswamy D, Gupta T: Assessment of the efficacy of an indigenously developed pulse oximeter dental sensor holder for pulp vitality testing—an in vivo study, *Indian J Dent Res* 17:111–113, 2006.

58. Gopikrishna V, Tinagupta K, Kandaswamy D: Comparison of electrical, thermal and pulse oximetry methods for assessing pulp vitality in recently traumatized teeth, *J Endod* 33:531–535, 2007.

SUGGESTED READINGS

Darby ML, Walsh MM: *Dental hygiene theory and practice*, ed 3, Philadelphia, 2010, Saunders.

Harris NO, Garcia-Godoy F: *Primary preventive dentistry*, ed 7, Upper Saddle River, NJ, 2008, Pearson Prentice Hall.

Hodges KO: *Foundations of periodontics for the dental hygienist*, ed 2, Philadelphia, 2007, Lippincott Williams & Wilkins.

Ibsen OAC, Phelan JA: *Oral pathology for the dental hygienist*, ed 5, St Louis, 2009, Saunders.

Petrou I, Heu R, Stranick M, et al: A breakthrough therapy for dentin hypersensitivity: How dental products containing 8% arginine and calcium carbonate work to deliver effective relief of sensitive teeth, *J Clin Dent* 20(1):23–31, 2009.

Beauchamp J, Caufield PW, Crall JJ, et al: Evidence-based clinical recommendations for the use of pit-and-fissure sealants: a report of the American Dental Association Council on Scientific Affairs, *J Am Dent Assoc* 139(3): 257–268, 2008.

Ahovuo-Saloranta A, Hiiri A, Nordblad A, Mäkelä M, Worthington HV: Pit and fissure sealants for preventing dental decay in the permanent teeth of children and adolescents, *Cochrane Database Syst Rev* CD001830, 2008.

Niederman R: Glass ionomer and resin-based fissure sealants—equally effective? *Evid Based Dent* 11(1):10, 2010.

Wilkins EM: *Clinical practice of the dental hygienist*, ed 10, Philadelphia, 2009, Lippincott Williams & Wilkins.

M. Anjum Shah and the publisher acknowledge the past contributions of Mary Catherine Dean and Jacquelyn L. Fried to this chapter.

CHAPTER 16 REVIEW QUESTIONS

Answers and Rationales to Chapter Review Questions are available on this text's accompanying Evolve site. See inside front cover for details.

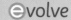

1. What behavioral theory explains that clients with the internal desire to change a behavior strive to accomplish it and the behavior usually lasts longer?
   a. Attribution
   b. Locus of control
   c. Motivation
   d. Self-efficacy

2. Which of the following categories of prevention within the agent–host–environment theory is exemplified by scaling and root planing for a client with periodontal disease?
   a. Primary
   b. Secondary
   c. Tertiary
   d. Action

3. Effective oral health education programs should include all of the following EXCEPT one. Which one is the EXCEPTION?
   a. Assess the client's risk for oral disease
   b. Include strategies for effective control of plaque biofilm
   c. Address current disease activity
   d. Unwillingness of patient to practice preventive behavior

4. What is the MOST commonly used product to control plaque biofilm?
   a. Antimicrobial mouthrinses
   b. Dental floss
   c. Power toothbrush
   d. Toothbrush

5. Power toothbrushing should be recommended to clients with all of the following EXCEPT one. Which one is the EXCEPTION?
   a. Meticulous oral hygiene
   b. Gingivitis
   c. Orthodontic appliances
   d. Abrasion

6. Which of the following methods would be MOST appropriate to disinfect a toothbrush for a client with candidiasis?
   a. Rinse thoroughly with water, and allow to air-dry
   b. Spray liberally with chlorine bleach
   c. Soak in 0.12% chlorhexidine
   d. Coat with a slurry of hydrogen peroxide and baking soda

7. Floss holders should be recommended for clients with which one of the following?
   a. Manual dexterity problems
   b. Excellent home oral care
   c. Dentinal hypersensitivity
   d. Inadequate exposure to fluoride

8. Which of the following professional fluoride agents is known for both its efficacy in caries prevention and control of dentinal hypersensitivity because of its high concentration of fluoride?
   a. Acidulated phosphate fluoride gel
   b. Stannous fluoride
   c. Sodium fluoride varnish
   d. Neutral sodium fluoride foam

9. Desensitizing agents for dentinal hypersensitivity disrupt pain transmission by preventing nerve depolarization or by blocking dentinal tubules; over-the-counter dentinal hypersensitivity products which occlude dentinal tubules contain potassium salts and products which affect nerve depolarization contain fluoride.
   a. Both statements are TRUE
   b. Both statements are FALSE
   c. The first statement is TRUE; the second statement is FALSE
   d. The first statement is FALSE; the second statement is TRUE

10. Which one of the following antimicrobial mouthrinses is available only as a prescription in the United States?
    a. 0.12% chlorhexidine gluconate mouthrinse
    b. 0.0 5% sodium fluoride mouthrinse
    c. Essential oils mouthrinse
    d. Cetylpyridinium chloride mouthrinse

11. A dental hygienists should recommend all of the following to a client struggling to control oral malodor EXCEPT one. Which one is the EXCEPTION?
    a. Refraining from using tobacco products
    b. Rinsing with antimicrobial mouthrinse
    c. Chewing on sugar-free gums or candies
    d. Drinking coffee without sugar

12. Which of the following should be recommended for a client at high to moderate caries risk?
    a. Fluoride varnish
    b. Products containing amorphous calcium phosphate
    c. Xylitol-containing chewing gum
    d. All of the above

13. **All of the following are true regarding oral irrigation devices EXCEPT one. Which one is this EXCEPTION?**
    a. Recommended for clients with fixed prosthetics
    b. Can be effectively used to treat periodontitis
    c. Helps reduce gingivitis
    d. Used for the delivery of antimicrobial agents subgingivally

14. **All of the following are true statements about 5% fluoride varnish EXCEPT one. Which one is the EXCEPTION?**
    a. Approved for caries control
    b. Can be applied to both children and adults' teeth
    c. Recommended for clients with high caries risk
    d. Available over the counter for caries prevention

15. **An interdental brush can be used to effectively remove plaque biofilm in all of the following situations EXCEPT one. Which one is the EXCEPTION?**
    a. Teeth with large diastemas
    b. Teeth with enamel erosion
    c. Type II embrasure space
    d. Fixed orthodontic appliances

16. **Which of the following dentifrice ingredients prevent separation by increasing the consistency of the mixture of liquid and solid ingredients?**
    a. Humectants
    b. Flavoring agents
    c. Preservatives
    d. Binding agents

17. **Which of the following ingredient in a dentifrice would a dental hygienist recommend to a client struggling to minimize supragingival calculus formation?**
    a. Potassium nitrate
    b. Pyrophosphate
    c. Hydrogen peroxide
    d. Triclosan

18. **A dry field is necessary for the long-term success of resin-based pit-and-fissure dental sealants; therefore, glass ionomer pit-and-fissure dental sealant material should be applied on the teeth of clients when moisture control is an issue.**
    a. Both statements are TRUE
    b. Both statements are FALSE
    c. The first statement is TRUE; the second statement is FALSE
    d. The first statement is FALSE; the second statement is TRUE

Use Case A to answer questions 19 to 29.

Case A

Ms. Ivory is a 45-year-old female who has just arrived for her first dental hygiene care visit in 11 years. Ms. Ivory recently acquired dental insurance and is interested in improving her oral health. Her physician is treating her for anxiety, hypertension, type 2 diabetes, and seasonal allergies. She takes Xanax (alprazolam) for anxiety and migraines; Atenolol (tenormin) for hypertension; Glucotrol (glipizide) for diabetes and an over-the-counter antihistamine product for seasonal allergy relief. She occasionally experiences dry mouth; she reports brushing twice per day, flossing occasionally, and using Parodontax® toothpaste without fluoride. In addition, she states that her gums bleed every time she brushes and flosses her teeth. Ms. Ivory has moderate levels of cervical plaque biofilm. She reports using a soft toothbrush but cannot remember the brand name. She also experiences sensitivity to cold, sweets, and pressure in the mandibular right posterior quadrant. She is missing teeth #1, #3, #14, #16, #17, and #32. A class I furcation involvement is present on the buccal surface of tooth #19, and generalized 2- to 3-mm recession throughout her mouth, with class II embrasure spaces. Radiographs show moderate horizontal bone loss and moderate subgingival and supragingival calculus, especially in the interproximal areas. She has three new class I and two class II and IV carious lesions. In five previously restored teeth, recurrent caries can be seen.

19. **To assist Ms. Ivory modify her current oral health behaviors and improve her oral health, it is important to determine her level on the learning ladder. What step of the learning ladder is Ms. Ivory currently on?**
    a. Unawareness
    b. Awareness
    c. Action
    d. Habit

20. **To address this client's dentinal hypersensitivity to cold, sweets, and pressure, all of the following** would be appropriate recommendations EXCEPT one. Which one is the EXCEPTION?
    a. Recommend an ADA-accepted or CDA-recognized dentifrice containing potassium nitrate and fluoride
    b. Evaluate the tooth vitality of the mandibular right molar and premolars
    c. Refer to a dental practitioner
    d. Obtain periapical radiographs of the mandibular molars and premolars

21. To help Ms. Ivory prevent future dental caries, the dental hygienist may suggest all of the following EXCEPT one. Which one is the EXCEPTION?
    a. An ADA-approved or CDA-recognized dentifrice containing fluoride
    b. Dental sealants on all permanent molars and premolars
    c. Xylitol-containing gums or candies
    d. Interdental brushing once per day

22. Reduction of future cervical plaque is best accomplished by the:
    a. Introduction of 0.12% chlorhexidine rinse
    b. Introduction of a soft bristle toothbrush
    c. Modification of the client's toothbrushing technique
    d. Modification of the client's flossing technique

23. When making recommendations regarding future caries control, the dental hygienist should consider all of the following EXCEPT one. Which one is the EXCEPTION?
    a. Plaque control behavior
    b. Xerostomia management
    c. Bleeding during toothbrushing
    d. Current fluoride exposure

24. Which of the following interdental aids would be MOST appropriate for this client's moderate horizontal bone loss?
    a. Power toothbrush
    b. Interdental brush
    c. Unwaxed floss
    d. Uni-tufted brush

25. Given this client's high caries incidence, systemic health issues, periodontal condition, and pharmacologic history, the inclusion of dietary analysis and counseling in the care plan would be appropriate:
    a. Both statements are TRUE
    b. The first part of the statement is TRUE, and the second part is FALSE
    c. The first part of the statement is FALSE, and the second part is TRUE
    d. Both statements are FALSE

26. All of the following factors may have contributed to Ms. Ivory's periodontal disease EXCEPT one. Which one is the EXCEPTION?
    a. Infrequent flossing
    b. Inclusion of fluoride in dentifrice
    c. Subgingival calculus
    d. Uncontrolled diabetes

27. Ms. Ivory can benefit from all of the following educational resources EXCEPT one. Which one is the EXCEPTION?
    a. Pamphlet explaining the value of oral products carrying the ADA Seal of Acceptance
    b. Pamphlet on the role of fluoride in dental caries prevention
    c. Methods to reduce dentinal hypersensitivity
    d. Tooth whitening methods

28. All of the following oral hygiene product ingredients can benefit Ms. Ivory's oral health EXCEPT one. Which one is the EXCEPTION?
    a. Triclosan
    b. Sodium lauryl sulfate
    c. Stannous fluoride
    d. Zinc chloride

29. What follow-up questions will the dental hygienist ask regarding Ms. Ivory's type 2 diabetes?
    a. What was your most recent A_{1c} (HbA_{1c}) test result?
    b. When did you last eat?
    c. Is your diabetes controlled or uncontrolled?
    d. All of the above

Use Case B to answer questions 30 to 37.

Case B

Mr. Jones, a 30-year old male, presents for his 6-month continued-care appointment. His health and pharmacologic histories reveal that he is taking an antidepressant drug. He has very tight contacts between his teeth and reports that flossing frustrates him. He smokes one-half pack of cigarettes daily. Intraoral assessment findings reveal a coated tongue, generalized brown extrinsic stains covering most of the lingual surfaces, generalized moderate gingivitis, and light interproximal calculus. Periodontal probe readings and radiographs reveal healthy teeth and periodontium with no bone loss. Recently separated from his long-time girlfriend, Mr. Jones is concerned about his self-image and wonders if he has "bad breath." He is interested in having his teeth whitened to improve his appearance and has requested your guidance in making his oral health care decisions.

30. To help Mr. Jones remove interproximal plaque biofilm, what should the hygienist recommend?
    a. Smoking cessation
    b. Power toothbrush
    c. Floss threader
    d. Floss holder

31. Which of the following is important for Mr. Jones to be aware of before a professional whitening procedure?
    a. Tobacco decreases the longevity of tooth whitening
    b. Professional tooth whitening will remove brown extrinsic stains
    c. Professional tooth whitening may cause dental erosion
    d. None of the above; clients who smoke should not have their teeth bleached

32. All of the following may be contributing to Mr. Jones's halitosis EXCEPT one. Which one is the EXCEPTION?
    a. Tight tooth contacts
    b. Coated tongue
    c. Necrotizing ulcerative gingivitis
    d. Smoking one-half pack of cigarettes daily

33. All of the following can be recommend to Mr. Jones for his halitosis EXCEPT one. Which one is the EXCEPTION?
    a. Tobacco cessation
    b. Tongue brushing
    c. Use of an ADA-accepted or CDA-recognized antimicrobial mouthrinse
    d. Daily fluoride mouthrinse

34. To assist Mr. Jones abstain from cigarette smoking, the dental hygienist should take all of the following actions EXCEPT one. Which one is the EXCEPTION?
    a. Recommend the use of pharmacologic adjuncts
    b. Refer him to a local tobacco cessation program
    c. Demonstrate interproximal cleaning
    d. Educate him on the consequences of smoking

35. Which of the following will help clients manage their nicotine withdrawal symptoms?
    a. Nicotine transdermal patch
    b. Referral to a tobacco cessation program
    c. Non-nicotine agent (e.g., SR bupropion HCl)
    d. All of the above

36. Recommendations to a client at high risk for oral cancer will include all of the following EXCEPT one. Which one is the EXCEPTION?
    a. Abstinence from tobacco products
    b. Abstinence from smoking
    c. Abstinence from excessive alcohol consumption
    d. Abstinence from essential oil mouthrinse

37. Clients need to be educated on mutable and non-mutable risk factors for oral cancer; alcohol and tobacco use falls under nonmutable risk factor.
    a. Both parts of the statement are TRUE
    b. The first part of the statement is TRUE; the second part is FALSE
    c. The first part of the statement is FALSE; the second part is TRUE
    d. Both parts of the statement are FALSE

38. All of the following are true regarding oral cancer diagnostic tools EXCEPT one. Which one is the EXCEPTION?
    a. Exfoliative cytology collects surface cells for microscopic evaluation
    b. Brush biopsy is indicated for unexplained clinically detectable lesions
    c. Brush biopsy is as effective as scalpel biopsy
    d. Use of topical anesthesia is contraindicated for brush biopsy

39. All of the following statements are true regarding oral cancer self-examination EXCEPT one. Which one is the EXCEPTION?
    a. All clients can potentially benefit from it
    b. A mirror and an adequate light source are essential for the procedure
    c. It is a substitute for professional evaluation
    d. Asymmetric, irregular lumps and sores indicate the need for professional evaluation

40. All of the following may contribute to oral malodor EXCEPT one. Which one is the EXCEPTION?
    a. Active periodontal disease
    b. Aphthous ulcer
    c. Use of tobacco products
    d. Lack of tongue brushing

41. Which toothbrushing method should be recommended for a client with plaque biofilm control problems around the cervical areas of the teeth?
    a. Stillman's method
    b. Charter method
    c. Bass method
    d. Leonard method

42. All of the following are true regarding the use of the oral irrigator EXCEPT one. Which one is the EXCEPTION?
    a. Used with cannula to irrigate to the base of the pocket
    b. Can be used as an adjunct to mechanical root debridement
    c. Delivers the antimicrobial mouthrinse subgingivally
    d. Eliminates the need for controlled release drug therapy

43. **All of the following should be recommended to a person with a dental implant EXCEPT one. Which one is the EXCEPTION?**
    a. Soft-bristled, multiple-tufted nylon toothbrush
    b. Interdental brushes with metal wire cores
    c. Floss containing a soft filament brush
    d. Flat and tapered end-tuft brush

Use Case C to answer questions 44 to 50.

Case C

Mr. Wilson, 28-years old, is a new patient at your dental office. His chief complaint is: "I have pinpoint white spots on my palate, and my front tooth is getting darker in color." Mr. Wilson smokes one pack of cigarettes per day. He has no known allergies. He has three 7-year-old implants with porcelain-fused-to-metal crowns on #5, #19, and #30. The gingiva around the implants are erythematous, with moderate plaque biofilm adhering to the implant fixtures. He has light calculus and stain accumulations on the linguals of mandibular and maxillary anterior teeth.

44. **Mr. Wilson's chief complaint is most likely caused by:**
    a. Candidiasis
    b. Allergy
    c. Smoking
    d. Implants

45. **All of the following should be initiated to assess the discoloration of the front tooth EXCEPT one. Which one is the EXCEPTION?**
    a. Take a periapical radiograph
    b. Obtain periodontal measurements
    c. Check for a widened periodontal ligament
    d. Conduct pulp vitality testing

46. **Mr. Wilson should be informed of all of the following EXCEPT one. Which one is the EXCEPTION?**
    a. Plaque biofilm, if left uncontrolled, will cause implant failure
    b. Smoking contributes to implant failure
    c. The reddish pinpoint lesions on his palate are caused by smoking
    d. A biopsy will be needed for his whitish pinpoint lesions on his palate

47. **For Mr. Wilson's dental implant maintenance, abrasive dentifrices should be avoided. Oral irrigation should also be avoided around the dental implants.**

    a. Both statements are TRUE
    b. The first statement is TRUE; the second statement is FALSE
    c. The first statement is FALSE; the second statement is TRUE
    d. Both statements are FALSE

48. **What is the most widely used method for oral cancer detection and screening?**
    a. Visual examination and palpation
    b. Brush biopsy and exfoliative cytology
    c. ViziLite®
    d. VELscope®

49. **Which one of the following statements is FALSE about the use of tobacco products?**
    a. Increase collagenase production
    b. Decrease collagen production
    c. Increase vascularity
    d. Impair helper lymphocytes

50. **Oral effects of tobacco use include all of the following EXCEPT one. Which one is the EXCEPTION?**
    a. Impaired healing
    b. Dental abrasion
    c. Migratory glossitis
    d. Nicotine stomatitis

Instrumentation for Client Assessment and Care

CHAPTER **17**

Jill S. Nield-Gehrig and Rebecca A. Sroda

This chapter focuses on the use of periodontal instruments for assessment and nonsurgical periodontal instrumentation. The primary objective of nonsurgical periodontal instrumentation is to restore periodontal tissue to health by removing dental plaque biofilm, its byproducts, and plaque-retentive factors from tooth surfaces and from within the tooth pocket space. Successful professional care depends on reducing plaque biofilm to a level that is acceptable to the tissue; therefore, instructing and supervising the client's daily self-care precedes, continues with, and follows instrumentation by the dental hygiene practitioner.

INSTRUMENT DESIGN

Parts of an Instrument

A. Handle—the part of a periodontal instrument that the clinician holds; various shapes, weights, sizes, and surface serrations (smooth, ribbed, or knurled) exist
   1. Types
      a. Single-ended—one working end
      b. Double-ended—two working ends; working ends may be unpaired (dissimilar working ends) or paired (mirror-image working ends)
   2. Handle design characteristics
      a. Small diameter ($\frac{3}{17}$-inch) handles, with smooth or flat texture, decrease the user's control and increase muscle fatigue
      b. Large diameter $\frac{3}{8}$-inch) handles that are lightweight and have bumpy texturing maximize the user's control and reduce muscle fatigue
B. Shank—connects the working end with the handle; usually bent in one or more places to facilitate placement of the working end against the tooth surface
   1. Functional shank—the part of the shank that allows the working end to be adapted to the tooth surface; begins below the working end and extends to the last bend in the shank nearest the handle
      a. Instruments with short functional shanks are used on teeth crowns
      b. Instruments with long functional shanks are used on both the crown and the root (Figure 17-1)
   2. Lower (terminal) shank—the bent portion of the functional shank nearest to the working end (see Figure 17-1)
   3. Extended lower shank—3 mm longer than a standard lower shank; provides additional leverage, acting like a fulcrum, and is ideal when using advanced levering techniques or for working in deep periodontal pockets
   4. Simple shank—bent in one plane (front to back); used primarily on anterior teeth; also called a *straight shank*
   5. Complex shank—bent in two planes (front to back and side to side) to facilitate instrumentation of posterior teeth; this design is necessary to reach around the crown and onto the root surface; also called an *angled shank* or *curved shank*
C. Working end—the part of the dental instrument that contacts the tooth or soft tissue to perform the work of the instrument; begins where the instrument shank ends; an instrument may have one or two working ends
   1. Parts of the working end—identified as the face, back, lateral surfaces, toe, and tip; on a hand-activated debridement instrument, a cutting edge is formed by the union of a lateral surface and the face of the working end
   2. Application of the working end—the tooth surfaces or areas of the mouth on which an instrument can be used
      a. Anterior use—one single-ended instrument (e.g., anterior sickle scaler, such as a Jacquette

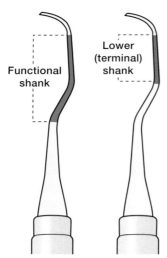

FIGURE 17-1 Functional shank and lower (terminal) shank. *(From Nield-Gehrig JS: Fundamentals of periodontal instrumentation and advanced root instrumentation, ed 6, Philadelphia, 2008, Lippincott Williams & Wilkins.)*

33) can be used to perform procedures on the facial, lingual, mesial, and distal surfaces of anterior teeth

   b. Posterior use—one double-ended instrument (e.g., posterior sickle scaler, such as a Jacquette 34/35) can be used to perform procedures on the facial, lingual, mesial, and distal surfaces of posterior teeth

   c. Universal use—one double-ended instrument (e.g., universal curet, such as a Columbia 13/14) can be used to perform procedures on both anterior and posterior teeth

   d. Area-specific use—an instrument that can be applied only to specific surfaces and areas of the mouth; a set of area-specific instruments (e.g., area-specific curets, such as the Gracey series) is needed for procedures on the entire dentition

3. Function of the working end

   a. Assessment of teeth, soft tissue, or both

   b. Debridement of tooth surfaces (the removal or disruption of calculus deposits, plaque biofilm, and their byproducts)

Design Characteristics

A. Instrument balance—a balanced instrument has working ends that are aligned with the long axis of the handle

   1. During a work stroke, for example, in calculus removal balance ensures that finger pressure applied against the handle is transferred to the working end, which results in pressure against the tooth

   2. An instrument that is not balanced is more difficult to use and increases stress on the muscles of the user's hand and arm

B. Instrument identification—the unique design name and number that identify each periodontal instrument

   1. Design name—identifies the school or individual responsible for the original design or development of an instrument or group of instruments (e.g., ODU 11/12 periodontal explorer, in which the ODU stands for Old Dominion University; and the TU-17, in which TU stands for Tufts University School of Dental Medicine)

   2. Design number—the number designation of the working end that, when combined with the design name, provides the exact identification of the working end (e.g., Gracey 11, in which Gracey is the design name, and 11 is the design number)

   3. Identification of the working ends of a double-ended instrument—a double-ended instrument will have two design numbers, one number for each working end of the instrument

      a. If the design name and number are stamped along the length of the handle, each working end is identified by the number closest to it

      b. If the design name and number are stamped across the handle, the first number identifies the working end at the top of the handle, and the second number identifies the working end at the bottom

HAND-ACTIVATED INSTRUMENTS

Classifications

A. Hand-activated nonsurgical periodontal instruments are classified as periodontal probes, explorers, sickle scalers, periodontal files, universal curets, area-specific curets, hoes, or chisels; hoes and chisels are rarely used because their functions have been largely replaced by mechanized instruments

B. Periodontal instruments are divided into classifications based on the specific design characteristics of the working end; design characteristics include:

   1. Design of the cutting edges, back, lateral surfaces, and shank

   2. Cross-section of the working end

   3. Relationship of the face to the lower shank (Table 17-1)

C. In selecting an instrument for a specific task, one of the most important considerations is the classification of the working end

TABLE 17-1 Use of Hand-Activated Instruments

Classification	Purpose
Calibrated probe	Measurement of pocket depths, clinical attachment level, width of attached gingiva, gingival recession, and intraoral lesions; evaluation of gingival tissue for consistency and presence of bleeding or exudate
Furcation probe	Detection of furcation involvement in multiple-rooted teeth
Explorer	Detection of calculus deposits, tooth surface irregularities, defective margins on restorations
Sickle scaler	Removal of medium-sized to large-sized calculus deposits from enamel surfaces; provides good access to the proximal surfaces on anterior crowns and the enamel surfaces apical to the contact areas of posterior teeth; usually confined to supragingival use; should NOT be used for root surface debridement
Periodontal file	Used to crush large calculus deposits and prepare burnished calculus before removal with another instrument; should NOT be used directly on cemental surfaces
Universal curet	Debridement of crown and root surfaces; removal of light to medium-sized supragingival and subgingival calculus deposits; some designs have long functional shanks that allow access to the cervical and middle thirds of root surfaces
Area-specific curet	Debridement of crown and root surfaces; removal of light supragingival and subgingival calculus deposits; some designs have extended shanks that allow access to the middle and apical thirds of root surfaces

From Nield-Gehrig JS: Fundamentals of periodontal instrumentation and advanced root instrumentation, *ed 6, Philadelphia, 2008, Lippincott Williams & Wilkins.*

Dental Mirror

A. Characteristics
  1. The working end has a reflecting (mirrored) surface
  2. Types
    a. Front surface—the reflecting surface is on the front surface of the glass; produces a clear mirror image with no distortion
    b. Concave—the reflecting surface is on the front surface of the mirror lens; produces a magnified but slightly distorted image

c. Plane—the reflecting surface is on the back surface of the mirror lens; this type of surface is less easily scratched than a front surface mirror but produces a double or "ghost" image
B. Uses
  1. Indirect vision—the mirror's reflecting surface provides a view of the tooth surface or intraoral structure that cannot be seen directly
  2. Retraction—using the mirror to hold the client's cheek or tongue to view tooth surfaces or other structures that are otherwise hidden by the cheeks or tongue
  3. Indirect illumination—reflecting light from the mirrored surface into a dark area of the mouth
  4. Trans-illumination—reflecting light from the mirrored surface through anterior teeth

Probe

A. Characteristics
  1. Assessment instrument that is used to evaluate the health of periodontal tissue
  2. Two types: calibrated and furcation probes
B. Types
  1. Calibrated probe (e.g., Williams, PSR screening probe) has a slender rod-shaped, blunt working end marked in millimeter increments; can be used as a miniature ruler for making intraoral measurements, such as for measuring sulcus and pocket depths, clinical attachment levels, width of attached gingiva, or the size of oral lesions; also used to assess for the presence of bleeding, or purulent exudate (pus)
  2. Furcation probe (e.g., Nabers 1N) is a curved, blunt-tipped instrument used to detect and assess bone loss in the furcation areas of bifurcated and trifurcated teeth
C. Calibrations—millimeter marks at intervals that are specific for each probe design
  1. Calibrated probes
    a. Probe designs may differ in millimeter markings (Table 17-2); only certain millimeter increments may be indicated on the probe (e.g., 1—2—3—5—7—8—9—10 mm), or each millimeter may be indicated (e.g., 1—2—3—4—5—6—7—8—9—10—11—12—13—14—15 mm)
    b. Color-coded probes are marked in bands (often black), with each band being several millimeters in width (e.g., 3–5 mm and 8–10 mm)
  2. Furcation probes
    a. Most furcation probes do not have millimeter markings
    b. Some furcation probes are marked in bands (usually black), with each band being several

TABLE 17-2 Examples of Probe Markings

Type	Marking Pattern	Increments (mm)
UNC15	All mm marked	1 to 15
Glickman 26G	No mark at 6 mm	1–2–3–5–7–8–9–10
Goldman Fox	No mark at 6 mm	1–2–3–5–7–8–9–10
Merritt	No mark at 6 mm	1–2–3–5–7–8–9–10
Williams	No mark at 6 mm	1–2–3–5–7–8–9–10
Maryland Moffitt	No mark at 6 mm; ball-end	1–2–3–5–7–8–9–10
Michigan "O"	Marks at 3, 6, and 8 mm	3–6–8
PSR Screening	Colored band from 3.5–5.5; marks at 8.5 and 11.5 mm; ball end	3.5–5.5–8.5–11.5
CP-18	Colored bands from 3–5 and 8–10	3–5–8–10
CP-11	Colored bands from 3–6 and 8–11	3–6–8–11
CP-12	Colored bands from 3–6 and 9–12	3–6–9–12
Hu-Friedy Novatech	Right-angled probe; available in a wide variety of designs	Available in various increments

From Nield-Gehrig JS: Fundamentals of periodontal instrumentation and advanced root instrumentation, ed 6, Philadelphia, 2008, Lippincott Williams & Wilkins.

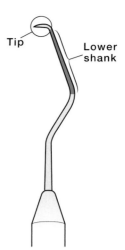

FIGURE 17-2 Design characteristics of a dental explorer. *(From Nield-Gehrig JS:* Fundamentals of periodontal instrumentation and advanced root instrumentation, *ed 6,* Philadelphia, 2008, Lippincott Williams & Wilkins.)

millimeters in width (e.g., 3–6 mm and 6–9 mm); these probes usually are used in research investigations to facilitate the investigator's calibration

Explorer

A. Characteristics
  1. Assessment instrument with a fine, flexible wire-like working end
  2. Provides the best tactile information to the clinician's fingers; used to locate calculus deposits, tooth surface irregularities, and defective margins on restorations
B. Design (Figure 17-2)
  1. The working end is 1 to 2 mm in length and is referred to as the *tip*; the side of the tip, rather than the actual point, is used for detecting calculus
  2. Circular in cross-section, the explorer may have paired or unpaired working ends

C. Types—available in a variety of design types; not all design types are well suited to subgingival use; therefore, the clinician must be knowledgeable about the recommended use of each design type
  1. Shepherd hook (e.g., #23 and #54 explorers)—an unpaired explorer with a short, highly curved shank and a sharp point; used for supragingival examinations to detect irregular margins of restorations; not recommended for calculus detection because subgingival use could result in tissue trauma
  2. Straight explorer (e.g., 6, 6A, 6L, 6XL)—an unpaired explorer with a short lower shank and a sharp point; used for examinations to detect irregular margins of restorations; not recommended for subgingival calculus detection
  3. Curved explorer (e.g., 3, 3A)—an unpaired explorer with a curved shank and a sharp point; limited for use in examining normal sulci or shallow pockets; may be used for calculus detection; however, care must be taken not to injure the junctional epithelium when the working end is used subgingivally
  4. Orban-type explorer (e.g., TU-17, Orban 20)—an unpaired explorer with a straight lower shank that can be used in deep pockets with only slight tissue displacement (stretching of the tissue wall away from the tooth); the explorer tip is bent at a 90-degree angle to the terminal shank, which allows the back of the tip (instead of the point) to be directed toward the junctional epithelium; useful for detecting subgingival calculus on anterior teeth or on the facial and lingual surfaces of posterior teeth; however, the straight lower shank makes it difficult to adapt to the

line angles and proximal surfaces of posterior teeth

5. Pigtail or cowhorn explorer (e.g., 3MI, 3CH, 2A)—a paired universal explorer with a short, broadly curved lower shank and a sharp point; the curved lower shank causes considerable tissue displacement; useful for detecting calculus in normal sulci or shallow pockets extending no deeper than the cervical third of the root

6. The 11/12-type explorer (e.g., ODU 11/12, 11/12 AF)—a paired universal explorer with an extended lower shank and a tip that is bent at a 90-degree angle to the terminal shank; the tip design allows the back of the tip to be applied to the pocket base without lacerating the junctional epithelium; this effective explorer design adapts well to all surfaces throughout the mouth and is equally useful when exploring a shallow sulcus or a deep periodontal pocket

Sickle Scaler

A. Characteristics
   1. Debridement instrument; limited for use on teeth crowns
   2. Anterior and posterior designs
B. Design (Figure 17-3)
   1. Cutting edges—two cutting edges that meet in a point
   2. Back—sharp, pointed back; some types of scalers are made with flattened backs
   3. Cross-section—triangular; lateral surfaces meet the instrument face at an internal angle between 70 and 80 degrees
   4. Face—perpendicular to the lower shank so that the cutting edges are level with each other; level cutting edges require that the lower shank be

tilted slightly toward the tooth surface to establish correct angulation

5. The anterior sickle scaler has an unpaired working end and a simple shank; primarily used on anterior teeth (e.g., Jacquette 33)

6. The posterior sickle scaler has paired working ends, with complex shanks; primarily used on posterior teeth but may be used on anterior teeth (e.g., Jacquette 34/35)

C. Uses
   1. Removal of medium-sized to large-sized supragingival calculus deposits
   2. Provides good access to the proximal surfaces on anterior crowns and to the enamel surfaces apical to the contact areas of posterior teeth
D. Limitations
   1. The pointed tip and the straight cutting edges do not adapt well to rounded root surfaces and concavities
   2. The pointed back is not suited to subgingival use (may injure the junctional epithelium)

Periodontal File

A. Characteristics
   1. Calculus removal instrument used to prepare calculus deposits before removal with another instrument
   2. Anterior and posterior designs
B. Design
   1. Cutting edges—multiple cutting edges at a 90- to 105-degree angle to the lower shank
   2. Working end—thin in width with a large circumference at the base; the base may be round, oval, or rectangular in shape
   3. Area-specific application—each working end is designed for use on a single surface (four working

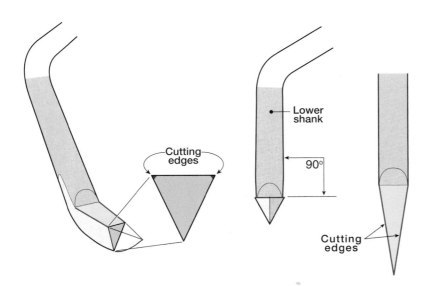

FIGURE 17-3 Design characteristics of a sickle scaler, consisting of two-level cutting edges that meet in a point and an instrument face that is at a 90-degree angle to the lower shank. *(From Nield-Gehrig JS: Fundamentals of periodontal instrumentation and advanced root instrumentation, ed 6, Philadelphia, 2008, Lippincott Williams & Wilkins.)*

ends are needed for procedures on all tooth surfaces); files with simple shanks work best on anterior teeth; those with complex shanks work best on posterior teeth

C. Uses

1. Preparation of burnished calculus deposit (a deposit with a smooth outer surface) before removal of the deposit with a curet; a file is used to scratch the surface of a burnished deposit so that it can be removed with another instrument

2. Crushing of a large calculus deposit; once a deposit has been crushed with a file, it is easier to remove with a curet

3. Smoothing overextended or rough amalgam restoration in sites where the file can be effectively adapted

D. Limitations

1. Limited to use on enamel surfaces or to applications on the outer surface of a calculus deposit; gouging could result if a file is used on root surfaces

2. The working ends have straight cutting edges on a flat base; do not adapt well to curved tooth surfaces

Universal Curet

A. Characteristics

1. One of the most frequently used and versatile of all the debridement instruments

2. Used both supragingivally and subgingivally; two curets usually are paired on a double-ended instrument (the paired working ends are mirror images of each other)

B. Design (Figure 17-4)

1. Cutting edges—two cutting edges that converge in a rounded toe

2. Back—the rounded back is ideal for subgingival use

3. Cross-section—semi-circular; lateral surfaces meet the instrument face at an internal angle between 70 and 80 degrees

4. Face—perpendicular to the lower shank so that the cutting edges are level with each other; the level cutting edges require that the lower shank be tilted slightly toward the tooth surface to establish correct angulation

5. Universal use—one double-ended instrument can be applied to all tooth surfaces in the anterior and posterior regions of the mouth

C. Uses

1. Debridement of the crown and root surfaces

2. Removal of small-sized to medium-sized calculus deposits

D. Limitations

1. The toe is wider than a pointed tip and, therefore, may be more difficult to adapt for use beneath the contact areas of anterior teeth

2. The level cutting edges require that the lower shank be tilted slightly toward the tooth for correct angulation

Area-Specific Curet

A. Characteristics

1. Debridement instrument with one cutting edge (only one cutting edge per working end is used for procedures); a set of curets is needed to perform procedures throughout the mouth

2. The curet is used supragingivally and subgingivally; especially well suited for root surface debridement within periodontal pockets

3. Designs include area-specific curets with miniature working ends, extended shanks, and flexible and rigid shanks

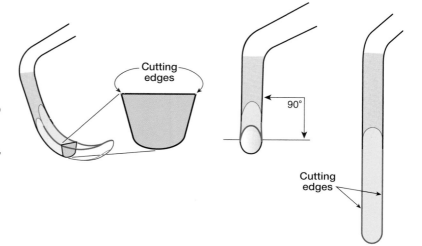

FIGURE 17-4 Design characteristics of a universal curet, consisting of two-level cutting edges and an instrument face that is at a 90-degree angle to the lower shank. *(From Nield-Gehrig JS:* Fundamentals of periodontal instrumentation and advanced root instrumentation, *ed 6, Philadelphia, 2008, Lippincott Williams & Wilkins.)*

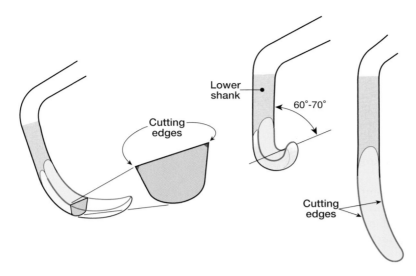

FIGURE 17-5 Design characteristics of an area-specific curet consisting of one cutting edge, an instrument face that is at a 70-degree angle to the lower shank, and one cutting edge positioned lower than the other nonworking cutting edge. *(From Nield-Gehrig JS: Fundamentals of periodontal instrumentation and advanced root instrumentation, ed 6, Philadelphia, 2008, Lippincott Williams & Wilkins.)*

B. Design (Figure 17-5)
1. Cutting edge—one working cutting edge per working end; only the lower, longer cutting edge is used
2. Back—rounded back; ideal for subgingival use
3. Cross-section—semi-circular; the lateral surfaces meet the instrument face at an internal angle between 70 and 80 degrees
4. Face—tilted at a 60- to 70-degree angle in relation to the lower shank, making one cutting edge (the working cutting edge) lower than the other; this tilted relationship makes the working cutting edge "self-angulated" (that is, when the lower shank is parallel to the tooth surface, the cutting edge is at the correct angulation)
5. Area-specific use—each working end is limited to use only on certain teeth and on certain surfaces

C. Uses
1. Debridement of crown and root surfaces
2. Removal of small deposits of calculus and plaque biofilm

D. Limitations
1. The toe is wider than a pointed tip and is, therefore, more difficult to adapt to the proximal surfaces of anterior crowns
2. A single working cutting edge per working end means exchanging instruments more frequently

Hand Instruments for Root Debridement

A. Characteristics
1. The treatment of clients with periodontitis requires specialized instruments with longer shank lengths and miniature working ends for instrumentation of root concavities and furcation areas

2. Designs include area-specific curets with miniature working ends, extended shanks, flexible and rigid shanks, and diamond-coated working ends

B. Examples of advanced root debridement instruments—a variety of periodontal instruments have been developed to increase treatment effectiveness on root surfaces within deep periodontal pockets
1. The 11/12-type periodontal explorer—an 11/12 AF (After Five) explorer has an extended shank and is ideal for use in deep periodontal pockets
2. Advanced curet designs—several curets are ideal for instrumentation within deep periodontal pockets
   a. Vision curvette curet series—have a working end that is shortened to half the length of a standard Gracey curet, a curved working end, and an extended lower shank
   b. Modified Gracey curets
      (1) Several varieties of modified Gracey curets—include modified Gracey curets with extended shanks, miniature Gracey curets, and micro Gracey curets
      (2) Design features for modified Gracey curets—include extended lower shank length, thinner working ends, and working ends that are shorter in length than in a standard Gracey curet
   c. Quetin Furcation curets—specialized instruments that are used to debride furcation areas and root concavities; each miniature working end has a single, straight cutting edge with rounded corners; the working ends are available in either 0.9-mm or 1.3-mm size
   d. O'Hehir debridement curets—area-specific curets that are designed to remove light

residual calculus deposits and bacterial contaminants from root surfaces
(1) The working end of an O'Hehir curet is a tiny circular disc; the entire working end is a cutting edge; the working end curves into the tooth for easy adaptation in furcation areas and developmental grooves
(2) These curets have extended lower shanks
e. Instruments with diamond-coated working ends
(1) The working ends of these instruments do not have cutting edges; instead, they are coated with a very fine diamond grit, for example, a version of the Nabers furcation probes are diamond coated
(2) Diamond-coated instruments can be used to remove light residual calculus deposits and bacterial contaminants from root surfaces
(3) Because of the abrasive nature of their working ends, these instruments should be used with light, even pressure against the root surface to avoid gouging or grooving

PRINCIPLES OF INSTRUMENTATION

Position of the Clinician

A. Neutral, seated position (Figure 17-6)
  1. Head—tilt of 0 to 15 degrees
  2. Shoulders—in a horizontal line
  3. Back—straight or leaning forward slightly from the waist or hips
  4. Thighs—hips slightly higher than the knees
  5. Upper arms—parallel to the long axis of the torso
  6. Elbows—at waist level; held slightly away from body
  7. Forearms—parallel to the floor; raised or lowered, if necessary, by pivoting at the elbow joint rather than by raising the elbows
  8. Feet—seat height should be positioned low enough so that the heels of the feet can rest on the floor
B. Relationship to the client and the dental unit
  1. The client's chair should be positioned such that the tip of the client's nose is at a lower level at a level slightly lower than clinician's elbows; clinician should not have to raise the elbows above his or her waist level to reach the client's mouth; lower arms should be in a horizontal position or raised slightly so that the angle formed between the lower and upper arm is slightly less than 90 degrees

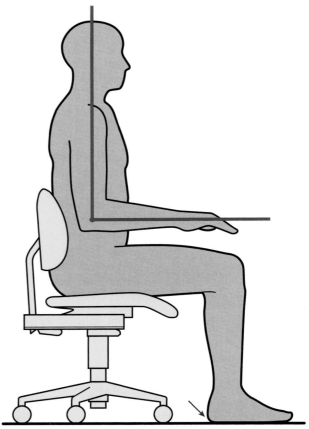

FIGURE 17-6 Neutral seated position for the clinician. *(From Nield-Gehrig JS: Fundamentals of periodontal instrumentation and advanced root instrumentation, ed 6, Philadelphia, 2008, Lippincott Williams & Wilkins.)*

  2. All instruments and equipment should be positioned within easy reach of the clinician

Stabilization During Instrumentation

A. Modified pen grasp—the recommended grasp for holding a periodontal instrument that allows precise control of the working end; precise placement of the fingers in the modified pen grasp is important to be successful in instrumentation technique
  1. Finger placement and function (Figure 17-7)
    a. Index finger and thumb—finger pads hold the instrument handle
    b. Middle finger—the side of the finger pad rests on the instrument's shank; the clinician's fingers should be able to feel the vibrations in the instrument's shank as the working end encounters roughness on the tooth surface
    c. Ring finger—fingertip rests on a stable surface, usually the occlusal or incisal tooth surface, which stabilizes the hand for control and strength

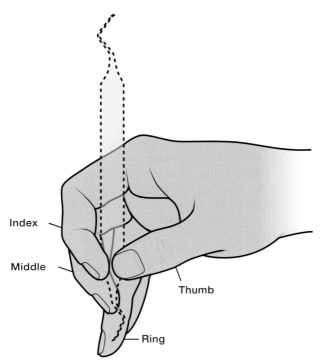

FIGURE 17-7 Finger placement in the modified pen grasp. The index finger and the thumb hold the instrument handle. The middle finger rests on the instrument shank. The ring finger acts as a support for the hand and instrument. *(From Nield-Gehrig JS: Fundamentals of periodontal instrumentation and advanced root instrumentation, ed 6, Philadelphia, 2008, Lippincott Williams & Wilkins.)*

2. Technique
  a. A light grasp is needed for increased tactile sensitivity during assessment procedures (e.g., subgingival use of explorer or probe)
  b. A firm grasp is used with hand-activated instruments during calculus removal
3. Glove fit—proper fit of sterile gloves is important in avoiding muscle strain during instrumentation
  a. Select right-hand and left-hand fitted gloves rather than ambidextrous gloves
  b. Select gloves that come in a range of numbered sizes, for example, 5½, 6, 6½, rather than those marked in size ranges of small, medium, and large
B. Fulcrum and finger rest
  1. Definitions
    a. Fulcrum—the point of support on which the clinician rests the hand; used to stabilize the clinician's hand during instrumentation; the pad of the ring finger serves as the fulcrum finger during instrumentation to control stroke pressure and length
    b. Finger rest—the place where the fulcrum finger rests during instrumentation

2. Types of fulcrums
  a. Basic intraoral fulcrum
    (1) The finger rest is placed on a tooth, close to the tooth being worked on; should not be positioned in the line of the instrument's stroke to prevent instrument stick
    (2) The intraoral fulcrum is considered the most desirable because it provides the greatest stability and strength for calculus removal
  b. Basic extraoral fulcrum—placed outside the client's mouth, usually on the chin or cheek
  c. Advanced fulcrums—variations of the basic fulcrum that may be required for access to posterior teeth or root surfaces within periodontal pockets; advanced fulcrums require greater skill and stroke control than the basic intraoral fulcrum
3. Advanced fulcrum techniques
  a. Piggy-backed—intraoral fulcrum in which the middle finger is stacked on top of the ring finger
  b. Cross-arch—intraoral fulcrum in which the finger rests on the side of the arch opposite the treatment area
  c. Opposite arch—intraoral fulcrum in which the finger rests on the arch opposite to the treatment area
  d. Finger-on-finger—intraoral fulcrum in which the finger of the nondominant hand serves as the resting point for the ring finger of the dominant hand
  e. Stabilized—intraoral or extraoral fulcrum in which a finger of the nondominant hand is used to concentrate lateral pressure against the tooth surface and to help control the instrument stroke

Adaptation

A. Definition—positioning the first 1 or 2 mm of the lateral surface of the working end of the instrument in contact with the tooth surface
B. Characteristics
  1. Explorer—the first few millimeters of the tip (not the point) are adapted to the tooth surface for calculus detection
  2. Probe—the side of the probe tip is maintained against the tooth surface, with the length of the probe almost parallel to the tooth surface being probed
  3. Sickles and curets—the leading one third of the cutting edge is positioned to conform to the tooth surface

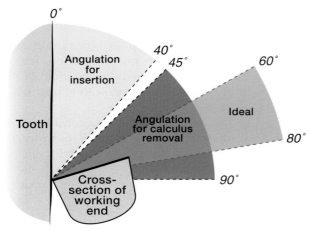

FIGURE 17-8 Angulation for calculus removal should be between 45 and 90 degrees. An angulation between 60 and 80 degrees is ideal for debridement. *(From Nield-Gehrig JS:* Fundamentals of periodontal instrumentation and advanced root instrumentation, *ed 6, Philadelphia, 2008, Lippincott Williams & Wilkins.)*

Angulation

A. Definition—the relationship between the face of a calculus removal instrument and the tooth surface to which the working end is applied
B. Principles
 1. For insertion beneath the gingival margin—the face-to-tooth surface angulation is between 0 and 40 degrees
 2. For debridement—the face-to-tooth surface angulation is between 45 and 90 degrees; a 60-degree angulation works well for removing plaque, whereas a 70- to 80-degree angulation is ideal for calculus removal (Figure 17-8)

Activation

A. Definition—moving an instrument to produce a stroke; it is the action of an instrument in the performance of the task for which it was designed
B. Types
 1. Hand–forearm activation
　a. Made by rotating the hand and forearm as a unit to provide the power for the instrumentation stroke; similar to the action of turning a doorknob
　b. Uses the power of the hand and arm to move the instrument; recommended for calculus removal with hand-activated instruments
 2. Digital (finger) activation
　a. Created by flexing the thumb, index, and middle fingers to move the instrument
　b. Used whenever physical strength is not required during a task, such as when using mechanized instruments, probes, and explorers

C. Stabilization and lateral pressure
 1. Definitions
　a. Stabilization—preparing for an instrument's stroke by locking the joints of the ring finger and pressing the fingertip against the tooth surface to provide control for the stroke
　b. Lateral pressure—applying pressure equally with the index finger and the thumb inward against the instrument's handle to engage the working end against a calculus deposit or the tooth surface before and throughout an instrument's stroke
 2. Stroke pressure
　a. Pressure during stroke activation—stroke pressure is applied in a coronal direction; the pressure ranges from light to firm, depending on the amount of pressure needed for the particular task (e.g., assessment, calculus removal)
　b. Pressure between strokes—finger muscles should be relaxed as the working end is repositioned, using light stroke pressure
D. Maintaining adaptation during stroke production
 1. Hand pivot—turning the hand and arm slightly while resting on the fulcrum to maintain adaptation; used when moving around line angles and onto proximal surfaces
 2. Handle roll—rolling the instrument handle slightly between the thumb and the index finger to maintain adaptation as the instrumentation strokes advance around the tooth surface; either the thumb or the index finger is used to roll the instrument
E. Neutral wrist position—correct wrist position is important to avoid muscle discomfort and injury during the procedure; the wrist should be aligned with the long axis of the forearm; bending the wrist up, down, or to the side should be avoided

Instrumentation Strokes

A. Types of strokes
 1. Placement stroke—used to position the working end at the base of the sulcus pocket or apical to a calculus deposit
 2. Assessment strokes—used to evaluate the tooth surface or the health of periodontal tissue
　a. Used with probes, explorers, curets
　b. Angulation—50 to 70 degrees
　c. Lateral pressure—in contact with the tooth surface; light pressure
　d. Character—fluid strokes of moderate length
　e. Number—many strokes used to cover the entire root surface

3. Calculus removal work strokes—used to remove calculus deposits
 a. Used with hand-activated sickle scalers, curets, and files
 b. Angulation—70 to 80 degrees
 c. Lateral pressure—moderate to firm
 d. Character—powerful strokes; short in length
 e. Number—the number of strokes should be limited to the areas where needed

4. Root debridement work strokes—used to remove residual calculus deposits, plaque biofilm, and plaque byproducts from root surfaces
 a. Used with hand-activated curets
 b. Angulation—60 to 70 degrees
 c. Lateral pressure—light to moderate
 d. Character—lighter strokes of moderate length
 e. Number—many strokes used to cover the entire root surface

B. Stroke direction
 1. Vertical—parallel to the long axis of the tooth; used on facial, lingual, and proximal surfaces of anterior teeth and on the mesial and distal surfaces of posterior teeth
 2. Oblique—diagonal to the long axis of the tooth; used most commonly on facial and lingual surfaces
 3. Horizontal—perpendicular to the long axis of the tooth; used at the line angles of posterior teeth, furcation crotch areas, and within pockets that are too narrow to allow vertical or oblique strokes
 4. Multidirectional—a combination of vertical, oblique, and horizontal strokes, one by one, used in succession; for assessment or debridement of a subgingival tooth surface

C. Stroke characteristics
 1. Length—short, powerful stroke for calculus removal; longer, lighter stroke for root surface debridement
 2. Overlap—strokes should overlap to ensure complete coverage; long ridges of calculus are treated in sections, in overlapping scaling zones
 3. Pattern
 a. Large calculus deposits should be removed in sections with a series of short, firm strokes
 (1) A calculus deposit should not be removed in layers because removing the outermost layer will leave the deposit with a smooth surface (burnished surface)
 (2) burnished calculus deposit may be indistinguishable (when explored) from the tooth surface
 b. For subgingival instrumentation, it is helpful to imagine that the root surface is divided into a series of narrow, diagonal instrumentation zones

 (1) Each instrumentation zone is only as wide as the toe-third of the cutting edge
 (2) Deposits are removed in each zone, from the junctional epithelium to the gingival margin, before progressing to the next zone

STEPS FOR CALCULUS REMOVAL WITH HAND-ACTIVATED INSTRUMENTS

A. Position the dental mirror, and establish a finger rest
B. Grasp the instrument in a modified pen grasp
C. Establish a finger rest
 1. Locate the finger rest near the site of instrumentation in the dental arch; precise control of the instrument's stroke becomes more difficult as the finger rest is moved farther away from the site of the procedure
 2. Select the correct working end of the instrument
D. Adjust the hand–wrist–forearm as a unit
 1. Position the thumb and the index finger across from each other on the instrument handle, near the junction of the handle and shank
 2. Lightly rest one side of the middle finger pad on the instrument shank
 3. Place the other side of the middle finger pad against the ring finger to allow the hand to function as a unit during the production of the stroke
 4. Balance the tip of the ring finger on an occlusal or an incisal surface to support the weight of the hand and instrument
 5. Position the wrist in a neutral position so that it is aligned with the long axis of the forearm (Figure 17-9)
E. Adapt the cutting edge
 1. If working subgingivally, close the face of the working end toward the tooth, and slide the

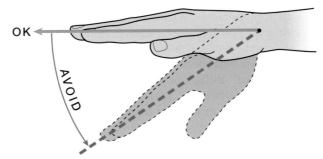

FIGURE 17-9 Neutral wrist position. The wrist should be aligned with the long axis of the forearm. *(From Nield-Gehrig JS: Fundamentals of periodontal instrumentation and advanced root instrumentation, ed 6, Philadelphia, 2008, Lippincott Williams & Wilkins.)*

working end to the junctional epithelium; use a light grasp while positioning the working end

2. Adapt the toe-third of the cutting edge to the tooth surface
3. Establish the instrument face-to-tooth surface angulation of 70 and 80 degrees
4. Fine-tune the grasp and the wrist position

F. Stabilize the grasp, and apply lateral pressure
   1. Press down with the ring finger against the finger rest
   2. Apply pressure against the instrument handle with the index finger and the thumb

G. Activate a pulling stroke away from the junctional epithelium
   1. Use hand–forearm activation for strength and control
   2. Activate pulling strokes in a coronal direction to prevent particles of calculus from being pushed into soft tissue
   3. Use vertical and oblique strokes in most areas; supplement these strokes with horizontal strokes, as needed
   4. Use short, powerful strokes for calculus removal and longer, lighter strokes for root surface debridement
   5. Use overlapping strokes to ensure complete coverage of the entire root surface

H. Pause briefly at the end of a stroke
   1. Relax the grasp, the finger rest, and the lateral pressure
   2. Use a relaxed grasp to reposition the working end of the instrument for the next stroke

I. Check the instrumentation area frequently with an explorer

INSTRUMENTATION FOR ASSESSMENT

Basic Concepts

A. Thorough assessment involves examining all aspects of the periodontium and teeth
B. Client preparation, based on information from the personal, comprehensive health and dental histories, is essential for safe instrumentation
C. Successful treatment depends on well-developed assessment skills, before instrumentation, for dental care planning, and during and after instrumentation for evaluating treatment outcomes

Assessments with Periodontal Probes

A. Purposes of the periodontal examination
   1. Aid in planning dental care by determining gingival characteristics, probing depth, level of attachment, and presence of bone loss

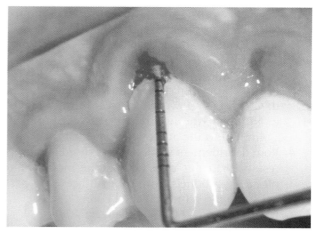

FIGURE 17-10 Assessment for the presence of bleeding. Bleeding upon probing is an early clinical sign of inflammation. *(From Nield-Gehrig JS: Fundamentals of periodontal instrumentation and advanced root instrumentation, ed 6, Philadelphia, 2008, Lippincott Williams & Wilkins.)*

   2. Determine the extent of inflammation in conjunction with the probing depth and attachment level; bleeding resulting from probing is an early clinical sign of inflammation (Figure 17-10)
   3. Evaluation of treatment outcomes according to:
      a. Tissue response to the client's self-care and nonsurgical periodontal therapy
      b. Evidence of health determined by the probe
         (1) No bleeding on gentle probing
         (2) Clinical attachment levels remain the same or decrease in depth

B. Factors that may affect probing accuracy
   1. Probe design
      a. Calibration—the probe must be clearly and accurately marked and easy to read; the clinician must be knowledgeable about the calibration pattern
      b. Thickness—a thinner probe causes less distention of the sulcus or the pocket wall; use a probe no larger than 0.5 mm in diameter
   2. Influence of tissue health and related factors
      a. Tissue resistance—with light pressure, the probe is inserted until it meets the physical resistance of the base of the sulcus or the periodontal pocket
         (1) Normal tissue—the junctional epithelium offers more resistance; probing is stopped by the coronal portion of the junctional epithelium
         (2) Gingivitis and early periodontitis—the junctional epithelium offers less resistance; the probe tip passes farther into the junctional epithelium
         (3) Advanced periodontitis—the junctional epithelium offers little or no resistance;

the probe tip may penetrate the junctional epithelium to reach the attached connective tissue fibers

  b. Dental calculus—large calculus deposits can hinder the placement of the probe

 3. Concepts of probing technique

  a. Adaptation—place the side of the probe tip against the tooth surface, with the length of the probe positioned as parallel as possible to the tooth surface; to assess the col region, tilt the probe so that the tip reaches under the contact area

  b. Stroke technique—strokes must be close to each other as the probe is "walked" along the entire circumference of the junctional epithelium

  c. Pressure—a light pressure of 10 to 20 g should be sufficient

Probing Technique

A. Parallelism—the probe is positioned as parallel as possible to the tooth surface being probed

B. Adaptation—the side of the probe tip is maintained in contact with the tooth at all times

C. Activation—digital (finger) activation may be used with the probe because only light pressure is used when probing

D. Walking strokes—a series of bobbing strokes made within the sulcus or the pocket while keeping the probe tip against the tooth

 1. The junctional epithelium is continuous around a tooth, and the probing depth may vary considerably on different surfaces; for complete evaluation, the entire circumference of the sulcus or the pocket base should be assessed with a series of probing strokes

 2. The probe is gently inserted under the gingival margin, holding the side of the tip against the tooth with a light lateral pressure; the probe tip is slid along the tooth until it encounters the resistance of the junctional epithelium

 3. The tip is moved up and down in short bobbing strokes of 1 to 2 mm while progressing forward in small 1-mm to 2-mm steps around the circumference of the tooth; with each downward stroke, the probe tip returns to gently touch the junctional epithelium

 4. The base of the sulcus or pocket will feel soft and resilient; if the resistance on the probe feels hard, the probe tip has encountered a large calculus deposit before reaching the junctional epithelium

 5. The probe should not be removed from the sulcus or the pocket after each measurement; repeated insertion and removal unnecessary and can cause trauma to the free gingival margin

E. Proximal surface probing—the probe is walked across the proximal surface until it touches the contact area; the probe is slanted slightly so that the tip reaches under the contact area; with the probe in this position, it is gently pressed downward to touch the junctional epithelium to take a reading

F. Sequence of steps for probing by quadrants

 1. Insert the probe at the distal line angle of the posterior-most tooth in the quadrant; walk the probe in a distal direction, adapting the probe around the line angle and across the distal surface, slightly past the midline of the distal surface (because this is the distal-most tooth in the quadrant, no contact area is present to contend with)

 2. Re-insert the probe at the distal line angle, and proceed in a mesial direction, across the distal surface, around the line angle, and across the mesial surface, slanting under the mesial contact area, as needed

 3. Remove the probe from the sulcus or the pocket, and re-insert at the distal line angle of the next tooth in the quadrant; assess each tooth in the quadrant in a similar manner, ending with the mesial surface of the central incisor

 4. After probing the facial aspect of the quadrant, assess the lingual aspect of the same quadrant

G. Calculus—when a large calculus deposit is encountered, the probe should be moved outward from the tooth and around the deposit and guided back to the tooth, proceeding in an apical direction

H. Recording probing depths—for the purpose of documentation, each tooth is divided into six areas (three on the facial aspect and three on the lingual aspect)

 1. The six areas are:

  a. Disto-facial line angle to the midline of the distal surface

  b. Facial surface

  c. Mesio-facial line angle to the midline of the mesial surface

  d. Disto-lingual line angle to the midline of the distal surface

  e. Lingual surface

  f. Mesio-lingual line angle to the midline of the mesial surface

 2. Only one reading per area recorded—if the probing depths vary within an area, the deepest reading obtained in that area is recorded (e.g., when readings for an area range from 3 to 6 mm, only the 6-mm reading is entered on the chart for that area)

3. Depths recorded in millimeters and rounded up (e.g., a reading of 4.5 mm is recorded as a 5-mm reading)

Clinical Measurements Using Periodontal Probes

A. Bleeding on probing
   1. Rationale
      a. Bleeding on probing is a significant clinical indicator of inflammation and is an earlier clinical sign than marginal redness
      b. Bleeding on probing correlates with increases in motile bacterial organisms, especially spirochetes, in the pocket
      c. No bleeding on probing is a criterion for healthy tissue
   2. Technique
      a. Insert the probe a few millimeters into the pocket (tip should not be in contact with the junctional epithelium)
      b. Make horizontal sweeping strokes along the pocket wall, using light pressure with the side of the probe
      c. Spongy tissue of a pocket wall will usually bleed near the gingival margin; firm chronic pocket linings usually do not bleed until sweeping strokes are made in the deep part of the pocket (bleeding may not be evident for a few seconds)
B. Measurement of recession of the gingival margin
   1. Definition and rationale
      a. Gingival recession—is the movement of the gingival margin from its normal position— slightly coronal to the cemento-enamel junction (CEJ), leading to exposure of a portion of the root surface to the oral cavity
      b. Gingival recession indicates the apical migration of the junctional epithelium
   2. Procedure
      a. Position a calibrated probe parallel to the tooth surface with the toe of the probe touching the gingival margin
      b. Measure the extent of recession in millimeters from the CEJ to the gingival margin with a calibrated periodontal probe
C. Measuring probing depths
   1. Definition—the distance in millimeters from the gingival margin to the base of the sulcus or the pocket, as measured with a calibrated probe
   2. Rationale
      a. Used in calculating clinical attachment levels
      b. Useful in prescribing client self-care regimens and in educating clients

3. Limitations—in the presence of gingival recession, probing depths are not an accurate indication of loss of attachment or level of bone support to the tooth
4. Technique
   a. With the probe in a vertical position and in contact with the attached tissue, record the distance from the gingival margin to the base of the sulcus or the pocket
   b. When the gingival margin contacts the probe between the millimeter marks, use the higher number for the final reading
D. Measuring clinical attachment levels (CALs)
   1. Definition—the position of the attached tissue at the base of the sulcus or the pocket, as measured from a fixed point, usually the CEJ
   2. Rationale
      a. Probing depths are not reliable indicators of the position of the junctional epithelium because the measurement is made from the gingival margin; the position of the gingival margin changes with recession and edema
      b. Measurements are taken from a fixed point on the tooth; the CEJ usually is used because it provides a more reliable indication of the level of the attached tissue
      c. When evaluating treatment outcomes, measurements taken from a fixed point provide a better way of monitoring whether the level of the attached tissue has remained the same, decreased, or increased in depth
   3. General concepts
      a. Two measurements are made and then used to mathematically calibrate the clinical attachment; the measurements include:
         (1) The probing depth
         (2) The distance from the CEJ to the gingival margin
      b. Three possible relationships exist between the CEJ and the gingival margin; the clinician must understand how to calculate the CAL for each of these relationships
         (1) Visible gingival recession (gingival margin is apical to the CEJ) (Figure 17-11)
         (2) Gingival margin is coronal to the CEJ
         (3) Gingival margin is approximately level with the CEJ
   4. Calculation technique in areas of visible gingival recession
      a. Measure and record the probing depth (distance from the gingival margin to the base of the pocket)
      b. Measure and record the amount of gingival recession (distance from the CEJ to the gingival margin)

Gingival Margin Below CEJ

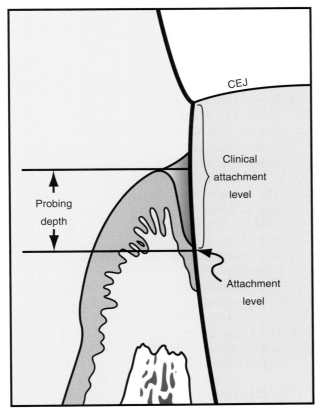

CEJ

Clinical
attachment
level

Probing
depth

Attachment
level

FIGURE 17-11 Comparison of the probing depth and the clinical attachment level when the gingival margin is apical to the CEJ. The clinical attachment level provides an accurate estimation of the level of the attached tissues. *(From Nield-Gehrig JS: Foundations of periodontics for the dental hygienist, ed 3, Philadelphia, 2010, Lippincott Williams & Wilkins.)*

  c. Calculate the clinical attachment level by adding the probing depth and the measurement of gingival recession
 5. Calculation technique in areas where gingival margin is coronal to the CEJ
  a. Measure and record the probing depth
  b. Apply the probe, and determine the location of the CEJ by tactile sensitivity; measure the distance from the gingival margin to the CEJ
  c. Calculate the clinical attachment level by subtracting the distance from the gingival margin to the CEJ from the probing depth
 6. Calculation technique in areas where the gingival margin is level with the CEJ—when the gingival margin is within 0.5 mm apical or coronal to the CEJ, the probing depth and the clinical attachment level are the same measurement
E. Mucogingival examination
 1. Rationale—to determine the width of the attached gingiva

 2. Procedure for determining the amount of attached gingiva
  a. On the external (outer) surface of the gingiva, measure the distance in millimeters from the gingival margin to the mucogingival junction; this is the total width of the gingiva (free and attached gingiva)
  b. Measure the probing depth
  c. Calculate the width of the attached gingiva by subtracting the probing depth from the total width of the gingiva
 3. Significance of finding
  a. If the probing depth is equal to or greater than the width of the total gingiva, no attached gingiva (NAG) exists
  b. If the probe tip passes the mucogingival junction, mucogingival involvement exists in this area
F. Furcation involvement
 1. Definition—furcation involvement occurs when periodontal infection invades the area between and around the roots of a bifurcated or trifurcated tooth, and the bone level is apical to the furcation crotch area
 2. Classification—furcation involvement is classified according to the extent of bone loss
  a. Class I—early, or incipient, involvement; the anatomy of the root surfaces can be felt by moving the probe from side to side, passing over the root into the concavity of the furcation area, and up the opposite side to the adjacent root
  b. Class II—moderate involvement; bone has been destroyed to an extent that allows the probe to partially enter the furcation, which extends approximately ⅓ of the width of the tooth between the roots
  c. Class III—severe, or advanced, involvement; in mandibular molars, the probe can pass between the roots, through the entire furcation; in maxillary molars, the probe can pass between the mesiobuccal and distobuccal roots to touch the palatal root
  d. Class IV—same as class III; also, the furca is visible clinically because of the presence of tissue recession
 3. Access to furcation area
  a. Bifurcated roots (two roots)
   (1) Mandibular molars—to examine between the mesial and distal roots, probe midfacial and midlingual aspects (Figure 17-12)
   (2) Maxillary first premolars—to examine between the buccal and palatal roots, probe from the mesial and distal aspects, under the contact area

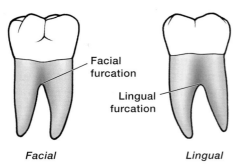

FIGURE 17-12 Furcation morphology on a mandibular molar (mesial and distal roots). The furcation can be examined from the facial and lingual aspects. *(From Nield-Gehrig JS: Fundamentals of periodontal instrumentation and advanced root instrumentation, ed 6, Philadelphia, 2008, Lippincott Williams & Wilkins.)*

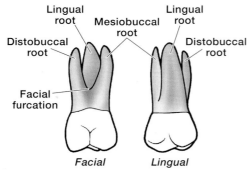

FIGURE 17-13 Furcation morphology on a maxillary molar (mesiobuccal, distobuccal, and palatal roots). The furcation can be examined from the facial, mesial, and distal aspects. *(From Nield-Gehrig JS: Fundamentals of periodontal instrumentation and advanced root instrumentation, ed 6, Philadelphia, 2008, Lippincott Williams & Wilkins.)*

  b. Trifurcated roots (three roots)—maxillary molars; to examine around the palatal root and the two facial roots, probe from the midfacial, mesial, and distal aspects (Figure 17-13)

G. Evaluation of oral deviations—a calibrated periodontal probe is used to determine the size of an oral lesion or deviation; when documenting measurements, anatomic terminology such as *anteroposterior* or *superoinferior*, is used, rather than terms such as *length* or *width*

Assessment with Dental Explorers

A. Purposes and uses
  1. Dental explorers detect, by tactile response, the texture and character of tooth surfaces before, during, and after treatment, to assess the progress and thoroughness of instrumentation

  2. Dental explorers examine tooth surfaces for:
    a. Dental calculus
    b. Cemental changes that may have resulted from pocket formation
    c. Anomalies
    d. Anatomic features such as grooves, curvatures, and furcation areas
  3. Dental explorers define the extent of instrumentation for treatment procedures of the tooth surface, including:
    a. Debridement
    b. Removal of overhanging restorations
    c. Sealant placement
B. Dental calculus (see the sections on "Bacterial plaque" in Chapter 9 and "Bacterial plaque biofilm" in Chapter 14)
  1. Definition
    a. Calcified or mineralized plaque biofilm; hard, tenacious mass that forms on tooth surfaces and on dental prostheses
    b. The surface of calculus is rough and is covered by a layer of plaque biofilm
  2. Types, distribution, and shape
    a. Supragingival (supramarginal) calculus
      (1) Located coronal to (above) the gingival margin
      (2) Distribution—localized, usually not generalized throughout the mouth
      (3) Most common locations include the lingual surfaces of mandibular anterior teeth, facial surfaces of maxillary molars, teeth out of occlusion, or overlapping teeth
    b. Subgingival (submarginal) calculus
      (1) Located apical to (beneath) the gingival margin
      (2) Distribution—may be localized or generalized; heaviest on proximal surfaces
      (3) Extends along the root surface almost to the base of the pocket; the newest, less calcified calculus is at the most apical area, near the soft tissue attachment
      (4) Shape—flattened to conform to pressure from the gingival pocket wall; forms may include combinations of the following:
        (a) Nodular deposits (spicules)
        (b) Ledge-like or ring-like formations
        (c) Thin, smooth veneers
        (d) Finger-like and fern-like formations
  3. Modes of attachment—calculus is more easily removed from some tooth surfaces than from others; the difficulty in removal usually is related to the manner in which the calculus is attached to the tooth; on any one tooth, more than one mode of attachment can occur

a. Attachment to acquired pellicle (thin acellular layer on tooth surface)—most common mode of calculus attachment to enamel; calculus may be removed readily because no interlocking of calculus to the tooth exists

b. Attachment by "locking" into minute irregularities in the tooth surface

c. Attachment of the calcified calculus matrix to the tooth surface by interlocking of inorganic crystals of the tooth with the mineralizing plaque

C. Calculus detection

1. Supragingival assessment—unnecessary supragingival exploration should be avoided; adequate light combined with the use of a dental mirror and compressed air will reveal most supragingival deposits

2. Subgingival adaptation
   a. Instrument grasp and lateral pressure—a relaxed grasp and light lateral pressure are used to enhance tactile sensitivity; pressure with the middle finger against the instrument shank should be avoided, as this reduces tactile sensitivity
   b. Activation—a combination of hand–forearm and digital activation
   c. Strokes—many, overlapping, fluid strokes are used to thoroughly cover the entire root surface

D. Carious lesions

1. Historically, the use of tactile examination of a tooth surface with a firm application of a sharp tip of an explorer into a suspected site of caries was a commonly used carious lesion detection method, but this method is no longer recommended

2. Research has shown this technique to be unreliable for carious lesion detection and to be potentially harmful

3. Firm application of a sharp explorer tip into a carious pit or fissure on a tooth surface may actually cause additional damage to the tooth surface that can interfere with subsequent attempts at remineralization of the caries lesion

DEBRIDEMENT CONCEPTS

Instrumentation Terminology

A. Instrumenting—using a periodontal instrument for a task

B. Deplaquing—the disruption or removal of subgingival plaque biofilm and its byproducts from cemental surfaces and the pocket spaces

C. Tactile sensitivity—the ability to feel vibrations transferred from the instrument's working end, shank, and handle to the clinician's fingers

D. Assessment—examination of a tooth and periodontium to determine anatomy and detect plaque-retentive factors, and oral disease status

E. Debridement—removal of hard and soft deposits from the tooth crown, root surfaces, and pocket space to the extent needed to re-establish periodontal health and restore a balance between the bacterial flora and the host's immune responses

F. Scaling—mechanical treatment of tooth surfaces for the removal of plaque biofilm and calculus deposits from coronal and root surfaces

G. Root planing—instrumentation procedure that may follow debridement; traditionally defined as the routine, intentional removal of cementum and the reduction of all root surfaces to a glassy, smooth texture; no longer recommended as a routine procedure to be performed on all root surfaces

H. Overhang removal—recontouring procedures that correct defective margins of restorations to provide a smooth surface that will deter bacterial accumulation

I. Supragingival—located coronal to (above) the gingival margin

J. Subgingival—located apical to (beneath) the gingival margin

K. Plaque-retentive factors—conditions that foster the establishment and growth of plaque biofilm, such as calculus deposits and overhanging restorations

Rationale for Periodontal Debridement

A. Arrests the progress of disease

B. Induces positive changes in the subgingival bacterial flora (count and content)

C. Creates an environment that permits the gingival tissue to heal, thereby eliminating inflammation

1. Converts the pocket from an area experiencing increased loss of attachment to one in which the clinical attachment level remains the same or decreases

2. Eliminates bleeding

3. Improves integrity of tissue attachment

D. Increases the effectiveness of client self-care

E. Permits re-evaluation of periodontal health status; surgery may then be unnecessary, lessened in extent, or confined to specific areas

F. Prevents recurrence of disease through supportive periodontal therapy

Rationale for Removal of Overhangs

A. Eliminates irregular surfaces where plaque biofilm can collect

B. Induces positive changes in the microflora of the pocket when the overhang extends subgingivally

C. Encourages resolution of inflammation

D. Facilitates interdental plaque removal and control by the client

Endpoint of Instrumentation

A. The goal of instrumentation is to render the root surface and pocket space acceptable to tissue so that healing occurs

B. Tissue healing occurs slowly, and it is not possible to assess tissue response for at least 1 month after completion of instrumentation

    1. The client's appointment for re-evaluation should be scheduled 4 to 6 weeks after completion of instrumentation

    2. During re-evaluation, a periodontal assessment that includes probing depths, clinical attachment levels, and bleeding on probing should be completed

    3. Nonresponsive sites are those that show continued loss of attachment and may exhibit clinical signs of inflammation or bleeding, or both, on probing; the following should be done to these sites:

        a. They should be thoroughly deplaqued, preferably with an ultrasonic instrument

        b. They should be thoroughly examined for residual calculus deposits or other plaque-retentive factors

    4. Rough areas may need root planing; consideration should be given to other risk factors that might be contributing to the disease process (host, environment, and dental factors)

Steps for the Preparation for Instrumentation

A. Protect client safety

    1. Review the client's personal and health histories for indications of special needs; prepare for a possible emergency

    2. Assess vital signs

    3. Observe the client for signs of stress

B. Use standard precautions (see Chapter 10)

    1. Postpone treatment for a client with a communicable disease or an open oral lesion

    2. Provide the means for lowering the bacterial count of the client's oral surfaces

        a. Provide the client with a pre-procedural antimicrobial mouthrinse or antimicrobial irrigation to lower the count of oral microorganisms

        b. Provide self-care instruction (e.g., plaque control) before any instrumentation

Sharpening of Hand-Activated Instruments

Sharp cutting edges are vital to achieve efficient debridement with minimal tissue trauma

A. Sharp cutting edges help provide more efficient treatment because of easier calculus removal, fewer strokes, improved stroke control, increased client comfort, and reduced clinician fatigue

B. To sharpen instruments correctly, the clinician must understand the design of the working end

    1. A sharp cutting edge is a line without width; a dull cutting edge is a rounded surface

    2. The internal angle formed between the face and lateral surface of a sickle scaler or curet is between 70 and 80 degrees

    3. Most sickle scalers have pointed tips and backs; curets have rounded toes and backs

    4. Sickle scalers and universal curets have two working cutting edges per working end; area-specific curets have one working cutting edge per working end

C. Instruments should be sharpened at the first sign of dullness—the cutting edge of the instrument dulls at various rates because of:

    1. Number of working strokes used

    2. Amount of lateral pressure used

    3. Hardness and tenacity of the deposit

    4. Composition of the metal of the instrument

D. Equipment

    1. A stable, well-lighted work surface

    2. Heat-sterilized rectangular sharpening stone or sharpening tool and plastic sharpening test stick (Table 17-3)

    3. Water or oil to lubricate the stone (depending on the type of stone)

    4. Protective eyewear, facemask, and household gloves (when sharpening contaminated instruments)

E. Principles of the moving-stone sharpening technique

    1. Grasp the instrument, and rest that hand on a stable countertop; or stabilize the hand by grasping the instrument against your torso

    2. Position the working end (sickle, universal curet, or area-specific curet) such that the face is parallel to the countertop (Figure 17-14)

    3. Grasp the lower third of the sharpening stone in the other hand, holding the edges of the stone so that your fingers do not get in the way during the sharpening

    4. Establish an angle of the stone at approximately 75 degrees to the face of the instrument's working end (see Figure 17-14)

    5. Sharpen the cutting edge in sections (heel, middle, and toe-thirds)

TABLE 17-3 Sharpening Stones and Tools

Type	Abrasiveness	Description	Purpose	Lubricant	Sterilization*
Ceramic	Fine	Synthetic stone	Routine sharpening of metal and some plastic implant instruments	Water	All methods
Arkansas	Fine	Natural stone	Routine sharpening of metal instruments	Mineral oil	All methods†
India	Medium	Synthetic stone	Sharpening of metal instruments that are dull	Water or oil	All methods
Composition	Coarse	Synthetic stone	Sharpening of metal instruments that are extremely dull or that need reshaping	Water	All methods
Nievert Whittler	—	Tungsten carbide steel	Routine sharpening of metal instruments	Water	All methods
Reciprocating honing device	—		Sharpening of metal instruments		

Includes autoclave, dry heat, or chemical sterilization.
†*Natural stones become brittle over time with heat exposure.*
Modified with permission from Nield-Gehrig JS: Fundamentals of periodontal instrumentation and advanced root instrumentation, *ed 6, Philadelphia, 2008, Lippincott Williams & Wilkins.*

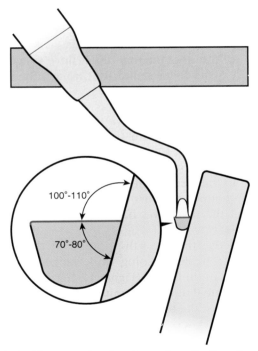

FIGURE 17-14 Preparation for sharpening. Position the instrument's working end so that the face is parallel to the countertop, and establish a stone-to-face angulation of approximately 75 degrees. *(Modified from Nield-Gehrig JS:* Fundamentals of periodontal instrumentation and advanced root instrumentation, *ed 6, Philadelphia, 2008, Lippincott Williams & Wilkins.)*

6. When sharpening a curet, recontour the toe and back of the working end
7. Use a sharpening stick to test for sharpness; it is common for one section of the cutting edge to be dull and another edge to be sharp
8. If appropriate, sharpen other cutting edges of the instrument

DEBRIDEMENT WITH MECHANIZED INSTRUMENTS

A. Description
1. Mechanized instruments use rapid vibrations of a fluid-cooled instrument tip to fracture and dislodge supragingival and subgingival calculus deposits from the teeth and to cleanse the environment within the periodontal pocket
2. Ultrasonic instruments (magnetostrictive and piezoelectric)
   a. High-frequency electrical energy is converted into mechanical energy in the form of ultrasonic vibrations; instrument tip vibrations range from 25,000 to 50,000 cycles per second (Hertz [Hz])
   b. Heat that is produced must be dissipated by a constant flow of water through the handpiece; antimicrobial solutions may be used instead of water in certain units
   c. Ultrasonic instruments provide efficient removal of all types of calculus deposits (old, new, supragingival and subgingival, light and heavy deposits)
3. Sonic instruments
   a. Air pressure also is used to create rapid mechanical vibrations; sonic instrument tip vibrations range from 3000 to 8000 cycles per second (Hz)

b. No heat is generated, so water cooling is not necessary; a water coolant is indicated, however, to obtain the benefits of water lavage

c. Because of the lower frequency of vibration, sonic instruments are less efficient in removing calculus deposits and have a limited ability to remove tenacious deposits; they function well for the removal of newly formed and light deposits

B. Definitions

1. Fluid lavage—the fluid stream within the periodontal pocket, produced by the constant flow of fluid through the handpiece, near the instrument's tip; when the fluid strikes the vibrating instrument tip, it creates a spray composed of millions of tiny bubbles

2. Cavitation—the energy release that occurs when the tiny bubbles in the fluid spray collapse; this energy can destroy bacteria by tearing the bacterial cell walls

3. Stroke—the maximum distance the instrument tip moves during one cycle of vibration

C. Instrument tip design

1. Working ends of mechanized instruments have no cutting edges to cut or tear tissue; less tissue trauma can result in faster healing rates for sites treated with ultrasonic or sonic instruments

2. The entire length of the working end is active; therefore, adaptation is not limited to a single region on the working end

3. Tip selection

a. Ultrasonic tip selection varies, depending on the manufacturer; the availability of a full range of tip designs is an important criterion when purchasing a mechanized instrument

b. Tips may range in size from large, broad tips (standard size), to medium-sized tips to slim-diameter slender tips

c. Standard tips (ultrasonic and sonic designs)

   (1) Broad, large tips are used to remove heavy, supragingival deposits

   (2) Medium-sized tips are used to remove medium and light deposits; some may be used subgingivally if the tissue permits easy insertion of the tip

d. Slim-diameter ultrasonic tips

   (1) Similar in diameter to periodontal probes, and significantly smaller in size than the working end of a curet

   (2) Approximately 40% thinner than a standard-sized ultrasonic tip

   (3) Available in straight, right-paired, and left-paired styles

   (4) Used for deplaquing and light calculus removal; provide excellent access to deep pockets and furcation areas

4. Energy dispersion—mechanized instrument tips are active on all surfaces; by adapting the appropriate tip surface, the clinician can control energy dispersion and client sensitivity during the procedure

a. Point—generates the most energy; should not be used directly against the tooth surface

b. Face (concave surface)—second most powerful surface (generates less energy than the point); usually not recommended for use against the tooth surface

c. Back (convex surface)—generates less energy than the face; follow the manufacturer's recommendations regarding direct use on the tooth surface

d. Lateral surfaces (sides)—generate the least amount of energy; may be used directly against the tooth surface

5. Fluid delivery—ultrasonic instruments require a constant stream of fluid running through the handpiece, which disperses in a fine spray at or near the instrument tip to prevent overheating of the vibrating instrument tip

a. Fluid delivery to the tip

   (1) The external flow tube is adjacent to the instrument's shank

   (2) In the internal fluid flow system, the fluid flows directly through the instrument tip

b. Water is the fluid most commonly used; some ultrasonic units have an independent fluid reservoir that can deliver distilled water or other fluid solutions (e.g., sterile saline, stannous fluoride, and chemotherapeutic agents) to the instrument tip

6. Tip frequency—the number of times per second that the tip moves back and forth during one cycle

a. Active tip area—the portion of the tip that is capable of doing work; ranges from 2 to 4 mm in length (Figure 17-15)

b. Manual ultrasonic units allow the clinician to adjust the tip frequency by turning an adjustment knob on the unit; automatic ultrasonic units control the tip frequency automatically; sonic instruments have a preset frequency that cannot be controlled by the clinician

D. Clinical power of mechanized instruments is the ability to remove calculus; several factors influence the force produced by the instrument tip

1. Exposure time—sufficient time must be allowed for the tip to do its work (e.g., ultrasonic instruments are effective, but even they do not instantaneously remove calculus); the tip should be moved back and forth over the deposit until it is dislodged

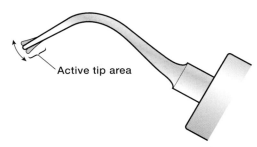

FIGURE 17-15 Active tip area of a mechanized instrument. The active tip area ranges in length from 2 to 3 mm and is the portion of the instrument tip that is capable of doing the work. *(From Nield-Gehrig JS: Fundamentals of periodontal instrumentation and advanced root instrumentation, ed 6, Philadelphia, 2008, Lippincott Williams & Wilkins.)*

2. Angle of adaptation—an angle of between 0 and 15 degrees is recommended for direct adaptation to tooth surfaces
3. Sharp or dull tip—only dull tips are recommended; sharpened tips emit high energy levels that could damage the tooth
4. Lateral pressure—tips function most effectively with light lateral pressure against the tooth or calculus deposit; moderate or firm lateral pressure decreases or even stops the vibrations of the tip

E. Uses of modern ultrasonic instruments
1. Removal of attached and unattached plaque biofilm (deplaquing) from root surface and pocket space
2. Disruption and destruction of bacteria
3. Removal of supragingival and subgingival calculus
4. Removal of toxins from root surfaces
5. Smoothing down overextended or rough amalgam restorations, removing extrinsic stains for aesthetic considerations, and removing orthodontic cement (using standard tips)

F. Contraindications
1. Client with a communicable disease that can be disseminated by aerosols
2. Immunocompromised client with high susceptibility to an infection who could be exposed to microorganisms in contaminated water, aerosols, or by other means (e.g., debilitated clients, those with uncontrolled diabetes, and clients who are immunosuppressed)
3. Client with respiratory disease or difficulty breathing (e.g., history of emphysema, cystic fibrosis, asthma); the client is at increased risk of respiratory infection if septic material or oral microorganisms are aspirated
4. Client who has difficulty swallowing or is prone to gagging (e.g., multiple sclerosis, amyotrophic lateral sclerosis, muscular dystrophy, or paralysis)
5. Client with a cardiac pacemaker; the dental clinician should check with the client's cardiologist if the device is shielded or unshielded
6. Client with primary or newly erupted teeth—danger of heat being conducted to large pulp chambers
7. Direct contact between the instrument tip and porcelain jacket crowns, composite resin restorations that could be damaged by the vibration or the tip, and demineralized enamel surfaces (conservation of demineralized enamel surfaces is indicated) should be avoided
8. Direct contact with titanium implant surface should be avoided, unless the instrument tip is covered with a specially designed plastic sleeve

G. Precautions
1. The handpiece and the working end of ultrasonic instruments must be cooled with constant flow of water to dissipate heat
2. Aerosols produced may be contaminated with pathogens; use of barriers, surface disinfectants, protective clothing, and laminar airflow systems is recommended
3. The client may experience sensitivity
4. Shifts in hearing sensitivity have been reported; the effect of ultrasonic and sonic equipment on the hearing of clinicians who frequently use these instruments has not been studied well

H. Preparation
1. Employ standard precautions, and ensure that protective attire is worn by the clinician, the assistant, and the client
2. Have the client use a pre-procedural antimicrobial mouthrinse, or irrigate the treatment area to reduce the number of airborne microorganisms in aerosols created by water spray
3. Monitor the condition of the equipment
4. Replace the instrument tip as soon as it shows signs of wear or damage
   a. Tip wear—1 mm of wear results in approximately 25% loss of efficiency; tips should be discarded at 2 mm of wear; some manufacturers offer wear guides that make it easy to determine tip wear; precision-thin tips must be replaced more frequently than standard tips
   b. Metal stacks of magnetostrictive insert—replace if the stacks are bent or separated or if the insert does not slide easily into the ultrasonic handpiece
5. Instrument tips and handpieces should be sterilized according to manufacturer's instructions; use surface disinfectant and barriers on an ultrasonic unit

I. Technique
   1. Biofilm control in water tubing—flush the water tubing of stagnant water for 2 minutes at the start of the day, and for 30 seconds between clients; use units with an independent fluid reservoir or waterline point-of-use filter, or both
   2. Tip selection—select the appropriate instrument tip for the task at hand
      a. Broad, standard tips for removal of heavy and medium-sized supragingival calculus
      b. Medium-sized standard tips for moderate and light supragingival use; also may be used subgingivally if the tissue permits easy insertion of the tip
      c. Slim-diameter tips for removal of light deposits and deplaquing
   3. Power—use standard instrument tips at medium-power or low-power setting, and slim-diameter tips at low-power setting; high-power setting is no more effective than medium power and is not recommended
   4. Grasp—use light, relaxed grasp, even during calculus removal
   5. Finger rest—use an intraoral or extraoral rest; advanced fulcrum techniques may be helpful for gaining access to posterior pockets
   6. Lateral pressure—use light stroke pressure for effective calculus removal
   7. Activation—use digital activation as recommended
   8. Fluid adjustment and containment
      a. Adjust the water spray around the instrument tip to create a light mist or halo effect, with no excess dripping of water; insufficient water flow over an ultrasonic tip can result in trauma to the pulp; a warm handpiece is a sign of inadequate fluid flow through the handpiece
      b. Use high-volume suction or a saliva ejector for fluid control; position the suction tip at the corner of the mouth where the fluid will pool; deactivate the instrument tip occasionally to prevent large amounts of fluid accumulation
      c. Use the client's lips and cheeks as barriers to deflect fluid back into the client's mouth
   9. Tip adaptation
      a. Adaptation to the tooth surface—position the tip with the point directed toward the junctional epithelium and the length of the tip at a 0- to 15-degree angle to the tooth surface; never apply the point of the tip directly to the tooth surface
      b. Adaptation to a calculus deposit—place the tip directly against the uppermost or outermost edge of the calculus deposit; the lateral surface of a tip may also be adapted to a calculus deposit
   10. Instrumentation strokes
      a. Motion—use a tapping motion against large-sized deposits and a sweeping, eraser-like motion against small deposits and to deplaque root surfaces
      b. Pressure—use light pressure; firm pressure decreases effectiveness
      c. Direction—use overlapping vertical, oblique, and horizontal strokes; subgingival strokes should cover the entire root surface for calculus removal and deplaquing
   11. Calculus removal
      a. Sequence—work in a coronal-to-apical direction, beginning at the gingival margin and working toward the junctional epithelium (this is the reverse of the sequence for calculus removal with a curet)
      b. Technique for removing stubborn deposits
         (1) Use an adequate number of strokes—move the tip repeatedly over the deposit or tap against the deposit; keep the tip in constant motion
         (2) Select the proper tip for the type of calculus; for example, do not use slim-diameter tips for medium-sized or large-sized deposits
         (3) Approach the deposit from different aspects (e.g., approach an interproximal deposit from both the facial and lingual aspects)
         (4) Do not apply firm stroke pressure; use of light pressure is most effective
         (5) Increase the frequency on a manually calibrated unit
         (6) Increase the power setting from low to medium

ADVANCED INSTRUMENTATION TECHNIQUES

Instrumentation of Dental Implants

A. Definitions
   1. Dental implant—a nonbiologic device surgically inserted into or onto the jaw bone to replace a missing tooth or to provide support for an implant superstructure (e.g., a fixed bridge or denture)
   2. Endosseous implant—most widely used type of implant; placed into alveolar or basal bone, or both
   3. Subperiosteal implant—placed on the surface of bone beneath the periosteum

4. Trans-osteal implant—placed through alveolar bone

B. General guidelines

1. Special instruments are recommended for assessing and debriding implants; plastic instruments are used most commonly because the plastic material is softer than the implant material

2. Metal instruments (e.g., stainless steel, carbon steel, and metal ultrasonic instruments) may leave scratches on the surface of the implant
   a. Scratches or surface roughness on an implant may promote accumulation of plaque
   b. Surface coating of an implant may be disturbed, thereby reducing the biocompatibility of the implant with the surrounding tissues

3. Some plastic instruments contain graphite fillers; these types of instruments may be used on the implant superstructure (prosthetic denture or bridge) but should not be used directly on the implant abutment (to avoid scratching of the abutment surface)

4. Some plastic instruments may be sterilized by autoclaving; follow the manufacturer's instructions for sterilization and reuse

C. Design of the working end of plastic instruments

1. Wrench-shaped, crescent-shaped, and hoe-shaped working ends—useful for the debridement of an implant's superstructure

2. Working ends that are similar in design to conventional metal probes, sickle scalers, and curets—useful for the assessment and debridement of an implant abutment

D. Use of plastic, calibrated probe for assessing peri-implant tissues (soft tissues that surround the dental implant)

1. Peri-implant probing depths are related to the thickness of the mucosa around the implant; deeper probing depths are found in conjunction with a thicker mucosa

2. Probing depths and clinical attachment levels are important parameters for the longitudinal monitoring of peri-implant tissue stability

3. Considerations
   a. Probing may be invasive because the probe may penetrate the weakly adherent biologic seal and could introduce bacteria into peri-implant tissue
   b. Accurate probing depths may be difficult to obtain owing to the constricted "cervical" area of some implants
   c. Radiographs are more accurate than probing depths for detecting the absence or presence of bone loss around implants

E. Instrumentation for calculus removal

1. Calculus is removed easily from implants because no interlocking or penetration of the deposit exists within the implant surface

2. Light lateral pressure with a plastic scaler or curet is recommended; care must be taken not to scratch the surface of the implant

3. Instrumentation should be restricted to supragingival deposit removal

SELECTIVE STAIN REMOVAL

A. Definitions

1. Intrinsic—stains that occur within the tooth substance; the process of removal is performed by a dentist using bleaching techniques or prosthetic coverage with a crown

2. Extrinsic—stains that occur on the external surface of the tooth; removed by client self-care and professional procedures such as scaling and rubber cup and brush scaling, rubber cup/brush, and air abrasion polishing

B. Significance of dental stains

1. No detrimental effects have been shown to result from the presence of dental stains; research shows that stains do not directly contribute to periodontal disease, dental caries, or any oral disease

2. Removal of unsightly dental stains on anterior teeth may contribute to the client's appearance and self-esteem

C. Rationale for selective stain removal

1. Polishing is viewed as a cosmetic procedure with limited application; stain removal provides no therapeutic benefit to the client and has numerous detrimental effects on teeth and soft tissue

2. Decision to include stain removal in a client's care plan can best be made after client self-care education and after complete periodontal debridement because much of the stain may be removed along with calculus deposits

D. Contraindications to polishing

1. Dental contraindications
   a. Tooth surfaces that have no extrinsic stains or have stains that are not visible when client smiles or engages in conversation
   b. Areas of dentinal hypersensitivity—application of fluoride is one treatment for tooth sensitivity; protective fluoride must be left undisturbed (see the section on "Control of dentinal hypersensitivity" in Chapter 16)
   c. Restored tooth surfaces—gold and other restorative materials may be scratched by the abrasive agent

d. Titanium implants—polishing could scratch the titanium abutment

e. Areas of demineralization—conservation of demineralized enamel surfaces is indicated

f. Gingiva that is enlarged, soft, spongy, or bleeds easily—polishing is not recommended because paste can enter the tissue, and the action of the rotating cup can further traumatize the tissue

2. Systemic contraindications

a. Client with a communicable disease that could be spread by aerosols

b. Client with a high susceptibility to infection who could inhale contaminated aerosols (e.g., client with respiratory or pulmonary disease; client who is debilitated)

c. Client who has a history of renal insufficiency, Addison's disease, Cushing's syndrome, or metabolic alkalosis; is taking mineralocorticosteroids, antidiuretics, or potassium supplements; air polisher use should be avoided

d. Client who has a history of hypertension or a sodium restricted diet; air polishing using a sodium-containing powder is contraindicated; air polishing can be used with one of the newer sodium-free polishing powder products such as those composed of aluminum trihydroxide or calcium carbonate

E. Adverse effects of polishing

1. Aerosol production and spatter from power-driven polisher

a. Contaminated aerosols present a hazard to the clinician, other dental personnel, and other clients in the oral health care environment

b. Spatter of polishing paste; protective eyewear is needed for clients and dental team members to protect eyes from splatter

c. Components of commercial prophylaxis pastes may include various chemicals that can cause a severe inflammatory response in the eye

2. Creation of bacteremia

a. Bacteremia can be induced during the use of a rotating cup; an assessment of client's health must be prepared initially and reviewed and updated at all appointments

b. New recommendations developed by the American Heart Association and the American Dental Association state that preventive antibiotics before dental procedures are advised for patients with artificial heart valves; a history of infective endocarditis; certain specific, congenital (present from birth) heart conditions; a cardiac transplant that develops a problem in a heart valve; total joint replacement

3. Iatrogenic damage to tooth surfaces

a. Enamel surfaces—stain removal with an abrasive agent removes the surface layer of tooth structure where the fluoride content is greatest and most protective; polishing the teeth for 3 minutes with pumice removes 3 to 4 micrometers (μm) of enamel; over time, the loss of enamel can be significant

b. Cemental surfaces—exposed surface near the CEJ has a thin cementum or dentin surface that can be abraded or removed with an abrasive agent

c. Heat production—care must be taken to use a wet polishing agent with minimal pressure and low speed to prevent overheating of a tooth, particularly the pulp tissues of small children; primary teeth have large pulp chambers, which make them particularly vulnerable to heat generated by power-driven handpieces

4. Tissue trauma—during polishing, abrasive paste is forced into the gingival sulcus and even into the tissue itself; some individuals experience a negative tissue response to abrasive particles or chemicals in the paste, which can delay tissue healing

F. Power-driven polisher

1. Description

a. Handpiece—connects to the dental unit's low-speed handpiece line

b. Prophylaxis angle—attaches to the handpiece; holds polishing cups and bristle brushes

c. Attachments

(1) Polishing cups—used for stain removal from tooth surfaces and for polishing restorations

(2) Bristle brushes—used for stain removal from occlusal surfaces; not for use near the gingival margin or on cementum or dentin, where the brush could denude the epithelium or remove cementum

2. Technique considerations

a. Application of polishing agent—apply agent only to individual teeth requiring stain removal for aesthetic purposes

b. Use the lowest possible handpiece speed

c. Apply the cup to the tooth with a light, intermittent pressure

(1) The edges of the cup should just barely flare from the tooth surface

(2) Use of continuous motion—avoid holding the cup on a single spot for too long to prevent buildup of frictional heat

G. Air polishing

1. Definition—an air-powered device using air and water pressure to deliver a controlled slurry of powder to the tooth surface

2. Technique
  a. Wear protective attire
    (1) Client—provide a plastic apron, hair cover, eye protection, and lip lubrication
    (2) Clinician and assistant—wear a paper or cloth long-sleeved garment, facemask, hair cover, eye protection, and gloves
  b. Administer a pre-procedural mouthrinse to lessen contaminated aerosols; have the client rinse with an antibacterial mouthrinse
  c. Establish the recommended angulation of the tip to the tooth surface
    (1) Facial and lingual surfaces of anterior teeth—position the nozzle tip at a 60-degree angle to the tooth
    (2) Facial and lingual surfaces of posterior teeth—position nozzle tip at an 80-degree angle to the tooth
    (3) Occlusal surfaces—position the nozzle at a 90-degree angle to the surface of the tooth
  d. Direct the spray in constant motion for only 3 to 5 seconds at any area on the enamel surface
H. Postoperative procedures for mechanical and air polishing
  1. Remove particles of abrasive at the contact areas with dental floss
  2. Loosen and remove particles in sulci or pockets by irrigation and aspiration with central suction

ETHICAL, LEGAL, AND SAFETY ISSUES

A. Provision of quality care by licensed dental hygienists includes ethical, legal, and safety issues
B. A comprehensive review of the client's medical health and pharmacologic histories is essential to assess the degree of client risk for dental procedures and to make necessary physician or specialty referrals
C. Adherence to the Health Insurance Portability Act (HIPAA) is necessary; thorough, accurate, and confidential chart documentation is essential
D. A comprehensive client assessment is essential to detect oral diseases and abnormalities and the degree of client risk for periodontal disease or disease progression
E. Failure to provide necessary care based on assessment findings constitutes supervised neglect; the licensed dental hygienist is accountable and responsible for client care
F. A thorough case presentation is essential so that the client can make an informed decision about recommended dental hygiene care; written informed consent should be obtained before beginning care; discussion of all procedures with clients using everyday language that the client can understand and encouragement of client participation essential
G. The dental hygienist has an obligation to provide evidence-based care
H. The dental hygienist has an obligation to protect the client from harm during care
I. The dental hygienist has an obligation to follow established protocol that protects the clinician and the client during treatment
J. It is essential to allow sufficient time during appointments for provision of adequate care
K. Nonsurgical periodontal instrumentation should be performed in an effective and responsible manner; use of sharp instruments and selection of appropriate instruments for the task is essential
L. It is essential to evaluate the success of nonsurgical periodontal instrumentation at appropriate continued-care intervals
M. The dental hygienist has a legal obligation to thoroughly and accurately document assessment, care plan, informed consent, services provided, and client response to care

@ WEB SITE INFORMATION AND RESOURCES

SOURCE	WEB SITE ADDRESS	DESCRIPTION
American Academy of Periodontology	http://www.perio.org	Parameters of care, position papers, scientific information, related links
Cochrane Collaboration	http://www.cochrane.org	Evidence-based health care database
National Center for Dental Hygiene Research	http://www.usc.edu/hsc/dental/dhnet	Current topics in dental hygiene; links
Hu-Friedy	http://www.hu-friedy.com	Online catalogue of periodontal instruments and ultrasonic tips; white papers, material safety data sheets (MSDS), instrument care, articles

Continued

@ WEB SITE INFORMATION AND RESOURCES—cont'd

SOURCE	WEB SITE ADDRESS	DESCRIPTION
Premier Dental	http://www.premusa.com	Online catalogue of periodontal instruments; fluoride; continuing education seminar information
Deldent Ltd. Air Polishers	http://www.deldent.com	Information about the products marketed by Deldent
Dentsply Ultrasonic Units	http://www.dentsply.com	News articles, career and legal information, and information about Dentsply products
KaVo America	http://www.kavousa.com	Information about KaVo dental products
ODONTO-Wave	http://www.odontoson.com	Information about Odonto-wave dental products and research supporting their value
Parkell Ultrasonic Scalers	http://www.parkell.com	Information about Parkell dental products
Tony Riso Company	http://www.tonyriso.com	Information about the company's ultrasonic instruments

SUGGESTED READINGS

Nield-Gehrig JS: *Fundamentals of periodontal instrumentation and advanced root instrumentation*, ed 6, Philadelphia, 2008, Lippincott Williams & Wilkins.

Darby ML, Walsh M: Instruments and instrumentation theory. In Darby ML, Walsh MM, editors: *Dental hygiene theory and practice*, ed 3, Philadelphia, 2010, Saunders.

CHAPTER 17 REVIEW QUESTIONS

Answers and Rationales to the Review Questions are available on this text's accompanying Evolve site. See inside front cover for details.
Use Case A to answer questions 1 to 9.

℮volve

SYNOPSIS OF PATIENT HISTORY			
Age	35		
Sex	F		
Height	5'4"		
CASE	A		
Weight	140 lbs / 64 kgs		

VITAL SIGNS
Blood pressure _110/72 mmHg_
Pulse rate _70 bpm_
Respiration rate _16 rpm_

1. Under Care of Physician
   Yes ☒   No ☐   Condition: _Obstetrician_
2. Hospitalized within the last 5 years
   Yes ☐   No ☒   Reason: _____
3. Has or had the following conditions
   Anemia
   _____
4. Current medications
   Prescription prenatal vitamins
   with extra iron due to history of
   anemia
5. Smokes or uses tobacco products
   Yes ☐   No ☒
6. Is pregnant
   Yes ☒   No ☐   N/A ☐   _Second trimester_

MEDICAL HISTORY:
History of anemia

DENTAL HISTORY:
Her last dental visit was 2 years ago with a history of sporadic recall visits.

SOCIAL HISTORY:
She works as a paralegal in a busy law firm. This is her first pregnancy and she plans to return to work after her maternity leave. Her law firm provides childcare for it employees.

CHIEF COMPLAINT:
"I would like to take better care of my teeth now that I am pregnant."

Adult clinical examination

Probe 2/1 — Facial: | 1 | 2 | 3 | 4 | 5 | 6 | 7 | 8 | 9 | 10 | 11 | 12 | 13 | 14 | 15 | 16 |

424 424 423   322 212 211 112 222 223   434 434 434

Palatal:
Probe 1/2: 433 434 433   221 111 111 111 112 223   334 434 434

Probe 2/1 — Lingual: 433 334 433   424 434 434 424 434 434   434 424 444

Facial:
Probe 1/2: 444 434 433   434 424 424 424 424 423   334 434 434
| 32 | 31 | 30 | 29 | 28 | 27 | 26 | 25 | 24 | 23 | 22 | 21 | 20 | 19 | 18 | 17 |

Case A

CURRENT ORAL HYGIENE STATUS:
1. Generalized tenacious black line stain on lingual aspect of both arches
2. Mandibular anterior sextant: marginal redness with papillary enlargement
3. Mandibular anterior sextant: moderate supragingival plaque biofilm and light subgingival calculus deposits
4. Maxillary and mandibular posterior sextants: moderate supragingival plaque biofilm and light subgingival calculus deposits on the proximal surfaces
5. Oral self-care is ineffective

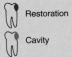 Restoration

Cavity

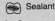 Sealant

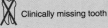 Clinically missing tooth

△ Furcation

▲ "Through and through" furcation

Probe 1: initial probing depth

Probe 2: probing depth 1 month after scaling and root planing

1. **The best way to remove the black line stain on the lingual aspects of both arches is to:**
   a. Polish with coarse grit pumice using a motor-driven handpiece
   b. Use a slim-diameter ultrasonic tip with a straight working end to remove the stain
   c. Use a Nabers diamond-coated file (This instrument has a similar design as a Nabers furcation probe and is diamond coated.)
   d. Use a universal curet to remove the stain

2. **Access to subgingival calculus deposits on the proximal surfaces of the mandibular anterior teeth is difficult because of papillary enlargement of the gingival tissue. Which of the following statements provides the BEST advice for thorough subgingival calculus removal?**
   a. Use a curet with a small, thin working end, and approach the deposit from both facial and lingual aspects
   b. Try to remove the deposit with an explorer using an assessment stroke
   c. Apply a topical anesthetic; then use a calculus removal stroke subgingivally with an anterior sickle scaler
   d. Use the ultrasonic with a universal insert applying heavy lateral pressure and working as quickly as possible

3. **Which one of the instruments listed below is the BEST choice for efficient removal of light subgingival calculus from the proximal surfaces of the client's posterior teeth?**
   a. A posterior sickle scaler
   b. A universal curet
   c. A set of standard Gracey curets
   d. An O'Hehir curet

4. **All of the following rationale statements for deplaquing plaque biofilm are correct EXCEPT one. Which one is the EXCEPTION?**
   a. Deplaquing may motivate the client's interest in performing better daily self-care
   b. Guiding the client as he or she removes plaque biofilm during the appointment provides an opportunity to teach better self-care skills
   c. Plaque biofilm causes inflammation of the gingival tissue
   d. Initial deplaquing will allow for easier removal of calculus deposits

5. **Blowing a stream of compressed air on mandibular anteriors reveals a sheet of light calculus covering the lingual aspect of tooth #22 to #27. Which of the following techniques would be BEST for calculus removal?**
   a. Use the pointed tip of an anterior sickle scaler
   b. Use the side of a Nabers diamond-coated file
   c. Use the toe-third of the lateral surface of a universal curet
   d. Use a rubber cup on a motor-driven handpiece

6. **While removing calculus deposits from mandibular anterior teeth, the presence of heavy bleeding makes the tooth surfaces slippery. Which of the following fulcrums would give the clinician the GREATEST stability and less chance for an occupational exposure while removing calculus deposits from the mandibular anterior sextant?**
   a. Basic intraoral fulcrum
   b. Opposite arch fulcrum
   c. Finger-on-finger fulcrum
   d. Stabilized extraoral fulcrum

7. **Because of her pregnancy, it is uncomfortable for the client to lie in the supine position with the back of the chair raised slightly. To ensure client comfort and facilitate the clinician's access to the maxillary arch, which of the following strategies would be helpful?**
   a. Ask the client to position her head in a manner that facilitates visualization of and access to the treatment area
   b. Ask the client to lie on her left side while she receives dental treatment
   c. Lower the back of the client's chair to enhance comfort
   d. All of the strategies listed above would improve client comfort and facilitate access to the maxillary arch

8. **The clinician is having difficulty accessing the lingual aspect of a maxillary posterior sextant. For right-handed clinicians, this is the maxillary right posterior sextant, lingual aspect. For left-handed clinicians, this is the maxillary left posterior sextant, lingual aspect. The client and clinician chairs are correctly positioned for the treatment area. Which of the following might allow better access?**
   a. Ask the client to turn her head away from you
   b. Ask the client to turn her head toward you
   c. Ask the client to lower her chin (chin down position)
   d. Lower the seat of the clinician chair

9. **While exploring the mandibular anterior sextant with the ODU 11/12 periodontal explorer, it is difficult to insert the explorer without unduly distending the tissue. Which of the following techniques might cause less tissue distension?**
   a. Switch to an Orban explorer
   b. Aim the point the tip of the ODU 11/12 explorer toward the base of the sulcus so less of the working end is inserted in the sulcus
   c. Switch to a cowhorn explorer
   d. Use a calibrated periodontal probe to explore for deposits

Use Case B to answer questions 10 to 19.

SYNOPSIS OF PATIENT HISTORY		
Age	88	
Sex	M	
Height	5'11"	
CASE	B	
Weight	154 lbs	
	70 kgs	

VITAL SIGNS
Blood pressure 135/95 mmHg
Pulse rate 100 bpm
Respiration rate 17 rpm

1. Under Care of Physician
   Yes ☒ No ☐ Condition: _Cardiologist and internal medicine specialist_
2. Hospitalized within the last 5 years
   Yes ☒ No ☐ Reason: _Hospitalized 6 months ago for placement of 2 arterial stents_
3. Has or had the following conditions
   Angina pectoris
4. Current medications
   Coreg; patient reports taking Coreg as prescribed but deliberately skips a day or two when he feels dizzy. (Dizziness is a common side effect of this medication.)
5. Smokes or uses tobacco products
   Yes ☐ No ☒ _Quit 1 year ago_
6. Is pregnant
   Yes ☐ No ☐ N/A ☒

MEDICAL HISTORY:
Angina pectoris
2 arterial cardiac stents

DENTAL HISTORY:
3 years since last dental visit due to poor health

SOCIAL HISTORY:
Reports having much more energy since the stents have been in place. Likes to read and play chess with his neighbor.

CHIEF COMPLAINT:
"Now that I am feeling better, I thought it was high time that I had a check-up. My mouth is very dry . . . it makes it difficult to talk and eat."

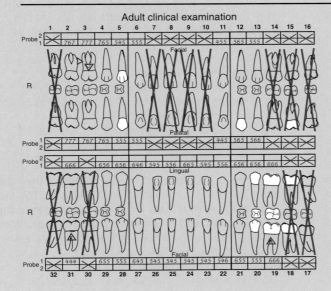

Adult clinical examination

Case B

CURRENT ORAL HYGIENE STATUS:
1. _Gingival description: generalized pale pink, fibrotic tissue with deep, narrow pockets._
2. _Xerostomia_
3. _Root caries_
4. _Generalized moderate, tenacious subgingival calculus deposits_

SUPPLEMENTAL ORAL EXAMINATION FINDINGS:

 Restoration

 Cavity

 Sealant

 Clinically missing tooth

△ Furcation

▲ "Through and through" furcation

Probe 1: initial probing depth

Probe 2: probing depth 1 month after scaling and root planing

10. The client has chronic periodontal disease with fibrotic tissue. Tenacious moderate black subgingival calculus is present on most tooth surfaces. Which of the instrument(s) listed below would be the BEST choice to initiate removal of the moderate calculus deposits?
    a. Ultrasonic beavertail tip
    b. Ultrasonic slim-diameter tip with a straight working end
    c. Set of rigid Gracey curets 1/2, 11/12, and 13/14
    d. Quetin (kee-tan) furcation curet

11. If the clinician decides to use ultrasonic equipment instead of hand instruments, she needs to keep contraindications for ultrasonic use in mind. Which of the following is NOT a contraindication for use of ultrasonic equipment?
    a. Client with a communicable disease
    b. Client with difficulty swallowing or who is prone to gagging
    c. Client with primary or newly erupted teeth
    d. Client with multiple amalgam restorations

12. One of the client's chief complaints is dry mouth. All of the following are useful suggestions for the client to minimize the effects of xerostomia EXCEPT one. Which one is the EXCEPTION?
    a. Increase the intake of caffeine-containing drinks to stimulate saliva production
    b. Take frequent sips of water throughout the day
    c. Use a humidifier in the bedroom at night
    d. Chew food slowly and thoroughly, and sip water with it before swallowing

13. The client has several areas of existing root caries and xerostomia. This combination places him at extreme risk for caries. All of the following are recommended management strategies for caries prevention EXCEPT one. Which one is the EXCEPTION?
    a. Professional application of fluoride varnish every 3 months
    b. Daily use of an antiseptic mouthrinse
    c. Twice daily brushing with a prescription sodium fluoride (NaF) toothpaste
    d. Twice daily topical application of calcium or phosphate paste

14. Which instrument would be BEST to detect furcation involvement on multiple-rooted teeth?
    a. ODU 11/12 explorer
    b. A periodontal file, such as an Orban file
    c. Nabers probe
    d. A calibrated periodontal probe, such as a UNC 15 probe

15. Tooth #3 has a class II furcation involvement on the facial aspect. Of the instruments listed below, which would be the BEST choice for smoothing the roof of the furcation area?
    a. Slim-diameter ultrasonic tip with a straight working end
    b. Nabers diamond-coated file
    c. Standard Gracey curet 11/12
    d. Universal curet with an extended lower shank

16. The clinician is using hand instruments to remove moderate calculus deposits. After 30 minutes, the clinician's hand muscles become noticeably fatigued. Potentially, all of the following can cause hand fatigue EXCEPT one. Which one is the EXCEPTION?
    a. Gloves that fit too tightly
    b. Using instruments with large-diameter, hollow handles
    c. Using an instrument that is not balanced
    d. Using finger motion instead of wrist motion activation

17. A full mouth radiographic survey indicates the presence of subgingival calculus in the mandibular right posterior sextant, but the clinician is unable to detect it with an ODU 11/12 explorer. All of the following may contribute to an inability to detect calculus EXCEPT one. Which one is the EXCEPTION?
    a. Not resting the middle finger lightly on the side of the instrument shank
    b. Grasping the instrument handle too tightly
    c. Keeping the anterior-third of the working end adapted to the root surface
    d. Not inserting the explorer to the base of the periodontal pocket

18. A clinician is having difficulty keeping the lower shank parallel to the long axis of tooth #3. The clinician is using a Gracey 13/14 curet with a miniature working end and an extended lower shank. Which of the following would MOST LIKELY improve access in this distolingual surface?
    a. Switch to an advanced fulcrum
    b. Use a straight, slim-diameter ultrasonic tip
    c. Use a universal curet with an extended shank
    d. Use a rigid Gracey curet instead

19. A large piece of burnished calculus is present on the distal aspect of tooth #2. Which instrument would be MOST effective in preparing the burnished deposit for eventual removal with another periodontal instrument?
    a. A beavertail ultrasonic tip
    b. A rigid Gracey 13/14
    c. A periodontal file
    d. A miniature Gracey 13/14 curet with an extended shank

Use Case C to answer questions 20 to 26.

SYNOPSIS OF PATIENT HISTORY		
Age	21	
Sex	M	
Height	5'9"	
CASE C		
Weight	151	lbs
	68	kgs

VITAL SIGNS
Blood pressure _118/78 mmHg_
Pulse rate _80 bpm_
Respiration rate _14 rpm_

1. Under Care of Physician
   Yes ☒   No ☐   Condition: _____
2. Hospitalized within the last 5 years
   Yes ☐   No ☒   Reason: _____
3. Has or had the following conditions
   Diabetes controlled by diet
   _____

4. Current medications
   none
   _____
   _____

5. Smokes or uses tobacco products
   Yes ☐   No ☒

6. Is pregnant
   Yes ☐   No ☐   N/A ☒

MEDICAL HISTORY:
Borderline diabetes controlled by diet

DENTAL HISTORY:
Last dental check-up was 18 months ago.

SOCIAL HISTORY:
Is a physically active member of a soccer team. Is studying architectural design at the local university.

CHIEF COMPLAINT:
"Sometimes my gums bleed on my lower front teeth."

Adult clinical examination

Case C

CURRENT ORAL HYGIENE STATUS:
1. _Class II division II occlusion; crowding of the mandibular anterior teeth; mandibular anteriors are in linguoversion._
2. _Mandibular anterior sextant: rolled gingival margins with heavy supragingival plaque biofilm on gingival third; heavy supragingival calculus deposits on lingual aspect_
3. _Posterior sextants: clinical attachment loss with moderate subgingival and subgingival calculus deposits_

- Restoration
- Cavity
- Sealant
- Clinically missing tooth
- △ Furcation
- ▲ "Through and through" furcation

Probe 1 : initial probing depth
Probe 2 : probing depth 1 month after scaling and root planing

20. **Which of the following instruments would be the MOST effective in removing a small subgingival calculus deposit on the lingual aspect of tooth #24?**
    a. A Gracey 1/2 curet with a miniature working end and an extended lower shank
    b. An anterior sickle scaler
    c. An periodontal file designed for use on the lingual aspect
    d. A standard Gracey 1/2 curet

21. **To determine if the client has calculus deposits on the proximal surfaces of the posterior teeth, the instrument of choice would be_____ and the instrumentation stroke used would be_____.**
    a. Orban explorer; a short, firm stroke
    b. Orban explorer; a light, flowing stroke
    c. ODU 11/12 explorer; a light, flowing stroke
    d. ODU 11/12 explorer; a short, firm stroke

22. **The client's mandibular anterior teeth are in linguo-version and are crowded. The clinician is having difficulty accessing the lingual surfaces of these mandibular anterior teeth. Which of the following patient positioning suggestions is BEST to ensure an ergonomic instrumentation technique?**
    a. Ask the client to lower his chin (chin-down position)
    b. Lower the back of the client's chair until it is parallel to the floor
    c. Ask the client to keep his chin in an upward position (chin-up position)
    d. Stand up and work, with the client in an upright seated position

23. **When the clinician puts a new mouth mirror in the client's mouth, she notices the image is distorted. What is the most reasonable explanation for this?**
    a. The client is breathing through his mouth, causing fog to form on mirror's reflecting surface
    b. The mirror has a concave reflecting surface
    c. The mirror has a plane reflecting surface
    d. The magnification of the reflecting surface is too extreme

24. **A periodontal instrument has the following design features: The face is perpendicular to the lower shank, the cutting edges are level with each other, and the working end has a rounded toe. Which of the following instruments also exhibits these design criteria?**
    a. A standard anterior Gracey curet
    b. An O'Hehir curet
    c. A posterior sickle scaler
    d. A universal curet

25. **When performing a coronal polish, all of the following areas should be avoided EXCEPT one. Which one is the EXCEPTION?**
    a. Areas of demineralization
    b. Extrinsic stain on maxillary anterior facials
    c. Gold crowns
    d. Areas with gingival enlargement and inflammation

26. **Which of the following ultrasonic tips would be MOST efficient for removing the heavy ledge of supragingival calculus on the client's mandibular anterior sextant, lingual aspect?**
    a. A bulky ultrasonic tip with a short shank, commonly called a *beavertail tip*
    b. A slim-diameter, straight ultrasonic tip with extended shank
    c. Paired right and left slim-diameter curved ultrasonic tips with extended shanks
    d. Ultrasonic tip with a rounded ball-end

Use Case D to answer questions 27 to 34.

SYNOPSIS OF PATIENT HISTORY		VITAL SIGNS	
Age	24	Blood pressure	108/60 mmHg
Sex	F	Pulse rate	60 bpm
Height	5'2"	Respiration rate	14 rpm
CASE	D		
Weight	108 lbs		
	49 kgs		

1. Under Care of Physician
   Yes ☒ No ☐   Condition: *Routine yearly check-up*

2. Hospitalized within the last 5 years
   Yes ☐ No ☒   Reason: _____

3. Has or had the following conditions
   none

4. Current medications
   none

5. Smokes or uses tobacco products
   Yes ☐ No ☒

6. Is pregnant
   Yes ☐ No ☒ N/A ☐

MEDICAL HISTORY:
none

DENTAL HISTORY:
Check-ups every 6 months.

SOCIAL HISTORY:
Social worker; engaged to be married in 6 months.

CHIEF COMPLAINT:
"I don't like the appearance of my front teeth"

Adult clinical examination

Case D

CURRENT ORAL HYGIENE STATUS:

1. *Tooth #8 was fractured as a child; restored with endodontic treatment and porcelain fused to metal crown*
2. *Carious lesion on occlusal of tooth #19*
3. *Tooth #7 exhibits red rolled margins and enlarged papillae on the facial aspect. Client reports that this tooth is very sensitive to toothbrushing*
4. *Generalized plaque biofilm on gingival thirds of teeth*
5. *Generalized moderate supragingival and subgingival calculus deposits*

SUPPLEMENTAL ORAL EXAMINATION FINDINGS:

- Restoration
- Cavity
- Sealant
- Clinically missing tooth
- Furcation
- "Through and through" furcation

Probe 1: initial probing depth
Probe 2: probing depth 1 month after scaling and root planing

27. The posterior sextants exhibit moderate supragingival and subgingival calculus deposits. Clinical attachment loss is present with periodontal pockets greater than 4 mm in depth. The clinician plans to complete calculus removal on the maxillary right posterior sextant. He plans to use a series of ultrasonic tips followed by hand instruments. Which sequence of ultrasonic tips would be MOST effective for calculus removal in this sextant?
    a. Beavertail tip, followed by a slim-diameter straight tip with extended shank length
    b. Standard-diameter universal tip with a curved shank, followed by paired right and left slim-diameter curved tips with extended shank length
    c. A slim-diameter straight tip, followed by paired right and left slim-diameter curved tips with extended shank length
    d. A standard-diameter universal tip with a curved shank, followed by a slim-diameter straight tip

28. A suspected carious lesion on the occlusal surface of tooth #19 is BEST detected by applying firm pressure with the sharp tip of an explorer to the occlusal grooves. Catching the tip of the explorer in the grooves of a tooth is a recommended method of caries detection.
    a. Both statements are TRUE
    b. The first statement is TRUE; the second FALSE
    c. The first statement is FALSE; the second TRUE
    d. Both statements are FALSE

29. Before beginning calculus removal, the clinician uses an explorer to determine the type, amount, and location of calculus deposits. Which of the following explorers is NOT recommended for calculus detection?
    a. ODU 11/12 explorer
    b. Shepherd's hook explorer
    c. Orban-type explorer
    d. Pigtail explorer

30. The clinician determines that many of the client's multiple-rooted teeth have loss of clinical attachment. This information should prompt the clinician to use the following instrument to assess for possible furcation involvement.
    a. An ODU 11/12 explorer
    b. Calibrated Nabers probes with curved working ends
    c. Calibrated periodontal probe with a straight working end
    d. Slim-diameter curved right and left paired ultrasonic tips with extended shanks

31. A posterior sickle is effective in removing moderate calculus deposits from the coronal surfaces of premolars and molars. A posterior sickle is a double-ended instrument that can be used on the facial, lingual, mesial, and distal surfaces of the crowns of posterior teeth.
    a. Both statements are TRUE
    b. The first statement is TRUE; the second FALSE
    c. The first statement is FALSE; the second TRUE
    d. Both statements are FALSE

32. Tooth #8 is restored with a porcelain-fused-to-metal crown. Which of the following instruments is contraindicated for use around tooth #8?
    a. A standard-diameter ultrasonic tip
    b. A universal curet
    c. An anterior Gracey curet
    d. An ODU 11/12 explorer

33. An intraoral fulcrum is accomplished by establishing a finger rest near the tooth to be instrumented. Establishing a finger rest as close as possible to the working end of the instrument is preferable so the fingers in the grasp will remain touching.
    a. Both statements are TRUE
    b. The first statement is TRUE; the second FALSE
    c. The first statement is FALSE; the second TRUE
    d. Both statements are FALSE

34. During periodontal instrumentation for calculus removal, the clinician's hand becomes fatigued. Self-assessment indicates he has been using finger motion with a hand instrument for calculus removal. Digital activation is acceptable for all of the following situations EXCEPT one. Which one is this EXCEPTION?
    a. Using an ultrasonic tip for calculus removal
    b. Using a calibrated probe to measure pocket depth
    c. Using an explorer to detect calculus
    d. Using a universal curet to remove calculus deposits

Use Case E to answer questions 35 to 44.

SYNOPSIS OF PATIENT HISTORY		
Age	70	
Sex	F	
Height	4'10"	
CASE E		
Weight	100	lbs
	45	kgs

VITAL SIGNS
Blood pressure _128/98 mmHg_
Pulse rate _78 bpm_
Respiration rate _15 rpm_

1. Under Care of Physician
   Yes ☒ No ☐ Condition: _____
2. Hospitalized within the last 5 years
   Yes ☐ No ☒ Reason: _____
3. Has or had the following conditions
   Hypertension _____
   _____
4. Current medications
   Lotensin for high blood pressure;
   herbal supplements, garlic,
   rosehips, and Co Q10
5. Smokes or uses tobacco products
   Yes ☐ No ☒
6. Is pregnant
   Yes ☐ No ☒ N/A ☐

MEDICAL HISTORY:
History of hypertension

DENTAL HISTORY:
Infrequent dental visits due to financial priorities

SOCIAL HISTORY:
Retired elementary school teacher; likes to garden and play cards with her friends

CHIEF COMPLAINT:
"My gums bleed when I brush"

Adult clinical examination

Case E

CURRENT ORAL HYGIENE STATUS:
1. _Gingival tissues: generalized marginal redness_
2. _Generalized moderate recession of the gingival margin_
3. _Generalized clinical attachment loss_
4. _Moderate plaque biofilm on gingival thirds of teeth and generalized moderate subgingival calculus deposits._
5. _Furcation involvement_
6. _Radiographs confirm generalized bone loss_

SUPPLEMENTAL ORAL EXAMINATION FINDINGS:

Restoration
Cavity
Sealant
Clinically missing tooth
Furcation
"Through and through" furcation

Probe 1 : initial probing depth
Probe 2 : probing depth 1 month after scaling and root planing

35. The posterior sextants exhibit moderate subgingival calculus deposits. The clinician plans to complete subgingival calculus removal on the mandibular left posterior sextant. Clinical attachment loss is present with periodontal pockets greater than 4 mm in depth. A class III furcation involvement is present on teeth #18 and #19. Which sequence of periodontal instruments would be MOST effective for subgingival calculus removal in this sextant?
    a. Posterior sickle scaler, Gracey curets with miniature working ends and extended shanks, periodontal files
    b. Posterior sickle scaler, standard Gracey curets
    c. Universal curet with an extended shank, Gracey curets with extended shank lengths, Gracey curets with miniature working ends and extended shanks, Nabers diamond-coated file
    d. Universal curet with a short lower shank, standard Gracey curets, Gracey curets with extended shank lengths

36. To remove light subgingival calculus from the furcation area of a mandibular molar, which of the following instruments would be MOST efficient?
    a. Standard anterior Gracey curet
    b. Universal curet with an extended shank length
    c. A Gracey curet with an extended shank and miniature working end
    d. Posterior sickle with a complex shank

37. A right-handed clinician is working on the buccal aspect of tooth #2. (For a left-handed clinician, this area would be equivalent to the buccal aspect of tooth #15.) The clinician is using a Gracey 13/14 curet and retracting the client's cheek with a mouth mirror. The clinician's neck is bent excessively as she works. What correction should the clinician make for more ergonomic positioning?
    a. Ask the client to turn her head slightly away from the clinician
    b. Turn the mirror head so that the reflecting surface can be used to view the distal surface
    c. Ask the client to turn toward the clinician and lower her chin down toward her chest (chin-down position)
    d. Raise the client's chair up to bring the working area level with the clinician's eye level

38. The client expresses great discomfort during periodontal probing. All of the following are true statements about periodontal probing technique EXCEPT one. Which one is the EXCEPTION?
    a. A thinner probe causes less distention of the sulcus or the pocket wall
    b. The junctional epithelium in healthy tissue offers more resistance against the probe than the junctional epithelium in diseased tissue
    c. Sufficient pressure for accurate reading is 30 to 50 g
    d. Probe tip should be in contact with the tooth at all times

39. The straight calibrated periodontal probe can be used for all of the following assessment procedures EXCEPT one. Which one is the EXCEPTION?
    a. Measuring the width of attached gingiva
    b. Assessment of dental restorations
    c. Measuring the extent of recession of the gingival margin
    d. Measuring the size of oral lesions

40. The client started gagging on the ultrasonic's water spray, so the clinician decides to use a hand instrument to remove a tenacious, moderate calculus deposit on the facial surface of tooth #31. The calculus deposit is located supragingivally on the crown of the tooth. Which of the following instruments would you choose?
    a. Universal curet with a short lower shank length
    b. Standard Gracey 13/14 curet
    c. A rigid Gracey curet
    d. A posterior sickle scaler

41. To minimize client discomfort during root surface debridement in periodontal pockets, the clinician should use caution when inserting a universal curet beneath the gingival margin. The face-to-tooth surface angulation during insertion of the working end beneath the gingival margin is between:
    a. 0 and 40 degrees
    b. 10 and 50 degrees
    c. 40 and 80 degrees
    d. 70 and 90 degrees

42. While removing calculus from the maxillary anterior tooth surfaces toward the clinician, good adaptation of the toe-third of the working end is facilitated by:
    a. Rolling the instrument handle
    b. Pivoting the hand
    c. Sitting to the side and front of the client
    d. All of the above contribute to proper adaptation

43. What type of instrumentation stroke uses a face-to-tooth angulation of 50 to 70 degrees, light lateral pressure, fluid, flowing strokes, and strokes of moderate length?
    a. Placement stroke
    b. Assessment stroke
    c. Root debridement stroke
    d. Calculus removal stroke

44. The suggested place to begin probing by quadrants is the distal line angle of the posterior-most tooth in the quadrant. The working end of the probe is removed from the sulcus or the pocket after each bobbing stroke.
    a. Both statements are TRUE
    b. The first statement is TRUE; the second FALSE
    c. The first statement is FALSE; the second TRUE
    d. Both statements are FALSE

Use Case F to answer questions 45 to 50.

SYNOPSIS OF PATIENT HISTORY		
Age	55	
Sex	F	
Height	5'6"	
CASE	F	
Weight	140 lbs	
	64 kgs	

VITAL SIGNS
Blood pressure _116/72 mmHg_
Pulse rate _80 bpm_
Respiration rate _20 rpm_

1. Under Care of Physician
   Yes No
   ☒   ☐   Condition: _Routine care_
2. Hospitalized within the last 5 years
   Yes No
   ☐   ☒   Reason: _____
3. Has or had the following conditions
   Thyroid
   _____
4. Current medications
   Synthroid 1.50 mcg per day
   (thyroid hormone replacement)
   _____
5. Smokes or uses tobacco products
   Yes No
   ☐   ☒
6. Is pregnant
   Yes No N/A
   ☐   ☒   ☐

MEDICAL HISTORY:
Hypothyroidism

DENTAL HISTORY:
Routine 6 month check-ups

SOCIAL HISTORY:
Surgical nurse at local hospital

CHIEF COMPLAINT:
Routine dental check-up

Adult clinical examination

Case F

CURRENT ORAL HYGIENE STATUS:
1. _Good self-care; no clinical attachment loss_
2. _Light plaque biofilm on mesial surfaces of #20 and #28_
3. _Light calculus deposits on proximal surfaces of posterior_
4. _Dental implants replace tooth #s 19 and 20_

SUPPLEMENTAL ORAL EXAMINATION FINDINGS:

Restoration

Cavity

Sealant

Clinically missing tooth

△ Furcation

▲ "Through and through" furcation

Probe 1 : initial probing depth

Probe 2 : probing depth 1 month after scaling and root planing

45. The working stroke used with an ultrasonic tip is in a coronal to apical direction (starting beneath the gingival margin and moving toward the junctional epithelium). The working stroke with a hand instrument moves in an apical to coronal direction (starting at the junctional epithelium and moving toward the gingival margin).
    a. Both statements are TRUE
    b. The first statement is TRUE; the second FALSE
    c. The first statement is FALSE; the second TRUE
    d. Both statements are FALSE

46. Teeth #19 and #20 have been replaced with dental implants. Which of the following instruments would be the BEST choice to remove light calculus from the prosthetic crowns of these dental implants?
    a. Plastic implant instrument with a curet-shaped working end
    b. Plastic implant instrument with a wrench-shaped working end
    c. Universal curet with a short lower shank length
    d. Standard-diameter ultrasonic universal tip with a curved working end

47. What type of stroke pressure usually is required to remove a calculus deposit from the prosthetic crown of a dental implant?
    a. Firm, scraping pressure
    b. Moderate, scraping pressure
    c. Light lateral pressure
    d. No pressure at all, use an assessment stroke

48. Periodontal probing of a dental implant may be invasive because the probe may penetrate the weakly adherent biologic seal and could introduce bacteria into peri-implant tissues. Accurate probing depths may be difficult to obtain because of the constricted "cervical" area of some dental implants.
    a. Both statements are TRUE
    b. The first statement is TRUE; the second FALSE
    c. The first statement is FALSE; the second TRUE
    d. Both statements are FALSE

49. Which of the following instruments would be the BEST choice for removing the light subgingival calculus deposits on the proximal surfaces of the posterior teeth?
    a. A set of standard Gracey curets
    b. A universal curet
    c. A posterior sickle scaler
    d. A set of Gracey curets with extended shank lengths

50. The client has porcelain veneers on the facial aspect of her maxillary anterior teeth. Which of the following polishing techniques for the removal of extrinsic stain would be considered the standard of care for a client with porcelain veneers and dental implants?
    a. Use of fine grit pumice with rubber cup on all teeth, including the porcelain veneers and dental implants
    b. Use of fine grit pumice on porcelain veneers only on maxillary anterior teeth and mandibular anterior teeth
    c. Use of an ultrasonic universal tip on all teeth with extrinsic stain, including the porcelain veneers and dental implants
    d. Selective polishing of only natural teeth with stain that is visible when the patient smiles or speaks

51. A clinician is removing calculus from the lingual aspect of the client's maxillary anterior tooth surfaces away from the 12 o'clock position. The clinician's head is bent forward, and the clinician is leaning toward the client. What correction should the clinician make for an ergonomic body position?
    a. Move around to the side of the client
    b. Raise the client's chair back to a 45-degree angle
    c. Ask the client to change from the chin-down to the chin-up position
    d. Raise the entire client chair so that the client's mouth is closer to the clinician

Management of Pain and Anxiety

Gwen I. Hlava and Todd N. Junge

As clinicians, dental hygienists must be able to manage the client's pain and anxiety. This requires mastery of head and neck anatomy, physiology, pharmacology, medical emergencies, and clinical technique. Local anesthetic agent administration is within the legal scope of dental hygiene practice in most legal jurisdictions in the United States. This chapter reviews four methods to relieve and manage pain and anxiety: (1) local anesthesia, (2) topical anesthesia, (3) computer-controlled local anesthesia, and (4) nitrous oxide–oxygen conscious sedation.

CHARACTERISTICS AND PHYSIOLOGY OF PAIN

A. Definitions
  1. Pain—sensation of discomfort resulting from the stimulation of specialized nerve endings called *nociceptors* (free nerve endings)
  2. Pain perception—process whereby the sensation of pain is transmitted from the periphery to the central nervous system (CNS)
  3. Pain reaction—result of pain perception; what a person will do about the perceived pain
  4. Pain-reaction threshold—amount of pain one must experience before exhibiting a reaction
B. Pain reactions and pain-reaction thresholds vary from individual to individual and within the same individual from day to day
C. Pain perception
  1. Functional unit—neuron, or nerve cell
  2. Types of nerve cells
     a. Unipolar
     b. Bipolar—transmits dental pain perception
     c. Multipolar
  3. Sensory neuron characteristics (Figure 18-1)
     a. Cell body
     b. Nucleus

  c. Axons (fibers, processors)
  d. Free nerve endings (nociceptors)
  4. Fiber diameter—varies; determines speed of impulse conduction and type of pain perceived
     a. A fibers—3 to 20 microns (μ)
        (1) Myelinated
        (2) Rapid conduction (rate of 100 meters per second [m/s])
     b. C fibers—0.5 to 1 μ
        (1) Nonmyelinated
        (2) Slow conduction (rate of 0.5 to 2 m/s)
  5. Nerve trunk versus ganglia—a nerve trunk is an extremely large bundle of nerve fibers or axons; a ganglion is the site where cell bodies are bundled
D. Resting nerve cell membrane
  1. Membrane potential—the difference in the electrical charges across the nerve membrane
  2. Membrane potential maintained by:
     a. The sodium–potassium pump
     b. The permeability of the cell membrane
  3. Ions essential to nerve conduction
     a. Potassium (K^+) ions
     b. Sodium (Na^+) ions
  4. Sodium–potassium pump; resting state polarized (unstimulated)

  Outside cell Na^+

  $\dfrac{+ + + + + + + + + + + +}{- - - - - - - - - - -}$ cell membrane

  Inside cell K^+

  5. Permeability of the cell membrane—impermeable to sodium (at rest)
E. Minimal threshold stimulus
  1. Stimulus—an environmental change that can be chemical, thermal, mechanical, or electrical in nature
  2. Minimal threshold stimulus—the magnitude of the stimulus required to initiate a nerve impulse

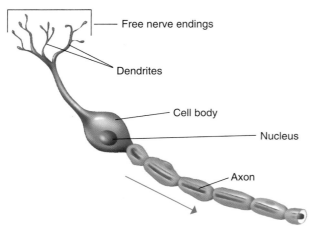

FIGURE 18-1 Sensory neuron showing the direction of impulse travel (*red arrow*). *(From Patton KT, Thibodeau GA:* Anatomy and physiology, *ed 7, St Louis, 2010, Mosby.)*

   3. All-or-none law—either the nerve fires as strongly as possible or it does not fire at all

F. Excitation

  1. When a minimal threshold stimulus excites the nerve:

    a. The permeability of the cell membrane changes

     (1) Influx—Na^+ enters the cell

     (2) Efflux—K^+ diffuses to the outside of the cell

    b. Reversed polarity

       Outside cell K^+

       $- - - - - - - - - - - -$

       $\overline{+ + + + + + + + + + + +}$ cell membrane

       Inside cell Na^+

  2. Depolarization—the time interval that exists while ionic concentrations are reversing

  3. Reversed polarity—the result of a reversal in ionic charges

  4. Repolarization—occurs after reversed polarity; the membrane becomes hyperpermeable to K^+ and impermeable to Na^+; polarity is re-established

  5. Action potential—rapid sequence of changes in the membrane potential (negative to positive, and positive back to negative); the stages are:

    a. Depolarization—resulting in reversed polarity

    b. Repolarization

  6. Absolute refractory period—the period during depolarization and reversed polarity when the cell membrane cannot be re-excited

  7. Relative refractory period—during repolarization, the nerve cell membrane can be re-excited, but it requires a greater stimulus than the stimulus required for excitation from the resting state

G. Pain intensity determined by:

  1. Number of fibers stimulated (depends on)

    a. Anatomy of the area

    b. Dimensions of the area being stimulated

  2. Frequency of excitation (depends on)

    a. Duration of the stimulus

H. Pain reaction—determined by a person's pain reaction threshold

  1. High pain reaction threshold produces hyporeactive behavior

  2. Low pain reaction threshold produces hyperreactive behavior

  3. Factors affecting the pain reaction threshold

    a. Emotional state—most consistently reported variable; greater anxiety and negativity results in lower pain-reaction threshold

    b. Fatigue—greater fatigue results in lower pain reaction threshold

    c. Age—younger people experience a lower pain reaction threshold

    d. Nationality

     (1) Latin Americans and southern Europeans experience lower pain reaction threshold than do North Americans or northern Europeans

     (2) American Indians experience the highest pain reaction threshold

    e. Gender—variable

ARMAMENTARIUM

A. Definition—all items essential for the administration of a local anesthetic agent

B. Armamentarium categories

  1. Needle

    a. Components (Figure 18-2)

    b. Composition—stainless steel

    c. Gauge (ga)—the diameter of the lumen is indicated by a number

     (1) The larger the gauge number, the smaller is the lumen diameter

     (2) The 25-, 27-, and 30-ga needles are the most common in dentistry

    d. Length—measured from hub to the point of bevel

     (1) Short = 1 inch

     (2) Long = $1\frac{5}{8}$ inches

    e. Method of sterilization—disposable needles come presterilized, with a security seal

  2. Anesthetic cartridge

    a. Components (Figure 18-3)

     (1) Metal cap end is directed toward the needle when the cartridge is loaded into the syringe

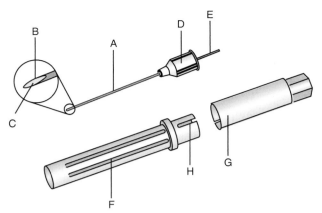

FIGURE 18-2 Components of a hypodermic needle. **A,** Shaft or shank, the working end of the needle. **B,** Bevel, or angulation, of the tip. **C,** Lumen, the hollow interior of the shaft. **D,** The hub holds the shaft and is threaded onto the adaptor of the syringe. **E,** The syringe end enters the anesthetic cartridge. **F,** The protective shield sleeve (*colored end*) covers the needle shaft. **G,** The protective shield guard (*clear or white*) covers the syringe end of the needle. **H,** The security seal holds the protective shield sleeve and guard together until the hub is assembled and attached to the syringe.

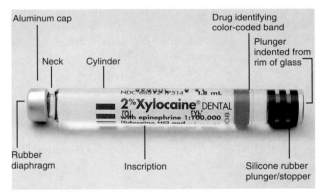

FIGURE 18-3 Components of the glass cartridge for the dental local anesthetic. *(Modified from Malamed SF: Handbook of local anesthesia, ed 5, St Louis, 2004, Mosby.)*

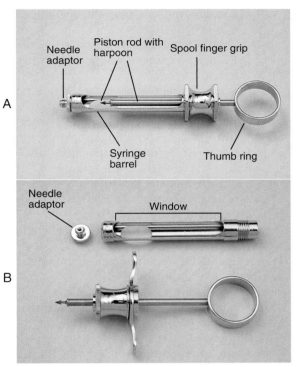

FIGURE 18-4 A, Assembled breech-loading, metallic, cartridge-type syringe. **B,** Disassembled local anesthetic syringe. *(Modified from Malamed SF: Handbook of local anesthesia, ed 5, St Louis, 2004, Mosby.)*

(2) Round rubber diaphragm—the syringe end of the needle penetrates this diaphragm and enters the cartridge
(3) Cylinder—glass tube containing the anesthetic solution
(4) Inscription—legally required information on the cartridge, which includes:
(a) Volume—1.8 mL
(b) Anesthetic agent—generic and brand names
(c) Percentage of drug
(d) Vasoconstrictor
(e) Concentration ratio of vasoconstrictor
(f) Manufacturer

(g) Lot number
(h) Expiration date
(5) Rubber stopper—seals the opposite end of cartridge; it is the movable component of the cartridge
b. Ingredients in the anesthetic solution
(1) Anesthetic drug
(2) Vasoconstrictor
(3) Preservative (sodium bisulfite)
(4) Sodium chloride—makes the solution isotonic
(5) Distilled water—inert ingredient
c. Method of storage—away from direct sunlight and ultraviolet light, and maintained at room temperature (68°F to 77°F; 20°C to 25°C) or slightly cooler
3. Anesthetic syringe (Figure 18-4)
a. Components
(1) Adapter—the hub of the needle is threaded onto this part of the syringe
(2) Barrel—holds the anesthetic cartridge
(3) Harpoon—the fish-hook–shaped tip is forced into the rubber stopper
(4) Piston rod—connects the harpoon to the thumb ring; can be advanced to expel the solution or retracted to aspirate

(5) Large window—faces the operator during injection; rubber stopper speed, positive aspirations, and volume are observable

(6) Small window—aids in removing the used cartridge

(7) Spool finger grip—place of rest for the index and middle fingers

(8) Thumb ring—enables the operator to aspirate or express fluid from the cartridge

b. Method of syringe sterilization—the bioburden is removed; the syringe is dried, packaged, and sterilized

c. Auxiliary materials—hemostat or cotton pliers; used if the needle breaks

C. Record keeping and documentation in client dental record

1. Documentation requirements vary by state law

2. Documentation includes:

a. Time of administration

b. Type and percentage of drug administered

c. Type and ratio of vasoconstrictor

d. Amount of drug administered

e. Name of injection(s) given and the side of the mouth in which the injection(s) is administered

f. Reactions to drug (if any)

g. The American Dental Association (ADA) code D9215 for health insurance reimbursement

▮ LOCAL ANESTHETIC AGENTS

Chemical Structure

A. Chemical components (Table 18-1)

1. Aromatic lipophilic group—for diffusion into the lipid nerve membrane

2. Intermediate chain—determines if the agent is an ester or an amide; also determines the potential for any allergic reaction

3. Hydrophilic group—required for diffusion into water-soluble tissues

B. Allergies related to chemical structure

1. A considerable amount of documentation on allergic reactions to esters is available; because of their potential for causing allergic reactions, esters are no longer used

2. Cross-reactivity occurs with esters; thus, if a client is allergic to one ester, an allergic reaction will occur with all other ester derivatives

3. No substantiated cases, to date, of allergic reactions to amides

4. Cross-reactive allergic reactions do not occur among amides

5. In cases where the agent cannot be identified, the client should be referred to an allergist for testing

Mechanism of Action

A. Physiologic effect—local anesthetics prevent cell membrane permeability to sodium

B. Injectable form

$$\begin{matrix} \text{Anesthetic drug} + \\ \text{(lipid soluble)} \end{matrix} \quad \begin{matrix} \text{HCl} \\ \text{ionized salt} \\ \text{(water-soluble)} \end{matrix} \quad \rightarrow \begin{matrix} \text{Anesthetic solution} \\ \text{ionized acidic salt} \\ \text{(water-soluble)} \end{matrix}$$

C. Dissociation—the ability of a drug to separate or part

$$\begin{matrix} \text{Anesthetic} \\ \text{solution} \\ \text{being injected} \end{matrix} \begin{matrix} \rightarrow\rightarrow \\ \text{at lipid nerve} \\ \text{membrane} \end{matrix} \begin{matrix} \text{Anesthetic} + \text{HCl} \\ \text{drug} \end{matrix}$$

$$\begin{matrix} \text{Ionized acidic} \\ \text{salt} \\ \text{(water-soluble)} \end{matrix} \quad \begin{matrix} \text{Lipid-} \\ \text{soluble} \end{matrix} \begin{matrix} \text{Ionized acidic} \\ \text{salt} \\ \text{(water-soluble)} \end{matrix}$$

D. Effects of inflammation—decreased anesthetic effect in areas of inflammation; caused by three factors:

1. Decreased pH of tissues—causes dissociation to occur more slowly

2. Edema—dilutes concentration of local anesthetic

3. Increased vascularity—facilitates rapid removal of drug from area

E. Nerve fiber susceptibility

1. Smaller, nonmyelinated fibers (C fibers) are the first to be blocked; however, sensation is regained last in these fibers

2. Large, myelinated fibers (A fibers) are the last to be blocked; however, sensation is regained first in these fibers

Potency

A. Definition—lowest concentration of drug needed to consistently produce adequate anesthesia

1. Potency is related directly to lipid solubility

2. If a local anesthetic drug is highly potent, lower concentrations are effective in achieving adequate anesthesia

3. Greater potency also equals greater chance of systemic toxicity

Toxicity

A. Definition—the amount of drug capable of causing adverse systemic reactions in normal persons; adverse reactions occur when the rate of drug absorbed is greater than the rate of biotransformation, the body's ability to metabolize the drug

B. True toxic reactions occur immediately—the most profound effects of toxic reaction are on the central

TABLE 18-1 Comparison of Frequently Used Local Anesthetic Agents in Dentistry

Generic Name	Commercial Name	Color Code	Concentration	Chemical Classification	Vasoconstrictor	Concentration of Vasoconstrictor	Onset of Action	APPROXIMATE DURATION — Without Vasoconstrictor	APPROXIMATE DURATION — With Vasoconstrictor	Toxicity	Method of Metabolism	Milligram/Cartridge	MAXIMUM SAFE DOSAGE FOR NORMAL ADULT CLIENT — Milligram/Milliliter	MAXIMUM SAFE DOSAGE FOR NORMAL ADULT CLIENT — Cartridge
Lidocaine	Xylocaine	Green	2%	Amide	Epinephrine	1/50,000	2–3 min		Pulpal = 60 min Soft tissue = 3–5 hr	2.0	Liver	36	300 mg 15 mL	8.3
		Red	2%	Amide	Epinephrine	1/100,000	2–3 min		Pulpal = 60 min Soft tissue = 3–5 hr	2.0	Liver	36	300 mg 15 mL	8.3
Mepivacaine	Carbocaine	Brown	2%	Amide	Neo-Cobefrin	1/20,000	1½–2 min		Pulpal = 60 min Soft tissue = 3–5 hr	1.5–2.0	Liver	36	300 mg 15 mL	8.3
		Tan	3%	Amide			1½–2 min	Pulpal = 20–40 min Soft tissue = 2–3 hr		1.5–2.0	Liver	54	300 mg 10 mL	5.5
Prilocaine	Citanest Forte	Yellow	4%	Amide	Epinephrine	1/200,000	2–4 min		Pulpal = 60–90 min Soft tissue = 3–8 hr	1.0	Liver and lung	72	400 mg 10 mL	5.5
	Citanest	Black	4%	Amide			2–4 min	Pulpal = 40–60 min Soft tissue = 2–4 hrs		1.0	Liver and lung	72	400 mg 10 mL	5.5
Articaine	Septocaine	Gold	4%	Amide	Epinephrine	1/100,000	2–2½ min		Pulpal = 60–75 min Soft tissue = 3–6 hrs	2.0	Plasma and liver	72	500 mg 12.5 mL	6.9

nervous system (CNS) and the cardiovascular system

1. Central nervous system
   a. CNS stimulation phase—the person becomes extremely talkative, restless, and anxious; convulsions may occur
   b. CNS depression phase—in extreme cases, unconsciousness may result
2. Cardiovascular effects
   a. During the stimulation phase—the person's blood pressure and pulse rise rapidly
   b. During the depression phase—the person's blood pressure and pulse drop significantly
3. Respiratory failure is the primary cause of death
4. Vital functions must be supported until the drug is eliminated by biotransformation (metabolism)

Biotransformation (Metabolism)

A. Definition—process whereby the drug is broken down, changed, or combined with other substances to render it physiologically inactive
B. Biotransformation (according to chemical group)
   1. Esters—metabolized in plasma through the process of hydrolysis; inactivated by plasma cholinesterase (an enzyme)
   2. Amides—metabolized in the liver; history of cirrhosis, alcoholism, liver disease or transplantation, and jaundice may affect the rate of biotransformation

Topical Anesthetic

A. Purpose—reduces the discomfort associated with the initial penetration of the needle through the mucosa
B. Controversy exists with regard to widespread use
   1. Dosage control—impossible to standardize because of variability in factors such as operator, client, and area of operation
   2. The concentration of the topical anesthetic used exceeds that which is administered by injection (e.g., 5%, 10%, 22% topical anesthetic versus 2%, 3%, or 4% local anesthetic)
   3. Except for 5% lidocaine (Xylocaine), all other topical anesthetics are esters
   4. Lidocaine or prilocaine periodontal gel (Oraqix) is an amide; used in adults who require limited pain control during root debridement in periodontal pockets
   5. Cetacaine—a combination of benzocaine, butamben, and tetracaine hydrochloride—is an ester topical indicated in adults who require pre-injection, deep scaling, and suture removal anesthesia (available in spray, liquid, or gel form)

C. Esters have a greater incidence of allergic reactions and cross-reactivity than amides
D. Topical agents have indications and contraindications; can interact with other medications; clinicians must always assess for potential allergies, side effects, and adverse effects and take appropriate precautions

Calculating the Amount of Local Anesthetic Drug in an Anesthetic Solution

A. Maximum recommended dose (MRD)—maximum amount of drug administered that does not produce a toxic reaction
B. Example of calculations
   1. Percentage of the anesthetic drug is the number of grams (g) of drug per 100 milliliters (mL) of solution (e.g., 2 g anesthetic drug/100 mL solution = 2% anesthetic solution). To find the number of milligrams of drug in 1 milliliter of solution, change the grams of drug to milligrams (mg) by multiplying by 1000 (e.g., 2 g drug/100 mL solution × 1000 mg/1 = 2000 mg/100 mL = 20 mg drug/1 mL solution). This calculation determines that 20 mg of anesthetic drug (e.g., lidocaine) are in each milliliter of this anesthetic solution
   2. To calculate the number of milligrams of anesthetic drug (e.g., lidocaine) that is administered, multiply the number of milligrams per milliliter of the drug by the number of milliliters of solution administered
      a. Anesthetic cartridges used in dentistry contain 1.8 mL of solution; if an entire cartridge of solution was injected, the calculation would be as follows:

$$20 \text{ mg/mL} \times 1.8 \text{ mL/cartridge} = 36 \text{ mg of anesthetic}$$
$$\text{drug (lidocaine)}$$
$$\text{per cartridge}$$

      b. If only ¼ of 1 cartridge was administered, the calculation would be:

$$1.8 \text{ mL} \div 4 = 0.45 \text{ mL},$$

   then

$$20 \text{ mg/1 mL} \times 0.45 \text{ mL/1} = 9 \text{ mg of anesthetic}$$
$$\text{drug (lidocaine)}$$
$$\text{per cartridge}$$

   3. To compute the MRD of an anesthetic drug in cartridges, divide the MRD in milliliters by the number of milliliters in 1 cartridge (1.8). The MRD of lidocaine 2% is 15 milliliters (15 mL/1.8 mL = 8.3 cartridges)

Vasoconstrictors (Table 18-2)

A. Definition—one of five ingredients in an anesthetic solution that functions to hold the anesthetic agent in the area where anesthesia is delivered

B. Description—all vasoconstrictors can be referred to as *adrenergic drugs* or *sympathomimetic amines*
  1. Adrenergic drug—capable of producing the same effects as those of adrenalin
  2. Sympathomimetic amine—mimics the sympathetic nervous system and contains an amine group within its chemical structure, which is characteristic of vasoconstrictors
  3. All vasoconstrictors can be produced synthetically; two naturally occurring vasoconstrictors, epinephrine and norepinephrine, are produced in the adrenal medulla and the sympathetic postganglionic nerve fibers

C. Function—hold the local anesthetic agent in the target site of analgesia by producing vasoconstriction; if absent from a local anesthetic agent, vasodilation will occur; the results of vasoconstriction are:
  1. Reduction of systemic absorption of the local anesthetic agent
  2. Reduction of chances of systemic toxicity
  3. Reduction of blood flow through the area (hemostasis)
  4. Prolongation of the action of the anesthetic
  5. Increase the effectiveness of the local anesthetic by decrease in diffusion
  6. Lower concentrations of the local anesthetic agents required

D. Mode of action—stimulate α-receptors located in the walls of arterioles
  1. α-receptors—responsible for arterial constriction

  2. β-receptors—responsible for dilation
  3. Each type of vasoconstrictor possesses varying degrees of response of both α- and β-activity (see Table 18-2); although epinephrine exhibits the most β-activity, to achieve the same amount of vasoconstriction as epinephrine, the concentration of all other vasoconstrictors must be increased

E. Biotransformation—metabolism of vasoconstrictors occurs in the bloodstream; the enzyme responsible for biotransformation is monoamine oxidase (MAO); persons taking MAO inhibitors have a decreased ability to metabolize vasoconstrictors

F. Pressor potency—the ability of a drug to produce vasoconstriction
  1. Epinephrine—the most potent vasoconstrictor; pressor potency value = 1
  2. Levonordefrin—another type of adrenergic vasoconstrictor; pressor potency value = $\frac{1}{6}$
  3. Concentrations of all vasoconstrictors must be increased to obtain the same vasoconstrictive potency as that of epinephrine

G. Vasoconstrictors in solution—unstable; preservative (e.g., sodium bisulfite) is added to prevent oxidation

H. Toxicity—toxicity resulting from vasoconstrictor overdose is caused by constriction of blood vessels, which raises blood pressure and cardiac rate from β-receptor stimulation
  1. Symptoms
     a. Increased blood pressure
     b. Increased heart rate (tachycardia >150 beats per minute)
     c. Talkativeness
     d. Restlessness
     e. Palpitations or irregular heart beat
     f. Headache

TABLE 18-2 Vasoconstrictors

Generic Name	Brand Name	Concentration Used In Dentistry	Pressor Potency	Milligram/ Milliliter (mg/mL)	Milligram/ Cartridge (Mg/Cart)	Maximum Safe Dose (MSD) (Normal Adult)		MSD (Cardiac)		Approximate % of α/β Activity
Epinephrine	Adrenalin	1:50,000	1	0.02	0.036	0.2 mg	5.5 cart	0.04 mg	1.1 cart	50/50
		1:100,000		0.01	0.018	0.2 mg	11.1 cart	0.04 mg	2.2 cart	
		1:200,000		0.005	0.009	0.2 mg	22.2 cart	0.04 mg	4.4 cart	
Levonordefrin	Neo-Cobefrin	1:20,000	$\frac{1}{6}$	0.05	0.09	1.0 mg	11.1 cart	1.0 mg	11.1 cart	75/25
Norepinephrine*	Levophed	1:30,000	$\frac{1}{4}$			0.34 mg		0.14 mg		90/10
Phenylephrine†	Neo-Synephrine	1:2,500	$\frac{1}{20}$			4.0 mg		1.6 mg		95/5
Felypressin‡	Octapressin									

*Was included with procaine/propoxycaine (withdrawn in January 1996).
†No longer available in dental cartridges.
‡Not available in the United States.

2. Prevention of cardiac emergencies—strict adherence to MRD in the case of persons with cardiac disease (see Chapter 21)

I. Dosage calculations (maximum recommended dose); for example, epinephrine 1:100,000

  1. 1:100,000 means 1 g epinephrine/100,000 mL solution

  2. Multiply 1 g × 1000 to determine the number of mg/100,000 mL of solution

  3. Divide the number of milliliters of solution by the number of milligrams of vasoconstrictor

$$1.0 \div 100 = 0.01 \text{ mg vasoconstrictor}/1 \text{ mL solution}$$

  4. If you administered more than 1 mL of solution, multiply the concentration in mg/mL by the number of mL administered

    a. Example: 1 cartridge; if there is 0.01 mg of epinephrine in each milliliter of solution and you administered 1 cartridge, then:

$$0.01 \text{ mg} \times 1.8 \text{ mL} = 0.018 \text{ mg epinephrine/cartridge}$$

    b. If you administered 2.5 cartridges of solution containing epinephrine 1:100,000, then:

$$2.5 \text{ cartridges} \times 1.8 \text{ mL} = 4.5 \text{ mL solution.}$$

Multiply mg/mL (0.01) times the number of milliliters of solution (4.50 mL)
Answer: $0.01 \text{ mg} \times 4.5 = 0.045$ mg epinephrine in 2.5 cartridges

J. Limiting factor (see Table 18-1)

  1. When determining the safety of administering a specific quantity of a particular anesthetic solution, you must compute both the MRD of the anesthetic drug and the MRD of the vasoconstrictor

  2. In any local anesthetic solution containing a vasoconstrictor, either the anesthetic drug or the vasoconstrictor drug will reach its MRD first; when you have determined which of the drugs limits the total amount of solution to be administered, you have determined the limiting factor

  3. Some of the questions are, for example: Can a dental hygienist administer five cartridges of lidocaine 2% containing epinephrine 1:50,000 to a normal healthy person? How many can be given? What is the limiting factor?

    a. Lidocaine 2%:

$$2\% = 2 \text{ g}/100 \text{ mL}$$
$$2 \text{ g}/100 \text{ mL} \times 1000 \text{ mg}/1 \text{ g} = 2000 \text{ mg}/100 \text{ mL} = 20 \text{ mg/mL}$$
$$20 \text{ mg/mL} \times 1.8 \text{ solution/cartridge} = 36 \text{ mg/cartridge}$$

The MRD for lidocaine 2% = 300 mg (300 mg ÷ 36 mg/cartridge = 8.3 cartridges); therefore, 8.3 is the number of cartridges that can be administered before reaching the MRD of lidocaine

    b. Epinephrine 1:50,000

$$1{:}50{,}000 = 1 \text{ g}/50{,}000 \text{ mL}$$
$$1 \text{ g}/50{,}000 \text{ mL} \times 1000 \text{ mg}/1 \text{ g} = 1000 \text{ mg}/50{,}000 \text{ mL}$$
$$= 0.02 \text{ mg/mL}$$
$$0.02 \text{ mg/mL} \times 1.8 \text{ solution/cartridge} = 0.036 \text{ mg/cartridge}$$

The MRD for epinephrine (normal adult) = 0.2 mg. 0.2 mg ÷ .036 = 5.5 cartridges Therefore, 5.5 is the number of cartridges of epinephrine 1:50,000 you can administer to a normal healthy person

    c. 5.5 is smaller than 8.3; therefore, the hygienist must limit the amount of lidocaine 2%, epinephrine 1:50,000 to 5.5 cartridges; the limiting factor is epinephrine

TRIGEMINAL NERVE: MAXILLARY DIVISION

See the section on "The nervous system" in Chapter 4.

Innervation

A. V2 branches given off in the middle cranial fossa—meningeal nerve

B. V2 branches given off in the pterygopalatine fossa

  1. Zygomatic nerve—divides further into:

    a. Zygomaticofacial nerve

    b. Zygomaticotemporal nerve

  2. Pterygopalatine nerves—divide further into:

    a. Orbital branches

    b. Nasal branches—nasopalatine (NP) nerve (relevant branch for local anesthesia)

    c. Palatine branches—subdivide into:

      (1) Greater palatine (GP) nerve (relevant branch for local anesthesia)

      (2) Lesser palatine nerve

    d. Pharyngeal branch

  3. Posterior superior alveolar nerve (PSA) (relevant branch for local anesthesia)

    a. External branch

    b. Internal branch

  4. Infraorbital nerve (IO) (relevant branch for local anesthesia)—divides further into:

    a. Middle superior alveolar (MSA) nerve

    b. Anter superior alveolar nerve (ASA)

    c. Lateral nasal nerve

    d. Superior labial nerve

    e. Inferior palpebral nerve

Maxillary Block Injections

See Table 18-3.

A. Anterior superior alveolar nerve block (ASA)
  1. Structures anesthetized (Figure 18-5)
    a. Facial gingiva of maxillary anterior teeth
    b. Maxillary anterior teeth
  2. Penetration site—mucolabial fold anterior and parallel to the canine eminence
B. Middle superior alveolar nerve block (MSA)
  1. Structures anesthetized (see Figure 18-5)

a. Facial gingiva of maxillary premolars and the mesiobuccal root of the first molar
b. Maxillary premolars and the mesiobuccal root of the first molar
  2. Penetration site—mucobuccal fold parallel to the apex of the second premolar
C. Infraorbital nerve block (IO)
  1. Structures anesthetized (see Figure 18-5)
    a. Facial gingiva of maxillary anterior teeth, premolars, and the mesiobuccal root of the first molar

TABLE 18-3 Maxillary Injections

Injection	Needle Length	Structures Anesthetized	Penetration Site	Terminal Deposition Site	Amount Deposited
ASA	Short needle	Facial gingiva of maxillary anterior teeth Maxillary anterior teeth	Mucolabial fold anterior and parallel to the canine eminence	Apex of the canine tooth	$\frac{1}{2}$–$\frac{2}{3}$ cartridge Wait 3–5 minutes
MSA	Short needle	Facial gingiva of maxilla, premolars, and mesial buccal root of the first molar Maxillary premolars and mandibular root of the first molar	Mucobuccal fold parallel to apex of second premolar	Bone superior to the apex of the second premolar	$\frac{1}{2}$–$\frac{2}{3}$ cartridge Wait 3–5 minutes
IO	Long or short needle	Facial gingiva of maxillary anterior teeth, premolars, and mesial buccal root of the first molar Maxillary anterior teeth, premolars, and mesial buccal root of the first molar Side of nose Upper lip Lower eyelid	Mucobuccal fold parallel to the apex of the first premolar	Infraorbital foramen.	$\frac{1}{2}$–$\frac{2}{3}$ cartridge Wait 3–5 minutes
PSA	Short needle	Facial gingiva of maxillary molars except for mesial buccal root of first molar Maxillary molars except for mesial buccal root of first molar	Height of mucobuccal fold over the maxillary second molar	Insert needle 45 degrees to the midsagittal plane and 45 degrees to the horizontal plane of the maxillary occlusal surfaces Approximately $\frac{1}{2}$ of short needle	$\frac{1}{2}$ cartridge Wait 3–5 minutes
GP	Short needle	Lingual gingiva of maxillary posterior teeth Palatal mucosa to the midline	Pressure anesthesia (1 min). 1–2 mm anterior to the greater palatine foramen	Approximately 2 mm (until the bevel is covered)	$\frac{1}{4}$–$\frac{1}{3}$ cartridge Wait 2–3 minutes
NP	Short needle	Lingual gingiva of maxillary anterior teeth Palatal mucosa in the premaxillary area	Pressure anesthesia (1 min). Incisive papilla at base and into the fattest portion	Approximately 5 mm (until bone is gently contacted)	$\frac{1}{4}$ cartridge Wait 2–3 minutes

ASA, anterosuperior alveolar; *MSA,* middle superior alveolar; *IO,* infraorbital; *PSA,* posterosuperior alveolar; *GP,* greater palantine; *NP,* nasopalantine.

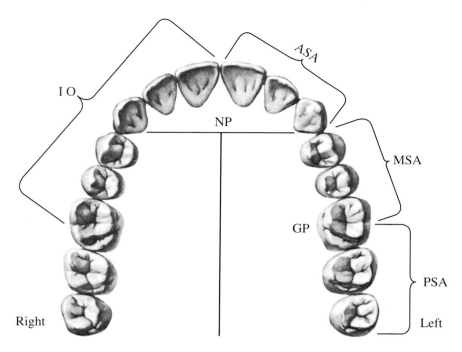

FIGURE 18-5 Structures anesthetized by maxillary injections (see also Table 18-3). *IO*, infraorbital nerve block; *ASA*, anterior superior alveolar nerve block; *MSA*, middle superior alveolar nerve block; *PSA*, posterior superior alveolar nerve block; *GP*, greater palatine nerve block; *NP*, nasopalatine nerve block. *(Modified from Massler M, Schour I: Atlas of the mouth in health and disease, ed 2, Chicago, 1975, American Dental Association.)*

    b. Maxillary anterior teeth, premolars, and the mesiobuccal root of the first molar
    c. Side of nose
    d. Upper lip
    e. Lower eyelid
  2. Penetration site—mucobuccal fold parallel to the apex of the first premolar
D. Posterior superior alveolar nerve block (PSA)
  1. Structures anesthetized (see Figure 18-5)
    a. Facial gingiva of maxillary molars, except the mesiobuccal root of the first molar
    b. Maxillary molars except the mesiobuccal root of the first molar
  2. Penetration site—height of mucobuccal fold over the maxillary second molar
E. Greater palatine nerve block (GP)
  1. Structures anesthetized (see Figure 18-5)
    a. Lingual gingiva of maxillary posterior teeth
    b. Palatal mucosa to the midline
  2. Penetration site
    a. Pressure anesthesia (1 minute)
    b. 1 to 2 mm anterior to the greater palatine foramen
F. Nasopalatine nerve block (NP)
  1. Structures anesthetized (see Figure 18-5)
    a. Lingual gingiva of maxillary anterior teeth
    b. Palatal mucosa in the premaxillary area
  2. Penetration site
    a. Pressure anesthesia (1 minute)
    b. Incisive papilla at the base and into the fattest portion

TRIGEMINAL NERVE: MANDIBULAR DIVISION

See the section on "The nervous system" in Chapter 4.

Innervation

A. V3 branches from the undivided nerve
  1. Meningeal nerve (sensory)
  2. Medial pterygoid nerve (motor)
  3. Tensor veli palatini nerve (motor)
  4. Tensor tympani nerve (motor)
B. V3 branches from the divided nerve
  1. Anterior division
    a. Lateral pterygoid nerve (motor)
    b. Masseter nerve (motor)
    c. Anterior deep temporal nerve (motor)
    d. Posterior deep temporal nerve (motor)
    e. Buccal nerve (sensory); relevant branch for local anesthesia
  2. Posterior division
    a. Auriculo-temporal nerve (sensory)
    b. Lingual nerve (sensory); relevant branch for local anesthesia
    c. Inferior alveolar nerve (mixed); relevant branch for local anesthesia
      (1) Mylohyoid nerve (motor)
      (2) Mental nerve (sensory)
      (3) Incisive nerve (sensory)

Mandibular Block Injections

See Table 18-4.
A. Inferior alveolar nerve block (IANB)
  1. Structures anesthetized (Figure 18-6)
    a. Mandibular teeth
    b. Facial gingiva of mandibular anterior teeth and the first premolar
    c. Skin of chin
    d. Lower lip
    e. Lingual gingiva of mandibular teeth
    f. Floor of mouth
    g. Anterior ⅔ of tongue
  2. Penetration site—pterygotemporal depression where the pterygomandibular raphe turns superiorly toward the maxilla
B. Buccal nerve block (B)
  1. Structures anesthetized (see Figure 18-6)
    a. Facial gingiva of mandibular molars
    b. Skin of cheek
  2. Penetration site—mucous membrane distal and buccal to the most distal molar
C. Mental nerve block (M)
  1. Structures anesthetized (see Figure 18-6)
    a. Facial gingiva of mandibular anterior teeth and the first premolar
    b. Skin of chin
    c. Lower lip
  2. Penetration site
    a. Vertical technique—mucobuccal fold between the first and second premolars
    b. Horizontal technique—mucobuccal fold at the apex of the first premolar

THE WAND/COMPUDENT: COMPUTER-CONTROLLED LOCAL ANESTHESIA DELIVERY SYSTEM

Wand/CompuDent Components

A. The Wand/CompuDent consists of three main components (Table 18-5):
  1. Drive unit
  2. Disposable plastic handpiece and tubing
  3. Foot control that activates the unit and controls the two flow rates:
    a. Fast rate
    b. Slow rate
B. The computer controls:
  1. The pressure of the fluid
  2. The flow rate of the anesthetic
C. Flow rates
  1. Slow
    a. Delivers one drop every 2 seconds
    b. 1.8 mL of anesthetic is delivered in 2 minutes

TABLE 18-4 Mandibular Injections

Injection	Needle Length	Structures Anesthetized	Penetration Site	Terminal Deposition Site	Amount Deposited
IANB	Long needle	Facial gingiva of mandibular anterior teeth and the first premolar Skin of chin Lower lip Mandibular teeth Lingual gingiva of mandibular teeth Floor of mouth Anterior ⅔ of tongue	Two thirds of the way up in the pterygotemporal depression. Penetration site is where the pterygomandibular raphe turns superiorly toward the maxilla. Place the thumb in the coronoid notch, and roll medial to temporal crest	The site is directly superior to the mandibular foramen between the sphenomandibular ligament and the ramus of the mandible. Bone should be contacted.	⅞ cartridge Wait 3–5 minutes
B	Long needle	1. Facial gingiva of mandibular molars 2. Skin of cheek	Mucous membrane distal and buccal to the most distal molar	2–3 mm. The needle is held parallel and inferior to the horizontal plane of occlusal surfaces when directed toward the penetration site	⅛ cartridge Wait 1 minute
M	Short needle	1. Facial gingiva of mandibular anterior teeth and the first premolar 2. Skin of chin 3. Lower lip	Vertical: mucobuccal fold between the first and the second premolars	Directly over the mental foramen (depth of penetration is 5–6 mm)	⅓ cartridge Wait 2–3 minutes

IANB, inferior alveolar nerve block; *B*, buccal nerve block; *M*, mental nerve block.

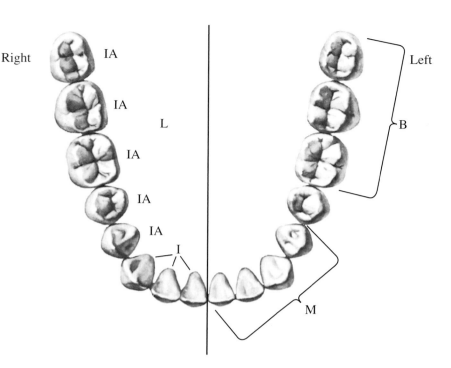

FIGURE 18-6 Structures anesthetized by mandibular injections (see also Table 18-4). *IA/L*, mandibular nerve block; *I*, incisive nerve block; *M*, mental nerve block; *B*, buccal nerve block. *NOTE*: The incisive and inferior alveolar nerves anesthetize *only* teeth and not lingual soft tissue. *(Modified from Massler M, Schour I: Atlas of the mouth in health and disease, ed 2, Chicago, 1975, American Dental Association.)*

2. Fast
    a. Delivers a steady stream (30 ga) or rapid drip (27 ga)
    b. Takes 1 minute to deliver the contents of a cartridge

Anesthetic Pathway

A. The two main causes of pain associated with dental injections are:
    1. Initial tissue puncture
    2. Depositing a volume of fluid too rapidly into a confined space
B. Purposes of the Wand/CompuDent
    1. Eliminates initial penetration pain by establishing an anesthetic pathway
    2. Eliminates pressure pain by constant pressure and controlled volume
C. Anesthetic pathway—the anesthetic drip precedes the path of the needle (used for all injections)
D. Technique used to establish anesthetic pathway
    1. Place the bevel of the needle against the tissue
    2. Use a cotton-tipped applicator on the top to seal the bevel to the tissue surface
    3. Initiate a slow flow of anesthetic for 2 to 3 seconds to force some of the anesthetic through the surface epithelium before actual penetration of tissue

Administering Injections Using the Wand/CompuDent Delivery System

A. Anterior middle superior alveolar (AMSA) nerve block—palatal approach
    1. Teeth anesthetized—central through second premolar
    2. Benefits
        a. Effective soft tissue anesthesia for scaling and root debridement of associated maxillary teeth
        b. Multiple tooth and pulpal anesthesia delivered from a single injection
        c. Simple and safe technique
        d. No numbness of lips and of the facial muscles of expression
        e. More comfortable palatal injection
    3. Injection site—spot on the palate that bisects the premolars in the palatine groove
    4. Amount—¾ to 1 cartridge
    5. Aspiration—not necessary
    6. Duration—60 to 90 minutes
    7. Flow rate—slow
    8. Needle—30 ga, ½ inch
B. Palatal–anterior superior alveolar (P-ASA) nerve block
    1. Teeth anesthetized—canine to canine
    2. Benefits
        a. Effective soft tissue anesthesia of associated maxillary teeth

TABLE 18-5 Comparison of Traditional Syringe to WAND™

	Traditional	Wand
Grasp and needle control	Palm grasp Relies on large muscles of wrist, forearm, and shoulder Weighs 80 g Held 9 inches from the insertion point	Pen grasp Control is transferred to the small muscles of the fingers and thumb Weighs a few grams Held within 2 inches of the insertion point
Fluid delivery	The thumb is used to start and stop the flow of solution	Uses a foot control to deliver a constant flow of solution
Fluid metering	Pressure and volume cannot be separated; thus is operator dependent	Maintains constant pressure and controlled volume
Aspiration	Relies on operator control	Aspirates automatically (on demand) by releasing the foot control
Needles	Threaded hub 25 ga, long and short 27 ga, long and short	Luer-Lok hub Smaller gauge and length preferred 30 ga, ½ inch 30 ga, 1 inch 27 ga, 1¼ inch
Path of insertion	Linear insertion (straight push through tissues, causing needle deflection)	Bi-rotational insertion (180 degrees) between the thumb and index finger to overcome needle deflection

    b. Multiple tooth and pulpal anesthesia delivered from a single injection (bilateral)
    c. Simple and safe technique
    d. No numbness of lips and of the facial muscles of expression
    e. More comfortable palatal injection
  3. Injection site
    a. The needle should penetrate laterally into the incisive papilla (tissue should be allowed to blanch)
    b. The needle should be reoriented to gain access to the incisive canal (advance needle to bony wall and aspirate)
  4. Amount—¾ to 1 cartridge
  5. Aspiration—required
  6. Duration—60 to 90 minutes
  7. Flow rate—slow
  8. Needle—30 ga, ½ inch

C. Periodontal ligament (PDL) injection
  1. Teeth anesthetized—single tooth
  2. Benefits
    a. Primary injection for pulpal anesthesia
    b. Supplemental injection to a block or infiltration
  3. Injection site—maxilla
    a. Molars have two sites—mesiobuccal and distobuccal line angles
    b. Premolars have one site—direct buccal
    c. Anterior teeth have one site—direct facial
  4. Injection site—mandible
    a. Molars have two sites—mesiolingual and distolingual line angles
    b. Premolars have one site—direct lingual
    c. Anterior teeth have one site—direct lingual
  5. Amount—½ cartridge at each site
  6. Aspiration—not necessary
  7. Duration—1 hour
  8. Flow rate—slow
  9. Needle
    a. 27 ga, ½ inch for premolars and molars
    b. 30 ga, ½ inch for incisors

CONSCIOUS SEDATION WITH NITROUS OXIDE–OXYGEN

A. Synonymous terms
  1. Conscious sedation
    a. The client is always awake and able to respond to verbal commands
    b. Protective reflexes are intact, including the ability to maintain an open airway, breathe automatically, and cough so that aspiration is avoided
  2. Inhalation sedation—nitrous oxide and oxygen gases are inhaled through the nose
  3. Nitrous oxide psycho-sedation—acts on the CNS in such a way that pain impulses are not relayed to the cerebral cortex or the interpretation of pain impulses is altered
  4. Relative analgesia
    a. Refers to the state of sedation produced
    b. Alters the mood and increases the pain reaction threshold but does not totally block pain sensations
B. Chemistry
  1. Nitrous oxide (N_2O) properties
    a. Stored as a liquid at 650 to 900 pounds per square inch (psi) in a blue cylinder and delivered as a gas
    b. The contents of the N_2O cylinder cannot be determined by the pressure gauge until it is almost empty
    c. Colorless

d. Tasteless

e. Sweet-smelling

f. Nonexplosive

g. Supports combustion

2. Oxygen (O_2)

a. Stored as a gas in a green cylinder and delivered as a gas

b. Contents of the O_2 cylinder can be determined by reading the pressure gauge (full = 2100 psi)

3. Blood–gas solubility coefficient

a. The blood–gas solubility coefficient of N_2O is 0.47, which means that 100 mL of blood dissolves 47 mL of N_2O

b. This blood–gas solubility coefficient accounts for the rapid onset and recovery from the effects of the analgesic

c. N_2O is 15 times more soluble in the blood than nitrogen; N_2O displaces nitrogen in blood

d. N_2O does not compete with O_2 and carbon dioxide (CO_2) in combining with the hemoglobin molecule

C. Pharmacology

1. N_2O has no effect on heart rate, blood pressure, and the liver or the kidneys, as long as an adequate amount of O_2 is delivered simultaneously

2. N_2O affects all sensations such as hearing, touch, pain, warmth

3. N_2O reduces the gag reflex but does not eliminate it

D. Physiology

1. N_2O works by depressing the CNS

2. The exact mechanism of action is unknown; however, the effect results in either altering the relay of nerve impulses to the cerebral cortex or causing them to be interpreted differently

3. The client experiences reduced anxiety and increased tolerance to pain

4. Pain perception is not blocked

5. N_2O does not combine with any body tissues; it is the only anesthetic that is not metabolized

6. The N_2O molecule enters the bloodstream through the lungs, where it displaces nitrogen and is eventually exhaled, unchanged, through the lungs

7. Toxic reaction associated with too much N_2O is hypoxia (lack of O_2 to the tissues), characterized by headache and nausea

E. Stages of anesthesia

1. Stage I: Analgesia stage—client feels pain but is not bothered by it; this stage has three planes; the first two planes are appropriate for dental hygiene care

2. Stage II: Delirium or excitement stage—hyperresponsiveness to stimuli; exaggerated inhalations and loss of consciousness

3. Stage III: Surgical anesthesia—used in oral and maxillofacial surgery; this stage has four planes

4. Stage IV: Respiratory paralysis—the patient is no longer breathing independently

F. Indications for use

1. Mild apprehension

2. Refusal of local and general anesthesia

3. Allergy to local anesthesia

4. Hypersensitive gag reflex

5. Intolerance for long appointments

6. Cardiac conditions

7. Hypertension

8. Asthma

9. Cerebral palsy

10. Intellectual and developmental disabilities

G. Relative contraindications to use

1. Pregnancy

2. Communication difficulties

3. Nasal obstruction

4. Emphysema

5. Multiple sclerosis

6. Emotional instability

7. Epilepsy

8. Negative response to past experience

H. Advantages and disadvantages of use

1. Advantages

a. History of cardiovascular disease—O_2 enrichment coupled with stress reduction

b. Simple, relatively safe procedure to perform

c. Minimal equipment

d. No restraining straps or pharyngeal airways

e. The client is awake and responsive

f. Rapid onset of and recovery from the effects of the anesthetic

g. No need for the client to be accompanied by someone to the appointment

h. No preoperative tests or food intake restrictions required

i. No need for the patient to spend time in a recovery room

2. Disadvantages

a. Oversedation causes vertigo, nausea, or vomiting

b. Difficult behavioral problems cannot always be managed

c. Instrumentation in the maxillary anterior region difficult because of the presence of the mask over the nose of the client

I. Signs and symptoms of nitrous oxide–oxygen sedation

1. Objective signs—directly observed by the clinician in the client

a. Being awake

b. Lessened pain reaction

c. Drowsy, relaxed appearance

d. Normal eye reaction and pupil size

e. Normal respiration

f. Normal blood pressure and pulse

g. Minimal movement of limbs

h. Flushing of skin

i. Perspiration

j. Lacrimation

k. Little or no gagging or coughing

l. Speech infrequent and slow

2. Subjective symptoms—reported by the client

  a. Mental and physical relaxation

  b. Indifference to surroundings and passage of time

  c. Lessened pain awareness

  d. Floating sensation

  e. Drowsiness

  f. Warmth

  g. Tingling or numbness

  h. Sounds seeming distant

J. Equipment

1. Cylinders—blue indicates N_2O; green indicates O_2

2. Gas machine

  a. Yokes

  b. Flowmeter

  c. Pressure gauge

  d. Reservoir bag

  e. Gas hose

3. Mask

  a. Only masks with two-hose scavenging systems reduce the N_2O exhaled into the air and breathed in by the operator

  b. Scavenging systems reduce environmental N_2O contamination from 900 to 30 parts per million (ppm)

  c. Maximum allowable contamination in health care environments is 50 ppm

K. Safety measures

1. Color-coded tanks—blue (N_2O) versus green (O_2)

2. Pin Index System—ensures that the N_2O cylinder does not fit into the yoke that holds the O_2 cylinder, and vice versa

3. Diameter Index System—the diameter of the hole at the top of the cylinder (O_2 or N_2O) fits only with corresponding cylinder head

4. Audible alarm system—emitted when O_2 runs out

5. Automatic turnoff—occurs when O_2 is depleted

6. Oxygen maintained at 2 to 3 L at all times in most units

7. Oxygen flush—fills the reservoir bag with 100% O_2

L. Record keeping and documentation in the client's dental record

1. Documentation will vary according to the laws of the state or the legal jurisdiction

2. Documentation includes:

  a. Tidal volume (TV) in liters (L)

  b. Amount of N_2O in liters (L) or percentage

  c. Amount of O_2 in liters (L) or percentage

  d. Duration of sedation

  e. Oxygenation period (5 minutes O_2/15 minutes N_2O delivered)

  f. Client's response

  g. ADA Code D9230 for health insurance reimbursement

SUGGESTED READINGS

Walsh MM, Darby ML: Local anesthesia. In Darby ML, Walsh MM, editors: *Dental hygiene theory and practice*, ed 3, Philadelphia, 2010, Saunders.

Walsh MM: Nitrous oxide-oxygen analgesia. In Darby ML, Walsh MM, editors: *Dental hygiene theory and practice*, ed 3, Philadelphia, 2010, Saunders.

Malamed SF: *Handbook of local anesthesia*, ed 6, St Louis, 2007, Mosby.

American Dental Association (ADA): Current dental terminology 2009-2010, Chicago, 2009, ADA.

Gwen I. Hlava, Todd N. Junge, and the publisher acknowledge the past contributions of Danielle Leigh Ryan to this chapter.

CHAPTER 18 REVIEW QUESTIONS

Answers and Rationales to Review Questions are available on this text's accompanying Evolve site. See inside front cover for details.

ℰvolve

1. Repolarization of the nerve after stimulation is primarily caused by:
   a. Active transport of potassium (K^+) out of the cell
   b. Active transport of sodium (Na^+) out of the cell
   c. Diffusion of Na^+ into the cell along the concentration gradient
   d. Diffusion of K^+ out of the cell along the concentration gradient

2. How does a nerve conduct an impulse?
   a. By blocking K^+ from leaving the inside of the cell membrane
   b. By sequential neuron cell membrane depolarization from segment to segment or node to node
   c. By rapid influx of chloride ions across the neuronal cell membrane
   d. By blocking Na^+ from entering the cell membrane

3. The two stages of an action potential are:
   a. Equilibrium/membrane potential
   b. Positive/negative
   c. Depolarization/repolarization
   d. Relative/absolute refractory period
   e. Myelinated/nonmyelinated

4. Local anesthetic agents prevent depolarization by:
   a. Blocking the sodium–potassium pump
   b. Preventing the transfer of K^+ ions from exiting the nerve cell membrane
   c. Preventing transfer of Na^+ ions from the interior of the nerve to the exterior
   d. Preventing transfer of Na^+ ions from the exterior of the nerve to the interior

5. Once the minimal threshold stimulus has been reached, the impulse will travel the entire length of the fiber without stimulation. This explains:
   a. Pain perception
   b. Pain reaction threshold
   c. Absolute refractory period
   d. Membrane potential
   e. All-or-none law

6. The gauge of a dental needle MOST recommended for intraoral injections with high risk of aspiration is:
   a. 18 gauge
   b. 30 gauge
   c. 27 gauge
   d. 25 gauge
   e. 23 gauge

7. All of the statements concerning local anesthetic needles are true EXCEPT one. Which one is the EXCEPTION?
   a. The term *gauge* refers to the diameter of the lumen of the needle
   b. The weakest portion of the needle is at its hub
   c. Larger needles provide more reliable aspirations
   d. Disposable needles will not normally become dull for at least 10 insertions
   e. Larger needles should be employed when a greater risk of positive aspiration exists

8. All of the statements concerning local anesthetic cartridges are true EXCEPT one. Which one is the EXCEPTION?
   a. The glass dental cartridge should not be autoclaved
   b. No alcohol should be present around the cartridges when they are stored outside the packaging container
   c. The rubber plunger is treated with silicone to decrease the incidence of "sticky stoppers"
   d. Cartridges exposed to extended periods of direct sunlight may have their contents undergo accelerated destruction
   e. Manufacturers recommend freezing cartridges so that they may be used beyond the posted expiration date

9. The purpose of aspirating before injecting a local anesthetic solution is to prevent:
   a. Allergic reactions
   b. Intravascular injections
   c. Traumatic injections
   d. Trismus

10. Why do local anesthetics NOT work well in infected tissues?
    a. The lower pH of infected tissue
    b. Increased edema
    c. Increased vascularity
    d. All of the above

11. Lidocaine is metabolized primarily in the:
    a. Liver
    b. Kidney
    c. Plasma
    d. Bloodstream

12. **Complete the sentence with the MOST accurate phrase. Local anesthetics_____.**
    a. Combine lipid-soluble acids and basic esters
    b. Form water-soluble salts with strong acids, which are unionized
    c. Dissociate in the tissues, liberating free base, which can diffuse through the nerve membrane
    d. Form amides, which transform to esters in tissues
    e. Are synthetic and do not contain amino groups

13. **Tissues with higher pH will cause:**
    a. Rapid hydrolysis of the anesthetic solution
    b. Decreased disassociation of the anesthetic drug
    C. Increased disassociation of the anesthetic drug
    d. None of the above

14. **The amount of anesthetic in a cartridge of 4% prilocaine is**
    a. 36 mg
    b. 30 mg
    c. 54 mg
    d. 72 mg
    e. 90 mg

15. **It takes 2 minutes to deliver 1.8 mL of anesthetic using the Wand fast flow rate; this is the ideal flow rate for a traditional injection according to Malamed (2007).**
    a. Both statements are TRUE
    b. Both statements are FALSE
    c. The first statement is TRUE; the second statement is FALSE
    d. The first statement is FALSE; the second statement is TRUE

16. **The maximum safe dose of carbocaine is 300 mg. How many cartridges of a 2% solution can be injected so as not to exceed the maximum?**
    a. 5 cartridges
    b. 6 cartridges
    c. 7 cartridges
    d. 8 cartridges
    e. 9 cartridges

17. **Which of the following would be the LONGEST lasting for inferior alveolar nerve block (IANB) anesthesia?**
    a. Prilocaine
    b. Lidocaine
    c. Mepivacaine
    d. Procaine
    e. Articaine

18. **How many milligrams of lidocaine does 1 mL of 2% lidocaine contain?**
    a. 2 mg
    b. 20 mg
    c. 200 mg
    d. 2 g
    e. 20 g

19. **All of the following statements about local anesthesia are true EXCEPT for one. Which one is the EXCEPTION?**
    a. Hemostasis is only achieved when the vasoconstrictor is deposited into the area of bleeding
    b. Maximum dosages of all drugs administered by injection should be calculated by body weight
    c. Children can tolerate adult doses of local anesthetics because of their faster metabolism, and overdose is of little concern
    d. The possible causes of decreased anesthetic effect include edema, pH, and vascularity
    e. Overdose reactions are dose related; allergic reactions are not dose related

20. **The maximum safe dose of 2% carbocaine for a normal adult client is:**
    a. 5.5 cartridges
    b. 8.3 cartridges
    c. 6.9 cartridges
    d. None of the above

21. **The maximum safe dose of 4% prilocaine is:**
    a. 300 mg
    b. 500 mg
    c. 400 mg
    d. None of the above

22. **The problem(s) with topical anesthesia is(are):**
    a. Dosage control
    b. All are esters except 5% lidocaine
    c. Concentrations used exceed concentrations administered by injection
    d. Topical anesthetic agents containing benzocaine are, by far, the most common
    e. All of the above

23. **Rapid biotransformation will result in:**
    a. Increased systemic toxicity
    b. Decreased systemic toxicity
    c. Increased disassociation of the anesthetic drug
    d. Decreased disassociation of the anesthetic drug

24. **Amides are inactivated by the enzyme:**
    a. Plasma cholinesterase
    b. Protease
    c. Lipase
    d. Monoamine oxidase
    e. Amylase

25. **Which of the following statements about the metabolism of local anesthetic agents is TRUE?**
    a. Amides undergo biotransformation by pseudo-cholinesterase
    b. Vasoconstrictors are broken down in the liver
    c. The rate of metabolism does not have any effect on potential toxicity
    d. The location of biotransformation is dependent on drug classification
    e. The metabolism of local anesthetic agents occurs in the kidneys

26. **The maximum safe dose of epinephrine for the healthy adult is 0.2 mg. How many cartridges of 1:100,000 epinephrine can be administered?**
    a. 2 cartridges
    b. 5 cartridges
    c. 9 cartridges
    d. 10 cartridges
    e. 11 cartridges

27. **How many milligrams of epinephrine are in a cartridge of local anesthetic with 1:200,000?**
    a. 0.005 mg
    b. 0.036 mg
    c. 0.009 mg
    d. 0.36 mg
    e. 0.01 mg

28. **The maximum safe dose (MSD) of epinephrine for clients with significant cardiovascular disease is:**
    a. 0.02 mg
    b. 0.04 mg
    c. 0.4 mg
    d. 0.02 mg
    e. 0.1 mg

29. **Inadvertent rapid intravenous injection of a local anesthetic containing a vasoconstrictor may cause:**
    a. Convulsions
    b. Palpitations
    c. Unconsciousness
    d. Depressed respiration
    e. All of the above

30. **Terminal deposition for the inferior alveolar nerve block is the:**
    a. Mental foramen
    b. Mandibular foramen
    c. Cingulum
    d. Infraorbital foramen

31. **What purpose(s) does epinephrine serve when added to a local anesthetic agent?**
    a. Prolongation of anesthesia
    b. Reduction of hemorrhage in field of operation
    c. Constriction of blood vessels in area of injection
    d. Prevention of toxic effects from too-rapid absorption
    e. All of the above

32. **What is(are) the overdose effect(s) of epinephrine?**
    a. Palpitation
    b. Tachycardia
    c. Hypertension
    d. Headache
    e. All of the above

33. **The following injection(s) should be administered when scaling and root debridement of a mandibular second molar:**
    a. Mental nerve block
    b. Buccal nerve block
    c. Inferior alveolar nerve block
    d. B and C
    e. None of the above

34. **What is the average adult depth of penetration for the mental nerve block?**
    a. 12 mm
    b. 6 mm
    c. 9 mm
    d. Until the bevel is covered
    e. Until bone is contacted

35. **During the administration of an inferior alveolar nerve block, the needle is inserted:**
    a. Medial to the pterygomandibular raphe
    b. Medial to the medial pterygoid muscle
    c. Lateral to the pterygomandibular raphe
    d. At the height of the maxillary tuberosity
    e. Lateral to the ramus of the mandible

36. **Trismus noted in a client the day following an inferior alveolar nerve block MOST likely results from:**
    a. Failure to use an aspirating syringe
    b. Irritation of the medial pterygoid muscle
    c. Accidental injection of the solution near a branch of the facial nerve
    d. Allowing the needle tip to rest beneath the periosteum during injection
    e. Accidental injection of the solution near a major branch of the trigeminal nerve

37. **All of the following statements about intraoral injections are false EXCEPT one. Which one is the EXCEPTION?**
    a. IANB does not block the mylohyoid nerve
    b. Periodontal ligament (PDL) injections are only administered using a specialized syringe
    c. Infraorbital injections block the entire maxillary nerve
    d. The success rate of the IANB is 80% to 85%

38. **All of the following statements about intraoral injections are false EXCEPT one. Which one is the EXCEPTION?**
    a. The incisive nerve block provides lingual soft tissue anesthesia
    b. An initial negative aspiration ensures no risk for intravascular injection, and additional aspiration is unnecessary during solution deposition
    c. The site of needle insertion for a posterior superior alveolar nerve block is the height of the mucobuccal fold above the maxillary second molar
    d. The recommended amount of time to inject a 1.8-mL cartridge with regard to client safety and comfort is 30 seconds

39. Which of the following nerves should be adequately anesthetized to scale and root-debride a maxillary first molar?
    a. GP/PSA
    b. LP/GP/NP
    c. PSA/MSA/GP
    d. ASA/MSA/GP
    e. PSA/MSA/LP

40. Within seconds following a posterior superior alveolar injection, a client's face becomes distended and swollen on the injected side. The appropriate action by the hygienist would be to:
    a. Have the dentist administer an antihistamine
    b. Have the dentist administer an antibiotic
    c. Have the dentist incise and drain
    d. Counsel the client, apply pressure to the site, and ice to the area
    e. Ask the client to exhale

41. Within seconds following a posterior superior alveolar injection, a client's face becomes distended and swollen on the injected side. The condition suspected in this situation is most likely a/an:
    a. Aneurysm
    b. Hematoma
    c. Angioedema
    d. Allergy
    e. Infection

42. A client develops paralysis of a half of his face and inability to close his eye on the side of an attempted inferior alveolar nerve block. The MOST logical explanation is that the injection was given into the:
    a. Parotid gland
    b. Masseter muscle
    c. Maxillary artery
    d. Posterior facial vein
    e. Pterygo-mandibular ligament

43. If the nitrous oxide (N_2O) flow rate is 2 liters/minute (L/min) and that of O_2 is 4 L/min, what is the percentage of the N_2O?
    a. 33%
    b. 67%
    c. 50%
    d. None of the above

44. What needs to be recorded in the client's treatment notes following the use of nitrous oxide–oxygen conscious sedation during nonsurgical periodontal therapy?
    a. Oxygenation period
    b. Duration of sedation
    c. Concentrations of N_2O and O_2 administered
    d. Tidal volume
    e. All of the above

45. Which of the following signs or symptoms may indicate the use of an excessive concentration of N_2O?
    a. Slight smile on the client's face
    b. Panicky look in the client's eyes
    c. The client feeling a sense of floating or sinking
    d. Mild diaphoresis (perspiration) experienced by the client

46. All of the following are relative contraindications to the elective use of nitrous oxide–oxygen conscious sedation EXCEPT one. Which one is the EXCEPTION?
    a. Communication difficulty
    b. Epilepsy
    c. Asthma
    d. Nasal obstruction
    e. Chronic obstructive pulmonary disease

47. All of the following statements about N_2O are false EXCEPT one. Which one is the EXCEPTION?
    a. The toxic reaction is associated with too much N_2O, which causes hypoxia.
    b. N_2O is metabolized in the lungs
    c. N_2O works by blocking pain perception
    d. N_2O affects heart rate, blood pressure, liver, and kidney
    e. N_2O makes the client perceive time as passing slowly

48. What structures are anesthetized with the AMSA (anterior middle superior alveolar) Wand injection?
    a. Muscles of facial expression
    b. Mandibular lingual gingiva and palatal mucosa
    c. Upper lip
    d. Mandibular facial gingiva from the central incisor to the second premolar
    e. Maxillary central incisor through the second premolar

49. Which statement regarding the Wand PDL injection is TRUE?
    a. Aspiration is required
    b. Anterior teeth have one injection site, and posterior teeth have two injection sites
    c. The penetration site on the maxilla is on the lingual aspect; it is on the facial aspect on the mandible
    d. One half cartridge is delivered at each site
    e. Fast or slow flow can be used

50. Which of the following regarding the palatal–anterior superior alveolar (P-ASA) Wand injection is TRUE?
    a. Anesthetizes six teeth
    b. Is a two-stage injection
    c. Requires aspiration
    d. Involves the administration of one cartridge
    e. All of the above

19 Dental Hygiene Care for Clients with Special Care Needs

Susan Lynn Tolle

Every person has unique abilities and needs. Two of every five clients treated in the oral health care environment may require a modified care plan because of special care needs. These special care needs may be transient, for example, pregnancy or a broken foot, or may be lifelong, for example, end-stage renal disease or intellectual and developmental disabilities. With ongoing health care reforms and better access to care for underserved populations, dental hygienists will be serving increased numbers of persons with special care needs in a variety of settings. The National Institute of Dental and Craniofacial Research describes persons with special care as those with genetic or systemic disorders that affect oral, dental, or craniofacial health; whose medical treatments cause oral problems; or whose intellectual or physical disabilities complicate oral hygiene or dental treatment.

GENERAL CONSIDERATIONS

Lifespan Approach to Care

A. Principles of growth, development, and maturation
   1. Growth includes physical and functional maturation
   2. Growth is generally a continuous and orderly process but can be modified by numerous factors (e.g., nutritional deficiencies)
   3. Different parts of the body grow and mature at different rates
   4. Critical periods exist in growth and development
   5. Hormonal changes can alter:
      a. Physical stature and function
      b. Mental state and mood
      c. Oral status
      d. Immunity and host response
   6. During growth and maturation, a person's perception of self and that of self in relation to others change
   7. Health status generally progresses from acute illness to chronic illness
   8. Transition from one life stage to another is gradual and not necessarily based on chronologic age
   9. Biologic age is not synonymous with chronologic age
   10. Signs of aging can appear at any age
B. The U.S. health care system (see the section on "Providing oral health care" in Chapter 20)
   1. The current system is categorical, with many gaps in services
   2. A continuum of services through people's life stages must ensure:
      a. Universal access
      b. Continuity of care
      c. Comprehensive philosophy of care
      d. System of planned change
   3. Health care providers should consider:
      a. Heterogeneity of persons bearing the same label
      b. Individualized approach to care
   4. Oral health needs and approaches to care can differ throughout a person's life cycle (Table 19-1)

Incidence and Prevalence of Individuals with Special Needs

A. National statistics on incidence and prevalence figures are difficult to compile because of:
   1. Unreliable reporting systems
   2. Variable and changing definitions of conditions
   3. Differences between acute conditions versus chronic conditions

TABLE 19-1 Life-Span Approach to Oral Health Care

Life Stage	General Care Concerns	Usual Oral Concerns
Early childhood	Teaching parents and caregivers oral care skills Preventing early occurrence of caries or trauma (protecting developing teeth) Controlling risk factors Preventing vertical and horizontal disease transmission	Oral infections Dental caries Dental development
Childhood	Developing positive dental attitudes and behaviors Teaching self-care skills Controlling risk factors Preventing vertical and horizontal disease transmission	Dental caries Dental development Gingivitis
Adolescence	Motivating toward self-responsibility for seeking and receiving care Controlling risk factors for disease Preventing oral injuries Tobacco use cessation	Dental caries Periodontal diseases Dental development
Young adult	Decreasing barriers and integrating oral health care into daily schedule Tobacco use cessation	Periodontal diseases
Midlife	Maintaining status and preventing deterioration Controlling risk factors Tobacco use cessation	
Older adult	Motivating to continue preventive care and accept new theories and interventions Decreasing barriers to care Controlling risk factors Tobacco use cessation	Periodontal diseases Dental caries Oral cancer
Elderly	Maintaining status and function and preventing infections and tooth loss Controlling risk factors Tobacco use cessation	Periodontal diseases Dental caries Oral cancer Fractures, tooth loss Oral infections

4. Overlap in data when dealing with multiple conditions
B. More than 60 million persons (1 in 5 persons) are considered disabled as defined by the Americans with Disabilities Act; of these, approximately 1 million are children younger than 6 years old
C. In the United States, 32.5 million persons are considered to have a severe disability
D. Table 19-2 identifies the most common chronic conditions in the older adult population
E. The most common disabilities in the United States are caused by cardiovascular disease, back problems, arthritis, asthma, and diabetes
F. The prevalence of disability increases with age
   1. Of persons in the United States age 5 to 15, 6% are disabled
   2. Of persons in the United States age 16 to 64, 12% are disabled
   3. Of persons in the United States age 65 and older, 41% are disabled
G. The most frequently reported chronic conditions that cause disability are diabetes, arthritis, cardiovascular disease, hypertension, cancer, spinal curvature, and back impairments

TABLE 19-2 Leading Chronic Conditions in the Older Adult Population

Noninstitutionalized	Nursing Home Residents
Arthritis	Arthritis
Hypertension	Heart disease
Hearing impairments	Mental illness
Heart disease	Paralysis

H. Of individuals with developmental disabilities, 80% live in community-based residences or at home with families

The Dental Hygienist and Individuals with Special Needs

A. Recognize physical, mental, medical, social, and oral needs
B. Communicate with clients and caregivers in a positive, appropriate, nondiscriminatory manner

C. Communicate with other professionals and team members to facilitate planning, implementation, and coordination of care

D. Plan, implement, and evaluate community-based and office-based programs

E. Adapt dental hygiene care plans, interventions, and evaluations to meet clients' special needs, considering:
1. Barriers to care
2. Resources
3. Personal skills and abilities
4. Cultural values and beliefs

F. Identify and eliminate potential barriers to care

G. Assess one's own attitudes, values, and commitment to provision of oral health services to these clients

H. Evaluate local, state, regional, and national trends for their potential impact on the provision of oral health care

I. Advocate oral health promotion and disease-prevention programs, full use of dental hygienists, and development of sound research so that evidenced-based care is provided in oral health care programs

General Definitions

These tend to change frequently and often overlap.

A. Labeling—the process of classifying persons for educational, medical, or financial reasons

B. Barrier-free environment—facilities that are physically accessible to everyone

C. Normalization—making available patterns and conditions of everyday life that are as close as possible to the norms and patterns of mainstream society

D. Mainstreaming—integration of persons with special needs into community-based programs and services

E. Access to oral health care—opportunity for each individual to enter into the oral health care system and use the needed services

Goals of Normalization for Persons with Special Needs

A. Ensure legal and civil rights

B. Guarantee appropriate education for continued learning

C. Increase or maintain social skills and problem-solving abilities

D. Increase employment options and decrease employer discrimination

E. Ensure comprehensive network of community resources

Potential Barriers to Oral Health Care

A. Accessibility
1. Financial
    a. One fourth of the older adult population has an inadequate income level; percentages are higher for women, ethnic minorities, and single heads of households
    b. Between 65% and 85% of disabled persons live near the poverty level
    c. Medicaid coverage for oral health care is extremely variable across states and often does not cover older adult care
    d. Medical and pharmaceutical expenses for many persons with disabilities consume a major portion of their incomes
    e. Many individuals with special needs who have limited incomes cannot afford standard private practice fees for dental care, have no health insurance, or are underinsured
2. Transportation and geography
    a. More than 50% of the disabled and older adult population lives in urban settings; the remainder lives in small rural communities or on farms
    b. Public transportation is often unreliable, confusing, unaffordable, or nonexistent
    c. Clients with special needs often rely on others for transportation to dental appointments, which increases their dependence and makes scheduling and compliance difficult
    d. Homebound, hospitalized, or institutionalized clients frequently cannot be transported for care in the community
3. Physical facilities
    a. Minimum standards for accessibility must be met by dentists according to the Americans with Disabilities Act of 1993
    b. External barriers include parking lots and spaces, walkways, curbs, stairs, narrow doors and entryways, heavy or pressurized doors, and small-print signs
    c. Internal barriers include narrow passageways or doors, cluttered rooms or hallways, loose rugs or heavy shag carpets, abrupt changes in floor textures, noncontrasting colors, and bathrooms without grab-bars or other modifications

B. Psychosocial concerns
1. More than 50% of persons in the United States express positive attitudes toward older adults and persons with disabilities, and yet most really perceive them as "different" and "inferior"
2. Society perceives disabilities, differences, and disease states before recognizing similarities

3. Feelings of guilt, anxiety, apathy, inadequacy, embarrassment, depression, anger, and resentment about special needs interfere with attempts to seek care
4. Fear of or inability to comprehend dental procedures, antisocial or atypical behavior, or dependency on oral health care providers interferes with provision of care
5. Basic daily needs and activities are often overwhelming and can lower the priorities for oral health care
6. Perception of self-image and worth can affect care planning

C. Provider philosophy and provision of care
1. The Americans with Disabilities Act requires that public and private dental offices serve persons with disabilities, that treatment is provided on the same basis as for nondisabled persons, and that dentists make reasonable modifications to facilitate access
2. Despite the Americans with Disabilities Act, surveys indicate that approximately 20% of dentists are unwilling to treat persons who are physically or mentally challenged
3. Reasons given for not treating individuals with special needs include:
   a. Inadequate facilities and equipment
   b. Inadequate training (knowledge and competencies)
   c. Not wanting to expose "normal" clients to "special" clients
   d. Inability to collect adequate fees
   e. Additional effort and time required
   f. Personal discomfort about perceived "differences" of special clients
   g. Treatment of medically complex persons increases insurance premiums

D. Communication and cultural concerns
1. Sensory impairments (hearing, visual) limit the client's ability to transmit and receive communications when scheduling or undergoing oral care or participating in oral health care education
2. The use of technical terminology or inappropriate language level may interfere with understanding
3. Differences in communication styles (eye contact, physical proximity and contact, formal versus informal speech, cultural variations, use of nonverbal cues and verbal language) can impair effective communication
4. Use of condescending voice tones or language levels closes off communication lines
5. Foreign language barrier may deter a client from seeking care or reduce effectiveness of care
6. Inadequate numbers of health care providers possess cross-cultural competence

E. Medical concerns
1. Situations compromising the provider or client
   a. Inadequate infection control procedures
   b. Inadequate or inaccurate health histories
   c. Inadequate precautions for potential emergencies
   d. Inadequate knowledge of systemic conditions and their treatments
F. Mobility and stability concerns
1. Impaired ambulation or use of assistive devices may hinder access to care
2. Uncontrolled or sudden movements may interfere with home care or dental hygiene interventions
3. Uncontrolled or aggressive behavior may endanger the care providers and the client
4. Spatial disorientation may interfere with client relaxation in the dental chair or with oral care procedures

SPECIFIC CONDITIONS

See Chapters 8 and 9.

Intellectual and Developmental Disabilities (IDD)

A. Definition
1. Subaverage intellectual functioning originating during the developmental period and associated with impairment in adaptive behavior (formerly known as *mental retardation*)
2. Not the same as mental illness
3. Label represents a highly heterogeneous group of persons
4. Most common developmental disability
B. Incidence—2% to 3% of the U.S. population (57.7 million total), depending on criteria
C. Categories
1. Mild—IQ 55 to 70 (89%)
2. Moderate—IQ 40 to 54 (6%)
3. Severe—IQ 25 to 39 (3.5%)
4. Profound—IQ below 25 (1.5%)
D. Etiology—acquired (12%), inherited (13%), unknown (75%)
1. Viral infections and toxemias (rubella, meningitis, lead poisoning)
2. Trauma and physical or chemical agents (child abuse; fetal alcohol syndrome)
3. Disorders of metabolism or nutrition (phenylketonuria—PKU)
4. Gross brain disease (atrophy or neoplasms)
5. Genetics

6. Gestational disorders (Rh incompatibility, anoxia, prematurity)
7. Environmental (lack of stimulation)

E. Signs, symptoms, and clinical manifestations
   1. Variable, depending on etiology
   2. Unusual difficulty in learning and applying what is learned to issues of daily living
   3. Skull or other craniofacial anomalies may exist
      a. Microcephaly—small cranium that restricts brain growth
      b. Hydrocephaly—expansion of the cranium from excessive accumulation of cerebrospinal fluid
      c. Malformation or asymmetry of growth
   4. General developmental delays
   5. Other possible manifestations include motor incoordination, visual or hearing disorders, specific learning disabilities, emotional disturbance, medical disabilities, seizure disorders

F. Oral manifestations
   1. Most oral health problems are not inherent to the disability but are related to extrinsic factors (e.g., neglect by caregivers or lack of coordination leading to poor oral disease control)
   2. Decayed-missing-filled surfaces (DMFS) scores comparable with those of the general population, but the "decayed" component may be higher because of lack of professional treatment (Figure 19-1)
   3. Higher prevalence of periodontal conditions, probably related to poor oral hygiene and lack of regular care
   4. Higher incidence of malocclusion and deviations in tooth eruption is associated with craniofacial syndromes or growth abnormalities (Figures 19-2 and 19-3)
   5. Some instances of enamel dysplasia, more commonly seen in those with severe mental deficiencies resulting from severe prenatal or perinatal defects or insults
   6. Some instances of physical self-abuse, if severely impaired

Fetal Alcohol Spectrum Disorders (FASD)

A. Definition—an umbrella term describing a pattern of malformations caused by maternal alcohol consumption during pregnancy, characterized by prenatal and postnatal growth deficiency, dysmorphic facial features, and central nervous system (CNS) dysfunction including fetal alcohol syndrome (FAS), alcohol-related neurodevelopmental disorders (ARND), and partial fetal alcohol syndrome (PFAS)

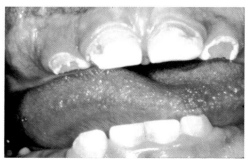

FIGURE 19-1 High incidence of dental caries is common and most likely related to neglect. *(From National Oral Health Information Clearinghouse, National Institute of Dental and Craniofacial Research: Oral conditions in children with special needs: A guide for health care providers, March 2011.)*

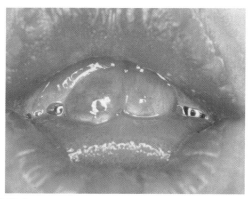

FIGURE 19-2 Delayed tooth eruption is a common oral condition in children with developmental disabilities. *(From National Oral Health Information Clearinghouse, National Institute of Dental and Craniofacial Research: Oral conditions in children with special needs: A guide for health care providers, March 2011.)*

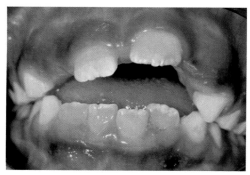

FIGURE 19-3 Malocclusion is a common oral finding in children with developmental disabilities. *(From National Oral Health Information Clearinghouse, National Institute of Dental and Craniofacial Research: Oral conditions in children with special needs: A guide for health care providers, March 2011.)*

B. Incidence and prevalence
   1. Incidence of fetal alcohol spectrum disorders is 1 in 100 live births or 40,000 infants each year in the United States
   2. Leading known preventable cause of mental impairments and birth defects in the United States

C. Etiology
   1. Severity of fetal alcohol effects is dose dependent
   2. Babies with fetal alcohol syndrome are born to women who are "heavy drinkers" during pregnancy (usually at least 45 drinks per month)
   3. Effects related to differences in blood alcohol content and differences in tissue susceptibility
   4. Alcohol affects the cell membrane and cell migration, thus altering the organization of embryonic tissue
   5. The fetal brain is most susceptible during the third trimester
   6. Metabolic disturbances can retard fetal cell division and growth

D. Signs, symptoms, and clinical manifestations
   1. Premature or postnatal (or both) growth retardation—results in short stature, slight build, small head
   2. Craniofacial dysmorphia—short eye openings, short upturned nose, smooth philtrum, flat midface, thin upper lip
   3. Nonspecific abnormalities in any organ system, depending on the time of alcohol insult
   4. Wide IQ range, many within the IDD range
   5. Limited ability to read and write, but with minimal comprehension; also language problems
   6. Poor social judgment and socialization skills
   7. Hyperactivity and short attention span
   8. Heart defects in more than 30%
   9. Skeletal and ear disorders
   10. Excessive hairiness at birth

E. Treatment—depends on specific anomalies and organ systems affected
   1. Surgery, if indicated for heart or other defects
   2. Infant stimulation programs
   3. Appropriate educational and vocational placements
   4. Nutritional and alcohol counseling for family

F. Oral manifestations
   1. The majority of children with IDD have oral problems related to tooth eruption, malformations, or malpositioning of teeth (usually class II or III malocclusion) (Figure 19-4)
   2. Some may have V-shaped or cleft palate
   3. Moderate to severe gingivitis is seen

Down Syndrome

A. Definition and etiology
   1. Mental or intellectual disorder
   2. Associated with an anomaly of chromosome 21 (trisomy 21) in all or some body cells

B. Incidence—most common chromosomal abnormality (1 in 800 live births; but varies with

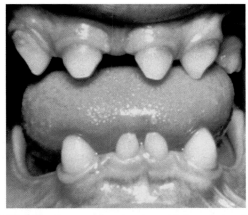

FIGURE 19-4 Tooth anomalies showing variations in eruption patterns and size and shape of the teeth. *(From National Oral Health Information Clearinghouse, National Institute of Dental and Craniofacial Research: Oral conditions in children with special needs: A guide for health care providers, March 2011.)*

maternal age); approximately 400,000 individuals in the United States affected

C. Signs, symptoms, and clinical manifestations
   1. Mild to profound IDD
   2. Poor muscular development, with hyperflexibility and hypotonia during childhood
   3. Short stature, with delay in skeletal maturation
   4. Short neck; extremities with broad stubby fingers
   5. High incidence of congenital heart defects (30% to 50%); language, vision (60%), and hearing problems (75%); risk of leukemia (less than 1% out of 100), thyroid problems, and immunologic defects
   6. Abnormal craniofacial features
      a. Small brachycephalic skull
      b. Round flat facies
      c. Small nasomaxillary complex
      d. Ocular hypotelorism (eyes closer together than normal)
      e. Epicanthal folds
      f. Strabismus (convergent eyes)
      g. Simian crease (single transverse palmar crease)
      h. More susceptible to infection due to poor immune response

D. Oral manifestations (Figure 19-5)
   1. Relative mandibular prognathism as a result of a small nasomaxillary complex
   2. Dry skin and thick, dry, fissured lips
   3. Open mouth posture, with a protrusive, fissured tongue
   4. Hyperplasia of the adenoids and tonsils
   5. Altered salivary gland mechanism (decreased flow)
   6. Increased susceptibility to severe periodontal disease of early onset, especially in anterior

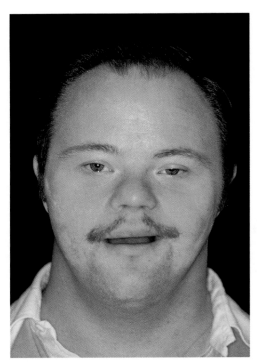

FIGURE 19-5 Common facial characteristics shown in a person with Down syndrome. *(From Regezi J, Sciubba J, Jordan R: Oral pathology: Clinical pathologic correlations, ed 5, St Louis, 2008, Saunders.)*

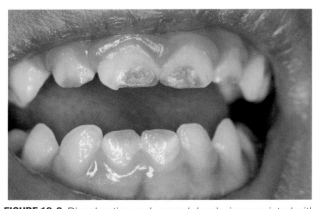

FIGURE 19-6 Discoloration and enamel dysplasia associated with developmental defects. *(From National Oral Health Information Clearinghouse, National Institute of Dental and Craniofacial Research: Oral conditions in children with special needs: A guide for health care providers, March 2011.)*

areas; may be related to host immune defects (e.g., periodontitis as a manifestation of a systemic disease)

7. Delayed eruption of teeth and abnormal tooth development

8. Higher incidence of congenitally missing teeth

9. Small tooth crowns with short crown–root ratio

10. Enamel dysplasia (Figure 19-6)

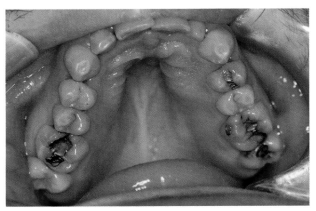

FIGURE 19-7 High-arched palate with decreased width and length. *(From Regezi J, Sciubba J, Jordan R: Oral pathology: Clinical pathologic correlations, ed 5, St Louis, 2008, Saunders.)*

11. Malocclusion—anterior open bite or cross-bite, posterior cross-bite, malocclusion common

12. Attrition

13. High palatal vault (Figure 19-7)

Autism Spectrum Disorders (ASD)

A. Definition
   1. A group of developmental disorders that affect the functioning of the brain, resulting in specific behavioral and communicative difficulties; speech, language and communication, social interaction, sensory impairments, play, and repetition of behaviors are key areas affected
   2. Wide range of symptoms and behaviors with considerable individual variation

B. Incidence and prevalence
   1. Incidence not completely known; prevalence rate of autism is increasing 10% to 17% annually
   2. Unclear if the increase is real or reflects better diagnostic practices
   3. Occurs in as many as 1 in 110 children
   4. Four times more common in males
   5. Appears during the first 3 years of life

C. Etiology—different theories
   1. Psychogenic theories
   2. Genetic theories
   3. Biochemical deficit theories
   4. Neurophysiologic theories

D. Signs, symptoms, and clinical manifestations
   1. Great variability in expression; no standard type
   2. Extreme aloneness; failure to develop eye contact, to cuddle as infants normally do, to develop social relationships, or to perceive others' feelings
   3. Language disturbances—repetitious speech, pronoun reversals, lack of ability to use gestures; failure to develop functional speech in 50%

4. Comprehension problems, especially with verbal directions

5. Obsessiveness about maintaining routines and sameness of the environment (resistance to change)

6. Abnormal response to stimuli; may not respond to pain; or may have constant movement and repetitious activity

7. Sensitivities to sight, hearing, touch, smell, and taste

8. May be aggressive or self-abusive

E. Treatment—variety of approaches tried with varying success

1. Psychotherapy and behavioral therapy

2. Sensory integration

3. Communication therapy

4. Pharmacologic treatments include antipsychotics such as risperidone, stimulants such as methylphenidate hydrochloride (HCl), antidepressants, and tranquilizers

F. Oral manifestations—none directly associated with the syndrome; difficult behaviors, feeding problems, and poor cooperation are challenges to dental care

Attention Deficit Hyperactivity Disorder (ADHD)

A. Definition

1. Developmental and behavioral disorder affecting specific areas of learning or impulse control that can cause problems in acquiring new skills

2. Relates primarily to vision, hearing, language, attention, and touch

B. Incidence and prevalence

1. Much controversy over diagnosis and treatment

2. Occurs in 7.8% of school-aged children; 4.5 million children aged 5 to 17 have been diagnosed in the United States

3. More common in boys

4. Affects up to 50% of adults who had ADHD in childhood

C. Etiology—unknown, but may be related to:

1. Neurologic deficits or neurochemical imbalances

2. Emotional factors

3. Environmental toxins

4. Genetic factors

D. Categories—areas of CNS function affected

1. Input—receiving, recognizing, and decoding messages (e.g., auditory-perceptual or visual-perceptual problems)

2. Organization—information storage, integration with other information, and prompt retrieval (e.g., short-term memory problem)

3. Output—management of movement or utterances (e.g., hyperactivity, apraxia)

E. Signs, symptoms, and clinical manifestations

1. Hyperactivity and inattentiveness

2. Irritability, impulsiveness, and need for immediate satisfaction

3. Problems with concentration and memory

4. Immaturity, clumsiness

5. Lack of sense of direction, position, or time

6. Problems in reading, writing, or math

F. Treatment

1. Behavioral management

2. Socialization training

3. Medications

4. Stimulants, nonstimulant therapy, antidepressants

G. Oral manifestations—none directly associated

Emotional Disturbance and Mental Illness

A. Definition

1. Any disease or condition affecting the brain that impairs thinking, feeling, behavior, or all of these functions

2. Second leading cause of disability and premature death in the United States

B. Incidence and prevalence

1. Approximately 44 million persons in the United States over the age of 18 affected (23% of the population)

2. At some point in life, 10% of all adults will need or benefit from some form of mental health intervention

3. Major depression, bipolar disorder, schizophrenia, and obsessive compulsive disorder are among top 10 leading causes of disability

C. Etiology—depends on the type of disturbance

1. Heredity (genetics)

2. Environmental stressors (e.g., death, divorce, financial problems, dysfunctional family life)

3. Biology (dysfunctional neurotransmitters and neurologic chemical imbalances)

4. Psychological trauma

D. Classifications (three common ones):

1. Psychoneuroses—anxiety, depressive, obsessive, or conversion reactions

2. Personality disorders—situational or adjustment reactions

3. Psychoses—schizophrenia

E. Signs, symptoms, and clinical manifestations (depend on the type of disorder)

1. Inner tensions create anxiety, frustration, fears, and impulsive behavior

2. Examples of behavior
   a. Translation of fears or anxieties into physical symptoms
   b. Regression to earlier forms of behavior
   c. Displays of hostility or aggression
   d. Withdrawal into fantasy (e.g., daydreaming)
   e. Fear of failure and criticism
   f. Development of substitute fears, phobias, or compulsions
F. Oral manifestations
   1. None directly associated
   2. May see intraoral trauma resulting from unusual habits or aggressive behavior
   3. May have xerostomia as a side effect of medications
   4. With compulsive behavior, may have immaculate oral hygiene

Disorders of Eating

See signs and symptoms of disordered eating in the section on "Energy balance and weight control" in Chapter 12.
A. Definition
   1. Anorexia nervosa
      a. Psychophysiologic condition characterized by suppression and denial of sensation of hunger
      b. May be socially isolated and relatively asexual
      c. Consumption of only 300 to 600 calories per day is common
      d. Often come from middle-class to upper-class families with high parental or societal expectations
      e. Perfectionists, competitive, and overachievers
      f. Deny their emaciated appearance
      g. Diagnosis based on person's refusal to maintain normal body weight for height and age; intense fear of becoming fat in spite of being underweight; denial of the seriousness of the starvation and a distorted body image
   2. Anorexia bulimia
      a. Syndrome involving episodic binge eating and purging
      b. Purging involves self-induced vomiting and use of laxatives, diuretics, or enemas
      c. Often occurs after failed attempts to lose weight through dieting
      d. May be of normal weight
      e. Usually outgoing and sexually active
      f. Calories consumed during bingeing range from 3500 to 20,000
      g. Vomiting episodes may last from 5 to 30 minutes
      h. Diagnosis of bulimia if there are at least two bulimic episodes per week for 3 months

B. Incidence and prevalence
   1. 90% are female; 0.6 to 4.5% of the U.S. population suffer from eating disorders in their lifetime
   2. Occurs in 1 in 200 white adolescent females
   3. Occurs in 3% to 20% of college students
   4. Most common age group is 12 to 35 years; also occurs in older adults
   5. 27% to 42% of persons with anorexia indulge in bulimia
   6. 9% mortality rate
C. Etiology—multiple interactive causes
   1. Depressive illnesses
   2. Fear of obesity
   3. Endocrine changes at puberty
   4. Feelings of low self-esteem and poor body image
D. Signs and symptoms
   1. Anorexia nervosa
      a. Intense fear of becoming obese; refusal to maintain normal weight
      b. Disturbance of body image
      c. Weight loss of at least 25% of original body weight not caused by any physical illness
      d. Downy growth of body hair (lanugo)
      e. Periods of overactivity
      f. Dry, flaky skin
      g. Lowered blood pressure, body temperature, and pulse
      h. Episodes of bulimia
      i. Complications include cardiac arrhythmia from reduced heart muscle mass and electrolyte imbalance from dehydration
   2. Anorexia bulimia
      a. Awareness that eating pattern is abnormal
      b. Depression and self-deprecating thoughts
      c. Repeated attempts to lose weight
      d. Recurrent bingeing (rapid intake of food in a short period), usually high-calorie, easily ingested food
      e. Inconspicuous eating
      f. Termination of episodes by purging via self-induced vomiting, laxatives, diuretics, enemas
      g. Weight fluctuation >10 pounds
      h. Dehydration
      i. Electrolyte imbalance
      j. Gastrointestinal disturbances
E. Treatment
   1. Physical stabilization of the seriously compromised patient
   2. Psychological and nutritional counseling
   3. Support groups
   4. Dental treatment
F. Oral manifestations
   1. Esophageal lacerations and chronic sore throat from repeated vomiting
   2. Parotid gland swelling and xerostomia

3. Burning sensation in the tongue
4. Perimyolysis (dental erosion), dentinal hypersensitivity, and margination of amalgams from acid erosion of vomiting; lingual surfaces of maxillary incisors most often affected
5. Rampant caries from high consumption of sucrose, xerostomia, and dehydration
6. Irritated soft tissues from vomiting, dehydration, and vitamin deficiencies
7. Dentinal hypersensitivity and vitamin deficiencies

Alzheimer's Disease

A. Definition
 1. Progressive irreversible brain disorder characterized by intellectual and cognitive disturbance, behavioral changes, and eventually a state of complete dependence
 2. Three types
  a. Early onset—diagnosis before age 65
  b. Late onset—occurs after age 65
  c. Familial—entirely inherited; onset often in the 40s
B. Incidence and prevalence
 1. 5.3 million cases in the United States
 2. Occurs in approximately 13% (5.1 million) of persons age ≥65, 50% of those age ≥85
 3. Occurs in 50% of all nursing home residents
 4. Sixth leading cause of death
C. Etiology
 1. Unknown
 2. Postulated theories
  a. Genetics
  b. Viral agents causing selective cell death
  c. Excessive accumulation of toxic agents
  d. Gene mutations identified on three chromosomes
  e. Age-related changes in the immune system
D. Signs, symptoms, and clinical manifestations—different parts of the brain affected in varying degrees but reflect neuronal degeneration
 1. Early
  a. Memory loss and inability to concentrate
  b. Anxiety, irritability, withdrawal, and petulance
  c. Abnormal sleep patterns
  d. Motor abnormalities, including exaggerated reflexes and gait disturbances
 2. Later
  a. Apathy, depression
  b. Disorientation and lack of judgment and understanding
  c. Incontinence

E. Treatment—no cures at this time
 1. Medications—cholinesterase inhibitors may slow progression
 2. Maintenance of current abilities and reality orientation; placement in structured, stress-free environment
F. Oral manifestations
 1. None specific to the condition
 2. Disease states usually are a result of neglect, the aging process, or any accompanying chronic illnesses

Seizure Disorders

See the section on "Seizures and convulsive disorders" in Chapter 21.
A. Definition
 1. Not a disease; the term is used to describe symptoms of recurrent or chronic brain dysfunction
 2. Characterized by discrete, recurring behavioral manifestations that include disturbances of balance, sensation, behavior, perception, or consciousness
 3. Should not be confused with one-time seizures that result from drug overdoses, brain tumors, or other problems
 4. Seizure—an episode of cerebral dysfunction produced by abnormal excessive neuronal discharge; not necessarily a recurring condition
 5. Convulsion—a broad range of behavioral manifestations, including seizure activity
 6. Aura—a specific sensation preceding a seizure, lasting from one to several seconds and manifested as:
  a. Numbness, tingling
  b. Unusual smell perception
  c. Peculiar sound perception
  d. Feeling of nausea or fear
 7. Status epilepticus
  a. Continuous convulsion lasting longer than 5 minutes
  b. May lead to death from heart failure, kidney failure, or both
  c. Constitutes a medical emergency
B. Incidence and prevalence
 1. Affects almost three million people in the United States
 2. 200,000 new cases of seizure and epilepsy are diagnosed in the United States each year
 3. Prevalence is highest among children, with occurrence of 5.2 to 7.3 per 1000 school-age children
C. Etiology
 1. Prenatal
  a. Maternal infections
  b. Fetal growth abnormalities or prematurity

c. Hormonal imbalances or Rh incompatibility
d. Chromosomal disorders
e. Toxicity or damage from drugs or radiation
f. Genetic influences

2. Perinatal
a. Delivery problems
b. Anoxia

3. Postnatal
a. Degenerative brain disease
b. Injury
c. Tumors
d. Prolonged high fever
e. Parasitic infections
f. Toxic agents (including alcohol and drugs)

4. Unknown

D. Types—can be classified by the origin of the seizure, the cause, or the type of seizure activity

E. Signs, symptoms, and clinical manifestations
1. Generalized tonic-clonic (grand mal)
a. May experience an aura
b. Loss of consciousness
c. Tonic movements (voluntary muscles experience continuous contractions)
d. Clonic movements (intermittent muscular contraction and relaxation)
e. Interruption of respiration and dilation of pupils
f. Loss of bladder or bowel control
g. Seizure activity usually lasts 1 to 3 minutes
h. Lethargy and disorientation follow the return of consciousness
i. May occur any time during the day or only during sleep

2. Generalized absence (petit mal)
a. Transient loss of consciousness
b. May have minor motor movements of the eyes, head, or extremities
c. Lasts 5 to 30 seconds
d. Person may not be aware of having had a seizure

3. Complex partial (psychomotor)
a. May be preceded by an aura
b. Transient clouding of the consciousness
c. Behavioral alterations
d. Purposeless, repetitive, and stereotypical movements or actions
e. Changes in affect or perception
f. May become antisocial
g. Person usually does not remember the incident

4. Mixed

F. Treatment
1. Drug therapy (70% of cases)
a. 50% of all patients with epilepsy gain complete control of seizures for substantial periods. 20% enjoy significant reduction in the number of seizures experienced
b. One or more anticonvulsants, for example, phenytoin (Dilantin), phenobarbital (Luminal), ethosuximide (Zarontin), valproic acid (Depakote), topiramate (Topamax), levetiracetam (Keppra), trimethadione (Tridione), carbamazepine (Tegretol)
c. Common side effects
(1) Drug-induced gingival enlargement (phenytoin)
(2) Drowsiness and headaches
(3) Vision and gait disturbances
(4) Loss of appetite, nausea
(5) Blood dyscrasias

2. Surgery
3. Avoidance of precipitating factors (fatigue, stress, abnormal sensory stimuli, drugs, inadequate medication compliance)

G. Oral manifestations
1. Orofacial trauma—lips, tongue, buccal mucosa, teeth, facial bones, or jawbone
2. Drug-induced gingival enlargement from phenytoin (Figure 19-8)
a. More marked in anterior regions and facial surfaces
b. Does not occur in edentulous areas
c. Correlated with poor oral hygiene
d. Characteristically pale, pink, and fibrous
e. Aesthetic concerns caused by gingival enlargement
f. Severe gingival enlargement may displace teeth, create malocclusion, and compromise aesthetics
g. Superimposed inflammation occurs from food retention or mouth breathing
h. Can sometimes be alleviated through meticulous oral hygiene, surgery, or pressure appliances

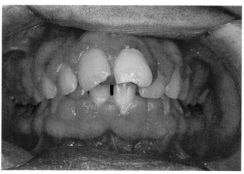

FIGURE 19-8 Drug-induced gingival enlargement associated with medication taken to control seizures. *(From Regezi J, Sciubba J, Jordan R: Oral pathology: Clinical pathologic correlations, ed 5, St Louis, 2008, Saunders.)*

Visual Impairment

A. Definition
  1. Visual impairment—when visual acuity in the best eye is no better than 20/200 after correction or if central or peripheral vision impairment is present
  2. Legally blind—visual acuity of less than 20/200 with correction
B. Incidence and prevalence
  1. Approximately 0.6 in 1000 persons in the United States is legally or totally blind
  2. Visual impairments occur in 12.2 in 1000 persons under age 18
  3. Five million persons in the United States > age 65 have severe visual impairments
  4. Leading cause of vision loss in the 25-to-74-year age group is diabetic retinopathy
C. Etiology—congenital, perinatal, postnatal, aging
  1. Trauma
  2. Disease (infections, inflammation, toxicity)
  3. Structural or developmental defects
    a. Nearsighted
    b. Farsighted
    c. Astigmatism
  4. Retrolental fibroplasia—high concentration of oxygen in the incubators of premature infants causes hemorrhage of retinal blood vessels, scarring, and retinal detachment
  5. Macular degeneration (loss of central vision)
  6. Retinitis pigmentosa—night blindness and loss of peripheral vision
  7. Diabetic retinopathy—retinal hemorrhages
  8. Glaucoma—failure of liquid in the eye to drain, resulting in increased pressure, pain, and destruction of the optic nerve
  9. Cataracts—clouding and opacity of the lens blocking light perception (mainly associated with aging or congenital problems)
D. Signs, symptoms, and clinical manifestations
  1. Wears glasses or contact lenses
  2. Awkward ambulation or bumping into objects
  3. Eye pain
  4. Constant tearing
  5. Unusual squinting or blinking
  6. Use of a guide dog or cane
  7. Deliberate, slow actions
  8. Attention to details and orderliness
  9. Cloudy or fuzzy vision
  10. Problems with glare
  11. Double vision
E. Treatment
  1. Cataracts—surgery: lens implants; contact lenses; cataract glasses
  2. Glaucoma—drugs or surgery
  3. Laser treatment
  4. Special education—auditory instruction and training in use of tactile senses (Braille)
  5. Corrective devices—telescopic or microscopic lenses
  6. Adaptive aids—large-print books, nonoptical filters
  7. Prevention—use of safety glasses, regular examinations
F. Oral manifestations
  1. No particular dental problems
  2. Gingivitis, if the person cannot see the gingiva to monitor gingival health
  3. Trauma to the orofacial area if the person experiences frequent accidents or falls

Hearing Impairment

A. Definition
  1. Hearing impairment—defective but functional hearing
  2. Deaf—unable to understand speech, even with the use of an aid
  3. Frequency—length of the sound wave (vibrations per second, or cycles per second [cps]; human range is 16,000 to 30,000 cps)
  4. Intensity—measured in decibels (dB); human range is 1 to 100 dB
B. Incidence and prevalence
  1. Approximately 31.5 million deaf and hearing-impaired persons in the United States (10% of the population); 66% of the affected are age ≥65; 1 in 6 persons aged 41 to 59 have a hearing impairment
  2. Two to three cases of congenital hearing loss in 1000 live births
  3. Hearing loss is associated with a number of other disabling conditions
    a. Cleft palate (90%)
    b. Cerebral palsy (20%)
    c. Down syndrome (70%)
  4. Environmental causes are increasing
C. Classifications—usually by severity of loss, as measured in decibel loss (Table 19-3)
D. Types of hearing loss (Table 19-4)
  1. Conductive hearing loss
    a. Injury or disease interferes with organs that conduct sound waves through the outer or middle ear
    b. Usually consistent over the entire range of sound
    c. The person benefits most from the use of a hearing aid (sound conducted by bone)
    d. Speech is soft and low; the person hears own voice louder than those of others
    e. Most commonly caused by obstruction of the ear canal by cerumen or a foreign object,

TABLE 19-3 Hearing Loss and Probable Outcomes

Classification	Loss (dB)	Hearing Status Without Amplification (Hearing Aid)
Normal range	0–15	All speech sounds
Slight loss	15–25	Hears vowel sounds clearly; may miss unvoiced consonant sounds
Mild loss	25–40	Hears only louder-voiced speech sounds
Moderate loss	40–65	Misses most speech at normal conversational level
Severe loss	65–95	Misses all speech at normal conversational level
Profound loss	>95+	Hears no speech or sounds

TABLE 19-4 Types of Hearing Problems

Type of Problem	Characteristics
Acoustic neurinoma	Benign tumor of the auditory nerve; causes gradual hearing loss, tinnitus, and dizziness
Mastoiditis	Inflammation of the air cells of the mastoid
Ménière's disease	Condition of the inner ear characterized by hearing loss, tinnitus, and vertigo
Otitis media	Inflammation of the middle ear caused by infection
Otosclerosis	Disease characterized by formation of spongy bone in bone surrounding the inner ear; results in gradual loss of hearing
Presbycusis	Progressive hearing loss that occurs with age
Tinnitus	Sensation of sound in the head (e.g., roaring, hissing, buzzing)
Transient	Temporary hearing shifts associated with noise exposure

perforated eardrum, otitis media, otosclerosis, or congenital malformations of the ear
   2. Sensorineural hearing loss
      a. Malfunction of organs that perceive sound (the sensory hair cells of the inner ear, the auditory nerve, the auditory center in the brain)
      b. Most common causes—aging process (presbycusis), hereditary disease, noise damage, childhood viral infections, skull fractures, intracranial tumors, oxytoxic drugs, and Rh incompatibility
      c. Involves loss of sensitivity and acuity in one or more frequencies (usually higher frequencies and consonants)
      d. If the individual wears a hearing aid, sound is conducted by air
      e. Speech is loud; the person cannot hear own voice
   3. Mixed hearing loss
      a. Combination of both conductive and sensorineural hearing problems
      b. Same causative factors as found in conductive and sensorineural hearing loss
   4. Central hearing loss
      a. Damage to the nuclei of the CNS in the brain
      b. Most commonly caused by pathologic conditions such as brain tumor, vascular deprivation of the inner ear, stroke, or erythroblastosis fetalis
E. Etiology
   1. Prenatal or congenital
      a. Genetic defects
      b. Infections (rubella accounts for 20% of congenital types), influenza, and syphilis
      c. Rh incompatibility
      d. Certain drugs, for example, thalidomide, streptomycin, aspirin, erythromycin, kanamycin, neomycin, indomethacin (Indocin), furosemide (Lasix)
      e. Unknown causes (10% to 20% of cases)
      f. Environmental noise (more than 30% of cases)
   2. Acquired
      a. Infections (e.g., mumps, measles, poliomyelitis, chronic serous otitis media)
      b. Hereditary conditions
      c. Trauma
      d. Chronic use of certain drugs (e.g., aspirin, streptomycin)
      e. Noise exposure
      f. Pathology (e.g., brain tumor, stroke)
F. Signs, symptoms, and clinical manifestations
   1. May lip-read or focus attention on other facial or nonverbal expressions (speechreading); but can generally only understand 26% to 40% of what is said
   2. Speech may be characterized by aberrant modulations, pronunciations, or grammatical structures
   3. May use sign language (American Sign Language [ASL]) or finger spelling (American or manual alphabet)
   4. May turn the head to one side if the loss is unilateral

5. May frequently ask others to repeat phrases or may provide an unrelated response to a question or comment

6. May not acknowledge having hearing loss

7. May fail to respond to conversation

G. Treatment

  1. Depends on the person's age at onset and type and cause of impairment

  2. Approaches

   a. Surgery

   b. Cochlear implants and infrared and frequency-modulating (FM) devices

   c. Hearing aid types

    (1) Conventional analog,

    (2) Analog programmable, and

    (3) Digital processing

   d. Hearing aid models—in-the-ear (ITE) or behind-the-ear (BTE), body, in-the-canal (ITC), or completely-in-the-canal (CIC)

   e. Education for development of communication skills

   f. Direct stimulation of the auditory nerve

H. Prevention of hearing loss

  1. Use of hearing protection devices (e.g., earplugs) to decrease noise exposure

  2. Prompt treatment of ear infections

  3. Reduction of risk of atherosclerotic plaque, which can affect blood flow to the inner ear

I. Oral manifestations

  1. Not generally seen with hearing impairments unless associated with a syndrome (e.g., rubella syndrome)

  2. Prematurity or rubella may result in enamel dysplasia

  3. Bruxism may be evident

Cleft Lip or Palate

A. Definition—disturbances in embryologic formation resulting in incomplete closure of the lip, the palatal area, or both

B. Incidence and prevalence

  1. Occurs in 1 in 1000 Caucasian live births in the United States; twice as common in Asian Americans; half as common in African Americans

  2. One of the most common congenital malformations of the face and mouth

  3. Cleft lip more common in males; cleft palate more common in females

  4. 1 in 2000 babies born with cleft palate, but without cleft lip

C. Classifications of cleft involvement

  1. Tip of the uvula

  2. Bifid uvula

  3. Soft palate

  4. Soft and hard palates

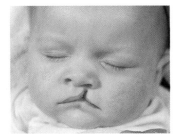

FIGURE 19-9 Cleft lip. *(From Regezi J, Sciubba J, Jordan R: Oral pathology: Clinical pathologic correlations, ed 5, St Louis, 2008, Saunders.)*

  5. Unilateral lip and palate (Figure 19-9)

  6. Bilateral lip and palate

D. Etiology

  1. Genetic in most cases

  2. Other risk factors include maternal nutritional deficiencies, alcohol use, infectious diseases, and smoking during pregnancy

  3. Cleft lip occurs during gestational weeks 4 to 7

  4. Cleft palate occurs during gestational weeks 8 to 12

  5. Folic acid supplementation for the mother during pregnancy may reduce risk

E. Signs, symptoms, and associated problems

  1. Oral–facial deformities

  2. Ear disease with resultant hearing loss

  3. Speech difficulties are a major disability caused by:

   a. Palatal insufficiency

   b. Missing or malpositioned teeth

   c. Hearing loss

  4. Feeding problems

  5. Predisposition to upper respiratory tract infections

F. Treatment

  1. Surgery—multiple operations at various developmental stages

  2. Taking of impression and insertion of an obturator or other appliance, if needed, for feeding or speech; appliance will need to be remade according to growth pattern

  3. Speech therapy

  4. Antibiotics to prevent infections

  5. Orthodontics

G. Oral manifestations

  1. High incidence of missing or maldeveloped teeth in the line of the cleft usually affects lateral incisors

  2. High incidence of malocclusion resulting from structural defects

  3. Oral–motor dysfunction

  4. Scar tissue from surgery

Cerebral Palsy

A. Definition—static, nonprogressive neuromuscular condition comprising a series of syndromes that result from damage to the brain

B. Incidence—approximately 800,000 persons in the United States have some degree of cerebral palsy; 2 to 3 out of 1000 babies are born with cerebral palsy; 40% to 50% of children born with cerebral palsy were premature, low birth weight, or both

C. Etiology
   1. Prenatal—genetic or congenitally acquired (e.g., anoxia, infections, alcohol or drug abuse, Rh incompatibility, metabolic disturbances, lack of folic acid)
   2. Natal—anoxia, hemorrhage
   3. Postnatal—head injury, infections, neoplasms, anoxia

D. Classification
   1. Motor disorders
      a. Spasticity (50% to 75%)—slight stimulus causes exaggerated muscle contraction; stiff and jerky movements
      b. Athetosis (15% to 25%)—muscles contract involuntarily; difficulty bringing the body to the upright position
      c. Ataxia (10%)—muscles respond to a stimulus but cannot complete a contraction; low muscle tone and poor coordination
      d. Hypotonia (<10%)—unable to respond to a volitional stimulus
      e. Rigidity (<10%)—increased initial muscle resistance; gives way with little force
      f. Mixed (5% to 20%)—two or more types appearing in the same person
   2. Limbs involved
      a. Monoplegic—one limb
      b. Hemiplegic—both limbs on the same side of the body
      c. Paraplegic—lower limbs
      d. Diplegic—like-parts on either side of the body (e.g., both lower limbs or both upper limbs)
      e. Quadriplegic—all four limbs
      f. Triplegic—three limbs

E. Signs, symptoms, and clinical manifestations (Figure 19-10)
   1. Characterized by paralysis, weakness, muscle spasms, incoordination, or other aberrations of motor function, especially involving voluntary muscles
   2. Joint immobility and contractures increase with age
   3. Retained primitive reflexes (e.g., asymmetrical or symmetrical tonic neck reflex)
   4. Other associated conditions

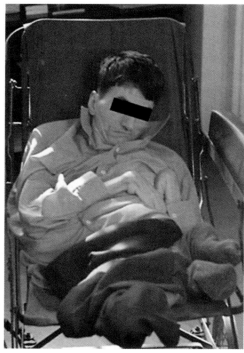

FIGURE 19-10 Person with spastic-type cerebral palsy, in which limbs are in a severe flexed posture. *(From Porter SR, et al: Medicine and surgery for dentistry, Philadelphia, 1999, Churchill Livingstone. In Darby M, Walsh M: Dental hygiene theory and practice, ed 3, Philadelphia, 2010, Saunders, p. 905.)*

      a. Speech and language disorders (60%)
      b. Hearing disorders (20%)
      c. Visual defects (40%)
      d. IDD (40%)
      e. Seizures (40%)
   5. Wide range of limitations, from mild to totally dependent

F. Treatment
   1. Magnesium sulfate may prevent the disorder in low-birth-weight babies
   2. Surgery for contractures
   3. Supportive therapies (physical therapy, occupational therapy, speech therapy)
   4. Assistive devices (braces, wheelchairs, walkers, mouth sticks, augmentative communication devices, voice synthesizers)
   5. Medications for control of seizures, muscle relaxation, and other manifestations
   6. Special education, if needed

G. Oral manifestations—marked variation among individuals
   1. Higher incidence of bruxism (Figure 19-11), dental caries, enamel dysplasia, malocclusion, and periodontal diseases
   2. Drug-induced gingival enlargement if phenytoin is used

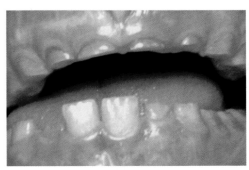

FIGURE 19-11 Example of extreme bruxism in a child with a developmental disability. *(From National Oral Health Information Clearinghouse, National Institute of Dental and Craniofacial Research: Oral conditions in children with special needs: A guide for health care providers, March 2011.)*

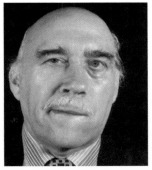

FIGURE 19-13 Person with Bell's palsy, in which the left side of the face is paralyzed. *(From Trend P, Swash M, Kennard C: Neurology: Color guide, Edinburgh, 1998, Churchill Livingstone. In: Darby ML, Walsh MM: Dental hygiene theory and practice, ed 3, St Louis, 2003, Saunders.)*

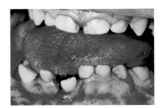

FIGURE 19-12 Example of oral trauma. *(From National Oral Health Information Clearinghouse, National Institute of Dental and Craniofacial Research: Oral conditions in children with special needs: A guide for health care providers, March 2011.)*

3. Oral–motor dysfunction (e.g., impaired swallowing), mouth breathing
4. Temporomandibular joint (TMJ) disorders
5. Increased gag reflex
6. Drooling
7. Trauma resulting from incoordination and frequent falls (Figure 19-12)
8. Attrition and possible TMJ disturbances from mouth sticks
9. Increased dental caries as a result of surgery to control saliva and drooling

Bell's Palsy

A. Definition—paralysis of facial muscles that are innervated by cranial nerve VII (facial nerve)
B. Incidence and prevalence
  1. 40,000 persons in the United States are affected annually
  2. After age 50; more common in males
C. Etiology
  1. Unknown
  2. Associated with bacterial and viral infections (herpes simplex), trauma from oral extractions, or surgery on the parotid gland

D. Signs, symptoms, and clinical manifestations (Figure 19-13)
  1. Abrupt paralysis without preceding pain
  2. Occurs unilaterally
  3. Corner of the mouth droops, causing drooling
  4. Eyelids will not close; lower eyelid droops; predisposes the eyes to infections
  5. Speech and chewing are difficult
  6. Spontaneous remission may occur in 2 to 8 weeks, or permanent paralysis
E. Treatment
  1. Corticosteroid therapy
  2. Heat and massage to maintain circulation and muscle tone
  3. Eyedrops or eye shield to prevent infections
  4. Surgery, if needed
F. Oral manifestations—oral–motor difficulties can cause food retention and the potential for increased caries or gingivitis

Myasthenia Gravis

A. Definition—autoimmune neuromuscular disease characterized by variable weakness or fatigue of striated, voluntary muscles
B. Incidence and prevalence
  1. Most commonly affects women under age 40
  2. If late onset after 60, men affected more often
  3. Affects approximately 2 in 10,000 persons
C. Etiology—autoimmune mechanism causing a defect in nerve impulse transmission at the neuromuscular junction
D. Signs, symptoms, and clinical manifestations
  1. First symptoms usually affect muscles of the eyes (blurred or double vision, drooping of one or both eyelids, weakness of muscles affecting the eyeball, facial expression, mastication, and swallowing)

2. Breathing and speech are disturbed (weak, muffled voice)
3. Fatigue and weakness of muscles vary widely but tend to be worse at the end of the day
4. Myasthenic crisis—weakness affects muscles that control breathing; usually transient but life threatening
   a. Precipitated by:
      (1) Emotional excitement, stress
      (2) Surgical procedures
      (3) Fatigue or loss of sleep
      (4) Infections
   b. Symptoms
      (1) Unable to clear secretions from the throat
      (2) Impaired breathing; assisted ventilation may be needed
      (3) Double vision

E. Treatment
1. Up to 20% of persons with myasthenia gravis may have remission of symptoms with no treatment; another 20% may improve with no treatment
2. Cholinergic drug therapy that blocks the action of cholinesterase at the myoneural junction, for example, neostigmine bromide (Prostigmin), pyridostigmine bromide (Mestinon), ambenonium chloride (Mytelase) (see the section on "Autonomic nervous system agents" in Chapter 11)
3. Thymectomy may lead to partial remission
4. Corticosteroids, immunosuppressive drugs, or adrenocorticotropic hormone (ACTH)
5. Plasma exchange to remove autoantibodies
6. High-dose intravenous (IV) immunoglobulin (Ig)

F. Medications that may cause muscle weakness and which must therefore be avoided:
1. β-blockers
2. D-penicillamine
3. α–interferon
4. Calcium channel blockers

G. Oral manifestations
1. Oral–motor dysfunction
2. Retention of food increases susceptibility to dental caries and periodontal problems
3. Weakness of masticatory muscles causes the mouth to continuously hang open
4. Chewing and swallowing difficulties
5. Furrowed and flaccid appearance of the tongue

Parkinson's Disease

A. Definition—progressive disorder of the CNS causing loss of postural reflexes, slowness of spontaneous movement, tremors, and muscle rigidity

B. Incidence and prevalence
1. Develops between ages 40 and 60
2. At age ≥60, 1 in 100 persons affected
3. Higher incidence in men than in women (2 to 1)
4. Approximately 1.5 million persons in the United States affected; four million worldwide

C. Etiology
1. Cause unknown
2. Imbalance of dopamine and acetylcholine

D. Signs, symptoms, and clinical manifestations
1. Mild, diffuse muscular pain
2. Tremors of the extremities, occurring mainly at rest
3. Shuffling, slow gait, with arms held to the side
4. Slurred, indistinct speech
5. Staring, mask-like facial expression
6. Excessive salivation or dryness of mouth (side effects of medications)
7. Intellect not usually affected
8. Tremors in the lips, tongue, or neck; difficulty swallowing; can lead to aspiration
9. Feelings of stiffness and rigidity (particularly of the large joints)
10. Sensitivity to heat

E. Treatment
1. Medications (see discussion about anticholinergic agents in the section on "Parasympathomimetic (cholinergic) agents" in Chapter 11)
   a. Levodopa or combination of levodopa and carbidopa (Sinemet) to alleviate dopamine deficiency, tremors, and rigidity
   b. Bromocriptine mesylate (Parlodel) and pergolide mesylate (Peramax) mimic the action of dopamine with fewer side effects than with levodopa
   c. Anticholinergic agents for rigidity
   d. Antispasmodic agents for tremors
2. Physical and occupational therapy
3. Surgery
4. Clinical trials for new therapies, including fetal brain cell transplants, are ongoing

F. Oral manifestations
1. Impaired oral–motor functions and home care skills may increase the incidence of dental caries, periodontal disease, and perioral skin irritation
2. Side effects of medications (e.g., xerostomia) may increase the incidence of dental caries and periodontal disease and negatively affect dental prosthesis retention
3. Rigidity and tremors can induce orofacial pain, TMJ discomfort, and trauma to soft and hard tissues

TABLE 19-5 Characteristics of Arthritis

	Osteoarthritis	Rheumatoid (Adult Type)	Rheumatoid (Juvenile Type)
Etiology	Unknown or from trauma, infection, or joint abnormality	Cause unknown; theories include autoimmunity, hereditary or psychosomatic factors, and infection	Same as adult type
Sites affected	Weight-bearing joints (hips, knees, vertebrae)	First affects fingers, hands, and knees; TMJ later	Involves many joints, especially fingers, knees, wrists, vertebrae, and TMJ
Signs and symptoms	Pain, aggravated by temperature changes; joint stiffness after inactivity; develops gradually; swelling rare; does not usually limit range of motion	Fatigue, loss of appetite, low-grade fever, migratory joint pain and swelling, stiffness after periods of inactivity, paresthesia, subcutaneous nodules, joint deformities, TMJ involvement, muscle atrophy near joints	Joint enlargement, stiffness, and pain; onset is acute with fever, rash, spleen and lymph node enlargement, tachycardia, and limited oral opening

TMJ, temporomandibular joint.

Arthritis

A. Definition
   1. Term used to describe more than 100 disorders that cause pain in the joints and connective tissue
   2. Joint inflammation
   3. The term *polyarthritis* refers to the involvement of many joints
B. Major types (Table 19-5)
   1. Osteoarthritis (affects 21 million adults in the United States)
   2. Rheumatoid (adult type) (affects three million adults)
   3. Rheumatoid (juvenile type)
   4. Others include gout, fibromyalgia, ankylosing spondylitis, lupus
C. Incidence and prevalence: common in all age groups
   1. One in five adults in the United States is affected
   2. Affects more than 22% of the U.S. population
   3. Affects 55% of the population age ≥65
   4. More common in women than in men
D. Etiology (see Table 19-5)
   1. Cause unknown
   2. Theories
E. Signs, symptoms, and clinical manifestations— these affect various sites in different ways; most are chronic (see Table 19-5)
F. Treatment
   1. Primarily involves relief of pain and maintenance of function
   2. Medications
      a. Nonsteroidal anti-inflammatory drugs (NSAIDs)
      b. Steroids
      c. Immunosuppressive medications
   3. Physical therapy and exercise to increase range of motion and prevent deformities
   4. Application of heat or hydrotherapy
   5. Surgery—joint replacement
G. Oral manifestations
   1. Bruxism and occlusal imbalances
   2. TMJ pain and limited ability to open the mouth
   3. Masking of inflammation by prolonged steroid therapy
   4. Malocclusion in the juvenile type
   5. Delayed healing with long-term aspirin therapy
   6. Mucosal ulcerations or secondary oral infections (especially of the gingiva) if gold salts are administered

Multiple Sclerosis

A. Definition—chronic degenerative disease of the CNS
   1. Myelin is destroyed through the formation of sclerotic tissue called *plaque*
   2. Nerve impulses to the brain are disrupted or not transmitted
   3. Scattered plaque accumulation causes inflammation and widespread and varied symptoms with periods of exacerbation and remission
B. Incidence and prevalence
   1. Approximately 500,000 persons affected in the United States; over 2.5 million worldwide
   2. Varies geographically; more common in northern regions

TABLE 19-6 Symptoms Associated with Lesions in the Central Nervous System

Location of Lesions	Possible Symptoms
Spinal cord	Numbness Loss of sensitivity in appendages Sensitivity to heat Unsteady gait; muscle stiffness Loss of strength in the legs Impaired eye–hand coordination resulting in difficulty in fine-motor movements
Brain stem	Blurred vision, double vision, or both Difficulty in swallowing or chewing Diminished gag reflex Slurred speech
Cerebrum (lesions in the cerebrum usually occur in the later stages of the disease process)	Disruptions in thinking Euphoria Depression Disruptions in behavior

From Lange BM, Enwistle BM, Lipson LF: Dental management of the handicapped: Approaches for dental auxiliaries, Philadelphia, 1983, Lea & Febiger.

3. Two to three times more common in women than in men
4. Onset occurs at any age, but usually between ages 20 and 50
C. Etiology
  1. Unknown, although genetic markers have been found
  2. Possibly an autoimmune reaction or associated with viral infections
D. Signs and symptoms
  1. Result from the location of lesions (Table 19-6)
  2. Precipitating factors
    a. Infections
    b. Stress and emotional trauma
    c. Injury
    d. Heavy exercise and fatigue
    e. Pregnancy
    f. Heat
  3. Periods of remission in some; chronic progression in others
  4. Death is usually the result of an infection
E. Treatment
  1. Currently no cure; treatment for reduction of symptoms and inflammation
  2. Physical and occupational therapies
  3. Alternating periods of rest and exercise
  4. Medications
    a. Corticosteroids used to control relapses
    b. Muscle relaxants to control spasms

  c. Pain medications and antidepressants to control pain and abnormal sensations
F. Oral manifestations
  1. Most are the result of poor oral hygiene or the side effects of drugs
    a. Ulcerations
    b. Xerostomia
    c. Drug-induced gingival enlargement (phenytoin administered for pain)
  2. Facial pain and TMJ dysfunction and pain

Muscular Dystrophies

A. Definition—group of progressive chronic diseases of the skeletal (striated) muscles characterized by the degeneration of muscle cells with replacement by fat or fibrous tissue
B. Incidence and prevalence
  1. Affects approximately 220,000 persons in the United States
  2. Two thirds of cases are children; 400 to 600 males are born with this disease each year in the United States
C. Etiology—inherited; defective gene leading to a protein abnormality
D. Types (Table 19-7)
  1. Duchenne's disease
  2. Limb-girdle
  3. Facio-scapulo-humeral
  4. Myotonic
E. Signs, symptoms, and clinical manifestations—vary by site and type (see Table 19-7)
F. Treatment—goal is to maintain the person's activity and involvement; no cure has been found yet
  1. Surgery for contracted tendons
  2. Medications—corticosteroids
  3. Orthopedic devices
  4. Nutritional counseling, if the person is overweight
  5. Physical therapy involves muscle-stretching exercises and use of adaptive aids to:
    a. Improve muscle strength
    b. Prevent and correct contractures
    c. Increase efficiency in the activities of daily living
  6. Speech therapy, if needed
G. Oral manifestations
  1. Weakness in masticatory muscles leads to decreased maxillary biting force
  2. Higher incidence of mouth breathing, open bite, and overexpansion of the maxilla
  3. In facio-scapulo-humeral type, the lips appear thick because of involvement of the orbicularis oris muscle
  4. Increase in dental disease if oral hygiene has been neglected

TABLE 19-7 Types and Characteristics of Muscular Dystrophies

	Duchenne's	Limb-Girdle	Facio-scapulo-humeral	Myotonic
Onset	Mainly affects boys; occurs before age 10	Occurs later (average age 20); affects both males and females	Males and females equally affected; usually occurs around puberty	Both sexes affected; appears in early adulthood
Severity	Most severe and destructive form	Slower progression in most cases	Least destructive and progresses at slower rate; least common type	Weakening spreads steadily; shortened lifespan
Etiology	Sex-linked recessive trait with high mutation rate	Autosomal recessive trait	Autosomal dominant trait	Autosomal dominant trait
Sites affected	Pelvis, abdomen, hip, and spine affected first; spreads to trunk, extremities, and myocardium (cranial nerves not affected); osteoporosis also noted	Initial weakness in pelvic girdle, then in shoulder	Facial muscles affected first; weakness is asymmetrical; progresses to shoulder girdle and upper arm	Weakness of lower legs and arms and facial muscles
Limitations	Becomes confined to wheelchair and bed within a few years of diagnosis; may develop scoliosis, obesity, and cardiopulmonary problems; death usually occurs during adolescence	May be severely disabled by midlife, with decreased lifespan	May remain in a state of indefinite remission, with some people living symptom-free, normal lifespan	Walking difficult; may be severely disabled; cataracts may develop
Signs and symptoms	Clumsiness, frequent falls resulting from precarious balance, toe-walking, weakness of hips, lordosis, cramping of legs and abdomen, Gowers' sign, enlargement of calves, decreased stamina	Begins as pain after exercise; then total muscle involvement	Mask-like, wrinkle-free, expressionless facial features; difficulty in closing eyes; muscles above elbow atrophy, below elbow are normal (Popeye effect); difficulty in raising arms	Stiffness, drooping eyelids and jaw, frequent tripping and falling

Spinal Cord Injuries

A. Definition
  1. Fracture, dislocation, hyperextension, compression, or severance of components of the spinal column
  2. Occurs most often in the cervical and lumbar curves
  3. Cord damage can occur above or below the level of bone injury
B. Incidence and prevalence
  1. Affects approximately 450,000 persons in the United States
  2. Approximately 14,000 new cases per year
  3. 82% of cases are males between ages 16 and 30
C. Etiology—acquired injury from accidents
  1. Automobile or motorcycle accidents cause 50% of injuries
  2. Occupational accidents cause 25% of injuries
  3. Sporting accidents cause 18% of injuries
  4. Falls, gunshot wounds, or other trauma cause 7% of injuries

D. Signs, symptoms, and clinical manifestations
  1. Depend on severity and level of injury
  2. Prognosis
    a. First-aid measures performed at the site of the accident
    b. Type and level of injury to the spinal cord
    c. Survival is increasing with advances in emergency care and rehabilitation
    d. Restoration of function still very limited
  3. *Paraplegia* refers to an injury below the cervical level that results in paralysis of the lower portion of the body
  4. *Quadriplegia* refers to an injury occurring in the cervical region that results in paralysis of all four limbs and the trunk
  5. Most frequent cause of death is kidney stones or infection
  6. Functional limitations and specific manifestations depend on the level of the lesion (Tables 19-8 and 19-9)

TABLE 19-8 Clinical Manifestations of Spinal Cord Injuries

Area Affected	Clinical Manifestations
Muscles (limb and trunk)	Innervation and perception of pain and touch disturbed; leads to muscle atrophy Concerns for safety around varying temperatures Formation of decubitus ulcers (pressure sores) caused by breakdown of tissue from immobilization, bruises, or braces Decreased or absent self-care skills Spasticity and tremors Adaptive equipment required, especially for: — Wrist stability — Pencil grasp — Arm movements
Respiration	Intercostal muscles may be paralyzed, resulting in need for diaphragmatic breathing or tracheostomy and total or partial dependence on a respirator
Bowel and bladder	Limited innervation, resulting in incontinence and encopresis or retention Can lead to infections, particularly of kidneys Autonomic hyper-reflexia can occur (medical emergency) Caused by sudden constriction of blood vessels Symptoms—rapid increase in blood pressure (e.g., 280/80 mmHg), low pulse, pounding headache, skin blotching and sweating above site of injury, cold goose bumps below site of injury
Bones/joints	Contractures from spasticity and immobilization Heterotopic ossifications (bony accumulations) may develop around joints
Metabolism	Regulation of body temperature impaired
Social and emotional status	Problems associated with coping with a debilitating acquired injury May experience stages of shock, denial, anger, depression, mobilization, and coping

TABLE 19-9 Functional Significance of Cervical, Thoracic, and Lumbar Lesion Levels

Lesion Level	Functional Expectations for Complete Lesions
Cervical Lesions	
C–1–3	Respirator dependent; totally dependent
C–4	Incapable of voluntary function in arms, trunk, or legs; poor respiratory reserve; totally dependent
C–5	Can stabilize and rotate neck; has function of rhomboids and deltoids, allowing some shoulder movement, elbow flexion; biceps and brachioradialis partially innervated
C–6	Can move shoulders well; strong elbow flexion; wrist muscles allow weak closure of hand; can use large-handled, lightweight objects; can sit up in bed with help and roll over; still needs attendant; can drive van with hand controls
C–7	Can lift own body weight; can use hands, which are weak and lack dexterity; can eat independently, with some assistance; confined to wheelchair; can live independently and manage self-care in a wheelchair- accessible environment without attendant
Thoracic Lesions	
T–1	Independent in bed, self-care (short of lifting weights); lacks trunk stability, respiratory reserve, and trunk fixation of arm prime movers
T–6	Capable of heavy lifting (because of thoracic musculature); increased respiratory reserve; independent transfers, self-application of braces
T–12	Can ambulate with crutches and braces, but still uses wheelchair as primary means of mobility
Lumbar Lesions	
L–4	Complete independence in all phases of self-care and ambulation—usually aided by crutches or canes

From Schubert MM, Snow M, Stiefel DJ: DECOD series: Dental management of patients with CNS and neurologic impairment: Spinal cord injury, Seattle, 1989, University of Washington.

E. Treatment
   1. Four phases of rehabilitation
      a. Physical—functional exercises to increase specific skills
      b. Equipment—selection of adaptive devices to allow for maximum independence
      c. Environment—implementation of structural and other changes in the home and work environment to accommodate the person's limitations
      d. Life—vocational counseling–training and reintegration into daily activities

2. Long-term medical management to prevent or control complications such as septicemia, pulmonary embolism, and pneumonia

3. Neural stem cell research on spinal cord regeneration is ongoing

Spina Bifida

A. Definition
 1. Neural tube defect of the spinal column
 2. Vertebrae fail to close completely around the spinal cord
B. Incidence and prevalence
 1. Affects 166,000 persons in the United States in some form
 2. Occurs in 1 in 1000 live births
 3. A major cause of paraplegia in children
C. Etiology—specific cause unknown; but multiple factors, including genetic and environmental factors, are suspected; folic acid supplements taken during pregnancy can prevent this
D. Types (Figure 19-14)
 1. Spina bifida occulta
  a. Small defect in a vertebra not involving the spinal cord
  b. Often undetected
 2. Meningocele—bony defect that allows meninges and cerebrospinal fluid to form a sac that protrudes from the vertebral column
 3. Meningomyelocele (also myelomeningocele)—severe defect in which the spinal cord also protrudes into the sac
E. Signs, symptoms, and clinical manifestations
 1. Potential exposure of the nervous system to the external environment results in an increased chance for further damage from trauma or infection
 2. Loss of motor function in the lower half of the body

  a. Differential involvement of muscle groups causes muscle imbalance, leading to spinal and limb deformities
  b. Loss of sensation to pain, touch, and temperature creates safety hazards and pressure sores
  c. Loss of bladder and bowel control
  d. Ambulation may be affected, creating a need for orthopedic devices or a wheelchair
 3. Deformity of the brain
  a. Most have normal intelligence but experience learning disabilities, especially visual–perceptual problems
  b. Some develop seizure disorders
  c. 65% will develop hydrocephalus and 70% to 90% will develop hydrocephalus with; if the person has third-stage spina bifida, or with myelomeningocele
   (1) Cerebrospinal fluid accumulates in the ventricles of the brain
   (2) Pressure expands the brain and skull
 4. Latex allergy is common in this population
F. Treatment
 1. Surgical correction of the defect
 2. Insertion of ventriculo-peritoneal or ventriculo-atrial shunt if hydrocephalus is present (Figure 19-15)
 3. Orthopedic management through surgery, bracing, and physical therapy
 4. Assisted urination or evacuation, catheterization
 5. Medications to prevent or treat infections
 6. Avoidance of decubitus ulcers
 7. Weight control, if fairly inactive
G. Oral manifestations—none directly associated

Viral Hepatitis

See the section on "Infections of the gastrointestinal tract" and Table 9-10 in Chapter 9.

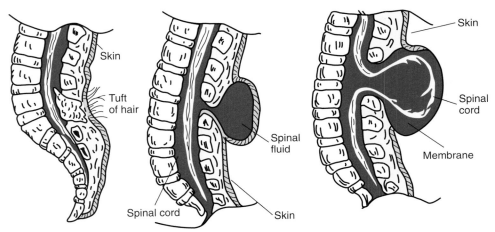

FIGURE 19-14 Types of spina bifida.

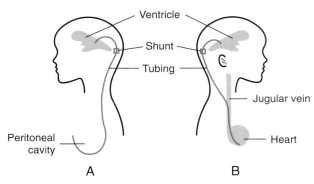

Ventricle
Shunt
Tubing
Jugular vein
Peritoneal cavity
Heart
A   B

FIGURE 19-15 Types of shunts.

Acquired Immunodeficiency Syndrome

See the sections on "Human immunodeficiency virus" in Chapter 8 and "Immunodeficiency" in Chapter 9.

Sexually Transmitted Diseases

See the section on "Infections of the reproductive and urinary systems" in Chapter 9.

Tuberculosis

See the section on "Infections of the respiratory tract" and Table 9-9 in Chapter 9.

Cystic Fibrosis

A. Definition—inherited disorder of the exocrine glands
B. Incidence and prevalence
   1. Occurs in 1 in 3000 live births in the United States
   2. Between 2% and 5% of the population are carriers
   3. Affects approximately 30,000 persons in the United States; 10 million or more are carriers of the gene for cystic fibrosis
   4. Most common cause of chronic lung disease in Caucasian children
   5. Mean survival about 37.4 years
C. Etiology—autosomal recessive disorder; defect in gene on chromosome 7 that results in phenylalanine deletion and problem with chloride ion transport
D. Signs, symptoms, and clinical manifestations—include increased viscosity of mucus (obstructs the pancreatic ducts, leading to cyst formation, impaired metabolism, and progressive deterioration)
   1. Accumulation of mucus in the lungs interferes with oxygen exchange
      a. Interferes especially with exhalation, causing a barrel-chested appearance

      b. Air sacs collapse and infections occur, often leading to suppurative bronchitis, pneumonia, and obstructive emphysema
      c. Clubbing of fingers and toes
      d. Chronic cough
   2. Sweat glands affected, leading to high levels of sodium in the sweat ("salty sweat")
   3. Salivary glands also affected
   4. Other findings and complications include a small gallbladder, cirrhosis of the liver, and sterility in males
   5. Delayed linear growth and bone development
   6. Insufficient pancreatic function can lead to diabetes
   7. Death usually occurs in early adulthood
E. Treatment
   1. Antibiotics to eliminate lung infection
   2. Bronchial dilators and mucolytics to assist with breathing and mucous secretions
   3. Dietary regimen
      a. High-calorie dense foods (20% to 40% greater caloric need)
      b. Increases in fat, protein, salt, and fat-soluble vitamins
      c. Pancreatic enzyme supplements
   4. Respiratory and exercise therapy
   5. General prevention of infections
   6. Gene therapy
   7. Early detection of gene carriers
   8. Possible lung transplant
F. Oral manifestations
   1. Lower dental caries rate and plaque accumulation with increased calculus deposits; probably a result of alterations in saliva and long-term use of antibiotics
   2. Enlargement of the salivary glands
   3. Intrinsic staining of the teeth, if tetracycline is administered during the formative years
   4. Mouth breathing, if sinuses are occluded

Chronic Obstructive Pulmonary Disease (COPD)

A. Definition
   1. General term for pulmonary disorders characterized by obstruction of airflow during respiration
   2. Consists of two or more disease processes that may coexist
   3. Bronchitis—obstruction caused by narrowing or loss of airways
   4. Emphysema—loss of elasticity and collapse of overinflated air sacs; loss of gas exchange surface area; causes obstruction during expiration
B. Incidence, prevalence, and etiology
   1. Chronic bronchitis affects 10% to 25% of adults in the United States

2. More common in males and in persons age ≥60

3. Most important risk factor is smoking, accounting for 80% to 90% of persons with COPD

4. Can be a hereditary defect in pulmonary tissue; may be caused by severe respiratory illnesses during childhood

C. Signs, symptoms, and clinical manifestations

1. Dyspnea and wheezing on exertion or at rest; orthopnea

2. Chronic cough, mucus, respiratory infections, and cyanosis in bronchitis

3. Use of accessory muscles of respiration

4. Chest pain

5. Advanced complications are heart failure and pulmonary failure

D. Treatment

1. Elimination of risk factors (e.g., smoking, environmental pollution)

2. Medications, including β-adrenergic agonists, mucolytics, bronchodilators, corticosteroids, anticholinergics

3. Lung transplantation

E. Oral manifestations—no associated oral manifestations unless a side effect of the medications

Bronchial Asthma

See the section on "Asthma" in Chapter 21.

A. Definition

1. Chronic clinical state of hyper-reactivity of the tracheobronchial tree characterized by recurrent paroxysms of dyspnea and wheezing

2. Results from bronchospasm, bronchial wall edema, inflammation, and hypersecretion by mucus glands

3. Status asthmaticus—persistent exacerbation of asthma despite drug therapy (life-threatening); causes excessive strain on the circulatory and respiratory systems

B. Incidence and prevalence

1. Affects approximately 30.2 million persons in the United States

2. Initial symptoms usually occur in the first 5 years of life

3. Approximately 50% of affected children become asymptomatic before adulthood

4. 75% to 85% also have allergies

C. Etiology—unknown, but precipitating factors and their effects are known

1. Extrinsic factors—smoking, dust, mold, pollen, smoke, animal dander, household sprays, wool, certain foods, air pollutants, sulfiting agents

2. Other factors—respiratory tract infections, aspirin and other anti-inflammatory drugs, overexertion

D. Signs, symptoms, and clinical manifestations

1. Wheezing, dyspnea, coughing, chest pain, sneezing, sputum production, fatigue, anxiety

2. Expiratory phase of breathing is slower and more pronounced

3. Facial (sinus) pain, conjunctivitis, otitis media

4. More severe symptoms—syncope, respiratory failure, cyanosis, hyperexpansion of the chest

E. Treatment

1. Avoidance of precipitating factors; monitoring of airflow with a peak flow meter

2. Immunotherapy (allergy shots)

3. Medications—inhaled or oral

a. Bronchodilators such as β-adrenergic agonists to stop the attacks

b. Anti-inflammatory agents such as corticosteroids to help prevent attacks

c. Development of sensitivity to many medications, including NSAIDs, β-blockers, and angiotensin-converting enzyme (ACE) inhibitors, may cause a fatal attack

4. Exercise program

F. Oral manifestations

1. β-Adrenergic agonists may impair salivary secretions, increasing caries risk

2. Mouth breathing

3. *Candida* infections from inhalant use

Congenital Heart Disease

A. Definition

1. Anomalies of heart structure

2. Usually develops during the first 9 weeks in utero

B. Incidence and prevalence

1. Occurs in 8 to 10 of 1000 births in the United States

2. Affects approximately 500,000 adults

C. Etiology

1. Generally unknown

2. Genetic (e.g., Down syndrome)

3. Environmental (maternal)

a. Fetal hypoxia, endocarditis, or immunologic abnormalities

b. Rubella infection (German measles) or other viruses

c. Nutritional deficiencies (especially vitamin deficiencies)

d. Drugs (e.g., lithium, alcohol, cocaine)

e. Radiation

f. Metabolic disorders (PKU or diabetes)

D. Types of malformations

1. Cause initial left-to-right shunting of blood (e.g., atrial septal defect, ventricular septal defect, patent ductus arteriosus)

2. Initial right-to-left shunting (e.g., tetralogy of Fallot)—causes significant cyanosis

3. Malformations that obstruct blood flow (e.g., pulmonary stenosis)

E. Signs, symptoms, and clinical manifestations
   1. Dyspnea, fatigue, weakness (most common symptoms)
   2. Cyanosis, dizziness, syncope, or ruddy color, leading to congestive heart failure
   3. Clubbing of fingers or toes
   4. Heart murmurs
   5. Delayed growth and development
   6. Complications—brain abscesses, bacterial endocarditis, congestive heart failure, acute pulmonary edema, bleeding problems

F. Treatment
   1. One fourth to one half of infants with these defects require treatment during the first year of life
   2. Surgery for others usually between ages 4 and 6
   3. Medications
      a. Digitalis
      b. Anticoagulants
   4. Variety of treatments for complications

G. Oral manifestations
   1. Bluish mucosa, if cyanotic; ruddy color, if the person has polycythemia
   2. Developmental defects of teeth sometimes seen
   3. Slight hemorrhage secondary to trauma, if bleeding problems are present
   4. May have decreased ability to fight oral infections

Rheumatic Fever and Heart Disease

See the section on "Infections of the circulatory system" in Chapter 9.

Cardiac Arrhythmias and Dysrhythmias

A. Definition
   1. Irregular heartbeat manifested as abnormal pulse rates or rhythms
   2. Produces alterations in the normal sequence of contractions, leading to inadequate blood flow
   3. Produces aberrant electrical depolarization
   4. Adversely affects the ventricular rate

B. Etiology
   1. Primary cardiovascular disease
   2. Pulmonary disorders
   3. Autonomic disorders
   4. Systemic disorders
   5. Side effects of drugs
   6. Electrolyte imbalance

C. Types and etiology
   1. Bradycardias—slowed heart rate (<60 beats per minute)
   2. Tachycardias—increased heart rate (>100 beats per minute)
   3. Isolated ectopic beats—premature impulses resulting in premature atrial beats
   4. Pre-excitation syndrome
   5. Cardiac arrest

D. Signs, symptoms, and clinical manifestations (may also be asymptomatic)
   1. Abnormal pulse
   2. Palpitations
   3. Breathlessness, pallor, fatigue
   4. Syncope or dizziness
   5. Cyanosis
   6. Pain
   7. Cardiac failure

E. Treatment
   1. No treatment required in some
   2. Antiarrhythmic drugs
   3. Pacemakers; most are the demand type, which stimulates the heart only when the rhythm deviates from a predetermined norm
   4. Cardioversion through defibrillation

F. Oral manifestations—may have side effects from medications or cyanotic oral tissues

Hypertensive Disease

See the section on "Vital signs" in Chapter 21.

A. Definition
   1. Hypertension—abnormal elevation of arterial blood pressure when constricted blood vessels increase resistance to blood flow, causing an increase in pressure against blood vessel walls
   2. Hypertensive heart disease—sustained elevation of the blood pressure, creating an increased workload for the heart, resulting in left ventricular hypertrophy and in late stage kidney disease
   3. Four hypertension categories (see Table 15-5 in Chapter 15; see the section on "Cardiac emergencies" in Chapter 21)
      a. Normal—less than 120/80 mm Hg
      b. Prehypertension—(120 to 139)/(80 to 89) mm Hg
      c. Stage 1—(140 to 159)/(90 to 99) mm Hg
      d. Stage 2—160/100 mm Hg or higher in either number
      e. Hypertensive crisis—higher than 200/120 mm Hg in either number

B. Incidence and prevalence
   1. Incidence is increasing, with hypertension affecting approximately 1 in 3 (or 74.5 million) persons in the United States; more remain undiagnosed

2. Prevalence increases with age and is greater in men before age 55 and in women after age 55

C. Etiology

1. Most cases are of unknown cause (essential hypertension)

2. 5 to 10% are secondary to other conditions such as renal disease or endocrine disorders

3. Risk factors include prehypertension, race (African American), age, stress, smoking, overweight and obesity, oral contraceptives, and excess salt and fat in the diet

4. Chronic hypertension causes cardiac enlargement and eventual congestive heart failure

D. Signs, symptoms, and clinical manifestations

1. Early—occipital headache, dizziness, tingling of the extremities, vision changes, tinnitus, dyspnea

2. Advanced—cardiac enlargement, ischemic heart disease, congestive heart failure, renal failure, stroke

E. Treatment (see the section on "Cardiac emergencies" in Chapter 21)

1. Approaches and therapies vary

2. Lifestyle changes in terms of stress reduction, avoidance of alcohol and tobacco, diet, and reduction of other risk factors

3. Drug management with antihypertensives—usually a combination used in a step care approach

    a. Diuretics

    b. β-blockers

    c. Vasodilators

    d. Angiotensin-converting enzyme (ACE) inhibitors

    e. Calcium channel blockers (also called *calcium blockers* or *calcium antagonists*)

4. Many side effects and precautions associated with drugs; some calcium channel blockers cause drug-induced gingival enlargement

F. Oral manifestations

1. Generally no direct oral manifestations

2. Facial palsy from some drugs

3. Oral lesions or xerostomia from drugs

Ischemic Heart Disease (Coronary Heart Disease)

A. Definition—coronary atherosclerotic heart disease that is symptomatic

B. Incidence and prevalence

1. Affects 17.6 million persons in the United States

2. Leading cause of death after age 40

3. Incidence and severity increase with age; more than 50% who die suddenly have no previous evidence of disease

C. Etiology

1. Risk factors are the same as for hypertensive disease

2. Periodontitis may be a significant risk factor related to elevated levels of cross-reactive protein and growth acceleration of lipids in blood vessels because of increased inflammatory mediators associated with periodontal gram-negative bacteria

3. Accumulation of atherosclerotic plaque inside blood vessels impairs blood flow and thus the oxygen supply to the heart

D. Signs, symptoms, and clinical manifestations

1. Angina pectoris—transient and reversible oxygen deficiency; classified as stable or unstable

    a. Pain—crushing or paroxysmal, usually <10 minutes; often mistaken for indigestion

    b. Sweating, anxiety, pallor, difficulty breathing

    c. Relieved by administration of nitroglycerin or rest

2. Myocardial infarction—an infarct or ischemic necrosis caused by a sudden reduction or arrest of blood flow

    a. Pain in the sternum, radiating to the left arm; lasts longer than angina

    b. Not relieved by nitroglycerin

    c. Same symptoms as angina, with nausea and vomiting, palpitations, and lowered blood pressure

    d. Often leads to sudden death from ventricular fibrillation

E. Treatment (see the section on "Cardiac emergencies" in Chapter 21)

1. Same management as for hypertensive disease

2. The earlier the treatment, the better is the prognosis; unfortunately, 50% wait 2 hours before going to the emergency department

3. Drug therapy—often in a step sequence

    a. Nitroglycerin and other nitrate

    b. βeta-adrenergic blockers and calcium channel blockers

    c. Aspirin

4. Coronary artery bypass graft surgery or percutaneous transluminal coronary angioplasty, if indicated

5. Rest

F. Oral manifestations

1. None directly associated

2. Oral lesions or xerostomia may result as a drug side effect

3. Pain may be radiated to the mandible, palate, or tongue

4. Drug-induced gingival enlargement may result as a side effect of some calcium channel blockers

Congestive Heart Failure (CHF)

A. Definition
   1. Represents a symptom complex that involves the failure of one or both ventricles (usually the left ventricle)
   2. Imbalance between the demand placed on the heart and its ability to respond
   3. Results in an inadequate supply of blood and oxygen throughout the body and in congestion of blood within the vascular system
B. Incidence and prevalence
   1. Most common cause of death in the United States
   2. Prevalence is 4.8 million persons; incidence is 400,000 cases each year; incidence of 5% occurs in persons under age 40
C. Etiology
   1. Underlying causes
      a. Heart valve damage; ventricular failure; overload of blood in the ventricles
      b. Obstructive lung disease
      c. Damage to the walls of the heart muscle
   2. Precipitating causes that place an additional demand on the heart
      a. Hypertensive crises
      b. Pulmonary embolism
      c. Arrhythmia
D. Signs, symptoms, and clinical manifestations
   1. Dyspnea, irregular breathing pattern, coughing, weakness; the person cannot breathe unless sitting up
   2. Swollen ankles late in the day, pitting edema, ascites
   3. Cyanosis, anxiety, fear
   4. Paleness, sweating, cold skin
   5. Decreased urine output
   6. Frothy pink or white sputum
   7. Weak pulse
   8. Confusion from decreased cardiac output, hence decreased oxygen to the brain
E. Treatment (see the section on "Cardiac emergencies" in Chapter 21)—depends on the type of underlying disease and initial responses to treatment
   1. Rest and limitation of activities
   2. Reduction in weight and other risk factors
   3. Dietary control (limit sodium intake)
   4. Medications
      a. Diuretics decrease congestion and eliminate water
      b. Digitalis glycosides increase the force of contractions
      c. Vasodilators (e.g., hydralazine) reduce resistance to the flow of blood
   5. Heart transplantation

F. Oral manifestations—infections, gingival bleeding, and petechiae if displaying polycythemia

Cerebrovascular Disease (Stroke)

A. Definition—sudden loss of brain function resulting from interference with the blood supply to a portion of the brain
B. Incidence and prevalence
   1. Affects 4.6 million persons in the United States; incidence of 75% occurs in persons age 66 or older
   2. Third leading cause of death in the United States; leading cause of serious disability
   3. African Americans are at greater risk than Caucasians
   4. Males are at greater risk than females
   5. Likelihood of having a stroke increases with age
C. Etiology
   1. Intracranial hemorrhage
   2. Blockage of vessels by thrombi or emboli (most common cause)
   3. Vascular insufficiency
   4. Predisposing conditions and risk factors
      a. Cerebral arteriosclerosis
      b. Dehydration
      c. Trauma
      d. Hypertension
      e. Diabetes
      f. Cigarette smoking
      g. Periodontitis
D. Signs, symptoms, and clinical manifestations—depend on the area of the brain involved and the extent of damage (Table 19-10)
   1. Immediate
      a. Syncope, headache, chills, convulsions, nausea, and vomiting
      b. Changes in level of consciousness
      c. Transient paresthesias
      d. Mood swing
   2. Residual or chronic
      a. Paralysis—hemiparesis or localized paralysis
      b. Speech problems and aphasia (reduced capacity for interpretation and formulation of language)
      c. Alterations in reflexes, especially the oral–motor reflexes
      d. Functional disorders of the bladder or bowel
      e. Visual impairments
      f. Seizures
E. Treatment (see the section on "Cerebrovascular accident (stroke, brain attack)" in Chapter 21)
   1. Reduce risk factors (e.g., high cholesterol levels, obesity, lack of exercise, smoking)
   2. Surgery, if needed

TABLE 19-10 Functional Limitations in Stroke Victims

Right Hemiplegia (L-CVA*)	Left Hemiplegia (R-CVA)
Language problems	Spatial–perceptual task difficulties—inability to judge distance, size, position, rate of movement, form, and relation of parts to a whole
Decreased auditory memory (cannot remember a long series of instructions)	Often thought to be unimpaired because able to speak and understand
Vocabulary problems	Visual field cuts; angles, etc. cannot be perceived
Slow, cautious, disorganized	Cannot use mirrors
Anxious	Cannot sequence tasks (such as toothbrushing)
	Decreased visual memory (loses place when reading)
	Cannot monitor self (keeps talking even though answered questions already)
	May neglect left side
	Tendency to be impulsive and unaware of deficits; spatial-perceptual difficulties are easy to miss

*CVA, cerebrovascular accident.
From Schubert MM, Snow M, Stiefel DJ: DECOD series: Dental management of patients with CNS and neurologic impairment: Spinal cord injury, *Seattle, 1989, University of Washington.*

3. Medications
   a. Anticoagulant therapy to prevent clot formation
   b. Antihypertensive therapy to reduce blood pressure
   c. Aspirin therapy to thin blood
4. Physical, occupational, and speech therapy
5. Rehabilitation services or program, if needed
F. Oral manifestations
   1. Oral–motor dysfunction
   2. Increased incidence of dental caries or periodontal disease caused by oral–motor problems and poor oral hygiene

Sickle Cell Disease

A. Definition
   1. Defect of hemoglobin that causes red blood cells to become sickle shaped

2. Sickle cell trait—individual shows no symptoms unless experiencing abnormally low concentration of oxygen
3. Sickle cell disease—progressively deteriorating and complex disease with multiple symptoms
B. Incidence and prevalence
   1. Found in African Americans and other nonwhite persons; occurs in both genders
   2. Two million persons in the United States are carriers of the sickle cell trait
   3. Approximately 80,000 persons in the United States have full-blown sickle cell anemia
   4. 1 in 1400 Hispanic American children is born with sickle cell anemia
   5. Babies do not show symptoms until age 6 months
C. Etiology
   1. Mutation in the globin gene of hemoglobin
   2. Sickle cell trait—the person has half normal hemoglobin and half sickled hemoglobin
   3. Sickle cell anemia—the person receives a sickle hemoglobin gene from both parents; sickle cell anemia is autosomal recessive
   4. Sickled cells clog blood vessels
D. Signs, symptoms, and clinical manifestations
   1. Young children
      a. Can develop enlarged spleen, septicemia, and meningitis
      b. Swelling of the feet and hands, anemia, pallor, tiredness, fever, pneumonia
      c. Severe pain crises affecting the extremities
      d. Stroke occurs in 10% of those affected
   2. Children and adolescents
      a. Can develop gallstones, enlarged hearts, and lung infarctions
      b. Bones degenerate as a result of repeated sickling
      c. Delayed growth and late puberty
      d. Increased chance for stroke, impaired kidney and liver functions, with jaundice, and arthritis
      e. Continued pain crises
   3. Adulthood
      a. Hemorrhage in the eye, or detached retina
      b. Pain crises—variable in each person
      c. Lung and kidney damage, gallstones
      d. Leg ulcers and bone changes
      e. Infection is a major cause of death and also precipitates crises
   4. High altitude, chilling temperatures, stress, psychological pressures, or infections can precipitate attacks
E. Treatment
   1. Bone marrow transplantation
   2. Prevention of complications with oral fluids, oxygen, ibuprofen, and transcutaneous electrical nerve stimulation for pain

3. Frequent transfusions (every 3 weeks) in some to prevent strokes; deferoxamine (Desferal) is administered to prevent iron toxicity
4. Hydroxyurea is also prescribed to increase the concentration of fetal hemoglobin, which is resistant to sickling

F. Oral manifestations
1. Sore, painful, red tongue
2. Loss of taste sensation
3. Osteoporosis
4. Decreased radiodensity with coarse trabecular bone pattern with large marrow spaces
5. Mucosal pallor
6. Delayed eruption of teeth
7. Hypoplastic enamel
   a. Pain in the mandible
   b. Periodontal involvement can precipitate a crisis
8. Bone loss can be significant in children

Cancer

A. Definition—cells that multiply at an abnormally rapid rate, invading and destroying healthy tissue
1. Metastasis—spread of cancer to distant sites
2. Invasion—spread of cancer to local sites

B. Incidence and prevalence
1. 1,248,900 new cases of oral cancer per year; less than 50% alive after 5 years
2. 201 in 100,000 persons will die of cancer each year in the United States
3. 75% of all head and neck cancers begin in the oral cavity
4. The tongue is the most common intraoral location (30%) (Figure 19-16)
5. Tonsils, tonsillar pillars, and oropharynx areas increasing most rapidly in incidence rates

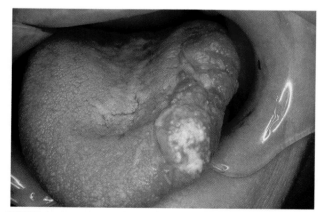

FIGURE 19-16 Squamous cell carcinoma on the lateral border of the tongue. *(From Regezi J, Sciubba J, Jordan R: Oral pathology: Clinical pathologic correlations, ed 5, St Louis, 2008, Saunders.)*

C. Etiology of oral cancer
1. Tobacco
2. Alcohol
3. Human papillomavirus 16–18
4. Ultraviolet light
5. Genetics

D. Warning signs of oral cancer
1. Unexplained swelling, lump, or growth with or without pain
2. White scaly patches or red areas
3. Any sore that does not heal in 2 weeks
4. Unexplained numbness or tingling
5. Difficulty opening mouth or swallowing
6. Prolonged hoarseness

E. Oral cancer screening tests
1. Brush cytology
2. Toluidine blue staining
3. Light-based detection systems (Vizilite)
4. Narrow emissions tissue fluorescence (VELscope)

F. Treatment—depends on type of cancer and stage of disease
1. Early detection through screening tests; survival related to stage when diagnosed
2. Surgery usually when tumor is localized
3. Radiation to shrink the tumor
4. Chemotherapy to kill the cells or stop their multiplication; can reach metastasized sites
5. Maintaining protective practices, including diet, exercise, sun protection, and avoidance of alcohol and tobacco
6. Combination of above therapies

G. Oral manifestations—depend on type of cancer and treatment
1. Oral ulcerations and mucositis
2. Candidiasis
3. Anemia
4. Xerostomia
5. Radiation caries (Figure 19-17)
6. Loss of taste
7. Osteoradionecrosis (Figure 19-18)
8. Tooth sensitivity
9. Muscular dysfunction and trismus
10. Spontaneous gingival bleeding
11. Cosmetic disfigurement

Leukemia

A. Definition
1. Progressive malignant neoplasms characterized by an overproduction of abnormal leukocytes
2. Abnormal leukocytes displace hematopoietic tissue in the bone marrow, leading to decreased production of platelets, erythrocytes, and normal leukocytes

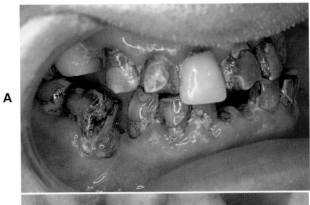

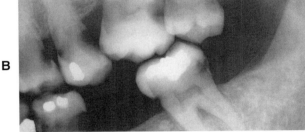

FIGURE 19-17 A and B, Radiation-associated cervical caries. *(From Regezi J, Sciubba J, Jordan R: Oral pathology: Clinical pathologic correlations, ed 5, St Louis, 2008, Saunders.)*

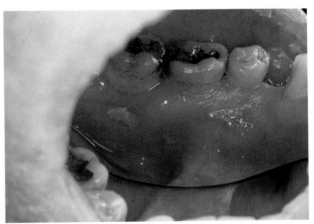

FIGURE 19-18 Osteoradionecrosis of the lingual mandible. *(From Regezi J, Sciubba J, Jordan R: Oral pathology: Clinical pathologic correlations, ed 5, St Louis, 2008, Saunders.)*

B. Classification
1. Chronicity
   a. Acute form (A)—large numbers of immature nonspecific leukocytes are produced; accounts for 25% more of the cases than the chronic form
   b. Chronic form (C)—leukocytes are well differentiated and able to mature; but immunologic capacity is decreased
2. Type of white cell predominating
   a. Myeloid
   b. Lymphoid
   c. Monocytic

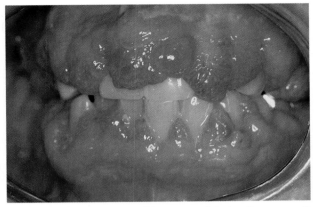

FIGURE 19-19 Gingival conditions associated with monocytic leukemia. *(From Regezi J, Sciubba J, Jordan R: Oral pathology: Clinical pathologic correlations, ed 5, St Louis, 2008, Saunders.)*

C. Incidence and prevalence
1. 44,790 new cases each year in the United States
2. 33% of cancers in children are leukemia
3. Seventh leading cause of cancer death in adults; leading cause of cancer death in children
4. Five-year survival rate is approximately 46%

D. Etiology
1. Specific cause unknown
2. Predisposing factors—genetic factors, ionizing radiation, chemical agents, exposure to human T cell lymphotrophic virus type I

E. Signs, symptoms, and clinical manifestations
1. Acute form appears suddenly and severely; chronic form is insidious
2. Fatigue, weakness, pallor, weight loss
3. Ecchymosed skin and nosebleeds
4. Fever
5. Headache, nausea, and vomiting

F. Treatment
1. Chemotherapy with blood transfusions and antibiotics
2. Irradiation
3. Bone marrow transplantation, when indicated
4. Interferon therapy

G. Oral manifestations (Figure 19-19)
1. Initial
   a. Leukemic infiltrate of the pulp and gingiva
      (1) Causes pain in teeth
      (2) Enlarged bluish-red, spongy, blunted papilla
      (3) Ulceration and necrosis
   b. Mucositis, mucosal atrophy, and mucosal pallor
   c. Areas of spontaneous hemorrhage (intermittent oozing) and petechiae
   d. Loss of lamina dura, resorption of alveolar bone, cancellous bone destruction

  2. Secondary
    a. Mucosal infections (*Candida, Pseudomonas*) and periapical infections
    b. Necrotizing ulcerative gingivitis
    c. Viral infections
    d. Osteomyelitis
  3. Tertiary (treatment effects)
    a. Painful oral ulcerations
    b. Stomatitis
    c. Xerostomia and dental caries
    d. Jaw pain with Bell's palsy
    e. Secondary infections

Hemophilias

See the section on "Hemophilia" in Chapter 8.
A. Definition—congenital disorder of the blood-clotting mechanism
B. Incidence and prevalence
  1. More than 18,000 persons in the United States have hemophilia; 400 births yearly
  2. Hemophilia A accounts for 80% to 85%; hemophilia B accounts for 10% to 15%
  3. 90% are under age 25
  4. Vast majority of those affected are men
C. Classification
  1. Type
    a. Hemophilia A (factor VIII deficiency)—1.9 in 10 persons with hemophilia have type A
    b. Hemophilia B (factor IX deficiency)—Christmas disease
    c. von Willebrand's disease (lack of plasma)—von Willebrand's factor is required for primary hemostasis
  2. Severity—level of clotting factor (normal level is 50% to 100%)
    a. Severe—have less than 1% of clotting factor; may bleed spontaneously or from minor trauma
    b. Moderate—have 5% to 25% of clotting factor; hemorrhage only with trauma
    c. Mild—have 25% to 50% of clotting factor; bleed only after severe injuries and surgery
D. Etiology
  1. Hemophilia A and B
    a. Sex-linked recessive mode of inheritance (female carrier and manifested in males)
    b. High mutation rate
  2. von Willebrand's disease—transmission by dominant autosomal gene; occurs with equal frequency in both genders
E. Signs, symptoms, and clinical manifestations
  1. Bleeding and bruising from minor cuts or pressure
    a. Ecchymoses and hematomas

    b. Oozing
    c. Intramuscular bleeding causes pain
  2. Hemarthroses—bleeding into the soft tissues of joints, leading to pain, swelling, and permanent joint contractures
  3. Renal function is impaired; exposure to hepatitis during transfusions
  4. Intracranial hemorrhages can cause seizures or other neurologic disorders
  5. Chronic complications include osteoarthritis, irregular growth, muscular atrophy, and tumor formation
  6. Inhibitor to antihemophilic factor can develop in hemophilia A, making the person resistant to replacement therapy
  7. Complications from bleeds include airway obstruction, intestinal obstruction, and compression of nerves and paralysis
F. Treatment
  1. Factor replacement therapy
  2. Amicar (antifibrinolytic) used to decrease oral bleeds; needed for periodontal debridement and root planing
  3. Desmopressin acetate used in von Willebrand's disease and mild hemophilia
  4. Prevention of bleeds
  5. Joint replacement; antibiotics for invasive procedure
  6. Recombinant antihemophilic factor
G. Oral manifestations
  1. Ecchymoses, hematomas, and gingival oozing can be problems
  2. Oral trauma is more evident and can be serious

Diabetes Mellitus

See the section on "Diabetes mellitus" in Chapter 21.
A. Definition—hereditary disease of metabolism with:
  1. Inadequate production and action of insulin from the pancreas
  2. Disorders in carbohydrate, protein, and fat metabolism
  3. Body cells unable to use glucose, leading to hyperglycemia
  4. Alternating extremes of hypoglycemia and hyperglycemia found in the person with "brittle" (very poorly controlled) diabetes
B. Incidence and prevalence
  1. Diabetes mellitus affects 23.6 million persons in the United States with approximately 8 million undiagnosed
  2. Third leading cause of death in the United States
  3. Much higher in Hispanic Americans and Native Americans
  4. Approximately 800,000 new cases diagnosed yearly

TABLE 19-11 Comparison of Type 1 and Type 2 Diabetes Mellitus

Characteristic	Type 1	Type 2
Age of onset	Young, usually before or during puberty, but may appear later	Adult, usually after 30 years, but may occur at younger age
Body weight	Normal or thin	Obesity is most important risk factor
Ethnicity	More common in Caucasians	More common in African Americans, Asian Americans, Hispanic Americans, and Native Americans
Hereditary	Yes, but less frequent occurrence in families than type 2	Much more frequent occurrence in families
Lifestyle	Restrictions very difficult for young persons	More frequent in sedentary individuals with high-fat diets
Onset of symptoms	Rapid, abrupt symptoms of hyperglycemia	Slow, insidious progression over years
Symptoms	Weight loss; weakness; polyuria; polydipsia; polyphagia; blurred vision; mimic flu; frequent/recurrent infections; slow healing; tingling/numb extremities; fatigue; eye/kidney/cardiovascular problems	Any type 1 symptom kidney/cardiovascular problems
Severity	Severe, life-threatening	Early mild but progressively serious
Complications	Acute hypoglycemic or hyperglycemic emergencies and chronic long-term complications common	Acute complications rare; chronic long-term complications common
Stability	Unstable, difficult and much effort to control	More stable, easier to manage
Exogenous insulin required	All	Some
Chronic manifestations	Uncommon before 20 years, prevalent and severe by 30 years	Develop slowly at later ages
Ketoacidosis	Common	Rare
Prevention	None (because of multiple factors)	Prevent or delay with lifestyle changes

Adapted from Wilkins EM: Clinical practice of the dental hygienist, ed 10, Philadelphia, 2009, Lippincott Williams & Wilkins.

C. Major types (Table 19-11)
  1. Type 1—insulin-dependent
  2. Type 2—non–insulin-dependent (92% of cases)
  3. Pre-diabetes—impaired glucose tolerance; higher than normal levels but not yet diagnostic for diabetes; at risk for atherosclerotic disease
  4. Gestational diabetes—occurs in 2% of pregnant women during the second or third trimester; the condition returns to normal after delivery in most cases, but 30% to 40% may develop type 2 diabetes later in life
D. Etiology
  1. Genetic disorder
  2. Destruction of the insulin-producing cells of the pancreas resulting from inflammation, viruses, cancer, or surgery
  3. Secondary to endocrine disorders (e.g., hyperthyroidism)
  4. Iatrogenic disease following the administration of steroids
  5. Obesity
E. Signs, symptoms, and clinical manifestations (Table 19-12)
  1. Cardinal symptoms are those associated with hyperglycemia
  2. An overdose of insulin or inadequate glucose intake to balance the insulin intake can result in insulin shock (hypoglycemia)
  3. Chronic complications include:
    a. Atherosclerosis and other cardiovascular problems
    b. Renal failure
    c. Motor, sensory, and autonomic neuropathies
    d. Glaucoma and cataracts leading to blindness

TABLE 19-12 Clinical Manifestations of Diabetes Mellitus

Hyperglycemia	Hypoglycemia
Polydipsia	Early stage
Polyphagia	— Diminished cerebral function
Polyuria	— Changes in mood
Loss of weight	— Decreased spontaneity
Fatigue	— Hunger
Headache	— Nausea
Blurred vision	More severe stage
Nausea and vomiting	— Sweating
Tachycardia	— Tachycardia
Florid appearance	— Piloerection
Hot and dry skin	— Increased anxiety
Kussmaul respiration	— Bizarre behavior patterns
Mental stupor	— Belligerence
Loss of consciousness	— Poor judgment
	— Uncooperativeness
	Later severe stage
	— Unconsciousness
	— Seizure activity
	— Hypotension
	— Hypothermia

Adapted from Malamed SF: Medical emergencies in the dental office, *ed 6, St Louis, 2007, Mosby.*

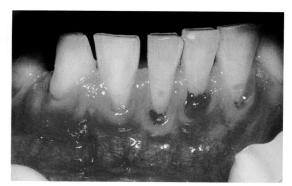

FIGURE 19-20 Gingival tissues exhibiting spontaneous bleeding, inflammation, and edema in an adult client with diabetes. *(From Newman, Takei:* Carranza's clinical periodontology, *ed 11, St Louis, 2012, Saunders.)*

e. Associated with increased incidence of large babies, stillbirths, miscarriages, neonatal deaths, and congenital defects

F. Treatment—no known cure
  1. Management of acute symptoms
  2. Exercise and diet plan (food exchange system)
  3. Medications
    a. Insulin therapy (injection or pump)
    b. Oral hypoglycemic agents (sulfonylureas) for type 2 diabetes
    c. Drugs to slow the digestion of carbohydrates to decrease rise in blood glucose are metformin (Glucophage), miglitol (Glyset), and acarbose (Precose)
    d. Insulin sensitizers are pioglitazone (Actos) and rosiglitazone (Avandia)
    e. Aspirin
  4. Control of blood pressure
  5. Maintenance of a delicate balance between diet, exercise, and insulin

G. Oral manifestations
  1. Seen more often in persons with uncontrolled diabetes
  2. Delayed wound healing and inability to manage oral infections (e.g., *Candida* infections), periodontal abscesses
  3. Decreased salivary flow may lead to increased caries; may have parotid gland enlargement
  4. Predisposition to aggressive periodontal disease in both types of diabetes, even in children and adolescents; magenta hue with edematous glassy tissue, enlarged papilla, mobility, alveolar bone loss (Figure 19-20)
  5. Periodontitis can make blood glucose levels more difficult to control
  6. Poor blood glucose control greatly increases risk for periodontal breakdown, bone loss and loss of attachment
  7. Children with diabetes may have accelerated tooth eruption and enamel hypoplasia

Thyroid Disease

A. Definition
  1. Hyperthyroidism (thyrotoxicosis)—excess of thyroid hormones in the bloodstream
  2. Graves' disease—type of hyperthyroidism; toxic goiter
  3. Hypothyroidism—inadequate thyroid hormones in the bloodstream
    a. Cretinism—childhood onset (congenital)
    b. Myxedema—adult onset (acquired)
B. Incidence and prevalence
  1. Thyroid disease affects 28 million persons in the United States, with up to one half undiagnosed
  2. Hyperthyroidism—disease is seven times more common in women; especially manifested during puberty, pregnancy, or menopause

TABLE 19-13 Clinical Features of Thyroid Disease

HYPOTHYROIDISM		Hyperthyroidism
Cretinism	**Myxedema**	
Dwarfism and obesity	Obesity	Weight loss
Coarse hair	Hair loss	Fine, friable hair
Eyes set apart	Puffy eyelids	Puffy eyelids
Muscle weakness	Muscle weakness	Exophthalmos
Dry, cold skin	Dry, cold skin	Tremors
Decreased sweating	Decreased sweating	Warm, moist skin
Cold intolerance	Cold intolerance	Increased sweating
Lethargy	Lethargy	Heat intolerance
Bradycardia	Bradycardia	Hyperactivity
Delayed tooth eruption		Tachycardia
Small jaws and malocclusion		Accelerated tooth eruption
		Large jaws
		Osteoporosis of alveolar bone
		Rapidly developing dental caries and periodontal disease

   3. Hypothyroidism
      a. Rare
      b. Myxedema is five times more common in females; most common between ages 30 and 60
      c. Permanent congenital hypothyroidism occurs in 1 in 3500 to 4500 births
C. Etiology
   1. Hyperthyroidism (Graves' disease)
      a. Cause is unknown
      b. Autoimmune cause or familial tendency is postulated
   2. Hypothyroidism
      a. Disease of the thyroid gland
      b. Myxedema may follow thyroid gland or pituitary gland failure resulting from irradiation, surgery, or excessive antithyroid drug therapy
D. Signs, symptoms, and clinical manifestations—results of underproduction or overproduction of thyroid hormone (Table 19-13)

E. Treatment
   1. Hyperthyroidism
      a. Antithyroid drugs, radioactive iodine, or iodides; may produce side effects
      b. Surgery
   2. Hypothyroidism—daily thyroid supplement
F. Oral manifestations—primarily delayed or accelerated dental development or deterioration of alveolar bone (Figure 19-21, *A* and *B*; see Table 19-13)

Chemical Dependency

See the section on "Substance abuse" in Chapter 11.
A. Definition
   1. State of psychological or physical dependence (or both) after administration of a drug on a periodic or continuous basis
   2. Drug use—when the effects of a drug can be realized with minimal hazard
   3. Drug misuse—when the drug or amount taken makes it more dangerous than necessary to produce the desired effect
   4. Drug abuse—continual misuse of a drug, loss of control over its use, or disruption of family, social, or job responsibilities
   5. Tolerance—use of larger doses of a drug to experience the same effects over time
   6. Recovery—overcoming physical and psychological dependence; commitment to drug-free life
B. Incidence and prevalence
   1. Several drugs or drug categories cause the most concern: cocaine, heroin and other opiates, marijuana, stimulants, barbiturates and other depressants, hallucinogens (psychedelics), tranquilizers, volatile solvents, and other inhalants
   2. Alcohol is a major problem (see the section on "Chronic alcohol abuse and dependence"); 70% of persons in the United States drink at least on a social basis
   3. Nitrous oxide and prescription drug abuse is of most concern to dental professionals
   4. Routes of administration—oral ingestion, inhalation, injection, snorting, buccal, suppositories
   5. In the United States, 41.7% of those over age 12 have used illegal drugs at least once
C. Etiology
   1. Stressful social, psychological, or economic environments
   2. Peer pressure
   3. Gateway drugs—alcohol, tobacco, marijuana
D. Signs and symptoms—vary with the agent involved and route of administration
   1. Affect autonomic, central, and peripheral nervous systems
   2. Drug interactions have additive, inhibitory, and synergistic effects

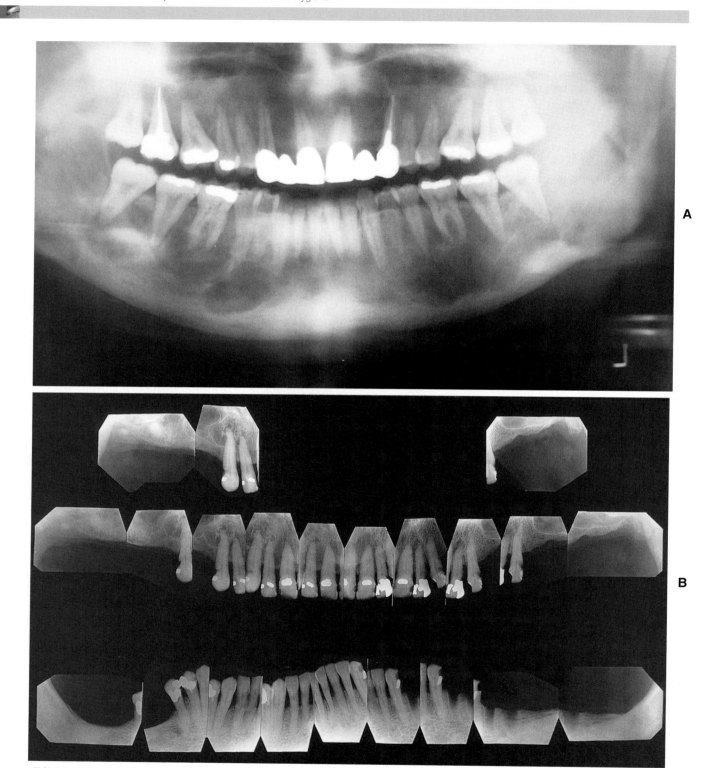

FIGURE 19-21 A, Radiograph of mandibular radiolucencies associated with hyperparathyroidism. **B,** Radiograph of loss of lamina dura associated with hyperparathyroidism. *(From Regezi J, Sciubba J, Jordan R: Oral pathology: Clinical pathologic correlations, ed 5, St Louis, 2008, Saunders.)*

3. Duration of effects ranges from 1 hour to many days
4. Withdrawal symptoms reported for all drug categories except hallucinogens
5. Possible effects of some drug categories
   a. Narcotics—euphoria, drowsiness, respiratory depression, constricted pupils, nausea
   b. Depressants—slurred speech, disorientation, intoxicated behavior
   c. Stimulants—alertness, excitation, euphoria, increased pulse rate and blood pressure, insomnia, loss of appetite
   d. Hallucinogens—illusions and hallucinations, poor perception of time and distance
   e. Marijuana—euphoria, relaxed inhibitions, increased appetite, disoriented behavior
E. Treatment
   1. Abstinence
   2. Educational programs, mentoring and drug-free activities
   3. Confrontational and family-oriented approaches; team also may involve employers and health care professionals
   4. "Lifelong recovery" approach
F. Oral manifestations
   1. Oral trauma—if the person engages in aggressive behavior or fights or has accidents
   2. Xerostomia—if dehydrated
   3. Mucosal lesions and leukoplakia from irritants smoked or used orally
   4. Increased caries commonly seen at the cervical area; periodontal disease prevalent if oral hygiene is neglected or the person consumes high-carbohydrate diet
   5. Advanced cervical caries associated with heavy methamphetamine use
   6. Tooth abrasion
   7. Increased risk for oral and esophageal cancers
   8. Reduced tolerance to pain
   9. Bruxism

Chronic Alcohol Abuse and Dependence

A. Definition and etiology
   1. Chronic impairment in physical, mental, or social functioning caused by frequent ingestion (more than two drinks per day) of alcohol
   2. Can become dependent on alcohol ingestion and develop a tolerance to increasing amounts
   3. Genetically transmitted susceptibility to alcoholism
   4. Often induced by a psychiatric disorder or stress
B. Incidence and prevalence
   1. 5.1 million persons in United States suffer from alcohol abuse

2. 1 in 13 adults in the United States abuses alcohol or is an alcoholic (7.42% of persons age 18 and older)
3. Alcohol problems are higher among young adults age 18 to 29
4. Normal activities are maintained by 90%
5. 80% are heavy smokers
C. Signs, symptoms, and clinical manifestations
   1. Alcoholic breath
   2. Unexplained tremors
   3. Nausea and vomiting, gastrointestinal problems, ulcers
   4. Cutaneous lesions (redness, acne, spider angiomas)
   5. Edema of the eyelids and other parts of the body
   6. Nutritional deficiencies (vitamin B, protein, calcium)
D. Long-term complications
   1. Hypertension and other types of heart disease
   2. Increased risk for various types of cancers
   3. Hepatitis, cirrhosis, and hypoglycemia
   4. Interference with secretion of pancreatic enzymes
   5. Bleeding tendencies
   6. Altered enzyme functioning and malabsorptive syndromes of the small intestine
   7. Irritation of the gastric mucosa leading to bleeding, inflammation, and ulceration
   8. Fetal alcohol syndrome (pregnant women)
E. Treatment
   1. Only about 10% of alcoholics receive treatment
   2. Some alcohol abuse programs involve use of disulfiram (Antabuse), which causes physical discomfort if alcohol is consumed
   3. Dietary modifications
   4. Counseling and support groups
   5. Abstinence is an overriding goal
F. Oral manifestations—increased incidence of:
   1. Caries caused by nausea and vomiting, neglected oral hygiene, and xerostomia
   2. Periodontal disease caused by an impaired immune system and the effects on white blood cells
   3. Glossitis and angular cheilitis from nutritional deficiencies
   4. Leukoplakia and oropharyngeal cancer (note that use of alcohol and tobacco products increases risk of oropharyngeal cancer)
   5. Swelling of the parotid glands leads to decreased salivation and increased caries incidence
   6. Trauma during inebriated states (accidents or fights)
   7. Attrition secondary to bruxism

End-Stage Renal Disease

A. Definition
   1. Progressive bilateral deterioration of renal function, resulting in uremia and eventual death
   2. Uremia is the toxic condition produced by retention of urinary constituents in the blood
B. Incidence and prevalence
   1. Chronic kidney disease affects approximately 20 million persons in the United States or 1 in 9 adults; over the past 5 years, the number of patients with kidney failure has averaged 90,000 annually
   2. More than 485,000 persons in the United States are being treated for end-stage renal disease; of these, more than 341,000 are patients receiving dialysis and 140,000 have a kidney transplantation
   3. More common in Caucasians (61%), African Americans (31.7%), Hispanic (14%), Asians (4.5%), Native Americans (1.3%) and other (1.5%)
C. Etiology
   1. Infectious diseases (e.g., nephritis, viral and fungal infections)
   2. Hypersensitivity states (e.g., glomerulonephritis)
   3. Developmental defects of the kidneys
   4. Circulatory disturbances (e.g., hypertension, hemorrhages)
   5. Metabolic diseases (e.g., diabetes)
   6. 10% of new cases may occur as a result of analgesic misuse
D. Signs, symptoms, and clinical manifestations
   1. Mental slowness or depression
   2. Swelling and edema
   3. Muscular hyperactivity
   4. Hyperpigmentation of the skin (brownish yellow)
   5. Anorexia, vomiting, and diarrhea
   6. Anemia
   7. Possible functional defect in factor VIII protein, leading to hemorrhagic episodes
   8. Hypertension, congestive heart failure
E. Treatment
   1. Potassium regulation
   2. Sodium regulation
   3. Maintenance of water balance (depends on urine output, edema, and weight change)
   4. Protein balance
   5. Acid–base balance—correct acidosis with calcium carbonate (also administer vitamin D)
   6. Sedatives and hypnotics to manage neuromuscular complications
   7. Dialysis when other methods alone are not effective
      a. Peritoneal—usually for acute renal failure
         (1) Injection of hypertonic solution into the peritoneal cavity
         (2) Draws out urea and other solutes
         (3) Less costly, easier to perform, but less effective than hemodialysis
         (4) More persons using ambulatory type, where continuous dialysis is performed by the patient, with drainage into a bag
      b. Hemodialysis for chronic renal failure
         (1) Creation of an arteriovenous fistula
         (2) Blood runs from the artery to the dialysis machine, is filtered, and then is returned to the vein
         (3) Heparin is added to prevent blood clotting
         (4) Patient is at risk for acquiring hepatitis B, hepatitis C, and hepatitis D viruses from commercial blood products
   8. Kidney transplantation—problems with graft rejection and infection; use steroids, antibiotics, and immunosuppressives such as cyclosporine
F. Oral manifestations
   1. Painful oral ulcerations and stomatitis from drugs
   2. Candidiasis or herpetic lesions from immunosuppression
   3. Increased calculus deposits
   4. Anemic mucosa
   5. Oral petechiae and hemorrhage
   6. Ground-glass appearance of alveolar bone caused by leaching of calcium (uremic bone disease)
   7. Bad taste and halitosis from urea in saliva
   8. Enamel hypoplasia
   9. Immunosuppressed patient who has received a transplant may have increased risk for cancer
   10. Drug-influenced gingival enlargement from cyclosporine (an immunosuppressant) or nifedipine (a calcium-channel blocker)
   11. Delayed eruption in primary teeth

Older Adults

A. Definition
   1. Age ≥55
   2. Older adults age ≥68
B. Incidence and prevalence
   1. 13% of the U.S. population age ≥66; fastest-growing segment of population
   2. It is estimated that 20% of the population will be age ≥65 by 2030
   3. 47% of older population lives in nursing homes
      a. 1% of persons age 65 to 74
      b. 20% of persons age 85 or older

C. Systemic manifestations
   1. Disease response—increased severity, longer course, and slower healing
   2. Decreased metabolism
   3. Reduced elasticity of tissues, diminished reparative ability
   4. Thin, dry, wrinkled skin; delayed healing
   5. Special senses
      a. 13% of persons age 70 to 74 and 31% of persons age ≥85 have a visual impairment
      b. 26% of persons age 70 to 74 and 49% of persons age ≥85 have a hearing impairment
   6. Musculoskeletal changes
      a. Osteopenia and osteoporosis
      b. Osteoarthritis
      c. Loss of muscle function and tone
   7. Increase in cardiovascular diseases
      a. High blood pressure
      b. Coronary heart disease
      c. Valvular disease
D. Common chronic conditions
   1. Arthritis
   2. Hypertension
   3. Cardiovascular disease
   4. Diabetes
E. Oral manifestations
   1. Soft tissues
      a. Dry, purse-string lips with opening difficulties, angular cheilitis (Figure 19-22)
      b. Capillary fragility, hyperkeratosis of oral mucosa
      c. Fissures, sublingual varicosities, reduced taste from loss of taste buds of tongue
      d. Increased incidence of oral cancer
   2. Hard tissues
      a. Abrasion, attrition, dark color of teeth
      b. Root caries
      c. Decreased tooth sensitivity
      d. Decreased pulp chamber size

DENTAL MANAGEMENT

A. Personal and professional prerequisites (Table 19-14)
   1. Interview the client in a sensitive manner to gather accurate data; initiate dental hygiene process
   2. Analyze and summarize data in oral or written formats
   3. Use problem-solving skills to develop alternative strategies to manage problems
   4. Evaluate client and professional goals and progress for appropriateness and effectiveness
   5. Remain current of new conditions, new protocols for medical management, and advances in dental and dental hygiene care
   6. Apply new knowledge or techniques from other areas to dental management of special clients
   7. Apply research principles and techniques to acquire clinical data that serve as the basis for care planning and decision making
B. Office management issues
   1. Stress a team concept with cooperation among members and coordination of information and activities; dental hygiene procedures may require the help of a dental assistant
   2. Identify and anticipate client needs and problems before initiation of care; use of a previsit questionnaire is helpful (Figure 19-23)
   3. Obtain informed consent for treatment from the client or an appropriate representative
   4. Explain office policies, procedures, and philosophy to the client or guardian before or at the first appointment
   5. Determine financial limitations that may affect care planning or payment procedures
      a. Assess additional resources available from other sources (e.g., community organizations)
      b. Attempt to provide flexible payment alternatives
   6. If the client is unable to receive care in the office because of physical limitations or geographic distance, determine if care can be provided in

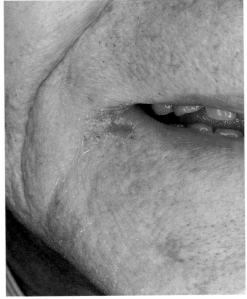

FIGURE 19-22 Angular cheilitis is a common oral finding in older adults because of nutritional deficiencies. *(From Ibsen OAC, Phelan JA:* Oral pathology for the dental hygienist, *ed 5, Philadelphia, 2009, Saunders.)*

Text continued on page 748.

TABLE 19-14 Dental Management Considerations for Clients with Special Needs

Condition	Medical Issues	Barriers to Care	Other Associated Health Issues	Treatment Considerations*	Prevention/Education/ Health Promotion Issues
Intellectual and developmental disabilities (formerly called *mental retardation*)	Syndrome Associated medical conditions and other disabilities Treatment regimens	Limited financial resources Degree of reliance on others Limited mental ability	Oral–motor dysfunction General incoordination Cariogenic foods and reinforcers Self-abuse Resistant behavior	Short appointments Gagging: radiographs, instrument placement, positioning Consult caregiver for behavioral management approaches Mental impairment: communication, cooperation, stability in chair, limited attention span, minimize distractions Limited finances: alternative treatment plans	"Tell, show, do" approach Simple language Frequent repetition and positive reinforcement Frequent continued care intervals, minimize distractions Alternatives for snacks and food reinforcers Chlorhexidine mouth rinses or spray, sealants ADA-approved or CDA-recognized antimicrobial mouthrinse daily
Fetal alcohol syndrome	Which organs affected? Heart? Brain? Growth deficiency	Family may be dysfunctional Behavioral problems May have mental disabilities	Attention deficit disorders Dental malformations	Behavior and attention: short structured appointments Family problems: ensure that follow-up care is understood Compliment cooperative behavior	Ensure adequate supervision for oral hygiene care Use same methods as for children with learning disabilities or intellectual and developmental disabilities ADA-approved or CDA-recognized antimicrobial mouthrinse daily based on level of cooperation
Down syndrome	Possible congenital heart defect (prophylactic antibiotic premedication) Hearing and vision problems Decreased resistance to infection; frequent respiratory infections	Same as for intellectual and developmental disabilities	Same as for intellectual and developmental disabilities	Same as for intellectual and developmental disabilities plus small oral area: oral access for procedures Hearing and vision disorders: communication Avoid use of air polisher and ultrasonic scaler Consult with physician about need for prophylactic antibiotic premedication	Same as for intellectual and developmental disabilities plus stress oral hygiene and periodontal maintenance care
Autism	No major problems unless self-abusive	Behavior Degree of reliance on others Communication, minimal Language skills	Disordered eating or fetishes Resistant behavior	Dependence on "routines"; procedure sequencing, desensitization appointment Lack of useful language: communication Learning disabilities and sensitivity to stimuli: communication, limit distractions Avoid light in eyes	Combine verbal and nonverbal communication techniques and positive reinforcers Teach toothbrushing as a "motion" rather than a function Avoid metaphors and complex language structures

Learning disabilities/attention-deficit hyperactivity disorder	Medications and potential side effects	Depends on type of disability	Depends on disability Oral–motor dysfunction General incoordination Hyperactive behavior	Depends on disability Disorientation/hyperactivity stability in chair, short: appointments, physical contact can be alarming Minimize distractions	Focus on strengths Use combination of teaching approaches Maintain attention through eye contact and physical contact; involve caregiver Consistency important
Emotional disturbance or mental illness	Medications and potential side effects Psychological causes of reported symptoms or diseases, fears	Limited financial resources in some cases Emotional concerns and fears Disturbed thought processes	Depends on nature of disturbance Inadequate diet or strange food practices Phobias about oral care Self-abuse Side effects of medications	Anxiety, fear, aggression: stability in chair, cooperation, communication, safety for patient and clinician	Reality orientation techniques Possible dietary counseling Involve caregivers Positive reinforcement and repetition For xerostomia, recommend a dry mouth management protocol that includes saliva substitutes, ice chips and drinking water, daily use of xylitol-containing products, fluoride therapy and calcium phosphate therapy ADA-approved or CDA-recognized antimicrobial mouthrinse daily
Disordered eating	Symptoms Amount of weight loss Presence and frequency of bulimia Medical and psychological interventions Eating patterns	Psychological status Denial of symptoms Length of treatment Compliance with appointments	Eating patterns Frequent vomiting Xerostomia Depression Life-threatening risk factors: conflict, life crises, major life changes, need for control and approval	Plan for referral and coordinated care with physicians, nutritionist, and psychologist Carious or eroded teeth: restorations, margination of restorations Anxiety: psychosedation Pit-and-fissure sealants if appropriate Study models to monitor progression of tooth structure loss	Rinsing with sodium bicarbonate after vomiting rather than using toothbrush Neutral pH sodium fluoride rinses or stannous fluoride gels used daily Frequent continued-care intervals For xerostomia, recommend a dry mouth management protocol that includes saliva substitutes, ice chips and drinking water, daily use of xylitol-containing products, fluoride therapy and calcium phosphate therapy ADA-approved or CDA-recognized antimicrobial mouthrinse daily
Alzheimer's disease	Multiple medical problems Medications Reduced bowel and bladder control Fatigue from abnormal sleep patterns Wheelchair	Behavior: uncooperative Finances may be limited by disability and medical problems Dependence on others	Oral–motor dysfunction Depression or disorientation leading to oral neglect General motor dysfunction Potential for injury	Dental consult as soon as possible after diagnosis Fluctuating moods and disorientation: short appointments, communication, cooperation, safety Motor problems: oral access, radiographs, stability in chair Memory loss: data collection Never leave unattended May need sedation Do not force client to have treatment	Involve caregivers Involve client when most lucid and positive Simple instructions and frequent repetition Positive reinforcement Frequent continued-care intervals Prevent oral injury Aggressive preventive program Powered oral hygiene aids

Continued

TABLE 19-14 Dental Management Considerations for Clients with Special Needs—cont'd

Condition	Medical Issues	Barriers to Care	Other Associated Health Issues	Treatment Considerations*	Prevention/Education/ Health Promotion Issues
Seizure disorders	Medications and side effects Seizure information Type of disorder Specific manifestations Presence of aura Frequency and how well controlled General management History of status epilepticus	Disturbance in self-image Transportation if cannot drive Embarrassment	Side effects of medications Potential for orofacial trauma during seizures	Seizure activity: precipitating factors, treatment planning, appointment scheduling, stability in chair, communication; stop procedures if seizure occurs Drug-influenced gingival enlargement from phenytoin Prolonged bleeding time from valproic acid Assess if medications are taken as directed	Optimal oral hygiene and frequent continued care intervals to control gingival enlargement from phenytoin First-aid instructions for oral trauma Positive reinforcement and self-image building Chlorhexidine mouth rinses or spray For xerostomia, recommend a dry mouth management protocol that includes saliva substitutes, ice chips and drinking water, daily use of xylitol-containing products, fluoride therapy and calcium phosphate therapy
Visual impairment	Degree of impairment? Sensitivity to light Treated versus untreated conditions	Degree of dependence on others Attitudes and stereotypes about disability and toward guide dogs Physical obstacles to or in office	Difficulty monitoring oral status	Determine level of assistance needed Sight impairment: appointment scheduling, explanation of procedures, communication, positioning of light, mobility in clinic, data collection, noise level Guide dog: role and placement in office Use other senses to connect with client	Large print with written instructions Demonstrate procedures on finger Tell-Show-Do approach Precede actions with clear verbal descriptions Have client explore own mouth prior to oral hygiene instructions Involve caregiver when necessary Use audio aids or physical models for teaching ADA-approved or CDA-recognized antimicrobial mouthrinse daily
Hearing impairment	Degree of impairment? Use interpreter or other assistive devices? Functioning of hearing aid	Degree of dependence on others Communication: sign language, lip reading, inaccurate pronunciation	No specific factors	Hearing impairment appointment scheduling, explanation of procedures, clinician position, use of normal tone of voice for lip reader, communication, data collection, noise interference, use of hearing aid during appointment Many pretend to hear out of embarrassment Remove mask when talking or use clear face shield as may be lip reader	Determine appropriate communication techniques Provide paper and pencil, if desired Involve interpreter if needed Watch facial expressions Demonstrate when possible Make cards with frequently used phrases Use physical models for teaching ADA-approved or CDA-recognized antimicrobial mouthrinse daily
Cleft lip or palate	Hearing impairment? Upper respiratory tract infections Prosthetic appliances Medications Diet	Fear of health care providers Self-image problems	Missing or malaligned teeth Oral-motor dysfunction Feeding disorders	Cleft: clear communication, instrument positioning or fulcruming, suctioning and prevention of aspiration Fear: dental procedures, cooperation	Instruct in cleaning any prosthetic aids Involve caregiver, when necessary Nutritional counseling, if needed

Condition					
Cerebral palsy	Associated disorders Medications Other therapies Respiration impaired? Presence of primitive reflexes Degree of impairment	Communication Transportation if in wheelchair or cannot drive May have limited financial resources Degree of dependence on others for care Mobility issues if in wheelchair Provider attitudes toward condition Self-image problems	Oral–motor dysfunction General-motor dysfunction Special diets	Primitive reflexes: client or clinician position, stability, instrument positioning or fulcruming, oral access, suctioning and amount of water used Treatment based on what they can tolerate Avoid use of air polisher or ultrasonic scaler Radiographs (few at a time) Wheelchair transfers calm treatment environment: relaxation needed to avoid muscle spasms Do not force arms and legs in unnatural positions May need sedation or muscle relaxants for extensive treatment Minimize distractions Softly cradle client's head during treatment	Modified or powered toothbrush Involve caregivers as appropriate Be patient with slowness of responses and progress Use combination of communication methods with consistency and repetition Assess need for adaptive aids for home care Frequent continued care Fluoride therapy, sealants, and antimicrobials if needed Simple, concrete instructions Involuntary movements and safety issues, may need restraints (consent necessary) ADA-approved or CDA-recognized antimicrobial mouthrinse daily
Bell's palsy	Therapies, especially prednisone Duration of condition Possible surgery to achieve facial symmetry	Language skills Self-image problems	Oral–motor dysfunction anesthesia used or opposite side affected precautions needed	Lack of eye closure: protection of eyes (goggles) Oral–motor dysfunction: protection of airway Corticosteroid therapy	Caution regarding effects of anesthesia Frequent rinsing or toothbrushing for food retention of affected side ADA-approved or CDA-recognized antimicrobial mouthrinse daily
Myasthenia gravis	Medications History of radiation therapy or surgery History of myasthenic crises	Communication Client may hold chin to help during speaking	Oral–motor dysfunction Choking risk myasthenia crisis from stress	Weakness increases during day: schedule short appointments in morning Drug interaction Amide types of local anesthetics used Oral–motor dysfunction, paralysis, and impaired breathing: protection of airway, use of rubber dam, suctioning, chair position, mouth props Difficulty retaining dentures Be prepared for emergency Avoid use of air polisher and ultrasonic scaler	Frequent continued-care intervals to prevent infection Frequent rinsing or toothbrushing for food retention Fluoride therapy, if needed Modified toothbrush or powered oral hygiene aids ADA-approved or CDA-recognized antimicrobial mouthrinse daily

Continued

TABLE 19-14 Dental Management Considerations for Clients with Special Needs—cont'd

Condition	Medical Issues	Barriers to Care	Other Associated Health Issues	Treatment Considerations*	Prevention/Education/Health Promotion Issues
Parkinson's disease	Medications and side effects Rigidity of larger joints Sensitivity to heat	Mobility to and in office Communication Embarrassment about condition	Oral–motor dysfunction Side effects of drugs Possible inadequate diet Hypersalivation	Tremors: stability, instrumentation, radiographs Sensitivity to heat: temperature of operatory Muscular pain and joint rigidity: chair position, appointment length Slurred speech: communication	Frequent continued care Frequent rinsing and toothbrushing Adaptive equipment or assistance if needed Fluoride therapy Counseling about side effects of medications ADA-approved or CDA-recognized antimicrobial mouthrinse daily
Arthritis	Medications Degree of impairment Joints affected; pain Joint replacement (premedication may be needed) Heberden's nodes	Mobility to and in office Limited finances, if disabled Weakness or fatigue decreases motivation to seek care	General motor impairment Drug-related complications such as prolonged bleeding, adrenal suppression, and bone marrow suppression	Steroid therapy Joint pain: chair position, appointment length Limited oral opening: positioning, instrumentation, radiographs, temporomandibular joint assessment Joint replacement: antibiotic premedication Long-term aspirin therapy: prolonged bleeding	Adaptive equipment or assistance is needed Counseling about side effects of medications Prevent sources of oral infection
Multiple sclerosis	Medications and side effects Degree of facial pain Degree of impairment Sensitivity to heat	Mobility to and in office, especially if in wheelchair Depression or moodiness Limited finances if disabled	Special diets Side effects of drugs Fine-motor coordination problems Oral–motor dysfunction Infection Fatigue, stress, and pain	Weakness and numbness: wheelchair transfer, stability, appointment length Oral–motor dysfunction: protection of airway Mood changes: communication, acceptance of treatment, cooperation Sensitivity to heat: room temperature Periods of exacerbation or remission: appointment scheduling	Adaptive equipment or assistance may be needed More frequent rinsing and brushing Assistance in dietary counseling Fluoride therapy ADA-approved or CDA-recognized antimicrobial mouthrinse daily More frequent continued-care intervals to prevent infections Refer for temporomandibular disorder (TMD) assessment Importance of healthy periodontium as infection can cause exacerbation of MS
Muscular dystrophies	Medications Other therapies Type and degree of involvement Prognosis Obesity, scoliosis, or cardiopulmonary involvement?	Depends on type Mobility to and in office, especially if in wheelchair Limited financial resources Weakness and possible decreased lifespan	Balance issues Oral–motor dysfunction General motor weakness and incoordination Dietary inadequacies Mouthbreathing	Facial muscle weakness can interfere with appointment length and self-care Depends on type and degree of involvement Muscle weakness: stability in chair, wheelchair transfers, radiographs, instrumentation, appointment length Oral–motor dysfunction: protection of airway, communication Incoordination: restorative treatment planning and possible emergency care Limited lifespan: treatment planning, motivation	Frequent continued care More frequent brushing and rinsing Fluoride therapy ADA-approved or CDA-recognized antimicrobial mouthrinse daily Adapted equipment or physical assistance for oral care Powered oral hygiene aids

Spinal injuries	Depends on level of injury Medications Respiratory involvement Decubitus ulcers Incontinence and encopresis Contractures Heterotopic ossifications Body temperature regulation Potential for autonomic hyperreflexia Type of adaptive equipment	Mobility to and in office, especially if in wheelchair or on respirator Limited financial resources Psychosocial concerns or depression Poor self-image	Depends on level of injury Oral–motor dysfunction Limited or total dependence on others Special diets	Psychological state: communication, cooperation Spasticity, tremors: stability Paralysis: mobility, wheelchair transfers, stability in chair, length of appointment, graphs Impaired respiration and oral–motor dysfunction: chair position, use of rubber dam, protection of airway, instrumentation Mouthstick appliance	Powered or adaptive equipment or physical assistance needed Fluoride therapy ADA-approved or CDA-recognized antimicrobial mouthrinse daily Emphasize self-care to degree possible
Spina bifida	Depends on type and degree of impairment Similar to spinal injuries Shunt for hydrocephalus (antibiotic premedication) Seizure disorders	Depends on type and degree of impairment Similar to spinal injuries	Similar to spinal injuries, except oral–motor dysfunction not apparent	Similar to spinal injuries, although psychological state not as poor Antibiotic premedication required for clients with shunts Latex sensitivity	Learning disabilities influence dental health education methods Powered oral hygiene aids
Viral hepatitis (see Chapters 8 and 9)	Type Degree of liver impairment Immunity versus active state versus carrier state Follow up with physician if status unclear Good history Need for antigen or antibody test to verify carrier state	Weakened state during acute illness No known barriers	Potential for transmission of virus Potential for abnormal bleeding in cases of significant liver damage Potential for altered drug metabolism Carrier may be asymptomatic High-carbohydrate diet	No treatment if active state Avoid use of aerosol-producing equipment (airpolishing, air-water syringe, ultrasonic scaler)	No specific concerns unless a chronic carrier Isolation of toothbrush from others if a carrier Counseling regarding transmission Discuss blood testing to determine carrier state if unknown Dietary counseling and fluoride therapy while on special diet ADA-approved or CDA-recognized antimicrobial mouthrinse daily

Continued

TABLE 19-14 Dental Management Considerations for Clients with Special Needs—cont'd

Condition	Medical Issues	Barriers to Care	Other Associated Health Issues	Treatment Considerations*	Prevention/Education/Health Promotion Issues
AIDS (see Chapters 8 and 9)	Systems involved Degree of impairment Consult with physician Kaposi's sarcoma Treatment regimens Predisposition to multiple opportunistic infections Immunosuppressive medications	Finding dentist who will treat Fear of rejection and discrimination Stigmas associated with disease Decreased motivation or depression Limited finances if unemployed, underinsured, or uninsured	Oral infections Debilitated state	Oral infections (e.g., candidiasis): palliation, transmission potential Kaposi's sarcoma: treatment planning Psychological state: communication, motivation Gingivitis should be treated to prevent necrotizing ulcerative periodontitis Povidone-iodine—use with initial debridement with necrotizing ulcerative periodontitis (NUP) Antibiotic may be needed	Palliative care for oral infections and oral ulceration Increased attention to oral hygiene Antimicrobial mouth rinses Frequent recare
Sexually transmitted diseases (see Chapters 8 and 9)	Determine status: history of disease, active disease reported or observed, in high-risk group Treatment regimen and compliance Follow-up care Medication sensitivity Complications from longstanding untreated cases	Psychosocial stigma of diseases	Potential for disease transmission	Oral lesions: palliative care	Counseling regarding disease transmission concerns
Tuberculosis (see Chapters 8 and 9)	Good history Treatment regimen (compliance and effectiveness) Appropriate follow-up care Instances of reinfection Organ systems affected	Stigma of condition	Potential for disease transmission Potential problem if it is multidrug-resistant type of tuberculosis	Disease transmission: same as for any infectious disease, especially if not sure if it is active Do not treat if active infection Avoid use of aerosol-producing equipment	Counseling regarding disease transmission

Continued

Condition					
Cystic fibrosis	Degree of impairment and prognosis Dietary changes Treatment regimens Chronic pulmonary disease Abnormal viscous secretions causing damage to major organs such as lungs, pancreas, and liver	Small stature may cause embarrassment Prognosis may decrease motivation Finances may be limited Short lifespan	Decreased resistance to infections Pulmonary complications compounded by problems of malabsorption and malnutrition Recurrent attacks of pneumonia, bronchiectasis	Mucus accumulations and impaired breathing: chair position, appointment scheduling and length, coughing, protection of airway, use of rubber dam Avoid use of air polisher and ultrasonic scaler Cooperation and scheduling issues Susceptibility to infections: appointment scheduling Tetracycline staining: aesthetics, treatment planning	For xerostomia, recommend a dry mouth management protocol that includes saliva substitutes, ice chips and drinking water, daily use of xylitol-containing products, fluoride therapy and calcium phosphate therapy Frequent oral care because of mouth-breathing Low-fat diet Recommend tartar-control products ADA-approved or CDA-recognized antimicrobial mouthrinse daily
Chronic obstructive pulmonary disease	Single or coexisting conditions Degree of impairment Medications or need for oxygen	Portable oxygen Fear of procedures that impair breathing	Side effects of medications	Impaired respiration: upright position, suctioning and coughing, rubber dam, orthopnea Medications: avoid those that depress respiration, nitrous oxide-oxygen is okay, drug interactions Avoid use of air polisher and ultrasonic scaler	Same as for bronchial asthma
Bronchial asthma	Type and severity of asthma Frequency and severity of attacks Precipitating factors Treatment regimens History of hospitalizations or status asthmaticus Instruct patient to bring inhalers if used Screen for sensitivity to nonsteroidal anti-inflammatory drugs	Fear of medical and dental environments Allergens in office	No specific risk factors	Anxiety: possible premedication or relaxation techniques Type of asthma, history of attacks Medications and precipitating factors: contraindications to prescribing or using certain drugs such as aspirin or β-blockers Avoid use of air polisher and ultrasonic scaler Medical emergency preparedness, eliminate allergens Have bronchodilator present Use of local anesthetic without epinephrine or levonordefrin in some cases; nitrous oxide–oxygen (N_2O-O_2) contraindicated Avoid aspirin-containing medications and nonsteroidal anti-inflammatory drugs	Model relaxed, stress-free environment For xerostomia, recommend a dry mouth management protocol that includes saliva substitutes, ice chips and drinking water, daily use of xylitol-containing products, fluoride therapy and calcium phosphate therapy ADA-approved or CDA-recognized antimicrobial mouthrinse daily
Congenital heart disease	Type and if repaired Extent of limitations Medications Prognosis Need for antibiotic premedication Physician consult	Financial constraints from medical bills Frequent illness Possibly debilitated state Overprotective attitude of parents	Decreased resistance to infections	Bleeding potential in some cases: treatment planning, need for laboratory tests, possible referral to specialist Prophylactic antibiotic premedication, stress management protocols, chair position	Emphasize danger of intraoral infections in terms of aggravating heart condition Frequent continued-care intervals Prevention of infective endocarditis ADA-approved or CDA-recognized antimicrobial mouthrinse daily

TABLE 19-14 Dental Management Considerations for Clients with Special Needs—cont'd

Condition	Medical Issues	Barriers to Care	Other Associated Health Issues	Treatment Considerations*	Prevention/Education/ Health Promotion Issues
Rheumatic fever and heart disease	Residual effects of rheumatic fever	No specific barriers	Rheumatic fever Pharyngeal infection with group A streptococci	Consult with cardiologist Antimicrobial rinse before treatment	Stress oral hygiene to prevent oral infections and self-induced bacteremias ADA-approved or CDA-recognized antimicrobial mouthrinse daily
Cardiac arrhythmias and dysrhythmias	Symptoms Medications and side effects Presence of pacemaker and type	Avoidance of certain electromagnetic equipment with older pacemakers	No specific risk factors Development of dysrhythmias or arrhythmias from cocaine–epinephrine interactions in cocaine abusers	Pacemaker: if not shielded may need to avoid electromagnetic equipment; check with physician Set up right—minimize x-rays Arrhythmia: stress-management protocol, drug precautions, bleeding potential from medications	No specific preventive regimens For xerostomia, recommend a dry mouth management protocol that includes saliva substitutes, ice chips and drinking water, daily use of xylitol-containing products, fluoride therapy, and calcium phosphate therapy
Hypertensive disease	Vital sign monitoring Physician consult or referral Medications and side effects and other treatment regimens Cause: primary or secondary Predisposing or general risk factors Severity, symptoms Possibility of orthostatic hypotension	Anxiety about oral health care	Side effects of medications Potential for stroke, myocardial infarction, and renal failure Potential for adverse drug interactions between vasoconstrictors and antihypertensive drugs Limit use of vasoconstrictor in anesthetics	Hypertension: stress-management protocols, chair position, treatment planning, monitoring vital signs, short appointment Overly stressed; terminate appointment Medications: drug interactions, gag reflex, bleeding potential, pain control, xerostomia, gingival enlargement; BP 180/110 mm Hg, delay treatment and refer to physician	Counseling regarding reducing general risk factors Palliative care for oral infections from medications For xerostomia, recommend a dry mouth management protocol that includes saliva substitutes, ice chips and drinking water, daily use of xylitol-containing products, fluoride therapy, and calcium phosphate therapy Create stress-free environment Prevent postural hypertension
Ischemic heart disease (coronary atherosclerotic heart disease)	Physician consult Angina or myocardial infarction episodes Hospitalizations Medications and side effects Surgery	Possible debilitated state Medical and other expenses Anxiety about dental treatment	Side effect of medications Susceptibility to infections if debilitated Limit use of vasoconstrictor in anesthetics	Heart condition: same considerations as for hypertensive disease and preparation for medical emergency, contraindications to treatment if unstable or recent attack (within 6 months) Medications: same as for hypertensive disease; pain control Aspirin use—bleeding concerns	Palliative care for side effects of medications Counseling regarding decreasing general risk factors Special oral hygiene instructions if hospitalized or bedridden Frequent maintenance visits Create stress-free environment Educate about increased risk for myocardial infarction in clients with periodontitis ADA-approved or CDA-recognized antimicrobial mouthrinse daily

Congestive heart failure	Same as for severe ischemic or hypertensive heart disease	Mobility Debilitated Labored breathing	Pulmonary congestion and edema Limit use of vasoconstrictor in anesthetics	Avoid use of air polisher and ultrasonic scaler Prone to nausea and vomiting during oral health care Keep client upright in chair	Frequent continued care intervals Create stress-free environment ADA-approved or CDA-recognized antimicrobial mouthrinse daily
Cerebrovascular accident (stroke)	Type of involvement, degree of limitation Seizures? Medications and side effects Other therapies	Communication Accessibility if need adaptive equipment or wheelchair Degree of dependence on others	Oral-motor dysfunction Side effects of medications Impaired general-motor coordination Dietary inadequacies Transient ischemic attacks Previous stroke, hypertension, cardiac abnormalities, atherosclerosis, diabetes mellitus, elevated blood lipids	Memory and speech impairment: communication, data collection Oral-motor dysfunction or paralysis: instrumentation, jaw stability, radiographs, treatment planning Impaired emotional control: cooperation, communication Evaluate calcifications in the carotid artery via panoramic radiographs Short morning appointments General paralysis: mobility, possible wheelchair transfers, stability in chair Minimize use of vasoconstrictors	Use combination of teaching approaches Reinforce and repeat instructions Frequent continued care Fluoride therapy, if needed ADA-approved or CDA-recognized antimicrobial mouthrinse daily Adaptive aids or supervision for oral care Avoid sensory overload Reorient client to situations, rinsing difficult or impossible Use one-step instructions Educate about increased risk for cerebrovascular accident in clients with periodontitis
Sickle cell disease	Precipitating factors for crises Symptoms and severity Associated conditions Transfusions? Lab tests needed? Physician consult regarding need for antibiotic premedication	Periods of pain Debilitated condition at times Fear of dental environment Limited financial resources because of medical bills	Susceptibility to infections Low stress tolerance	Sickle cell crises: emergency care only Susceptibility to infections: periodontal maintenance, physician consult for prophylactic antibiotic premedication Reduce patient stress Consultation with physician Avoid medications that depress respiration	Dietary counseling Frequent maintenance care because of associated alveolar bone problems and need to control oral infection Involvement of others in care Create a stress-free oral health care environment Emphasis on optimal oral health care behaviors as periodontitis can cause a crisis ADA-approved or CDA-recognized antimicrobial mouthrinse daily

Continued

TABLE 19-14 Dental Management Considerations for Clients with Special Needs—cont'd

Condition	Medical Issues	Barriers to Care	Other Associated Health Issues	Treatment Considerations*	Prevention/Education/Health Promotion Issues
Cancers	Parts of body affected, treatment regimens, medications and side effects, potential for bleeding and anemia Physician consult regarding need for antibiotic premedication	Frequent hospitalizations or medical appointments Debilitated states Financial burdens Reliance on others Depression	Side effects of medications Oral infections and ulcerations Metastasis to oral cavity Weakness for self-care	Radiation therapy: care before and after Prevention and palliative care for oral infections and ulcerations Short appointments and frequent active follow-up Potential bleeding problem Prompt treatment of dental-related infections Evaluate need for antibiotic premedication	With cues, if bleeding is a problem Fluoride therapy ADA-approved or CDA-recognized antimicrobial mouthrinse daily Oral hygiene aids Help with oral care, if needed Monitor removable appliances Frequent maintenance care For xerostomia, recommend a dry mouth management protocol that includes saliva substitutes, ice chips and drinking water, daily use of xylitol-containing products, fluoride therapy, calcium phosphate therapy, and antifungals, as needed
Leukemias	Type Treatment regimens, frequency Presence of anemia, thrombocytopenia, and infection Immunosuppression from therapy	Stages of acute disease versus remissions Fear of dental environment	Side effects of chemotherapy or radiation therapy Susceptibility to infections Oral hemorrhage	Bleeding potential: platelet count status needed—avoid treatment if less than 50,000 mm³, appointment scheduling, physician consult, surgical procedures Susceptibility to infections: periodontal maintenance, antibiotic premedication Ideally, provide invasive care before chemotherapy or radiation therapy Acute versus remission stages: treatment planning, appointment scheduling Chemotherapy or radiation therapy: treatment planning Consultation with oncologist	Palliative care for oral lesions Frequent continued-care intervals Fluoride therapy program Involvement of others in care program For xerostomia, recommend a dry mouth management protocol that includes saliva substitutes, ice chips and drinking water, daily use of xylitol-containing products, fluoride therapy, and calcium phosphate therapy Eliminate potential sources of oral infection Meticulous oral hygiene ADA-approved or CDA-recognized antimicrobial mouthrinse daily
Hemophilias	Type and severity Frequency and location of bleeds Treatment regimens Joint replacements? Hepatitis? AIDS? Seizures? Inhibitor status Laboratory tests needed?	Finding dentist who will treat Resources for emergency care	Potential for oral bleeds Potential to acquire hepatitis, cirrhosis, or AIDS associated with frequent clotting factor replacement therapy	Bleeding potential: preappointment laboratory tests, surgery, physician consult, factor replacement therapy, instrumentation, radiographs, use of rubber dam, suctioning, use of Amicar or Cyklokapron Joint replacements: prophylactic antibiotic premedication Hepatitis carrier: disease transmission procedures Avoid use of aspirin	Use extra soft-bristled brush ADA-approved or CDA-recognized antimicrobial mouthrinse daily Counseling regarding first aid for oral trauma Frequent continued care intervals Educate about role of oral infection and increased bleeding

Condition					
Diabetes mellitus	Type and severity Medication regimens Dietary regimen Complications Hypertension and other heart conditions Frequency of episodes of hypoglycemia or hyperglycemia	Finding dentist who will treat if have chronic complications	Susceptibility to infections (e.g., oral candidiasis) Decreased salivary flow Recalcitrant periodontal disease Slow healing Complications associated with disturbances in vision and kidney function	Insulin–sugar balance: potential for medical emergency, appointment scheduling, stress-management protocol Susceptibility to infection: periodontal maintenance, possible antibiotic premedication Avoid elective treatment, if uncontrolled	3- to 6-month continued-care intervals Dietary analysis For xerostomia, recommend a dry mouth management protocol that includes saliva substitutes, ice chips and drinking water, daily use of xylitol-containing products, fluoride therapy, and calcium phosphate therapy Need for excellent bacterial biofilm control ADA-approved or CDA-recognized antimicrobial mouthrinse daily Minimize stress Control of oral infections Prevention of insulin shock or diabetic coma Role of periodontitis in blood glucose control
Thyroid disease	Type and cause Symptoms and severity Medications Cardiac arrhythmias/dysrhythmias	No specific barriers Swelling of tongue in hypothyroidism may cause difficulty in speech communication	Abnormal dental development Thyroid crisis is life threatening	Sensitivity to drugs: treatment planning, postoperative instruction, preparation for medical emergency Intellectual and developmental disabilities in some (see "Management for intellectual and developmental disabilities") Abnormal dental development: treatment planning Heat or cold intolerance: room temperature, length of appointment "Thyroid storm" or thyroid crisis precipitated by surgery, infection, trauma, or uncontrolled thyroid disease Exaggerated response to central nervous system depressants	Prevention of infection ADA-approved or CDA-recognized antimicrobial mouthrinse daily Prevention of thyroid crisis Create a stress-free environment
Chemical dependency	Obtaining adequate history Types of drugs used Symptoms Treatment interventions Potential for drug interactions or overdose Emotional stability during appointment At risk for AIDS, hepatitis	Emotional state Denial of drug problem Demanding requests for use of nitrous oxide or pain medications Disoriented behavior	Neglect personal hygiene Potential for oral trauma Potential link (not documented) to oral cancer Potential drug interaction if local anesthetic with epinephrine is injected into blood vessel	Coordinated care: professional team and family if in treatment program Use of drugs for procedure: restrict Strict guidelines for keeping appointments necessary Avoid local anesthesia with epinephrine for 6 hours after cocaine use Complete as much treatment as possible per visit	Frequent brushing and flossing Teach oral self-examinations Avoid mouthrinses containing alcohol Topical fluoride program

Continued

TABLE 19-14 Dental Management Considerations for Clients with Special Needs—cont'd

Condition	Medical Issues	Barriers to Care	Other Associated Health Issues	Treatment Considerations*	Prevention/Education/ Health Promotion Issues
Chronic alcoholism	Client's perception of severity of problem Symptoms Treatment program Nutritional deficiencies Chronic complications Degree of liver impairment At risk for tuberculosis	Potential for no-show appointments or intoxication at appointment Limited finances, if unemployed	Susceptibility to infection Nutritional deficiencies Nausea and vomiting Potential for oral trauma	Liver impairment and bleeding potential: preappointment laboratory testing, drug metabolism, instrumentation, treatment planning Inebriated states: emergency care, appointment scheduling, treatment planning, data collection Use only alcohol-free medicaments Recommend alcohol-free mouthrinses	Nutritional counseling Frequent continued care intervals Fluoride therapy and alcohol-free antimicrobials Frequent soft tissue evaluation for oral cancer Counseling regarding oral trauma For xerostomia, recommend a dry mouth management protocol that includes saliva substitutes, ice chips and drinking water, daily use of xylitol-containing products, fluoride therapy and calcium phosphate therapy Instill responsibility for oral care Counsel to avoid alcohol prior to premedication
Chronic renal failure	Symptoms and severity Hypertension Dialysis? Transplantation? Special diets Need for antibiotic premedication Excretion of drugs Electrolyte and fluid imbalance	Finding dentist who will treat Debilitated condition at times Limited finances Fear of oral health care environment	Susceptibility to oral infection Dietary inadequacies Viral hepatitis Drug-influenced gingival enlargement from cyclosporine	Hypertension and kidney failure: vital signs, drug interactions, avoid use of drugs metabolized by the kidney Bleeding tendency: preappointment blood tests, consult with patient's physician Schedule dental treatment the day after dialysis Screen for bleeding disorder Hemostatic measures Atrioventricular fistula: antibiotic premedication, take blood pressure in arm without fistula Dialysis: scheduling, hepatitis precautions Transplants: prophylactic antibiotic premedication, complete all care	3- to 6-month continued-care interval because of increased calculus Prevent infection Palliative care for oral lesions Daily home fluoride therapy Tartar control dentifrices Chlorhexidine mouthrinses

| Pregnancy | Trimester
Side effects
Nutritional status
Rise in progesterone levels
Significant changes in the immune response | Frequent sickness
Physical comfort
Nausea and sensitivity to various odors | Possible dietary inadequacies
Vulnerability of fetus during first trimester
Increased incidence of gingivitis | Fetal sensitivity: avoidance of drugs, elective dental procedures
Pressure of fetus on mother's vena cava: chair position, orthostatic hypotension (turn on left side to alleviate pressure)
Safest period to provide routine care is second trimester
Short appointments | Prenatal counseling
Meticulous oral hygiene to decrease response to local irritants
Education on the relationship between bacterial plaque, hormone level, and periodontal disease
Education on increased risk for preterm and low-birth-weight delivery in clients who are pregnant and have periodontitis
Education on the relationship between caries process and gastric acids from vomiting
Education on vertical and horizontal disease transmission, care of infant's oral cavity and causes of early childhood caries (may need to initiate a xylitol protocol)
Daily home fluoride therapy and sodium bicarbonate mouth rinses (before toothbrushing if episodes of vomiting)
ADA-approved or CDA-recognized antimicrobial mouthrinse daily |
| Older adult | Medications and potential side effects
Chronic diseases
Joint replacements
Sensory impairments
Reduced disease resistance | Transportation problems
Finances may be limited
Person may be depressed | Side effects of medications
Physical side effects of chronic diseases
Anatomic changes of gingiva | Identify side effects of medications
Sensory impairments
Short appointments in mid-morning
Increased risk for root caries
Assess need for sodium fluoride therapy (home and in office)
Assess need for antibiotic premedication | Instruct person about oral cancer self-examination and risk factors
Instruct in oral hygiene and modifications of oral hygiene devices
For xerostomia, recommend a dry mouth management protocol that includes saliva substitutes, ice chips and drinking water, daily use of xylitol-containing products, fluoride therapy and calcium phosphate therapy
Make suggestions gradually
ADA-approved or CDA-recognized antimicrobial mouthrinse daily |

AIDS, acquired immune deficiency syndrome; *ADA,* American Dental Association, *CDA,* Canadian Dental Association.
Standard precautions for infection control are used at each appointment.

Name_____ Telephone_____

Address_____ Age _____

Name and address of contact person (if different) Telephone _____

_____

_____

_____

Physician _____ Specialty _____ Telephone _____

Physician _____ Specialty _____ Telephone _____

Medical problems or disabling conditions _____

_____

Potential barriers:

Transportation _____

Finances _____

Communication _____

Psychosocial _____

Cultural _____

Medical _____

Mobility/stability _____

Other _____

Scheduling limitations _____

Other data _____

FIGURE 19-23 Previsit questionnaire for gathering preliminary data about individuals with special needs.

the home or community setting with portable equipment

7. If office facilities do not comply with accessibility guidelines, discuss ways to:
   a. Make them physically accessible
   b. Accommodate client needs or refer the client to a provider who can provide the needful
8. Ensure that office layout and environment are not safety hazards or health hazards for some clients
9. Keep scheduling somewhat flexible to allow for transportation or other problems; block appointments are helpful when dealing with groups
10. Be prepared to implement wheelchair transfers

C. Medical issues
   1. Obtain a health history from the client or caregiver, with supplemental information from other professionals or agency records
   2. Update the health history at each visit
   3. Because many standard health history forms are inadequate for the multiple conditions and problems of some clients, ask supplemental questions
   4. Obtain specifics regarding medical treatment regimens or other therapies that may affect scheduling or treatment

5. Obtain names, addresses, and phone numbers for all the client's physicians who might provide helpful data (e.g., generalist, cardiologist, orthopedist, endocrinologist) with permission to release information
6. Be particularly alert to the client's physical status during initial assessment
7. Monitor vital signs, as indicated
8. Record all medication information; update at each visit
9. Note any indications or contraindications to treatment or premedication
10. Maintain records of all medical advice, prescriptions, or drugs given
11. If clients refuse to disclose medical information or do not follow recommended standard procedures for their own protection (e.g., antibiotic premedication), have them sign a statement to that effect for the records

D. Treatment adaptations
1. Demonstrate understanding and acceptance of conditions or problems to the client and to caregivers or family
2. Determine which special needs require provider adaptations versus client adaptations

3. Demonstrate empathy, not sympathy
4. Discuss before implementation:
   a. Behavioral expectations
   b. Overview of the entire care plan
   c. Procedures that will be performed at the appointment
   d. Approximate time required
   e. Communication techniques to be used during the appointment
5. Introduce clients to the oral health care setting gradually by using desensitization, modeling, "show-tell-do," or other methods
6. Ensure client comfort in the dental chair through frequent assurance, positioning, and supportive measures as needed (e.g., pillows)
7. Explain carefully any need for client body restraint or stabilization for behavioral or stability purposes to ensure the clinician's safety and the client's safety while in the chair; Velcro® straps similar to safety belts are helpful for stability (Figure 19-24, *A* to *D*); ensure the following:
   a. Obtain informed consent to use these
   b. Ensure least restrictive restraint is used
   c. Clearly document restraint used

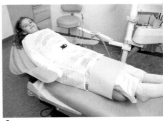

A

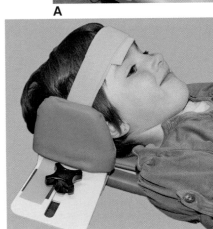

C

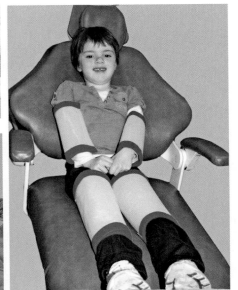

B

D

FIGURE 19-24 The Rainbow® Stabilizing System. **A,** Adult on large hinged board. **B,** Child with elbow and knee stabilizers that prohibit movement of joints. **C,** Head stabilizer. **D,** Safety belts for securing the client safely in the dental chair. *(Used with permission from Specialized Care Co., Hampton, NH.)*

d. Check state regulations to ensure proper compliance

8. Pharmacologic restraints such as oral, intramuscular, intravenous, or inhalation sedation may be needed; general anesthesia is sometimes necessary when a client is not easily stimulated or has partial or complete loss of protective reflexes

9. Be aware that adaptations for specific procedures require problem solving and experimentation among the provider, client, and caregiver, if appropriate; Figure 19-25 displays a variety of mouth props

10. Discuss the mechanisms for wheelchair transfers with each client, as preferences and techniques vary

11. Protect the client's airway through use of a rubber dam, adequate suctioning, and other means; this is of paramount importance because of the frequency of impaired oral reflexes

12. Some pediatric clients' behavior may improve if they bring comfort items such as a stuffed animal or a blanket; asking the caregiver to sit nearby or hold the client's hand may be helpful as well

13. For the most part, keep appointments short and positive

14. Fluoride therapies (varnishes) and antimicrobial rinses are important preventive measures

15. Stress the importance of good oral health being part of good general health

E. Preventive measures
1. Identify risk factors for oral disease to plan preventive programs that:
   a. Maximize positive health behaviors
   b. Eliminate risk factors
   c. Eliminate existing disease
2. Common risk factors include:
   a. Inappropriate nursing and feeding habits
   b. Transfer of oral pathogens from mother or caregiver to infant (vertical transmission); usually from sharing food and eating utensils; can also occur among siblings or playmates (horizontal transmission)
   c. Nutritionally inadequate diet
   d. Frequent intake of cariogenic foods
   e. Suboptimal fluoride supplementation
   f. Oral–motor dysfunction (e.g., hyperactive gag reflex or impaired tongue control)
   g. General motor dysfunction interfering with oral hygiene care
   h. Crisis orientation to care
   i. Preoccupation with one's disability; depression
   j. Previous negative experience with health care
   k. Limited income and education
   l. Different cultural values and beliefs
3. Develop individualized programs to reduce or eliminate the risk factors and increase the protective factors

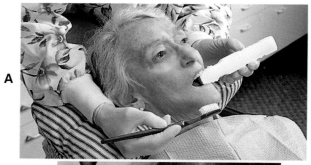

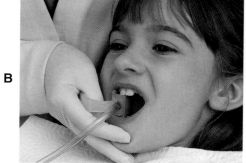

FIGURE 19-25 **A,** Clinician shown using the OpenWide® Disposable Mouth Prop on an adult. **B,** Clinician shown using the OpenWide® Re-Usable Mouth Prop that allows for a saliva ejector to be kept in place with the bite block. *(Used with permission from Specialized Care Co., Hampton, NH.)*

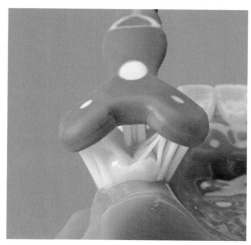

FIGURE 19-26 The Surround® Toothbrush has a unique head that surrounds the tooth to clean all surfaces at the same time; ideal aid for caregiver brushing someone else's teeth. *(Used with permission from Specialized Care Co., Hampton, NH.)*

4. Consider the client's limitations when recommending home care procedures
   a. Problems with fluoride or antimicrobial rinses or disclosing tablets if the client has oral–motor problems
   b. Problems performing the sequence of toothbrushing strokes if the client has memory or general motor impairment; Figure 19-26 displays a modified toothbrush for easier accessibility
   c. Problems picking up and using a toothbrush and toothpaste if the client has paralysis or control problems

   d. Power toothbrushing and flossing devices can work well, but some patients may respond poorly since they can be frightened by the noise
5. Provide anticipatory guidance to parents on milestones and preventive measures at each developmental stage
6. Schedule frequent maintenance care appointments
7. Coordinate preventive efforts in the home, school, daycare, workplace, or oral health care settings
8. Encourage the establishment of a dental home

@ WEB SITE INFORMATION AND RESOURCES

SOURCE	WEB SITE ADDRESS	DESCRIPTION
American Academy of Pediatric Dentistry	http://www.aapd.org	Information, education, policies, and guidelines on working with all children, including those with special care needs
National Maternal and Child Oral Health Resource Center	http://www.mchoralhealth.org/default.html	Information on working with children with disabilities
National Institute of Dental and Craniofacial Research	http://www.nidcr.nih.gov	Information, education, and strategies on providing care to patients with special care needs
The Center for Children with Special Needs	http://www.cshcn.org/	Health information and resources for families and professionals caring for children with special health care needs and chronic health conditions
National Institute on Disability and Rehabilitation Research	http://www.ed.gov/programs/nidrr	Support related to rehabilitation of individuals with disabilities

---

SUGGESTED READINGS

American Dental Education Association: *Oral health for independent older adults.* Available at http://www.adea.org/publications/Documents/CurriculumResourceGuide.pdf: Accessed June 12, 2010.

Cawson RA, Odell EW: *Cawson's essentials of oral pathology and oral medicine,* ed 8, Philadelphia, 2008, Elsevier.

Darby M, Walsh M: *Dental hygiene theory and practice,* ed 3, Philadelphia, 2010, Saunders.

Dils ES: Management strategies for the patient with a developmental disability, *J Prac Hyg* 16(9):6–8, 2007.

Little JW, Falace DA: *Dental management of the medically compromised patient,* ed 7, St Louis, 2008, Mosby.

Mayo Clinic Website: Diseases and conditions, Available at www.mayoclinic.com/invoke.cfm: Accessed April 24, 2010.

National Oral Health Information Clearinghouse: Practical oral care for people with developmental disabilities, *Making a Difference Series, NIH Publication* 04-5193, July 2009.

National Oral Health Information Clearinghouse: Oral health care for older adults. Information for patients and professionals, *Publication OP-41,* July 2009.

CHAPTER 19 REVIEW QUESTIONS

1. Each of the following is a common oral manifestation of end-stage renal disease EXCEPT one. Which one is the EXCEPTION?
   a. Glossitis
   b. Petechia
   c. Urea in saliva
   d. Ground glass appearance of alveolar bone

2. Failure of the liquid in the eye to drain resulting in increased pressure and optic nerve destruction defines:
   a. Cataract
   b. Retrolental fibroplasia
   c. Retinitis pigmentosa
   d. Glaucoma

3. Which of the following disabling conditions often occurs with hearing loss?
   a. Cleft palate
   b. Multiple sclerosis
   c. Thyroid disease
   d. Blindness

4. Perimyolysis of the maxillary anterior lingual teeth is associated with:
   a. Epilepsy
   b. Anorexia nervosa
   c. Cleft palate
   d. Bulimia

5. An autoimmune neuromuscular disease characterized by muscle weakness caused by problems with nerve transmission describes:
   a. Muscular dystrophy
   b. Myasthenia gravis
   c. Parkinson's disease
   d. Arthritis

6. A client with a spinal cord injury at the level of C-6 would be a quadriplegic. Power scaling devices are CONTRAINDICATED for clients with paralysis.
   a. The first statement is TRUE; the second is FALSE
   b. The first statement is FALSE; the second is TRUE
   c. Both statements are TRUE
   d. Both statements are FALSE

7. Antibiotic premedication prior to invasive dental services is often required for clients with all of the following conditions EXCEPT one. Which one is the EXCEPTION?
   a. Sickle cell anemia
   b. Kidney transplantation
   c. Hip replacement
   d. Heart murmur

8. The high incidence of dental caries in patients with an intellectual impairment is MOST likely caused by:
   a. Oral neglect
   b. Genetic defects
   c. Abnormal oral musculature
   d. Swallowing problems

9. A client's blood pressure reading is 140/90 mm Hg. The dental hygienist should inform the patient that this reading indicates:
   a. Normal blood pressure
   b. Prehypertension
   c. Stage 1 hypertension
   d. Stage 2 hypertension

10. A. supine position during dental hygiene treatment is CONTRAINDICATED in clients with:
    a. Multiple sclerosis
    b. Congestive heart disease
    c. Intellectual impairments
    d. Cleft palate

11. A client with diabetes with a glycated hemoglobin assay (Hb_{A1c}) test value of 9% means that his or her diabetes is:
    a. Well controlled
    b. Slightly under control
    c. Moderately controlled
    d. Uncontrolled

12. Clients with diabetes are CONTRAINDICATED for dental implants, since the implantation of foreign bodies is commonly rejected in persons with diabetes.
    a. The first part of the statement is TRUE; the second part is FALSE
    b. The first part of the statement is FALSE; the second part is TRUE
    c. Both parts of the statement are TRUE
    d. Both parts of the statement are FALSE

13. A client undergoing dialysis should have the dental hygiene visit scheduled:
    a. Immediately after dialysis
    b. Within 12 hours of dialysis
    c. The day after dialysis
    d. 3 days after dialysis

14. Which of the following is a common oral finding in persons who are addicted to methamphetamine?
    a. Rapid gingival recession
    b. Rampant cervical caries
    c. Leukoplakia
    d. Increased rate of occlusal caries

15. To be in compliance with the Americans with Disabilities Act, all doorways in a dental office must be:
    a. 32 inches wide
    b. Affixed with a lever-type handle
    c. 8 feet tall
    d. Posted for disability access

16. Which one of the following medical emergencies is MOST likely to occur in a client with diabetes mellitus?
    a. Ketoacidosis
    b. Hypoglycemia
    c. Hyperglycemia
    d. Seizure

17. Which of the following medications is BEST recommended for oral pain management in clients with asthma?
    a. Nonsteroidal anti-inflammatory drugs (NSAIDs)
    b. Acetaminophen
    c. Aspirin
    d. Procardia

18. Which of the following is a common oral side effect of radiation to the head and neck area?
    a. Occlusal caries
    b. Fissuring of the tongue
    c. Cervical caries
    d. Periodontal abscesses

19. The type of seizure where consciousness begins and ends abruptly in 5 to 30 seconds followed by a quick resuming of activities describes:
    a. Simple seizure
    b. Tonic clonic (grand mal) seizure
    c. Absence (petite mal) seizure
    d. Complex-focal seizure

20. A chronic immunologic systemic disease in which joint inflammation occurs during periods of exacerbation and remission defines:
    a. Progressive systemic sclerosis
    b. Rheumatoid arthritis
    c. Tubular sclerosis
    d. Lupus erythematosus

21. Angle's classification of malocclusion commonly found in clients with Down syndrome is:
    a. Class I
    b. Class II, division one
    c. Class II, division two
    d. Class III

22. Which of the following patient conditions would require antibiotic premedication for invasive dental hygiene procedures?
    a. Mitral valve prolapse
    b. Stent placement
    c. Functional heart murmur
    d. Valvular prosthesis

23. The MOST common location of oral cancer is the:
    a. Floor of the mouth
    b. Lateral border of the tongue
    c. Lip
    d. Pharynx

24. Clients over age 60 who smoke are the fastest growing segment of the oral cancer population. Human papilloma virus 16 (HPV 16) is responsible for the increased risk for oral cancer especially in the tonsillar area.
    a. The first statement is TRUE; the second is FALSE
    b. The first statement is FALSE; the second is TRUE
    c. Both statements are TRUE
    d. Both statements are FALSE

25. All of the following oral conditions are common in clients with cerebral palsy EXCEPT one. Which one is this EXCEPTION?
    a. Open bite
    b. Facial asymmetry
    c. Nerve paralysis
    d. Swallowing problems

26. Which of the following professional fluoride treatments would be BEST for a special-care child client?
    a. Paint on stannous fluoride
    b. Sodium fluoride varnish
    c. Acidulated phosphate fluoride gel
    d. Sodium fluoride foam

27. Antibiotic premedication is commonly needed in clients with Down syndrome because of the high incidence of:
    a. Congenital heart valve defects
    b. Obstructive airway problems
    c. Impaired leukocyte function
    d. Chromosomal abnormalities

28. Each of the following is important to teach a caregiver about oral home care for a special care client EXCEPT one. Which one is the EXCEPTION?
    a. Tongue blades taped together can make a safe at-home mouth prop
    b. Toothpaste with fluoride always should be a part of the home care regimen
    c. Only attempt to teach flossing if toothbrushing can be mastered
    d. Caregivers' legs can be placed over the arms of a child to restrain long enough for oral home care

29. **Delayed and abnormal tooth eruption patterns are common in clients with Down syndrome. The lips are thin, and the tongue is very small, and this contributes to the delayed eruption of teeth.**
    a. The first statement is TRUE; the second is FALSE
    b. The first statement is FALSE; the second is TRUE
    c. Both statements are TRUE
    d. Both statements are FALSE

30. **A power scaling instrument would be contraindicated in clients with:**
    a. Human immunodeficiency virus (HIV) infection
    b. Epilepsy
    c. Cystic fibrosis
    d. Hypertensive disease

31. **Each of the following conditions is associated with paralysis EXCEPT one. Which one is the EXCEPTION?**
    a. Bell's palsy
    b. Graves' disease
    c. Stroke
    d. Spinal cord compression

32. **Elective dental treatment should be postponed until ___ months after a stroke.**
    a. 1
    b. 2
    c. 4
    d. 6

Use Case A and Figures 19-27 through 19-30 to answer questions 33 to 42.

SYNOPSIS OF PATIENT HISTORY		
	Age _58_	VITAL SIGNS
	Sex _M_	Blood pressure _180/90 mmHg_
	Height _5'11"_	Pulse rate _96 bpm_
	Race _African American_	Respiration rate _14 rpm_
CASE _A_	Weight _____ lbs _____ kgs	

1. Under Care of Physician — *Renal transplant hypertension Parkinson's disease GERD*

   Yes No
   ☒   ☐   Condition: *Hyperlipidemia*

2. Hospitalized within the last 5 years
   Yes No
   ☒   ☐   Reason: _____

3. Has or had the following conditions

   _____
   _____
   _____

4. Current medications
   Nifedipine (Procardia®)
   Cyclosporin (Neoral®)
   Clopidogrel (Plavix®)
   Levodopa (Dopar®)
   Omeprazole (Prilosec®)

5. Smokes or uses tobacco products
   Yes No
   ☒   ☐

6. Is pregnant
   Yes No N/A
   ☐   ☐   ☒

MEDICAL HISTORY:
Patient had a kidney transplant two years ago after 4 years of dialysis.
Patient reports an allergy to penicillin.

DENTAL HISTORY:
Patient's physician recommended he get his teeth cleaned. Scaling and root debridement was started on the mandibular right side 6 months ago but was not completed because he could not afford to complete care at that time. He has never received regular dental care.

SOCIAL HISTORY:
Patient is on disability and lives with his wife. He taught high school for 20 years. Patient reports smoking about a pack of cigarettes a day and reports he has tried to quit unsuccessfully several times.

CHIEF COMPLAINT:
I need my teeth cleaned; my gums bleed when I brush.

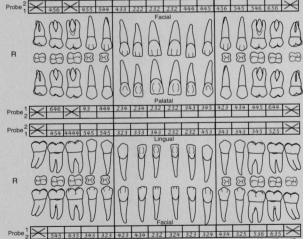

Adult clinical examination

Case A

CURRENT ORAL HYGIENE STATUS:

SUPPLEMENTAL ORAL EXAMINATION FINDINGS:

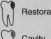

Restoration

Cavity

Sealant

Clinically missing tooth

Furcation

"Through and through" furcation

Probe 1: initial probing depth

Probe 2: probing depth 1 month after scaling and root planing

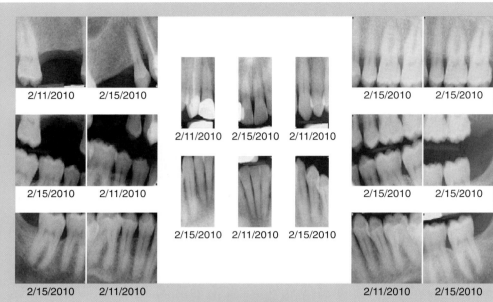

2/11/2010   2/15/2010

2/15/2010   2/11/2010

2/15/2010   2/11/2010

2/11/2010   2/15/2010   2/11/2010

2/15/2010   2/11/2010   2/15/2010

2/15/2010   2/15/2010

2/15/2010   2/15/2010

2/11/2010   2/15/2010

FIGURE 19-27

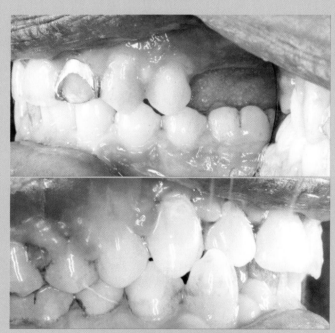

FIGURE 19-28

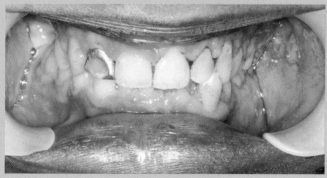

FIGURE 19-29

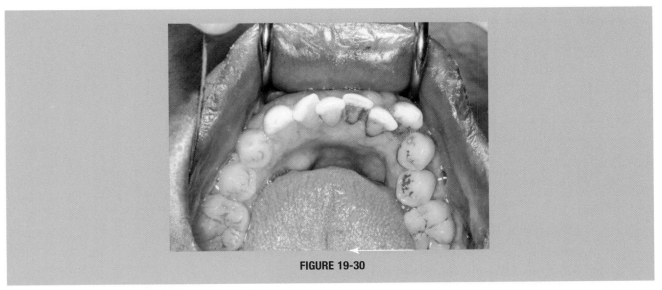

FIGURE 19-30

33. The technique error associated with the left molar bitewing could be corrected by changing the:
   a. Film holder
   b. Position of the film packet
   c. Vertical angulation
   d. Beam indicating device alignment

34. Which of the client's conditions is a degenerative disorder of the central nervous system that often impairs motor skills, speech, and postural stability?
   a. Gastroesophageal reflux disease (GERD)
   b. Hyperlipidemia
   c. Parkinson's disease
   d. Hypertension

35. In which of the American Society of Anesthesiologists (ASA) Physical Status Classifications would you place this client?
   a. I
   b. II
   c. III
   d. IV

36. The arrow in the mandibular right premolar radiograph is indicating the:
   a. Mandibular canal
   b. Internal oblique ridge
   c. Genial tubercles
   d. Hamular notch

37. What client condition places him or her at risk for dental erosion?
   a. Hypertension
   b. GERD
   c. Hyperlipidemia
   d. End-stage renal disease

38. Local anesthestic agents with epinephrine are contraindicated on this client because clients with hypertension cannot adequately metabolize anesthetic agents.
   a. The statement is CORRECT, but the reason is INCORRECT
   b. Both the statement and the reason are CORRECT
   c. Both the statement and the reason are INCORRECT
   d. The statement is INCORRECT, but the reason is CORRECT

39. The raised hard asymptomatic area in the mandibular area on the photograph visible by the arrow is MOST likely a(an):
   a. Fistula
   b. Exostosis
   c. Pyogenic granuloma
   d. Cementoma

40. Which of the following contributing factors is the MOST likely reason for the condition of this client's gingiva?
   a. Smoking
   b. Medications
   c. Poor self-care
   d. Vitamin deficiency

41. Which of the following premedication regimens would be recommended for this client?
   a. None
   b. 2.0 g of amoxicillin
   c. 2.0 g of ampicillin
   d. 600 mg of clindamycin

42. The technique error associated with the right maxillary canine radiograph can be attributed to improper:
   a. BID alignment
   b. Placement of film holding device
   c. Horizontal angulation
   d. Placement of film packet

Use Case B and Figures 19-31 through 19-36 to answer questions 43 to 50.

SYNOPSIS OF PATIENT HISTORY

Age __22__
Sex __M__
Height __5'8"__

CASE __B__

Weight _____ lbs
_____ kgs

VITAL SIGNS
Blood pressure __150/90 mmHg__
Pulse rate __70 bpm__
Respiration rate __20 rpm__

1. Under Care of Physician
   Yes ☒ No ☐   Condition: *Seizure disorder / Hypertension / Anxiety disorder*
2. Hospitalized within the last 5 years
   Yes ☐ No ☐   Reason: _____
3. Has or had the following conditions
   Mild intellectual impairment; prosthetic mitral valve placed as an infant; Hearing impairment, functional with hearing aids; Anxiety disorder
4. Current medications
   Valium® diazepam
   Lasix® furosemide
   Cardizem® diltiazem
   Tegretol® carbamazepine
5. Smokes or uses tobacco products
   Yes ☐ No ☒
6. Is pregnant
   Yes ☐ No ☐ N/A ☒

MEDICAL HISTORY:

DENTAL HISTORY:
Patient has not been to a dentist in over 10 years. Patient reports only occasionally brushing his teeth and does not floss.

SOCIAL HISTORY:
Patient lives in a group home for adults and is employed at a linen service company.

CHIEF COMPLAINT:
Patient reports pain in his bottom right side.

Adult clinical examination

	1	2	3	4	5	6	7	8	9	10	11	12	13	14	15	16
Probe 2/1	✕	✕	423	423	444	424	324	444	223	233	334	434	424	445	✕	544

Facial

R

Palatal

	1	2	3	4	5	6	7	8	9	10	11	12	13	14	15	16
Probe 1/2	✕	✕	434	534	333	434	434	323	333	342	223	434	554	334	✕	445
Probe 2/1	✕	544	434	434	434	333	333	334	333	343	233	344	335	534	✕	435

Lingual

R

Facial

	32	31	30	29	28	27	26	25	24	23	22	21	20	19	18	17
Probe 1/2	✕	534	434	343	434	333	432	234	345	243	23	343	334	545	✕	434

Case B

CURRENT ORAL HYGIENE STATUS:
Patient has heavy generalized supra and sub gingival calculus; generalized BOP

SUPPLEMENTAL ORAL EXAMINATION FINDINGS:

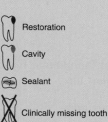

Restoration

Cavity

Sealant

Clinically missing tooth

Furcation

"Through and through" furcation

Probe 1: initial probing depth

Probe 2: probing depth 1 month after scaling and root planing

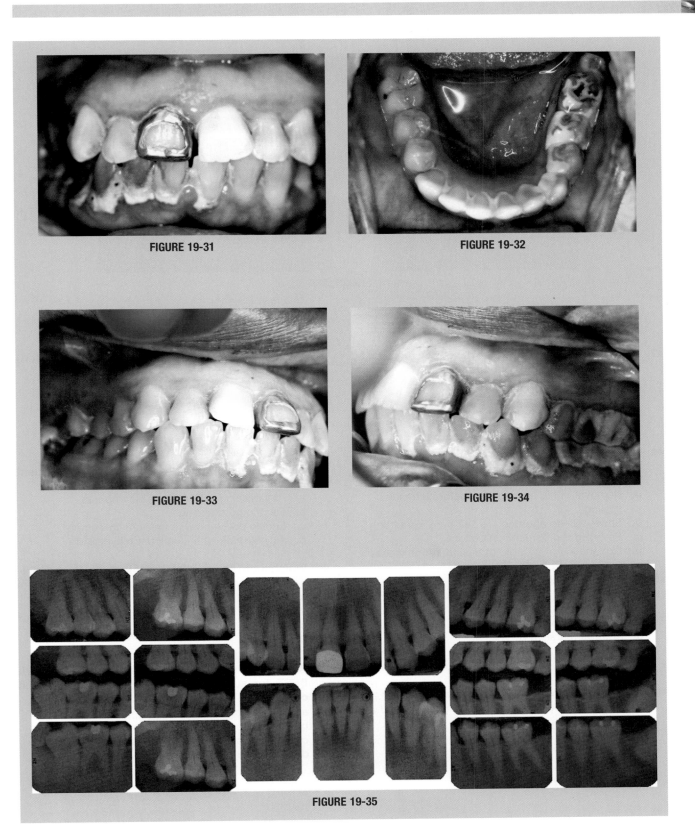

FIGURE 19-31

FIGURE 19-32

FIGURE 19-33

FIGURE 19-34

FIGURE 19-35

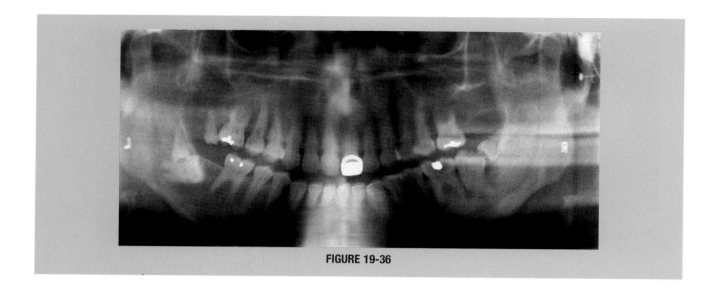

FIGURE 19-36

43. **Which of the following BEST describes the area by the arrow in the panoramic radiograph?**
    a. Unerupted third molar
    b. Odontoma
    c. Supernumerary tooth
    d. Fibrous dysplasia

44. **Each of the following should be considered when treating this client EXCEPT one. Which one is the EXCEPTION?**
    a. Removal of his hearing aids before ultrasonic scaling
    b. Show–tell–do approach to self-care instruction
    c. Powered toothbrush instructions
    d. Explanation of the role of biofilm in oral disease

45. **Tegretol is being used to treat:**
    a. Anxiety
    b. Seizures
    c. Hypertension
    d. Artificial mitral valve

46. **What is the MOST likely explanation for the white areas on occlusal surfaces of teeth #30 and #31?**
    a. Sealants
    b. Composite restoration
    c. Calculus
    d. Decalcification

47. **Which of the following describes the client's periodontal condition?**
    a. Gingivitis
    b. Chronic periodontitis
    c. Generalized aggressive periodontitis
    d. Necrotizing ulcerative gingivitis

48. **All of the following could safely be used un the client EXCEPT one. Which one is the EXCEPTION?**
    a. Air polishing with sodium bicarbonate
    b. Electric pulp testing
    c. Engine polishing with calcium carbonate
    d. Air polishing with aluminum trihydroxide

49. **Which tooth shows radiographic signs of a periapical lesion?**
    a. #3
    b. #14
    c. #17
    d. #30

50. **Which of the following instrument would work BEST for supragingival calculus removal in this client?**
    a. H6/H7 sickle scaler
    b. Beaver-tail ultrasonic scaling tip
    c. Straight slim-line ultrasonic scaling tip
    d. Universal curved ultrasonic scaling tip

Community Oral Health Planning and Practice

Christine French Beatty

Assessment, diagnosis, planning, implementation, and evaluation—the dental hygiene process of care—are used in community oral health practice, program development, and outcomes assessment. Community health extends the role of the dental hygienist from the traditional health care setting to the community as a whole. In a sense, the community can be viewed as the client and the oral care environment as the neighborhood health center, extended care facility, hospital, school, agency, or country. With increased emphasis on improving public access to oral health care, the responsibilities of the dental hygienist to promote oral health in the community take on renewed importance.

BASIC CONCEPTS

A. Health—community health practice requires a broad view of health: "a state of complete physical, mental, and social well being and not merely the absence of disease or infirmity; a state characterized by anatomic, physiologic, and psychological integrity; ability to perform personally valued family, work, and community roles; ability to deal with physical, biologic, psychological, and social stress; freedom from the risk of disease and untimely death; the extent to which an individual or a group is able to realize aspirations and satisfy needs and to change or cope with the environment; a positive concept, emphasizing social and personal resources as well as physical capabilities";[1] a state of health may be described as a state of physical and mental well-being that facilitates the achievement of individual and societal goals

B. Oral health—status of the oral cavity, encompassing all features, normal and abnormal, of the oral, dental, and craniofacial complex

C. Determinants of health—consist of social and economic factors, the physical environment, and the person's individual characteristics and behaviors; many determinants are nonmodifiable; risk factors are modifiable determinants; the study of public health focuses on attempts to modify risk factors through education and preventive therapies and to control other determinants through policy and changes to the structure of health care delivery[2]

D. Public health—"the science and art of preventing disease, prolonging life, and promoting physical and mental health and efficiency through organized community efforts";[3] the combination of sciences, skills, and beliefs directed at the maintenance and improvement of the health of all persons through collective or social actions; characteristics include a teamwork approach, preventing rather than curing disease, dealing with population-level health rather than individual-level health, social responsibility for oral health, use of epidemiology and a multi-factorial approach to controlling and preventing disease, and application of biostatistics
  1. Aggregate health of a group, community, state, nation, or group of nations
  2. Public health seen as people's health
  3. Concerned with four broad areas:
     a. Lifestyle, behavior, and culture
     b. Environment
     c. Human biology
     d. Organization of health programs and systems

E. Dental public health—"science and art of preventing and controlling oral diseases and promoting oral health through organized community efforts; that form of dental practice that serves the community as a client rather than the individual; concerned with the oral health education of the public, with applied dental research, and with the administration of group oral health care programs, as well as the prevention and control of oral diseases on a community basis";[4] the application of public health and all its characteristics to oral health

F. Community—any group with common traits, shared features, or communal experiences; not strictly defined by traditional geographic boundaries; as broad as a region of a state or as focused as a nursing home community, including administrators, staff, residents, and caregivers

G. Community health—generally synonymous with public health; full range of health services, environmental and personal, including major activities such as health education of the public and the social context of life as it affects the community; efforts that are organized to promote and restore the health and quality of life of the people; uses a population-based approach for identifying and addressing community-based problems

H. Community oral health—services directed toward developing, reinforcing, and enhancing the oral health status of people, either as individuals or as groups and communities

I. Access—an individual's or group's ability to obtain appropriate health care services

J. Prevention—primary focus of community oral health is prevention; the wellness model focuses educational and behavioral efforts and programs toward prevention of disease and maintenance of an optimum state of well-being; three levels of prevention:
  1. Primary—prevention of disease before it occurs
  2. Secondary—early disease control, including early identification and prompt treatment
  3. Tertiary—provision of services that prevent further disability

K. Comparison of private health versus community health—steps are presented in Table 20-1; the focus of public health is to function as an interdisciplinary health team rather than as an individual practitioner to serve people in community settings, rather than the individual in private offices; a public health practitioner needs knowledge and skills in public health administration, research and epidemiological methods, prevention and control of oral diseases, provision and financing of oral health care, the availability of resources, and the adaptation of care and programs to diverse people from a variety of cultures

L. Criteria for the traditional approach to a public health problem
  1. A disease or other threat to health is widespread
  2. The disease is one that can be prevented, alleviated, or cured
  3. Such knowledge is not being applied

TABLE 20-1 Comparison of Private Dental Practice and Community Oral Health Practice*

Private Dental Practice	Community Oral Health Practice
Assessment of client's dental, health, pharmacologic, and sociocultural history and oral health status	Survey of community oral health status; situation analysis including assessment of population demographics, culture, mobility, economic resources, and infrastructure
Diagnosis of client's oral health needs	Analysis of survey data to determine the oral health needs of the population
Treatment plan based on diagnosis, professional judgment, client's needs, and priorities	Program plan based on data analysis, community priorities, and resources available
Treatment plan initiated; primary dentist may coordinate treatment with other providers (e.g., dental hygienists, specialists)	Program operation implemented; the group will comprise varied, sometimes interdisciplinary, personnel
Payment methods determined	Financing takes place throughout process; may be combination of local, state, and federal funds, philanthropic or community agencies
Evaluation during treatment, at specific intervals, on completion of treatment, or at all these times	Evaluation and appraisal is ongoing and varied, conducted in terms of effectiveness, efficiency, appropriateness, and adequacy

Education occurs at all levels to facilitate anticipated outcomes.

M. Current approach to the criteria of a public health problem
  1. Condition, practice, or situation that is widespread and an actual or potential cause of morbidity (disease) or mortality (death)
  2. Public, nongovernmental agency (NGO), government, or public health personnel perceive that the condition is a public health problem

N. Public health solution—solutions to public health problems that are directed to the community at large; possess seven characteristics:
  1. Safe; not hazardous to life or function
  2. Effective in reducing or preventing a targeted disease, condition, or practice
  3. Easily and efficiently implemented
  4. Potency maintained for a substantial time period
  5. Attainable regardless of socioeconomic status (SES), education, or income

6. Effective immediately on application
7. Affordable; cost effective and within the means of a community

O. Core functions of public health—nationally identified; form the foundation of all community health activities[5]

   1. Assessment—regular and systematic collection, assembling, and analysis of data related to the health of the population and making the data available for use by various agencies

   2. Policy development—development of comprehensive public health policies based on scientific evidence

   3. Assurance—provision of services necessary to achieve agreed-upon health goals related to improving the health of the public

P. Levels of public health—each level provides various services and meets different needs of the population; various levels support the activities of other levels, but one level is not directly controlled by another; programs at lower levels are often funded by grants from higher levels

   1. Local—responsible for direct administration of educational, preventive care, and patient care programs

   2. State—consultation to the local level and other agencies; channels federal and state funds such as Medicaid and Children's Health Insurance Program (CHIP); conducts programs in rural areas that do not have local public health agencies

   3. National—numerous national public health government agencies are involved in public health issues of national significance; some of the more significant ones that are a resource in community programming are:

     a. NIH (National Institutes of Health)—conducts epidemiologic research, provides science transfer, and publishes and distributes educational materials; several are relevant to oral health, such as National Institute of Dental and Craniofacial Research (NIDCR), National Cancer Institute (NCI), and National Institute on Aging (NIA)

     b. CDC (Centers for Disease Control)—provides expertise, information, tools, and community collaboration to assist agencies with community programming; formulates recommendations for evidence-based practice (e.g., infection control and use of F varnish), develops educational programs (e.g., tobacco cessation) for local implementation, and provides surveillance data (e.g., fluoridation)

     c. PHS (Public Health Service)—commissioned officer core led by the Surgeon General that staffs clinics (e.g., in federal prison programs

and Indian Health Service programs) and responds to national crises

     d. IHS (Indian Health Service)—provides direct patient care and community health programming for Native American populations

     e. DOD (Department of Defense) and VA (Veteran's Administration) provide direct care for specific populations

   4. International—World Health Organization (WHO) is the best-known and largest international health agency; primarily serves developing countries but also monitors health conditions and establishes programs to coordinate health care throughout the world; also Pan-American Health Organization (PAHO)

Q. National documents relevant to community oral health programming—classic documents continue to provide a basis to prioritize programs and target specific population groups;[5] these documents complement each other as they categorize community oral health needs of the population and strategies to address those needs; are based on the three core public health functions:

   1. *Oral Health in America: A Report of the Surgeon General*[6]—the key points of the publication are:

     a. Oral health is more than just healthy teeth

     b. Oral health is integral to general health for all Americans

     c. General health factors (e.g., tobacco use, poor diet, obesity, diabetes, etc.) affect oral and craniofacial health

     d. Oral health can be achieved by all Americans

     e. Currently, disparities exist in the oral health of Americans

   2. *A National Call to Action to Promote Oral Health*[7]—includes five principles and implementation strategies designed to result in programs that will more effectively contribute to the goal of optimum oral health for all Americans:

     a. Change perceptions about oral health

     b. Build the science, and accelerate the transfer of the science

     c. Increase collaborations (partnerships, coalitions)

     d. Increase workforce diversity, capacity, and flexibility

     e. Overcome barriers by replicating effective programs

   3. *Healthy People 2020*[8]—a comprehensive list of disease prevention and health promotion objectives including developmental objectives that have no baseline data source (see Box 20-1 for detailed list of oral health and related objectives); establish priorities for community programming for the decade 2010 to 2020; similar

BOX 20-1 *Healthy People 2020* Oral Health and Related Objectives

Oral Health (OH) Objectives

Oral Health of Children and Adolescents

OH-1 Reduce the proportion of children and adolescents who have dental caries experience in their primary or permanent teeth

OH-1.1 Reduce the proportion of young children aged 3 to 5 years with dental caries experience in their primary teeth; target 30.0 percent; baseline 33.3 percent

OH-1.2 Reduce the proportion of children aged 6 to 9 years with dental caries experience in their primary and permanent teeth; target: 49.0 percent; baseline 54.4 percent

OH-1.3 Reduce the proportion of adolescents aged 13 to 15 years with dental caries experience in their permanent teeth; target: 48.3 percent; baseline 53.7 percent

OH-2 Reduce the proportion of children and adolescents with untreated dental decay

OH-2.1 Reduce the proportion of young children aged 3 to 5 years with untreated dental decay in their primary teeth; target: 21.4 percent; baseline 23.8 percent

OH-2.2 Reduce the proportion of children aged 6 to 9 years with untreated dental decay in their primary and permanent teeth; target 25.9 percent; baseline 28.8 percent

OH-2.3 Reduce the proportion of adolescents aged 13 to 15 years with untreated dental decay in their permanent teeth; target: 15.3 percent; baseline 17.0 percent

Oral Health of Adults

OH-3 Reduce the proportion of adults with untreated dental decay

OH-3.1 Reduce the proportion of adults aged 35 to 44 years with untreated dental decay; target 25.0 percent; baseline 27.8 percent

OH-3.2 Reduce the proportion of older adults aged 65 to 74 years with untreated coronal caries; target: 15.4 percent; baseline 17.1 percent

OH-3.3 Reduce the proportion of older adults aged 75 years and older with untreated root surface caries; target: 34.1 percent; baseline 37.9 percent

OH-4 Reduce the proportion of adults who have ever had a permanent tooth extracted because of dental caries or periodontal disease

OH-4.1 Reduce the proportion of adults aged 45 to 64 years who have ever had a permanent tooth extracted because of dental caries or periodontitis; target 68.8 percent; baseline 76.4 percent

OH-4.2 Reduce the proportion of older adults aged 65 to 74 years who have lost all of their natural teeth; target 21.6 percent; baseline 24.0 percent

OH-5 Reduce the proportion of adults aged 45 to 74 years with moderate or severe periodontitis; target: 11.4 percent; baseline 12.7 percent

OH-6 Increase the proportion of oral and pharyngeal cancers detected at the earliest stage; target 35.8 percent; baseline 32.5 percent

Access to Preventive Services

OH-7 Increase the proportion of children, adolescents, and adults who used the oral health care system in the past year; target 49.0 percent; baseline 44.5 percent

OH-8 Increase the proportion of low-income children and adolescents who received any preventive dental service during the past year; target: 29.4 percent; baseline 26.7 percent

OH-9 Increase the proportion of school-based health centers with an oral health component

OH-9.1 Increase the proportion of school-based health centers with an oral health component that includes dental sealants; target 26.5 percent; baseline: 24.1 percent

OH-9.2 Increase the proportion of school-based health centers with an oral health component that includes dental care; target 11.1 percent; baseline: 10.1 percent

OH-9.3 Increase the proportion of school-based health centers with an oral health component that includes topical fluoride; target: 32.1 percent; baseline: 29.2% Health Care (NASBHC)

OH-10 Increase the proportion of local health departments and Federally Qualified Health Centers (FQHCs) that have an oral health component

OH-10.1 Increase the proportion of Federally Qualified Health Centers that have an oral health care program; target 83 percent; baseline 75 percent

OH-10.2 Increase the proportion of local health departments that have oral health prevention or care programs; target 28.4 percent; baseline 25.8 percent

OH-11 Increase the proportion of patients who receive oral health services at Federally Qualified Health Centers each year; target 33.3 percent; baseline 17.5 percent

Oral Health Interventions

OH-12 Increase the proportion of children and adolescents who have received dental sealants on their molar teeth

OH-12.1 Increase the proportion of children aged 3 to 5 years who have received dental sealants on one or more of their primary molar teeth; target 1.5 percent; baseline 1.4 percent

OH-12.2 Increase the proportion of children aged 6 to 9 years who have received dental sealants on one or more of their permanent first molar teeth; target: 28.1 percent; baseline 25.5 percent

OH-12.3 Increase the proportion of adolescents aged 13 to 15 years who have received dental sealants on one or more of their permanent molar teeth; target 21.9 percent; baseline 19.9 percent

OH-13 Increase the proportion of the U.S. population served by community water systems with optimally fluoridated water; target 79.6 percent; baseline 72.4 percent

OH-14 (Developmental) Increase the proportion of adults who receive preventive interventions in dental offices

BOX 20-1 *Healthy People 2020* Oral Health and Related Objectives—cont'd

OH–14.1 (Developmental) Increase the proportion of adults who received information from a dentist or dental hygienist focusing on reducing tobacco use or smoking cessation in the past year

OH–14.2 (Developmental) Increase the proportion of adults who received an oral and pharyngeal cancer screening from a dentist or dental hygienist in the past year

OH–14.3 (Developmental) Increase the proportion of adults who are tested or referred for glycemic control from a dentist or dental hygienist in the past year

Monitoring, Surveillance Systems

OH–15 (Developmental) Increase the number of States and the District of Columbia that have a system for recording and referring infants and children with cleft lips and cleft palates to craniofacial anomaly rehabilitative teams

OH–15.1 (Developmental) Increase the number of States and the District of Columbia that have a system for recording cleft lips and cleft palates

OH–15.2 (Developmental) Increase the number of States and the District of Columbia that have a system for referral for cleft lips and cleft palates to rehabilitative teams.

OH–16 Increase the number of States and the District of Columbia that have an oral and craniofacial health surveillance system; target: 51 (50 States and the District of Columbia); baseline 32 States

Public Health Infrastructure

OH–17 Increase health agencies that have a dental public health program directed by a dental professional with public health training

OH–17.1 Increase the proportion of States (including the District of Columbia) and local health agencies that serve jurisdictions of 250,000 or more persons with a dental public health program directed by a dental professional with public health training; target: 25.7 percent; baseline 23.4 percent

OH–17.2 Increase the number of Indian Health Service Areas and Tribal health programs that serve jurisdictions of 30,000 or more persons with a dental public health program directed by a dental professional with public health training; target: 12 programs; baseline 11 programs

Other Objectives That Relate to Oral Health

Access to Health Services (AHS)

AHS--1.2 (Developmental) Increase the proportion of persons with dental insurance

AHS--6.3 Reduce the proportion of individuals who are unable to obtain or delay in obtaining necessary dental care; target: 5.0 percent; baseline 5.5 percent

Cancer (C)

C–6: Reduce the oropharyngeal cancer death rate; target 2.3 deaths per 100,000 population; baseline 2.5 oropharyngeal cancer deaths per 100,000 population

C–12 Increase the number of central, population-based registries from the 50 States and the District of Columbia that capture case information on at least 95 percent of the expected number of reportable cancers; target: 51 (50 States and the District of Columbia); baseline 42

C–13 Increase the proportion of cancer survivors who are living 5 years or longer after diagnosis; target 72.8 percent; baseline 66.2 percent

Diabetes (D)

D-8 Increase the proportion of persons with diagnosed diabetes who have at least an annual dental examination; target 61.2 percent; baseline 55.6 percent

Educational and Community-Based Programs (ECBP)

ECBP-1 (Developmental) Increase the proportion of preschool Early Head Start and Head Start programs that provide health education to prevent health problems in ... dental health ...

ECBP--2.5 Increase the proportion of elementary, middle, and senior high schools that provide comprehensive school health education to prevent health problems in ... tobacco use and addiction ...; target 89.1 percent; baseline 81 percent

ECBP--2.8 Increase the proportion of elementary, middle, and senior high schools that provide comprehensive school health education to prevent health problems in ... unhealthy dietary patterns; target: 92.7 percent; baseline 84.3 percent

ECBP--4.2 Increase the proportion of elementary, middle, and senior high schools that provide school health education to promote personal health and wellness in ... oral health ...; target 71.3 percent; baseline 64.8 percent

ECBP--7.5 Increase the proportion of college and university students who receive information from their institution on ... tobacco use and addiction ...; target 36.7 percent; baseline 33.4 percent

ECBP--10.4 Increase the number of community-based organizations providing population-based primary prevention services in ... tobacco use ...; target 96.7 percent; baseline 88.0 percent

ECBP-11 (Developmental) Increase the proportion of local health departments that have established culturally appropriate and linguistically competent community health promotion and disease prevention programs

Health Communication and Health Information Technology (HC/HIT)

HC/HIT-1: (Developmental) Improve the health literacy of the population

HC/HIT–2: Increase the proportion of persons who report that their health care providers have satisfactory communication skills

HC/HIT–2.1 Increase the proportion of persons who report that their health care provider always listened carefully to them; target 65 percent; baseline 59 percent

HC/HIT–2.2 Increase the proportion of persons who report that their health care provider always explained

Continued

BOX 20-1 *Healthy People 2020* Oral Health and Related Objectives—cont'd

things so they could understand them; target: 66 percent; baseline 60 percent

HC/HIT–2.3 Increase the proportion of persons who report that their health care provider always showed respect for what they had to say; target 68.2 percent; baseline 62 percent

HC/HIT–2.4 Increase the proportion of persons who report that their health care provider always spent enough time with them; target: 54 percent; baseline 49 percent

HC/HIT–3: Increase the proportion of persons who report that their health care providers always involved them in decisions about their health care as much as they wanted; target: 56.8 percent; baseline 51.6 percent

Older Adults

OA–7.4: Increase the proportion of dentists with geriatric certification; target 0.22 percent; baseline 0.20 percent

Tobacco Use (TU)

TU–1 Reduce tobacco use by adults

TU–1.1 Cigarette smoking; target 12.0 percent; baseline: 20.6 percent

TU–1.2 Smokeless tobacco products; target 0.3 percent; baseline 2.3 percent

TU–1.3 Cigars; target: 0.2 percent; baseline 2.2 percent

TU–2 Reduce tobacco use by adolescents

TU–2.1 Tobacco products (past month); target 21.0 percent; baseline 26.0 percent

TU–2.2 Cigarettes (past month); target 16.0 percent; baseline 19.5 percent

TU–2.3 Smokeless tobacco products (past month); target 6.9 percent; baseline 8.9 percent

TU–2.4 Cigars (past month); target 8.0 percent; baseline 14.0 percent

TU–3 Reduce the initiation of tobacco use among children, adolescents, and young adults

TU–3.1 Children and adolescents aged 12 to 17 years—Tobacco products; target 5.7 percent; baseline 7.7 percent

TU–3.2 Children and adolescents aged 12 to 17 years—Cigarettes; target 4.2 percent; baseline 6.2 percent

TU–3.3 Children and adolescents aged 12 to 17 years—Smokeless tobacco products; target 0.5 percent; baseline 2.5 percent

TU–3.4 Children and adolescents aged 12 to 17 years—Cigars; target 2.8 percent; baseline 4.8 percent

TU–3.5 Young adults aged 18 to 25 years—Tobacco products; target 8.8 percent; baseline 10.8 percent

TU–3.6 Young adults aged 18 to 25 years—Cigarettes; target 6.3 percent; baseline 8.3 percent

TU–3.7 Young adults aged 18 to 25 years—Smokeless tobacco products; target 0.2 percent; baseline 2.2 percent

TU–3.8 Young adults aged 18 to 25 years—Cigars; target: 4.1 percent; baseline 6.1 percent

TU–4 Increase smoking cessation attempts by adult smokers

TU–4.1 Increase smoking cessation attempts by adult smokers; target: 80.0 percent; baseline 48.3

TU–4.2 (Developmental) Increase smoking cessation attempts using evidence-based strategies by adult smokers

TU–5 Increase recent smoking cessation success by adult smokers

TU–5.1 Increase recent smoking cessation success by adult smokers; target 8.0 percent; baseline 6.0 percent

TU–5.2 (Developmental) Increase recent smoking cessation success using evidence-based strategies by adult smokers.

TU–6 Increase smoking cessation during pregnancy; target 30.0 percent; baseline 11.3 percent

TU–7 Increase smoking cessation attempts by adolescent smokers; target 64.0 percent; baseline 58.5 percent

TU–10.3 (Developmental) Increase tobacco cessation counseling in dental care settings

Data from U.S. Department of Health and Human Services: Healthy People 2020: *Available at http://www.healthypeople.gov/:* Accessed March 28, 2011.

to *Healthy People 2010* objectives, with more topic areas, some objectives remaining the same, some revised, and some new ones and more realistic targets set[9] based on progress made toward *Healthy People 2010* objectives;[10] oral health objectives are organized into six major categories:

a. Oral health of children and adolescents
b. Oral health of adults
c. Access to preventive services
d. Oral health interventions
e. Monitoring, surveillance systems
f. Public health infrastructure

R. Roles of the dental hygienist reflect the various activities in public health[11]

1. Clinician—provides direct client care based on sound scientific information
2. Educator—uses valid educational theories to present scientific information to individuals and groups to prevent disease and promote oral health
3. Advocate—promotes change and advances the health of the public through legislation and public policy
4. Researcher—determines which procedure, products, and programs most effectively promote

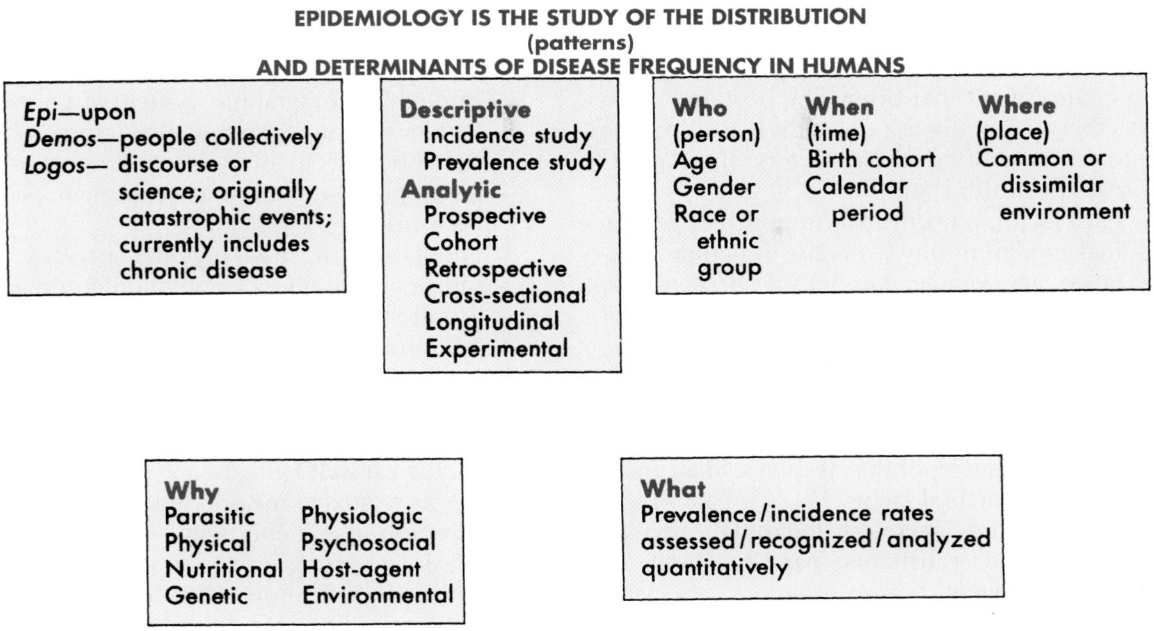

EPIDEMIOLOGY IS THE STUDY OF THE DISTRIBUTION
(patterns)
AND DETERMINANTS OF DISEASE FREQUENCY IN HUMANS

Epi—upon
Demos—people collectively
Logos— discourse or
    science; originally
    catastrophic events;
    currently includes
    chronic disease
	Descriptive
	  Incidence study
	  Prevalence study
	Analytic
	  Prospective
	  Cohort
	  Retrospective
	  Cross-sectional
	  Longitudinal
	  Experimental
		Who **When** **Where**
		(person) (time) (place)
		Age Birth cohort Common or
		Gender Calendar dissimilar
		Race or period environment
		  ethnic
		  group

Why Parasitic Physiologic Physical Psychosocial Nutritional Host-agent Genetic Environmental	**What** Prevalence / incidence rates assessed / recognized / analyzed quantitatively

FIGURE 20-1 The study of epidemiology.

oral health and prevent disease, and communicates those findings

5. Administrator/manager—administers and manages programs aimed at promoting oral health

EPIDEMIOLOGY

A. Definitions
 1. Epidemiology—study of health-related states in human populations and how these states are influenced by the environment and ways of living, including the nature, cause, control, and determinants of health and disease as well as related factors; concerned with factors and conditions that determine the occurrence and distribution of health, disease, defects, disability, and deaths among individuals and groups; characterized by the use of statistical and research methods to focus on comparisons between groups or defined populations (Figure 20-1)
 2. Applied epidemiology—the application or practice of epidemiology to address public health issues
B. Uses of epidemiology
 1. Study patterns among groups; establish a history of disease in a population
 2. Collect data to describe normal biologic processes
 3. Understand the natural history of disease

4. Test hypotheses for prevention and control of disease in populations
5. Plan and evaluate health care services
6. Study nondisease entities such as accidents, suicide, or injury
7. Measure the distribution of diseases in populations
8. Identify risk factors, risk indicators, risk markers, and other determinants of disease such as health literacy
9. Estimate risk of diseases among population groups
10. Evaluation of intervention and preventive strategies to control disease
11. Evaluate trends in chronic disease and social epidemiology
12. Identify syndromes and precursors
13. Evaluate the appropriateness and utility of health services
C. Characteristics of epidemiology
 1. Groups rather than individuals are studied
 2. A multi-factorial approach is used to study disease (multiple causation); modifiable risk factors are controlled to control the disease or condition
 3. Determinants—risk factors or events that are capable of bringing about a change in health; the various factors that make up the multi-factorial approach to a disease or health condition
 4. Epidemiologic triad (epidemiologic triangle)—the traditional model of infection or disease

causation that is used to study the occurrence and distribution of disease; includes an external agent (etiologic agent), a susceptible host, and an environment that brings the host and agent together so that disease occurs; it is the ongoing interaction among these factors that affects disease or health status:[12]

  a. Host factors—intrinsic factors such as genetic makeup, immunity to disease or natural resistance, age, gender, race, ethnic background, physiologic state, gender, culture, level of immunity, physical or morphologic factors; fitness, personal lifestyle and habits, attitudes, and behaviors that influence an individual's exposure; dietary excesses and nutritional deficiency, susceptibility, response to an agent or environmental factor

  b. Agent factors—chemical, microbial, physical or mechanical irritants; parasitic, viral, or bacterial agent whose presence, excessive presence, or absence, in the case of immunodeficiency diseases, is essential for the occurrence of disease

  c. Environment factors—extrinsic factors, such as climate or geography, culture, food and water sources, socioeconomic conditions, pollution and sanitation, animal hosts and vectors that provide an opportunity for exposure to disease

  d. Time dimension—exposure to factors occurs over a period of time; the time required for the disease or condition to occur varies according to the other factors

5. Burden of disease—cumulative effect of a broad range of harmful disease consequences on a community, including the health, social, and economic costs to the individual and to society

6. Preventive intervention—strategies to eliminate risk factors and to reduce occurrence of disease

D. Related epidemiology concepts

1. Acute disease—beginning abruptly with marked intensity or sharpness, and then subsiding after a relatively short period; often treatable

2. Chronic disease—developing slowly and persisting for a long period, often for the remainder of the lifetime of the individual

3. Cluster—an aggregate of cases of a disease, or other health-related conditions, particularly cancer or birth defects, closely grouped in time or space; the number of cases may or may not exceed the expected number; frequently, the expected number is not known

4. Endemic—continuing problem involving normal disease prevalence; the expected number of cases indigenous to a population or geographic area

5. Epidemic—a disease of significantly greater prevalence than normal; more than the expected number of cases; a disease that spreads rapidly through a demographic segment of a population

6. Pandemic—an epidemic that crosses international borders to affect a large proportion of the geographic population of a continent, people, or the world

7. Population at risk—includes persons in the same community or population group who can acquire a disease or condition

8. Mortality—death from a disease or condition

9. Morbidity—presence of disease; any departure, subjective (personal) or objective (clinically measurable), from a state of physiologic or psychological well-being

E. Concepts related to measurement of disease and its distribution in epidemiology

1. Basic screening—a rapid assessment accomplished in a short time by visual detection and providing information about gross dental and oral lesions; can be accomplished with a tongue blade, dental mirror, and appropriate lighting

2. Epidemiologic examination—a detailed visual–tactile assessment accomplished with dental instruments and a light source in a survey; provides more detailed information than basic screening; differs from a clinical examination in that it does not involve a clinical diagnosis and resulting treatment plan

3. Surveillance—ongoing, constant, systematic observation, persistent watching over, scrutiny, analysis, and evaluation of health data to assess changes in populations related to disease, conditions, injuries, disabilities, or death trends, for the purpose of program planning; essential feature of epidemiology

4. National Oral Health Surveillance System (NOHSS)—a collaborative effort between the CDC Division of Oral Health and the Association of State and Territorial Dental Directors (ASTDD) to track oral health indicators on a state and national level using a variety of clinical and nonclinical methods, including the National Health and Nutrition Examination Survey (NHANES); nine oral health indicators are routinely assessed, based on the *Healthy People* objectives:

  a. Dental visits
  b. Teeth cleaning
  c. Complete tooth loss
  d. Partial tooth loss of 6 or more teeth
  e. Cancer of the oral cavity and pharynx
  f. Dental caries experience
  g. Untreated dental caries

h. Dental sealants

i. Fluoridation status

5. Monitoring—intermittent measurement to detect changes in the environment or in the health status of populations; less accurate than surveillance

6. Status—current state of a disease or health-related condition in the population

7. Trend—long-term changes or movements in disease patterns and health-related conditions in the population identified by examining surveillance data

8. Validity—the accuracy of a measure; produced by measuring what is supposed to be measured

9. Sensitivity—the ability of a test to accurately identify the presence of a disease or condition when the disease is, in fact, present

10. Specificity—the ability of a test to accurately identify the absence of a disease or condition

11. Predictive value—ability of a diagnostic test to accurately measure both the presence and absence of disease

12. Reversal—also called *negative reversal*; a change of diagnosis in an illogical direction over a period; a positive reversal is a change of the measurement made in error in a logical direction

13. Reliability—consistency or reproducibility of a measurement over time

14. Inter-examiner reliability—the agreement among two or more examiners as they apply an index or instrument to measure a disease or condition

15. Intra-examiner reliability—the consistency of a single examiner in the application of an index or instrument over time to measure a disease or condition

16. Calibration—the standardization of examiners to increase reliability as they apply epidemiologic measurements

17. Count—simplest measure of a disease or condition occurring in a population; the actual number of cases

18. Rate—the numeric expression of disease in a population in which the number of disease occurrences appears as the numerator and the number of possible occurrences (entire population) appears as the denominator; usually expressed as a standardized denominator such as 100 or 1000, and includes a time dimension, usually a year; allows for valid comparisons from year to year or population to population; for example, the number of deaths of newborn infants within the first year of life per 1000 births or the percentage of people diagnosed with oral cancer during a specific year

19. Incidence—the rate of new cases of a disease during or over a specific period; incidence is a rate

20. Prevalence—the numeric expression of the total number of all existing cases of a disease or health condition in a population measured at a given time, in relation to the number of individuals in the population; expressed as a proportion; can be expressed as a percentage; does not include a time dimension like incidence does

21. Occurrence—general term of frequency of disease that does not distinguish between incidence and prevalence

22. Ratio—expression of the magnitude of one occurrence of disease exposure in relation to another with a fraction; in contrast to a proportion, a relationship between the numerator and denominator, for example, ratio of dentists to hygienists, does not exist

23. Eradication—the elimination of the infectious disease agent through surveillance and containment; contrasted to control, which is to keep the disease at a minimum level so that it no longer poses a health problem

24. National Health and Nutrition Examination Survey (NHANES)—routinely conducted national health surveys carried out by the National Center for Health Statistics of the Centers for Disease Control and Prevention (NCHS/CDC) to monitor the health and nutritional status of U.S. adults and children of all ages; conducted through interviewing and direct physical and dental examinations; began in the 1960s and has evolved to the current continuous program that has a changing focus on a variety of health and nutrition measurements to meet emerging needs; the survey examines a nationally representative sample of about 5000 persons each year, located in counties across the United States, 15 of which are visited each year; oral health is one of the areas of diseases and health indictors monitored by NHANES[12]

25. Socioeconomic status (SES)—includes education, income, occupation, attitudes, and values; frequently evaluated as it relates to distribution of disease and health-associated characteristics in the population

EPIDEMIOLOGY AND RESEARCH

A. Evidence-based practice[13,14]

1. Involves the conscientious, explicit, and judicious use of current best evidence to make decisions about the care of individual clients

2. Evidence alone is not sufficient to make decisions; the clinical expertise of the professional and client preferences and values are combined with the best available external clinical evidence from a body of rigorous research findings to make evidence-based practice decisions[15]

3. Evidence is ranked in the following order:[16]
   a. Systematic reviews, preferably with meta-analysis; Cochrane reviews
   b. Randomized controlled clinical trials
   c. Nonrandomized controlled clinical trials
   d. Cohort studies
   e. Case-control and cross sectional studies
   f. Case series, case reports, other descriptive studies
   g. Editorials, reports of expert committees, opinions of respected authorities
   h. Studies that do not involve human participants (laboratory or animal model studies)

4. The gold standard of evidence (best clinical evidence available) is at least one published systematic review of multiple, well-designed randomized controlled trials

5. Evidence-informed practice relates to the practice of the dental hygienist in all roles and settings, not just clinical; has implications for all aspects of community oral health practice

6. All oral health care must be evidence informed; lifelong learning and access to quality research findings are critical to evidence-based practice

B. Research—continual search for truth using the scientific method; systematic and objective inquiry through laboratory, field, and clinical investigations that lead to discovery or revision of knowledge, resulting in improvements in health and health care delivery

C. Scientific method—methods used in any type of research that increase the likelihood that information gathered will be relevant, reliable, and unbiased; steps of the method include:
   1. Identification and statement of the problem
   2. Formulation of a hypothesis
   3. Collection, organization, and analysis of data
   4. Formulation of conclusions
   5. Verification, rejection, or modification of the hypothesis

D. Categories of community oral health research
   1. Epidemiologic research to determine the presence and distribution of disease in the population and factors that relate to the occurrence of disease within the population
   2. Clinical trials and tests of techniques and products to prevent and control disease
   3. Research in educational techniques and the behavioral sciences related to oral health education
   4. Evaluation of community oral health programs

E. Risk versus causality[12]
   1. Risk identifies attributes that are associated with a disease (from case-control and cohort studies); causality identifies factors that have been demonstrated to be causally related (from randomized controlled clinical trials)
   2. Risk is established with analytic studies; causality is established with experimental studies
   3. Types of risk attributes—different types are identified with different types of analytic studies (Table 20-2)
      a. Risk factors—strong indication of risk, causality is inferred; can be modified; should be an important consideration in making recommendations to clients
      b. Risk indicators—weaker indication of risk; causality may be incorrectly assumed; can be modified; should be applied with care when making recommendations

TABLE 20-2 Types of Non-experimental Studies and Risk

Type of Study	Number of Groups	Number of Measures	Classification of Study	Used to Identify	Modifiability	Causal Role
Descriptive	1	1	Prevalence	Not applicable (N/A)	N/A	N/A
Cohort	1	2 or more	Longitudinal, prospective, incidence	Risk factor	Modifiable	Inferred
				Risk indicator	Modifiable	Assumed
Case control	2	1	Retrospective	Risk predictor	Nonmodifiable	None
				Risk indicator	Modifiable	Assumed
Cross-sectional	1	1	Cross-sectional	Risk predictor	Nonmodifiable	None

Data from CF Beatty: Oral epidemiology. In Nathe CN: Dental public health and research, ed 3, Upper Saddle River, NJ, 2011, Pearson.

c. Risk predictor—also called *risk marker* or *demographic risk factor*; nonmodifiable; has no role in making recommendations to clients but has importance in identifying target populations for community oral health programs

F. Three classifications of epidemiologic research:

1. Descriptive research—involves description, documentation, analysis, and interpretation of data to evaluate a current event or situation; does not test specific hypothesis but helps increase understanding of diseases; uses survey method with a cross-sectional design (Table 20-3)

2. Analytic research—observation of a disease or condition to identify determinants of the disease by showing relationships or associations between diseases and other factors (risk factors or risk indicators); does not establish a cause-and-effect relationship; analytic studies are also called *observational* or *development studies*; noninterventional; types of analytic studies (see Table 20-2):

a. Cohort—a well-defined group (*cohort* means homogeneous group) is observed over time to determine the natural progression of a disease or condition after exposure without controlling any factors; the cohort can be compared with a homogeneous group not exposed to the disease; longitudinal; prospective; establishes incidence; used to confirm risk factors

b. Case-control—two groups are compared, one group with a disease or condition (called *cases*) and a second group without it (called *controls*), to identify factors in their history that can be associated with the disease or condition; retrospective; used to identify risk indicators and risk predictors but cannot be used to confirm risk factors; usually used to examine relationships among variables that cannot be studied prospectively because of ethical concerns about research participants

c. Cross-sectional—representative cross-section of the population (one group, but several subgroups) is observed at one point in time, and disease attributes and potential risk attributes are assessed at this same point in time to associate them with each other; used to identify risk indicators and risk predictors but cannot be used to confirm risk factors; used to identify prevalence

d. Related terminology
(1) Prospective—study planned before data are collected; observations made forward (into the future)

TABLE 20-3 Comparison of Clinical Trials and Epidemiologic Surveys

	Clinical Trial	Epidemiologic Survey
Populations	Experimental and control groups are specially constituted as representative samples from appropriate populations	Naturally occurring samples of target populations are usually studied
Sample size	Sample sizes are often small, particularly when "treatments" are more complicated	Fairly large sample sizes are used
Time frame	Trials are conducted over a period, usually varying from 1 week to 6 months to several years (e.g., dental caries research), depending on treatment involved and disease or condition measured, to compare treatment outcomes	Surveys are usually cross-sectional in design, using only one period; longitudinal designs are used occasionally
Methods	Although assessment methods may include indices, biomedical instruments, or physiologic measures, methods have validity, reliability, and clinical significance	Indices used for assessment and to establish the disease level of selected populations; these indices are, in general, used for comparison of data for different populations
Data	Data generated from clinical trials are applicable to specific hypothesis testing	Data generated from surveys are used to establish underlying etiologic factors and derive possible preventive methods, leading to the development of hypotheses to be tested by controlled clinical trials

(2) Longitudinal—conducted over a long period to observe the progression of a disease or condition (length of time depends on condition being studied)

(3) Retrospective—study using data collected in the past; also termed *ex-post facto* or *causal-comparative*

3. Experimental research—a carefully designed study to test a hypothesis after analytic studies have inferred the cause of the disease; deliberate application or withholding of the supposed cause or controlling agent of a condition and observation of the result (longitudinal); used to determine the effectiveness of altering some factor or factors to establish cause-and-effect relationships (causality); a randomized clinical trial is a well-controlled experimental study with humans; an experimental study that is not well controlled is called *quasi-experimental* (see Table 20-3)

a. Requirements for an experimental study
   (1) Use of a control group
   (2) Control of extraneous variables
   (3) Randomization (random assignment to groups)
   (4) Control of errors in measurement to increase validity and reliability
   (5) The independent variable is manipulated
   (6) The dependent variable is measured
   (7) The independent variable occurs before the dependent variable in design

b. A representative sample is required to allow for generalization (also called *inference*); replication studies (repeated studies with different samples) are frequently done to compensate for the poor generalizability (low external validity) resulting from the use of small convenience samples; multiple-site studies broaden the representation of the population and improve the generalizability of findings

c. Experimental study designs
   (1) Pretest/post-test—the dependent variable is measured before and after introducing the independent variable; provides a baseline measure for comparison
   (2) Post-test only—the dependent variable is measured only after introducing the independent variable; controls any possible effect of the pretest procedure on the dependent variable
   (3) Split mouth—procedure unique to oral health research, in which each side of the mouth receives a different intervention; controls subject-related variables

(variables that can vary from one participant to another)

(4) Cross-over—each group receives a different intervention or control and after a period, they are switched over to the opposite treatment, with an intervening washout period, during which no treatment is given, to eliminate the possibility of the first treatment affecting the second one; controls subject-related variables

(5) Time-series (repeated measures)—design in which the dependent variable is measured several times over a specific period, to determine whether its effect on the dependent variable holds over time

(6) Blind (or masking)—this refers to examiners measuring the dependent variable without knowing the group assignment, to eliminate bias; if *both* examiners and participants are unaware of their group assignments, it is called *double-blind*

(7) Designs can be combined; for example, a study can combine double-blind, pretest/post-test, split mouth, and repeated measures designs to test the effectiveness of an antimicrobial to reduce or control periodontal pocket depths over a long period

G. Hypothesis—a predictive statement of the expected outcome or relationship among variables; answers the research question in a manner that is observable and measurable

1. Null hypothesis—negative statement of the hypothesis that assumes the absence of statistically significant differences between the sample groups, for example, statement that no difference exists in the effectiveness of the two treatments; this is the hypothesis that is statistically tested

2. Research hypothesis—also called the *positive* or *alternative hypothesis*; positive statement of the hypothesis is in terms that express the opinion or prediction of the researcher, for example, statement that a difference exists in the effectiveness of the two treatments

H. Variables—state, condition, concept, construct, or event whose value is free to vary, for example, height, dental caries rate, IQ, creativity

1. Independent variable—the treatment or intervention under study; condition that is manipulated or controlled by the investigator; the experimental variable; the experimental treatment; in a non-experimental study, it is the factor studied to explain or predict the dependent variable or the outcome of interest

2. Dependent variable—measure that is expected to change as a result of the manipulation of the independent variable; it is measured to observe the effect of the independent variable; in a non-experimental study, it is the factor or the outcome that is thought to be changed by the independent variable

3. Extraneous variables—uncontrolled variables that may influence the dependent variable and influence (or confound) the outcome, thus interfering with accurate interpretation and producing invalid research results

I. Sampling
1. Population—portion of the universe to which the researcher wants to generalize findings; all members of a specific group who possess a clearly defined set of characteristics

2. Sample—a portion of a specific population that, if properly selected, can provide meaningful information about the entire population; a sample is examined when the researcher has no time, money, or resources to study an entire population; a sample may be random or nonrandom and may be representative or nonrepresentative

   a. Random sample—composed of study participants who are chosen independently of each other, with known opportunity or probability for inclusion; increases external validity by controlling differences in study participants, which allows for valid generalization of results to the population (reduced bias); results in a representative sample with a homogeneous population

   b. Stratified random sample—study participants randomly selected from an existing, known subdivided population; results in the sample proportionately and accurately representing the subgroups in the population; most representative sample for a heterogeneous population

   c. Systematic random sample—selection of every n^{th} member of the population from a list or file of the total population; the n depends on the size of the sample desired in relation to the population, for example 10% is every tenth member of the population; not a strictly random sample; the first one is selected randomly and considered to be random if the list or file is in random order

   d. Convenience sample—study participants chosen on the basis of availability; used when access to the total population is not feasible for random sample selection; introduces bias, which reduces validity of the sample and limits the generalizability of study results

   e. Judgment or purposive sample—study participants are chosen by the researcher or someone else who has knowledge of the population; biased; least valid method; generalization of results not possible

3. Table of random numbers—a table composed of numbers that have been generated by a random technique used to select a random sample; done by computers

4. Sample size
   a. Large sample; if selected properly:
      (1) Accurately represents the defined population
      (2) Increases the precision and accuracy of collected data
      (3) Reduces the standard error of the sample mean
      (4) Larger samples are required for descriptive research
   b. Small sample
      (1) May be necessary, depending on the purpose of the research, for example, a pilot study (conducting a study on a small sample as a trial run to work out the research design and methods before initiating the full-scale study)
      (2) May lead to inaccurate conclusions when inappropriate for the type of research
      (3) Small samples require specialized statistics (nonparametrics)

5. Group assignment—the assignment of participants to the groups of the research study
   a. Experimental group—sample group in an experimental study that is exposed to the experimental variable under study; the group that receives the independent variable
   b. Control group—sample group in an experimental study that does not receive the experimental treatment (independent variable) but, rather, receives a placebo treatment, traditional or standard treatment, or no treatment at all
   c. Assignment should be accomplished with random procedures to ensure equivalency of groups (called *randomization* or *randomized group assignment*)

EPIDEMIOLOGY OF ORAL DISEASES AND CONDITIONS

Targets for various oral health diseases and conditions and the strategies to address them were set in the *Healthy People 2020* objectives (Box 20-1) for the U.S. population;[8] these targets will drive community oral health programming for the decade 2010 to 2020.

Progress was made on most of the targets for *Healthy People 2010*, although some ground was lost on four targets[11] (Table 20-4), resulting in the establishment of more realistic targets in *Healthy People 2020*.[9] The *Healthy People 2020* targets form the foundation for the oral health priorities for the U.S. population and should be considered when developing community oral health programs. Study of the current status of oral diseases and conditions should include trends and progress in relation to targets of *Healthy People* objectives.

A. Dental caries

    1. Over the past few decades, the trend has been substantially declining rates in the incidence of cumulative caries in all age groups

        a. Lower cumulative caries rates, less severe caries, substantially fewer carious lesions in anterior teeth; fewer teeth lost to caries

        b. Factors that have contributed to lower caries rates

            (1) Fluoride is the most significant factor in the long term, primarily reducing smooth-surface caries: water fluoridation, fluoride dentifrices, and fluoride supplements

            (2) More recently, dental sealants have contributed to reductions in pit and fissure caries

            (3) Greater emphasis on preventive care and increased dental utilization

    2. Although the trend is a decline in caries rates, dental caries is still widespread

        a. 22% of 2- to 4-year-olds, 51% of 6- to 8-year-olds, and 57% of 15-years-olds have experienced dental caries in at least one primary or permanent tooth[11] (see Table 20-4).

        b. Prevalence increases with age; 85% of adults age ≥18 years have experienced dental caries[7]

        c. 28% of 2- to 5-year-old children have early childhood caries (ECC) and represent a slight increase in caries; the number of untreated caries remains the same compared with the previous NHANES;[17] the term *early childhood caries* (*ECC*) replaces terms such as *baby-bottle tooth decay, nursing caries, baby-bottle mouth,* and *baby-bottle caries*; ECC and S-ECC (severe early childhood caries) are classified on the basis of months of age and number of dmfs[18] (Table 20-5).

        d. 25% of the adult dentate population age > 18 years has root caries; rates increase with age

        e. 17% of 2- to 4-year-olds, 28% of 6- to 8-year-olds, 18% of adolescents, and 26% of adults age > 18 years have untreated decay

        f. Dental caries is the most common chronic childhood disease; among 5- to 17-year-olds, dental caries is five times more common than asthma and seven times more common than hay fever[7]

        g. Dental caries is one of the major reasons for hospitalization of children; costly to treat[19]

    3. Decrease in caries rates over past decade (see Table 20-4)[11]

        a. Caries rates have continued to decrease during the past decade in all age groups except among 2- to 4-year-olds

        b. An increase in caries experience has been reported among 2- to 4-year-olds over the past decade

        c. Small decreases in disparities of dental caries have been demonstrated[20]

    4. Distribution of dental caries in the population

        a. State and regional differences exist, although not as pronounced as in the past because of the widespread use of fluorides

        b. Rates are similar for male and female children in all age groups, although adult females have slightly higher DMFT (decayed, missing, and filled permanent teeth) rates and lower rates of untreated decay for both coronal and root caries, most likely because of higher dental care utilization rates

        c. Disparities continue to occur; compared with all other groups, the non-Hispanic Caucasian cohort has more caries-free individuals and less untreated decay[7,11] regardless of the type of caries (primary teeth, permanent teeth, ECC, root caries) and regardless of the age group; greatest disparities occur in preschool-age children; differences relate to SES and dental care utilization

        d. Caries rates and unfilled tooth decay rates are higher for lower SES cohorts at all ages; approximately 75% of dental caries is seen in 25% of children from lower SES groups; poorest children age 2 to 4 years experience three times as many dental caries

        e. Caries patterns have changed, showing a greater percent reduction for smooth-surface caries; thus, proportionately fewer smooth-surface lesions than pit-and-fissure lesions are seen on occlusal and faciolingual surfaces

        f. First and second molars are the most frequently affected teeth

        g. Most commonly occurring type of caries is pit-and-fissure caries, followed by smooth-surface coronal caries and root caries

    5. Risk and associated factors for dental caries

        a. Caries is a multi-factorial, infectious, transmissible disease

        b. Microbial cause includes *Lactobacillus* spp. and *Streptococcus mutans* that are transmitted,

TABLE 20-4 Progress Made on *Healthy People 2010* Oral Health and Related Objectives

Number	Oral Health Objective	Baseline Age	Baseline Data 2000 (%)	*Healthy People 2010* Goal (%)	Mid-decade Data (%)	% of Target Achieved
21-1	Reduce dental caries experience in children and adolescents					
	Young children	2–4	18	11	22	−57 ↓
	Children	6–8	52	42	51	10 ↑
	Adolescents	15	61	51	57	40 ↑
21-2	Reduce untreated dental decay in children and adults					
	Young children	2–4	16	9	17	−14 ↓
	Children	6–8	29	21	28	14 ↑
	Adolescents	15	20	15	18	40 ↑
	Adults	35–44	27	15	26	8 ↑
21-3	Increase adults with teeth who have never lost a tooth as a result of dental caries or periodontal disease	35–44	30	40	38	80 ↑
21-4	Reduce complete tooth loss in adults	65–74	29	22	24	71 ↑
21-5	Reduce gingivitis and destructive periodontal disease in adults					
	Gingivitis	35–44	48	41	NDA	NDA
	Destructive periodontal disease	35–44	22	14	20	25 ↑
21-6	Increase detection of oral cancer lesions at stage 1	All	36	51	35	−7 ↓
21-7	Increase number of adults who report having received an oral cancer examination	40+	13	20	NDA	NDA
21-8	Increase dental sealants					
	In first molars	8	23	50	31	30 ↑
	In first and second molars	14	15	50	20	14 ↑
21-9	Increase persons on public water receiving fluoridated water	All	62	75	67	38 ↑
21-10	Increase annual use of oral health care system by children and adults	2+	44	56	44 (adults)	0
21-11	Increase annual use of dental services by residents of long-term care facilities	All	19	25	NDA	NDA
21-12	Increase number of low-income children and adolescents who receive preventive services	2–18	25	66	29	10 ↑
21-13	Increase number of school-based health centers with oral health component					
	Dental sealants	K–12	12	15	NDA	NDA
	Dental care	K–12	9	11	NDA	NDA

Continued

TABLE 20-4 Progress Made on *Healthy People 2010* Oral Health and Related Objectives—cont'd

Number	Oral Health Objective	Baseline Age	Baseline Data 2000 (%)	*Healthy People 2010* Goal (%)	Mid-decade Data (%)	% of Target Achieved
21-14	Increase number of community health centers and local health departments with oral health component	N/A	52	75	64	52 ↑
21-15	Increase number of states and the District of Columbia with a system to record and refer clefts and other craniofacial anomalies	N/A	16	51	NDA	NDA
21-16	Increase number of states and the District of Columbia with a state-based oral and craniofacial health surveillance system	N/A	0	51	NDA	NDA
21-17	Increase number of dental health programs directed by a public health trained dental professional					
	Tribal	N/A	9	9	8	−11 ↓
	State and local	N/A	39	41	NDA	NDA

↑, *moved toward target;* ↓, *moved away from target; NDA,= No data available; N/A = Not applicable.*
Note that targets were neither met nor exceeded for any objectives.
Data from U.S. Department of Health and Human Services: Progress toward Healthy People 2010 targets: Available at http://www.healthypeople.gov/publications/: Accessed August 26, 2010.

TABLE 20-5 Categorizing Early Childhood Caries (ECC) and Severe Early Childhood Caries (S-ECC)

Age (months)	ECC	S-ECC
<12	>1 dmfs	>1 smooth dmfs
12–23	>1 dmfs	>1 smooth dmfs
24–35	>1 dmfs	>1 smooth dmfs
36–47	>1 dmfs	>1 cavitated maxillary anterior smooth dmfs OR < 4 dmfs
48–59	>1 dmfs	>1 cavitated maxillary anterior smooth dmfs OR < 5 dmfs

dmfs, decayed, missing, and filled primary tooth surface.
Note: Age 72 months (6 years) is no longer considered early childhood for classification of ECC.
Data from American Academy of Pediatric Dentistry (AAPD): Policy on early childhood caries (ECC): Classifications, consequences, and preventive strategies, Oral health policies, pp 40–43. Chicago: Author, 2008: Available at http://www.aapd.org/media/Policies_Guidelines/: Accessed August 27, 2010.

primarily within families and from caregivers of young children
c. Risk is increased by sugar and other fermentable carbohydrates as well as by highly acidic foods in the diet, especially in childhood
   (1) Both the total amount and the frequency of sugar intake relate to the incidence of dental caries
   (2) The bacteria present in dental plaque biofilm ferment dietary carbohydrates to produce organic acids that demineralize the tooth structure
   (3) Plaque biofilm bacteria use fermentable carbohydrates to produce the sticky polysaccharide matrix of plaque biofilm
d. Fats and proteins have demonstrated minor protective characteristics against caries
   (1) Fats may decrease caries activity by altering the surface properties of enamel, reducing sugar solubilization, being toxic to oral bacteria, or simply replacing dietary carbohydrates
   (2) Proteins may reduce caries by a direct effect on plaque biofilm metabolism, by replacement of dietary fermentable carbohydrates, or by increasing salivary urea levels
e. The tooth's resistance to acid attack is increased by fluorides, calcium, and phosphate: their presence in the saliva and plaque biofilm bring about remineralization during the continual demineralization–remineralization process of dental caries production (see discussion on fluorides in Chapters 13 and 16)
f. Severe and chronic caries in early childhood is a risk factor for future caries

g. Low SES is the most powerful predictor of caries in young children; caries control programs should be targeted to low SES populations

h. Population-based research continues to evaluate whether familial tendencies toward dental caries have a genetic basis or are simply related to familial transmission, dietary habits, and behavioral traits

i. Primary risk factors are bacteria, fermentable carbohydrates in the diet, and tooth susceptibility; primary preventive measures are to reduce bacteria with good oral hygiene and antimicrobials; reduce the amount and frequency of fermentable carbohydrates and other acidic foods and drinks in the diet; use fluorides and other chemotherapeutic measures to increase the resistance of the enamel to acid attack and enhance the protective nature of saliva; and place dental sealants to increase the caries resistance of pit and fissure surfaces; secondary preventive measures are to eliminate carious lesions and restore cavitated teeth to eliminate bacteria and improve the ability to remove plaque biofilm

6. Additional risk factors for ECC

   a. Infant feeding practices, including the infant falling asleep during feeding and on-demand feeding, whether the infant is breastfed or bottle fed, and delayed weaning from bottle feeding or breastfeeding

   b. High cariogenic diet, including sugar drinks in the bottle or sippy cup and high sugar in other components of the diet

   c. Transmission of cariogenic bacteria from the caregiver to the young child

   d. ECC is more prevalent not only in low SES populations but also in circumstances in which child care is provided by individuals with little education or understanding of disease prevention; a caregiver from the low SES group who does not have oral health literacy can create risk for children from middle and upper SES groups

7. Other risk and associated factors for root caries

   a. Root caries increases with age because of a greater likelihood of exposed cementum and other risk factors

   b. Increasing age of the population and decreasing tooth loss result in more available root surfaces to become carious

   c. Greater use of medications that cause xerostomia among older adults; multiple medications are especially a major risk factor; saliva loses its protective capacity in such cases

d. Increased sugar intake as sense of taste diminishes and eating habits change with age create a greater risk for older individuals

e. History of coronal caries and smoking are risk factors for root caries

f. Root caries rates are higher in males, lower SES cohorts, and groups that have lower dental attendance rates

B. Dental sealants

1. Approximately 31% of 8-year-old children had one or more first molars sealed, and 20% of 14-year-old children had one or more first and second molars sealed; these rates have improved during the past decade[11]

2. Disparities occur in the rates of sealants in children, with greater numbers of non-Hispanic Caucasian children receiving sealants because of SES differences and resulting higher dental care utilization rates; parents' educational level is associated with children's sealant rates

3. Permanent molar teeth are most frequently sealed and are targeted in community-based sealant programs because of their greater susceptibility to caries

4. Prevalence of dental sealants decreases with increasing age because they are targeted at children; placement as soon as possible after tooth eruption is recommended

C. Periodontal diseases (see the section on "Epidemiology of periodontal diseases and related risks" in Chapter 14)

1. Periodontal diseases manifest as different clinical entities, depending on aggressiveness, severity, rate of progression, systemic diseases present, hormonal influences, genetics, and other factors

2. A decline in dental caries has resulted in increased attention to periodontal diseases by both the public and the oral health professions

3. Prevalence of periodontal diseases

   a. The presence of periodontal diseases, either gingivitis or periodontitis or both, is almost universal, with over 70% of adults in all countries affected; worldwide data collected indicate the prevalence of severe periodontitis in the range of 7% to 15% in almost all populations, regardless of economic development, oral hygiene, or dental care available; increased levels of prevalence and severity of periodontal diseases are found in areas of the world where generalized malnutrition is common; differences in periodontal disease levels between peoples of the developed countries and the developing countries are attributed to differences in oral hygiene levels

b. Variations in data related to the prevalence of periodontal diseases can be attributed to differences in study designs and measurement

c. According to U.S. national data, approximately 20% of the population suffers from severe destructive periodontitis, but the rates have improved during the past decade;[11] periodontitis is observed even in well-treated patients because of the influence of genetics and immune response; the presence of severe destructive periodontitis is uncommon in young children

d. Mild and moderate forms of periodontitis are more common; over 90% of persons 13 years of age or older show signs of some clinical attachment loss (CAL) while still maintaining a functioning dentition; mild and moderate CAL in young children is <10%

e. Although gingivitis has declined in recent years because of greater attention to oral hygiene, it is still present in the majority of the population; approximately 48% of 35- to 44-year-olds showed signs of gingivitis; gingivitis of varying severity is a universal finding in children and young adolescents because of hormonal changes and poorer oral hygiene; the prevalence of gingivitis does not vary by age in adults

4. Distribution of periodontal diseases in the population

a. Prevalence and severity of periodontal disease are higher in rural areas than in urban areas

b. At all ages, men are more likely than women to have recession, deeper pockets, and at least one site of severe CAL and to experience severe destructive periodontitis; women experience more gender-related temporary periodontal conditions related to hormonal changes; women have better oral hygiene than men

c. The prevalence of moderate and severe CAL, gingival recession, and pocket depth increases with age; the risk for disease increases for older adults who keep their teeth and with many environmental factors such as smoking, poorly controlled diabetic status, and genotype-positive status

d. Disparities exist in the rates of CAL and gingivitis, with lower rates in non-Hispanic Caucasian groups; major disparities exist in treatment rates with more treatment in non-Hispanic Caucasians; disparities are a result of SES and health literacy differences that influence the values and behaviors relating to prevention and dental care utilization

e. The presence of periodontal diseases is inversely related to increasing education and increasing family income (SES)

5. Risk and associated factors

a. Smoking—one of the strongest risk factors

b. Systemic conditions

c. Psychosocial stress

d. Host response mechanism—especially in severe destructive periodontitis

e. Genetics—especially in severe destructive periodontitis

f. Previous periodontal condition, the strongest clinical observable determinant

g. Oral hygiene—plaque biofilm containing specific microbes that are the etiologic agents for periodontal diseases are more strongly associated with specific forms of periodontal disease

   (1) Most forms of gingivitis are a direct result of growth and accumulation of oral microorganisms, hence the term *dental plaque–induced gingivitis*

   (2) Mild to moderate forms of periodontitis are also strongly associated with the presence of plaque biofilm

   (3) The etiologic role of oral hygiene in severe destructive periodontitis is weaker; the critical factors are the type of bacteria present in plaque biofilm and the individual's susceptibility

h. Calculus is an associated factor and is almost universally present in the population; in a U.S. national survey, 84% percent of the employed group and 89% of older adults had calculus

D. Tooth retention and tooth loss

1. Rate of edentulism for adults age ≥65 years is 18% percent, and 43% of adults age ≥65 years have lost six or more teeth because of periodontal disease or dental caries;[21] rates increase with age

2. Rates are decreasing in spite of the aging population in the United States because of increased emphasis on preventive dentistry, greater use of fluorides, improved success with periodontal therapy, and higher dental care utilization rates; 38% of adults age 35 to 44 years have never lost a tooth as a result of dental caries or periodontal disease[11]

3. Overall health literacy, health, and health beliefs and values are associated with edentulism

4. Smoking and early tooth loss are risk factors for edentulism

5. Disparities exist in both edentulism and partial tooth loss; non-Hispanic Caucasian cohorts have lower rates, again because of SES and dental care utilization rates

6. Complete tooth loss does not vary by gender; rates are higher for lower SES groups

7. Dental caries is the principal cause of tooth loss at almost all ages, with the exception of adults age >80 years

E. Denture use

1. One in five persons 18 to 74 years of age wears a removable prosthodontic appliance to replace some or all teeth

2. Removable prosthodontic appliances are worn disproportionately more often by women than by men

3. Differences in denture use by ethnic group are not clear

4. In spite of reductions in tooth loss, the number of denture wearers will remain significant because of the aging population; the need for denture fabrication and related patient education will continue

F. Oral and pharyngeal cancers

1. Prevalence

a. In the United States, over 30,000 new cases of oral and pharyngeal cancers are diagnosed each year, with over 8000 deaths;[21] occurrence and site distribution within the mouth vary widely in different parts of the world

b. Oral and pharyngeal cancers (cancers of the lips, tongue, buccal mucosa, floor of the mouth, and pharynx) account for 3% of all cancers in the United States; the sixth most common cancer in the developed world

c. The mortality rate for oral cancers in the United States is 2.5 out of 100,000; the rate has not improved in the past few decades;[11] 5-year survival rates are 50%[21]

2. Distribution

a. Oral cancers are 2.6 times more prevalent among males, and twice as many deaths occur among males as among females; except in the case of cancer of the pharynx, the male–female ratio for oral cancer is 1.8 to 1; the gender gap between males and females is narrowing, which is attributed to increased and prolonged use of tobacco products by women

b. The prevalence of oral cancers increases with age; males 40 to 65 years of age have the highest number of lip and tongue cancers; 95% of oral cancers occur in individuals age ≥35 years

c. Disparities occur with lower rates of oral cancers and higher survival rates in non-Hispanic Caucasians and higher SES groups; related to differences in high-risk behaviors and dental care utilization

3. Causal and risk factors

a. Evidence is sufficient to infer a causal relationship between the use of tobacco and cancers of the larynx, esophagus, oral cavity, and pharynx; a dose–response relationship exists between cigarette smoking and cancers of the lung, larynx, oral cavity, and urinary bladder in women

b. Risk factors for oral cancers are alcohol consumption, excessive exposure to ultraviolet light (lip cancer), and chronic inflammation; combining tobacco use and alcohol consumption increases the risk two to four times compared with either factor alone

c. Other determinants include viral infections, immunodeficiency, poor nutrition, occupational exposures, and genetics

4. *Healthy People 2020* goals directed at improving oral and pharyngeal cancer morbidity and mortality rates include increased screening by dentists and dental hygienists, increased detection of oral and pharyngeal cancers in the early stage, and increased tobacco cessation counseling by dentists and dental hygienists; no progress was made on these objectives during the past decade 2000 to 2010[11]

G. Cleft lip and palate

1. Prevalence—1 in every 500 to 750 live births; ranging from 0.18 to 4.04 per 1000 live births for different ethnic groups

a. Oral clefts are the most common class of congenital malformations in the United States; cleft lip is more common than cleft palate

b. The rates are higher in the non-Hispanic Caucasian cohort compared with African American and Hispanic cohorts and are the highest in the Asian and Native American populations

c. More isolated cleft palates are seen in girls, and more facial clefts are seen in boys

2. Clefts are associated with threatened spontaneous abortion during the first and second trimesters of pregnancy, diminished oxygen supply, and maternal influenza, fever, drug consumption (e.g., opiates, penicillin, and salicylates), infectious diseases, nutritional deficiencies (e.g., folic acid deficiency), alcohol consumption, use of teratogenic agents (e.g., corticosteroids, drugs of abuse), and smoking during the early stages of pregnancy; the Human Genome Project outcomes have led to a better understanding of genetic risk factors

3. A positive relationship exists between clefts and premature births; infants with clefts are of lower birth weight than the general population of infants

4. In the United States, 32 states have oral and craniofacial health surveillance systems; a *Healthy People 2020* objective is to include all 51 states, including Washington, D.C.; a developmental objective is to increase the states that have recording and referral systems for clefts

H. Malocclusion

1. Malocclusions can occur from congenital or acquired crowding of the teeth or jaws; prolonged bottle feeding, thumb sucking, and other behaviors during development are attributed

2. Current data are not available; the NHANES III indicated most of the racial and ethnic groups have noticeable incisor irregularity; only 35% of adults exhibit well-aligned mandibular incisors; in 15%, the irregularity is severe enough to affect social acceptability and function; 57% to 59% of the population need at least some degree of orthodontic treatment; disparities occur in treatment, depending on the SES of the groups[22]

3. Rates can be reduced by education of young mothers regarding feeding practices and the habits of young children

I. Craniofacial injuries and tooth trauma

1. An estimated 25% of the U.S. population experiences injury that damages one or more anterior teeth; more injuries occur in children, and the rates decrease with age[23]

2. The leading causes of head and face injuries are accidental falls, assaults, sports-related and recreational activities, bicycle and automobile collisions, and work-related tasks and projects around the house; one in six sports-related injuries is to the craniofacial area[24]

3. Injury rates can be reduced by promoting the use of seat belts, air bags, helmets, protective gear, mouth guards, facemasks, and goggles; a *Healthy People 2010* objective was to increase use of mouth protection during school-sponsored physical activities

4. Most injuries are treated in emergency rooms; education of medical personnel will increase the success of treatment of dental-related injuries

J. Temporomandibular disease

1. Epidemiologic study results vary on the basis of measurements; this has resulted in prevalence rates ranging from 35% to 72%; studies include signs and symptoms in various population groups and almost universally in orthodontic patients[25]

2. The prevalence of conditions such as pain in the joint or masseter muscles during joint movement, mandibular deviations in opening, and joint clicking or crepitus is high, even among individuals who do not perceive a problem

K. Dental fluorosis

1. Description—chronic endemic form of enamel hypoplasia caused by ingesting large amounts of fluoride during the time of tooth formation in the late secretory to early maturation stage of enamel development; starts for central incisors as early as age 22 months, usually occurs at 24 months, and may occur as late as age 4 years (critical period for permanent centrals is ages 1 to 4 years);[26] defective calcification of teeth produces a white, chalky appearance that may undergo brown discoloration and change of surface texture; characterized by retention of enamel proteins and change in enamel matrix structure

2. Dean's classification of dental fluorosis in Table 20-6 provides a description of the appearance of fluorosis

3. Prevalence of dental fluorosis

a. About 22% of school children exhibit fluorosis, distributed across the following classifications: 17% very mild, 4% mild, 1% moderate, and 0.3% severe; 78% of the population is fluorosis free; the prevalence of fluorosis in young children may be increasing in the very mild to mild categories as a result of widespread use of fluorides; actions and recommendations related to fluoride dentifrices and supplements and judicious use of other fluorides are in response to the need to control fluorosis; future assessment will determine the results of current measures to prevent fluorosis

b. Occurs in some children in all communities; 7% to 16% of children born and raised in an optimally fluoridated community exhibit mild or very mild dental fluorosis in the permanent dentition

c. Occurs in many parts of the world; a public health problem in East Africa, India, and Eastern Europe; not considered a public health problem in the United States at this time

4. Causes

a. Ingesting water with naturally occurring excessive fluoride

(1) 1 to 2 parts per million fluoride (ppm F) results in mild fluorosis; 2 to 4 ppm F results in moderate to severe fluorosis

(2) The Environmental Protection Agency (EPA), which is responsible for the safety and quality of water, has set the maximum allowable limit for fluoride at 4-ppm and secondary limit at 2-ppm (defluoridation is required at the 4-ppm level and recommended at the 2-ppm level)

TABLE 20-6 Common Dental Indices Used in Community Oral Health and Oral Health Research

Dental Index	Procedure for Use	Interpretation
Dental Caries Indices Decayed-Missing-Filled Teeth (DMFT) index: An irreversible index used to measure past and present caries experience of a population with permanent teeth; D indicates a carious tooth; M indicates a tooth missing as a result of dental caries; F indicates a filled tooth	Count and record the D, M, and F teeth in each member of the sample or population	Complex index; requires careful calibration Total DMF indicates cumulative caries experience, D provides information about morbidity and specific treatment needs, F and M provide information about dental utilization; programming needs can be determined by the total score as well as the scores within each category, e.g., high caries experience (DMF) indicates need for programs to prevent and control caries, high D indicates need for treatment programs, high M indicates need for education and earlier intervention, high F score indicates dental utilization; scores can be compared to evaluate program success, e.g., reduction of D and increase in F indicates a successful caries treatment program, marked increase in D, DMF, or both indicates failure of caries prevention program
	DMF and def can be scored on teeth (DMFT and deft) or surfaces (DMFS and defs); scoring on surfaces provides more sensitivity for research purposes, but greater variability; scoring on surfaces is recommended for clinical trials, and scoring on teeth is recommended for survey work	
	Regardless of the index (DMF or def), and regardless of whether teeth or surfaces are scored, if both a restoration and a carious lesion are present in the same area, it is scored as D	
deft index: A variation of the DMFT; is used to measure observable caries experience in primary teeth; the d and f symbols are the same as in the DMFT; however, e indicates the need for extraction (not extracted), and missing teeth are not considered	Scores can be expressed as follows: 1. The total DMFT or DMFS (D+M+F) count is an indication of caries experience in the individual 2. Individual DMFT or DMFS counts are averaged to indicate the caries experience of the population 3. The total number of individuals in the population with a DMF count is also used as an expression of the caries experience of the population 4. The total DT can be divided by the total DMFT to express a percentage of decayed teeth; this percentage is an indication of caries morbidity and treatment needs 5. The total FT or the total FT+MT can be divided by the total DMFT to express a percentage of filled teeth or filled and missing teeth; this percentage of filled teeth is referred to as "filling needs met," and both are an indication of dental utilization	
		To control for variability of scoring missing teeth in children at the age of exfoliation, the deft index does not score exfoliated or extracted teeth, thus possibly under-representing caries experience
Root Caries Index (RCI): A method for reporting root caries that measures the severity of disease and delineates the true intraoral population at risk (exposed root surfaces) as the denominator	Only root surfaces exposed to the oral environment are at risk Scoring is relatively straightforward; four surfaces of the root are evaluated: mesial, distal, facial, and lingual; if multiple surfaces are exposed, the most severely affected surface is recorded for the tooth The index is expressed as a percentage and computed as follows: 1. D and F root surfaces are summed 2. The sum is then divided by the total number of exposed root surfaces 3. The result is then multiplied by 100 for a percentage	Scored only on root surfaces; assumes that gingival recession is a necessary antecedent condition before root caries can develop and that gingival recession must be evident at the time of examination

Continued

TABLE 20-6 Common Dental Indices Used in Community Oral Health and Oral Health Research—cont'd

Dental Index	Procedure for Use	Interpretation
Gingivitis Indices		
Gingival Index (GI): A reversible index based on severity of inflammation and location; can be used to determine prevalence and severity of gingivitis in epidemiologic surveys as well as individual dentition; GI often used in controlled clinical trials of preventive or therapeutic agents	A score of 0 to 3 is assigned to four gingival scoring units: mesial, distal, buccal, and lingual surfaces of teeth; a blunt instrument, such as a periodontal probe, is used to assess bleeding potential; totaling the four area scores around each tooth and dividing by 4 yields a GI score for the tooth; totaling all tooth scores and dividing by the number of teeth examined provides a GI score per person; these scores can be averaged for a mean score for the population; can be used on selected or all erupted teeth; criteria include: 0—Normal gingiva 1—Mild inflammation: slight change in color; slight edema; no bleeding on probing 2—Moderate inflammation: redness, edema, and glazing; bleeding on probing 3—Severe inflammation: marked redness and edema, ulceration; tendency to spontaneous bleeding	0.1–1.0: Mild gingivitis 1.1–2.0: Moderate gingivitis 2.1–3.0: Severe gingivitis Difficult to replicate; calibration difficult
Sulcus Bleeding Index (SBI): designed to detect early symptoms of gingivitis; useful in short-term clinical trials	Scored on maxillary and mandibular anterior teeth; a score is assigned for each of four gingival areas or teeth: labial and lingual marginal gingival areas and mesial and distal papillary gingival areas for a total of 64 units; each area is probed with a blunt periodontal probe and observed for 30 seconds to detect bleeding; scores and criteria include: 0—Healthy appearance of papillary and marginal gingiva; no bleeding on sulcus probing 1—Apparently healthy papillary and marginal gingiva showing no change in color and no swelling; but bleeding from sulcus on probing 2—Bleeding on probing and change of color caused by inflammation; no swelling or microscopic edema 3—Bleeding on probing; change in color; and slight edematous swelling 4—Bleeding on probing; obvious swelling; may have change in color 5—Bleeding on probing; spontaneous bleeding; change in color; and marked swelling with or without ulceration	Calibration of examiners critical; results reported by frequency of score
Gingival Bleeding Index (GBI): A simple measure of the presence or absence of bleeding (dichotomous measure) with the use of floss	Bleeding is measured by inserting waxed floss into each interproximal space using a normal C-shaped flossing technique and moving the floss up and down for one stroke; the area is observed for 30 seconds to detect bleeding; scored as bleeding present or absent	Easy to implement; only provides information about bleeding; dichotomous measure lacks sensitivity
Eastman Interdental Bleeding Index (EIBI): a simple measure of the presence or absence of bleeding (dichotomous measure) with the use of an interdental stimulator	Bleeding is measured by inserting a triangular wooden interdental stimulator into each interproximal space; the stimulator is inserted and removed four times, inserted horizontally with 1 to 2 mm of depression of interdental papilla; each area is observed for 15 seconds to score bleeding as either present or absent	Easy to implement; easy to calibrate; measures only bleeding

TABLE 20-6 Common Dental Indices Used in Community Oral Health and Oral Health Research—cont'd

Dental Index	Procedure for Use	Interpretation
Periodontal Disease Indices		
Periodontal Disease Index (PDI): Used to measure the presence and severity of periodontal disease; measures reversible and irreversible disease within the same index	Six teeth are examined: Numbers 3, 9, 12, 19, 25, and 28; the PDI assesses gingivitis, gingival sulcus depth, calculus, plaque, occlusal and incisal attrition, mobility, and lack of contact.	The six teeth are sensitive for partial mouth scoring of periodontal conditions with other indices; the teeth are referred to as the Ramfjord teeth (after Dr. Ramfjord, who developed the index); current method of combining recession and pocket depth to determine clinical attachment loss (CAL) was first introduced with this index; no longer recommended because of current understanding that gingivitis and periodontitis are two different disease entities; the various components are currently measured separately with other indices or measures
Community Periodontal Index of Treatment Needs (CPITN): Three indicators of periodontal status are used for this assessment: (1) presence or absence of gingival bleeding, (2) supragingival or subgingival calculus, and (3) periodontal pockets subdivided into shallow (4–5 mm) and deep (≥6 mm) Requires specially designed lightweight probe with a 0.5-mm ball tip bearing a black band between 3.5 and 5.5 mm (list of probes available from the World Health Organization)	The mouth is divided into sextants defined by teeth numbers 1–5, 6–11, 12–16, 17–21, 22–27, and 28–32; a sextant is examined only if 2 or more teeth are present and not indicated for extraction; for adults age ≥20 years, tooth numbers 2, 3, 8, 14, 15, 18, 19, 24, 30, and 31 are used; two molars in each posterior sextant are paired for recording; if one is missing, there is no replacement; if an index tooth in a sextant is not present or does not qualify for examination, all remaining teeth are examined; for individuals up to age 19, tooth numbers 3, 8, 14, 19, 24, and 30 are examined; each index tooth is probed using the probe as a sensing instrument to determine pocket depth and detect subgingival calculus; the probe tip is inserted gently, and the depth is read against the color coding; six areas on each tooth are examined: mesiofacial, mid-facial, distofacial, and corresponding lingual sites. One recording is made for each sextant reflecting the highest probe reading in the sextant; the highest code determines assessment and treatment planning needs; in epidemiologic surveys, recording is based on examination of 2 molars in each posterior sextant and 1 central incisor in each of 2 anterior sextants; in individual screenings, the worst condition is recorded around any one of 4 or 6 teeth comprising the sextant CRITERIA FOR CODES Code 0—Line at colored area visible; no rough areas, no bleeding Code 1—Line at colored area visible with bleeding after probing Code 2—Line visible with bleeding and rough areas (calculus) Code 3—Colored area only partially visible (>3.5 mm) Code 4—Colored area completely disappears (>5.5 mm) * by code for furcation involvement, mobility, mucogingival problem, marked recession, or all INTERPRETATION OF CODES 0—Preventive care; biofilm control 1—Preventive care; biofilm control 2—Preventive care and calculus removal; biofilm removal 3—Comprehensive periodontal assessment and treatment plan (TP); counseling regarding TP; biofilm control 4—Comprehensive periodontal assessment and TP for non-surgical periodontal therapy; counseling regarding TP; biofilm control	Index is used as part of the Oral Health Surveys by the World Health Organization; facilitates rapid assessment of mean disease status of a population of various grades of periodontal involvement; the Periodontal Screening and Recording (PSR) index developed by the American Dental Association for use in clinical practice uses the same codes and criteria

Continued

TABLE 20-6 Common Dental Indices Used in Community Oral Health and Oral Health Research—cont'd

Dental Index	Procedure for Use	Interpretation
Community Periodontal Index (CPI): Adapted by the World Health Organization from the CPITN to measure periodontal status of a community; treatment need codes from the CPITN are eliminated	Measured by epidemiologic examination using a special probe bearing a black band between 3.5 and 5.5 mm and with a ball at the end to help feel calculus (same probe used for CPITN); scores gingival health, presence or absence of gingival bleeding, supragingival or subgingival calculus, periodontal pockets categorized as 4 to 5 mm or 6 mm or more, and loss of attachment (LOA; same as CAL); each sextant receives a code that represents the worst probe depth found in that sextant; highest code determines assessment category CRITERIA FOR CPI PERIODONTAL STATUS CODES Code 0—Entire black band visible; healthy periodontal tissues: no bleeding Code 1—Entire black band visible; bleeding upon probing Code 2—Entire black band visible; calculus present Code 3—Black band partially hidden: 4–5 mm pockets Code 4—Black band entirely hidden: >6 mm pockets If the cemento-enamel junction (CEJ) is visible or the CPI is 4, LOA codes 1 to 4 are used CRITERIA FOR LOA (CAL) CODES Code 0— 0–3 mm LOA—CEJ covered by gingival margin and CPI score of 0 to 3 Code 1— 3.5 to 5.5 mm LOA; CEJ within the black band on probe Code 2—6 to 8 mm LOA; CEJ between top of black band and 8.5 mm mark on probe Code 3—9 to 11 mm LOA; CEJ between 8.5 and 11.5 marks on probe Code 4—LOA >12 mm; CEJ beyond highest mark (11.5 mm) on probe	Measures periodontal status in contrast to the CPITN, which measures periodontal treatment needs as well as periodontal status
Oral Hygiene Indices Simplified Oral Hygiene Index (OHI-S): A reversible index used to measure oral hygiene status; scores six teeth—first fully erupted tooth distal to the second premolar in each quadrant (facial surfaces on maxilla and lingual surfaces on mandible) and maxillary right and mandibular left central incisors (labial surface of each)—are assessed separately for debris and calculus; assessment yields a DI-S score (debris index-simplified) and a CI-S score (calculus index-simplified); scores are combined for the OHI-S score.	Surfaces are examined for debris and scored by using the DI-S system: 0—No debris or stain present 1—Soft debris covering not more than one third of tooth surface being examined or presence of extrinsic stains without debris regardless of surface area covered 2—Soft debris covering more than one third but not more than two thirds of exposed tooth surface 3—Soft debris covering more than two thirds of exposed tooth surface Surfaces are examined for calculus and scored by using the CI-S system: 0—No calculus present 1—Supragingival calculus covering not more than one third of exposed tooth surface being examined 2—Supragingival calculus covering more than one third but not more than two thirds of exposed tooth surfaces or presence of individual flecks of subgingival calculus around cervical portion of tooth 3—Supragingival calculus covering more than two thirds of exposed tooth surface or a continuous heavy band of subgingival calculus around cervical portion of tooth	OHI-S: 0.0–1.2: Good oral hygiene 1.3–3.0: Fair oral hygiene 3.1–6.0: Poor oral hygiene DI-S or CI-S: 0.0–0.6: Good oral hygiene 0.7–1.8: Fair oral hygiene 1.9–3.0: Poor oral hygiene Useful to survey oral hygiene in a population

TABLE 20-6 Common Dental Indices Used in Community Oral Health and Oral Health Research—cont'd

Dental Index	Procedure for Use	Interpretation
Plaque Index (PII): Used to assess extent of soft deposits; measures differences in thickness of debris at gingival margin; used in conjunction with GI; useful in longitudinal studies and clinical trials	Four gingival scoring units: mesial, distal, buccal, lingual; examined by using mouth mirror, dental explorer, and air-drying; PII for a tooth is obtained by totaling these four plaque scores and dividing by 4; PII score per person is obtained by adding the tooth PII scores and dividing by the number of teeth examined; the score may be obtained for a segment or group of teeth SCORING CRITERIA 0—No plaque in gingival area 1—Film of plaque adhering to free gingival margin and adjacent area of tooth; plaque only noticed by running probe across tooth surface 2—Moderate accumulation of soft deposits within gingival margin, on adjacent tooth surface, or in both areas can be seen with the naked eye 3—Abundance of soft matter within gingival pocket, gingival margin, or both, and adjacent tooth surface	0: Excellent 0.1–0.9: Good 1.0–1.9: Fair 2.0–3.0: Poor Useful index for clinical trials; plaque is assessed only at the gingival margin in relation to gingival and periodontal conditions
Patient Hygiene Performance (PHP): Developed to assess individual's performance in removing debris after oral hygiene instruction, including effectiveness of interdental cleaning	Teeth are disclosed; six teeth are evaluated: numbers 3, 8, 14, 19, 24, and 30; each tooth is divided into 5 areas: three longitudinal thirds: distal, middle, and mesial; the middle third is subdivided horizontally into incisal, middle, and gingival thirds; score per person is obtained by totaling these five subdivision scores per tooth surface and dividing by number of tooth surfaces examined	0: Excellent 0.1–1.7: Good 1.8–3.4: Fair 3.5–5.0: Poor Provides overall assessment of oral hygiene; has advantage that interproximal areas are scored separately to evaluate interdental cleaning; simple to use; can be performed quickly
Turesky modification of Quigley Hein Plaque Index (TPI): Provides an overall assessment of oral hygiene similar to the OHI-S	Teeth are disclosed; all teeth except third molars are evaluated on the mesial, distal, and mid-aspects of the buccal and lingual surfaces; each buccal and lingual surface is scored on a scale of 0 to 5 0—No plaque 1—Separate flecks of plaque at the cervical margin 2—A thin continuous band of plaque (up to 1 mm) at the cervical margin 3—A band of plaque wider than 1 mm but covering less than one third of the tooth surface 4—Plaque covering at least one third but less than two thirds of the surface 5—Plaque covering two thirds or more of the surface All surface scores are totaled and divided by the number of surfaces examined to determine the TPI for the individual person	Similar to the OHI-S but more sensitive because (1) the scale has more differentiation at the lower end, (2) all teeth are scored, and (3) disclosant is used; recommended for clinical trials of preventive and therapeutic agents; requires careful calibration
Modified Navy Plaque Index (MNPI): Detailed assessment of individual's oral hygiene, including effectiveness of interdental cleaning	Disclosed plaque is scored on tooth numbers 3, 9, 12, 19, 25, and 28; buccal and lingual surfaces are divided into 9 areas: 3 at the gingival margin extending to the distal and mesial, 3 on area just incisal–occlusal to the marginal area and extending into the contact areas, 3 in the area just incisal/occlusal to that extending to distal and mesial contacts, and 1 on the incisal/occlusal one quarter of the surface; plaque is scored as present (1) or absent (0) in each of the 9 areas; the area scores are added for a total score; the highest total score for any of the 6 teeth assessed is the individual person's MNPI score; area plaque scores can be grouped and designated as: Whole mouth (all 9 areas) Marginal (mesial, distal, and mid-aspect of the marginal area) Approximal (mesial and distal of the area just above the marginal areas, i.e., the contact areas)	Index is similar to the PHP with more sensitivity as a result of the surfaces being divided into 9 instead of 5 areas; practical to evaluate interdental cleaning as well as overall oral hygiene; requires careful calibration; useful to assess the value of oral health education programs and individuals' oral hygiene practices

Continued

TABLE 20-6 Common Dental Indices Used in Community Oral Health and Oral Health Research—cont'd

Dental Index	Procedure for Use	Interpretation
Volpe-Manhold Index (VMI): Measures extent of supragingival calculus for calculus clinical trials	Calculus is measured on the gingival, distal, and mesial planes of the lingual surfaces of the mandibular anterior teeth only (numbers 22–27) the height of the calculus is measured with a periodontal probe in increments of 0.5 mm up to 5.0 mm; scores on each plane are summed for a tooth score, and tooth scores are summed for the whole mouth VMI score; the possible high score for a tooth is 15, and the possible high score for the whole mouth is 90	This index was developed for tartar control dentifrice clinical trials; useful for any trials related to calculus control; large range of scores allows for more valid statistical analysis

Dean Fluorosis Index (Community Fluorosis Index)

Description	Classification & Score	Criteria	Interpretation
The same categories are used for Dean Fluorosis Index and Community Fluorosis Index	Normal (0)	The enamel presents the usual translucent semi-vitriform type of structure; the surface is smooth, glossy, and usually of a pale, creamy white color	An individual is categorized by classification; prevalence of each category is reported in a population; the Community Fluorosis Index (CFI) is assigned based on the mean of all scores of the study population
Dean developed the classification as categories only, referred to as Dean Fluorosis Index; later numbers ranging from 0–4 were added to denote the categories for research purposes, and the index was referred to as the Community Fluorosis Index	Questionable (0.5)	The enamel discloses slight aberrations from the translucency of normal enamel, ranging from a few white flecks to occasional white spots; this classification is used in those instances in which a definite diagnosis of the mildest form of fluorosis is not warranted and a classification of "normal" not justified	Community Fluorosis Index (CFI) scores: **Range — Significance of scores** 0.0–0.4 — Negative 0.4–0.6 — Borderline 0.6–1.0 — Slight 1.0–2.0 — Medium 2.0–3.0 — Marked 3.0–4.0 — Very marked
Classifies the severity of dental fluorosis based on the two most severely affected teeth	Very mild (1)	Small, opaque, paper-white areas scattered irregularly over the tooth but not involving as much as approximately 25% of the tooth surface; frequently included in this classification are teeth showing no more than about 1–2 mm of white opacity at the tip of the summit of the cusps of the premolars or second molars	A classification of mild or less is not considered a cosmetic problem; a CFI score of less than 0.6 is not considered a problem for the community
	Mild (2)	The white opaque areas in the enamel of the teeth are more extensive but do not involve as much as 50% of the tooth	
	Moderate (3)	All enamel surfaces of the teeth are affected, and surfaces subject to attrition show wear; brown stain is frequently a disfiguring feature	
	Severe (4)	All enamel surfaces are affected, and hypoplasia is so marked that the general form of the tooth may be affected; the major diagnostic sign of this classification is the discrete or confluent pitting; brown stains are widespread, and teeth often appear as if corroded	

Data from Burt B, Eklund S: Dentistry, dental practice, and the community, *ed 6, St Louis, 2005, Saunders; Reddy S:* Essentials of clinical periodontology and periodontics, *ed 2, New Delhi, India, 2008, Jaypee Brothers: Available at http://googlebooks.com: Accessed September 1, 2010; Vandersall DC:* Concise encyclopedia of periodontology, *Hoboken, NJ, 2007, John Wiley & Sons; Wilkins EM:* Clinical practice of the dental hygienist, *ed 10, Philadelphia, 2008, Lippincott, Williams & Wilkins; World Health Organization:* Oral health Country/Area Profile Programme (CAPP), methods and indices: *Available at http://www.whocollab.od.mah.se/: Accessed August 29, 2010.*

(3) Some communities do not have a community water supply; some members of the population depend on well water; fluoride levels of well water vary

b. Children swallowing excessive amounts of fluoride-containing dentifrices—swallowing or overenthusiastic use of fluoridated toothpaste by young children is a concern; prudent use is a "pea-size" or "smear" amount on the brush, placement of toothpaste by an adult, and use of children's dentifrices with lower levels of fluoride; currently manufacturers have limited the fluoride content of children's dentifrices

c. Inappropriate supplementation with fluoride tablets or fluoride-containing vitamins—mild to moderate fluorosis is associated with use of fluoride supplements, especially in the higher SES groups

d. Halo effect of secondary fluoride exposures to fluoride in processed foods and beverages, especially those that vary by water source, can be significant even in nonfluoridated areas

   (1) Infant formula, especially soybean-based formulas, should be used in moderation in fluoridated communities

   (2) Fruit juices and drinks with moderate to high concentrations of fluoride consumed by children may contribute to fluorosis; in the United States, water and processed beverages can provide approximately 75% of a person's fluoride intake

   (3) Some bottled water manufactured in the United States contains an optimal concentration of fluoride (1 ppm); most contain <0.3 ppm fluoride

e. Consumption of fluoridated water in combination with other significant dietary sources of fluoride

   (1) Combining systemic fluorides will increase the fluoride level above the optimum and will cause fluorosis in children who are still in the stages of enamel development (up to age 8 years); education is needed to inform the public of the need to control early consumption of fluoride

   (2) Care must be taken to control young children inadvertently swallowing other sources of fluoride such as gels, mouthrinses, and foams

5. Prevention of dental fluorosis

a. Box 20-2 presents the Centers for Disease Control and Prevention (CDC) recommendations designed to balance dental caries prevention with risk of fluorosis

---

BOX 20-2 Recommendations to Balance Dental Caries Prevention with Risk of Fluorosis

- Counsel parents and caregivers regarding the use of fluoride toothpaste by young children, especially those age <2 years
- Supervise use of fluoride toothpaste among children age <6 years
- Promote use of low-fluoride toothpaste for children age <6 years
- Target mouthrinsing and application of high-concentration fluoride products to persons at high risk for dental caries
- Target and judiciously prescribe fluoride supplements
- Know the fluoride concentration in the primary source of drinking water to be able to make appropriate recommendations
- Use an alternative source of water for children age ≤8 years whose primary drinking water contains >2 parts per million fluoride (ppm F)
- Label the fluoride concentration of bottled water
- Collaborate to educate health care professionals and the public
- Re-evaluate the method of determining optimal fluoride concentration of community drinking water to take into account current consumption patterns of water, processed beverages, and processed foods
- Identify effective strategies to promote adoption of recommendations for using fluoride

Data from U.S. Department of Health and Human Services, Centers for Disease Control and Prevention, Community Water Fluoridation Web site: Reducing the risk for enamel fluorosis: Available at http://www.cdc.gov/fluoridation/safety/reducing_risk.htm: Accessed August 29, 2010.

---

b. The U.S. Department of Health and Human Services (HHS) and the U.S. Environmental Protection Agency (EPA) have recommended reduction of the amount of fluoride per liter of water from 0.7–1.2 milligrams to 0.7 milligrams to reduce the possibility of children receiving too much fluoride. This updated recommendation is based on recent EPA and HHS scientific assessments, which will also guide the EPA in determining whether to lower the maximum amount of fluoride allowed in drinking water. (U.S. Department of Health and Human Services: News Release: HHS and EPA announce new scientific assessments and actions on fluoride, January 7, 2011. Available at http://www.hhs.gov/news. Accessed March 30, 2011.)

c. Prior to promoting a fluoride modality or combination of modalities, one must consider the group's risk for dental caries, fluoride history, current fluoride sources, and potential for dental fluorosis

L. A link exists between oral health and systemic health; inflammation may be the common denominator
1. The mouth reveals significant information about the general health of an individual
2. Periodontitis, tooth mobility, and tooth loss share genetically determined risk factors with other chronic degenerative diseases such as ulcerative colitis and rheumatoid arthritis
3. The oral cavity can reveal signs of disease, drug use, domestic physical abuse, harmful habits, and addictions
4. Radiographs of the oral and craniofacial structures can reveal skeletal changes such as osteoporosis and developmental disorders
5. Oral epithelial cells and fluids such as saliva can be tested for a range of substances unrelated to oral health and deoxyribonucleic acid (DNA)
6. The oral cavity can reveal a range of conditions such as sexually transmitted diseases, blood diseases, tuberculosis, and infectious diseases
7. Research has linked oral infections with diabetes, cardiovascular disease, and adverse pregnancy outcomes; some research has linked oral pathogens with pneumonia, dementia, and certain cancers
8. Functional, psychosocial, and economic quality of life is influenced by an individual's oral health and orofacial image
9. This oral–systemic connection emphasizes the importance of the interdisciplinary team approach in public health

MEASUREMENT OF DISEASES AND CONDITIONS IN ORAL EPIDEMIOLOGY

A. Dental index—abbreviated measurement of the presence or degree of intensity of a disease or condition in a population that aids in collection of data; graduated numerical scale with defined upper and lower limits designed to facilitate summarizing the disease or condition in the population and comparison with other populations classified by the same criteria and methods; a higher number on the scale indicates more or more severe disease or condition; measured by clinical observation with an epidemiologic examination

B. Attributes of an ideal index
1. Validity—measures what is intended to be measured
2. Reliability—measures consistently at different times; reproducibility, stability of measurement

3. Utility—clear, simple, and objective
4. Sensitive to shifts in disease in either direction
5. Acceptable to the subjects involved
6. Quantifiable; amenable to statistical analysis
7. Clinically significant and meaningful

C. The index may assess disease that is a reversible condition, an irreversible condition, or a combination; therefore, indices are classified as:
1. Reversible index—measures conditions that can be reversed (e.g., gingivitis is reversible)
2. Irreversible index—measures cumulative conditions that cannot be reversed (e.g., dental caries, fluorosis)

D. Some common dental indices that are used in community oral health and oral health research are presented in Table 20-6

E. Index selection is determined by:
1. Type of condition to be assessed, specific to the information of interest or the needs of the client
2. Age of the population to be studied
3. Purpose of the assessment, for example, survey or clinical trial

F. Other approaches to measurement in a population
1. A disaggregated approach rather than an index was used on the NHANES III and more recent national surveys to assess periodontal conditions: gingival bleeding, recession, pocket depth, CAL, and calculus as contributing risk factors
2. Basic Screening Survey (BSS)
   a. The BSS, developed by the ASTDDs, is a simple survey method for use with adults, school age children, and preschool age children; the BSS has been used on the NHANES III and other national surveys
   b. Oral screening and an optional questionnaire are included in the BSS; screeners may be non-dental to improve access to the population and reduce the cost of screening
   c. A variety of oral health conditions are assessed; data levels are consistent with the *Healthy People* oral health objectives to be able to monitor the success of the objectives and compare population groups
   d. The BSS is an efficient method to assess dental caries in a survey; it uses dichotomous measures (e.g., yes or no) to assess the absence or the presence of untreated dental caries and dental caries experience (at least one decayed, restored, or missing tooth) on a per-person basis
   e. The following categories are used to assess need and referral for dental care, regardless of condition being measured:
      (1) None—no obvious oral health problem; routine care recommended

(2) Early—Observable oral health problem; early dental care (within several weeks) recommended

(3) Urgent—signs or symptoms present (pain, infection, swelling, soft tissue ulceration) of >2 weeks' duration; emergency dental care (within 24 hours) recommended

G. Examiners or raters should use calibrated or standardized observational criteria in their use of the index or the BSS criteria; training on use and interpretation of evaluative criteria and repeated use of the index are required to produce examiner reliability

1. Intra-rater (intra-examiner) reliability—each examiner is scoring equivalently time and time again; extent to which an investigator remains consistent within himself or herself

2. Inter-rater (inter-examiner) reliability—consistency exists between examiners; degree to which different investigators obtain the same results when using the same data collection instrument

H. Potential errors in assessing disease

1. Errors in sampling technique that result in a nonrepresentative sample—use of nonrandom samples, use of incorrect sampling technique, nonparticipation of a segment of the target population, nonresponse on a survey, and too-small sample size

2. Errors in collecting and recording data—variation in assessment, lack of calibration, inconsistent or inaccurate data collection by the examiners, known or unknown bias, intended or unintended misleading or untruthful responses, lack of compliance of participants, incorrect recording of data by recorders, inaccurate data entry into the computer

3. Errors in analyzing data—incorrect computation, incorrect selection of statistical tests, incomplete analysis, and invalid interpretation

---

PREVENTING AND CONTROLLING ORAL DISEASES AND CONDITIONS

Public Health Measures

A. Community-focused strategies to alleviate, reduce, or eliminate a health problem or issue that is an actual or potential cause of morbidity or mortality

B. Selection of strategy is based on the seven characteristics of an effective public health solution (see the section on "Basic concepts" earlier in this chapter)

BOX 20-3 Ten Great Public Health Achievements—United States, 1900–1999

1. Control of infectious diseases
2. Decline in deaths from coronary heart disease and stroke
3. Family planning
4. Fluoridation of drinking water
5. Healthier mothers and babies
6. Motor vehicle safety
7. Recognition of tobacco as a health hazard
8. Safer and healthier foods
9. Safer workplaces
10. Vaccination

Data from Centers for Disease Control and Prevention: Ten great public health achievements in the 20th century, 1900–1999, August 20, 2008: *Available at http://www.cdc.gov/mmwr/preview/mmwrhtml/00056796.htm: Accessed August 26, 2010.*

C. Examples of public health measures include vaccination, water purification, and water fluoridation (Box 20-3)

Measures for Preventing and Controlling Dental Caries

A. Water fluoridation

1. Adjustment of the natural fluoride concentration to approximately 1 part fluoride to 1 1 ppm water; range 0.7 to 1.2 ppm, depending on average mean daily temperature of the area (1 ppm same as 1 mg/L); HHS and EPA have recommended reduction of the recommended level to 0.7 (see section on "Dental fluorosis" earlier in this chapter)

   a. The hotter the climate, the lower the recommended fluoride concentration because of increased water consumption

   b. The colder the climate, the higher the recommended fluoride concentration because of decreased water consumption

   c. The suggested level of 0.7 to 1.2 ppm F is a non-enforceable recommendation from the U.S. Public Health Service

      (1) Partial exposure (lower than the recommended level of fluoride) provides partial protection

      (2) Level must be maintained; benefits are lost when fluoridation is discontinued

2. Community water fluoridation—dentistry's most significant contribution to solving a public health problem; meets the requirements of a public health solution

a. Fluoridation does not have specific targets; by reaching everyone in the community, it has the potential to reduce disparities

b. It is the most practical form of preventing caries in communities with established community water systems

3. Effectively prevents and controls dental caries in children and adults

a. Incidence of dental caries—reduced by 20% to 40% in the mixed dentition of children (8 to 12 years of age), and 15% to 35% in the permanent dentition of adolescents (14 to 17 years of age); reduced by 20% to 40% of coronal caries in adults

(1) Benefits primary and permanent teeth equally

(2) Primarily benefits smooth surface caries; as DMFS (decayed, missing, and filled permanent surfaces) rates in a population are reduced by fluoride, the proportion of pit-and-fissure caries increases, even though the absolute number is reduced

(3) Quantifying benefits for adults is challenging because of varied histories

b. Controls both coronal and root caries in older adults

c. Helps control caries resulting from reduced salivary flow caused by medications

d. No known prenatal benefits

e. Critical period for benefits in children is immediately after tooth eruption so that immature enamel of newly erupted teeth can uptake the fluoride (ages 6 months to 13 years)

f. Benefits of fluoride accumulate; combination of water fluoridation with topical fluoride provides additional benefits (systemic programs should not be combined to avoid increase in fluorosis in the population)

g. Fluoride is the most effective means to prevent and control dental caries; a common misconception is that oral hygiene is the most effective means

h. Indirect benefits include fewer missing teeth resulting in improved self-image, less complicated restorative procedures, pain reduction, decreased malocclusion, and decreased periodontal problems related to tooth loss, all of which lead to improved quality of life for the public; indirect benefits also include positive influence on the practice of dentistry and dental hygiene

4. Although fluoride is obtained through ingestion of water, the primary benefit of fluoridated water occurs after tooth eruption as a result of topical effects; pre-eruptive effects are minor

a. Post-eruption benefits rely on the fluoride being available in solution at the surface of the tooth;[27] systemic fluoride is released into saliva and is available in saliva and plaque fluids

(1) Fluoride inhibits demineralization by adsorbing to the carbonated hydroxyapatite crystals, protecting the enamel surface from dissolution by acids

(2) Fluoride enhances remineralization of incipient caries by adsorbing during the continual demineralization–demineralization process; this is the primary action of fluoride for control of dental caries

(3) When fluoridated water is consumed, saliva has a constant level of fluoride, making it continually available for uptake by the enamel

(4) Bound fluoride in plaque biofilm is released in response to the lowered pH level and taken up more readily by the demineralized enamel

b. Pre-eruption benefits—once thought to be the primary action, this is now understood to be a minor effect compared with the posteruptive action of fluoride; fluoride is incorporated into the mineralized tooth structure during tooth development by the replacement of hydroxyapatite with fluorapatite during enamel formation

5. Most cost-effective and efficient method of bringing fluoride benefits to a community

a. A *Healthy People 2020* oral health objective calls for 79.6% of the U.S. population served by community water systems to have optimally fluoridated water; 72.4% of the population currently has fluoridated water (see Box 20-1)

b. The cost varies with the size of the community, water system, labor costs, and chemicals used; smaller communities experience higher costs because equipment and supplies required for smaller water systems are more costly

c. The approximate annual per-person cost of water fluoridation is 50 cents for communities of over 20,000 residents, $1 for communities of 10,000 to 20,000 residents, and $3 for communities of less than 5,000[28]

d. Annual per-person savings of dental treatment costs range from $16 in small communities to $19 in large communities; every $1 invested yields $38 in savings of dental treatment costs; the approximate cost of providing fluoridation to an individual for a lifetime is equivalent to the national average cost to restore one carious lesion[28]

e. Fluoridation is compatible with other water-treatment processes; quality-assurance protocol, including recommended annual training of personnel to prevent spills, is necessary; equipment or machinery used for community water fluoridation resembles that used to add other agents to water systems, making training of water treatment personnel easier

6. Compounds used for water fluoridation
   a. Any compound that forms fluoride ions in aqueous solution can be used; the selection depends on the number and accessibility of water sources and water quality
   b. Most popular compounds used in fluoridation of water supplies include:
      (1) Sodium silicofluoride (solid)
      (2) Sodium fluoride (solid)—most commonly used and least expensive; byproduct of fertilizer manufacturing; results in the claim of those opposed to fluoridation that it is a ploy to use waste
      (3) Hydrofluorosilicic acid (liquid)—most expensive

7. Extensive research has demonstrated the safety of fluoridation
   a. It does not cause cancer or other conditions as claimed by its opponents
   b. It is safe to the fetus; the U.S. Food and Drug Administration (FDA) does not recommend the use of fluoride during pregnancy because no known benefits exist, not because it is considered unsafe
   c. Kidney failure is the only condition that requires consideration; kidney dialysis requires the use of mineral-free water

8. Role of government agencies
   a. The Public Health Service (PHS) provides funding through block grants and consultation to states
   b. The CDC provides education to public and water operators and monitors water fluoridation
   c. State oral health departments provide consultation and assistance to cities attempting to fluoridate, training and monitoring for water system operators, and monitoring of water fluoridation within the state
   d. Local governments decide whether or not to fluoridate, implement water fluoridation, and pay the ongoing costs of equipment and supplies

9. Legality of fluoridation—courts have upheld the constitutionality of water fluoridation

10. Promotion of water fluoridation
    a. Ongoing education of individuals is required to encourage their continual support of fluoridation; fluoridation continues to be an issue with regard to wider public acceptance; individuals should be aware of their community fluoride water levels (information is available at My Water's Fluoride at http://apps.nccd.cdc.gov/MWF/Index.asp) and of the ways in which they have benefited from fluoridation in their communities
    b. Three methods of implementation of fluoridation:
       (1) Administrative decision—a community leader introduces the idea of community water fluoridation through appropriate government channels, and the idea is approved by the appropriate governing body (i.e., water board, public services director, mayor, city council)
       (2) Initiative petition or referendum—allows members of the community to vote for or against fluoridation of the water supply; the referendum should be a last resort to avoid a politically charged situation
       (3) Legislative action—mandate passed by state legislators that requires specified public water supplies to be fluoridated or allows health departments to order public water supplies to be fluoridated under certain conditions; it is generally recommended that the decision to fluoridate be made at the local level although some states have mandatory fluoridation laws
    c. Oral health care professionals are responsible for promoting water fluoridation within a community (Box 20-4)
    d. Public attitudes toward water fluoridation are both positive and negative
       (1) Only 20% of population is opposed to fluoridation; the majority of Americans support fluoridation; the lack of organization and passivity on the part of the supporters of fluoridation make it easier for well organized anti-fluoridationists to block its implementation or adoption
       (2) Opponents' arguments—questionable effectiveness, environmental issues, government over-regulation, loss of individual choice, and suspicion of government programs or officials

---

BOX 20-4 Strategies to Increase Water Fluoridation in the United States

The 2008 Water Fluoridation Statistics indicated 72.4% of the U.S. population on public water systems received optimally fluoridated water.*

Healthy People 2020 has set a goal that 79.6% of the population on public water systems should receive optimally fluoridated water by 2020.

Strategies
- Develop and implement a plan of action to maintain the efficacy of water fluoridation as a proven public health measure
- Organize and enlist the support of other state and federal organizations that have an influence in guiding the development of health policies bringing about social change
- Effectively translate fluoridation information into the languages of all racial and ethnic groups
- Develop new and innovative strategies to meet the challenge of fluoridation opponents, past and present
- Develop a national clearinghouse for fluoridation materials
- Develop a national surveillance system to collect, analyze, and evaluate risk factor data related to fluorides
- Support legislation to fund community water fluoridation

Data from U.S. Department of Health and Human Services, Centers for Disease Control and Prevention, Community Water Fluoridation Web site: Available at http://www.cdc.gov/fluoridation/: Accessed August 26, 2010; U.S. Department of Health and Human Services, Centers for Disease Control and Prevention: 2008 Water Fluoridation Statistics: *Available at http://www.test.cdc.gov/fluoridation/statistics/2008stats.htm: Accessed August 26, 2010; and U.S. Department of Health and Human Services:* Healthy People 2020: *Available at http://www.healthypeople.gov/2020/: Accessed April 7, 2011*

e. Anti-fluoridationists' tactics used to oppose fluoridation:
   (1) Using emotion and scare tactics
   (2) Associating fluoridation with concerns about poor health, disease, and aging
   (3) Implying that water fluoridation is poisonous and causes health hazards such as allergies, cancer, heart disease, increased death rates, and Alzheimer's disease
   (4) Claiming that it causes fluorosis
   (5) Suggesting that water fluoridation is unconstitutional and violates individual freedom of choice
   (6) Creating suspicion of government programs, officials, or both

   (7) Claiming that adults do not benefit and that it only benefits a portion of the population, making it inappropriate to spend tax dollars to implement it
   (8) Creating an illusion of scientific controversy where none exists and challenging the benefits of fluoridation
   (9) Using invalid research results to support their claims
  (10) Some Internet sites offer additional sources of misinformation and negative rhetoric
f. Strategies used to support water fluoridation:
   (1) Outcomes from rigorous studies that provide the evidence base for fluoridation
   (2) Knowledge of the community (e.g., past efforts to either introduce water fluoridation or discontinue water fluoridation)
   (3) Working with all community leaders, organizations, stakeholders, and members of the community having influence such as newspaper editors or radio or television personalities; collaboration with other health care professionals
   (4) Creating awareness of the methods, tactics, and nonscientific materials used by fluoridation opponents; recognition of the impact of incorrect information presented in print and electronic media
   (5) Steps to implement a fluoridation campaign are presented in Box 20-5
B. Dietary fluoride supplements
  1. Dosage and age recommendations from the American Dental Association (ADA) and the American Academy of Pediatric Dentistry are based on the concentration of fluoride in drinking water and the weight of the child (Table 20-7); other available fluoride and related factors such as risk, cooperation, age, and ability of the child should also be considered
  2. Current public health recommendation to prevent fluorosis is to use fluoride supplements only with children age ≥6 years and only when fluoridated water is not being consumed; these recommendations suggest judicious use of fluoride supplements because of other sources of fluoride and the risk of fluorosis; a targeted approach is necessary to balance caries reduction benefits of fluoride for high-risk children and its potential to cause fluorosis
  3. Requires a prescription from a physician or dentist; can be administered at home or in a school-based program

BOX 20-5 Steps to Implement Water Fluoridation in a Local Community to Avoid a Referendum

- Form a citizen's community such as "Citizens for Healthy Teeth"; consider hiring a consultant or arrange for consultation from the state dental public health department
- Know the facts: Scientific basis for fluoridation, physiology, effectiveness, safety, cost of fluoridating community, anti-fluoridationists' tactics, charges and answers, legality of fluoridation, and history of local fluoridation
- Identify and contact key community leaders to educate them and get support for the issue
- Gather endorsements from key community leaders to document support when meeting with the city council
- Form a broad base of support beyond the dental and medical professions through the committee and endorsements
- Educate the city council members on the issue, one-on-one, before the issue is brought before council meetings
- Bring the issue formally before the city council only after support has been received from community leaders and individual council members
- Attend council meetings to show support of the issue
- Be prepared to testify at the city council meetings

TABLE 20-7 Dietary Fluoride Supplementation Schedule (in mgF/day*)

	CONCENTRATION OF FLUORIDE IN THE WATER (PPM)		
Age	<0.03 ppm	0.3 ppm to >0.6 ppm	>0.6 ppm
0–6 months	0	0	0
6 months–3 years	0.25 mg	0	0
3–6 years	0.50 mg	0.25 mg	0
6–16 years	1.0 mg	0.50 mg	0

*2.2 mg sodium fluoride (NaF) contains 1 mg fluoride ion; ppm, parts per million; 1.0 ppm, 1 mg/liter.
Data from American Academy of Pediatric Dentistry (AAPD): Guideline on fluoride therapy, clinical guidelines (pp 128–131). Chicago: Author, 2008: Available at http://www.aapd.org/media/Policies_Guidelines/: Accessed August 27, 2010.

4. Includes tablets, lozenges, drops, liquids, and fluoride–vitamin preparations containing sodium fluoride (NaF) (more common) or acidulated phosphate fluoride (APF); tablets are intended to be chewed, swished, and swallowed; drops are used with infants

5. Daily use at home results in caries reduction comparable with water fluoridation; effectiveness is neither enhanced nor reduced when combined with vitamins; increased client compliance may be achieved with combined fluoride–vitamin supplements; difficulties may include incorrect prescription, client or parental compliance, and overprescribing when other sources of fluoride are available, all of which contribute to fluorosis; questionable benefits have been demonstrated in studies, possibly because of study designs and potential effect of strong motivation of dentally aware volunteer study participants to comply with good oral health practices

6. Dietary supplements are not recommended for infants who are breastfed; breast milk contains 0.0004 ppm F

7. Prenatal supplementation with fluoride is not recommended, although it is not harmful to the fetus; even though it crosses the placental barrier and enters the circulation of the fetus, benefits are minor, since mineralization of enamel is not advanced until after birth and primary benefit of fluoride occurs after tooth eruption

8. School-based fluoride supplement programs were initiated when multiple sources of fluoride were not available; programs yielded 30% reduction in dental caries; they were initiated at the earliest grade (kindergarten) for maximum effectiveness and provided topical and systemic benefits; they were cost effective and efficient but required parental consent and ongoing cooperation of highly motivated administrators, teachers, parents, and others; because of increased water fluoridation and other sources of fluoride, these programs are no longer emphasized in public health

C. Sodium fluoride varnish is recommended by the ADA, the Canadian Dental Association (CDA), and the CDC for use in preschool-age children; recommended as a public health program through Head Start programs and preschools as well as through well-baby clinics in local health departments

1. Studies have demonstrated 45% percent reduction in caries with public health varnish programs

2. Advantages of public health fluoride varnish programs (Box 20-6)

3. Child positioning is key to public health varnish programs[29]

   a. Infants are held by parents in their laps, with the child's head on the parent's knees and the child's legs around the parent's waist, and the operator is knee to knee with the parent, treating the infant from behind; an alternate is to

BOX 20-6 Advantages of Public Health Fluoride Varnish Programs

- No special dental equipment required
- Professional dental cleaning not required before application
- Ease of application
- Dries immediately on contact with saliva
- Safety
- Well tolerated by all; especially convenient for use on infants, young children, and individuals with special needs
- Inexpensive
- Minimal training required for placement; non-dental personnel can be trained
- Allows the ability to eat or drink immediately after application
- Prevents and reverses decay
- Shows caries reduction up to 45% compared with 30%–35% for other fluoride systems

Data adapted from Texas Department of State Health Services: Happy Child, Bright Smile Fluoride Varnish Manual, Publication #E08-13077, December 2009: Available at http://www.dshs. state.tx.us/dental/default.shtm: Accessed September 23, 2010.

place the infant on an examination table and work from behind

b. Young children are seated in small school chairs and the operator is seated directly facing the child, tilting the child's head back for good visualization; alternative positions are the child standing in front of the seated operator or the operator standing behind the seated small child and working from above

4. The varnish should be re-applied every 3 months in high-risk children and every 6 months in moderate-risk children

5. Inclusion of an educational component is critical

D. School water fluoridation
1. Once recommended in areas with suboptimal fluoride, particularly rural areas where community water fluoridation was impossible because of absence of community water supplies; no longer recommended by the CDC because of increased community water fluoridation, availability of other sources of fluoride, and disadvantages of this method
2. This reduced caries among schoolchildren by approximately 40%; more recent studies have indicated that the effect was not as significant as a result of multiple sources of fluoride ingested; the extent of current practice is unknown
3. School water is fluoridated at 4.5 times the optimum concentration recommended for the

community in which the school is located; the increase is to compensate for children drinking fluoridated water only when school is in session
4. Disadvantages—children do not receive benefits until they begin school; exposure occurs only during the school year and school days, not during weekends, breaks, and summer vacation; benefits only schoolchildren; equipment for these small water systems have logistical problems and greater risk of spills

E. Fluoridated salt
1. Addition of fluoride to table salt is a feasible way to deliver systemic fluoride (with topical benefits also), particularly in countries lacking widespread municipal water systems; studies indicate 250 ppm is a suitable concentration
2. Reduction in caries parallels rates found with water fluoridation
3. The World Health Organization (WHO) criteria for salt fluoridation include the inability to implement water fluoridation, low levels of fluoride in the diet and environment, lack of political will to introduce water fluoridation, centralized salt production, and appropriate package labeling
4. Disadvantages—a fixed concentration may not be appropriate for all persons; difficult to use in areas where naturally occurring fluoride concentrations vary; salt's role in aggravating hypertension is suspected, although no evidence exists to support this concern
5. Sold in Switzerland and France, and a few countries in Central and South America; never used in the United States or Canada; not appropriate because of extent of water fluoridation

F. Fluoridated milk
1. The addition of fluoride to milk consumed in schools has been studied in several countries; outcomes have shown protection from caries comparable with water fluoridation at the same concentration; however, milk is not an ideal vehicle for fluoride delivery
2. Disadvantages—only provides a single fluoride exposure on school days, requires refrigeration, milk consumption declines with increasing age of child, and inability to control dairy production
3. Not used in the United States and Canada; not appropriate because of extent of water fluoridation

G. Professionally applied topical fluoride (see the sections on "Topical fluorides and fluoride varnishes" in Chapter 13 and "Fluorides" in Chapter 16)
1. Professional application of topical fluoride is least cost effective as a public health measure;

low concentration and frequent use of fluoride, as with fluoridated dentifrices, is more effective

2. NaF, stannous fluoride (SnF$_2$), and APF in gel, foam, and mouthrinse forms are no longer recommended as a population-based strategy, although they may be indicated in high-risk populations in targeted programs such as institutions for high-risk, special-needs groups

H. Fluoride mouthrinses in school-based public programs

1. Widely used at one time as a public health measure in both fluoridated and nonfluoridated communities; studies indicated a 20% to 35% reduction in caries; not cost effective in combination with systemic fluoride; most common compound was NaF in a 0.2% concentration for weekly rinsing or a 0.05% concentration for daily use

2. Although highly successful, their use is limited today because of expansion of water fluoridation, availability of other sources of fluoride, dependence on teachers and school nurses to administer the program, and level of parental compliance required

3. Current over-the-counter mouthrinses have the same concentration as the daily school-based rinse; they are useful as a targeted approach to reduce caries in people who have xerostomia and have moderate to high risk for caries

I. Fluoride dentifrices

1. Fluoride dentifrices are the most important fluoride vehicle on a global scale; they provide 15% to 30% reduction in children over a 3-year period without water fluoridation; they add to the effectiveness of water fluoridation and other sources of fluoride

2. Their use is institutionalized in the United States, Canada, and other developed countries, accounting for over 90% of the market; distribution as a public health measure is unnecessary in the developed countries but has value in the developing countries where the population does not have access to fluoride dentifrices

3. Higher concentration fluoride dentifrices are recommended for people with high risk for caries

J. Other chemical therapies

1. Xylitol

a. Used in food and snack items as a noncariogenic sweetener; because of its evidence-informed anticariogenic and cariostatic properties; also used to control dental caries in people with moderate or higher risk for caries

b. Studies have shown that xylitol reduces growth of *S. mutans*, new caries formation, the incidence of tooth decay, and caries risk

by destroying the bacteria and reducing the quantity of bacterial plaque, making plaque biofilm less adhesive, stimulating saliva, and raising the pH, thus allowing the enamel surface to remineralize

c. Some studies have shown it to be superior to other chemical therapies to interrupt the vertical transmission of dental caries from parent or caregiver to infants and the horizontal transmission among siblings;[30] maternal consumption of 5 to 9 g of xylitol per day (e.g., chewing xylitol gum three to five times per day) for the first 2 years of a child's life has been shown to reduce *S. mutans* colonization and hence reduce the incidence of childhood caries in the child 6 years later;[27] pregnant women infected by *S. mutans* are encouraged to begin use of xylitol during the last months of pregnancy and the first 3 months postpartum[30]

d. Therapeutic doses of xylitol gum, lozenges, or mints contain 1.55 g of xylitol used four or five times daily throughout the day

e. Should be used in combination with topical fluorides

2. Chlorhexidine gluconate

a. Effective against *S. mutans*

b. Recommended for individuals who are at high or extreme risk for caries[27]

c. 0.12% chlorhexidine gluconate rinsed for 1 minute daily for 1 week each month[31]

d. Loses effectiveness in the presence of lauryl sulfate or fluoride; should be used about 30 minutes after toothbrushing with dentifrices that contain either compound[30]

3. Iodine

a. Limited research has shown a potential for in-office one-time swabbing with 10% povidone-iodine to control ECC in young children[27]

b. Not recommended for home use

4. Amorphous calcium phosphate (ACP)—also known by the name *Novamin*

a. Calcium and phosphate ions in ACP will seek out areas of demineralization and enhance enamel remineralization, occlude dentinal tubules, increase fluoride uptake, and prevent caries progression[30]

b. Recommended for use by individuals who are at high risk for caries or who experience sensitivity

c. Should be used in combination with fluoride

d. Contained in dentifrices and sensitivity relief products as well as professional use products such as polishing paste and sealants

5. Casein phosphopeptides–amorphous calcium phosphate (CPP–ACP)—also known by the name *Recaldent*
  a. Enhances the effects of fluorides and provides a supersaturated environment of calcium and phosphate for remineralization; not a substitute for fluoride therapy[30]
  b. Recommended for use by individuals who are at high risk for caries or who experience sensitivity
  c. Studies suggest long-term caries prevention effects[32]
  d. Contained in chewing gum and pastes for professional application
6. Sodium bicarbonate
  a. Neutralizes acids produced by acidogenic bacteria and has antibacterial properties[30]
  b. Recommended for individuals with xerostomia
  c. Contained in chewing gum and dentifrice; can be rinsed by mixing two teaspoons baking soda with 8 ounces of water[27]
  d. Aggressive use of fluoride dentifrice, mouthrinse, and in-office treatments should be continued
K. Dental sealant programs[33] (see the sections on "Pit-and-fissure sealants" in Chapter 13 and "Dental sealants" in Chapter 16)
  1. Sealants recommended for all children and teenagers living in fluoridated and nonfluoridated communities; differences in percentage of effectiveness, retention, and caries incidence not apparent between studies in fluoridated versus nonfluoridated communities; however, slightly greater benefit for sealants has been found in fluoridated communities
  2. Sealant and fluoride programs are the most beneficial community-based dental disease–prevention programs; efficacy and effectiveness are well recognized; critical component of disease-prevention programs
  3. Especially targeted at schools with high rates of children from low SES groups who are at high risk of dental caries, as determined by the percentage of students eligible for free or subsidized lunch programs; limited resources require that sealant programs use criteria that include risk of dental caries, availability of care, grade level of the targeted group (e.g., second and sixth grades), and teeth with deep pits and fissures; sealants should be placed within 6 months of eruption of first and second molars; education of the targeted community is critical
  4. The cost-effectiveness of community-based sealant programs is a result of the pattern of

dental caries; 90% of dental caries in school children occurs in pits and fissures
  5. Use of fluorides in conjunction with sealants is recommended so that both smooth surfaces and pit-and-fissure surfaces benefit
  6. Retention rates are comparable, whoever applies sealant; key for retention is a competent operator; cost-effectiveness depends on the use of non-dentists to place sealants
  7. Most third-party payers cover sealants
  8. Sealant program settings may include schools, clinics, and day-care facilities; a team approach is necessary for screening and treatment, including necessary support and cooperation from school administrators, teachers, parents, caregivers, and volunteers
  9. Based on epidemiologic evidence, sealant programs are justified for children and young adults, but not other age groups
  10. An educational component is critical
L. Caries management by risk assessment (CAMBRA)[27,30,31,34,35]
  1. The process of dealing with dental caries as an infectious disease by risk assessment and planned intervention or treatment (caries risk management) on that risk
    a. Risk is based on the balance of pathologic factors (bacteria, high-sucrose diet, absence of saliva) and protective factors (salivary components of calcium, phosphate, salivary antibacterial agents, enzymes, acid buffers, and protective proteins; sealants, fluoride, effective diet
    b. Caries risk assessment involves a quantitative measurement of the pathologic and protective components and a professional judgment of their balance; client intake and interviewing provides information about caregiver SES, dental home, developmental problems, recent restorations, parental caries experience, amount and frequency of fermentable carbohydrate intake, use of fluorides and other chemical therapies, and presence of saliva-reducing factors, for example, medications; clinical examination reveals presence of active carious lesions, white spots or decalcification, plaque biofilm, and xerostomia; salivary testing provides quantitative analysis of the stimulated salivary flow rate and bacterial loading for *S. mutans* and lactobacilli
  2. Three risk levels exist; treatment and intervention are based on the level of risk; the level is determined by professional judgment of the balance of pathologic and protective factors; parent or caregiver of a child belonging to a low SES group automatically results in high risk;

current or recent caries experience places any age individual at a high risk level; xerostomia or special needs automatically places an individual at extreme risk

a. Health and low risk—oral hygiene instruction, dietary counseling, twice-daily fluoridated dentifrice (1000 ppm) for over age 6 years; use of xylitol gum or mints and use of fluoride varnish for root exposure or sensitivity are optional for those over age 6 years

b. Moderate risk—everything recommended for the low-risk individual with the addition of fluoridated dentifrice for children under age 6 years, addition of 0.05% NaF rinse daily for over age 6 years, and addition of professional fluoride application for both age groups; use of xylitol gum or mints added for over age 6 years

c. High risk—everything recommended for moderate risk plus use of chlorhexidine and more frequent professional fluoride applications; addition of paste that combines calcium phosphate with fluoride for under age 6 years; increase in concentration of fluoride in dentifrice for over age 6 years

d. Extreme risk (high risk plus xerostomia or special needs)—everything recommended for the moderate- to high-risk individual plus the use of a baking soda product (rinse, gum, dentifrice) to neutralize acid immediately after a snack and the use of a dentifrice that delivers calcium and phosphate combined with fluoride for adults

e. Cavitated lesions are restored with appropriate restorative material using minimally invasive procedures; noncavitated lesions are managed with chemical rather than surgical treatment to reduce pathogens, inhibit demineralization, and enhance remineralization and are monitored closely with short recall intervals

f. Sealants are recommended for individuals at moderate or higher risk level

g. Frequency of recall caries examinations and bitewing radiographs increases as risk level increases

h. Salivary testing is optional for low-risk and moderate-risk individuals to establish baseline and is recommended at every recall caries examination for high-risk and extreme-risk individuals

Measures for Preventing and Controlling Periodontal Disease

A. No parallel to water fluoridation exists for the prevention of periodontal disease

B. A combination of meticulous self-care by individuals on a regular basis, elimination of negative behaviors such as smoking, control of systemic diseases, and periodic periodontal maintenance therapy leads to improved gingival health, decreased attachment loss, and maintenance of natural dentition

1. Various mechanical and chemical interventions prevent and control periodontal diseases

2. Gingivitis is controllable with mechanical oral prophylaxis and instruction in oral hygiene to reduce or disrupt dental plaque biofilm

3. Personal oral hygiene practices such as regular toothbrushing and interdental cleaning can be supplemented by over-the-counter and prescription antimicrobial mouthrinses

4. Tobacco cessation aids in periodontal disease prevention, control, and progression

5. Educational strategies to inform persons about the relationship of systemic diseases (diabetes, heart disease, stroke, osteoporosis, stress, respiratory disease) and pregnancy to periodontal health

C. Community activities should include:

1. Public education to increase health literacy, e.g., personal oral hygiene and regular professional oral care

2. Support of funding for and promotion of population-based research

3. Tobacco cessation programs

Measures for Preventing and Controlling Other Oral Diseases and Anomalies

A. Oropharyngeal cancers

1. On average, 3000 children and teenagers become regular smokers each day; rise in the prevalence of hookah smoking

a. School-based prevention programs are important; Medicaid and some health insurance coverage for tobacco dependence therapy

b. Focus on restricting social influences and environments that lead to smoking

2. A primary prevention technique for cancer does not exist; avoiding known risk factors such as alcohol and tobacco is recommended; decline of cigarette use in the United States has been reported; however, the use of "spit" tobacco and hookahs has increased

3. Secondary prevention or control consists of early detection (screening) and treatment; also oral health education

4. Recommendations for education of students—for example, programs and information from the CDC and the American Dental Hygienists'

Association (ADHA) Smoking Cessation Initiative Project:

a. Develop and enforce a school policy on tobacco use prevention, control, and cessation

b. Provide instruction on the short-term and long-term negative physiologic and social influences of tobacco, peer norms regarding tobacco use, and refusal skills

c. Provide tobacco-use prevention education in kindergarten through twelfth grade; this instruction should begin as early as fifth grade, be especially intensive in middle school, and reinforced in high school

d. Provide program-specific training and dialog scripts to teachers and school nurses

e. Involve parents and families in support of school-based programs to prevent tobacco use

f. Support cessation efforts among students and all school staff who use tobacco; involve other associations and organizations such as parent–teacher associations (PTAs), American Association of Retired Persons (AARP), employers, and health insurers

g. Evaluate outcomes of tobacco-use prevention program at regular intervals

5. Other recommended strategies:

a. Prevent and reduce use of "spit" tobacco (e.g., focus on little league teams)

b. Emphasize health warnings on posters, brochures, Web sites, products, and public service announcements that warn of hazards

c. Promote regular visits to the professional oral health care provider for examination and for advice and assistance with quitting tobacco use

d. Mass screening for oral cancers is costly; professionals should include oral cancer examinations as part of their assessment, teach self-examination techniques to clients, and provide tobacco cessation counseling; no progress was made during the past decade on related *Healthy People 2010* objectives

e. Provide public education regarding signs and symptoms of oral cancer; promote regular self-examination

f. Promote use of QUIT lines such as Take Control 1-800-QUIT-NOW (http://www.quitline.com/), which includes multicultural and multi-language advice

g. Promote use of online smoking cessation assistance, for example, www.quitnet.com, www.smokefree.gov, www.smoking-cessation.org/, www.cdc.gov/tobacco/quit_smoking/how_to_quit/index.htm, and www.cancer.org/

Healthy/StayAwayfromTobacco/Guideto QuittingSmoking/index

h. Support population-based research efforts and lobbying strategies

i. Additional information on tobacco cessation is available from the ADHA's Smoking Cessation Initiative at www.askadviserefer.org

B. Craniofacial birth defects

1. Include cleft palate and cleft lip syndromes

2. Public health programs should emphasize awareness of risk and protective factors during pregnancy

a. Prenatal care

b. Good nutrition

c. Cessation of tobacco use

d. Cessation of alcohol use

e. Cessation of all forms of drug abuse

f. Knowledge about the effects of teratogenic prescription drugs (e.g., drugs used to treat acne)

C. Facial injury or trauma (see the section on "Mouth protectors [athletic mouthguards])" in Chapter 13)

1. Oral health education that focuses on preventive behaviors

2. Increased public attention to the importance of head and facial protection, including headgear and athletic mouth protectors, during contact-sports activities, with special emphasis on the education of parents and coaches; safety restraints in automobiles, and helmets for bicycling, skateboarding, roller blading, and motorcycle use

3. Increased safety measures to prevent injuries from falls in the home, including good lighting, nonskid flooring materials, and handrails

COMMUNITY PROGRAMMING

A. Steps of dental hygiene process of care are followed in community programming in a circular approach to continually improve programs

1. Assessment

2. Problem identification

3. Planning

4. Implementation

5. Evaluation

B. Community groups vary

1. Programming principles can be applied to all groups and types of programs, regardless of size or diversity of community

2. Factors to consider—current health care system, resources, funding, geography, sociocultural background, SES, cultural and political climates, and oral health knowledge and literacy

B. Community programming uses various strategies[5,36]
  1. Surveillance—an ongoing systematic collection, analysis, and interpretation of outcome-specific data for use in the planning, implementation, and evaluation of public health practice
  2. State oral health programs engage in surveys, needs assessment, and surveillance efforts
    a. Survey—a snapshot estimate of the defined population at a point in time
    b. Needs assessment identifies:
      (1) Extent and types of existing and potential problems in a community
      (2) Current system of services available
      (3) Extent of unmet needs and under-utilized resources
    c. Surveillance systems
      (1) Provide information necessary for public health decision making
      (2) Collect data on health outcomes, risk factors, and intervention strategies for the whole population, segment of the population, or representative sample
      (3) May link current databases and address identified data gaps
      (4) Identify public health issues requiring immediate action
      (5) Measure and monitor trends in the burden of disease
      (6) Guide planning, implementation, and evaluation of programs
      (7) May influence public policy, allocation of funds
      (8) Important qualities of a surveillance system include simplicity, flexibility, data quality, representativeness, and timeliness
C. Dental hygienists' roles in community health planning and practice
  1. Program planner or initiator
  2. Consultant and resource person
  3. Service provider
  4. Administrator, manager of a particular program or division, or both
  5. Researcher and data collector
  6. Educator and oral health promoter
  7. Consumer advocate
  8. Politician
D. Community oral health programming framework (education, financing, and evaluation are ongoing through the entire process)
  1. Identify target population
  2. Assess the target population
  3. Collect, organize, and analyze data
  4. Determine priorities
  5. Develop a program plan

  6. Implement the plan
  7. Evaluate the program

Assessment and Problem Identification

A. Definition—multi-faceted, organized, and systematic approach to identify a target group and define the extent and severity of the oral health care needs that are present
  1. Target group—group of individuals who are the focus of a particular oral health care service or program
    a. Health professional may identify the target group
    b. Target group with a defined need may contact health care professionals
  2. Community-oriented primary care (COPC) philosophy of health planning, where community identifies its perceived needs and assigns priorities
B. Data collection
  1. Important to complete before planning
    a. Identify ongoing oral health programs, services, or projects
    b. Assess oral health status and needs; use primary or secondary data
    c. Develop a community profile of the area where the target population is located
  2. Identify ongoing types of programs or projects
    a. Purpose: provision of oral health services, education, disease prevention, research, or combination
    b. Community individuals and groups responsible for programs and success
    c. Locations or facilities where oral health care activities can occur
    d. Individuals, special equipment (e.g., mobile vans or portable equipment), facilities, coalitions, funding opportunities, and other resources to meet the oral health care needs of the target population
  3. Assess current oral health status and needs
    a. Three methods for documenting oral health status and needs:
      (1) Identify and use an assessment method to obtain specific data related to the proposed project or program
      (2) Coordinate assessment with an agency or group such as an academic center or community-based agency that is seeking similar data about the target population
      (3) Research and collect secondary data from records of state or local health care agencies, dental or medical programs, and public health or related agencies

b. Assessment methods
  (1) Baseline data—data collected before program implementation; used for planning and evaluating a program; also known as *pretest data*
  (2) Used to identify the extent and severity of need and in determining project aims and objectives; influenced by the type of information needed
  (3) Assessment methods can be used in combination with each other
4. Various assessment methods can be used (Table 20-8)
  a. Types of data collected for assessment
    (1) Primary data—use various techniques for data collection (e.g., questionnaire, interview, direct observation, indices, records, and documents)
    (2) Secondary data—collected by federal or state agencies, public policy organizations or other sources, for example, Census Bureau, Gallup polls, Oral Health America
  b. Surveys—used to assess knowledge, oral health status, oral health behavior, interests, values, and attitudes; can be done by use of questionnaire or interview
  c. Oral health surveys—used to collect information about oral health, disease status, and treatment needs for planning or monitoring oral health care needs
    (1) Clinical examination or review of dental records
    (2) Existing survey data available for comparisons of comparable groups and geographic regions
      (a) National data from federal agencies responsible for monitoring health and oral health status, for example, CDC and NOHSS
      (b) State-level data available from the CDC through the Behavioral Risk Factor Surveillance System (BRFSS) and Youth Behavior Risk Surveillance System (YBRSS)
    (3) Special considerations for planning oral health surveys because of characteristics of the primary diseases studied: dental caries and periodontal diseases
      (a) Disease is age related
      (b) A significant percentage of the population is affected
      (c) Dental caries and loss of clinical attachment are irreversible; thus, data on current status include the amount of disease present and of previous disease

(d) Trends in disease prevalence exist
(e) Common oral diseases exist in all populations; high prevalence in underserved and minority populations
(f) Extensive documentation on variation of profiles of dental caries and periodontal diseases exists for populations with different socioeconomic levels, health insurance status, and environmental conditions
(g) Many observations have been made in standard measurements for each subject
(4) Surveying requires planning, calibration of examiners, and possibly pilot testing if a large survey is conducted before implementation
(5) The ASTDD and the WHO are resources for guidelines for conducting and reporting an oral health survey
(6) Four types of examinations and inspections are used in oral health surveys to measure dental caries:
  (a) Type I—complete examination using a mouth mirror and explorer, adequate illumination, thorough radiographic survey, and, when indicated, percussion, pulp vitality tests, transillumination, study models, and laboratory tests; because of time, expense, and personnel required, seldom used in public health
  (b) Type II—limited examination using a mouth mirror, explorer, adequate illumination, and posterior bitewing radiographs (when indicated, periapical radiographs); useful when program may include dental treatment for individuals; helpful where time and money permit
  (c) Type III—inspection using a mouth mirror, explorer, and adequate illumination; used in the BSS
    [1] Advantages—basis for oral health instruction, opportunity for establishing rapport and planning motivational strategy, provides baseline information on dental needs of target group
    [2] Disadvantages—inspection may be erroneously relied on as an examination and need for complete assessment overlooked; of no value unless follow-up occurs; parents or guardians not present

TABLE 20-8 Some Data Collection Methods and Applications

Data Collection Methodology	Instrument	Indications	Advantages	Limitations
Direct observation of events, objects, people	Checklist, content analysis, evaluation forms, camera, tape recorder, videotape, thermometer, sphygmomanometer, rating and ranking scales	1. Used when subject recall may affect accuracy of data collection 2. Used to study behavior 3. Used to study psychomotor activity 4. Used in experimental research	1. Observations can be made as they occur in the "natural" setting 2. Observations can be made of behaviors that might not be reported by respondents	1. Time consuming 2. Difficulty in recording 3. Factors that may interfere with the situation 4. Difficulty in quantification of observations 5. Expensive 6. Observer–respondent interaction
Interview; face-to-face or telephone survey	Interview guide (interview schedule)	1. Used for obtaining information on attitudes, beliefs, and opinions 2. Used in a survey 3. Used to gain information on past or present events 4. Face-to-face method can be used for focus groups or one-on-one	1. Flexibility 2. Questions can be clarified and explained 3. Complete data can be collected 4. Subjects do not have to read or write	1. Respondents may be inhibited to respond accurately and truthfully 2. Time consuming 3. Expensive 4. Interviewer may affect the responses 5. Language barriers
Question-based survey—written or oral	Questionnaire, opinionnaire, email source; asking questions to seek specific information	1. Used for obtaining information on attitudes, beliefs, and opinions 2. May be used to gain information on present conditions and past events 3. Used to obtain information about existing status 4. Used in planning	1. Ease of administration 2. Relatively inexpensive 3. Standardization of instructions and questions 4. Economy of time 5. Data can be gathered from a wide geographic area 6. Data can be gathered to reflect public opinion 7. Vast amount of data can be collected 8. Cross-sectional, generalized statistics can be obtained	1. Misinterpretation of questions by respondents 2. If written, low return may bias results 3. Superficiality of responses 4. Incomplete data collection 5. Honesty of respondent 6. Control of extraneous variables is lacking
Epidemiologic survey, screening survey	Dental indices	1. Used to study disease patterns in a population 2. Used to evaluate the effectiveness of therapeutic or preventive treatments in a specific geographic area	1. Vast amount of data can be collected 2. Cross-sectional, generalized statistics can be obtained 3. Data are quantifiable 4. Provides actual measure of health status	1. Difficulty in determining causation because of complexity of variables 2. Time consuming 3. Expensive; requires trained and calibrated examiners
Records, documents	Reports of legislative bodies and state or city officials, deeds, wills, appointment records, dental charts, report cards	Used to study past events	1. Unbiased in terms of the investigator 2. Inexpensive 3. No subject–investigator interaction 4. Convenience and economy of time	1. Incomplete records 2. Accuracy of records may be unknown

Modified from Geurink, KV: Community oral health practice for the dental hygienist, ed 3, St Louis, 2012, Saunders.

to observe outcomes if inspection occurs in school

(d) Type IV—screening with a tongue depressor and available illumination; identifies glaring needs for assessment in program planning; type III and IV are the most common methods used in dental public health and in the developing countries

C. Development of a community profile

1. Community profile—provides information essential in planning a community health program; the rationale is to understand the environment in which the target population is located

2. Size, location, and type of community dictate the type, amount, and comprehensiveness of information necessary for a community profile

3. General areas for inclusion can consist of:

a. Community overview

(1) Number of individuals in the population

(2) Population distribution by income, age, education, employment rate, health and dental insurance rates, public assistance, percentage of population on Medicare, Medicaid, or CHIP

(3) Geographic location and boundaries

(4) Population setting and density (urban or rural); standard of living; homelessness

(5) Ethnic background, cultural heritages, languages, customs, behaviors, beliefs

(6) Diet, nutritional levels, nutrition programs

(7) Amount, types, and influence of public services and utilities

(8) Transportation schedules, routes, fares, reliability

(9) Informed consent procedures and confidentiality of health records

(10) Distribution of public and private schools and religious or faith-based organizations

(11) Extent and type of community fluoride and sealant programs; fluoridation history

(12) State and local statutes, public health codes, and related administrative rules and regulations

b. Community leadership and organization; political atmosphere (health care being a right versus a privilege)

(1) Community, financial, and religious leaders, liaisons, and councils and their attitudes toward oral health, acquired through interviews or surveys

(2) Community power base for policy formulation

(3) Governance structure (e.g., health council, city government, advisory board, school board, union); political environment

(4) Grassroots individuals with political influence

(5) Educational institutions providing professional education, resources, and support

c. Financing and funding of health services

(1) Local and state budget allocation procedures for oral health care programs

(2) Mechanism for requesting the necessary funding; the importance of the need for collaborative partners to successfully obtain funding must be determined

(3) Funding sources (e.g., federal, state, or local funding; individual or third-party payment; private funds, foundations, grants, or endowments)

d. Facilities, resources, and person power

(1) Location of space and facilities in the community or institution; U.S. Department of Labor Occupational Safety and Health Administration (OSHA) standard compliance

(2) Availability and adequacy of equipment

(3) Location of medical and health science centers, clinics, community health centers, and dental laboratories; ease of access

(4) Number of licensed practicing dentists, dental hygienists, dental assistants, laboratory technicians, medical personnel, or others experienced in working with target population

(5) Consortia of health professionals, facilities, and resources (collaboration is important)

(6) Barriers that limit access to oral health care, for example, cost, transportation, and so on

D. Analysis of data

1. Analysis includes organizing, tabulating, and interpreting data

2. Data analysis can range from simple to complex

a. Planner alone tabulates

b. Statisticians, oral and social epidemiologists, and statistical tests are used

c. Computers and other technologies are used

d. Inclusion of qualitative observations and perceptions (e.g., perceptions of need for oral health care services)

e. Economic analysis including cost–benefit ratio

3. Following analysis, needs and priorities can be identified
   a. Target group input is solicited; for example, focus groups
   b. Community representatives, partners, and advisory groups consulted
      (1) Provides an opportunity for dialogue and support
      (2) May include consumers, political, religious, and financial leaders, and health care professionals
   c. Scheduling input
      (1) Meetings with formal or informal input
      (2) Dissemination (by email, Web site, facsimile, or mail) requesting input
      (3) Focus groups
      (4) Internet discussion group
   d. Population groups identified with high-risk oral needs should be included in the community assessment
      (1) Preschool and school-age children
      (2) Intellectually, developmentally, and physically challenged persons
      (3) Chronically ill and medically compromised persons
      (4) Older adults
      (5) Pregnant women and infants
      (6) Low-income and minority groups
      (7) Residents of inner-city and rural communities

Program Planning

A. Definition—organized response to reduce or eliminate one or more problems; organized effort that includes the objective of reducing or eliminating one or more problems, performance of one or more activities, and use of resources
B. Elements of a program plan:[37,38]
   1. Identification of program goals and objectives
   2. Strategies and specific activities to meet objectives
      a. Sequence of activities
      b. Individuals responsible for each activity
   3. Resources required
      a. Location and facilities
      b. Equipment and materials
      c. Personnel (employed and volunteer)
      d. Criteria used to determine resources required
         (1) Appropriateness—most suitable to accomplish tasks
         (2) Adequacy—extent or degree to which the resources would complete tasks
         (3) Effectiveness—how capable or plentiful the resources to complete tasks are

      (4) Efficiency—dollar cost and time expended to complete tasks
   4. Timetables and deadlines clearly outlined, with some flexibility
   5. Projected budget and budget justification
   6. Program promotion and marketing
   7. Identification of Strengths, Weaknesses, Opportunities, and Threats (SWOT analysis)
C. Goals and objectives
   1. For each need prioritized, a goal with related objectives must be determined
      a. Goal—broadly based statement of what changes will occur as a result of the program; provides direction
      b. Objectives—specific statements that describe, in a measurable manner, the desired outcomes from program activities
      c. SMART formula for developing objectives
         (1) Specific: Clearly states the objectives
         (2) Measurable: Objectives can be evaluated
         (3) Appropriate: Taking the identified needs of target population into consideration
         (4) Realistic or Related: Objectives that are achievable and related to anticipated outcomes
         (5) Time bound: Establishment of a timeline
   2. Categories of goals and objectives
      a. Ultimate or long-term
      b. Intermediate
      c. Short-term or immediate (*Note*: Most activities may deal with immediate goals, but intermediate and long-term goals must also be considered)
   3. Immediate objectives are stated in specific, measurable terms; factors considered:
      a. What—identify the condition or situation to be attained
      b. Extent—scope and magnitude of situation or condition to be attained
      c. Who—target group or portion of the community in which attainment is desired
      d. Where—geographic area or physical boundaries of the program
      e. When—time "at or by" which the desired situation or condition is to exist
D. Activities
   1. Program activities—the dynamic, energy-using procedures carried out to achieve program objectives; might be preventive, educational, treatment oriented, or research oriented
   2. To meet objectives, personnel, location, equipment, materials, resources, and costs are determined
E. Promotion or marketing of program
   1. Necessary for participation, recognition, and success of project

2. Promotion techniques—an advisory committee composed of stakeholders (those who have a stake in the outcome of the program) and key leaders from the community, liaison groups, mass media (television and radio), printed media, banners, billboards, Web-based and special-interest publications and programs; smaller programs may use posters, flyers, invitations, newsletter announcements, and email

F. Implementation
   1. Operationalizing the plan
   2. Monitoring plan for activities, personnel, equipment, resources, and supplies
   3. Feedback mechanism from personnel and participants
   4. Ongoing evaluation mechanisms

G. Evaluation plan—the evaluation plan should be in place to ensure its successful implementation throughout and on completion of the program

IMPLEMENTATION

Health Education and Health Promotion

Also see the sections on "Oral health education" and "Prevention-oriented health models" in Chapter 16.

A. Related concepts
   1. Health promotion—any planned combination of strategies designed to facilitate voluntary adaptations of behavior conducive to health; includes educational, political, regulatory, organizational, economic, and environmental (e.g., programs encouraging persons of all ages to stop using tobacco, or product labeling indicating the amount of sugar in a product); changing the lifestyles of people to attain optimal health and to improve the quantity and quality of life
   2. Health education—health information delivered in such a way that people apply it in everyday living; designed to predispose, enable, and reinforce voluntary healthy behaviors in individuals, groups, or communities; a process with intellectual, psychological, and social dimensions relating to activities that increase the abilities of persons to make informed decisions affecting their personal, family, and community well-being; an evidence-influenced process that facilitates learning and behavioral change in both health care personnel and consumers; voluntary adaptations of behavior occur
   3. Health continuum—conceptualization of health status as perceived on a continuous scale from optimal health through illness and death
   4. Prevention—dimension of health education that endows individuals and groups with the

tools and know-how to lead a long and productive life free of disease and disability

5. Theories of health education and health promotion (Table 20-9)
   a. Approaches to health promotion and health education strategies and interventions should be based on sound theories that will result in changes in oral health status of individuals and communities
   b. No single theory applies to all situations; theories can be combined to meet the needs of the situation; multi-dimensional approaches may be more effective for conditions with multiple social, behavioral, and biologic risk factors, like most of the oral health conditions, for example, Stages of Change could be combined with the Health Belief Model to provide the factual information related to the oral health behavior and the Social Cognitive Model to provide motivation and self-efficacy to progress through the stages of behavior change[39]
   c. These theories can help the professional move individuals through the stages of the Learning Ladder (progression of learning): unawareness, awareness, self-interest, involvement, action, and habit
   d. Individual models should be used to design community oral health education programs; community models should be used to develop oral health promotion strategies that may include health education

6. Communication skills are critical to the effective implementation of health promotion and health education programs, regardless of the type of program, community being served, or health education or health promotion model followed (see the section on "Client management with effective communication" in Chapter 15)

7. Health education and health promotion programs must demonstrate cultural sensitivity to meet the needs of varied groups within the population; programs should be adapted to the culture of the target population[40]

8. The health literacy of the target population must be considered for successful outcomes; many groups within the U.S. population have low health literacy, especially groups with lower levels of education[41]

B. Goals of health education
   1. Learning factual information
   2. Providing motivation
   3. Outcomes: behavior change

C. Both direct and indirect processes impact oral health education

TABLE 20-9 Health Education and Promotion Theories

Theory	Key Points	Application Examples	Limitations
Individual Theories			
Health Belief Model (HBM)	Underlying foundation: when individuals have accurate information, they will make better health choices Four health perceptions (beliefs) accepted in order: - Susceptibility to disease - Seriousness of disease - Effectiveness of intervention to control disease - Possibility of overcoming barriers (self-efficacy)	Presentations that provide health information Providing clients with brochures and handouts of health information	Just knowledge is not enough: information is essential but not sufficient Does not provide tools needed for behavior change to occur Behavior change is not so linear
Trans-theoretical Model (Stages of Change)	State of readiness is required to change Follows step-by-step, orderly process of change through predictable stages Precontemplation Contemplation Preparation—think about making change at this stage Action Maintenance—more than 6 months of behavior change Termination—like old behavior never existed at all	Assessing one's state of readiness and position in the stages; then adapting education to the appropriate stage Smoking cessation programs	Behavior change is not so linear Research shows more success in immediate change (early stages) than in long-term change (maintenance and termination stages)
Theory of Reasoned Action	People make rational decisions based on knowledge, values and attitudes (multi-dimensional) Person's intent to change is strongest predictor of action Intentions and behavior are affected by personal behavioral beliefs and normative beliefs (social norms)	Focus on or establishment of social norms for desired oral health behavior: children brushing at school, mom brushing with child, expression of concern for oral health by authority figures Appeal to social acceptability for teens	Does not deal with factual information; focuses only on the emotional aspects and motivation of behavior
Social Cognitive Theory (SCT)	Knowledge, behavior, and environment act in a reciprocal (circular) manner to continually affect each other (multi-dimensional) and increase self-control over personal actions Self-efficacy is belief that personal actions affect outcomes; predicts health status Self-efficacy is acquired through enactive attainment, verbal persuasion, observational learning, behavioral capability, and reinforcements	Using small successes to motivate behavior change Counseling that failure is part of the learning process Using credible role models to tie learning to someone else's experience Providing ongoing counseling Reinforcing behavior Encouraging self-initiated rewards and incentives Personally modeling desired oral health behaviors and outcomes	Not a step by step model; sloppy Self-efficacy varies for different health conditions
Locus of Control (LOC)	Perception of personal control over health status Internal LOC: personal actions determine health status External LOC: others strongly influence health decisions and health status; can negate positive influence of knowledge One's LOC tends to relate to all health issues	Counseling that focuses on individual's personal power over health decisions and health status	Perceptions can be deeply ingrained and emotionally driven

Continued

TABLE 20-9 Health Education and Promotion Theories—cont'd

Theory	Key Points	Application Examples	Limitations
Sense of Coherence (SOC)	The extent to which one has confidence that one's environment is predictable and that things will work out as well as can reasonably be expected Application to health is based on concept that disease is a continuum Stressors and tension (problems) move one along the continuum toward disease Individuals develop resources to reduce or manage stressors to move along the continuum toward health Resources consist of heredity, knowledge, finances, physical resources, friends, family, faith, etc. that help one view problems as manageable (have resources to cope), understandable (make sense), and meaningful (willing to use or spend resources to manage stressors) Higher SOC is associated with better oral health	Helping people identify resources that are available to manage the stressors that relate to their oral health, e.g., dental insurance, source of accurate information, trusted oral health care provider, access to healthy food, belief that oral health is important	Is cognitive, perceptual, and social; does not include a focus on expanding knowledge of factual oral health information
Community Theories			
Community Organization	Represents several theories that describe how community groups are assisted in identifying common problems or goals, mobilizing resources, and implementing strategies to reach the goals they have set collectively Accomplished through empowerment, community competence, participation and relevance, issue selection, and critical consciousness	Application on a small scale to help a school or other community group improve the oral health of the members of that population	Requires time and effort to identify key influencers and involve the members of the community in the assessment, planning, and implementation processes
Diffusion of Innovation	Addresses how new ideas, products, practices, and services spread within a society Diffusion process consists of a spread of planned efforts to make the innovation become routine, taking into account the society's communication channels and social system Strategies are planned that address the characteristics of the innovation: relative advantage, compatibility, complexity, triability, and observability	Adoption of sealants, fluoride varnish, CAMBRA (caries management by risk assessment), and other innovative dental procedures by our society, including the profession	Requires a complex and comprehensive approach
Organizational Change Theory	A wide variety of forces make an organization resistant to change; these forces include how it operates, and its structure, culture and control systems A wide variety of forces also push an organization toward change; these include changing of tasks and the environment of the organization These two sets of forces always oppose each other For an organization to change, it is necessary to find ways to increase the forces for change, decrease the resistance of change, or do both at the same time	Reorganizing the structure of the health system in the nation Reorganizing a community-based clinic to meet the changing needs of the population it serves Reorganizing a professional organization to influence its members in the direction of meeting population needs	Theory relates to the infrastructure of community oral health practice, not to health promotion Requires a complex and comprehensive approach Requires time and effort to change an organization

Data from Hollister MC: Health education and promotion theories. In Harris NO, Garcia-Godoy F, Nathe CN, editors: Primary preventive dentistry, ed 7, Upper Saddle River, NJ, 2009, Pearson; Bray KS, Gluch JI: Health promotion: a basis of practice. In Daniel SJ, Harfst SA, Wilder RS, editors: Mosby's dental hygiene concepts, cases, and competencies, ed 2, St Louis, 2008, Mosby; Oliver HE: Communication and behavioral change theories. In Darby ML, Walsh MM, editors: Dental hygiene theory and practice, ed 3, St Louis, 2010, Saunders.

1. Formal activities include the deliberate provision of oral health education designed to elicit specific health promotion or disease-prevention behaviors, for example, the curricula of elementary and secondary schools, community-focused preventive education events, health professionals conducting in-service workshops and programs, health care agencies providing education and service

2. Informal activities include the indirect acquisition of oral health–related information that may lead to specific health promotion or disease-prevention behaviors; accidental or vicarious learning, for example, the environment and its support of oral health behaviors; policies related to oral health behaviors; interaction with colleagues, family, oral health care professionals, and the oral health care environment; many of these activities are designed as health promotion and impact health education as well

D. Health education and promotion are integral parts of community activities; may be directed to:
1. Health care professionals
2. Elementary, secondary, and college students
3. Educators
4. Special population groups and caregivers
5. Adult and senior citizen groups
6. Institutionalized populations
7. Diverse population groups recently settled in the community

E. Health education topics are not limited to oral hygiene instruction; topics might include
1. Preventive measures, for example, appropriate use of fluorides, xylitol, dental sealants
2. Periodontal disease, malocclusion, oropharyngeal cancers, and risk factors such as tobacco use, diet, systemic diseases, and poor oral self-care behaviors
   a. Assessment, prevention, and treatment
   b. Self-examination techniques
3. Dental safety and dental emergencies (e.g., use of mouth protectors, procedures for avulsed tooth)
4. Roles of various health professionals and their inter-relationships
5. Care of the oral cavity and dental prostheses
6. Careers in dentistry and dental hygiene
7. Becoming a discriminating dental consumer; oral health care products
8. Effects of tobacco use on oral and systemic health
9. Environmental factors affecting oral health (e.g., occupation-related concerns)
10. Prenatal and postnatal oral health issues; parent programs; early childhood caries
11. How to provide oral health care to those unable to care for themselves
12. Oral and systemic disease links
13. *Healthy People 2020* national promotion and disease-prevention topics (see Box 20-1); *Healthy People 2020* Interventions and Resources Web site and ADHA Smoking Cessation Initiative are some of the resources

Methods of Oral Health Education

A. Instructional methods
1. Lecture—informative talk, prepared beforehand and given to a group; useful to introduce new topics, arouse interest in a subject, or review concepts
   a. Advantages
      (1) Can present many facts and ideas in a short period
      (2) Can convey information to large numbers of individuals
      (3) Preparation takes place before presentation
      (4) Allows instructor to determine aims, content, organization, pace, and direction of presentation
      (5) Integrates diverse materials and pulls various ideas and concepts in an orderly fashion; uses media
      (6) Builds on foundation knowledge in subsequent presentations; allows for gradual development of complex or difficult concepts and theories
   b. Disadvantages
      (1) No active participation by the learner; encourages one-way communication; stifles creativity
      (2) Instructor must have effective writing, speaking, and modeling skills; poor presentation technique is a barrier to learning
      (3) Difficult to monitor student learning; requires a considerable amount of unguided student time outside the classroom
2. Lecture-demonstration—informative talk that presents information supplemented by a demonstration to reinforce learning; can be used to introduce information and to demonstrate skills or techniques to supplement information
   a. Advantages
      (1) Illustrates information visually
      (2) Sets forth information in a complete format
      (3) Allows for concentration of attention and economical use of time

(4) Useful for reinforcing material

(5) May use models, computer-generated presentation, slides, videotapes, or other teaching tools; technology may allow larger number of participants to view a demonstration, for example, viewing computer monitors

b. Disadvantages

(1) Difficult for large groups to see a demonstration unless appropriate technology is used

(2) Requires careful preparation for success; requires adequate equipment and facilities

3. Discussion—group activity in which the student and teacher define a problem and seek a solution; an interaction between teachers and students to promote divergent thinking where closure is not expected; promotes understanding and clarification of concepts, ideas, and feelings; includes use of questions by the leader to stimulate interaction

a. Advantages

(1) Allows interaction among participants

(2) Provides two-way communication between the group leader and members

(3) Encourages individuals to contribute to the discussion

(4) Engages participants in problem solving (higher order learning)

(5) Encourages teamwork, tolerance of divergent opinion, and development of interpersonal skills

(6) Assists leader in directing the discussion

(7) Can be focused on both cognitive and affective learning

b. Disadvantages

(1) Strong personalities can influence a group

(2) Poor discussion leader may contribute to failure of the discussion

(3) Nothing may be achieved; discussion may go in many directions without closure

(4) May not be profitable if group members do not have appropriate background

4. Discovery learning—uses a less direct questioning format to prod the learner into using logic or common sense to discover ideas or concepts; useful to build on foundation knowledge and to introduce new concepts

a. Advantages

(1) Requires learner involvement

(2) Requires application of knowledge (higher level learning)

(3) Promotes critical thinking; motivates student to discover the "right answer"; several answers may be plausible

b. Disadvantages

(1) May be interpreted as guessing

(2) Need to guide learner so that correct information is concluded

5. Brainstorming—free sharing of ideas generated by unstructured group interaction; may have a well-defined, clearly stated problem to address; ideas recorded for future discussion but never analyzed for merit during session; useful for group identification of an issue or problem

a. Advantages

(1) Useful for youth and adult groups

(2) Encourages creativity

(3) Encourages application of knowledge

(4) Encourages contribution by all participants with no fear of a "wrong answer"

(5) Encourages people to build on others' ideas

b. Disadvantages

(1) Group dynamic may be influenced by stronger personalities

(2) Needs to be carefully managed so the purpose is not lost

(3) Not useful for actual sharing of information, just for problem identification or issue clarification

6. Web-based resource—uses a computer to present information in a method that can be interactive; includes use of the monitor to present photos, animation, video, print, and sound for lecture-demonstration and cases, discussion groups, online testing, and other online teaching methods

a. Advantages

(1) Provides an alternative medium to present information

(2) Accessible at all times if learner has access to a computer

(3) Can be updated

(4) Provides enhanced printed material

(5) Provides ready access to wealth of resources on the Web

b. Disadvantages

(1) Some older adults and institutionalized persons may not have computer skills or access to appropriate technology

(2) Cost of equipment and linkages

7. Cooperative and collaborative learning activities—occur both inside and outside the classroom or learning environment, for example, group activities and projects

8. Additional options
   a. Field trips; virtual field trips
   b. Panel discussions and debates
   c. Problem-solving assignment
   d. Symposium reporting
   e. Distance learning
   f. Computer simulations and modeling
   g. Library research
   h. Independent study
9. General principles for selection of oral health instructional methods
   a. Oral health education should be focused on education and intervention, stressing skill acquisition and adoption of risk-reducing behaviors (evidence-based)
   b. Oral health education is more successful when characterized by active involvement of participants
   c. A combination of teaching techniques should be used to meet the needs of various learning styles and to keep the interest of the audience

B. Selection of media—vehicles of communication
   1. Major categories
      a. Web sites and links as sources of communication
      b. Written, electronic, and mediated materials used in teaching individuals or groups
      c. Mass media (e.g., television, radio, newspapers)—effective for creating awareness
      d. Distance education technologies (e.g., Internet, computerized instruction, Web-based tutorials, telecommunications, teleconferencing, iPods, discussion boards, etc.)
   2. Criteria for selection of media for instruction
      a. Material presented at an opportune time
      b. Material presented at participants' level of understanding
      c. Size of participant group conducive to the instructional medium chosen
      d. Educational technology available and familiarity with operation
      e. Environment conducive to use of media and technology (e.g., lighting, seating, equipment)
   3. Educational aids
      a. Printed materials (e.g., pamphlets, books)
      b. Photos, overheads, charts, posters, models, puppets, mobiles
      c. Electronic, computer-generated presentations, slides, videotapes, CD-ROMs, DVDs,
      d. Boards—story, flannel, bulletin, magnetic
      e. Science experiments
      f. Computer-generated media
      g. Distance education technologies

4. Mass media—useful to increase awareness
   a. Printed materials
   b. Radio and television (including cable)
   c. Newspaper and magazine
   d. Billboards
   e. Advertisements
5. World Wide Web
   a. Use of Internet for oral health information (see "Web site information and resources" at the end of this chapter and on the textbook Web site)
   b. Scientific accuracy is an issue; Internet can be a source of misinformation
6. General principles for evaluation and selection of media
   a. Specific purpose—arouse interest, provide information, develop attitudes, change behavior
   b. Accuracy and relevancy
   c. Based on scientific principles and rigorous research (evidence-informed)
   d. Target audience—appropriateness, attractiveness, audience appeal, racially inclusive, culturally sensitive
   e. Complexity of information; readability
   f. Physical properties—illustrations, color, continuity, and style

Characteristics of Different Types of Learners

A. Groups of learners share commonalities; all groups are made up of individuals, so care must be taken not to generalize
B. Characteristics of adult learners[42,43]
   1. Goal orientation and relevancy orientation; need to know the reason to learn something
   2. Driven by intrinsic motivation to learn
   3. Interested in the immediacy of its application
   4. Bring knowledge and experience to the learning situation
   5. Come to the learning situation ready to learn
   6. Possibly shy and apprehensive; do not respond as quickly as children do
   7. Used to an authority system and can take direction
   8. Enjoy a fun, warm, friendly and humorous learning environment
   9. Respond well to personal attention, compliments, and reinforcement
   10. Value being treated as equals; are put off if talked down to, embarrassed, or kept waiting
   11. Are social; like to share stories and get to know each other

12. Prefer hands-on, practical, tangible, orderly and predictable activities that include active involvement

13. Need a focus on transference of information (ability to use information in a new setting)

C. Suggestions for oral health education programs for low-literacy learners[42,44]

1. Assess level of knowledge

2. Provide new information, building on and relating to what is already known

3. Have meaningful interactions; ask questions related to responses

4. Provide information via familiar modes; use television, radio, personal experience, demonstration, and oral explanation

5. Provide explicit information that is relevant to current needs

6. Limit the amount of information taught at one time

7. Use basic terminology; maintain a fifth grade level, especially for written materials

D. Characteristics of young children as learners[45]

1. Have undeveloped intrinsic motivation; respond to reinforcement and behavior modification

2. Have limited attention and concentration spans; a variety of activities are required to maintain attention

3. Have undeveloped problem-solving skills

4. Have a weak memory; repetition is required

5. Have limited life and learning experience; tend to accept information being presented at face value

6. Use concrete reasoning; are unable to understand abstract concepts; learning is better with hands-on and visual activities related to the tangible, for example, demonstration and practice

7. Very young children are unable to read and write; lessons must use pictures

8. Have varied interests at different ages, based on their physical and emotional development and life experiences

9. Motivations are current interests and needs (e.g., young children's need for approval by teacher; adolescents' need for peer acceptance)

10. Respond well to oral health education geared to current level of development, for example, tooth eruption, orthodontic treatment

11. Do not possess fine motor coordination skills required for flossing; skill can be introduced

12. Possess a social nature and interest in sharing stories when asked questions

13. Show lack of self-control; classroom management is required to control behavior

Oral Health Education Plan Development

A. Health education plan (lesson plan)—organization of topics and learning experiences so that they relate to a central theme or problem; provides educators with an organized approach to present specific topics and ideas to achieve stated objectives; provides a basic foundation on which teaching and learning can be assessed, planned, implemented, and evaluated; should include an organized plan with objectives, activities, materials required, and evaluation techniques; vital in dynamic teaching for both student and teacher; concept should be used in all oral health education activities to provide conceptual framework for presentations

B. Assessment of needs—learner needs, oral health status, interests, and developmental level; teaching environment; availability of media; resources available to support the lesson; previous oral health learning experiences and current oral health knowledge and behavior

C. Prioritization of the learning needs of the audience to determine the purpose, aim, and rationale of the lesson

D. Planning the lesson

1. Goals—one or two recommended; general, broad statements of direction for the lesson

2. Instructional objectives—statement that describes the intended outcome, aim, or product of instruction; what a successful learner is able to do at the end of instruction; expected behavior; should be precise and measurable; useful for guiding instruction and evaluation; components of an effective, precise instructional objective

a. Performance—what a learner is expected to be able to do or demonstrate when the instructional event ends, using a verb that denotes an observable behavior or action, for example, "The client will demonstrate the modified Bass toothbrushing technique"

b. Conditions—the important conditions (if any) under which the performance is to occur, for example, "Given a soft-bristled toothbrush, the client will demonstrate the modified Bass toothbrushing technique on all tooth surfaces and on the tongue"

c. Criterion—the criterion of acceptable performance; a description of how well the learner must perform to be considered acceptable, for example, "Given a soft-bristled toothbrush, the client will demonstrate the modified Bass toothbrushing technique and remove all clinically visible plaque biofilm, as measured by the Plaque Index"

3. Identifying teaching strategies and learning experiences—should be based on the objectives and on the principles of learning and strategy selection elsewhere in this section
4. Identifying materials and media needed based on criteria elsewhere in this section; identifying resources for materials; allowing preparation time
5. Identifying and arranging for equipment required to present lesson
6. Planning follow-up activities and materials, for example, handouts to send home to parents or caregivers

E. Implementing the lesson
  1. Introduction, main activity or activities, closure or conclusion, and follow-up activities
  2. Considering the learning needs of the audience during presentation
  3. Preparing and practicing beforehand to control anxiety

F. Evaluation of learning outcomes—should relate to objectives and to pretest and assessment procedures to provide basis for comparison

Health Education and Promotion Programs in the School Setting

A. The program should focus on a combination of strategies and efforts to reach parents, students, school personnel, and the community
B. The programs in school settings have the potential to reach significant numbers of participants
C. The school environment supports learning and reinforcement, ideally through an integrated curriculum, not isolated instances
D. The school program should be comprehensive, including efforts directed to improving the environment, providing education, and providing or promoting services (e.g., referrals, school-based sealant and fluoride programs)
E. Teachers can serve as role models
F. Success is enhanced by identifying responsible individual(s) (decision makers); involving parents for reinforcement at home; using community resources and personnel (e.g., agencies, other oral health care professionals); evaluating and revising the program, when appropriate
G. The primary role of the dental hygienist is to be a resource, train teachers, work with the various groups to enhance the overall program, and manage and support the program, not to provide all the classroom instruction

EVALUATION

General Principles

A. Program evaluation is a key element of community oral health programs; should take place at all stages; consists of both formative and summative evaluation
  1. Formative evaluation—ongoing evaluation during the program to assess processes; can lead to revisions to improve program success
  2. Summative evaluation—evaluation of outcomes based on program objectives; provides comparison to needs assessment data to determine success of the program
B. Program evaluation is applied research; research methods are used (see the earlier section on "Epidemiology and research")
C. Points to evaluate
  1. Quality of program and personnel (formative)
  2. Progress and effectiveness of activities—identify problems and solutions to assist in revisions and modifications to meet goals and objectives (formative)
  3. Perceptions, attitudes, and participation of recipients of program (formative)
  4. Systematic and regular evaluation of goals and objectives by using specific measurement instruments; outcome assessment (summative)
  5. Health status indicators of recipients of program (summative)

Use of Statistics[46]

Data
A. Data—numbers collected from measurements or counts
  1. Continuous data—numerical data capable of being any value along a continuum, for example, periodontal probe readings, blood pressure, time, temperature; can be expressed meaningfully as a fraction
  2. Discrete data—numerical variables or data that are counted only in terms of whole numbers, for example, number of clients examined, number of children who had teeth sealed, number of teeth with caries experience
  3. Categorical data—division of data into categories with no numeric representation, for example, SES, ethnic group, gender, school attended, grade in school
  4. Dichotomous data—categorical variable with only two groups, for example, male/female, yes/no, bleeding/no bleeding, pass/fail
B. Scales of measurement—data fall in one of four scales:

1. Nominal scale—observations belong to mutually exclusive classes or categories, for example, Republicans/Democrats; smokers/nonsmokers; normal/abnormal; place of residence
2. Ordinal scale—classes or categories that have ranking of characteristics in some empirical order, for example, class rankings of high school graduates; Likert scales such as strongly disagree, disagree, agree, strongly agree for patient satisfaction and other measures; most dental indices; periodontal classification; Periodontal Screening and Recording (PSR) codes; SES
3. Interval scale—measurement scale characterized by equal intervals along the scale; has no absolute zero, for example, a Fahrenheit thermometer; not useful in oral health research
4. Ratio scale—measurement scale characterized by equal intervals along the scale and the presence of an absolute zero, for example, age, weight, height, DMF, number of sealants, test scores; most dental indices are treated as ratio data

Statistics

A. Statistics—science that describes, summarizes, analyzes, and interprets numerical data for the purpose of making an inference about a population
   1. Statistic—numerical characteristic of a sample derived from the data collected
   2. Parameter—numerical characteristic of a population
B. Descriptive statistics—statistics used to numerically describe and summarize data collected
   1. Measures of central tendency—used to describe what is typical (the mid-point) in the sample group based on the data gathered
      a. Mean ($\bar{x}$)—the arithmetic average; the sum of the values (Σx) divided by the number of items (n)

$$\bar{x} = \sum x/n$$

      (1) Incorporates the value of each score
      (2) Affected by extreme scores
      (3) Interval or ratio statistic
      b. Median—mid-point of a distribution with 50% of the scores falling above it and 50% of the scores falling below it; arrange scores of distribution in either ascending or descending order to locate the mid-point
      (1) When the total number of scores is odd, the median is the middle score
      (2) When the total number of scores is even, take the two middle scores, add them, and divide by 2; median can be a decimal
      (3) Not affected by extreme scores

      (4) Ordinal statistic, for example, first, second, third; can be used with ratio data to avoid effect of extreme scores
      c. Mode—the most frequently occurring score in a distribution
      (1) Distribution may be unimodal, bi-modal, multi-modal, or have no mode
      (2) Nominal statistic
   2. Measures of dispersion—used to describe variability of scores in a distribution
      a. Range—the spread between the highest and the lowest scores in a distribution
      (1) Easily determined
      (2) Somewhat unreliable because it is determined by only two scores of the distribution
      (3) Can be used with ordinal data
      b. Variance—measure of average deviation or spread of scores around the mean; sum of the squared deviations from the mean divided by n; requires ratio data

$$\text{Variance} = \sum (x - \bar{x})^2 / n$$

      c. Standard deviation (SD)—the positive square root of the variance
      (1) The greater the dispersion of scores from the mean of the distribution, the higher is the value of the standard deviation and variance
      (2) Small standard deviation indicates that the distribution of scores is clustered around the mean; a large standard deviation indicates that scores are dispersed widely around the mean
C. Correlation statistics—statistical measure for determining the strength of the linear relationship between two or more variables
   1. Analysis yields a measure called a correlation coefficient (r), ranging from +1.0 to −1.0; the sign indicates the direction of the correlation, and the number indicates the strength of the correlation
   2. Directions of correlations
      a. Positive—value of one variable increases as the value of the second variable also increases, for example, presence of plaque and gingivitis; expressed as a positive number; perfect positive correlation is a +1.0
      b. Negative—inverse relationship between two variables, for example., fluoride exposure and dental caries; expressed as a negative number; perfect negative correlation is a −1.0
   3. Various versions of r exist depending on number of variables and type of data

4. Interpretation of correlation coefficient (r), regardless of direction of relationship
   a. Very high: $r = 0.9$–1.0 (+ or −)
   b. High: $r = 0.70$–0.89 (+ or −)
   c. Moderate: $r = 0.50$–0.69 (+ or −)
   d. Weak: $r = 0.26$–0.49 (+ or −)
   e. Little if any: $r = 0$–0.25 (+ or −)
   f. Some statisticians interpret $r = 0.30$–0.70 (+ or −) as moderate; varies according to the variables and study design

5. Used in analysis of data from analytic studies to determine risk; does not demonstrate causality

D. Summary presentation of descriptive and correlation statistics
   1. Frequency distribution table—table that summarizes the frequencies of data in the distribution; data are entered into a frequency distribution table prior to creating a graph
   2. Bar graph (or bar chart)—two-dimensional diagram used to pictorially display data that are discrete in nature, regardless of scale of measurement; bars do not touch
   3. Histogram—type of bar graph used to represent interval-scaled or ratio-scaled variables that are continuous in nature; bars touch each other
   4. Frequency polygon—line graph used to represent data that are continuous in nature; a histogram and a frequency polygon can be used to represent the same data; frequency polygon can be easier to read when more than one distribution is presented for comparison
   5. Polygon—a line graph that does not represent frequency data, for example, a line graph showing the progression of a Plaque Index score over time in a repeated measures experimental study (this would also be called a *time series graph*)
   6. Pie graph (or pie chart)—used to display parts of a whole
   7. Scattergram (or scatter plot)—a graph in which scores are plotted to show the relationship or association of two variables; visually shows the relationship represented by r
   8. Advantages of tables and graphs are that they provide a neat and organized way to present data, facilitate understanding and analysis of data at a glance, expedite review of data, enable comparisons, and ease recall of data

E. Distributions of data
   1. Normal (bell) curve—symmetrical distribution of scores in which the mean, median, and mode have the same value, and the scores fall within a standard relationship to the mean
      a. 68% of the scores fall between +1 and −1 SD of the mean
      b. 95% of the scores fall between +2 and −2 SD of the mean
      c. 99% of the scores fall between +3 and −3 SD of the mean
   2. Skewed distribution is one in which the distribution is asymmetrical
      a. Positive skew—mean has a higher value than the median and mode; the bulk of the scores are at the lower end of the distribution and the tail of the curve is at the higher end
      b. Negative skew—mean has lower value than the median and mode; the bulk of the scores are at the higher end of the distribution and the tail of the curve is at the lower end

F. Inferential statistics—that branch of statistics used to infer research findings from the sample to the general population from which the sample was taken; used to test hypotheses, generalize results to a larger population of interest, and provide evidence of causality
   1. Parametric statistics—inferential statistical procedures that require the following assumptions about the population parameters:
      a. Data are interval or ratio scaled
      b. Population from which the data are taken is normally distributed (Bell curve)
      c. Sample is large, that is, $n \geq 30$, and randomized
   2. Nonparametric statistics—inferential statistical procedures used when the population parameters do not meet the assumption required for parametric statistics
      a. Data are nominal or ordinal in nature
      b. Population from which the sample is drawn does not have a normal distribution (skewed curve) or distribution is unknown
      c. May or may not be a small sample
      d. Variables are discrete

Statistical Decision Making

A. Statistical decision making—tool used by the researcher to aid in the interpretation of findings; based on statistical results
   1. Statistical decision making is not the sole means by which research findings are interpreted and applied
   2. Clinical significance—practical implications of research that may or may not be inherent in research results; findings may have statistical significance without having clinical significance, for example, the free gingival margin has a statistically significant resorption of 0.1 mm, but the pocket depth is still 0.6 mm

B. Null hypothesis is tested statistically to make the statistical decision
   1. Retaining the null hypothesis is equivalent to the rejection of the research or alternative hypothesis

2. Rejection of the null hypothesis is equivalent to the acceptance of the research or alternative hypothesis
3. Failure to accept the null hypothesis implies accepting the alternative hypothesis

C. Statistical significance—according to the probability established by the level of significance, the obtained result is less likely to be a chance occurrence and more likely the result of the independent variable; does not necessarily mean that data are important, valid, or meaningful (see "Clinical significance" above)

D. Probability level (p value)—researcher's acceptable odds for determining the operation of chance factors in producing the obtained research result; the cut-off point used to reject or accept the null hypothesis; also known as *significance level* and *alpha value*
1. Small p values indicate rare chance occurrences that lead to the rejection of the null hypothesis and provide more confidence that the decision is correct
2. Large p values indicate that chance occurrences are more likely to account for the result and therefore the null hypothesis should be accepted (the alternative hypothesis is rejected)
3. Maximum p value to reject the null hypothesis in oral health research is typically 0.05; p values of 0.01 and 0.001 indicate greater statistical significance
   a. If the probability is <0.05, the results obtained are reported as statistically significant
   b. A probability result of >0.05 (p >0.05) indicates data are not significantly different
   c. Test statistics used to make the statistical decision depend on the size of the sample, the number of samples, the type of data, and other factors, as explained later

E. Because statistical decision making is based on probability (chance), errors may occur
1. Type I error—based on statistical results, the researcher rejects the null hypothesis and concludes that a statistically significant difference exists when, in fact, no true difference is present; rejecting a null hypothesis that is true
2. Type II error—the researcher concludes that no statistically significant difference exists and accepts the null hypothesis when, in fact, a significant difference does exist; accepting a null hypothesis that is false
3. Relationship between two types of testing errors (Figure 20-2)
4. The p value is set to control the acceptable rate of error, which depends on the clinical importance or significance of the question being researched
   a. Type I errors lead to unwarranted change, for example, a client could receive ineffective treatment
   b. Type II errors maintain status quo, for example, a client could miss out on treatment that could have been helpful or even life saving
5. The potential for error is the reason why multiple randomized controlled trials (RCT) are critical for evidence-based decision making

F. Parametric inferential statistics (see "Assumptions" in the previous section)
1. t test—inferential statistical analysis of choice for determining if a statistically significant difference exists between two mean scores
   a. t test for independent samples—data are from two sample groups drawn independently from a population (two independent groups); commonly known as *Student's t test*
   b. t test for dependent samples—data are from two samples that are related (two groups that are matched for relevant variables or pretest and post-test from one group); also known as *t test for correlated samples* and *paired t test*; more sensitive than the t test for independent samples because groups are paired, eliminating a possible source of variance
2. Analysis of variance (ANOVA)—inferential statistic used to analyze the effects of two or more independent variables simultaneously within the same research design and to determine interactions among the variables in multiple sample groups; used to analyze three or more mean scores

FIGURE 20-2 Type I and type II statistical errors.

		Null hypothesis is	
		Accepted	Not accepted
Null hypothesis is actually	True	No error	Type I error ($p = \alpha$)
	Not true	Type II error ($p = \beta$)	No error

a. *F* ratio—value that results when ANOVA is computed
b. Result communicates if a difference exists somewhere among the mean scores; follow-up statistics are used to determine exactly where the difference lies
c. Variations of ANOVA include ANCOVA (analysis of covariance) to control for extraneous variables in the study design and MANOVA (multi-variate analysis of variance) when multiple dependent variables are measured

G. Nonparametric inferential statistics (see "Criteria for their use" in the previous section)
1. Chi-square test (χ^2)—statistical test to determine if a statistically significant difference exists between frequencies of data (versus comparing mean scores as is done with parametrics); used with nominal data from two or more distributions with >5 scores in each one; has different versions for special applications
   a. One version is used with a single distribution of data to determine whether or not a significant difference exists between the observed number of cases within designated categories and the expected number of cases within designated categories according to the hypothesis
   b. Another version is used with two data sets to test the differences in the distributions of data (versus the differences in the mean scores)
   c. Another version is used to test the statistical significance of a correlation coefficient result
2. Other similar nonparametic statistics exist to test differences of data distributions that represent ordinal data, come from groups with <5 in each one, come from more than two groups, or a combination

Evaluating Professional Literature[47]

A. Professional responsibility includes keeping current with new developments for evidence-informed decision making
B. Reviewing the professional literature is important for the contemporary dental hygienist in the roles of clinician, educator, administrator/manager, advocate, and researcher
1. Necessary to review and study the literature before and during community programming
2. Provides an impetus and evidence base for various types of community activities
3. Journal articles, particularly randomized clinical trials, systematic reviews, and meta-analyses, serve as a source of current information for evidence-informed decision making

C. Reviewing the professional literature is a valuable way of continuing education
D. Scientific writing should be comprehensible for the average reader who is knowledgeable about the general area

Criteria for Reviewing the Professional Literature

A. Overall description of the article
1. The title is concise and descriptive
2. The article is found in a reputable, peer-reviewed (refereed) journal
   a. The journal has an editorial review board; articles are peer reviewed prior to publication
   b. The journal is affiliated to a learned society, professional group, specialty group, or reputable scientific publisher
   c. The journal is not a "popular" magazine sponsored by a cause or published by a commercial firm
   d. The articles are concisely written using a scientific style
3. Data published indicate current knowledge and are not outdated by more recent research (5 years is a general guide)

B. The author is qualified to write the article
1. The author has appropriate credentials to have knowledge of the topic
2. The author's current or past position supports expertise in a particular area
3. The researcher has a satisfactory reputation for well-conducted research
4. If the report is of product research, the researcher is not affiliated with a commercial firm

C. Funding of research
1. If the article is reporting research results, evidence of finances and facilities to support the research is present
2. The funding of the research does not represent a conflict of interest

D. References are available for articles
1. References are comprehensive, accurate, and reputable
2. Given the topic, an appropriate number of current references are present, although older references may be indicated for historical purposes or because they are considered classic

E. The research problem is clearly, accurately, and completely described
1. The purposes of the study are clear
2. A thorough review of the literature has been done
3. Important terms and concepts are operationally defined in an adequate manner

4. Hypotheses or objectives are adequate and clearly stated and follow directly from the problem statement

F. Methods are appropriate for the type of study; descriptive, analytic and experimental studies require different methods[48]

   1. The characteristics of the population sampled are described; allocation of groups are outlined if it was a clinical trial

   2. The sampling techniques are described in an adequate manner

   3. No bias in the selection or assignment of objects or persons in the sample is evident

   4. The research design is described; control is indicated for variables that might influence the results; comparability of experimental and control groups is evident; bias is controlled by the design; the limitations of the design are pointed out

   5. Tests and instruments used give reasonable measures of the factors under study

      a. Tests and instruments used are valid and reliable; evidence of reliability is provided

      b. Conditions in which measurements are made are controlled

      c. The reliability of the examiners is controlled and reported

      d. The duration of the study is appropriate

   6. All the factors needed to test the hypotheses or achieve the objectives are included in the analysis

      a. Statistical tests are described; general-purpose computer programs for data analysis are specified

      b. Hypotheses are tested through statistical analysis

   7. Findings are presented in a clear manner

      a. Data tables and figures are clear, easy to understand, and titled

      b. Data are presented in a straightforward manner; authors report statistical method used and the reason for the selection

   8. The discussion highlights significant issues from the research

      a. Results are interpreted

      b. The importance or significance of the findings is clear

      c. The strengths and limitations of the study are explained

      d. Treatment or study complications and adverse effects are reported

      e. Results are related to the current literature

      f. Implications for practice or the profession are discussed

   9. Conclusions are supported by methods and findings

PROVISION OF ORAL HEALTH CARE

Diverse Modes of Dental Practice in the United States

A. Private sector

   1. Solo practice—dental practice which is a single proprietorship by a dentist who may employ dental hygienists, dental assistants, and other appropriate staff

      a. Advantages

         (1) Provider and client flexibility in terms of availability of services

         (2) Inherent economic incentive to be efficient because of investment involved

         (3) The provider can accept or refuse clients within acceptable legal parameters

         (4) The provider determines the practice location, office design, equipment, and personnel composition

         (5) The provider sets the practice policy and standards

      b. Disadvantages

         (1) Total responsibility for the care of clients lies with one practitioner; may limit the practitioner's off-work time

         (2) The practitioner assumes all the financial risk for expenses and overheads

         (3) The types of care available to clients are limited

         (4) The times when care is available to clients are limited

         (5) Quality assurance and quality improvement are difficult to monitor

   2. Solo group (cluster) practice—a variation of solo practice; day-to-day operations shared by two or more dentists (generalists or specialists); dentists share specified operational costs and equipment but retain autonomy; the practice is independent but the costs of office space, rent, utilities, and so on are shared; the dentists may share the services of employees

      a. Advantages

         (1) Each practitioner has his or her own clients; colleagues are close at hand for consultations, referrals, and emergency coverage

         (2) Sharing of expenses allows purchasing of highly specialized equipment for joint use

         (3) Practice management is more independent

         (4) The right to determine the decision-making process remains with individual practitioners

b. Disadvantages
  (1) Decision making about personnel, materials, products, equipment, expenditures, productivity, and office space has to be shared among partners
  (2) Each partner needs to have a legal contract to protect himself or herself
3. Group (non-solo) practice—dental practice in which dentists, sometimes in association with members of other health care professions, agree formally among themselves on certain arrangements to provide efficient dental services; may include a practice with at least one other dentist; a formally arranged and legally recognized entity that is organized to provide dental care through the services of three or more dentists; the group's expenses and incomes are shared in a systematic manner; equipment, records, facilities, and personnel in both client care and business management are shared
  a. Advantages
    (1) Greater leverage with banks and lending institutions is possible
    (2) Dentists in group practices generally enjoy higher levels of income than do their solo colleagues; each practitioner experiences less stress
    (3) The group practice affords personal freedom with regard to time because colleagues are available to substitute when needed
    (4) Emergency care is available to clients
    (5) Quality of care may improve because of built-in peer review and consultation
    (6) Fringe benefits are possible because of the number employed within the practice
    (7) Management responsibilities are shared or reduced; personnel, space, equipment, and supplies can be shared
    (8) The potential for a variety of specialties to be represented within the practice is present; various services can be provided to patients
    (9) The practice can be available to clients during nontraditional hours of the day or week
    (10) The practice grows more quickly and takes advantage of newer technology and marketing strategies
  b. Disadvantages
    (1) Personality conflicts may occur, affecting the practice; the philosophies of the practitioners may differ; personal goals need to be balanced against group goals

    (2) The practitioners experience loss of individuality; the identity of the practice belongs to the group, not to individual practitioners
    (3) More sophisticated and complex systems of management are necessary
    (4) The transfer of property from one partner to another may be complicated when a partner leaves the practice
  c. Prepaid group practice—a group practice that provides dental services on a prepaid basis by some agency (third party)
4. Dental department in a hospital
  a. Examples of hospital practice are county, community-based, private, military, and veterans' hospitals; funding depends on the type of hospital
  b. May operate a clinic for routine care and also use operating rooms for oral surgery
  c. Dental care is provided for special populations such as persons requiring general anesthesia or other hospital services
  d. Routine care is provided for persons with special needs such as individuals with cleft palate repair, medically compromising conditions, or physical and intellectual disabilities
  e. The department can be staffed by specialty dentistry residency programs, the U.S. Public Health Services (USPHS) core dental officers, or military dental officers, depending on the type of hospital
5. Corporate dental clinic—company-owned and company-operated dental care facility designed to meet the oral health care needs of employees
  a. Advantages—provides dental benefits to employees, retirees, and dependents; reduces employee absenteeism; providers are full-time salaried employees of the corporation
  b. Currently a rare model
6. Corporately managed models
  a. Examples
    (1) Dental clinic facilities owned by and located in retail establishments, for example, Walgreens and Wal-Mart
    (2) Franchised dental clinics—the franchise is purchased from the corporation by the dentist; a system of marketing dental practices under a trade name, for example, Cool Smiles™
  b. Some dental practice acts require ownership by a dentist, in which case the practice is owned by the dentist
  c. If state laws allow ownership by nondentists, corporations can own dental clinics and hire dental personnel as salaried employees

d. Advantages—high visibility, convenient locations, expanded hours, flexible appointment scheduling, advertising to attract clients, name recognition, discount volume purchasing abilities, management training; dentists have the advantages of being employees, rather than owners of a business; retail store clinics may accept in-house credit cards for ease of payment; large corporations can establish payment plans and manage Medicaid and CHIP reimbursement programs; clients may be drawn from segment of the population that would not otherwise seek routine dental care

e. Disadvantages—high initial and ongoing costs if buy-in is required; dentists will have to relinquish control; quality of care may be an issue when decisions are made by the corporation

f. This model is increasing as the weak economy and rising costs of dental school education make it difficult for dentists to establish traditional dental practices and as third-party payment systems and managed care increase

B. Public sector

1. Community health centers and migrant health centers are federally funded group practices; primarily medical with a dental component; located in underserved areas to provide services to communities where dental and medical practitioners are not found in adequate numbers; some community health centers are faith based and are funded through various sources, including federal and local grants, Medicaid, and CHIP

   a. Similar to a well-developed group practice with different financing arrangements

   b. Provide primary medical and dental care; referral services are based on income

   c. Include neighborhood health centers, family health centers, rural health initiative centers, and migrant health centers

   d. Can be staffed by employed or volunteer oral health care providers or by both types

2. U.S. Public Health Service (USPHS)—component of the Department of Health and Human Services (DHHS)

   a. Major responsibilities include health research and health promotion through public health efforts

   b. Federal, hospital, Indian Health Service (IHS), and community-based clinics are staffed to provide oral health care to Native Americans, federal prisoners, Coast Guard personnel, coast and geodetic survey personnel, Merchant Marine personnel, merchant seamen,

migrant and seasonal farm workers, the homeless, and individuals suffering from Hansen's disease

3. National Health Service Corps (NHSC)—federally sponsored program aimed at reducing maldistribution of health care providers

   a. Offers financial incentives, including scholarships, salaries, and pay-back programs, to encourage health care providers to practice in remote and underserved areas

   b. Dentists and dental hygienists are eligible

4. State and local programs—operated by state, county, or city government entities; aimed at providing care for indigent populations eligible to receive public welfare or special populations, for example, the intellectually and developmentally challenged, in publicly funded residential centers

Oral Health Care Personnel

A. Types—dentist, dental assistant, dental hygienist, expanded-function dental hygienists and assistants, dental laboratory technician, denturist, emerging mid-level practitioners in some states based on ADHA's ADHP model[49]

B. Supply and distribution of dentists

1. Supply is traditionally measured with a dentist-to-population ratio; currently, in the United States, the supply ratio is 80 dentists to 100,000 persons (0.8 to 1000)[50]

2. Dentist-to-population ratio—not always an accurate reflection of supply because of location, population involved, community need, and demand for dental services

3. The number of active dentists began to decline in 2000, influenced by retirement patterns and smaller annual number of graduates; 141,900 dentists in 2008, a decrease of 20,000 compared with 2006[51]

4. Relative supply and ratio are declining; predictions range from 52 to 100,000 to 54 to 100,000 by 2020, based on retirement of the large cohort of dentists who graduated in the 1970s and 1980s

5. Uneven distribution of dentists exists for various reasons

   a. Dentists have freedom to choose their practice location

   b. Location of dental schools provides an abundant number of dentists in some areas and few in other areas; 16 states have no dental school

   c. Dentists tend to locate their practices in areas of economic opportunity and in desirable environments

d. Popular areas are those with a high demand for services; demographic shifts and resulting demand for services will affect the choice of practice setting
  (1) Geographic population shifts result in changes in areas of high demand; portability of license from state to state is needed to be able to easily relocate; a national dental licensing examination would provide greater portability
  (2) Rapid growth is seen in southern and western regions; the growth is slower in the northeast and midwest regions
  (3) Suburban areas have higher demand; rural and urban areas have a lower demand

6. The dental profession has recognized the need to increase under-represented minorities in the oral health care professions and to develop programs to resolve maldistribution problems

7. Inadequate supply and maldistribution of dental personnel results in dental health professions shortage areas (DHPSA), as defined by the federal government
  a. Based on provider-to-population ratio; access to care according to distance, time, and incomes at poverty level
  b. In 2009, more than 49 million people were living in over 4000 DHPSAs; the number of practitioners needed to achieve a target ratio of 1 dentist per 3000 patients was 9579; the number of DHPSAs, the number of people living in DHPSAs, and the number of dentists required to remedy the shortage areas have increased steadily over the past decade[52]

8. Workforce issues should continue to be analyzed and adjustments made on the basis of retirement patterns of practicing dentists, productivity improvement, population and economic growth, and new models of mid-level oral health care practitioners

C. Gender and racial–ethnic composition of dentists
  1. The number of women graduating from dental schools has gradually increased; prediction is that by 2015, 40% of dentists will be female; need to evaluate the effect of this increasing shift of gender on the values, caring quality, patient orientation, and practice models of dentistry as well as the number and distribution needed to meet the needs of the population[53]
  2. A continuing need to increase the diversity of the dental profession exists; the IHS and the Health Resources and Services Administration (HRSA) programs are geared toward diversifying the health care professions workforce through scholarships, repayment programs, and other

incentives;[11] although *Healthy People 2010* targets for representation of the Asian or Pacific Islander population in dentistry were exceeded, the opposite is true for the black non-Hispanic population; and no change occurred in the representation of other minority groups in the dental profession[11]

3. Goal—diversity of oral health care personnel must be proportionate to the diversity of the population; U.S. Census Bureau data in 2010 were 72.4% white, 12.8% African American, 18.3% Hispanic (overlap with other groups), 0.2% Pacific Islanders, 4.8% Asian, 8.2% other, and 2.9% two or more races.

D. Dental school enrollment
  1. 59 U.S. dental schools, located in 36 states, the Commonwealth of Puerto Rico, and the District of Columbia, representing a very slight increase over the past 10 years[54]
  2. 4700 dental school applicants in 2008, representing a marked increase in applicants and three times as many applicants as enrollments[51]
  3. The number of dental school graduates has been increasing slowly since 1992; 4796 graduated in 2008[55]
  4. Current trends reflect an increase in the number of dental school applicants but not enough enrollments to keep up with the increasing dentist retirements and the increasing demand for services;[56,57] five new dental schools are under consideration in Illinois, Texas, Arkansas, Maine, and Nevada to address the anticipated shortage of dentists[56]

E. Supply of dental hygiene personnel
  1. 152,000 dental hygienists at the end of 2007; 130,000 were active practitioners; the trend is an increase[58]
  2. As an organized profession, dental hygiene has sought alternatives to help meet the oral health care needs of the population and improve access to care by:
    a. Developing programs to increase recruitment and retention of dental hygienists
    b. Improving dental hygiene care to society
    c. Promoting higher levels of education within dental hygiene, for example, baccalaureate, master's, and doctoral degree preparation
    d. Creating new models of practice to improve access to care for the underserved portions of the population, for example, ADHP[59]
      (1) Revision of scope of practice guidelines for dental hygienists and dental assistants
      (2) Development of the ADHP model, educational program to implement the model, and revision of state practice acts

to allow its implementation; currently being implemented in Minnesota

3. 314 dental hygiene programs in 50 states, Washington, D.C., and Puerto Rico in 2010, representing a marked increase (9.4% increase from 2006 to 2010)[55]

4. 58.1% increase in dental hygiene programs between 1986 and 2010, compared with 1.7% decrease in dental schools during the same period[54,55]

5. More dental hygienists than dentists have graduated every year since 1990; 6723 graduated in 2008, representing a 72.2% increase in dental hygiene graduates from 1989 to 2008 compared with an 11.2% increase in dentists graduated during the same period;[55] ratio of dental graduates to dental hygiene graduates in 2008 was 1 : 1.4

6. More and more states are revising their dental practice acts to provide for nontraditional practice models for dental hygienists, for example, collaborative practice and independent practice, that better meet the needs of community oral health care practice
   a. The trend of more dental hygienists than dentists graduating will result in a larger pool of dental hygienists; this can lead to the expansion of their scope of practice to accommodate for the decreasing numbers of dentists so that the increasing demand for dental care can be met cost effectively
   b. The master of science program in oral health care practice at the Metropolitan State University in Minnesota accepted its first class in 2009 to prepare licensed dental hygienists for advanced dental hygiene practice to enhance the oral health care of underserved and diverse populations; this could mark the beginning of a new era in dentistry in relation to the use of mid-level practitioners to increase access for underserved populations

F. Gender and racial–ethnic composition of dental hygienists
   1. Enrollment by gender in dental hygiene programs in 2008–2009—97% female[60]
   2. Inadequate minority group representation in the dental hygiene profession;[61] 78.6% enrolled in 2008–2009 were non-Hispanic white[60]

G. Enrollment in other oral health care programs
   1. Dental assisting programs: 266 accredited programs in 2010, representing a decrease; more will be needed to fill the needs of increasing numbers of dentists
   2. Dental laboratory technology programs: 20 programs in 2010, representing a decrease

H. Recruitment and retention efforts
   1. Total number of dentists and other oral health care personnel must be increased; number of dental and dental hygiene educators must be increased
   2. Focus on recruitment of under-represented minorities must be a collaborative effort among dental, dental education, and allied dental professional associations, government agencies, dental and allied dental educational institutions, and philanthropic groups, for example, Robert Wood Johnson Foundation, with three objectives: expansion of community-based dental education programs, recruitment and retention of under-represented minority and low-income students, and enhancement of cultural sensitivity among students and faculty
   3. Activities must begin at the K–12 level, with emphasis on science and mathematics
   4. Women and under-represented minorities must be introduced to health care professions and science careers
   5. Efforts must continue to focus on the recruitment of women and minorities as dental and allied dental educators to serve as role models and mentors for academic careers

FINANCING ORAL HEALTH CARE

Financing of oral health care in the United States is very complex because of the dual involvement of both the corporate sector and the public sector in financing, as well as the presence of varied and multiple mechanisms of payment, sources of payment, types of insurance plans, and providers of insurance plans. This pluralistic system results in greater emphasis on individual responsibility for oral health care.

Mechanisms of Payment

A. Barter system—the provider and the client negotiate payment by exchanging goods or services without using money; still evident in some rural areas and developing countries; two-party arrangement

B. Fee-for-service—arrangement in which fee scale is set for a service; charge or payment for performed services; traditional method of billing
   1. Declining method of payment as third-party payment becomes more prevalent
   2. Locality sensitive
   3. Examples of fee-for-service
      a. Full fee—the dentist provides service, and the client or a third party pays the fee

b. Usual, customary, and reasonable (UCR) fees—fees set by insurance companies; influenced by the fees dentists charge in various geographic areas and by population sizes; the Health Insurance Association of America (HIAA) surveys dentists every 6 months with regard to their fees to guide insurance companies on setting UCR fees; three components of the UCR fee are:
  (1) Usual—fee most often charged by a dentist for a specific dental procedure
  (2) Customary—fee level determined by the administrator of a dental benefit plan, that is, the insurance company, from actual fees submitted for a specific dental procedure; this is the maximum benefit payable for the procedure
  (3) Reasonable—the fee charged by a dentist for a specific dental procedure that has been modified because of complications or other unusual situations
c. Discounted fee—a decreased fee paid by a specifically identified group (students, senior citizens) or by participants in a prepaid group; becoming a more common approach to managed care in dentistry
d. Table of allowances—a system in which the insurance company establishes a list of covered services with an assigned dollar amount that will be reimbursed to the subscriber; the dentist can charge more, and the patient pays the difference
e. Sliding fee scale—a system in which the fee varies according to patients' ability to pay; used by some community programs
f. Cost-control mechanisms used by dental insurance plans
  (1) Co-payment—a portion of the cost of each service is paid by the client, stated as a flat amount, and the remainder of the fee is covered by the third-party or other agency; the purpose is to discourage overuse
  (2) Co-insurance—similar to co-payment, but it is a percentage rather than a fixed amount; used by most dental insurance plans
  (3) Deductible—the patient pays a required amount for an out-of-pocket expense before the insurance plan will pay
  (4) Annual limits (maximum coverage)—the insurance plan will pay only up to a specific dollar limit each year
  (5) Waiting period—the patient must wait a specified length of time before coverage begins

C. Fee schedule—a list of charges set by a dental plan administrator and agreed to by the dentist who enrolls as a provider; the dentist cannot charge more; this is the system used by Medicaid
D. Capitation—a form of contracted care, usually by a corporation, institution, or other group for its members; the provider receives a set fee per person per a given period and provides all or most of the services covered in the program to the subscribers of the program; payment is made to the provider regardless of use by enrollees; two financial arrangements are available:
  1. Fee—a fixed monthly or yearly payment to an individual dentist by a third party based on the number of clients assigned for treatment; the provider receives the fees whether or not clients use his or her services
  2. Premium—fixed yearly or monthly amount paid to an organization, for example, a prepaid group practice or health maintenance organization (HMO), to provide dental care to individuals participating in the plan
E. Encounter fee—a set fee each time a patient has a health care encounter (comes in for treatment), irrespective of what services are provided; used by many community programs as a discounted fee

Sources of Payment

A. Two-party system
  1. The dentist provides the service, and the client pays with cash, credit card, or check
  2. Post-payment or budget payment plans through bank loans or credit cards—initially proposed to bring the benefits of routine dental care to a large segment of the population
B. Third-party system
  1. Payment for health care services by some agency other than the beneficiary of those services (e.g., insurance company, employer) designed to improve access to care and increase use of care
  2. Characteristics
    a. The dentist and the client are the first and second parties; the administrator of the finances is the third party (also known as the *carrier, insurer, underwriter,* or *administrative agent*)
    b. The third party may collect premiums, assume the financial risk, pay claims, and provide administrative services
    c. The purchaser of a plan can be an organized private group such as a union or employer or a government agency
    d. Third-party plans can be private (a private insurance company or employer) or public

(government program, e.g., Medicaid, Medicare, or CHIP)

3. Direct reimbursement—beneficiaries are reimbursed by the employer or benefits administrator (e.g., insurance company) for a specified percentage of dental expenses on presentation of evidence of expenses

4. Third-party payments are called *prepayments* because the care is paid for ahead of time through premiums; this allows for the spread of the financial burden of dental care over a group because these insurance plans are provided as group insurance, usually by employers and unions

5. Reimbursement for prepayment plans is done by the UCR fee, capitation, discount, table of allowances, fee schedule, or other agreed-on mechanism

6. The percentage of patients covered by dental insurance increased from <5% in 1970 to >50% in 2000 and has remained similar since then with only minor fluctuations[11]

C. Public funding of dental care as a source of payment is addressed separately in a later section

Different Types of Dental Insurance Plans

A. Indemnity dental insurance plans (also called *fee-for-service plan* or *traditional plan*)
  1. Traditional form of dental insurance offered by most dental insurance providers
  2. Until a few years ago, was only offered to employee groups, not to individuals
  3. Benefits may be paid to the dentist or directly to the patient (direct reimbursement)
  4. The patient chooses any dental provider (open panel); any dentist can choose to participate and accept reimbursement from the insurance company
  5. Coverage amount usually ranges from 50% to 80% of the UCR, depending on the service
  6. The patient is responsible for the difference between the benefit paid and the fee charged
  7. Includes annual limits and deductibles and may exclude pre-existing dental conditions; deductible frequently higher than with a PPO (Preferred Provider Organization) plan
  8. Most expensive form of insurance; provides greatest choice of dental care providers

B. PPO plans
  1. The beneficiary is required to choose a dental care provider from within the network of providers on the plan (closed panel)
  2. The insurance company negotiates lower fees with these providers in exchange for their participation within the network, growth of their

client base, and promise of faster claims processing; dentists agree to utilization reviews

  3. Coverage varies among PPOs but usually ranges between 50% and 80% of dental costs
  4. The insurance company reimburses the patient, or the dentist accepts payment directly from the insurance company
  5. Co-insurance, annual limits, and deductibles apply
  6. The beneficiary can visit a dentist outside the PPO and pay the difference (amount above the discounted fee)
  7. PPO plan premiums are slightly less costly than traditional indemnity plan premiums
  8. The number of participating dentists is currently low but is growing

C. Exclusive Provider Organization (EPO), also known as Exclusive Provider Arrangement (EPA)
  1. Similar to a PPO in administration, structure, and operation, but more restrictive
  2. Does not cover out-of-network care (with some exceptions for emergency and out-of-area services); company self-insures

D. HMO plans
  1. A dentist contracts with an insurer to provide care at lower-than-average fees
  2. Dental care providers receive a certain portion of the premiums as pre-payment (capitation form of payment)
  3. Insurers selectively direct patients to specific providers (closed panel)
  4. Includes co-payment and possibly maximum coverage limits; no deductibles
  5. Because HMO plan premiums received by the dentist may not adequately cover the actual cost of providing treatment, many dentists set themselves a limit on the number of patients with HMO plans

E. Point-of-service (POS) plans
  1. POS plans have all the characteristics of the HMO plan, but the beneficiary may seek care out of network
  2. Mechanisms are in place to encourage the use of in-network providers

F. Direct reimbursement plans (EPO and EPA)
  1. Not a true insurance plan; many companies are beginning to use these plans for their employees' dental care to save the cost of the middle man, the insurance plan administrator
  2. The employer sets aside a certain amount of money in a savings fund to finance employees' dental expenses
  3. The employee chooses any dentist, is responsible to pay the dental fees on completion of services, submits receipts to the employer, and is reimbursed from the savings fund

4. The client negotiates directly with the provider about treatment decisions and the fee structure

5. Includes an annual limit on the amount the company sets aside for each employee

G. Discount dental plans

1. The client pays a low annual membership fee and receives a dental discount card

2. The card can be used at participating dental care providers (who also pay a fee to be on the plan) for a savings of 10% to 60%

3. No deductibles, no annual limits, no co-payments, no paperwork for the patient or the dentist, and no prequalifications

Providers of Dental Insurance Plans

A. Dental service corporations—legally constituted nonprofit organizations incorporated on a state-by-state basis and sponsored by a constituent dental society to negotiate and administer dental insurance plans, for example, Delta Dental Plans

1. Contractual agreement with dentists to provide care to eligible beneficiaries

2. Dentists on the plan must file a UCR fee structure with organization

3. Dentists accept payment at the 90th percentile of the UCR fee as payment in full

4. Regular fee audits are performed to ensure that all insured persons are charged the same

5. A small amount of each payment is withheld to build an insurance reserve; subject to state insurance laws

B. Health service corporations—offer limited dental coverage as part of their hospital-surgical-medical policies (e.g., Blue Cross/Blue Shield); not strictly dental insurance

C. Commercial insurance companies

1. Operate for profit

a. Compete with dental service corporations through promotion and marketing

b. Can provide attractive total health package plans to potential purchasers

2. Have no obligation to the oral health of the community; can be selective about groups to which they offer insurance

3. Use fee profiles developed from reported expenses, similar to the UCR fee profile

4. Reimburse enrollees or service providers

D. Prepaid group practice

1. Large group practices are involved

2. Contract directly to groups of subscribers

3. Payment mechanisms vary

4. Less common approach

E. Health Maintenance Organization (HMO)

1. Organization that provides a comprehensive prescribed range of services to a defined population during a defined period using an HMO insurance plan and a capitation payment mechanism

2. Primarily provides medical services; small proportion of HMOs also provide dental care

3. Three types of HMO organizations:

a. Staff model—the health care plan owns the health care facility and pays health care providers as salaried employees; enrollees are restricted to the HMO's providers

b. Group model—the HMO contracts with a group practice, partnership, or corporation to provide care; the provider group is managed independently and reimbursed on a capitation basis

c. Individual Practice Association (IPA)—a group of independent dental providers contracts with an HMO to provide services to their enrollees at discounted fees or through capitation arrangement; may have private patients as well; most common type of HMO

Public Financing of Care

A. The Social Security Amendments of 1965 to the Social Security Act removed barriers to health care for selected groups

1. Title XVIII Medicare—federal insurance program from trust funds to pay medical bills for insured persons; administered by the Centers for Medicare and Medicaid Services (CMS)

a. Persons age ≥65 years and certain disabled individuals are eligible; also persons with end-stage renal disease; no income limitations

b. Three parts—part A, hospital insurance; and part B, voluntary supplemental medical insurance; both have complex service benefits available; part B requires some payment by the client; Part C is a drug benefit

c. Dental care coverage is limited to services that have medical implications, for example, jaw reconstruction following accidental injury; dental expenditures have consistently been declining

2. Title XIX Medicaid—health insurance program that provides access to health care to low-income and other special groups, for example, children of lawfully admitted immigrants, newborn children without insurance, children under Child Protective Services, disabled individuals[62]

a. Federal and state governments form a partnership to finance health care; percentage of funds that comes from the state varies according to a formula based on the ratio of the state's per capita income to the national per capita income

b. The program is administered by the state; eligibility, designated expenditures, and authorized services vary from state to state

c. Dental care is only mandatory for persons under 21 years of age; all states must provide oral health care services to Medicaid-eligible children as specified by the Early and Periodic Screening, Diagnosis, and Treatment (EPSDT) program (medical, dental, and vision care are mandatory)

d. Dentists must enroll as providers; patients must be enrolled in Medicaid and can only seek care from Medicaid providers

e. Medicaid has been plagued by changing eligibility requirements, limitation of services, low allowable fees paid, delays in payment for services, and dentists' refusal to treat Medicaid clients

(1) Reasons given by dentists for not enrolling with Medicaid include low reimbursement rates, missed appointments by Medicaid clients, difficult treatment issues, too much bureaucratic paperwork, reluctance to have patients from low SES groups in the reception room with other patients, and preference to provide charity care rather than Medicaid services

(2) The services allowed and fees reimbursed by Medicaid have recently been increased

(3) Initiatives of public health departments to increase the number of dental providers have recently been instituted

f. The percentage of persons living in poverty in 2008 as determined by the poverty level guidelines set by the federal government was 19% for ages 18 and under, 11.7% for adults (28.7% for single-parent females), and 9.7% for age ≥65 years; rates were higher for foreign-born, noncitizen, and minority racial groups compared with the non-Hispanic white cohort; rates varied by geographic region (higher in the south and the west) and by metropolitan status (higher inside principal cities and in rural areas);[63] the low SES groups experience a greater number of factors that are associated with poor health (determinants of health)

g. 16.4 million (20%) children in the United States were covered by Medicaid in 2008, at a cost of $69.2 billion to taxpayers

h. The number of Medicaid recipients (children, adults, and older adults) increased from 2.4 million in 1972 to 41.4 million in 2003; an estimated 60% of low SES Americans are not covered by Medicaid; the aging baby-boomer generation is the fastest growing group on Medicaid, especially lower SES older adults

i. Dental coverage is inadequate: across the states, in 2007, only 21% to 43% of children covered by Medicaid received dental services; the percentage of total Medicaid dollars going to dental care dropped from 3% in 1972 to 1% in the early 2000s; expenditure per recipient dropped from $71 to $45 for the same period (adjusted for inflation); 16 million Medicaid-eligible low SES children do not receive dental care[64]

j. Medicaid reimbursement—also used to support local philanthropic, educational, and public programs that bill Medicaid for services; "safety net" for low SES groups

B. In 1997, the Social Security Act was amended through Title XXI, creating the State Children's Health Insurance Program (SCHIP); reauthorized in 1999 as CHIP[65]

1. Joint federal–state program that gives each state permission to offer health insurance to children up to 19 years of age who are not eligible for Medicaid but have an income too low to allow access to health care (generally up to 200% of federally determined poverty level)

2. All states participate; states administer the program and determine eligibility requirements and available services; the program varies from state to state

3. The program can be implemented as an expansion of a state's Medicaid program, through the state's existing health insurance program for state employees with benefits equivalent to those available to state employees, or using a combination of these strategies; some states have expanded their Medicaid program; others have created their own state program

4. Dental benefits must be at least equivalent to those provided under Medicaid; nearly all states provide CHIP coverage for dental benefits

5. Co-payments and co-insurance for certain treatments vary from state to state

6. Most public expenditures for dental care are from Medicaid or CHIP

C. Treatments for children with craniofacial deformities, cleft lip and palate, and certain other conditions are funded by other state and federal funds (e.g., Crippled Children's Program)

D. The federal government provides financing for dental treatments for children through Head Start, the federal preschool child development program

E. Civilian Health and Medical Program of the Uniformed Services (CHAMPUS)—health care services for military personnel and dependents; also voluntary dental insurance program; requires participants to pay part of premiums

F. Public Health Service (PHS)—care financed for defined groups such as prisoners, Native Americans, migrant and seasonal farm workers, and the homeless

G. Federal block grants, primarily the Maternal and Children's Health Services (MCHS) Title V Block Grant and the Preventive Health and Health Services (PHHS) Block Grant, usually referred to as *preventive block grants*

H. State programs—vary from state to state; use state funds to provide care to particular populations, for example, state prisoners and intellectually and emotionally challenged individuals; primarily provide programs to support health education and health promotion at state and local levels; various programs suggested to supplement health care costs (e.g., catastrophic health insurance) frequently fail or are modified by state or federal budget concerns

I. Indian Health Service (IHS)—responsible for medical and dental care for Native Americans and Alaska Natives who are members of federally recognized tribes; IHS clinics are staffed by PHS officers

J. Federal agencies responsible for the provision of dental services and oral health education to specific population groups such as military personnel and their dependents, the disadvantaged, and the incarcerated
  1. Department of Defense (DOD)
  2. Department of Veterans Affairs (VA)
  3. Department of Justice's Bureau of Prisons (BOP)
  4. DHHS (Department of Health and Human Services) Indian Health Service (IHS)
  5. DHHS Health Resources and Services Administration (HRSA)

K. Federal agencies providing additional oral health education and health promotion programs
  1. Department of Agriculture, Women, Infants and Children program (WIC)
  2. Health professional education through the Ryan White Comprehensive AIDS (acquired immune deficiency syndrome) Resources Emergency Act

L. State, county, and city programs
  1. Funded through a variety of sources, including local and state tax funds, Maternal and Child Health Bureau of the HRSA (MCHB) and federal PHHS Block Grants, WIC, Medicaid, and CHIP, as well as foundations and faith-based organizations
  2. Collaboration must occur among public health agencies, nongovernmental organizations (NGOs), dental and dental hygiene associations and educational programs, community agencies, and volunteer groups to fund local community oral health care programs

M. Involvement of the federal government in health care financing has increased steadily, especially since 1965; dental care has continued to be a small part, at best; demand for services for the low-income population has increased at a time when available services are declining; alternative health care plans may emerge as a result of the Healthcare Reform Act passed in 2010; future expectations for oral health care financing include a continuation of the current varied and complex financing systems, possible increase in publicly financed oral health care, and continuation of coverage for a large proportion of the population, primarily the poor, even though inadequate

N. Other community-based programs
  1. Faith-based programs—clinics and school dental programs operated by churches and other faith-based institutions
  2. Community clinics—funded by local foundations
  3. Programs operated by organized dental hygiene—Head Start varnish programs, school- and community-based sealant programs
  4. Programs operated by organized dentistry—Give Kids a Smile (free dental care events sponsored by the ADA); Donated Dental Services (direct dental care), Bridge (preventive education services and screening by hygienists in facilities for developmentally disabled individuals), and House Calls (homebound dental care) conducted by the National Foundation of Dentistry for the Handicapped, an affiliate of the ADA

Managed Care

A. The integration of health care delivery and financing; a cost-containment system that directs the use of benefits by restricting type, level, and frequency of treatment, limiting access to care, and controlling the level of reimbursement for services
  1. Characterized by a comprehensive set of health care services, selected providers (closed panel), and financial incentives to use selected providers
  2. Typified by internal programs to monitor the amount and quality of services provided (quality assurance)
  3. Providers receive compensation in a predetermined form, for example, fixed amount per program member or fixed amount per service
  4. Implementation—result of increased costs of health care, the need to control costs, and the need to improve access to care for a large segment

of the population without traditional dental insurance

B. Managed dental care has not yet evolved to the extent of managed medical care
  1. Major managed dental care entities are PPOs, HMOs, IPAs, and POSs, which reflect the key elements of managed care
  2. Indemnity private dental insurance plans have some of the characteristics of managed care
    a. Include prepayment review
    b. Require preauthorization and practice guidelines that may limit or discount payment for dental procedures
  3. Public financing mechanisms help provide managed care
  4. Views on managed care vary
    a. Dental professional groups have expressed concern about closed-panel third-party approaches because clients are denied freedom of choice of dentists[66]
    b. Another argument against the closed panel is related to the quality of care provided, although charges of poor quality cannot be substantiated
    c. Association of Managed Care Dentists[67]—a nonprofit volunteer organization of dentists with a mission to:
      (1) Educate dentists on issues related to managed care
      (2) Influence plan designs for managed care
      (3) Encourage quality assurance within managed care
      (4) Improve quality patient care in managed care plans
    d. Managed care is expected to increase; dental hygienists may contribute significantly in a managed care model because of the emphasis on prevention and on cost savings

NEED FOR, DEMAND FOR, AND UTILIZATION OF DENTAL SERVICES

Definitions

A. Need—normative, usually professional judgment about the amount and kinds of health care services or medical care services required by an individual to attain or maintain some standard level of health; normative need defined as professionally determined
  1. Expressed in terms of a population or individual
  2. Includes specific needs identified through clinical or community-based assessment procedures
  3. Perceived need or felt need—defined as determined by the client or the public; can differ from

normative need; clinically, can be referred to as a chief concern

B. Demand—volume and types of health care services that an individual or population desires to consume at some price level
  1. Effective demand—desire for care and ability to obtain care (has access to care)
  2. Potential demand—desire for care and inability to obtain care (lacks access to care)

C. Utilization—proportion of the population that uses dental services over a period of time; volume and types of services actually consumed

D. Wellness—high-level wellness is described as a dynamic process in which the individual is actively engaged in moving toward fulfillment of his or her human needs and potential
  1. Reflects a change in the perceptions of health and wellness from the medical model of health care that is treatment oriented
  2. Includes a prevention orientation that examines the relationships among the host, agent, environment, and preventive strategies
  3. Includes a health promotion orientation aimed at creating an environment that enables individuals to increase control over and improve current and future health status

Factors That Influence Utilization and Health Behaviors

A. Knowledge—influenced by SES and health literacy
B. Increase in public awareness of health and oral health, influenced by:
  1. New technologies such as telehealth, bioinformatics, and virtual reality
  2. Databases specifying the human, animal, and microbial genomes
  3. Strong emphasis on evidence-informed approaches to health care delivery
C. A person's level of adopting the wellness paradigm versus the health–disease paradigm
D. Compliance with recommendations as a result of:
  1. Beliefs—trust placed in a provider, a health custom, or a system of health care as a result of acceptance that something is true; personal or cultural beliefs about illness and wellness that may then influence health behaviors
  2. Attitudes—patterns of mental views based on judgments of likes and dislikes (about health care systems, providers, or utilization); established because of prior experience
  3. Values—the importance or worth placed on health care and health practices; beliefs, attitudes, and values are all inter-related and affect each other; although difficult to do, beliefs, attitudes, and values related to oral health care and

health practices can be changed over time through development of rapport, communication, persuasion, education, and new experiences

Dental Care Utilization Patterns

A. Measured as the number of persons who visit a health care provider during a given year; the rate was 68.5% for the general population in 2008 as measured through the Behavioral Risk Factor Surveillance System (BRFSS), an ongoing telephone health survey system conducted by the National Center for Chronic Disease Prevention and Health Promotion;[21] dental attendance of those from low SES groups is <50%

B. Shift in dental services used, for example, reported increase in examinations, preventive services, extractions, implants, and aesthetic dentistry; slight decline in dentures

C. Increase in demand for aesthetic, implant, prosthodontic, and periodontal treatments as a result of the changing demographics of the population; persons age >65 years are the fastest growing segment of the American population and have higher tooth retention rates, which has resulted in their increased utilization of dental services; dentate persons are more than four times as likely as edentulous persons to report a dental visit within the past year

D. Each generation demands a different variety of services, for example, older populations focus on restoration, periodontal treatment, prosthetics, and control and treatment of root caries; middle-aged persons need some restorative and periodontal services or orthodontic services; children need more primary prevention and orthodontic services

E. The success of preventive interventions affects the types of services needed by adults and seniors

F. General interest in prevention has caused an increase in preventive dentistry services

G. The American society's interest in appearance and aesthetics influences demand for restorative options, cosmetic dentistry, orthodontics, periodontal services, and dental implants

H. Varying economic patterns and availability of discretionary income and third-party payment have resulted in increased utilization

I. Age—rise in preschool use of services (about 50%); peak ages are school age and late teenage years; decreases among adults and older adults; seniors utilize more dental services than in the past

J. Gender—females have more dental visits than do males

K. Race and ethnicity—difficult to determine utilization of dental care because the status is closely related to income and education (SES), culture, and location[47]
  1. Hispanic Americans and African Americans have limited access to dental care, including available dental providers
  2. Native Americans residing on reservations receive care through the IHS; traditionally utilization has not been high; however, it varies from location to location

L. Higher education and income are associated with better dental care utilization rates

M. Traditionally, utilization of dental care is lower in rural communities (both farm and nonfarm) than in urban areas; a greater increase in utilization is being seen among rural residents than among city dwellers; suburbanites are the most frequent users

N. Access to dental insurance
  1. Utilization rates for individuals with private insurance are 38% higher than for individuals without dental insurance
  2. Dental coverage varies by race, ethnicity, age, income, and educational levels; higher rate of coverage is associated with being non-Hispanic white and having higher income and higher educational level; individuals age ≥65 years have the lowest coverage of dental insurance
  3. Dental insurance coverage influences the types of services used; concerns exist about insurance companies dictating the care provided based on guidelines for payment

O. Regional differences in utilization exist; lowest utilization rates in the United States are seen in the southern region

P. Most powerful predictors of dental utilization are gender, SES, dentate status, dental insurance, and overall economy

Q. Barriers to dental care
  1. Barriers not related to cost
     a. Lack of perceived need; for example, edentulism is a frequently reported reason for not seeking dental care
     b. Pain and discomfort associated with dental treatments
     c. Access to care being difficult or impossible
     d. Availability of providers, for example, office hours, maldistribution of personnel
     e. Types of services needed not being available because of practitioners' lack of skill or interest
     f. Geographic isolation
     g. Nonambulatory status (e.g., being homebound or institutionalized)
     h. Lack of public transportation
     i. Values, attitudes, and beliefs

j. Unfavorable view of dental personnel—not accommodating to or knowledgeable about special needs

2. Cost-related barriers
   a. Services not affordable
   b. Insurance issues
      (1) Coverage limited or not available; more than 131 million children and adults lack dental insurance, 2.5 times the number of those who lack health insurance
      (2) Lack of providers available to individuals with Medicaid and CHIP
      (3) A narrow insurance company definition of medically necessary dental care that sets limits on oral health care services available to many insured clients, especially seniors on Medicare
   c. Lost wages resulting from time away from work; more critical than the perceived need for services
3. Social and psychological barriers
   a. Dental care and facial appearance related to the oral cavity not valued
   b. Unpleasant prior experience resulting in anxiety
   c. Emotional factors such as fear of dental care
4. Cultural barriers
   a. Language—client unable to find a provider who speaks his or her language
   b. History and tradition—no importance given to dental care in the client's culture
   c. Basic cultural beliefs about health, illness, disease, and health care model
   d. Failure to understand the impact of a missed appointment that can be costly and disruptive
   e. Difficulty in understanding the recommendations for care or dietary changes
   f. Few health care providers from minority groups—research results show that members of minority or racial and ethnic groups respond better to health care personnel from their own backgrounds, especially if these clients have low SES or poor English-speaking skills

R. Reduction of disparities in oral health care services requires a multi-pronged approach that includes improvement of access to care for underserved populations, increased demand for oral health care, and reduction of barriers to oral health care; the need exists for a variety of interventions that address all the core functions of public health, assessment, policy development and assurance, using evidence-based approaches to health education, health promotion, and provision of services

CURRENT CHALLENGES IN ORAL HEALTH AND ORAL HEALTH CARE

A. Oral diseases are progressive and cumulative and become more complex over time
B. Significant burden of oral diseases and disorders
   1. Striking disparities exist in dental diseases and conditions, depending on income levels of clients
   2. Unintentional injuries commonly affect craniofacial tissues
   3. Tobacco-related oral diseases are prevalent among adolescents who use spit tobacco
   4. 25% of children in the United States have not seen a dentist before entering kindergarten
   5. Uninsured children are 2.5 times less likely than insured children to receive dental care
   6. 51 million school hours are lost each year because of dental-related illnesses
   7. Employed adults lose more than 164 hours of work each year because of dental visits or dental disease
   8. Less than two thirds of adults report having visited a dentist in the past 12 months
C. Trends in oral health care delivery
   1. Increasing numbers of people see a dentist each year; dental attendance in 2008 was 68.5%
   2. Expenditure for dental services makes up only 4.7% of the national health expenditure
   3. Medicaid and CHIP are unable to fill the gaps in the provision of dental care to poor children; fewer than 50% of children covered by Medicaid and CHIP receive dental care
   4. The focus needs to be on making those who do not seek care aware of available dental care services as well as implementing health promotion strategies to change their oral health behaviors
   5. Caries rates are declining except in the youngest age group (age 2 to 4); tooth-retention rates are increasing
   6. The public as well as professional focus needs to be on the control and prevention of caries in young children, prevention of periodontal disease, control of tobacco use by young people, and early detection of oral cancer
   7. Emphasis on aesthetics, adult orthodontics, and dental implants is broadening treatment options
   8. The current society in general is more oriented to oral disease prevention, as reflected in the increase in the marketing and sales of nonprescription dental products such as fluoridated dentifrices, power toothbrushes and interdental cleaners, and mouthrinses

9. Changes in oral disease patterns and a decline in total tooth loss in seniors are seen, increasing the optimism about the potential for increased utilization

10. Practitioners are cautioned not to provide services for which they are not qualified; the current litigious society demands skilled practitioners and high-quality services

D. The redirected focus of dental personnel is to:
1. Identify individuals currently not seeking care, for example, special population groups and low-income and minority individuals
2. Increase access to and availability of care, for example, vary office hours, offer care in non-traditional settings, improve payment and financing mechanisms, and explore the use of mid-level practitioners
3. Educate the public with a focus on periodontal disease, caries, oral cancer, tobacco cessation, systemic–oral health connection, and preventive interventions
4. Encourage professional lifelong learning to address the changing oral health care needs of the population, cultural competence and sensitivity, and technologies to assess and treat populations
5. Develop strategies to educate other health care professionals about the demographic and ethnic changes in the population; educate and sensitize professionals about cultural perception of health and disease
6. Recognize dentistry's changing role, with an emphasis on diagnostic skills and evaluation
7. Accept dental hygienists' changing role as more autonomous, interdependent practitioners and as collaborators with other members of the oral health care team as well as interdisciplinary health care teams
8. Employ appropriate oral health care personnel; recognize the capabilities of all team members
9. Make changes in oral health care delivery and oral health promotion that address recommendations made in the *Surgeon General's Report on Oral Health, A National Call to Action to Promote Oral Health, Healthy People 2020,* and *Advancing Oral Health in America*
10. Incorporate scientific evidence into all aspects of oral health care practice
11. Use innovative collaborations and partnerships to promote oral health and solve oral health problems

E. Actions recommended to reduce disparities in oral health and oral health care[7]
1. Through research, identify biomarkers that will facilitate early detection and diagnosis of disease
2. Conduct epidemiologic studies of populations to establish baselines for the incidence and prevalence of specific oral health problems; assist in tracking, reducing or eliminating identified health disparities
3. Conduct randomized controlled clinical trials to provide an evidence base for the effective prevention and management of health disparities
4. Carry out population-based research to understand the basis of health disparities
5. Place a high priority on efforts to reduce widespread disparities in oral health status and access to care

F. Focus of oral health care professional educational programs to meet the critical requirement of preparing a qualified workforce[68]
1. Continue to expand the scientific bases of health professional schools
2. Restructure the missions and organizational structures of education programs to focus on local community needs
3. Focus curriculum on multiple skills (training in various appropriate tasks to function in many roles) and interdisciplinary core curricula
4. Improve articulation and career advancement opportunities
5. Strengthen linkages with diverse care delivery environments
6. Improve recruitment of students from minority and disadvantaged groups and those with disabilities
7. Improve faculty leadership skills and competence in clinical outcomes
8. Establish innovative collaborations among professional associations and community organizations and improve integration with parent institutions to better serve the needs of the public
9. Improve the collection, evaluation, and dissemination of data related to allied health education, training, practice, and regulations
10. Focus on serving all Americans, regardless of SES, gender, and ethnic or racial group representation, in the recruitment of students and faculty, design and implementation of curricula, conduct of research, provision of services, and participation in community outreach
11. Focus on the development of health oriented, socially aware practitioners who will seek innovative solutions for issues related to access to care
12. Continue to seek ways to prepare a culturally competent workforce
13. Make curricular changes in professional education to better prepare oral health care practitioners for the needs and types of services required to treat all clients according to their needs and on the basis of risk assessment

14. Improve the communication of efforts and successes to the public

CHALLENGES FOR THE TWENTY-FIRST CENTURY

A. Unprecedented changes in demography, patterns of disease and disorders, and health care financing and delivery, including greater involvement of public financing
B. Changes in science and technology
C. Access to multiple information systems, including the Internet, computer-assisted technology, telehealth care, and distance education technology
D. Improved technology and therapeutics; new biomaterials and biotechnology
E. Access to genetic information that will influence assessment of risk factors and care planning
F. A philosophy of "best practices," that is, determining which treatment will work for which clients and under what circumstances; an evidence-informed approach to dental and dental hygiene care based on risk assessment
G. Paradigm shift to a treatment model that focuses on nonsurgical, noninvasive, biologic, and pharmacologic interventions that are guided by genetics and risk assessment, requiring a shift in oral health care education, teaching, and outcome methodologies and a greater focus on lifelong learning for oral health care personnel
H. Oral health education and promotion for preventive strategies; individual and community-based focus with greater emphasis on the use of validated health education, health promotion, and organizational theories
I. Coordination and collaboration of dental care and medical care
J. Decreasing health disparities; increasing access to care for underserved populations
K. Emphasis on research and community oral health promotion programs that will result in decreasing incidence and prevalence rates of oral diseases and conditions for the entire population as well as special emphasis on populations at high risk for these conditions
L. Need for creative solutions to meet increasing demands for dental care personnel during a period of natural retirement of an older dental profession; decreasing numbers of dental schools and dental assisting programs; increasing numbers of dental hygiene programs and emergence of mid-level oral health care practitioners to improve access to care for underserved populations
M. The need to increase measures to ensure oral health and access to care for children by correcting inadequate government policies; for example, increasing Medicaid funding, implementing school sealant programs, and fluoridating community water supplies, all of which could make dramatic differences in the oral health of children[69]
N. The increasing complexity of the oral health care delivery system because of the numerous, multifaceted arrangements for delivering services and financing care, the changes in supply and distribution of provider personnel, and the varying laws from state to state regarding mid-level dental personnel
O. Funding and implementation of changes in response to the Health Care Reform Act passed in 2010

ETHICS

A. Ethics—guiding framework for professional decision making and subsequent actions to achieve outcomes related to improving community health (see Chapter 22)
   1. Applied to community as a "client";[70] weighing the needs of the individual and the community[71]
   2. Principles of social justice, common good, and human dignity, confidentiality, informed consent, nonmaleficence, beneficence, integrity and totality, competence and capacity, autonomy and surrogacy apply to community oral health practice[72-74]
   3. Encompass professionalism, personal and professional ethics, and the role of the profession and the educational system in the context of the greater society[71]
B. Ethical practices in action
   1. Focus by educational institutions to develop skilled, ethically and socially sensitive graduates committed to their professional obligation to community education and service
      a. Development and implementation of community-based models of education and service that may include alumni participation, local professional society participation, or both
      b. Commitment of educational institutions to incorporate community outreach activities as part of the professional curriculum; emphasis on a multi-disciplinary approach with other health care students and providers
      c. Reinforcement of a lifelong commitment to the professional codes of ethics (ADHA, ADA) that suggest an ethical obligation to community oral health and well-being

d. Development of strategies to develop cultural and linguistic competence through lifelong learning

e. Expansion of minority representation in the profession

f. Education of students about the career opportunities in federal, state, and local public health agencies and in other community organizations that provide oral health care services to various population groups (e.g., IHS, VA, local hospitals)

2. Develop mechanisms that encourage and support a perspective of social responsibility

a. Identification and development of mechanisms, such as scholarships and pay-back programs, to encourage minority and other health care providers to serve the underserved

b. Increasing knowledge and awareness of community oral health issues, best practices, skills, and resources by obtaining information from journals, conferences, seminars, Web sites, and other means

c. Promotion of evidence-informed decision making in relation to all aspects of community oral health practice, including scientific bases for disease control and prevention, as well as application of tested theories of organization, health promotion, and health education

d. Setting standards of ethical conduct that reflects social responsibility to the community through oral health promotion, education, and practice

3. Focus of individual practitioners on social responsibility in their dental hygiene practice

a. Serve on advisory boards to community oral health programs

b. Volunteer in community service activities sponsored by local professional societies, educational institutions, and community organizations

c. Participate in, encourage the development of, and organize community outreach events through the private offices of employment

d. Commit to lifelong learning and evidence-based practice in relation to community oral health practice as well as clinical practice

e. Provide leadership in the solution of local public health problems to improve the oral health of the local community

@ WEB SITE INFORMATION AND RESOURCES

SOURCE	WEB SITE ADDRESS	DESCRIPTION
American Dental Hygienists' Association, Smoking Cessation Initiative	http://www.askadviserefer.org	Resource for practitioners for information on smoking cessation
Association of State and Territorial Dental Directors	http://www.astdd.org	Access to state and territorial public health agencies of the United States, U.S. territories, and the District of Columbia; engaged in legislative, scientific, educational, and programmatic issues and activities on behalf of public health; makes recommendations for current, effective community oral health programming
National Maternal and Child Oral Health Resource Center	http://www.mchoralhealth.org/index.php	A variety of resources to develop community oral health programs for young children, including publications, "how-to" guides, tool boxes, Head Start information, and grants
U.S. Department of Health and Human Services, Office of Disease Prevention and Health Promotion, Healthy People initiative	http://www.healthypeople.gov	Overview of *Healthy People 2020*, history and development, objectives, baseline measures, target outcomes, suggestions for interventions and resources, and methods to measure outcomes
World Health Organization	http://www.who.int	Oral health resource for information on international programs and health status of people in various countries
Advancing Oral Health in America	http://www.iom.ed/Reports/2011/Advancing-Oral-Health-in_America.aspx	Comprehensive report by the federal government on how to improve oral health in the U.S.

REFERENCES

1. World Health Organization: Health action in crisis: definitions: Available at http://www.who.int/hac/about/definitions/en/: Accessed August 16, 2010.
2. World Health Organization: The determinants of health, 2010: Available at http://www.who.int/hia/evidence/doh/en/: Accessed October 7, 2010.
3. Winslow, CE: The untitled field of public health, Mod Med 2:183, 1920. In Geurink KV, editor: *Community oral health practice for the dental hygienist*, ed 2, St Louis, 2012, Saunders.
4. American Board of Dental Public Health: Guidelines for graduate education in dental public health, Ann Arbor, MI: Author, 1970. In Nathe CN, editor: *Dental public health and research*, ed 3, Upper Saddle River, NJ, 2011, Pearson.
5. Association of State and Territorial Dental Directors: *Guidelines for state and territorial oral health programs* [revised 2010]: Available at http://www.astdd.org/state-guidelines/: Accessed August 26, 2010.
6. U.S. Department of Health and Human Services: *Oral health in America: A report of the Surgeon General.* Rockville, MD, 2000, Author: Available at http://www.surgeongeneral.gov/library/oralhealth/: Accessed March 10, 2010.
7. U.S. Department of Health and Human Services: *A national call to action to promote oral health, NIH Publication No. 03-5303*, Rockville, MD, Spring 2003, U.S. Department of Health and Human Services, Public Health Service, National Institutes of Health, National Institute of Dental and Craniofacial Research.
8. U.S. Department of Health and Human Services: Healthy People 2020: Available at http://www.healthypeople.gov/2020/: Accessed April 7, 2011.
9. U.S. Department of Health and Human Services: Healthy People 2010: Available at http://www.healthypeople.gov/2010: Accessed April 7, 2011.
10. Beatty CF: Oral epidemiology. In Nathe CN, editor: *Dental public health and research*, ed 3, Upper Saddle River, NJ, 2011, Pearson.
11. U.S. Department of Health and Human Services: Healthy People 2010 mid-course review, 2007: Available at http://www.healthypeople.gov/data/midcourse/default.htm: Accessed March 15, 2010.
12. Centers for Disease Control and Prevention: National Health and Nutrition Examination Survey, July 21, 2009: Available at http://www.cdc.gov/nchs/nhanes.htm: Accessed October 7, 2010.
13. Hackshaw A, Paul E, Davenport E: *Evidence-based dentistry: An introduction*, Hoboken, NJ, 2007, John Wiley.
14. Forrest JL, Miller SA: Evidence-based decision making. In Daniel SJ, Harfst SA, Wilder RS, editors: *Mosby's dental hygiene concepts, cases, and competencies*, ed 2, St Louis, 2008, Mosby.
15. Darby ML, Walsh MM: The dental hygiene profession. In Darby ML, Walsh MM, editors, *Dental hygiene theory and practice*, ed 3, St Louis, 2010, Saunders.
16. Library of the Health Sciences, University of Illinois at Chicago: Evidence-based dentistry: Available at http://ebp.lib.uic.edu/dentistry/?q=node/12: Accessed September 24, 2010.
17. Dye BA, et al: Trends in oral health status, United States, 1988–1994 and 1999–2004. National Center for Health Statistics, *Vital Health Stat* Series 11(248):1–92, 2007: Available at http://www.cdc.gov/nchs/data/series/sr_11/sr11_248.pdf: Accessed October 7, 2010.
18. American Association of Pediatric Dentistry: Policy on early childhood caries classifications, consequences, and preventive strategies, 2008: Available at http://www.aapd.org/media/Policies_Guidelines/P_ECCClassifications.pdf: Accessed August 28, 2010.
19. KIDS COUNT: Rhode Island kids count factbook, 2010: Available at http://www.rikidscount.org/matriarch/documents/10_Factbook_Indicator_18.pdf: Accessed October 7, 2010.
20. U.S. Department of Health and Human Services, Centers for Disease Control: Trends in oral health status United States, 1988–1994 and 1999–2004. *Vital Health Stat*, Series 11, Number 248, April 2007: Available at http://www.cdc.gov/nchs/data/series/sr_11/sr11_248.pdf: Accessed September 23, 2010.
21. U.S. Department of Health and Human Services, Centers for Disease Control, National Center for Chronic Disease Prevention and Health Promotion, Division of Oral Health: National oral health surveillance system oral health indicators, 2010: Available at http://www.cdc.gov/nohss/: Accessed September 23, 2010.
22. Proffit WR, Fields HW, Moray LJ: Prevalence of malocclusion and orthodontic treatment need in the United States: Estimates from the NHANES III survey, *Int J Adult Orthodon Orthognath Surg* 13(2):97–106, 1998.
23. U.S. Department of Health and Human Services, Centers for Disease Control and Prevention: Promoting oral health: Interventions for preventing dental caries, oral and pharyngeal cancers, and sports-related craniofacial injuries, November 30, 2001, Vol. 50, No. RR-21: Available from http://www.cdc.gov/mmwr/PDF/rr/rr5021.pdf: Accessed September 23, 2010.
24. American Dental Association, Councils of Access, Prevention and Interprofessional Relations, and Scientific Affairs: Using mouthguards to reduce the incidence and severity of sports-related oral injuries, *J Am Dent Assoc* 137(12):1712–1720, 2006.
25. Farrell C: TMJ disorder and orthodontics, *Dent Tribune*, April 20, 2010: Available at http://www.dental-tribune.com/: Accessed October 7, 2010.
26. Franzman MR: Fluoride dentifrice ingestion and fluorosis of the permanent incisors, *J Am Dent Assoc* 137(5):645–652, 2006.
27. Young DA, Featherstone JDB, Budenz AW: Dental caries and caries management. In Daniel SJ, Harfst SA, Wilder RS, editors: *Mosby's dental hygiene concepts, cases, and competencies*, St Louis, 2008, Mosby.
28. U.S. Department of Health and Human Services: Community water fluoridation: Frequently asked questions: Available at http://www.cdc.gov/fluoridation/: Accessed August 29, 2010.
29. Texas Department of State Health Services: Happy child, bright smile fluoride varnish manual, Publication #E08-13077, December 2009. Available at http://www.

dshs.state.tx.us/dental/default.shtm: Accessed September 23, 2010.

30. Darby ML: Caries management: Fluoride, chlorhexidine, xylitol, and amorphous calcium phosphate therapies. In Darby ML, Walsh MM, editors: *Dental hygiene theory and practice*, ed 3, St Louis, 2010, Saunders.

31. Jenson L, Budenz AW, Featherstone JD, Ramos-Gomez FJ, Spolsky VW, Young DA: Clinical protocols for caries management by risk assessment, *CDA J* 35(10):714–723, 2007: Available at http://www.cda.org/library/cda_member/pubs/journal/jour1007/jenson.pdf: Accessed September 24, 2010.

32. Yengopal V, Mickenautsch S: Caries preventive effect of casein phosphopeptide-amorphous calcium phosphate (CPP-ACP): A meta-analysis, *Acta Odontol Scand* 21:321–332, 2009.

33. Bertness J, Holt K, editors: *Dental sealants: A resource guide*, ed 3, Washington, D.C., 2010, National Maternal and Child Oral Health Resource Center: Available at http://www.mchoralhealth.org/: Accessed October 7, 2010.

34. Young DA, Buchanan PM, Lubman RG, Badway NN: New directions in interorganizational collaboration in dentistry: The CAMBRA coalition model, *J Dent Edu* 71(5):595–600, 2007.

35. Ramos-Gomez FJ, Crall J, Gansky SA, Slayton RL, Featherstone JD: Caries risk assessment appropriate for the age 1 visit (infants and toddlers), *CDA J* 35(10):687–702, 2007.

36. Association of State and Territorial Dental Directors: Proven and promising best practices for state and community oral health programs, 2010: Available at http://www.astdd.org/best-practices/: Accessed September 23, 2010.

37. National Maternal and Child Oral Health Resource Center: *A guide for developing and enhancing community oral health programs*: Available at http://www.aacdp.com/Guide/: Accessed September 1, 2010.

38. Tomar SL: Planning and evaluating community oral health programs, *Dent Clin N Am* 52(2):403–421, 2008.

39. Hollister MC: Health education and promotion theories. In Harris NO, Garcia-Godoy F, Nathe CN, editors: *Primary preventive dentistry*, ed 7, Upper Saddle River, NJ, 2009, Pearson.

40. Darby DL, Darby ML: Cross-cultural practice. In Darby ML, Walsh MM, editors: *Dental hygiene theory and practice*, ed 3, Philadelphia, 2010, Saunders.

41. Dickinson A: Community oral health education. In Mason, J, editor: *Concepts in dental public health*, ed 2, Philadelphia, 2010, Lippincott, Williams & Wilkins.

42. Gagliardi L: *Dental health education lesson planning and implementation*, ed 2, Upper Saddle River, NJ, 2007, Pearson Prentice Hall.

43. Nnolim N: Understanding the traits of adult learners, February 4, 2010: Available at http://www.suite101.com/educationandcareer: Accessed September 24, 2010.

44. Andrulis DP, Brach C: Integrating literacy, culture, and language to improve health care quality for diverse populations, *Am J Health Behav* 31(Suppl 1):S122–S133, 2007.

45. Young learner characteristics, November 15, 2008: Available at http://knol.google.com/k/young-learner-characteristics#: Accessed September 24, 2010.

46. Beatty CF: Biostatistics. In Nathe CN: *Dental public health and research*, ed 3, Upper Saddle River, NJ, 2011, Pearson.

47. Nathe CN: *Dental public health and research*, ed 3, Upper Saddle River, NJ, 2011, Pearson.

48. Nathe CN, McKinney BE, Beatty CF: Research approaches and designs. In Nathe CN, editor: *Dental public health and research*, ed 3, Upper Saddle River, NJ, 2011, Pearson.

49. American Dental Hygienists Association (ADHA): Minnesota passes legislation allowing mid-level oral health provider, May 18, 2009: Available at http://www.adha.org/media/releases/05182009_MN_mid-level.htm: Accessed September 24, 2010.

50. Kaiser Family Foundation Web site: Available at http://www.statehealthfacts.org/comparemaptable.jsp?ind=691&cat=8: Accessed September 27, 2010.

51. American Dental Association Web site: Available at http://www.ada.org: Accessed January 15, 2010.

52. ADEA: Dental Health Professions Shortage Areas [data from Health Resources and Services Administration], March 31, 2009: Available at http://www.adea.org/policy_advocacy/federal_legislative_regulatory_resources/Pages/DentalHealthProfessionsShortageAreas.aspx: Accessed September 27, 2010.

53. Carlisle LD: The gender shift, the demographics of women in dentistry: What impact will it have? ADA, Survey Center, n.d. Available at http://www.spiritofcaring.com/public/488.cfm: Accessed September 27, 2010.

54. American Dental Association: 2008–09 Survey of dental education academic programs, enrollment, and graduates—Volume 1, February 2010: Available at http://www.ada.org/sections/professionalResources/pdfs/survey_ed_vol1.pdf: Accessed September 25, 2010.

55. American Dental Hygienists' Association, Division of Education: Dental hygiene education facts, April 2010: Available at http://www.adha.org/downloads/edu/dh_ed_fact_sheet.pdf: Accessed September 25, 2010.

56. Moulton WB: New trend in dental school applications, Mesquite, NV, *Desert Valley Times*: Available at http://moultonddsmesquite.com/wordpress/?p=179: Accessed September 25, 2010.

57. U.S. Department of Labor, Bureau of Labor Statistics: Occupational outlook handbook, 2010–2011 Edition, December 17, 2009: Available at http://www.bls.gov/oco/ocos072.htm: Accessed September 27, 2010.

58. American Dental Hygienists' Association (ADHA): Survey of dental hygienists in the United States: Executive summary, 2007: Available at http://www.adha.org/research/index.html: Accessed October 15, 2010.

59. American Dental Hygienists' Association Web site: Available at http://www.adha.org: Accessed September 15, 2010.

60. American Dental Association, ADA Survey Center: 2008–09 survey of allied dental education. Chicago: Author, November 2009: Available at http://www.ada.org/sections/professionalResources/pdfs/survey_allied.pdf: Accessed September 27, 2010.

61. Onik E: Missing persons: African Americans in dental hygiene, *J Dent Hyg* 83(2):62–69, 2009: Available at http://findarticles.com/p/articles/mi_hb6368/is_2_83/ai_n39302210/?tag=content;col1: Accessed September 27, 2010.

62. Texas Health and Human Services Commission: CHIP/Children's Medicaid: Available at http://www.chipmedicaid.org/: Accessed March 10, 2010.

63. U.S. Census Bureau: Income, poverty, and health insurance coverage in the United States: 2008, September, 2009: Available at http://www.census.gov/prod/2009pubs/p60-236.pdf: Accessed January 30, 2010.

64. U.S. Department of Health and Human Services, Centers for Medicare and Medicaid Services: 2008 National dental summary, January 2009: Available at http://www.cms.hhs.gov/MedicaidDentalCoverage/Downloads/natdensum011209.pdf: Accessed March 10, 2010.

65. U.S. Department of Health and Human Services, Centers for Medicare and Medicaid Services: Children's Health Insurance Program: Available at http://www.cms.hhs.gov/home/chip.asp: Accessed March 10, 2010.

66. American Dental Association: ADA current policies 1954–2008, 2009: Available at http://www.ada.org/prof/resources/positions/doc_policies.pdf: Accessed March 10, 2010.

67. Association of Managed Care Dentists Web site: Available at http://www.amcd.org/: Accessed March 12, 2010.

68. Davis EL, Stewart DC, Guelmann M, et al: Serving the public good: Challenges of dental education in the twenty-first century, *J Dent Educ* 71(8):1009–1019, 2007: Available at http://www.jdentaled.org/cgi/reprint/71/8/1009: Accessed October 7, 2010.

69. Pew Charitable Trusts: Pew report finds majority of states fail to ensure proper dental health and access to care for children, February 23, 2010: Available at http://www.pewtrusts.org/news_room_detail.aspx?id=57449: Accessed September 27, 2010.

70. American Dental Hygienists' Association: Code of ethics, June 28, 2010: Available at http://www.adha.org/downloads/ADHA-Bylaws-Code-of-Ethics.pdf: Accessed October 7, 2010.

71. Public Health Leadership Society: Principles of the ethical practice of public health, version 2.2, 2002: Available at http://www.apha.org/about/: Accessed October 12, 2010.

72. Munte C: The goals of public health: An integrated, multidimensional model, *Public Health Ethics* 1(1):39–52, 2008: Available at http://phe.oxfordjournals.org/content/1/1/39.full: Accessed October 12, 2010.

73. Zarkowski P: Ethical principles. In Mason J, editor: *Concepts in dental public health*, ed 2, Philadelphia, 2010, Lippincott Williams & Wilkins.

74. Ascension Health: Key ethical principles, 2009: Available at http://www.ascensionhealth.org/: Accessed October 12, 2010.

SUGGESTED READINGS

Association of State and Territorial Dental Directors: Best practices for state oral health programs and guidelines for state and territorial oral health programs, 2010: Available at http://www.astdd.org/: Accessed September 23, 2010.

CDC, National Center for Chronic Disease Prevention and Health Promotion, Division of Oral Health: National oral health surveillance system oral health indicators, 2010: Available at http://www.cdc.gov/nohss/: Accessed September 23, 2010.

Darby DL, Darby ML: Cross-cultural practice. In Darby ML, Walsh MM, editors: *Dental hygiene theory and practice*, ed 3, Philadelphia, 2010, Saunders.

Darby ML: Caries management: Fluoride, chlorhexidine, xylitol, amorphous calcium phosphate therapies. In Darby ML, Walsh MM, editors: *Dental hygiene theory and practice*, ed 3, Philadelphia, 2010, Saunders.

Gagliardi L: *Dental health education: Lesson planning and implementation*, ed 2, Upper Saddle River, NJ, 2007, Pearson Prentice Hall.

Hollister MC: Health education and promotion theories. In Harris NO, Garcia-Godoy F, Nathe CN, editors: *Primary preventive dentistry*, ed 7, Upper Saddle River, NJ, 2009, Pearson.

IOM (Institute of Medicine): *Advancing Oral Health in America*, Washington, D.C., 2011, The National Academies Press.

Jenson, L, Budenz AW, Featherstone JD, Ramos-Gomez FJ, Spolsky VW, Young DA: Clinical protocols for caries management by risk assessment, *CDA J* 35(10):714–723, 2007. Available at http://www.cda.org/library/cda_member/pubs/journal/jour1007/jenson.pdf: Accessed September 24, 2010.

Mason J: *Concepts in dental public health*, ed 2, Philadelphia, 2010, Lippincott Williams & Wilkins.

Nathe CN: *Dental public health and research*, ed 3, Upper Saddle River, NJ, 2011, Pearson.

National Maternal and Child Oral Health Resource Center: A guide for developing and enhancing community oral health programs: Available at http://www.aacdp.com/Guide/: Accessed September 1, 2010.

U.S. Department of Health and Human Services: Healthy People 2010 mid-course review, 2007: Available at http://www.healthypeople.gov/publications/: Accessed September 26, 2010.

Christine French Beatty and the publisher acknowledge the past contribution of Pamela Zarkowski to this chapter.

CHAPTER 20 REVIEW QUESTIONS

Answers and rationales to Review Questions are available on this text's accompanying Evolve site. See inside front cover for details.
Use Testlet A to answer questions 1 to 5.

TESTLET A

You have been employed as a public health dental hygienist in a local health department to provide educational presentations for the participants in the WIC (Women, Infant, and Child) program in a nonfluoridated community. The natural fluoride concentration of the community water supply is 0.3 ppm F. One of your first assignments is to present an educational program on basic oral health practices for culturally diverse pregnant teens in three alternative high schools that have day-care facilities

1. **Which of the following roles of the dental hygienist is illustrated by this activity?**
   a. Administrator
   b. Advocate
   c. Clinician
   d. Educator

2. **How much additional fluoride would be required to bring the fluoride concentration of the water supply to the optimal level?**
   a. 0.7 ppm F
   b. 1 ppm F
   c. 0.4 to 0.9 ppm F
   d. 0.7 to 1.2 ppm F

3. **What would be the first step in conducting this program?**
   a. Develop a lesson plan for the educational session for the pregnant teens
   b. Meet with the people involved to determine program goals and objectives
   c. Plan an educational presentation for the day-care children

   d. Request funding for oral hygiene supplies from the local health department
   e. Select teaching strategies for the educational program

4. **Which index would be BEST to determine the rate of pregnancy gingivitis in this population?**
   a. CPI
   b. CPITN
   c. GI
   d. PSR

5. **Which of the following agencies would be the BEST resource for program planning for this population?**
   a. National Maternal and Child Oral Health Resource Center
   b. U.S. Department of Health and Human Services (DHHS) Center for Medicare and Medicaid
   c. U.S. Public Health Service
   d. U.S. DHHS Human Resources and Services Administration

Use Testlet B to answer questions 6 to 11.

TESTLET B

The director of the Vintage Retirement Center contacts the local dental hygienists' society to provide a seminar on oral health. The facility has a population of 100 well residents between the ages of 60 and 78 years who have a middle SES. Twenty percent of the residents are edentulous, and the remaining 80% have varying numbers of teeth present. The oral health assessment results revealed a mean PlI of 2.1, mean DMFT of 5.2, mean D of 0, RCI of 2.1, and untreated root caries of 1.5. Correlation analysis revealed a correlation coefficient of $r = +0.81$ for the relationship between the RCI and PlI in this group. Seventy percent of the residents have a dental home and report having regular dental care. Less than 10% of them report mild signs and symptoms of xerostomia.

6. **What relationship does the correlation between the RCI and PlI demonstrate between root caries and plaque biofilm in this target population?**
   a. Moderate positive
   b. Strong negative
   c. Strong positive
   d. Weak negative
   e. Weak positive

7. **All of the following are established potential risk factors for root caries in this population EXCEPT one. Which one is the EXCEPTION?**
   a. Diabetes and heart disease
   b. Medications
   c. Plaque biofilm accumulation
   d. Smoking
   e. Xerostomia

8. **What level of oral hygiene is revealed by the mean PlI?**
   a. No plaque present
   b. Slight plaque present
   c. Moderate plaque present
   d. Severe plaque present
   e. Cannot be determined from the information provided

9. **Which of the following programs should be planned to address one of the *Healthy People 2020* oral health objectives for this target population?**
   a. Denture marking and educational presentation on denture care
   b. Oral cancer screening and referral, as needed
   c. Referral to a Medicaid provider for dental treatment
   d. Screening of periodontal condition and referral, as needed
   e. Treatment with fluoride varnish to control dentinal hypersensitivity

10. **Which of the following is the MOST precise instructional objective for the seminar?**
    a. Residents will be able to explain the systemic–oral health connection
    b. Residents will be able to demonstrate correct toothbrushing, flossing, and use of other aids on a typodont
    c. Residents will be able to list in the correct order all steps of oral cancer self-assessment as they were presented in the seminar
    d. Residents will understand the importance of daily oral hygiene

11. **All of the following preventive programs are indicated by the assessment results EXCEPT one. Which one is the EXCEPTION?**
    a. Educational presentation on basic oral hygiene
    b. Referral for restorative treatment
    c. Use of a 0.12% chlorhexidine rinse daily
    d. Daily use of a higher concentration fluoride dentifrice

---

Use Testlet C to answer questions 12 to 17.

TESTLET C

A public health dental hygienist has been contacted by the local farm bureau because of a large number of worker absences caused by oral health issues. The population has low SES, is homogeneous, and does not have access to a community water supply. The hygienist decides to gather information via oral screenings conducted on a sample of the population. Findings indicate a mean DMFT score of 13.4, a mean OHI-S of 2.5, and a mean CPI of 3.1 with no clinical evidence of recession.

12. **Which sampling technique would be BEST to use to ensure a representative sample for this target population?**
    a. Convenience sampling
    b. Judgmental or purposive sampling
    c. Random sampling
    d. Stratified random sampling
    e. Systematic random sampling

13. **Which step of program planning is BEST represented when the hygienist conducts the oral screenings for this program?**
    a. Analysis of needs
    b. Collection of data
    c. Determination of priorities
    d. Implementation strategy development
    e. Program evaluation

14. **What is the BEST interpretation of the reported CPI score of 3.1?**
    a. The average score of the population was 3.1
    b. The majority of scores were within 3.1 of the mean
    c. The middle score was 3.1
    d. The most commonly occurring score was 3.1
    e. The range of scores was 0 to 3.1

15. **What is the first line of defense to prevent future caries in this population?**
    a. Daily exposure to low-dose topical fluoride
    b. High-concentration professional fluoride applications every 6 months
    c. Pit-and-fissure sealants
    d. Water fluoridation

16. **What change in the DMFT scores would indicate that the needs are being met 5 years after implementation of a program?**
    a. A decrease in the total DMFT score
    b. A decrease in D, increase in F, and no change in M
    c. An increase in F, decrease in M, and no change in D
    d. An increase in F, increase in M, and no change in D

17. **After a program is in place, the oral health indicators are monitored for 5 years. Which term BEST describes any new dental caries resulting in an increase in DMFT 5 years later?**
    a. Count
    b. Incidence
    c. Prevalence
    d. Proportion
    e. Rate

Use Testlet D to answer questions 18 to 26.

TESTLET D

The director of a local nursing home has approached a public health dental hygienist to design an oral health protocol for the 300 residents. Currently, a registered nurse is performing the intake oral examination, and the nursing home has an "on call" dentist. The majority of residents are partially edentulous, have partial removable dentures, and require assistance with daily hygiene practices. The caregivers state that the residents have severe halitosis, trouble eating, and frequently lose their removable partial dentures. The dental hygienist observes that the caregivers are neglecting daily oral hygiene care and are not expected to conduct oral cancer screenings. On the basis of these observations, the dental hygienist determines to carry out oral hygiene and oral cancer screening of all residents and introduce an educational component to be used by the facility's caregivers and interested family members. Flashlights, disposable mouth mirrors, masks, gloves, protective eyewear, and 2 × 2 gauze are required for the screening. The educational component will consist of six weekly 1-hour sessions and will focus on knowledge of the risk of oral cancer, the benefits of periodic oral screenings, recognition of signs and symptoms of common oral lesions, daily oral hygiene care, and other oral health procedures to meet the needs of the residents. A pretest and post-test will be used to evaluate change in knowledge.

18. **Which of the following would be an effective teaching strategy to raise the caregivers' value of oral hygiene?**
    a. Demonstrate proper oral hygiene procedures
    b. Lecture on the importance of oral hygiene
    c. Show them pictures of oral cancer
    d. Train them in personal oral hygiene skills

19. **What type of study is represented by evaluating the change of knowledge as a result of the educational component?**
    a. Case control
    b. Correlational
    c. Pretest/post-test
    d. Time series

20. **How can you determine the caregivers' compliance with providing daily oral hygiene care for the residents?**
    a. Assess a change in the values of caregivers by conducting focus groups
    b. Assess the caregivers' knowledge with a post-test
    c. Measure the plaque and gingivitis scores of residents over time
    d. Observe the caregivers' ability to brush correctly at the last session
    e. Survey the beliefs and attitudes of caregivers with a questionnaire

21. **Which of the following would be the BEST use of the dental hygienist in this program?**
    a. Conduct an educational program over daily oral hygiene care for the residents
    b. Make available dental hygiene services for the residents using portable equipment
    c. Present an in-service training program to the nursing home staff
    d. Provide daily oral hygiene care for the residents in their rooms

22. **What type of data are being collected with the screening?**
    a. Qualitative and primary
    b. Qualitative and secondary
    c. Quantitative and primary
    d. Quantitative and secondary

23. **If the data reveal lesions that have not been identified previously, the dental hygienist plans to work with the director of nursing to establish a new protocol for routine oral cancer screening by the registered nurses on staff. What core public health function would this exemplify?**
    a. Assessment
    b. Assurance
    c. Policy development
    d. Tertiary prevention

24. **What is the BEST method of evaluating the caregivers' ability to conduct oral cancer screening on completion of the educational program?**
    a. Administer a post-test over the cancer screening procedure
    b. Interview the residents about the caregivers' technique
    c. Observe the caregivers conducting oral cancer screening
    d. Survey the family members about the caregivers' technique

25. **The success of the program is evaluated by screening the residents again a year later to identify any lesions that have not been found previously. What type of study would this exemplify?**
    a. Cross-over
    b. Prospective
    c. Retrospective
    d. Time series

26. **What would be the BEST measure of the success of the program?**
a. Administrative support for the program
b. Improved oral health indicators of the residents
c. Increased availability of oral hygiene supplies for use by the residents
d. Increased oral health knowledge of the staff

Use Testlet E to answer questions 27 to 31.

TESTLET E

A high dental caries rate has been reported by the school nurses in Kern County Head Start children on the basis of the rate of toothaches and absences. The families are primarily Spanish-speaking Hispanic and East Indian migrant farm workers. They reside in predominantly rural settings with individual well water supplies. A team of dental hygiene students from the local college has been asked to design a comprehensive program to address the problem of dental caries in this population. They begin by collecting baseline data using the deft, OHI-S, and GI.

27. **Which of the following is indicated by the e component of the def index as used in this program?**
a. A decayed surface
b. A decayed tooth
c. A tooth that needs to be extracted because of the severity of decay
d. A tooth that has been extracted because of decay
e. A tooth that has naturally exfoliated

28. **At an informational meeting, the dental hygiene coordinator introduces the goal of the program to the Head Start family advocates. Which of the following would be MOST appropriate to explain during this session?**
a. The benefits of community water fluoridation
b. The cause of early childhood caries
c. The effectiveness of daily brushing
d. The value of healthy food choices

29. **All of the following EXCEPT one would be an appropriate source of funding for this program. Which one is the EXCEPTION?**
a. CHIP
b. Head Start grant
c. Medicare
d. Medicaid
e. Private funding from a local foundation

30. **Which preventive program is indicated for this target population?**
a. Distribution of fluoridated dentifrice
b. Fluoride varnish
c. Pit-and-fissure sealants
d. Water fluoridation

31. **On the basis of the baseline OHI-S scores, the dental hygiene students present oral hygiene education programs to the Head Start children, staff, and parents. Which index would be appropriate to evaluate the improvement in the children's oral hygiene as a result of these programs?**
a. OHI-S
b. PHP
c. PlI
d. Any of the above would be appropriate

Use Testlet F to answer questions 32 to 37.

TESTLET F

Dental hygiene students from a local program visit a geriatric day care called Camp Sunshine to implement a service learning project. These campers are functionally independent, although they are medically compromised. Under faculty supervision, the students screen the seniors to identify denture cleanliness and teach them how to clean their dentures daily. The goals are to improve their oral health by cleaning their dentures or partial dentures, increase their awareness of the need for daily oral care, and empower them to clean their dentures. The students compute the mean scores of the denture cleanliness measure for future evaluation of the program outcomes.

32. The program had to be rescheduled because of a sudden increase in absences from the camp—a large number of participants came down with the flu that week. Which of the following terms BEST describes this flu situation?
a. Cluster
b. Endemic
c. Epidemic
d. Occurrence
e. Pandemic

33. Which of the following is an ethical responsibility of the students and faculty who are implementing this program?
a. Communicate oral findings to the staff of the facility
b. Prepare a formal report of findings to submit to the health department
c. Refer clients who have suspicious lesions identified during the program
d. Take the dentures back to the dental hygiene clinic to clean them more thoroughly

34. What is the purpose of the screening for denture cleanliness?
a. To collect data requested by the Camp Sunshine administrative staff
b. To give students practice in the techniques of screening
c. To individualize the education provided
d. To motivate the clients

35. What is the BEST teaching method for this program?
a. Demonstration
b. Guided practice
c. Lecture
d. A video presentation

36. To evaluate the success of the program, the students return in 6 months to measure denture cleanliness. What statistic would be used to compare the mean baseline and post-test scores of denture cleanliness?
a. Analysis of variance (ANOVA)
b. Chi-square
c. Correlation coefficient
d. t test

37. The next class of students volunteers to repeat the program with a new group of campers. The students decide to request that Camp Sunshine provide funding for supplies to conduct the program. They prepare a proposal to submit to the camp director. What is the BEST way for the students to communicate the positive quantitative outcomes of the previous program to the camp director in an easy-to-understand format?
a. Discuss the results at a meeting in which they provide a written proposal of the funding request
b. Include in the written proposal a list of the campers with their baseline and post-test cleanliness scores
c. Include in the written proposal tables and graphs that summarize the pretest and post-test denture cleanliness data
d. Write a few paragraphs in the proposal that describe the statistical analysis of the pretest and post-test denture cleanliness data

Use Testlet G to answer questions 38 to 45.

TESTLET G

A local dental hygienists' association and a local faith-based organization collaborate to target a school in a nonfluoridated area for a comprehensive oral disease prevention program. The school serves a population that consists of 50% Medicaid-eligible children, and 75% of them are on the school lunch program. The ethnic group representation is 15% Hispanic American, 5% African American, and 80% non-Hispanic white. The community water supply naturally contains 0.3 ppm F. Children in grades 2 and 6 are screened annually by a public health dentist who uses a mirror, an explorer, and dental light. Preschool and grade K children are screened twice a year with a tongue blade and light. Data for 2011 indicate a 20% urgent decay rate across all ages. A sealant program is conducted in grades 2 and 6, and a fluoride varnish program is conducted with the preschoolers and grade K, including two applications annually. A pizza party is planned for each classroom that has a 100% return rate of parental consent forms for the sealant and fluoride varnish programs. Educational presentations are made in classrooms and with parent groups twice a year. Three portable dental units are borrowed from the regional office of the state health department to conduct the program. The program is funded with a grant and staffed with volunteer hygienists and students from a local dental hygiene program.

38. **Which of the following is a required action for this program?**
    a. Phone call to each family to describe the program
    b. Presence of a dentist while the fluoride varnish is placed by hygienists
    c. Radiographs before placing sealants
    d. Written informed consent form signed by parents or legal guardians of all children who participate

39. **What assessment classification is done with pre-schoolers and grade K in this program?**
    a. Type I
    b. Type II
    c. Type III
    d. Type IV

40. **What would have been the BEST index to identify the reported decay rate?**
    a. Basic Screening Survey (BSS)
    b. deft
    c. DMFT
    d. RCI

41. **The same education materials can be used with participants in the other schools in the district BECAUSE the cultural diversity of this population represents the cultural diversity of the general population of the United States**
    a. Both the statement and reason are correct and related
    b. Both the statement and reason are correct but NOT related
    c. The statement is correct, but the reason is NOT
    d. The statement is NOT correct but the reason is correct
    e. NEITHER the statement NOR the reason is correct

42. **What is the basis for deciding to target this school with this program?**
    a. Convenience
    b. Cultural diversity of the school
    c. Random selection of the school
    d. SES of the children in the school

43. **Which factor should be considered to determine the optimal level of water fluoridation for this community?**
    a. Children's decay rate
    b. SES of the target population
    c. The average daily air temperature
    d. The brand of dentifrice used by the population
    e. The current level of fluoride in the water supply

44. **What would be the first step to organize a fluoridation campaign for this community?**
    a. Contact key community leaders to obtain a broad base of support for fluoridation
    b. Organize a massive community educational program about the benefits and safety of fluoridation
    c. Schedule a referendum to allow the citizens to express their opinion about fluoridation
    d. Testify before the city council to convince them to fluoridate the water

45. **Which of the following programs has the HIGHEST priority to further meet the needs of this population?**
    a. Conduct a daily classroom fluoride rinse program
    b. Establish dental homes and refer children for treatment
    c. Make plans to implement school water fluoridation
    d. Plan a health fair for children and their families

Use Testlet H to answer questions 46 to 50.

TESTLET H

A dental hygiene U.S. Public Health Services (USPHS)–commissioned core officer is assigned to an Indian Health Service (IHS) clinic to improve the oral care of pregnant women in an American Indian rural community with a population of 26,000. Approximately 20% of the pregnant women in this population develop gestational diabetes. When a woman first sees the physician in the clinic for prenatal care, she is referred to the dental clinic for a dental examination. Only 25% of the patients referred over the previous 6 months complied with the dental referral, scheduled an appointment, and received treatment. As a result of this, the community is not classified a dental manpower shortage area. A survey of the pregnant women served by this clinic reveals poor health literacy, that is, the women do not realize their risk for diabetes, are unaware of the relationship between oral health status and diabetes, and do not understand the benefits of an oral health assessment in relation to their overall health and the health of their babies.

46. **Which would be the BEST intervention to implement first to increase compliance with the dental referral?**
    a. Conduct a mailing program to remind pregnant women to schedule an appointment for a dental examination
    b. Develop an oral health screening program to be implemented during prenatal care visits
    c. Develop written educational materials for distribution during prenatal visits
    d. Document the oral condition of the women who have complied and received a dental examination
    e. Plan an educational presentation for the pregnant women on the relationship among oral health, systemic health, and the risks and consequences of diabetes

47. **On the basis of the results of the survey, which health education theory is indicated as the foundation for an oral health education intervention to improve compliance with the dental referral?**
    a. Health Belief Model
    b. Learning Ladder
    c. Social Cognitive Theory
    d. Theory of Reasoned Action
    e. Transtheoretical Model Stages of Change

48. **Lack of compliance with the dental referral could be a result of all the following factors EXCEPT one. Which one is the EXCEPTION?**
    a. Cost of dental care
    b. Lack of available appointments
    c. Lack of transportation to the dental clinic
    d. Low dentist-to-population ratio

49. **Which characteristic of public health is exemplified by the dental referral by the medical clinic?**
    a. Application of biostatistics to analyze population health problems
    b. Community rather than the individual as the client
    c. Multi-disciplinary team approach to solving public health problems
    d. Social responsibility for oral health

50. **For the purpose of discussing the problem and possible solutions, the dental hygienist arranges a meeting of the medical clinic director, the dental clinic director, the medicine man of the Indian tribe, and a dental clinic staff member who is a member of the tribe. Which theory of health promotion is exemplified by this action?**
    a. Community Organization
    b. Diffusion of Innovation
    c. Organizational Change
    d. Sense of Coherence

CHAPTER 21 Medical Emergencies

Heidi A. Schlei

Dental hygienists must be prepared to manage medical emergencies that may occur in the oral health care environment. Careful client observation and questioning during assessment will enable the dental hygienist to identify, prepare, and care for the client who experiences a medical complication. Knowledge of the principles of first aid, cardiopulmonary resuscitation (CPR), and basic life support is essential. Equally important is the ability to measure, assess, and record vital signs; recognize signs and symptoms of medical disorders; and prevent further complications through appropriate intervention.

GENERAL CONSIDERATIONS

A. Medical emergency
   1. A medical emergency means a client experiencing an unforeseen, immediate, health-related difficulty that is potentially life threatening
   2. Medical emergencies require prompt recognition and action by the dentist and the dental hygienist to maintain the client's health and, at times, life
B. Dental hygienist's legal responsibility
   1. To provide quality care according to the standards of practice
      a. According to the established standards of care, dental hygienists may be held liable if they are inadequately prepared for medical emergencies within the oral health care environment
      b. Standards require current training in medical emergency management and CPR
   2. To maintain complete records of medical emergencies in the health care setting
      a. Complete records describe the onset and management of the emergency, the client's vital signs, type of and response to treatment

performed, type and dose of drugs administered, and time treatment is rendered
      b. Complete records document the incident and protect the oral health care team in the event of legal action
C. Preventing medical emergencies
   1. A thorough health history reveals conditions that predispose a client to medical complications; the health history is taken at the first appointment and updated at each subsequent appointment
   2. Information obtained from the health history is used to modify the client's care plan and reduce the likelihood of the client experiencing a medical complication or emergency in the oral health care setting
   3. If more information regarding the client's health status is needed, the dentist or the dental hygienist should consult the client's general physician
   4. The assessment and documentation of the client's vital signs (generally blood pressure, body temperature, pulse, respiration rate) provide information regarding the client's health status
   5. The probability of a stress-induced medical emergency in the oral health care environment may be reduced by careful appointment planning, stress management protocol, good client rapport, and stress reducing premedication
D. Preparing for medical emergencies
   1. Every health care setting should maintain a basic medical emergency kit that is accessible to all treatment areas; staff should be familiar with the kit's contents and location
   2. Basic medical emergency kit (Table 21-1)
      a. Emergency drugs and equipment available in the oral health care setting should reflect the training of the dentist and the staff
      b. Drugs and equipment that the dentist, the dental hygienist, and the staff are not trained

TABLE 21-1 Basic Medical Emergency Kit*

Drug	Route	Indication	Comments
Oxygen	Inhaled (nasal cannula, face mask, bag–valve–mask)	Respiratory distress, cardiac disease	Do not use in hyperventilation
Aromatic ammonia	Inhaled	Syncope	
Nitroglycerin	Sublingual	Angina pectoris	No more than three doses in 15 minutes; may cause a drop in blood pressure
Epinephrine pen	Subcutaneous	Acute allergic reaction; acute bronchospasm (asthma)	
Bronchodilator (e.g., Albuterol)	Inhaled	Bronchospasm (asthma)	
Antihistamine (e.g., Benadryl)	Oral	Allergic reaction	May cause drowsiness in adults; may excite children
Glucose (nondiet soft drink; glucose tablet, honey sticks)	Oral	Hypoglycemia	
Aspirin	Oral (chewable)	Analgesic, antipyretic, anti-inflammatory	Potentiates bleeding problems

*The drugs and equipment available in the dental office should reflect the training of the dentist and the staff. Only drugs and equipment that the dentist, the dental hygienist, and the staff are trained to use should be included in the medical emergency kit.

to use should be excluded from the medical emergency kit contents

3. Each member of the dental staff should be currently certified in basic life support (BLS) and the recognition and management of common medical emergencies
4. Certain states may require dental hygienists to have successfully completed and to be current in BLS for license eligibility
5. Each oral health care team member should have delegated responsibilities in the event of a medical emergency; periodic staff drills are essential

VITAL SIGNS

Basic Concepts

A. Vital signs—the numerical values given to blood pressure, body temperature, pulse rate, respiration rate, and body height and weight
B. Vital signs and health history are used to determine a client's fitness to undergo oral health care
C. Abnormal values and significant findings should be brought to the attention of the dentist, the client, and the client's physician
D. Vital sign values (blood pressure, body temperature, pulse rate, respiration rate) should be recorded on the client's chart at each dental visit
E. Dental hygienists should explain the purpose of and the method for measuring vital signs to the client before initiating these procedures

Blood Pressure

A. Definition—force exerted by the blood on the walls of the blood vessels during the contraction and relaxation of the heart
1. Systolic pressure—force exerted during ventricular contraction (heart beat); the highest pressure in the cardiac cycle
2. Diastolic pressure—resting pressure; occurs during ventricular relaxation (heart rest) and is the lowest pressure of the cardiac cycle
3. Pulse pressure—value obtained when diastolic pressure is subtracted from systolic pressure
4. Hypertension—sustained, abnormally high blood pressure
5. Hypotension—sustained, abnormally low blood pressure
B. Factors that affect blood pressure values
1. Blood pressure depends on the heart's contractile force, peripheral vascular resistance, and vascular volume
2. Blood pressure may increase with age or in response to exercise, stress, certain medications, smoking, and illness
C. Normal values for adults and children
1. The client's blood pressure should be measured at each dental visit and recorded on the chart
2. Blood pressure is recorded as millimeters of mercury (mm Hg), with the systolic pressure over the diastolic pressure; systolic (mm Hg)/diastolic (mm Hg)

3. Properly calibrated and validated equipment should be used, with the client seated quietly for at least 5 minutes in a chair and the arm supported at chest level

4. Normal systolic values for adults are <120 mm Hg;

5. Normal diastolic values for adults are <80 mm Hg; older adults (≥70) may have normal values up to 90 mm Hg

6. Normal blood pressure values for children should also be <120 mm Hg systolic and <80 mm Hg; the values are adjusted for age, height, and gender

D. Abnormal values for adults and children

1. Prehypertension—values of 120 to 139 mm Hg (systolic) and 80 to 89 mm Hg (diastolic) are considered prehypertension; lifestyle changes that promote health are recommended; routine dental and dental hygiene care can proceed after assessment

2. Stage I hypertension—a systolic reading of 140 to 159 mm Hg, diastolic reading of 90 to 99 mm Hg, or both; should be rechecked at three consecutive appointments; if readings at all three appointments remain elevated, the client should be referred to a physician for further medical evaluation; dental and dental hygiene care can proceed after assessment or if the treatment is only routine

3. Stage II hypertension—a systolic reading of ≥160 mm Hg, a diastolic reading ≥100 mm Hg, or both; should be rechecked in 5 minutes; the decision to proceed with routine dental and dental hygiene care can be made based on this re-evaluation; stress-reduction protocol should be used; the client should be referred to a physician for further evaluation

4. Hypertensive crisis (emergency care needed) a systolic reading ≥180 mm Hg, a diastolic reading ≥110 mm Hg, or both; should be rechecked in 5 minutes; if still elevated, do not treat the patient. An immediate medical evaluation is recommended to assess for possible organ damage; activate the EMS if the person is experiencing chest pain, shortness of breath, back pain, numbness/weakness, changes in vision or difficulty speaking.

E. Measuring blood pressure

1. Equipment
   a. Sphygmomanometer—device used to measure blood pressure; consists of an inflatable cuff (available in different sizes), a central bladder, pressure gauge, tubing, bulb, and valve
   b. Cuff width should be 20% greater than the diameter of the upper arm (a cuff that is too

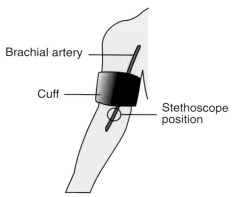

FIGURE 21-1 Stethoscope position for blood pressure measurement.

small will result in an artificially elevated blood pressure)
   c. Stethoscope is used to listen to the sounds of the blood as it passes through the brachial artery (Figure 21-1)

2. Technique—palpatory–auscultatory method
   a. The client is seated upright with an arm (palm up) at chest level and with legs uncrossed
   b. The cuff is placed snugly around the upper arm so that it is one inch above the antecubital fossa; the bladder of the sphygmomanometer is placed around the upper arm and thus on the brachial artery
   c. The radial artery is palpated, and the cuff is inflated until the radial pulse disappears; the cuff is then inflated by an additional 30 mm Hg
   d. The cuff is deflated at a rate of 2 to 3 mm Hg per second until the radial pulse returns; this value is the palpatory systolic pressure
   e. The diaphragm of the stethoscope is placed over the brachial artery; the stethoscope's earpieces are turned forward
   f. The cuff is inflated again to a level 30 mm Hg above the palpatory systolic pressure
   g. The cuff is deflated at a rate of 2 to 3 mm Hg per second
   h. The first sound heard through the stethoscope is the systolic blood pressure; Korotkoff sounds, which are vibrations of an artery under pressure, are heard through the stethoscope; the sound intensity decreases as the cuff pressure decreases
   i. The last distinct sound heard is the diastolic blood pressure
   j. Blood pressure is recorded as a fraction—systolic/diastolic; on the right or left arm; with the client standing or sitting

Body Temperature

A. Basic concepts
  1. Body temperature should be measured orally in the oral health care setting
  2. Body temperature of 99.5°F (orally measured) is considered elevated and may suggest the presence of infection or disease
  3. A client with an elevated temperature should see the dentist or the physician for further evaluation
B. Factors that affect body temperature
  1. Body temperature elevation may be caused by exercise, ingestion of hot food or drink, smoking, or a pathologic condition
  2. Body temperature may be decreased because of starvation or shock
  3. Body temperature may vary during the day
C. Normal values
  1. Normal oral temperature for an adult is 96.0° to 99.5°F (35.5° to 37.5°C); rectal temperature is approximately 0.5° to 0.7°F (0.27° to 0.38°C) higher than oral temperature; axillary temperature is 1.0°F less than oral temperature
  2. Values higher than 101°F may indicate an active disease process; values 99.5°F indicate a fever
D. Measuring body temperature
  1. Several different types of thermometers exist; most common are oral, rectal, and external thermometers; mercury, electronic, and chemical thermometers are available; disposable barriers decrease the risk of cross-contamination
  2. Oral thermometers are contraindicated for small children and unconscious or unstable clients
E. Technique for measuring body temperature with a mercury-column thermometer
  1. The thermometer should be shaken until the mercury level is below the mark indicating 96°F
  2. If the client has been eating, smoking, or drinking recently, the temperature should not be measured for 15 minutes
  3. The thermometer bulb is placed under the client's tongue for 3 minutes
  4. Temperature scale measurements are given at 0.2 (two tenths) of a degree; the highest temperature reading should be recorded
F. Conversion equations
  1. $°C = (°F - 32) \times 5/9$
  2. $°F = (°C \times 9/5) + 32$

Pulse

A. Basic concepts
  1. Pulse is the force of the blood through an artery created by the heart's contraction; each contraction creates a wave of blood that can be felt by

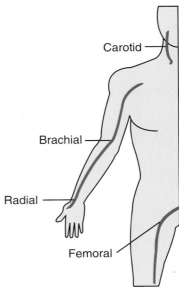

FIGURE 21-2 Location of pulse points.

gently pressing a superficial artery against underlying tissue
  2. Pulse is evaluated by rate (fast, slow), rhythm (regular, irregular), and quality (full or strong, thready or weak)
  3. Pulse rate is measured as the number of heart beats per minute
B. Factors that affect the pulse rate
  1. Pulse rate may increase because of exercise, certain drugs, anxiety, heat, eating, or disease
  2. Pulse rate may decrease because of sleep, certain drugs, fasting, or disease
C. Normal resting heart rate ranges
  1. Adult—60 to 100 beats per minute (beats/min)
  2. Infant—100 to 160 beats/min
  3. Child—80 to 120 beats/min
D. Determining the pulse rate
  1. Sites (Figure 21-2)
    a. Brachial pulse—located on the medial aspect of the antecubital fossa of the elbow
    b. Radial pulse—located on the lateral aspect of the wrist (thumb side) on the ventral surface
    c. Carotid pulse—located in the neck groove, just anterior to the sternocleidomastoid muscle
    d. Femoral pulse—located on the medial aspect of the upper thigh
  2. In nonemergency situations, the brachial or radial pulse is monitored; in emergency situations, the carotid pulse (which indicates that blood is flowing to the brain) is monitored; care is required in carotid palpation because vagal stimulation may occur, resulting in a decrease in blood pressure or syncope; also, it is important

not to palpate the carotid arteries simultaneously as one or both may be partially occluded

E. Technique for palpating the radial pulse
  1. The first three fingers are used to locate the radial pulse on the thumb side of the wrist
  2. Count the number of beats in 1 minute (pulse rate)
  3. Record the pulse rate, rhythm, and quality

Respiration Rate

A. Basic concepts
  1. Respiration is inspiration and expiration of air by the body
  2. Respiration rate is the number of breaths per minute
  3. Evaluate the depth (shallow, deep), rhythm (regular, irregular), rate, quality (labored, easy), breathing sounds (wet/noisy, clear), and client position during respiration
B. Factors that affect respiration
  1. Respiration rate may be increased as a result of exercise, pain, certain drugs, anxiety, shock, or disease
  2. Respiration rate may be decreased as a result of sleep, certain drugs, or disease
C. Normal respiration rate ranges
  1. Adult—12 to 20 respirations per minute
  2. Child—approximately 20 respirations per minute
D. Evaluating respiration
  1. After determining the pulse rate, continue to hold the client's wrist for 60 seconds and count the number of times the chest rises and falls
  2. Record the respiration rate, rhythm, depth (shallow, deep), quality (labored, easy), sounds, and client position (sitting, lying)

EMERGENCY CARDIAC CARE

Definition

A. Emergency cardiac care (ECC)—includes recognition, prevention, reassurance, and the ability to monitor and treat a person in need of BLS, advanced cardiac life support, and the transferring of the stabilized person to a medical care facility for definitive treatment
B. Basic life support (BLS)—maintains an individual's heart and lung functions through prompt recognition, intervention, CPR, or all of these actions
C. Advanced cardiac life support (ACLS)—BLS with use of additional equipment; an intravenous access; administration of fluids or medications, or both; defibrillation; arrhythmia control; and continued care following resuscitation

D. Cardiopulmonary resuscitation (CPR)—a basic life support technique with the goal of providing oxygen to the brain, heart, and other vital organs until definitive medical treatment can be given; CPR requires assessment and basic skills in the management of the airway, breathing, and circulation
E. Emergency medical system (EMS)—a coordinated community system that uses communication, transportation, prevention, education, trained personnel, emergency medical facilities, and other elements in providing emergency medical care
F. "Successful" completion of an American Heart Association (AHA) or other approved course in CPR, BLS, or ACLS may be required for dental hygiene licensure in some states
G. Advances in scientific knowledge and clinical research have resulted in frequent changes in the ECC technique and protocol; therefore, the most current literature should be consulted for up-to-date information

Basic Concepts

A. CAB Sequence of CPR
  C Circulation—assess and provide cardiac support by external cardiac compressions
  A Airway—assess and establish a clear air passage
  B Breathing—assess and provide respiration through rescue breathing
B. Respiratory arrest—a sudden cessation of breathing
C. Cardiac arrest—a sudden, unexpected cessation of the heart and circulation
D. Clinical death—cessation of the heart and breathing; may be reversible through life support measures, especially if initiated within 4 to 6 minutes, or it may progress to biologic death
E. Biologic death—permanent cellular damage, particularly of the oxygen-sensitive brain cells, resulting from an inadequate supply of oxygen

Cardiopulmonary Resuscitation by the Health Care Provider

Single-Rescuer Cardiopulmonary Resuscitation

A. Determining consciousness
  1. Determine the victim's level of consciousness by gently shaking the shoulder and shouting, "Are you okay?" At the same time the health care provider should determine if there is no breathing or no normal breathing (agonal gasps which sometimes sound like a snore or snort may be present)
  2. Activate the EMS if the victim does not respond; dial or direct a bystander to dial 9-1-1; give the

location of the emergency, the phone number you are calling from, what happened, how many persons need help, the condition of victim(s), and what is being done for the victim(s)

   a. Do not hang up until directed to do so by the EMS dispatcher

3. Obtain an automated external defibrillator (AED), if one is available; send a second rescuer to do this if possible

4. Carefully place the person in the supine position. Roll the body as a unit, avoiding any twisting motion; caution is needed if you suspect a back or neck injury. If the victim is not on a firm surface, place the spine board under the victim or move the victim to a firm surface

B. Check for a pulse, taking no longer than 10 seconds; use the carotid artery for adults; use the carotid or the femoral artery for children ages 1 to puberty; use the brachial artery for infants (child and infant CPR guidelines)

   1. If no pulse is present, begin performing cardiac compressions at a rate of at least 100 compressions per minute pushing hard and fast; compress the sternum at least 2 inches with each compression and allow the chest to completely recoil between compressions

   2. To perform external cardiac compressions, place the heel of one of your hands on the center of the victim's chest between the nipples

   3. Place the heel of one hand on top of the other hand; fingers may be extended or interlaced

   4. Use both hands to alternately depress the sternum at least 2 inches; push hard and fast; fully release pressure on the sternum and allow the chest to recoil after each compression

   5. The compression rate is at least 100 per minute with a count of "one and two and three and …" and so on

   6. Continue the cycle for a compression : ventilation ratio of 30 : 2

   7. Administer two breaths (about 1 second each) after every thirtieth compression; refer to rescue breathing techniques following the AED section

   8. Check the pulse after four cycles and every few minutes thereafter; if a pulse is evident, continue rescue breathing at 10 to 12 breaths per minute; if no pulse is evident, continue the CPR

   9. To perform cardiac compressions on a child, (age 1 year to puberty) depress the lower half of the sternum at least $\frac{1}{3}$ the depth of the chest or about 2 inches with the heel of one or both hands; the compression : ventilation ratio is 30 : 2, with a rate of at least 100 compressions per minute; if you did not witness the arrest and you are alone, give 2 minutes of CPR before leaving to call the EMS

10. To perform cardiac compressions on an infant, use two fingers placed just below the infant's nipple line; compress the chest at least $\frac{1}{3}$ the depth of the chest or about $1\frac{1}{2}$ inches, using a ratio of 30 : 2 and a rate of at least 100 per minute; if you did not witness the arrest and you are alone, give 2 minutes of CPR before leaving to call the EMS

11. Because early defibrillation and ACLS measures increase the chance of survival, it is important to emphasize activation of the EMS system by calling 9-1-1 as soon as possible

Two-Rescuer Cardiopulmonary Resuscitation

A. The rescuers kneel on either side of the victim, one at the victim's head to perform ventilations, the other at the victim's chest to perform compressions

B. One rescuer provides compressions at a rate of at least 100 per minute with a count of "one and two and three and …" and so on

C. The second rescuer administers two breaths (about 1 second each) after every thirtieth compression; breaths should take no longer than 5 seconds

D. The cycle is continued for a compression : ventilation ratio of 30 : 2

E. The rescuers should switch positions every 2 minutes, limiting the switch to <5 seconds; pulse rate should be checked every few minutes and at every rescuer switch

F. The rescuer performing ventilations should monitor the effectiveness of the CPR by assessing the carotid pulse and air exchange

G. If an advanced airway has been placed, two rescuers deliver compressions at a rate of at least 100 per minute without pausing for breaths; the person providing breaths administers 8 to 10 per minute, avoiding excessive ventilations

H. For children (ages 1 year to puberty) and infants, two rescuers working together use a compression to ventilation ratio of 15 : 2; compressions for infants are performed with the thumbs placed over the infant's chest just below the nipple line and the hands encircling the infant's chest

AUTOMATED EXTERNAL DEFIBRILLATORS

A. Computerized devices that analyze cardiac rhythms and deliver an electric shock when appropriate; if an AED is available, they should be used as soon as possible in the CPR sequence, since early defibrillation increases the chances of survival for victims of sudden cardiac arrest

B. AEDs are available in a variety of models; if an AED is present in the office, the dental hygienist should become familiar with its operation (by studying the manufacturer's instructions) and follow current recommended CPR/AED techniques; standard AEDs may be used on children >8 years and adults

C. Universal steps in AED operation (victim is unresponsive, without pulse, and not breathing)
1. Power on the AED
2. Attach the electrode pads to the victim's chest (the pads may or may not already be connected to the cables, the machine, or both)
3. "Clear" the victim by ensuring that no one is touching the victim
4. Press the "Analyze" button
5. "Clear" the victim and allow the machine to "Analyze" the rhythm; make sure that no one is touching the victim, and press the shock button if a shock is indicated by the machine; once the shock has been delivered, resume CPR by starting with chest compressions; the AED will provide additional prompts
6. If no shock is indicated, resume CPR; the AED will provide additional prompts

D. Precautions
1. AEDs may be used on infants and children ages 1 to 8
2. Child pads and a pediatric-capable AED should be used for children (1 to 8 years); if the child becomes pulseless suddenly and the emergency event has been witnessed, activate the EMS and begin CPR; an AED should be attached and used as soon as possible; if the collapse of the child who has no pulse has not been witnessed, about 2 minutes of CPR should be performed before using an AED; if an AED with child capability is not available, a standard AED may be used; take care that the pads do not touch each other
3. Manual defibrillators are preferred for use on infants; if neither a manual defibrillator nor a pediatric-capable AED is available, a standard AED may be used; take care that the pads do not touch each other
4. The victim should be kept dry
5. The defibrillator pads should not be placed over implanted pacemakers; the pads should be placed at least 1 inch to the side
6. The defibrillator pads should not be placed over transdermal medication patches (remove the medication patch, wipe the area, and attach the AED pad)

Rescue Breathing Technique

A. Determine the need for rescue breathing
1. Follow the steps used for CPR to determine consciousness and presence of adequate breathing

2. After notifying the EMS and obtaining an AED, check for a pulse
3. If a pulse is present, the victim is breathing adequately, and no spinal injury is suspected, place the victim on his or her side, monitor vital signs until help arrives
4. If a pulse is present and the person is not breathing or not breathing adequately, open the airway and give 2 breaths, continue with 1 breath every 5 to 6 seconds (10 to 12 breaths per minute); recheck for a pulse every 2 minutes
5. If a pulse is not present, follow the guidelines presented in the CPR section
6. The basic technique for opening the airway is the head-tilt-chin lift; use a jaw-thrust in the trauma victim with suspected neck injury
7. Airway technique
   a. The head-tilt is performed by placing one palm on the forehead of the victim and pressing backward to gently tilt the head back
   b. The chin-lift is achieved by placing the fingers of the other hand under the victim's mandible near the chin and raising the chin gently forward; care is required to avoid pressing into soft tissue and to avoid using the thumb to lift the chin
   c. The jaw-thrust is used for extra forward displacement of the mandible; it may be the safest method for opening the airway in a victim with a suspected neck injury; to perform the jaw-thrust, use both hands (one on each side), gently grasp the angles of the mandible, and carefully lift to move the jaw forward; the rescuer may need to provide support for the victim's head to avoid head movement

B. Performing rescue breathing for an adult
1. The rescuer's position is at the victim's shoulders
2. Open airway or maintain open airway by using the head-tilt-chin-lift (or in the case of a neck injury, use the jaw-thrust)
3. Rescue-breathing techniques—because disease transmission is a concern, mouth-to-mouth resuscitation should be performed, when possible, using ventilation devices such as pocket masks with one-way valves or resuscitation bags; however, the value of ventilation devices rather than mouth-to-mouth resuscitation in the prevention of disease transmission is unknown; rescue breathing should not be delayed while waiting for adjunct ventilation or oxygen delivery devices. Current American Heart Association CPR guidelines note that although the risk of transmissions of infection during CPR is

considered very low, OSHA requires the use of Standard Precautions for healthcare workers providing CPR in the workplace

    a. Mouth-to-mask—a transparent mask with mouthpiece and one-way valve may be used for assisted ventilation; the technique includes placing the mask around the victim's mouth and nose, placing the heel and thumb of each hand on the borders of the mask to firmly seal the margins; grasping the mandible with the index, middle, and ring fingers with gentle pressure upward; and ventilating through the mouthpiece

    b. Mouth-to-mouth—uses the rescuer's exhaled air to inflate the victim's lungs; an airtight seal is created by pinching the victim's nostrils closed (use the thumb and index finger of the hand involved in the head-tilt) and by placing the mouth around the victim's mouth after taking a breath; the rescuer then breathes into the victim's mouth

    c. Mouth-to-nose—may be needed if it is not possible to ventilate through the victim's mouth; the victim's mouth should be closed; the rescuer takes a deep breath and places his or her mouth around the victim's nose and exhales; the rescuer must remove his or her mouth from the victim's nose after each exhalation to allow the victim to exhale; periodic opening of the victim's lips may be necessary if nasal blockage occurs

    d. Mouth-to-stoma technique—used in a person who has undergone laryngectomy and has a stoma (opening at the base of the neck connecting to the trachea); assess for breathing at the stoma site; after taking a breath, place your mouth over the stoma, exhale, and remove your mouth to allow the victim to exhale after each breath

  4. Give two breaths into the victim's mouth (nose or stoma)

  5. Watch for chest to rise; allow 1 second per breath to provide visible chest expansion and to decrease the possibility of gastric distention

  6. Take a normal breath after each ventilation; adequate volume produces visible chest rise

  7. If ventilations are unsuccessful, reassess and reposition the victim's head; repeat the attempt to ventilate

  8. Rescue breathing is performed at 12 to 20 breaths per minute for adults, one breath every 5 or 6 seconds

C. Performing rescue breathing for a child or infant—the following modifications must be made:

  1. Seal the child's mouthpiece or mouth (and nose) with your mouth, inflate the lungs with less force and volume than in the case of an adult, and give two breaths (1 second per inflation) with a pause between breaths

  2. Rescue breathing is performed at 12 to 20 breaths per minute, approximately one breath every 3 to 5 seconds

Basic Life Support in Late Pregnancy

A. Oxygen intake progressively increases during pregnancy (averages 20% to 30% higher) to meet the needs of the fetus, the uterus, and the increased demands on the respiratory and circulatory systems of the mother; the functional residual capacity of the lungs is decreased because of the upward displacement of the diaphragm; the oxygen reserve is further compromised when the pregnant woman is in the supine position; also, in this position, the enlarged uterus may compress the abdominal aorta and the inferior vena cava, resulting in hypotension and reduced cardiac output by as much as 25%

B. To help alleviate the effects of the supine position on circulation (as during CPR), the uterus should be shifted toward the left side by placing a folded towel or wedge under the right hip

C. Aspiration caused by delayed gastric emptying is also a concern, because of the enlarged uterus compressing the stomach and possibly a decrease in the tone of the lower part of the esophagus

D. Chest compressions for CPR should be performed higher on the sternum, just above the center of the sternum to accommodate the upward displacement of the diaphragm

E. For severe foreign-body airway obstruction in a conscious woman in her last trimester of pregnancy, chest thrusts rather than abdominal thrusts are recommended. For severe foreign-body airway obstruction in an unconscious pregnant woman, the EMS should be activated and CPR started (see the section on "Management of an obstructed airway" below)

Duration of Basic Life Support

BLS should continue until effective and spontaneous ventilation and circulation or until the resuscitation efforts have been transferred to another person trained in BLS; until a physician is available or EMS personnel arrive and assume responsibility; until the victim is transferred to trained personnel accepting responsibility for emergency medical services; or until the rescuer becomes exhausted and is unable to continue BLS.

MANAGEMENT OF AN OBSTRUCTED AIRWAY

A. Basic concepts
1. Obstructed airway occurs when an object or foreign body prevents exchange of air during breathing
2. Foreign-body obstruction may occur when eating, when unconscious (the tongue may block the pharynx), during resuscitation (aspiration of vomitus or blood), or during other events

B. Recognizing an obstructed airway in a conscious client
1. Mild airway obstruction with good air exchange—the victim can cough forcefully; encourage spontaneous coughing and deep breathing
2. Severe airway obstruction with poor air exchange—the victim has a weak cough, may be cyanotic, makes high-pitched noises, has increased difficulty breathing, is unable to speak or breathe, and may clutch at the neck

C. Treating an obstructed airway in a conscious client
1. Determine if the victim has a severe airway obstruction by asking victim, "Are you choking?" If the person indicates otherwise, do not interfere with the person's own attempts to dislodge the object but remain with client until it is dislodged, or summon help
2. Subdiaphragmatic abdominal thrusts (the Heimlich maneuver) are recommended to manage severe foreign-body airway obstruction; in a conscious victim who is standing or sitting, the rescuer stands behind the victim, wraps an arm around the victim's waist, places the thumb side of the fist between the victim's xiphoid process and navel, supports the fist with the other hand, and presses the fist into the victim's abdomen with a brisk inward and upward motion; each motion should be distinct and repeated until the foreign body is removed or the victim loses consciousness; for conscious infants (<1 year old) with severe airway obstruction, the rescuer holds the infant's body so that the infant is face down (supporting the infant's body with forearm and thigh) and performs five back blows; the rescuer rotates the infant (still supporting the infant's body) and performs five chest thrusts; this sequence is continued until the object is removed or the infant becomes unconscious
3. In an obese or pregnant victim with severe airway obstruction, the rescuer stands behind the victim with arms wrapped around the victim's chest; the thumb side of the fist is centered on the midsternum; the other hand is used to support the fist, and backward motions (chest thrusts) are administered until the foreign body is expelled or the victim loses consciousness

D. Treating an obstructed airway in an unconscious client
1. If a choking victim becomes unconscious, activate the EMS, carefully lower the victim to the ground, and begin CPR starting with chest compressions
2. If an object is observed when giving rescue breaths, and can be easily removed, remove it
3. If the obstruction has been removed, ventilate the lungs twice, and continue BLS, as indicated
4. If a choking child becomes unconscious follow the same procedure as for an adult; begin CPR, look into the child's mouth each time the airway is opened for rescue breaths; do not perform blind finger-sweeps, but observe for an object and finger-sweep only if the object can be visualized
5. If a choking infant becomes unconscious, call for someone to activate the EMS, and begin CPR; look into the infant's mouth each time the airway is opened for rescue breaths, and finger-sweep only if a foreign body can be visualized; if the EMS has not been activated after 2 minutes of CPR, do so
6. Do not perform blind finger-sweeps on an unconscious person of any age
7. If an unconscious victim is found and it is not known if the victim has choked, follow the standard C-A-B CPR sequence

ADMINISTRATION OF OXYGEN

A. Basic concepts
1. Purpose
   a. Oxygen is essential for most chemical reactions in the body; carbon dioxide is the major waste product of these reactions
   b. Circulatory and respiratory systems transport these gases
   c. During a medical emergency, the body's increased need for oxygen or its diminished ability to obtain or use oxygen may call for the administration of a higher concentration of oxygen than exists in regular air
   d. A system for delivering this oxygen to a client is essential in the management of emergency situations
2. Indications for oxygen administration include syncope, cardiac problems, and respiratory difficulties (with the exception of hyperventilation)

B. Equipment—portable oxygen unit consists of an oxygen tank (an E cylinder is recommended), regulator, tubing, a self-inflating resuscitation bag (Ambu bag used for high-flow oxygen, 10 to 15 liters per minute [L/min]), a clear oxygen mask with a reservoir bag (covers face and nose, used for high-flow oxygen, 8 to 15 L/min), and a nasal cannula (used for low-flow oxygen, up to 6 L/min)

C. Technique for administering oxygen to an unconscious client
 1. Place the client in the supine position, and open the airway
 2. Start the oxygen flow from the cylinder, and adjust the rate such that the flow inflates the positive-pressure reservoir bag on the mask
 3. Secure the mask over the client's face to cover the nose and mouth
 4. Observe for chest movement and exhalation
 5. If the client is breathing but the breaths appear to be weak or shallow, or if respirations are decreased in number, provide additional ventilations with an Ambu bag to equal about 10 to 12 breaths per minute

D. Technique for administering oxygen to a conscious client
 1. Place the client in the supine position, or encourage the client to assume a comfortable position
 2. Determine the appropriate oxygen delivery device for the client and attach it to the oxygen cylinder; adjust the rate to provide an appropriate amount of oxygen based on the client's needs
 3. Allow the client to breathe at his or her own rate
 4. If using a non-rebreather mask with a reservoir bag, prevent the reservoir bag from completely deflating during inspiration by increasing oxygen flow as needed; monitor the client's breathing and vital signs

UNCONSCIOUSNESS

A. Unconsciousness—the inability to respond to stimuli, make purposeful movements, or gain awareness of events taking place
B. Levels of unconsciousness range from syncope (transient, simple fainting) to coma (prolonged, deep unconsciousness)
C. Causes
 1. Unconsciousness may result from diminished blood supply to the brain (inadequate cerebral circulation), altered quality of blood flow to the brain (metabolic disorder), central nervous system disorder, or emotional disturbance
 2. Common causes of unconsciousness in the dental setting are psychogenic factors (fear, anxiety); treatment for this type of unconsciousness is aimed at increasing the amount of oxygenated blood received by the brain

D. Preventing loss of consciousness
 1. To decrease the probability of a client's becoming unconscious, the dental hygienist should obtain a complete health history, evaluate vital signs, and determine the dental stress level for every client
 2. Stress reduction, premedication, and pain management may be of value in treating the anxious client
E. Managing unconsciousness
 1. If a client becomes unconscious, the dental hygienist should initiate BLS and summon help. If the client is in the dental chair, the chair back may be lowered to facilitate cerebral blood flow
 2. Procedures for emergency management should be initiated immediately, according to a pre-established plan

MANAGING OTHER MEDICAL EMERGENCIES

Syncope (Fainting, Vasodepressor Syncope)

A. Syncope—a sudden, transient loss of consciousness; most common medical emergency encountered in dental settings
B. Causes
 1. Syncope is caused by decreased cerebral function resulting from impaired circulation or altered metabolism
 2. Syncope may result from psychogenic (anxiety, fear) or nonpsychogenic (hypoglycemia, position change, heat) factors
C. Preventing syncope
 1. The dental hygienist should obtain from each client a complete health history to determine previous syncopal episodes, dental stress level, and other pertinent information
 2. Anxiety-reduction measures may include good client rapport, a low-stress environment, and premedication
 3. Clients who "feel faint" may be aided by reclining the dental chair to the Trendelenburg position (head lower than legs)
D. Signs and symptoms—three stages of syncope: presyncope, syncope, and postsyncope
 1. Presyncope stage—the client may be subjectively weak and nauseated, with a feeling of lightheadedness and tingling in the toes and fingers and increased pulse rate; objectively, the dental hygienist may observe pallor and sweating; the attack may be aborted if the client is placed in the Trendelenburg position

2. Syncope stage—subjectively characterized by flaccid muscles and impaired consciousness; objectively, the client is pale, with a weak pulse and shallow breathing; the duration is less than 5 minutes

3. Postsyncope stage—the client wakens, blood pressure and pulse rate return to normal, the client may report feeling weak and disoriented; the client should remain supine and rest for a time sufficient to prevent another episode

E. Managing syncope
1. A client who appears "faint" should be placed in the supine position, and dental or dental hygiene treatment should be discontinued
2. Syncope management protocol
   a. Assess and open the airway
   b. Determine the client's breathing status; if the client is breathing, monitor the vital signs, and provide BLS, as needed; if the client is not breathing, initiate BLS immediately, and activate the EMS
   c. Keep the client warm
   d. Administer oxygen, if needed
   e. An ammonia ampule, if available, may be administered; gently pass the crushed capsule under the client's nose; use care, as ammonia ampules emit a strong odor
   f. A client who has experienced syncope generally will return to consciousness within 5 minutes; when the client regains consciousness, reassure the client that he or she will be fine, and keep the client in the supine position; it is advisable to discontinue dental treatment and make arrangements for the client to be escorted home
   g. If it is likely that the client became unconscious from causes other than simple fainting, medical follow-up may be necessary

Shock

A. Shock—a condition in which the circulatory system does not adequately circulate blood through body tissues; a lack of oxygen in the cells results

B. Causes and pathophysiology—five commonly accepted categories, or causes, of shock:
   1. Hypovolemic shock—caused by inadequate blood volume
   2. Anaphylactic shock—caused by an acute allergic reaction
   3. Septic shock—caused by an infectious agent
   4. Cardiogenic shock—caused by heart failure
   5. Neurogenic shock—caused by psychologic or neurologic disorder

C. Signs and symptoms
   1. The client may complain of thirst, restlessness, or anxiety
   2. Blood pressure may decrease; pulse and respiratory rates may increase; and skin may be pale, cool, and clammy; in severe cases, the victim may go into a coma

D. Treatment
   1. Place the client in the Trendelenburg position
   2. Call for medical assistance, and be prepared to administer BLS; activate the EMS
   3. Monitor the vital signs and skin signs
   4. Administer oxygen

Asthma

A. Asthma attacks may be prevented by identifying the client at risk through thorough history taking and by reducing stress during dental hygiene care

B. Signs and symptoms of asthma include the onset of an unproductive cough, dyspnea (shortness of breath), anxiety, wheezing, and cyanosis

C. Treatment for an asthma attack
   1. Encourage the client to assume a position that facilitates breathing (usually sitting)
   2. Allow the client to administer his or her own prescribed medications (bronchodilators), if available; encourage clients with asthma to bring their inhalers to all dental appointments
   3. Administer oxygen if the episode continues
   4. Seek the assistance of the dentist or a physician, or activate the EMS if the episode continues

Hyperventilation

Hyperventilation is characterized by rapid breathing and is often brought about by pain, anxiety, or drugs; rapid breathing causes an excessive elimination of carbon dioxide, which results in respiratory alkalosis

A. Signs and symptoms of hyperventilation include the client's subjective report of tingling, giddiness, lightheadedness, dizziness, and heart palpitations; the dental hygienist may observe rapid respirations and a rapid pulse

B. To assist the hyperventilating client, the dental hygienist should reassure the client that he or she will be all right, terminate dental procedures, and place the client in the upright position; tight clothing should be loosened, if necessary; and the client should be encouraged to breathe slowly and deeply (only 4 to 6 breaths per minute)

C. It may be helpful to have the client breathe into his or her cupped hands; oxygen should not be administered

Cardiac Emergencies

See the sections on "Infections of the circulatory system" in Chapter 9 and "Congenital heart disease," "Rheumatic fever and heart disease," "Cardiac arrhythmias and dysrhythmias," "Hypertensive disease," "Ischemic heart disease (coronary heart disease)," and "Congestive heart failure" in Chapter 19.

A. Cardiac emergencies have many causes and require immediate, definitive medical treatment; sudden unexpected cessation of cardiac activity is called *cardiac arrest*; unless CPR or other ECC is promptly performed to maintain the heart's function, biologic death may result (review earlier section on ECC and other current literature); a cardiac emergency may be caused by accidents (electric shock, drowning, trauma, asphyxiation) or coronary disease, which is the focus of this section

B. Causes and pathophysiology—coronary disease and emergencies may result from a change in the heart's function (arrhythmia, hypertrophy, ischemia), blood vessels (atherosclerosis, arteriosclerosis), blood volume (shock, hemorrhage), or blood composition (anemia)

C. Prevent cardiac emergencies in the oral health care setting by identifying clients at risk with thorough history taking, recognizing present signs and symptoms, and prompt referral to a physician; if coronary symptoms develop in the dental office, then rapid access of the EMS is indicated

D. Cardiovascular diseases
   1. Hypertension—a persistent elevation of blood pressure, which indicates that the heart is working harder to supply blood through the arteries; the probability of a stroke, myocardial infarction, congestive heart failure, and kidney disease may be increased as a result of a consistently elevated blood pressure
      a. Cause and pathophysiology
         (1) 90% of clients with high blood pressure have primary hypertension; primary hypertension is of unknown origin; risk factors include heredity, race, gender, age, diet (e.g., high sodium), obesity, stress, nicotine, and lack of exercise
         (2) 10% of clients with high blood pressure have secondary hypertension; secondary hypertension has a specific cause such as kidney disease
      b. Signs and symptoms
         (1) May include headaches, dizziness, or no symptoms
         (2) Consistent, elevated blood pressure readings
      c. Treatment
         (1) The client with hypertension needs referral to a physician

         (2) Primary hypertension is controlled by reduction of risk factors, medications, and continued medical care
         (3) Secondary hypertension is controlled by identifying and treating the underlying disease
   2. Angina pectoris
      a. Angina pectoris—a transient (temporary) ischemia (lack of oxygenated blood) of the myocardium (heart muscle), usually manifested by chest pain or discomfort
      b. Signs and symptoms
         (1) Chest pain or discomfort may be described as pressing, crushing, burning, or squeezing; may radiate to the shoulders, arms, neck, mandible, or epigastrium; may last 1 to 10 minutes; may be precipitated by exertion; and may be accompanied by weakness and shortness of breath
         (2) The dental hygienist may observe that the client has labored breathing or is sweating
      c. Treatment
         (1) Discontinue dental hygiene care, and alert the dentist and other staff
         (2) Allow the client to rest; if the client uses nitroglycerin and it is available, he or she may take one nitroglycerin tablet every 3 to 5 minutes with no more than three doses within a 15-minute period (refer to current literature for protocol); nitroglycerin should not be taken unless the systolic blood pressure is greater than 100 mm Hg (it lowers blood pressure)
         (3) Administer oxygen by nasal cannula
         (4) Monitor the client's vital signs
         (5) If the pain is relieved by rest and nitroglycerin, encourage rest, discontinue oral health services for that appointment, and refer the client for further evaluation by a physician
         (6) If the pain is not relieved by rest and nitroglycerin and if the pain persists, activate the EMS immediately
   3. Myocardial infarction
      a. Myocardial infarction—a diminished or interrupted supply of oxygenated blood to the heart that causes death (necrosis) of part of the heart muscle, resulting in impaired heart function and diminished cardiac output; if a large area of the heart is affected, the heart may be unable to function and may stop beating
      b. Signs and symptoms
         (1) A common presentation of a myocardial infarction is chest pain or discomfort that

may radiate to the arm, neck, or mandible, lasts for more than 15 to 20 minutes, and is not relieved by nitroglycerin or rest; may have various presentations and may also include sweating, nausea, shortness of breath, and weakness; women do not always present with these classic signs but rather experience more vague warning signs before a heart attack, such as indigestion, nausea, vomiting, dizziness, breathlessness, back pain, or deep throbbing in the left or right bicep or forearm

(2) The dental hygienist should be aware that in a case of myocardial infarction, the client may not look "sick," and the pain is not necessarily severe

c. Treatment

(1) Discontinue dental hygiene care, alert the dentist, and immediately activate the EMS

(2) The client should be in a comfortable position and able to rest

(3) Monitor the client's vital signs, administer high-flow oxygen and BLS, as needed, and continue support until definitive treatment is available

(4) If the client uses nitroglycerin and the medication is available, he or she may take one nitroglycerin tablet every 3 to 5 minutes with no more than three doses within a 15-minute period; nitroglycerin should not be taken unless the systolic blood pressure is greater than 100 mm Hg (it lowers blood pressure); if pain is not relieved, the hygienist should suspect myocardial infarction

4. Congestive heart failure (CHF)

a. Congestive heart failure results when the heart is unable to meet the body's demands; precipitating factors include hypertension, coronary artery disease, congenital and valvular heart disease, toxins, inflammatory disorders, and endocrinopathies

b. Signs and symptoms

(1) The client may complain of weakness, shortness of breath, cough; swelling of the ankles may be present

(2) The dental hygienist may note edema, cyanosis, tachycardia, and prominent jugular veins

c. Treatment

(1) The client with CHF needs continued medical care; the client's physician on record should be consulted before dental or dental hygiene care

(2) In the dental setting, the client with CHF may feel more comfortable with the back of the dental chair in the upright position

(3) If the client with CHF has a medical emergency, discontinue dental treatment, ensure a comfortable client position, administer oxygen and BLS, as needed, monitor vital signs, alert the dentist, and activate the EMS

5. Sudden cardiac death

a. Sudden cardiac death (SCD) is the unexpected cessation of heart and lung functions

b. The causes of SCD may include coronary artery disease, respiratory arrest, shock, drugs, arrhythmias, accidents, or anaphylaxis

c. Signs and symptoms include unconsciousness and absence of a pulse, blood pressure, and respirations

d. Treatment is immediate activation of the EMS; ECC procedures, including BLS; ACLS; and definitive medical treatment

Allergic Reactions

A. Allergic reactions—wide range of physiologic responses caused by hypersensitivity to an allergen

B. Causes and pathophysiology

1. Allergic responses may be evoked by drugs, pollens, foods, chemicals, insect bites, and other factors

2. When the body comes into contact with these substances, an antigen–antibody reaction occurs and results in an inappropriate response of the body's immune system

C. Preventing allergic reactions

1. Thorough health history should reveal a previous history of allergic reactions to drugs or materials used in dental therapeutics

2. Ask the client who has a prior history of an allergic reaction to describe its type and severity

3. Refer the client with a suspected allergy for evaluation by a physician

D. Types

1. Delayed allergic reactions

a. Signs and symptoms include skin manifestations (such as erythema, urticaria, angioedema) or respiratory reactions (respiratory distress, wheezing, dyspnea, angioedema) that occur hours or even days after contact with an allergen

b. Treatment

(1) Delayed reactions may be mild and necessitate no treatment

(2) If the allergic reaction is severe, the dentist may administer medications (antihistamine, epinephrine), oxygen, or both, as needed for each client

(3) If the reaction persists, the client should be accompanied to a physician; if a delayed reaction becomes severe, the EMS should be activated

2. Immediate reaction or anaphylaxis
   a. Immediate allergic reactions—characterized by urticaria, nausea, angioedema, and respiratory distress; may progress to cardiovascular collapse; the client may have a very rapid and weak pulse as well as heart palpitations and may become cyanotic
   b. Treatment
      (1) Anaphylaxis is a serious life-threatening emergency; immediately activate the EMS and provide BLS until definitive medical treatment is available
      (2) Place the client in the supine position, if possible; keep the client warm
      (3) Administer high-flow oxygen
      (4) Monitor the vital signs
      (5) The dentist or a physician may administer epinephrine
      (6) Continue BLS, as needed

Drug-Related Emergencies and Poisoning

Basic Concepts

A. Drug-related emergencies—include allergic response, overdose, psychogenic response (syncope or hyperventilation), idiosyncratic reaction, drug interactions, and complications in a client who is chemically dependent
B. Thorough health history should reveal the client's drug allergies, previous adverse reactions, or chemical dependency; these agents, materials, and drugs must be avoided during dental and dental hygiene care
C. Dental hygienists should be prepared to manage reactions to a local anesthetic agent or fluoride therapy

Specific Reactions

A. Local anesthetic agent reactions may be the result of psychogenic or allergic response, toxic overdose, or chemical intoxication
   1. Psychogenic response usually manifests as syncope or hyperventilation, which is generally the result of fear of the injection rather than a reaction to the local anesthetic agent; syncope and hyperventilation should be managed

according to the criteria described in related sections of this chapter
   2. Allergic reactions, which occur more often with ester-type anesthetics (procaine), are very rare and should be managed by the criteria established under the section on "Allergic reactions" in this chapter
   3. Toxic overdoses of local anesthetic agents may occur as a result of delayed biotransformation or elimination of the agent, excess total dose, or intravascular injection of the agent
      a. The client who experiences a toxic overdose may be anxious and confused; may have a rapid pulse and respirations, followed by shock, respiratory arrest, and cardiovascular collapse
      b. Toxic overdose is managed by discontinuing the injection, monitoring vital signs, administering oxygen, activating the EMS, and providing BLS, as needed
   4. Chemically dependent client
      a. Prevent emergencies by identifying the chemically dependent client and adjusting the dental treatment accordingly
      b. If a local anesthetic agent with epinephrine is injected into the vascular system of a cocaine-intoxicated client, cardiovascular compromise may result, necessitating activation of the EMS; begin BCLS, as necessary, until ACLS-trained personnel arrive
B. Fluoride poisoning by ingestion may be acute (caused by a single large dose of an agent) or chronic (caused by long-term ingestion)
   1. Acute toxic reactions to fluoride are rare, although fatal fluoride poisoning may be caused by accidental ingestion of large quantities of fluorides such as those contained in insecticides with sodium fluoride; ingestion of a certainly lethal dose (CLD) of fluoride is based on kilograms of body weight; for adults 5 to 10 g of sodium fluoride taken at one time; for children 0.5 to 1 g (500 to 1000 mg) of sodium fluoride taken at one time, depending on weight and size; safely tolerated dose (STD) is ¼ the CLD (based on weight and size) (Figure 21-3 and Table 21-2)
   2. Some oral health care products contain enough fluoride to be hazardous, especially to children; 1 ounce of topical fluoride gel or one 8-ounce tube of fluoridated toothpaste could be life threatening to a small child
   3. Signs of acute fluoride toxicity include nausea, abdominal pain, excessive salivation, thirst, vomiting, and diarrhea; in severe cases muscle cramping, bronchospasm, and cardiac arrest may occur

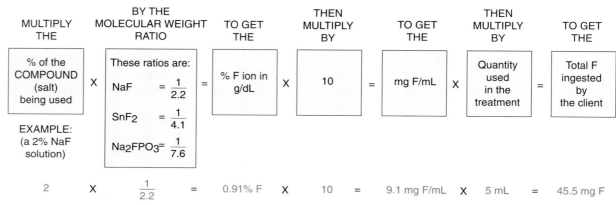

FIGURE 21-3 Flowchart depicting the method for calculating the amount of fluoride ingested by a client from a compound used in professional care. *(Modified from Heifetz SB, Horowitz HS: The amounts of fluoride in current fluoride therapies: Safety considerations for children, ASDC J Dent Child 51:257, July–August, 1984.)*

TABLE 21-2 Certainly Lethal and Safely Tolerated Doses of Fluoride

Age	Body Weight (lb)	CLD (mg)	STD (mg)
2	22	320	80
4	29	422	106
6	37	538	135
8	45	655	164
10	53	771	193
12	64	931	233
14	83	1206	301
16	92	1338	334
18	95	1382	346

From Heifetz SB, Horowitz HS: The amounts of fluoride in current fluoride therapies: Safety considerations for children, ASDC J Dent Child 51:257, July–August, 1984.

4. Treatment of acute fluoride poisoning (for adults and children age ≥6 years)
   a. Induce vomiting through digital stimulation of the soft palate or posterior tongue; or with ipecac syrup (only if client has a gag reflex, is conscious, and is not convulsing)
   b. Administer milk or 1% calcium gluconate or calcium chloride orally
   c. Activate the EMS or admit the client into a medical care facility for definitive treatment as soon as possible
   d. Support the client with BLS, if necessary
   e. Medical personnel will administer calcium gluconate intravenously, perform gastric lavage, and institute other advanced interventions, depending on the client's condition

Bleeding and Hemorrhage

A. Client may have a bleeding problem in the oral health care setting because of a dental procedure, accident, or spontaneous bleeding (such as a nosebleed)

B. Clients taking certain types of medications, such as heparin and warfarin (Coumadin), may be more susceptible to bleeding problems; such clients may be identified by a thorough health and pharmacologic history

C. Modifications in the client's medication regimen may be necessary to reduce the likelihood that the client will have a bleeding problem as the result of oral health care; the physician of record must be consulted before any modifications are suggested

D. Bleeding may be arterial or venous; arterial bleeding is usually redder in color and "spurts" with the contraction of the heart; venous bleeding is darker in color and "oozes"

E. Treatment of hemorrhage usually can be managed by direct pressure on the bleeding area; use sterile gauze to apply pressure
   1. If bleeding is from a dental extraction or surgical site, pack the area with gauze, and have the client stay nearby for observation until the bleeding stops
   2. For nosebleed, apply cold compresses to the nose, and apply pressure to the bleeding side; bleeding also may be reduced if the nostril is gently packed with gauze; have the client tilt his or her head forward and down to prevent swallowing the blood
   3. If bleeding is severe or cannot be controlled, watch for signs of shock, administer oxygen, be ready to administer BLS, and activate the EMS

Cerebrovascular Accident (Stroke, Brain Attack)

A. Pathophysiology and causes
1. Cerebrovascular accident (CVA), or stroke, results when the supply of oxygen to the brain cells is disrupted by ischemia, infarction, or hemorrhage of the cerebral blood vessels; referred to as a *brain attack* to highlight the importance of early recognition and prompt treatment
2. Factors contributing to a CVA include tobacco use, hypertension, diabetes mellitus, and coronary disease

B. Prevention
1. To decrease the probability of a CVA, the client is advised regular medical examinations; control of high blood pressure, dietary fat, and diabetes; elimination of tobacco use; and reduction in risk factors such as a sedentary lifestyle
2. The dental hygienist should take a thorough health history and evaluate the vital signs to help identify clients at risk for a CVA

C. Signs and symptoms
1. Signals suggestive of a stroke include sudden weakness on one side (hemiparesis), difficulty of speech, temporary loss of vision (especially in one eye), unexplained dizziness, altered level of consciousness, shortness of breath, nausea, sudden severe headache, and confusion
2. A client experiencing CVA may have an elevated blood pressure and cardiac arrhythmias (irregular heart beats)

D. Treatment
1. Conscious client
   a. Discontinue oral health care, alert the dentist, and activate the EMS
   b. Assist the client in assuming a comfortable position
   c. Monitor the client's vital signs, and administer oxygen and BLS, as needed
   d. Continue support and monitoring until medical assistance arrives
2. Unconscious client
   a. Alert other staff, and activate the EMS
   b. Place the client in the supine position (or in the recovery position with the affected side down), monitor the vital signs, administer oxygen, initiate BLS as indicated, and continue support until medical assistance arrives

E. Transient ischemic attacks (TIAs) or mini-strokes can present with similar symptoms as stroke; however, the client recovers relatively quickly; because of a high risk for future strokes, this condition requires immediate referral to a physician for preventive treatment

Seizures and Convulsive Disorders

See the section on "Seizure disorders" in Chapter 19.

A. Seizures and convulsive disorders are the result of changes in brain function
1. Seizures—characterized by alterations in consciousness, motor function, and sensory perceptions; usually have a rapid onset and brief duration (usually 1 to 3 minutes)
2. Convulsions—involuntary contractions of the voluntary muscles
3. Epilepsy or seizure disorder—a condition characterized by recurrent seizures and convulsions

B. Causes and pathophysiology
1. Seizures and convulsions result from a disturbance of the brain's electrical activity
2. Seizures may be the result of tumors, congenital abnormalities, injuries, drugs, infections, fever (especially in young children), and idiopathic causes

C. Preventing seizures
1. Thorough health history should identify an individual with a history of seizures or convulsive disorders
2. If a client has a history of seizures, determine if medications have been prescribed to control seizures and if the client has taken the required medication before the appointment
3. Short appointments scheduled early in the day may reduce the likelihood of a susceptible client having a seizure in the oral health care setting
4. The use of nitrous oxide is contraindicated in clients with seizure disorders

D. Types of seizures
1. Convulsive—generalized tonic–clonic (grand mal) seizure; signs and symptoms include an aura (change in taste, smell, or sight precedes the seizure), loss of consciousness (a few to several minutes), an epileptic cry (sudden expulsion of air through glottis), involuntary tonic–clonic muscle contractions, altered breathing, and sometimes involuntary defecation or urination; after the seizure, respirations should spontaneously return, muscles relax, and consciousness returns; the person may have a headache, muscle aches, and be drowsy or disoriented
2. Nonconvulsive—absence (petit mal) seizure; signs and symptoms are sudden momentary loss of awareness without loss of postural tone and a blank stare for a duration of several to 90 seconds; although individual may twitch, he or she is usually unaware of the seizure
3. Complex partial (psychomotor) seizure; signs and symptoms may include an aura, purposeless movements, and loss of awareness lasting for only a few minutes

E. Treatment
1. Convulsive seizure in the oral health care setting
   a. Terminate the dental procedure, and lower the dental chair so that the client is supine with legs elevated; clear the area of all sharp and dangerous objects
   b. Make no attempts to restrain the client or place any objects in the mouth
   c. Protect the client's head, if needed, by placing a soft item under the head
   d. Assess and establish an airway
   e. Monitor the vital signs, and initiate BLS, as needed; activate the EMS, if needed
   f. If the breathing does not spontaneously return, evaluate for a foreign body (review earlier section on "Foreign bodies"), associated myocardial infarction, or neck and back injury
   g. After the seizure is over, position the client on his or her side for drainage of secretions; care is required if a back or neck injury is suspected
   h. Allow the client to rest
   i. After the seizure, assess for injuries to teeth or oral tissues, and assist the client in leaving the oral health care facility; arrange for medical evaluation
2. Nonconvulsive seizure in the oral health care setting
   a. Terminate the dental procedure, and closely observe client; clear area of all sharp objects
   b. Monitor the vital signs, and initiate BLS, as needed
   c. Furnish supportive treatment; the client may need further medical evaluation

Diabetes Mellitus

See the section on "Diabetes mellitus" in Chapter 19.
A. Diabetes—characterized by elevated levels of blood glucose resulting from an impaired ability to produce or use the hormone insulin
B. Clients with diabetes mellitus will exhibit a number of clinical manifestations of the disease and have an increased susceptibility to infection and diseases of the blood vessels
C. Cause and pathophysiology
1. Insulin is normally produced by beta cells of the islets of Langerhans in the pancreas
2. Cells of the body need insulin to take in glucose, and the liver uses insulin to store glucose as glycogen
3. If glucose and glycogen are unavailable to the body as energy sources, the body must break down other materials for "fuel"

4. Emergencies related to diabetes may occur as the result of two different situations:
   a. The client has too much insulin (hyperinsulinism), resulting in hypoglycemia (low blood sugar)
   b. The client has inadequate insulin, resulting in hyperglycemia (high blood sugar)
D. Types
1. Type 1, or insulin-dependent, diabetes mellitus usually occurs in the young and is more likely to precipitate a diabetic emergency
2. Type 2, or non–insulin-dependent, diabetes mellitus usually occurs in adulthood and rarely results in an emergency situation (clients with type 2 diabetes may become insulin dependent; review their health histories)
E. Preventing diabetic emergencies
1. A thorough health history is essential to prevent diabetic emergencies in the oral health care setting; factors to determine when taking the health history include the type and severity of diabetes; medications and their frequency, duration, and dosage; medical consultation may be necessary
2. Client whose diabetes is not under control should postpone dental and dental hygiene care except for emergency procedures
3. Dental hygienist should establish that the client's medications have been taken according to prescriptions and that the client has eaten meals according to schedule on the day of the appointment
4. Efforts should be made to minimize the client's stress and anxiety
5. Appointments should be scheduled to ensure that the client is rested and that the client's meal and medication schedules are not interrupted; morning appointments are best, 1 to 1½ hours after breakfast
F. Diabetic emergency—insulin reaction resulting from too much insulin (hypoglycemia or hyperinsulinism)
1. Insulin reaction occurs when too much insulin is present, with the result that the client's blood glucose is abnormally low (<50 mg/dL); this reaction may occur when the client increases insulin dosage, omits a meal, vomits, or engages in excessive exercise
2. Signs and symptoms of hypoglycemia may occur suddenly and include altered level of consciousness (confusion, anxiousness, incoherence, uncooperative or bizarre behavior), hunger, headache, pale moist skin, and feelings of dizziness and weakness; the client experiencing an insulin reaction will not be thirsty and will have normal breath odor

3. Treatment for insulin reaction includes the administration of sugar in the form of a sugar drink or sugar; this will usually bring about a rapid recovery (when recovered, the client should be encouraged to eat a complex carbohydrate with protein to ensure sufficient blood sugar levels to prevent a recurrence of the hypoglycemia); determine the need for EMS activation; if the client becomes unconscious, seek assistance through the EMS, monitor the vital signs; perform BLS, as necessary (including high-flow oxygen); do not give an unconscious client any substance by mouth

G. Diabetic emergency and diabetic coma (hyperglycemia, diabetic ketoacidosis)
1. Diabetic coma occurs when insufficient insulin is present, with the result that some cells cannot metabolize blood glucose
2. Signs and symptoms of impending diabetic coma in a conscious client include the "classic" signs of polydipsia (excessive thirst), polyuria (excessive urination), polyphagia (excessive hunger), nausea, dry flushed skin, deep and rapid respirations, weak and rapid pulse, and a "fruity" breath odor; unconsciousness may follow
3. Treatment for a client having symptoms of impending diabetic coma includes discontinuing oral health care, accessing the EMS, and support through BLS (including oxygen via nasal cannula), if necessary
4. If the dental hygienist has doubts regarding the origin of a diabetic-related problem, it is advisable to administer a small amount of sugar if the client is conscious; because hypoglycemia is more common than diabetic coma, the administration of sugar may improve the client's condition

Acute Adrenal Insufficiency, or Adrenal Crisis

A. Acute adrenal insufficiency (adrenal crisis)—occurs when the adrenal gland produces insufficient amounts of cortisol, a glucocorticosteroid that enables the body to respond to stress
B. Dental and dental hygiene care may induce considerable stress for some clients, causing this serious complication
C. Adrenal crisis is a life-threatening situation, and clients having adrenal insufficiency may go into cardiac arrest or shock
D. Cause and pathophysiology—the adrenal gland is unable to produce enough cortisol to enable the body to respond to a stressful situation (may be caused by abrupt withdrawal of exogenous

administration of glucocorticosteroid medications; may also result from disease)
E. Signs and symptoms
1. Client undergoing acute adrenal insufficiency may experience confusion, weakness, lethargy, and abdominal pain
2. Pulse may be rapid and weak; client may develop hypotension, followed by shock-like symptoms and unconsciousness
F. Treatment
1. Alert other staff, and activate the EMS
2. Discontinue dental or dental hygiene care
3. Place the client in the Trendelenburg position
4. Monitor the vital signs
5. Administer high-flow oxygen
6. The dentist or a physician may administer a glucocorticosteroid
7. If the client becomes unconscious, BLS may be necessary until definitive EMS treatment is available

Foreign Body in the Eye

A. Having a foreign body in the eye may happen to the dental hygienist or to the client in the oral health care environment
B. Safety glasses with side shields should be worn by both the dental hygienist and the client to prevent injury from spatter of materials used during dental hygiene care
C. Foreign material in the eye usually causes tearing, pain, and blinking
D. Procedure for removing a solid particle from the eye
1. While client looks down, pull the upper eyelid down over the lower lid
2. If the particle is not removed, turn the lower eyelid down, and examine it for irritants
3. Irrigate the eye with an eye cup or with gently running water for non-embedded foreign material; irrigation should start at the medial corner of the eye and flow toward the lateral corner
4. If the particle cannot be easily removed, refer the client to a physician for prompt treatment; it may be necessary to cover the eye with sterile gauze to prevent the client from further damaging eye by rubbing
E. Procedure for removing a caustic solution from the eye—check the MSDS forms for chemicals; when a chemical solution is splashed into eyes, immediate, copious irrigation with water from the medial toward the lateral corner of the affected eye may be required; activation of the EMS and prompt evaluation by an ophthalmologist may be necessary

MANAGING DENTAL EMERGENCIES

Dislocated Mandible

A. Dislocated jaw, or mandible, may occur from trauma or forced movement
B. The client with a dislocated jaw cannot return the mandible to the normal position because the head of the condyle is anterior to the articular eminence
C. The client with a dislocated mandible may experience considerable pain and anxiety
D. To return the mandible to its normal position, wrap both your thumbs in a cloth or towel to protect them and place the thumbs directly on the occlusal surfaces of the client's mandibular teeth; fingers should be placed under the client's mandible at the curve; to move the mandible back into place, make sure that the client's head is firm against the headrest; press firmly down and guide backward with your thumbs; pull up and forward with your fingers; the mandible should slip into place (use care to prevent injury to your thumbs)

Avulsed Tooth

A. Avulsed tooth—a tooth that is forcibly removed from the mouth by trauma
B. Avulsed teeth should be handled by the crown only; do not remove any tissue from the root surface
C. The tooth should be rinsed with milk or normal saline solution and gently placed into the socket while the client is transported for emergency care
D. If the tooth cannot be placed into the socket, the client should place the tooth in low-fat milk or in an optimal storage environment such as a Save-A-Tooth system for transportation to the oral health care setting for emergency treatment
E. The client should receive immediate emergency treatment in the oral health care setting

Aspirated Materials

A. Dental materials and instruments may be aspirated during oral health care because of the client's position, diminished responses caused by drugs, and diminished "oral awareness" caused by local anesthesia
B. Prevention of aspiration of materials can be accomplished through use of a rubber dam during many dental procedures

C. If a client is already reclining in the dental chair and aspirates an object into the oropharyngeal area, lower the back of the chair, and place client on his or her left side, using gravity to assist the client's efforts to dislodge the object; encourage coughing; however, the client may wish to sit upright
D. If an object is aspirated into the trachea, activate the EMS; manage as mild or severe obstruction; the client may wish to sit upright to facilitate breathing and coughing
E. If an object that has been swallowed cannot be located, the client must be escorted to seek further medical evaluation; a chest x-ray may be indicated to rule out aspiration into a lung

Broken Dental Hygiene Instruments

A. Instrument breakage can be minimized by careful sharpening, frequent inspection, and regular instrument replacement
B. If an instrument breaks, stop the procedure immediately
C. Inform the client of the situation
D. Do not use suction; have the client spit into a cup if he or she feels the need to swallow
E. Isolate and dry the area, and examine it for the broken piece of the instrument (e.g., the tip); if it is believed to be in a sulcus or periodontal pocket, use gentle instrumentation to explore the area; take care to avoid pushing the broken piece farther into the sulcular tissue
F. If the piece cannot be located, inform the dentist of the situation; use dental radiographs and transillumination to locate the broken piece; if unable to locate the piece, chest radiography should be performed to rule out aspiration of the broken piece
G. Follow-up by a dentist or a physician may be necessary

This chapter is only an approximate guideline for some common medical emergencies encountered in dental hygiene practice. Dental professionals should use standard operating protocols to manage emergencies and review or practice them regularly. Please consult current textbooks and journals for detailed information, and the American Heart Association and the American Red Cross for current protocol and training in BLS, ACLS, and EMS (see the box "Web site information and resources" below).

@ **WEB SITE INFORMATION AND RESOURCES**

SOURCE	WEB SITE ADDRESS	DESCRIPTION
eMedicine, Inc.	http://www.emedicine.com	Medical emergency reference
American Academy of Family Physicians	www.aafp.org	Health topic search and health information handouts and links to health-related sites
American College of Emergency Physicians	www.acep.org	Links to other emergency sites and fact sheets about diverse subjects, including emergency treatment
American Heart Association	www.americanheart.org	National directory of resources related to heart diseases
EMBBS (Emergency Medicine Bulletin Board System) Emergency and Primary Care	www.embbs.com	Educational resources for emergency and health care providers
Nemours Center for Children's Health Media	www.kidshealth.org	First aid and safety section; also contains articles and fact sheets on a variety of health topics

SUGGESTED READINGS

Hazinski F, editor: *American Heart Association guidelines for CPR and ECC 2010*, Dallas, 2010, American Heart Association.

American Heart Association: *BLS for healthcare providers student manual*, 2011, American Heart Association.

Little J, Falace D, Miller C, Nelson R: *Dental management of the medically compromised patient*, ed 7, St Louis, 2008, Mosby.

Pickett F, Gurenlian J: *Preventing medical emergencies use of the medical history*, Baltimore, 2009, Lippincott Williams & Wilkins.

U.S. Department of Health and Human Services: *Seventh report of the joint national committee on prevention, detection, evaluation, and treatment of high blood pressure (JNC7)*, NIH publication no. 03-5231, May 2003.

Walsh MM: Medical emergencies. In Darby ML, Walsh MM, editors: *Dental hygiene theory and practice*, ed 3, Philadelphia, 2010, Saunders.

CHAPTER 21 REVIEW QUESTIONS

Answers and rationales to the Review Questions are available on this text's accompanying Evolve site. See inside front cover for details. Use Case A to answer questions 1 to 5.

eVolve

CASE A

A 7-year-old patient arrives for an afternoon appointment with the dental hygienist. The vital signs are recorded. A blood pressure reading is not obtained, but pulse rate is 110 beats per minute, regular and strong. Respirations are 18 per minute, regular and easy. At the end of the appointment, it is determined that sodium fluoride (NaF) treatment would be beneficial. Using trays, 2 mL of 2% NaF (cherry flavor) gel is administered. During the fluoride treatment, the child swallows some of the fluoride gel. The mother is advised that the child should not eat or drink for 30 minutes and that some fluoride gel has been ingested. The dental hygienist does not anticipate any problems but informs the mother of symptoms to watch for and that she should contact her physician if she has any concerns after the appointment.

1. **Which of the following statements concerning the client's vital signs are correct?**
   a. Pulse rate is within normal limits, but respirations are high
   b. Respirations are within normal limits, but pulse rate is normal
   c. Both pulse rate and respirations are high
   d. Both pulse rate and respirations are within normal limits

2. **When obtaining the pulse rate for this client, which location is used?**
   a. Brachial pulse
   b. Carotid pulse
   c. Radial pulse
   d. Femoral pulse

3. **How safe is the maximum amount of fluoride potentially ingested by the child?**
   a. Any amount of fluoride ingested is considered safe
   b. The amount ingested is above the certainly lethal dose (CDL)
   c. The amount ingested is below the safely tolerated dose (STD)
   d. The amount was only a single dose and only long-term ingestion is of concern

4. **Treatment for acute fluoride toxicity includes all of the following EXCEPT one. Which one is the EXCEPTION?**
   a. Administration of glucose orally
   b. Administration of 1% calcium gluconate orally
   c. Administration of calcium chloride orally
   d. Administration of milk

5. **Which of the following is NOT a sign or symptom of acute fluoride toxicity?**
   a. Nausea
   b. Excessive salivation
   c. Nosebleed
   d. Thirst

Use Case B to answer questions 6 to 11.

CASE B

At the end of a periodontal debridement appointment, a 63-year-old female client becomes shaky, pale, and weak. The client is under a physician's care for diabetes, which she states is controlled by oral medication. Vital signs obtained at the start of the appointment included a blood pressure of 138/88 mm Hg; pulse rate of 76, regular and strong; and regular respirations of 16. The client states that she ate breakfast about 2 hours before her appointment; her most recent blood glucose reading is 100 mg/dL. The hygienist notifies the dentist, and together they reassure the client while managing the emergency.

6. Which of the following actions would be the MOST important one in managing this potential emergency safely?
   a. Administration of the client's oral medication
   b. Administration of insulin
   c. Administration of sugar
   d. Administration of a sugar-free energy drink

7. Before the emergency, the blood pressure reading obtained would be classified as:
   a. Normal
   b. Prehypertension
   c. Stage I hypertension
   d. Stage II hypertension

8. Insulin is normally produced in the:
   a. Gall bladder
   b. Liver
   c. Pancreas
   d. Small intestine

9. Prevention of a diabetic emergency would include all of the following steps EXCEPT one. Which one is the EXCEPTION?
   a. Medications are taken according to prescription
   b. Minimize stress and anxiety during treatment
   c. Schedule appointments after meals
   d. Schedule appointments before meals

10. Before treatment, the client's blood glucose levels were:
    a. High, hyperglycemic
    b. Low, hypoglycemic
    c. Within a normal range
    d. Not a factor in treatment

11. If this client becomes unconscious, which of the following actions would be CONTRAINDICATED?
    a. Activation of the EMS
    b. Application of high-flow oxygen
    c. Administration of orange juice
    d. Monitoring vital signs

Use Case C to answer questions 12 to 16.

CASE C

A 61-year-old male client expresses concern over receiving an injection of local anesthesia for periodontal debridement. The client explains that he had a bad experience many years ago. The client has a history of smoking, high blood pressure, and coronary atherosclerosis. He takes a calcium channel blocker medication. Vital signs obtained at the start of the appointment were blood pressure of 146/92 mm Hg; pulse rate of 66, regular; and respirations at 16 per minute. The hygienist begins treatment but stops when the client states that the procedure hurts during debridement. After a discussion with the client and the dentist, the hygienist administers a posterosuperior alveolar (PSA) nerve block depositing ¾ of a cartridge of lidocaine with epinephrine 1:100,000. The dental hygienist reassures the client while administering the anesthetic and monitors him during the onset of anesthesia. After a few minutes, the client complains of a squeezing pressure or tightness in his chest. The dental hygienist discontinues treatment and raises the chair to a semi-sitting position for client comfort. The client is experiencing some difficulty breathing.

12. Which of the following choices is MOST likely the cause of the client's symptoms?
    a. Allergic reaction
    b. Angina pectoris
    c. Congestive heart failure
    d. Shock

13. This client will benefit from administration of:
    a. Insulin
    b. Glucocorticosteroid
    c. Oxygen
    d. Nitroglycerin
    e. Both oxygen and nitroglycerin

14. Symptoms being experienced by the patient are also associated with:
    a. Aspiration of a foreign object
    b. Asthma
    c. Cerebrovascular accident
    d. Myocardial infarction

15. Decreasing the risk of an emergency related to toxic overdose of a local anesthetic can be accomplished by all of the following EXCEPT one. Which one is the EXCEPTION?
    a. Aspiration before the injection
    b. Blood pressure not assessed before treatment
    c. Staying within the maximum safe dose
    d. Use of a vasoconstrictor

16. If this victim loses consciousness and is not breathing, which one of the following actions should occur first?
    a. Activate the EMS, and open the airway
    b. Activate the EMS, obtain a defibrillator, check for a pulse, and begin chest compressions if no pulse is present
    c. Activate the EMS, and begin CPR starting with respirations
    d. Check radial pulse, and begin chest compressions if no radial pulse is present

Use Case D to answer questions 17 to 21.

CASE D

The dental hygienist observes an older adult client as he walks toward her. She notes that he uses a cane, walks slowly, and appears to be short of breath. As she reviews the health history with him, the client tells her that he takes a diuretic and a "drug for his heart," which she recognizes as an angiotensin-converting enzyme (ACE) inhibitor. His respirations are 26 per minute and shallow. Pulse rate is 90 beats per minute and regular. After consultation with the client's physician, who confirms that the client is being treated for congestive heart failure (CHF) but is healthy enough for routine dental treatment, the dental hygienist begins an initial assessment.

17. **Other signs of CHF that the hygienist might expect to observe in this client include:**
    a. Confusion, sudden severe headache, and hemiparesis
    b. Cyanosis, prominent jugular veins, and swollen ankles
    c. Hyperglycemia, pale skin, and hyperventilation
    d. Hyperventilation, aura, and involuntary muscle contractions

18. **Treatment modifications for this client would include:**
    a. Having a source of sugar available
    b. Placing a folded towel under the right hip when supine
    c. Treating the client in the semi-supine or upright position
    d. Treat client in the Trendelenburg position

19. **The respiratory rate for this patient falls into:**
    a. Faster than the normal range
    b. Slower than the normal range
    c. Within the normal range
    d. No normal range for respirations

20. **If it becomes necessary to administer oxygen to this client, which of the following oxygen delivery devices would be the BEST choice?**
    a. Ambu bag
    b. Nasal cannula
    c. Non–rebreather mask
    d. Pocket mask

21. **All of the following dental care strategies should be avoided when treating this client EXCEPT one. Which one is the EXCEPTION?**
    a. Scheduling long appointments
    b. Using anesthetics containing vasoconstrictors
    c. Making frequent quick chair position changes
    d. Using stress management protocols

22. **Cardiopulmonary resuscitation (CPR) is being performed on a 73-year-old client who is not breathing and has no pulse. Choose the statement that BEST describes the correct compression technique.**
    a. With both hands, depress the sternum to at least 2 inches, release pressure fully, and push hard and fast providing at least 100 compressions per minute
    b. With both hands, depress the sternum $1\frac{1}{2}$ inches to 2, release pressure fully, and push hard at 60 compressions per minute
    c. With both hands, depress the sternum 1 to $1\frac{1}{2}$ inches, release pressure fully, and push hard at 80 compressions per minute
    d. With both hands, depress the sternum $\frac{1}{2}$ to 1 inch, release pressure, and push hard at any rate possible

23. **Use of a blood pressure cuff that is 20% larger than the diameter of the client's arm will most likely result in a blood pressure reading that is:**
    a. Artificially elevated
    b. Artificially low
    c. Correct
    d. Difficult to hear

24. **If the tip of a curet breaks during subgingival scaling, the hygienist should follow all of the following procedures EXCEPT one. Which one is the EXCEPTION?**
    a. Asking the client to spit into a cup
    b. Informing the client and advise him or her not to swallow
    c. Isolating, drying, and examining the area where breakage occurred
    d. Suctioning the area carefully to remove the broken tip

25. **A 26-year-old female client is 7 months pregnant. During treatment, client positioning should include:**
    a. Placing the head lower than the feet
    b. Placing a folded towel under the middle of her back
    c. Placing a folded towel under her left hip
    d. Placing a folded towel under her right hip

26. What is the MOST likely adverse reaction that may occur in a client who has an excessive fear of a dental injection?
    a. Acute allergic reaction
    b. Decreased pulse and respiratory rates
    c. Psychogenic shock
    d. Toxic overdose

27. A dental client becomes unconscious but is breathing and has a pulse. The EMS has been activated. While monitoring respirations, the dental hygienist notices that the rate has dropped to three respirations per minute. The BEST treatment while waiting for the EMS to arrive would be to:
    a. Allow the client to continue breathing at three respirations per minute
    b. Apply a face mask with low-flow oxygen
    c. Use an Ambu bag to administer supplemental high-flow oxygen and ventilate at about 10 to 12 times per minute
    d. Use an Ambu bag to administer supplemental high-flow oxygen and ventilate at least 20 times per minute

28. A dental client reports that he feels weak, light-headed, and has a slight tingling in his fingers during treatment. His skin appears flushed, and it is dry and warm. Which action should be taken?
    a. Administer epinephrine
    b. Administer sugar
    c. Raise the chair to the upright position
    d. Recline the client into the Trendelenburg position

29. Low-flow oxygen is administered to a conscious client through a(n):
    a. Ambu bag
    b. Nasal cannula
    c. Non–rebreather mask
    d. Pocket mask

30. The compression rate for CPR for a 9-year-old child is:
    a. At least 40 compressions per minute
    b. At least 60 compressions per minute
    c. At least 80 compressions per minute
    d. At least 100 compressions per minute

31. In which of the following emergency situations would you NOT administer oxygen to a conscious client?
    a. Anaphylactic allergic reaction
    b. Angina
    c. Hyperventilation
    d. Toxic overdose of anesthetic

32. A 3-year-old child in the waiting room begins choking on a pretzel. He cannot speak and has poor air exchange. Emergency treatment should begin with:
    a. Abdominal thrusts until the pretzel is expelled or the child becomes unconscious
    b. Blind finger-sweeps until the pretzel is removed or the child becomes unconscious
    c. CPR
    d. Five back blows until the pretzel is expelled or the child becomes unconscious

33. Assessment and documentation of pretreatment vital signs is essential in care planning. If the client states that he or she is healthy and no medical problems were noted at the last dental visit 6 months ago, no complications should occur during treatment.
    a. The first statement is TRUE; the second statement is FALSE
    b. The first statement is FALSE; the second statement is TRUE
    c. Both statements are FALSE
    d. Both statements are TRUE

34. Which statement concerning management of convulsive seizures in the dental setting is MOST accurate?
    a. After the seizure is over, place the client in the Trendelenburg position
    b. Terminate procedures, and place the client in a semi-supine position
    c. Terminate procedures, and place the client in a supine position
    d. Terminate procedures, and restrain the client to prevent injury

35. Reimplantation of an avulsed tooth will have the best chance of success if:
    a. The tooth is thoroughly cleaned of all debris before re-implantation
    b. The tooth is placed back into the socket after good clot formation has occurred
    c. The tooth has been placed in low-fat milk and left out of the socket for at least 24 hours
    d. The tooth has been transported in low-fat milk and re-implanted as soon as possible

36. A 142/92 mm Hg blood pressure reading has been obtained for a 32-year-old male client. This is the third consecutive appointment that the diastolic reading has been above 90 mm Hg. The blood pressure for this client would be categorized as:
    a. Normal
    b. Prehypertension
    c. Stage I hypertension
    d. Stage II hypertension

37. When measuring blood pressure, how many additional mm Hg above the disappearance of the radial pulse should the cuff be inflated?
   a. 10 mm Hg
   b. 20 mm Hg
   c. 30 mm Hg
   d. 40 mm Hg

38. An apparently healthy 34-year-old female client begins to complain of sudden severe headache. She smokes 10 cigarettes a day. The only medication listed in the health history is a birth control pill. The client becomes extremely anxious and confused. She states she has slightly blurred vision in her left eye. She is MOST likely undergoing:
   a. An asthma attack
   b. A stroke
   c. A nonconvulsive (petit mal) seizure
   d. Syncope

39. Which of the following symptoms would the dental hygienist observe in a client undergoing acute adrenal insufficiency?
   a. Abdominal pain, altered level of consciousness, weakness, hypotension
   b. Aura, purposeless movements, blank stare
   c. Hypoglycemia, anxiousness, pale moist skin, bizarre behavior
   d. Nausea, dizziness, hemiparesis

40. Determining if a pulse is present in a 15-year-old client before initiation of CPR is accomplished by palpation of the:
   a. Aortic artery
   b. Brachial artery
   c. Carotid artery
   d. Radial artery

41. A male dental client with a history of heart disease has experienced chest pain during treatment. Treatment is discontinued. The client self-administers one nitroglycerin tablet, which relieves his discomfort. Because the nitroglycerin relieves the symptoms, the client MOST likely suffered a(n):
   a. Angina attack
   b. Asthma attack
   c. Myocardial infarction
   d. Transient ischemic attack

42. Severe bleeding from a dental extraction is BEST managed by:
   a. Direct pressure applied to the carotid artery
   b. Direct pressure applied to the facial artery
   c. Direct pressure applied with gauze over the bleeding extraction site
   d. High-volume suction applied over the bleeding extraction site

43. The BEST course of action during any emergency situation in which the client's medical condition fails to improve is to:
   a. Activate the EMS
   b. Ask a family member to transport the client to the emergency room
   c. Initiate CPR
   d. Transport the client with a staff member to the emergency room

44. A 5-year-old boy playing in the reception area "swallows" his older brother's Lego block. Shortly afterward, the 5-year-old stops breathing and becomes unconscious. After the EMS has been activated, which of the following sequences of care should be initiated?
   a. Give five back blows followed by five chest thrusts repeated until the object is expelled
   b. Perform subdiaphragmatic abdominal thrusts until the object is removed
   c. Activate the EMS, lower the child to the ground, and begin CPR with chest compressions by compressing the chest about $1\frac{1}{2}$ inches.
   d. Open the airway, perform blind finger-sweeps, attempt to ventilate, reposition the head, re-attempt ventilations, and start CPR by beginning with chest compressions, compressing the chest about 1 inch.

45. The ratio of compressions to breaths and compression rate for one rescuer providing CPR for a 9-month-old infant would be:
   a. 30 compressions to 2 breaths at a rate of 80 compressions per minute
   b. 30 compressions to 2 breaths at a rate of at least 100 compressions per minute
   c. 15 compressions to 2 breaths at a rate of 60 compressions per minute
   d. 15 compressions to 2 breaths at a rate of at least 100 compressions per minute

46. When it is necessary to perform CPR for an infant, which of the following would be correct?
   a. The heel of one hand is placed on the center of the infant's chest between the nipples
   b. The heel of one hand is placed on the center of the infant's chest between the nipples and the heel of the other hand is placed on top of the first hand
   c. Two fingers are placed in the center of the infant's chest just below the nipple line
   d. The hands encircle the infant's chest with the thumbs of both hands placed over the middle of the chest just below the nipple line when two rescuers are performing CPR
   e. Both C and D

47. **An automated external defibrillator (AED) has been used on a client who is not breathing and has no pulse. From the following scenarios, choose the one that is MOST correct.**
    a. If a shock is indicated, "clear" the client and press the "shock" button, following recommended CPR/AED techniques
    b. If a shock is indicated, press the "shock" button as quickly as possible regardless of other rescuers or bystanders
    c. If no shock is indicated, press the "shock" button anyway
    d. If no shock is indicated, then CPR is not necessary

48. **A dental patient experiencing a toothache learns that endodontic treatment is necessary. After discussing the procedure, the patient reports feeling dizzy and begins to breathe rapidly. Her respirations are 30 and her pulse is 100. She states that she feels like she is having heart palpitations. Which of the following procedures would NOT be recommended when assisting this patient?**
    a. Reassure the patient
    b. Place the dental chair in the upright position
    c. Encourage the patient to breathe slowly and deeply
    d. Administer high-flow oxygen
    e. Terminate dental procedures

49. **Clinical death may be reversible. This is more likely if life support measures are initiated within 6 to 10 minutes.**
    a. The first statement is TRUE; the second statement is FALSE
    b. The first statement is FALSE; the second statement is TRUE
    c. Both statements are FALSE
    d. Both statements are TRUE

50. **While waiting for his mother to complete her dental treatment, a 17-year-old male with a history of breathing difficulties begins to complain of pressure in his chest. Audible wheezing becomes apparent when he breathes. He states that it feels like he is unable to breathe. The young man's condition should improve after administration of:**
    a. An anticonvulsant medication
    b. A prescribed bronchodilator
    c. Nitroglycerin
    d. Oxygen
    e. Both B and D

22 Ethical and Legal Issues

Pamela Zarkowski

Understanding and applying legal and ethical principles protects the provider (dental hygienist), the client, the employer, and the employee. Dental hygienists make decisions that are influenced by laws and ethics. At times, these decisions are clear; other times ethical dilemmas create conflict with employers, colleagues, or clients. Dental hygienists must be cognizant of the laws governing the employer–employee relationship and influencing the responsibilities and rights of the parties involved. This chapter reviews the laws and ethics most closely associated with the dental hygiene profession.

ETHICAL CONSIDERATIONS

A. Definitions
  1. Ethics—the science of human duty; correlate motives and attitudes with moral actions and values
  2. Professional ethics—rules or standards governing conduct of members of a profession
  3. Bioethics—ethical and moral implication of new biologic discoveries and biomedical advances
B. Ethical theories
  1. Are the foundation of ethical analysis; explain moral principles
  2. Provide a basis for ethical rule, policy development, or both
  3. Assist in the resolution of ethical dilemmas
C. Three major theories
  1. Teleologic/utilitarian ethics (John Stuart Mill)—comprise rules for conduct based on consequences of action; an action is considered right or wrong on the basis of its usefulness; useful actions bring about the greatest good for the greatest number of individuals
    a. Act utilitarianism—examines a situation and determines which course of action will bring

about the greatest happiness or least harm and suffering to an individual regardless of personal feelings or societal constraints such as laws
    b. Rule utilitarianism—searches for the greatest happiness and seeks public agreement to define nature of happiness; considers the law and fairness; an action is considered right if it conforms to a rule; the rule should have positive results in a wide range of situations
  2. Deontologic ethics (Immanuel Kant)—focus on the morality of the act rather than the situation or consequences of actions; one would say, "It's the principle of the thing"; a person's intention, not the consequences of the action, is key; three important elements: applied universally to all individuals, unconditional, demand an action
    a. Act deontology—based on personal moral values of the individual making the decision and considers the ethical principles involved in an action in light of the circumstances—for example, avoid the truth if it is harmful
    b. Rule deontology—based on the belief that certain standards for ethical decisions are of greater value than an individual's moral values; considers the principles and rules in general as they apply to types of actions
  3. Virtue ethics (Aristotle and Plato)—focus on character traits and excellence of character; evaluate ethical dilemma by asking, "Is this what a virtuous person would do?"
  4. Other theories
    a. Situational ethics—course of action determined by:
      (1) The unique characteristics of each individual
      (2) The relationship between the health care provider and the client

(3) The most humanistic action in a given circumstance

b. Principalism—focuses on ethical principles, including autonomy, beneficence, nonmaleficence, and justice

c. Professional codes of ethics—designed in a rule-making format; usually direct decision making among professionals more than ethical theories

D. Universal principles

1. Veracity—truthfulness; mutuality for the client and the provider, for example, the client must be truthful to receive appropriate care, and the provider must provide truthful information so that the client can exercise his or her autonomy

2. Autonomy—personal liberty; individuals are free to make decisions regarding their own health; respect for the individual autonomy of others is basic to the health care provider–client relationship; informed consent and informed refusal is basic to autonomy (see discussion on informed consent in the section on "Legal issues for the dental hygienist" later in this chapter)

3. Beneficence—the provider's duty is a commitment to the health and welfare of the client above all other considerations; duty to prevent or remove harm and promote good

4. Nonmaleficence—the provider's duty not to use the treatment to injure or wrong the client; inflict no harm

5. Fidelity (role fidelity)—health care providers are required to provide services within the scope of their practice; ethics require that health care providers practice within the constraints of the role assumed within the health care environment; the provider is expected to follow through with commitments

6. Confidentiality—based on an individual's right to privacy, for example, client has the right to expect all his or her medical records and communications to be kept confidential

7. Justice—fair and equitable treatment of clients

PROFESSIONALISM

Defining a Profession

A. Characteristics of a profession

1. Special advanced education or preparation
2. Identifiable membership
3. Strong service orientation
4. Promotion of a body of knowledge in the field (research and theory development)
5. Autonomy of practice
6. Self-regulation
7. The recognized authority with societal sanction

8. Primarily intellectual nature of the work
9. Adherence to a code of ethics

B. Code of ethics

1. Historical evidence of Western medical ethics traced to guidelines outlining the duties of physicians

2. Early evidence included oaths and rabbinic and Christian sources

3. Common themes include:
   a. Respecting autonomy
   b. Preventing harm
   c. Protecting confidentiality

4. Oath of Hippocrates—fifth century B.C.E.; statement of principles guiding the professional conduct of physicians
   a. Stated "Above all, do no harm"
   b. Protected the rights of the patients
   c. Admonished physicians to keep the confidence of patients
   d. Placed needs of patient above those of society
   e. Placed an obligation on physicians to teach the next generation of physicians

5. Ethical codes for health care professionals continue to be evaluated and revised to reflect:
   a. Current practice issues
   b. Protections for population groups that are subjects in research investigations
   c. Identification of impaired health care providers
   d. Professional responsibilities

6. Common elements of codes
   a. Self-imposed—the health care professional self-assesses and determines compliance; range of sanctions from a professional organization or licensing agency for lack of compliance
   b. Set rules governing behavior—the professional uses them as a framework for action
   c. Serving to protect the public—on the basis of ethical principles that support actions to benefit the client and prevent harm
   d. Striving to enhance the profession—adherence to code characterizes a profession
   e. Providing a framework for ethical decision making

7. American Dental Hygienists' Association (ADHA) Code of Ethics and the Canadian Dental Hygienists' Association (CDHA) Code of Ethics
   a. Identify and describe ethical principles to guide the oral health care provider
   b. State the obligations and responsibilities of the dental hygienist
      (1) Personal and professional obligations and responsibilities

(2) Obligations and responsibilities to the public and the scientific community
8. Codes of Ethics—compare all codes
   a. For the ADHA's Code of Ethics, visit the Web site at http://www.adha.org/downloads/ADHA-Bylaws-Code-of-Ethics.pdf (also see Appendix C)
   b. For the CDHA's Code of Ethics, visit the Web site at http://www.cdha.ca/pdfs/Profession/Resources/CDHA_Code_of_Ethics_public.pdf
   c. For the American Dental Association's Code of Professional Responsibility and Conduct (revised January 2010), visit the Web site at http://www.ada.org/ethicsconduct.aspx
9. Client's Bill of Rights—outlines client expectations and provides guidelines for provider conduct; the client has the right to:
   a. Respectful, competent, and considerate care irrespective of ethnicity, gender, national origin, age, or disability
   b. Receive current, accurate, and complete information regarding diagnosis, treatment, and prognosis
   c. Receive information necessary to give informed consent or informed refusal before treatment; be informed of the consequences of refusing treatment.
   d. Confidentiality regarding all communications, consultations, and records except when permission has been granted to submit this information to others
   f. Obtain information relating to the credentials of all providers rendering services
   g. Reasonable continuity of care
   h. Examine and receive accurate copies of professional services and fees
   i. Receive treatment from health care professionals who act within the limits of their professional licenses (scope of practice) and adhere to the standard of care in delivering services
10. Types of professional credentials
    a. Licensure—state regulation of professionals
       (1) Granted by a state agency or board
       (2) Limits practice to:
          (a) Responsibilities and behaviors prescribed by law in the state practice act in the United States or determined by the provincial practice act in Canada
          (b) Responsibilities and behaviors delineated by rules and regulations
       (3) Authorized practice by professionals meeting specified qualifications

(4) Failure to meet responsibilities and expected behaviors may result in fines, suspension, or removal of license
(5) Status of license available to public; may indicate current license status (e.g., active, pending, suspended)
(6) The purpose is to protect the public from unqualified or unethical providers
   b. Registration—qualified professionals listed in a directory
      (1) Dental hygiene is a self-regulated profession in most Canadian provinces, and registration is a provincial responsibility (e.g., College of Dental Hygienists of Ontario http://www.cdho.org/indexmain.htm)
      (2) A certificate of registration to practice is issued only to those who meet established standards of qualification and practice
   c. Certification—state or national recognition
      (1) Recognition by a nongovernmental agency (e.g., a professional association)
      (2) Identification of professionals who have met specified qualifications

ETHICAL ISSUES IN PUBLIC POLICY

A. Ethical issues and public policy
   1. Distributive justice—fair allocation of resources involved
      a. Macro-allocation of resources—based on public needs (e.g., water fluoridation)
      b. Micro-allocation of resources—based on individual needs (e.g., fluoride varnish treatment)
   2. Distributive justice or allocation of scarce resources—determination of who should receive treatment when all cannot be treated; services may be allocated on basis of:
      a. Equity—all persons receive equal treatment
      b. Need—treatment allocated on the basis of prioritized needs
      c. Effort—treatment allocated to those who have earned it
      d. Contribution—treatment allocated to those who are making a contribution to society
      e. Merit—treatment allocated to those who are most deserving
   3. Influenced by principles of human dignity and human rights and contributing to the common good
   4. Current health policy debates
      a. Question of whether public health funds should be used for:

(1) Financial assistance and care of the disadvantaged or seniors

(2) Financial assistance and care for undocumented immigrants

(3) Financial support for victims of:

(a) Acute or chronic diseases

(b) Personal choices (e.g., tobacco use, risky lifestyle)

(4) Provision of health care services

(a) Appropriate range of services provided

(b) Impact of public versus private funding on the:

[1] Consumer and taxpayer

[2] Provider

[3] Third-party payer

[4] Government (local, state, federal, or all)

(c) Concerns about authority in treatment decisions

(d) Tele–health care

b. Research

(1) Identification of appropriate decision makers to identify and prioritize research agendas, especially for controversial topics (e.g., stem cell research)

(2) Identification of sources of financial support (e.g., what proportion of the national budget should be allocated to health care and research

B. Public policy

1. A system of plans of action, regulatory measures, laws, and funding priorities concerning a specific topic or issue

2. Promulgated by a governmental entity or its representatives

3. Public policy is commonly embodied in constitutions, legislative acts, and judicial decisions

C. Creating public health policy

1. Goal—assessment of a variety of actions and consequences to solve identified societal problem

2. Action—a decision by all members of society or their elected representatives (e.g., public vote versus state legislature passing statute regarding mandatory use of seat belts)

3. Analysis—determining which policy among alternatives best achieves the goal, how policy should be implemented, or how to evaluate what is currently being done

D. Policy makers—usually legislators, members of executive branch of government, and government officials who write regulations

E. Policy analysts—provide policy makers with information required to determine the impact of past and current public policies; determine whether new policy should be implemented or present policy or nonpolicy should continue

F. Examples of community-based programs requiring public policy analysis

1. Federal or state partnerships to provide oral health services

2. Fluoridation initiatives (e.g., community water fluoridation and school fluoride programs)

3. Caries prevention programs such as dental sealant or fluoride varnish programs in public health settings

4. Provision and funding of oral health care services by nondental personnel

G. Policymakers may seek input from professionals or professional associations; health-related professional associations frequently hire lobbyists to influence government policy makers

H. Distinctions between ethics and law

1. Laws are societal mandates, whereas ethics are professionally based

2. Ethical principles and legal doctrine are related

a. Ethical principles integral to federal and state legislation that is enacted

(1) Obligation to get informed consent (client autonomy)

(2) HIPAA (Health Insurance Portability and Accountability Act) regulations (confidentiality)

(3) Discrimination protections for clients suffering from specific disease states such as human immunodeficiency virus (HIV) infection (justice)

(4) Tort regulation (nonmaleficence)

b. Ethical issues inherent in the litigation of cases

3. Ethical duties are usually greater than legal duties; for example, a health care provider who is acquitted in civil or criminal court after being charged with illegal conduct did not necessarily act ethically

4. Compliance with the law sometimes mandates unethical conduct—health care providers are ethically and legally bound to keep confidential all client communications and records; however, the law makes exceptions and requires disclosure to appropriate authorities in specific situations (e.g., in cases of suspected child or elder abuse or threats of inflicting bodily harm to another person or self)

5. Personal values not necessarily congruent with professional ethics or the law—under law, individuals have a right to control their own bodies; this includes the right to refuse medical or dental treatment; health care providers must honor this right despite their own personal values

TABLE 22-1 Differentiating Between Ethics and Law

	Ethics	Law
Definition	Individual interpretation of the nature of right and wrong and rules of conduct	Rules and regulations by which society is governed set forth in a formal and legally binding manner
Source	Internalized; individual nature and beliefs	Externalized rules and regulations of society
Emphasis	Individual moral behavior for the good of the individual within society	Social behaviors that are good for society as a whole
Conduct	Motives and reasons why the individual behaves the way he or she does	Overt conduct of the individual; what a person actually did or failed to do
Sanctions	Professional organization—expulsion from the organization	Judicial and administrative bodies—criminal sanctions such as fines and imprisonment imposed by the courts; civil sanctions such as monetary damages imposed by the courts; disciplinary sanctions such as fines, license suspension, or license revocation by a board of dentistry

6. Differentiating between ethics and law (Table 22-1)

LEGAL CONCEPTS

A. Law defined
  1. Rules and regulations that govern society
  2. Reflects society's attitudes, mores, and needs; therefore, law is constantly changing to meet the requirements and expectations of society
B. Sources of law
  1. U.S. Constitutional law
    a. Constitutional law—supreme law of the land; both state and federal laws must be consistent with the U.S. Constitution
    b. The U.S. Constitution establishes the organization of the federal government and places limitations on the federal government through the Bill of Rights (first 10 amendments to the U.S. Constitution)
    c. Delineates the specific powers of the federal government to the:
      (1) Executive branch (Office of the President)
      (2) Legislative branch (U.S. Congress)
      (3) Judicial branch (U.S. Supreme Court)
    d. Powers not specifically granted to the federal government are the powers of state government
    e. Each state has its own constitution that grants powers and places limitations on the powers of the state government
  2. Statutory law
    a. Laws made by the legislative branch of government (federal, state, and local governments)
    b. State dental practice acts are examples of statutory laws
  3. Administrative law
    a. Administrative agencies are given the authority to oversee the specific laws or statutes to ensure that the intent of the law is enforced
    b. Administrative laws are the results of decisions of administrative agencies, for example, state boards of dentistry or the College of Dental Hygienists of Ontario implement rules and regulations to enforce the law
    c. Administrative agencies may conduct investigations and hearings and may issue decisions that suspend or revoke the license of a dentist or a dental hygienist; decisions of administrative agencies may be appealed through the state court system to determine whether:
      (1) The agency complied with the regulation
      (2) Evidence supports the agency's decision
      (3) The agency exceeded its authority
      (4) The delegation of power to the agency was proper
      (5) The agency followed proper procedures
      (6) The agency acted in an arbitrary or capricious manner
  4. Judicial law
    a. Determined by courts (state, provincial, and federal), which interpret legal issues in dispute
    b. Stare decisis[1] (Latin, meaning "let the decision stand")—doctrine of law whereby the court will base its decision on previous case law (a prior case with similar facts); the previous case must be from the same jurisdiction (state); emphasizes the importance of legal precedent
    c. Landmark decisions—court decision that departs from precedent, for example, new technology may require different conclusions based on the same facts
    d. Res judicata[1] (Latin, meaning "a thing or matter settled by judgment")—legal doctrine

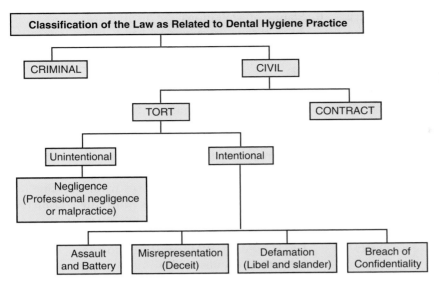

```
Classification of the Law as Related to Dental Hygiene Practice
         │
   ┌─────┴─────┐
CRIMINAL     CIVIL
              │
        ┌─────┴─────┐
      TORT       CONTRACT
        │
   ┌────┴────┐
Unintentional  Intentional
   │
Negligence
(Professional negligence
or malpractice)
```

Assault and Battery │ Misrepresentation (Deceit) │ Defamation (Libel and slander) │ Breach of Confidentiality

FIGURE 22-1 Classifications of law as it relates to dental hygiene practice.

that applies when a legal ruling has been made by a competent court of jurisdiction, and no appeals are possible; prevents parties from taking the same issues to different courts

C. Classifications of law (Figure 22-1)
   1. Common law and civil law—two concepts of legal thought, one from England (common law) and one from Europe (civil law)
      a. Common law—general principles derived from decisions in case law using the concept of precedent
      b. Civil law—civil code system developed by legislature, based on rules and regulations; enforced through the court system and protects the legal rights of private persons
      c. Level of proof—preponderance of evidence; the greater weight of the evidence required in a civil (non-criminal) lawsuit for jury or judge without a jury to decide in favor of one side or the other
   2. Criminal law—relates to acts considered offensive to society as a whole
      a. Classifications of crimes
         (1) Misdemeanors—usually involve fines of less than $1000 or imprisonment for less than 1 year, or both; examples include vandalism, trespassing, and reckless driving
         (2) Felonies—serious crime; usually involve punishment ranging from fines of more than $1000 or imprisonment of more than 1 year (or both); receiving a death sentence depending on the crime committed and the jurisdiction (state); examples include robbery, illegal drug use or sale, and battery

      b. Certain violations of law may be considered both criminal and civil, for example, if a client loses his or her life resulting from gross negligence of a dental hygienist, the dental hygienist could suffer loss of professional license, the estate of the deceased person could bring civil charges such as wrongful death against the hygienist, and the state may bring criminal action such as manslaughter against the hygienist
      c. Level of proof required to determine innocence or guilt beyond a reasonable doubt; the level of certainty a juror must have to find a defendant guilty of a crime
D. Primary individuals involved in a lawsuit
   1. Plaintiff—party bringing the lawsuit
   2. Defendant—party against whom the lawsuit is filed
   3. Attorney—individual serving as an advocate for either the plaintiff or the defendant
   4. Expert witness—explains specialized information to jurors; possesses appropriate credentials and expertise
   5. Lay witness—testifies as to facts for judge and jury
   6. Dental hygienist as a witness (lay or expert)
      a. Expert qualifications based on education, licensure or certification, experience, and publications
      b. Expertise to testify as to standard of care for dental hygiene
      c. Familiarity with the state or provincial dental practice act
      d. Knowledgeable about all written records relating to the controversy

e. Knowledge of office or institutional policy and procedure where (and at the time) the incident occurred

7. Cannot be lay witness if named in lawsuit

E. Due process and equal protection

1. Due process—protects the public from arbitrary actions of the state; the law must apply to all persons equally; elements of due process
   a. The law, as applied, must be reasonable and definite
   b. Fair procedures must be followed in enforcing the law, for example, the state may not arbitrarily take away a license to practice dental hygiene; the hygienist must first be given notice of the violation, a hearing, and an opportunity to respond before license revocation or suspension is imposed

2. Equal protection—equal protection clause of the Fourteenth Amendment to the U.S. Constitution protects individuals from state action; states may not enforce laws based solely on classification of persons such as race, age, gender, religion, national origin, or disability

F. Judicial process

1. Questions of law or fact—usually the jury determines what is fact from the evidence admitted by the court; the judge determines questions of law

2. Jurisdiction of the courts—authority of the court to determine the controversy, for example, the bankruptcy court may not hear divorce cases

3. State courts
   a. Trial courts—courts with trial jurisdiction; usually handle cases such as traffic, probate, family matters, arraignments for felonies, small claims, juvenile, and criminal misdemeanors
   b. Appellate courts—courts with trial, appellate, civil, and criminal jurisdiction; usually with a monetary restriction (plaintiff must request a fair minimum amount)
   c. State supreme court—appellate jurisdiction only

4. Federal courts
   a. Federal district courts—courts with trial jurisdiction; hear only matters that involve federal law or parties with diversity of citizenship (residents of different states)
   b. U.S. Courts of Appeal—courts with appellate jurisdiction only
   c. U.S. Supreme Court—court with appellate jurisdiction only; decisions cannot be overturned by any other court (state or federal); decisions can only be changed by new congressional legislation or subsequent Supreme Court decisions

G. Statute of limitations

1. Each state (or province) has a statute (law) that delineates specific periods within which a lawsuit must be filed after the event that caused the action; after that period, the right to initiate a lawsuit is lost

2. In tort actions, time may be measured from the time of the injury or harm or may be measured from when the plaintiff discovers the injury; periods vary from state to state

H. Case law—case law comprises the decisions, or the interpretations made by judges while deciding on the legal issues before them which are considered common law or as an aid for interpretation of a law in subsequent cases with similar conditions; case law is used by attorneys to support their views to favor their clients; it also influences the decisions of the judges; it is public record (occasionally court records are sealed)

1. Legal decisions available in publications appropriate for the level of the court where the case was tried; most decisions of state appellate courts are published in regional reports

2. Citations—references to legal authority that provide key information about the case, for example, in the following citation, *Edwards v Penn. Dental Examining Board*, 454, A2d 218 (1983): Edwards is the plaintiff (party bringing the lawsuit), the Dental Board is the defendant (party against whom the lawsuit is filed), 454 is the volume number of A2d (second series of the Atlantic Regional Reporter); 218 is the page number; and 1983 is the year the case was decided

CIVIL LAW AND THE DENTAL HYGIENIST

A. A lawsuit can be filed against an oral health care provider in two areas of civil law:

1. Contract violation
2. Tort violation

B. Contract law[1]—a contract is an agreement between two or more consenting and competent parties to do or not to do a legal act for which sufficient consideration exists; breach of contract occurs if either party fails to comply with the terms of the contractual obligations

1. Two methods to create a contract:
   a. Implied contract through signs, inaction, or silence; also called *apparent*
   b. Express contract entered through oral or written communication

2. The contract exists between a client and a health care provider when the client agrees to a specific treatment

3. Contractual responsibilities of the provider to the client
   a. Possess proper license and certification
   b. Exercise reasonable skill, care, and judgment in diagnosis and treatment
   c. Use standard drugs, materials, and techniques
   d. Complete the treatment in a reasonable time
   e. Never abandon the client
   f. Complete procedures consented to by the client
   g. Provide adequate instructions
   h. Refer appropriately
   i. Maintain confidentiality and client privacy
   j. Maintain an appropriate level of knowledge
   k. Practice within the scope of practice never exceed the defined scope
   l. Maintain accurate records
   m. Comply with all laws regulating practice
   n. Practice in a manner consistent with a code of ethics
4. Contractual obligations of the client
   a. Pay a reasonable fee in a reasonable time
   b. Cooperate in care
   c. Keep appointments
   d. Provide accurate history; information
   e. Follow instructions
   f. Keep the dental provider aware of status
   g. Follow home care instructions
5. Client–practitioner relationship—contractual; both are free to enter or decline the relationship; the practitioner may decline to undertake treatment of a client unless he or she has agreed to treat the client by participating in a specific dental insurance plan or the practitioner is employed by another who makes treatment decisions; if the practitioner offers services to the public, he or she may not refuse to treat clients because of race, color, gender, religion, national origin, disability, or any other basis that would constitute invidious discrimination; being bound to the code of ethics assumes a preexisting relationship of the client-practitioner
6. Termination of the client–practitioner relationship may be by:
   a. The client
   b. The practitioner, after giving the client notice and an opportunity to secure an alternative source of future treatment
7. Abandonment[1]—failure of a health care professional to provide services after the health care professional has established a relationship with the client; duty to the client to complete all treatment started; clients may be dismissed from future treatment

C. Tort law[1]—deals with civil wrongs committed against a person or a person's property; wrongful conduct
1. Unintentional torts
   a. Negligence and malpractice
      (1) Negligence—failure to use such care as a reasonable person would use under similar circumstances
      (2) Malpractice—wrongful acts of professional persons; usually failure to meet the standard of care or failure to foresee consequences that one with his or her particular skills and education should foresee
   b. Elements of negligence or malpractice, which must be shown in order for a lawsuit to go forward
      (1) Duty owed to the client (the plaintiff)
      (2) Breach of the duty by the professional or the defendant
      (3) Harm to the client (the plaintiff)
      (4) Causation—harm must be caused by breach of duty; foreseeability, that is, the event may reasonably be expected to cause the result
   c. Standard of care—the degree of care that a reasonably prudent professional should exercise; minimum requirements of acceptable client care, for example, practicing within the rules and regulations of the state or provincial dental practice act
   d. Damages (awarded to the defendant; to restore injured party)
      (1) Special damages—actual expenses
      (2) Nominal damages—at the court's discretion (could be $1)
      (3) General damages—part of harm; difficult to determine (e.g., can include pain and suffering)
      (4) Contract damages—for breach of contract
      (5) Punitive damages—to punish deliberately wrongful conduct (usually not covered by liability insurance)
      (6) States may place a cap on the maximum allowable damages that can be paid
   e. Res ipsa loquitur[1] (Latin, meaning "the thing speaks for itself")—legal doctrine that permits the plaintiff to prove negligence or malpractice without proving fault; no expert testimony required if the plaintiff shows a particular result occurred and would not have occurred but for someone's negligence
      (1) The type of injury does not occur unless negligence has occurred

(2) The injury is caused by something or someone under exclusive control of defendant

(3) The injury was not caused by plaintiff by contributing to own injury in any way (no contributory negligence)

f. Defenses to unintentional torts (protect defendant from liability)—not limited to, but include:

(1) Statute of limitations—time limit for initiating lawsuit has passed

(2) Comparative or contributory negligence—injured party is held responsible for a portion or all of the injury (states or provinces differ regarding degree of responsibility)

(3) Release—signed during the settlement of claim to prevent future claims

(4) Immunity—protection from prosecution, for example, the action may fall within a state's Good Samaritan law

(5) Defense of fact—no causation exists

2. Intentional tort—an act must be willful; the defendant must have intended to cause the harm or injury; the act must have been a substantial factor in bringing about the injury

a. Assault—any action that places one in fear of bodily harm (e.g., threatening behaviors)

b. Battery—intentional infliction of offensive or harmful bodily contact; unwanted touching

c. Defamation—communication to a third person of an untrue statement about another person

(1) Libel—written defamation (e.g., untrue or unflattering statement entered into a client's record)

(2) Slander—spoken defamation (e.g., discussing an employer in a derogatory manner while dining in a restaurant and being overheard by a third person)

d. Invasion of privacy—protects one's right to privacy

(1) Intrusion on seclusion—invasion of a private place or affairs of another; must be highly offensive to a reasonable person

(2) Appropriation—use of another's name or likeness for financial gain (e.g., unauthorized photographs of dental clients used in a research article or textbook)

(3) Publicity of private life—publicizing details of another person's private life; must be highly offensive to a reasonable person; health care professionals must not disclose a client's information without written authorization (e.g., no disclosure of client information over the phone or

to client's relatives, including spouse or friends)

(4) False light—putting another person before the public eye in a false light; highly offensive to a reasonable person

e. Infliction of mental distress—outrageous conduct that causes emotional distress; behavior must be beyond standards of rudeness; behavior was intended to cause mental distress and actually did cause mental distress (e.g., publicly revealing client's nonpayment; notifying neighbors or relatives of nonpayment)

f. Fraud or intentional misrepresentation—intentional perversion of truth (misrepresentation) for the purpose of gaining another person's trust and reliance whereby that person suffers harm or loss as a result of trusting and relying (e.g., never guarantee treatment outcomes)

g. Interference with advantageous relations—generally prevents an individual from interfering with the gainful employment of another; name and definitions may vary from state to state; giving a former employee a poor reference is not a basis for this tort

h. Wrongful discharge—illegal termination of an employee; most dental hygienists are hired without employment contracts and are employees-at-will; they can be fired for any reason except

(1) If reason for firing was against federal and/or state anti-discrimination laws, e.g., pregnancy of employee

(2) If firing is against public policy, e.g., sexual harassment or "whistleblower" cases

(3) Office policy and procedures (oral and written) may be considered an implied employment contract, e.g., office manual must address the issue in controversy

i. Defenses against intentional torts are not limited to, but include

(1) Statute of limitations—whether the time limit for initiating lawsuit has passed

(2) Privilege—person making the statement has the duty to do so; for instance, dental hygienists are often required by state law to report cases of suspected child abuse; in that case they are not held legally liable for doing so

(3) Disclosure statutes (state and federal)—permit access to client records by specific individuals or agencies without client consent, e.g., worker's compensation

statutes allow for such access to client information if a claim is filed

    (4) Consent: oral, implied by law, e.g., during emergencies (when a client is not capable of consent), or apparent, e.g., client sits in dental chair and opens his or her mouth for an examination

    (5) Self-defense or defense of others—behavior is justified to protect self or others from harm; if force is necessary, one may use only the amount of force necessary for protection (reasonable force)

    (6) Necessity—allows personal property to be confiscated, e.g., weapon

3. Informed consent—from concept of battery and individual rights to make choices regarding his or her own body

  a. Content—legal requirements vary from state to state; in general, a client must have information that a reasonable person would find material in making a decision regarding treatment

  b. Client should be told in a language or format that he or she can understand

  c. Specifically, client must be informed of the

    (1) Diagnosis

    (2) Proposed treatment and benefits

    (3) Risks regarding proposed treatment and chances of success

    (4) Alternative forms of treatment

    (5) Prognosis if treatment is refused

    (6) Provided with an opportunity to ask questions

    (7) Needs to sign a consent form indicating that he or she fully understands the information provided (no technical language on form)

  d. Competency of consent

    (1) Client must be of legal age and mentally competent (able to understand material facts)

    (2) Consent must be knowing and voluntary (cannot force someone to consent to a procedure)

    (3) Minors and incompetent adults

      (a) Parents or legal guardian may sign for a child; children of divorced parents may have specific requirements for consent related to divorce decree

      (b) Emancipated minor may sign for themselves; teenager can obtain emancipation by

        [1] Proving independence from parental control to the court; legal process involved

        [2] Legally marry

        [3] Enlist in one of the U.S. Armed Forces

      (c) Legal guardians or healthcare decision maker must sign for incompetent adults

  e. Informed refusal[2,3]—client may refuse treatment; to refuse

    (1) client must be provided with same type information as provided informed consent; include general and oral health risks

    (2) documentation of refusal including information provided to client must be placed in the client's record

    (3) client, operator, and witness signature recommended

D. Dental practice acts

  1. Statutes regulating the dental professions; in all legal jurisdictions (e.g., states and the District of Columbia or provinces)

  2. Enacted by state or provincial legislature; grant authority to a board of dentistry (board of dental examiners or other administrative agency) to adopt rules and regulations for dentistry, dental hygiene, and dental assisting and for dental laboratory technologists and denturists

    a. Rules and regulations must be consistent with the statute

    b. A board may not waive provisions unless specifically authorized to do so by statute

  3. Practice acts are enacted to protect the public; boards of dentistry or other agencies grant licenses to individuals to engage in a specific profession after demonstrating a minimal level of competence to perform the responsibilities required of the profession

  4. Composition of dental boards—usually elected or appointed officials who are:

    a. Dentists

    b. Dental hygienists (Figure 22-2)

    c. Consumers

    d. Others (e.g., lawyers, dental assistants, or denturists)

  5. Board duties

    a. Regulate applications for licensure

    b. Implement mechanisms for measuring competence of applicants, that is, credentials, examinations, mandatory continuing education

    c. Implement mechanisms for investigating complaints made against practitioners

    d. Grant and revoke licenses

    e. Draft laws pertaining to the dental professions for the legislature

DENTAL HYGIENISTS ON STATE DENTAL BOARDS

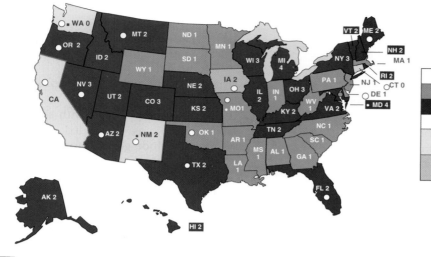

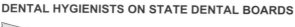

November, 2010

FIGURE 22-2 Dental hygienists on state dental boards. *(From the American Dental Hygienists' Association.)*

    f. Design rules and regulations pertaining to the dental professions

    g. Monitor educational standards

    h. Monitor other procedures related to licensure (e.g., licensure renewal, continuing education requirements)

6. Elements of dental practice act (vary from jurisdiction to jurisdiction)

    a. Requirements for licensure and renewal to show minimum competence

      (1) Minimum age and education

      (2) Character references

      (3) Examinations required

      (4) Continuing education requirements for re-licensure

      (5) Exemptions—"grandfather" clauses (e.g., licensure of dental hygienists trained in jurisdictions where preceptorship is legal)

      (6) Provisions for licensure across jurisdictions

        (a) Reciprocity—agreements between states for recognition of licensure from another state

        (b) Endorsement—grants of licensure if the applicant is licensed in another state and can present specific documents or credentials, and the states' requirements were the same or similar

        (c) Licensure by examination: when no reciprocity or endorsement is granted by states

        (d) Licensure by waiver—when a step toward licensure can be omitted (e.g., waiver of the clinical examination requirement)

      (7) Disciplinary action—boards have this authority with the power to enforce licensure requirements

        (a) License revocation or refusal to renew

        (b) License suspension

        (c) Probation

        (d) Reprimand—public or private

    b. Requirements for practice—defines scope of practice, that is, legally permissible tasks or procedures (Table 22-2)

      (1) List regulations—many states have a list of legal tasks delegated to dental hygienists

      (2) Open provision—some states have a general statement of what cannot be delegated; tasks delegated are at the discretion of the supervising dentist

    c. Legally problematic areas (scope of practice)

      (1) If a negligent act presents a scope-of-practice issue, a dental hygienist's actions should be within the scope of practice for the particular jurisdiction; procedures billed to the insurance company must be performed by the appropriately licensed professional, or the state insurance board also could take action

      (2) When the standard of care changes or increases because of the type of

TABLE 22-2 Dental Hygiene Practice Act Overview: Permitted Functions and Supervision Levels by State

FUNCTION	AL	AK	AZ	AR	CA	CO	CT	DE	DC	FL	GA	HI	ID	IL	IN	IA	KS
Prophylaxis	D	G/A	G/A	G/A[1]	G/A	A	G/A	G	G	G	D	D/G	G	G	D/G	G/A	G/A
X-Rays	D	G/A	G/A	G	G/A	A	G/A	G	G	G		D/G	G	G	D/G	G/A	G
Local Anesthesia		G/A	D	D	D	G	D	D	D		D	D		D	D	D	D
Topical Anesthesia	D	G/A	G/A		G/A	A	G/A	G	G	G	D	D/G	G	G	D	G/A	G/A
Fluoride	D	G/A	G/A	G/A[1]	G/A	A	G/A	G	G	G/A[4]	D	D/G	G	G	D/G	G/A	G/A
Pit/Fissure Sealants	D	G/A	G/A	G/A[1]	G/A	A	G/A	G	G	G	D	D/G	G	G	D	G/A	G
Root Planing	D	G/A	G	D	G/A	G	G/A	G	G	D	D	D/G	G	G	D	G/A	G
Soft Tissue Curettage	D	G	G	D	D	G		G	G	D	D	D/G		G	D		G
Administer N20	D	D	D	D	D	D			D		D		D	D	D	D	G
Study Cast Impressions	D	G	G	G	G/A	A	G/A	G	G	D	D	D/G	D	G	D	G	G
Place Perio Dressings	D	G	D		G/A	G	G/A	G	D	G	D	D/G	D	D	D	G	G
Remove Perio Dressings	D	G	D		G/A	G	G/A	G	D	G	D	D/G	G	G	D	G	G
Place Sutures			D									D/G					
Remove Sutures	D	G	G		G/A	G	G/A	G	D	G	D	D/G	G	G	D	G	G
DH Diagnosis/Assessment				G/A[1]	G/A	A	G									G/A	G/A
Treatment Planning					G/A	A	G									G	G/A

FUNCTION	KY	LA	ME	MD	MA	MI	MN	MS	MO	MT	NE	NV	NH	NJ	NM	NY	NC
Prophylaxis	G	D/G	G/A	G	G/A	G/A	G/A	D	G/A	G/A	G/A	G/A	G/A	D/G	G/A	G	D/G
X-Rays	G	D/G	G	G	G/A	G/A	G/A	D	G	G/A	G	G/A	G	D/G	G/A	G	D/G
Local Anesthesia	D	D	D	D	D	D	G		D	D	D	D/G	D	D	D/G	D	
Topical Anesthesia	D	D/G	G/A	G	G/A	G/A	G		G	G/A	G	G/A	G	D	D	G	D/G
Fluoride	G/A	D/G	G/A	G	G/A	G/A	G/A	D/G[4]	G/A	G/A	G/A	G/A	G/A	D/G	G/A	G	D/G
Pit/Fissure Sealants	G/A	D/G	G/A	G	G/A	G/A	G/A	D	G/A	G/A	G/A	G/A	G/A	D/G	G	G	
Root Planing	G	D	G/A	G	G/A	G/A	G/A	D	G	G/A	G	G/A	G/A	D/G	G	G	D/G
Soft Tissue Curettage			G/A	G		D	G	D		G/A	G/A	G/A			G		
Administer N20	D	D[1]				D	G		D			D/G	D	D		D	
Study Cast Impressions	G	D	G/A	G	G/A	G/A	G		G	G	G	G/A	G	D	G	D	D/G
Place Perio Dressings	G	D	D	G	G/A	G/A	G		G	G	G	G/A	D	D	D	D	
Remove Perio Dressings	G	D	G/A	G	G/A	G/A	G		D	G	G	G/A	G	D	G	D	D/G

Continued

TABLE 22-2 Dental Hygiene Practice Act Overview: Permitted Functions and Supervision Levels by State—cont'd

FUNCTION	KY	LA	ME	MD	MA	MI	MN	MS	MO	MT	NE	NV	NH	NJ	NM	NY	NC
Place Sutures																	
Remove Sutures	G	D	G/A	G	G/A	G/A	G	G	G	G	G	G/A	G	D		D	D/G
DH Diagnosis/Assessment	G														G/A		
Treatment Planning															G/A		

FUNCTION	ND	OH	OK	OR	PA	RI	SC	SD	TN	TX	UT	VT	VA	WA	WV	WI	WY
Prophylaxis	G	G/A[1]	G	G/A	G/A	G/A	G	G	G	G/A	G	G/A	G/A[5]	G/A	G/A	G/A	G
X-Rays	G	G	G	G/A	G/A	G/A	G	G	G	G/A	G	G/A	G	G	G	G	G
Local Anesthesia	D	D	D	G	D	D	D	D	D		D	D	D[3]	D	D	D	D
Topical Anesthesia	G	G	G	G/A	G/G	G/A	D	G	G	G/A	G	G/A	G	G	G	G	G
Fluoride	G	G/A[1]	G	G/A	G/G	G/A	G	G	G	G/A	G	G/A	G/A[5]	G/A	A	G	G
Pit/Fissure Sealants	G	G/A[1]	G	G/A	G/A	G/A	D/G	G	G	G/A	G	G/A	G/A[5]	G/A	G	G/A	D
Root Planing	G[2]	G	G	G/A	G/A	G/A	D/G	G	D	G/A	G	G/A	G	G/A	G	G/A	G
Soft Tissue Curettage	G[2]	D	G	G/A				G	D		G			D/A			
Administer N2O	D	D	D	D	D			D	D		D		D[3]	D	D	D	D
Study Cast Impressions	G	G	G	G/A	D	D	D	D	D	G/A	G	G	G	G	G	G	G
Place Perio Dressings	G	G	G	G/A	D	D				G/A	G	G	G	D	D	D	D
Remove Perio Dressings	G	G	G	G/A	D	D	D		D	G/A	G	G	G	D	D	D	D
Place Sutures																	
Remove Sutures	G	D	G	G/A	D	D	D	D	D	G/A	G	G	G	D	D	D	G
DH Diagnosis/Assessment				A													
Treatment Planning	G			A													

Key:

D   Direct Supervision Levels; dentist needs to be present

G   General Supervision Levels; dentist needs to authorize prior to services, but need not be present

A   Direct Access Supervision Levels; hygienist can provide services as she determines appropriate without specific authorization

Two letters denote separate supervision levels depending on setting Private/Public

1. Rules pending
2. Upon direct order
3. On patients 18 years or older
4. Public health supervision applies to fluoride varnish only
5. Participating in remote supervision pilot program

Footnotes apply to both settings if applicable.

Disclaimer: Information based on staff research. This document should not be considered a legal document.

States that Permit General Supervision in the Dental Office

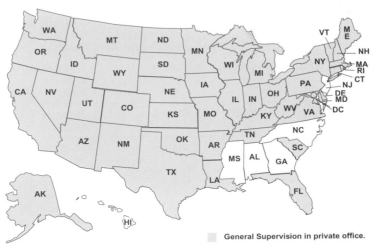

General Supervision in private office.

Direct Supervision means that a dentist must be present in the facility when a dental hygienist performs procedures.

General Supervision means that a dentist has authorized a dental hygienist to perform procedures but need not be present in the treatment facility during the performance of those procedures.   *August,2008*

American Dental Hygienists' Association

www.adha.org

FIGURE 22-3 States in which dental hygienists can perform prophylaxis in the dental office under general supervision. *(From the American Dental Hygienists' Association.)*

procedure performed or the addition of a legally recognized duty; for example, a dental hygienist administering a local anesthetic agent would be held to the same standard of care as a comparably trained professional such as a dentist

(3) When issues arise relating to use of new technology that may not yet be addressed in the dental practice act (e.g., use of lasers to fuse deep pits and fissures)

(4) Wide variations exist from state to state in the scope of dental hygiene practice; for example, practicing in a new jurisdiction where the dental practice act is more restrictive does not always allow the dental hygienist to deliver the treatment he or she was trained to perform or is competent to provide in another jurisdiction

d. Supervision (varies from state to state, and province to province)

(1) General supervision and assignment—licensed dentist authorizes the procedures on the basis of his or her diagnosis and treatment plan; need not be physically present when procedures are performed; some states require that the dentist or a designated dentist be available for consultation, if needed

(2) Indirect or close supervision—licensed dentist authorizes procedures and remains in dental facility while procedures are being performed

(3) Direct and immediate supervision—licensed dentist diagnoses the condition to be treated, authorizes procedures to be performed, and remains on premises while work is being performed, before the client is dismissed; some states do not require a dentist to approve the work before dismissal

(4) Personal supervision—licensed dentist provides a service for a client and authorizes an auxiliary to aid treatment by concurrently performing supportive procedures

(5) Unsupervised practice—services may be performed by a licensed dental hygienist without the supervision of a licensed dentist

(6) States are diverse in requirements for dental hygienists

(a) Forty-seven states allow general supervision, which does not require that a dentist be physically present during traditional dental hygiene procedures in offices (Figure 22-3)

(b) Forty-four states permit dental hygienists to administer a local anesthetic agent (Table 22-3 and Figure 22-4); all states except Oregon require the administration of a local

TABLE 22-3 Local Anesthesia Administration by Dental Hygienists State Chart

State & Year Implement	Supervision Required	Block and/or Infiltration	Education Required	Exam Required	Implement Language in Statute or Rules	Legal Requirements for Local Anesthesia Courses?
AK 1981	General	Both	Specific	Yes—WREB	Statute	16 didactic 6 clinical 8 lab
AZ 1976	Direct	Both	Accredited	Yes—WREB	Statute	36 hours, 9 types of injections
AR 1995	Direct	Both	Approved And Accredited	No	Statute	16 didactic 12 clinical
CA 1976	Direct	Both	Course taken as part of a dental hygiene program or course approved by the Dental Hygiene Committee of California	No	Rules	16 didactic 3 clinical 8 types of injections listed
CO 1977	General	Both	Accredited	No	Statute	12 didactic 12 clinical
CT 2005	Direct	Both	Accredited	No	Statute	20 didactic 8 clinical
DC 2004	Direct	Both	Board Approved	No	Rules	20 didactic 12 clinical
HI 1987	Direct	Both	Accredited	Yes—Exam given by course	Statute	39 didactic and clinical 50 injections
ID 1975	General	Both	Accredited	Yes—Board approved	Statute	No
IA 1998	Direct	Both	Accredited	No	Rules	
IL 2000	Direct	Both	Accredited	No	Statute	24 didactic 8 clinical
IN 2010	Direct	Both	Accredited	Yes—NERB Local anesthesia exam or equivalent state or regional exam.	Rules	15 didactic 14 clinical Permit required
KS 1993	Direct	Both	Accredited and board approved	No	Statute	12 hrs total
KY 2002	Direct	Both	Accredited and board approved	Yes—Written exam given by course	Statute	32 hour didactic 12 hours clinical
LA 1998	Direct	Both	Accredited	Yes—Board approved	Rules	72 total hours; minimum of 20 injections
MA 2004	Direct	Both	Accredited	Yes—NERB written exam by NERB	Statute	35 Total; No Less than 12 hours clinical

TABLE 22-3 Local Anesthesia Administration by Dental Hygienists State Chart—cont'd

State & Year Implement	Supervision Required	Block and/or Infiltration	Education Required	Exam Required for Certificate?	Implement Language in Statute or Rules	Legal Requirements for Local Anesthesia Courses?
ME 1997	Direct	Both	Accredited	Yes—Board administered	Rules	40 hrs total; minimum of 50 injections
MD 2009	Direct	Infiltration	Accredited/Board approved	Yes—NERB	Rules	20 didactic 8 clinical
MN 1995	General	Both	Accredited	No	Rules	No
MO 1973	Direct	Both	Accredited/Board approved	No	Rules	No
MI 2002	Direct	Both	Accredited	Yes—State or regional board-administered written exam (NERB)	Statute	15 didactic 14 clinical
MT 1985	Direct	Both		Yes—WREB	Statute	No
ND 2003	Direct	Both	Accredited	No	Rules	Course must include clinical and didactic components, but there are no specific hourly requirements.
NE 1995	Direct	Both	Approved	No	Statute	12 didactic 10 types of injections listed 12 clinical
NH 2002	Direct	Both	Accredited	Yes—NERB local anesthesia exam	Statute	20 didactic 12 clinical
NV 1982	Direct/ General	Both	Accredited and Approved	No	Rules	No
NM 1972	Direct	Both	Accredited and approved	Yes—WREB	Statute	24 didactic 10 clinical
NJ 2008	Direct	Both	Accredited/Board Approved	Yes—NERB local anesthesia	Rules	20 didactic 12 clinical Including a minimum of 20 hours monitored administration of local anesthesia
NY 2001	Direct	Infiltration	Accredited	No	Statute	30 didactic 15 clinical & lab
OH 2006	Direct	Both	Accredited	Yes—Written regional or state exam.	Statute	15 didactic 14 clinical
OK 1980	Direct	Both	Approved	No—Exam given by course	Rules	20 hours
OR 1975	General	Both	Accredited or approved	No	Rules	No
PA 2009	Direct	Both	Accredited/ Approved	No	Rules	30 hours Didactic and Clinical Permit, must renew
RI 2005	Direct	Both	Accredited	Yes—NERB	Statute	20 didactic 12 clinical

Continued

TABLE 22-3 Local Anesthesia Administration by Dental Hygienists State Chart—cont'd

State & Year Implement	Supervision Required	Block and/or Infiltration	Education Required	Exam Required for Certificate?	Implement Language in Statute or Rules	Legal Requirements for Local Anesthesia Courses?
SC 1995	Direct	Infiltration	Approved	Yes—Board	Statute	No
SD 1992	Direct	Both	Accredited Approved	No	Statute	No
TN 2004	Direct	Both	Accredited Approved	No	Rules	24 Didactic 8 Clinical
UT 1983	Direct	Both	Accredited	Yes—WREB	Statute	No
VT 1993	Direct	Both	Accredited	Yes—Board administered	Statute	24 hrs total
VA 2006	Direct	Both *Only on patients over age 18	Accredited	Yes—accredited program Board of another jurisdiction accepted	Statute	36 didactic-clinical
WA 1971	Direct	Both	Approved	Yes—WREB	Statute	10 listed injections
WI 1998	Direct	Both	Accredited	No	Statute	10 didactic 11 clinical
WV 2003	Direct	Both	Board Approved	NERB local anesthesia exam or equivalent state or regional exam	Statute	12 didactic 15 clinical
WY 1991	Direct	Both	Approved	Yes	Rules	No

Key:
Accredited—Course must be provided within a CODA accredited DH program or an institution housing a CODA program
Approved—Course must be approved by the state licensing agency
Specific—Course is specified in law. Data complied from 51 practice acts/rules
Direct Supervision—means the dentist must be present.
General Supervision—means dentist need not be present.

FIGURE 22-4 States in which dental hygienists can administer local anesthesia. *(From the American Dental Hygienists' Association.)*

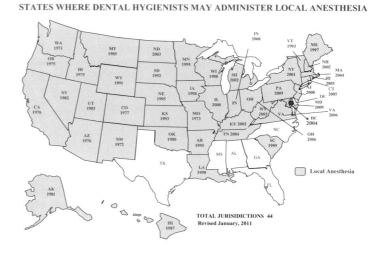

STATES WHERE DENTAL HYGIENISTS MAY ADMINISTER LOCAL ANESTHESIA

TOTAL JURISIDICTIONS 44
Revised January, 2011

American Dental Hygienists' Association

www.adha.org

anesthetic agent to be completed under direct supervision

(c) Twenty-eight states permit dental hygienists to administer nitrous oxide–oxygen analgesia (Table 22-4 and Figure 22-5)

(d) Thirty-two states allow direct access, which means that the dental hygienist can initiate treatment on the basis of his or her assessment of a client's needs without the specific authorization of a dentist to treat the client

TABLE 22-4 Nitrous Oxide Administration by Dental Hygienists

State	Year Enacted	Statute/ Rules	Education	Permit or Certificate
Alaska	1997	rules	3 clinical/3 didactic CPR	no
Arizona	1976	rules	36 hours Included in Local anesthesia course	no
Arkansas	1994	rules	Minimum of 4 hours	no
California	1974	rules	board approved course	no
Colorado	1997	statute	16 hours	yes
DC	2004	rules	32 hours total	yes
Idaho	1979	rules	degree completion or accredited	no
Illinois	1999	rules	14 hours	no board certification, but 12 hour course required. Must provide proof of completion.
Iowa	2001	rules	Board approved course or part of degree	no
Kansas	1994	statute	Board approved course 12 hours	no
Kentucky	2002	statute	2 hrs clinical, in addition to 32 hours of local anesthesia course and 12 hours of practical demonstration	yes
Louisiana	2010	Statute	Rules pending	yes
Michigan	2004	statute	4 didactic 4 clinical	yes
Minnesota	1995	rules	16 hours of clinical didactic CPR	no
Missouri	1994	rules	Course that provides proof of competence	yes
Maine	2006	rules	8 hours didactic 8 hours clinical CODA or board approved course and exit exam	yes
Nevada	1982	statute	Board approval course or part of degree	yes
New Hampshire	2006	statute	8 hours didactic 6 hours clinical	yes
New Jersey	2008	rules	7 didactic 7 clinical CPR	yes
New York	2001	statute	30 didactic 15 clinical	yes
Ohio	2010	Rules	4 didactic 2 clinical Written exam Clinical evaluation	yes
Oklahoma	1975	rules	12 hrs completion in board approved course	no

Continued

TABLE 22-4 Nitrous Oxide Administration by Dental Hygienists—cont'd

State	Year Enacted	Statute/ Rules	Education	Permit or Certificate
Oregon	1975	rules	14 hours in N20 CPR	yes
South Dakota	1992	rules	board approved course	yes
Tennessee	2000	rules	board approved course	yes
Utah	1983	statute		yes
Virginia *on patients aged 18 and older only	2006	statute	8 hours didactic &clinical	yes
Washington	1971	rules	didactic clinical competency	no
Wyoming		rules	Board approved course	yes

*Most states require dentist to be present. Please check with the state licensing agencies for specific information on any one state.

States Where Dental Hygienists Can Administer Nitrous Oxide

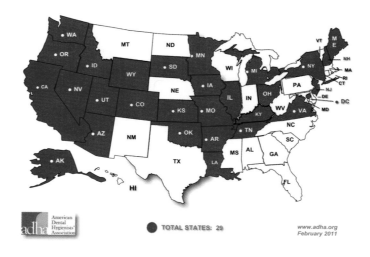

FIGURE 22-5 States in which dental hygienists can administer nitrous oxide–oxygen analgesia. *(From the American Dental Hygienists' Association.)*

TOTAL STATES: 29

www.adha.org
February 2011

without the presence of a dentist and can maintain a provider– client relationship (Table 22-5).
7. State dental hygiene committee
   a. Seventeen states have dental hygiene committees
   b. These committees assist in varying degrees in the regulation of dental hygiene practice (Box 22-1)
8. Alabama dental hygiene practice and education
   a. The state practice act allows only direct supervision of dental hygienists

   b. Prohibits performance of restorative functions by dental hygienists (see Table 22-5)
   c. Prohibits administration of a local anesthetic agent or nitrous oxide–oxygen analgesia by a dental hygienist
   d. Has unique educational and licensing procedures for dental hygienists
      (1) Alabama Dental Hygiene Program; since 1919
      (2) Only such preceptorship program in the United States
      (3) Eligibility—1 year employment as a dental assistant followed by an

TABLE 22-5 Dental Hygienists Restorative Duties by State

State	Apply Cavity-Liners & Bases	Place & Remove Temporary Restorations	Place/Remove Temporary Crowns	Place/Carve/Finish Amalgam Restoration	Place & Finish Composite Resin Silicate Restoration	Requirements
AK				Allowed*	Allowed*	Board Approved Course WREB or Equivalent Exam
AL	Allowed*	Allowed*	Place only*	Prohibited	Prohibited	
AR				Prohibited	Prohibited	Program
AZ		Place*				
CA				Allowed*	Allowed*	Requires Registered Dental Assistant in Expanded Functions (RDAEF) License
CO						
CT		Prohibited		Prohibited	Prohibited	
DC	Prohibited	Allowed		Prohibited	Prohibited	
DE		Prohibited	Prohibited	Prohibited	Prohibited	
FL	Allowed	Allowed	Allowed	Prohibited	Prohibited	
GA	Allowed*		Allowed*			
HI				Prohibited	Prohibited	
IA	Allowed*	Allowed*				
ID	Allowed*		Place only*	Allowed	Allowed	Restorative Endorsement; WREB or Equivalent Restorative Exam.
IL				Prohibited	Prohibited	
IN						
KS						
KY	Allowed*		Allowed*	Allowed*	Allowed*	Proof of competency.
LA				Prohibited	Prohibited	
MA	Prohibited	Remove only*	Allowed*	Prohibited	Prohibited	
MD		Allowed	Allowed	Prohibited	Prohibited	
ME		Allowed	Allowed*	Allowed*	Allowed*	Board approved EFDA program
MI	Allowed*	Allowed*	Allowed	Allowed*		Registered Dental Assistant took approved course
MN		Allowed*	Allowed*	Allowed	Allowed*	Board approved course to place & adjust permanent restorations.

Note: MN also permits RDH to place, contour and adjust glass ionomer.

State	Apply Cavity-Liners & Bases	Place & Remove Temporary Restorations	Place/Remove Temporary Crowns	Place/Carve/Finish Amalgam Restoration	Place & Finish Composite Resin Silicate Restoration	Requirements
MO		Allowed*		Allowed*	Place Only*	Proof of Competency
MS						
MT		Allowed*		Prohibited	Prohibited	
NC	Allowed*	Place Only*				
ND	Prohibited	Allowed*	Allowed*	Prohibited	Prohibited	

Continued

TABLE 22-5 Dental Hygienists Restorative Duties by State—cont'd

State	Apply Cavity-Liners & Bases	Place & Remove Temporary Restorations	Place/ Remove Temporary Crowns	Place/Carve/ Finish Amalgam Restoration	Place & Finish Composite Resin Silicate Restoration	Requirements
NE				Prohibited	Prohibited	
NH	Allowed	Allowed	Allowed*	Place		Expanded Duty Course
NJ		Allowed*				
NM		Allowed	Allowed	Allowed	Allowed	EFDA Certification
NV		Place Only	Allowed			
NY		Allowed*		Allowed*	Allowed*	Approved Course
OH		Allowed*		Place Only	Place Only	
OK		Place Only				
OR				Allowed*	Allowed*	Board Approved Course, WREB or Equivalent Exam, Restorative Function Endorsement.
PA	Allowed*			Allowed*	Allowed*	
RI		Allowed		Prohibited	Prohibited	
SC				Prohibited	Prohibited	
SD		Place Only		Prohibited	Prohibited	
TN	Allowed	Allowed		Place Only		Restorative Function Permit
TX	Prohibited	Prohibited	Prohibited	Prohibited	Prohibited	
UT						
VA						
VT						Trainings expanded function.
WA		Allowed*	Allowed*	Allowed*	Allowed*	Restorative services in curriculum of Washington Dental Hygiene programs. WREB restorative required for dental hygiene license.
WI		Place Only				Replacement of temporary restorations in emergency situations only.
WV	Allowed*	Allowed*	Allowed			
WY		Place Only		Allowed (with EP Certificate)	Allowed (with EP certificate)	Expanded function certificate no longer offered, but existing certificates honored.

This chart is for comparative purposes only. If information does not indicate whether one of the functions is prohibited or allowed, no assumptions should be made.
Disclaimer: Information based on staff research of state statutes and legislation. This document should not be considered a legal document.
*Can do services by virtue of inclusion in dental assistants scope of practice. Please check practice act for education requirements.

BOX 22-1 Dental Hygiene Participation in Regulation

The following states have dental hygiene advisory committees or varying degrees of self regulation for dental hygienists.

1. Arizona

The Arizona advisory committee consists of one dentist and one dental hygienist from the board, plus four additional dental hygienists and one public member. The committee serves as a forum for discussion of dental hygiene issues and advises the board on rules and proposed statute changes concerning dental hygiene education, regulation and practice. In addition the committee evaluates CE classes for expanded functions and monitors dental hygienists' compliance with CE requirements.

2. California

The Dental Hygiene Committee of California is a self-regulating dental hygiene committee in conjunction with the Department of Consumer Affairs. The committee consists of four dental hygienists, four public members and one dentist appointed by the governor.

3. Connecticut

Connecticut is unique. Dental hygiene is directly under the Department Public Health, and although there is no standing dental hygiene committee, if there is a need to address rules or disciplinary matters, the department director has the ability to appoint an ad hoc committee of dental hygienists.

4. Delaware

Delaware's Advisory Committee is appointed by the governor and consists of three dental hygienists. The Committee writes the examination for dental hygiene licensure (in conjunction with the dental board). In addition, the Committee votes with the board on issues of dental hygiene licensure by credentials, disciplinary decisions, continuing education requirements for dental hygiene licensure, disciplinary action involving dental hygienists and issues involving the policy and practice of dental hygiene but not the scope of practice.

5. Florida

Florida has both dental hygiene and dental assisting councils. The dental hygiene council is composed of four dental hygienists, one of whom sits on the board, and one dentist member of the board. The council is expected to develop all dental hygiene rules to submit to the board for its approval.

6. Iowa

Beginning in 1999, both dental hygienists on the dental board and one of the dentists became a dental hygiene committee of the board. This committee has the power to make all rules pertaining to dental hygiene. The board will be required to adopt those rules and enforce the committee rules.

7. Maine

Maine has a subcommittee on dental hygiene. The subcommittee consists of five members: one dental hygienist who is a member of the board; two dental hygienists appointed by the governor; two dentists who are members of the board and appointed by the president of the board. The duties of the subcommittee are to perform an initial review of all applications for licensure as a dental hygienist, submissions relating to continuing education of dental hygienists, and all submissions relating to public health supervision status of dental hygienists.

8. Maryland

Maryland's committee consists of three dental hygienists, one dentist, and one public member, all of whom are full voting members of the dental board. The committee was created during sunset review as a compromise to the creation of a separate dental hygiene regulatory board. According to statute, all matters pertaining to dental hygiene must first be brought to the committee for its review and recommendation.

9. Michigan

A five member advisory committee, comprised of four dental hygienists and one dentist, considers matters related to the dental hygiene profession and makes recommendations to the full board of dentistry. All members of the advisory committee are voting members on the board. The existence of the advisory committee is not mandated by state rules or statutes, but instead is a committee appointed by the chairperson of the board.

10. Missouri

A five member advisory commission, composed of the dental hygienist on the dental board and four dental hygienists appointed by the governor was created by the state legislature in 2001. The commission will make recommendations to the board concerning dental hygiene practice, licensure, examinations, discipline and educational requirements.

11. Montana

In 2002, the board assigned both dental hygienist members and one dentist member to be a standing committee to consider and address dental hygiene issues in a timely fashion. The committee will formulate specific recommendations to bring to the entire board for action.

12. Nevada

Legislation in 2003 added a third dental hygienist to the board, who together with a dentist appointed by the board, will constitute a dental hygiene committee that may formulate recommendations on dental hygiene rules for the board and be assigned additional duties by the board.

13. New Mexico

New Mexico has a board of dental health care comprised of five dentists, two dental hygienists and two public members. There is a dental hygiene committee comprised of five dental hygienists, two public members and two dentists. The committee selects two of its dental

Continued

BOX 22-1 Dental Hygiene Participation in Regulation—cont'd

hygiene members to serve as the dental hygienists on the board. The board's public members and two of its dentist members are the dentist and public members of the committee. The committee adopts all the rules pertaining to dental hygiene and is also responsible for the discipline of dental hygienists. The board enforces the dental hygiene committee's rules.

14. Oklahoma
The dental hygiene advisory committee is comprised of the dental hygiene board member and four additional dental hygienists appointed by the board.

15. Oregon
Under its authority to create standing committees, the Oregon dental board has appointed a committee comprised of three dentists, three dental hygienists, and one non-dental healthcare provider to advise the board concerning dental hygiene issues.

16. Texas
In 1995, a dental hygiene advisory committee comprised of three dental hygienists and two public members appointed by the governor and one dentist appointed by the board was established. All rules relating to the practice of dental hygiene must be submitted to the committee for review 30 days prior to board adoption. The committee has been responsible for researching and developing recent rules for licensure by credentials and the application of tetracycline fibers. Legislation in 2003 gave the committee the authority to propose specific rules for board action.

17. Washington
The state of Washington has a uniform disciplinary code which applies to all health professions and creates the regulatory bodies to implement each practice act. Dentistry and dental hygiene have separate practice acts. Dentists are regulated by the Dental Quality Assurance Commission (an independent dental board with no dental hygiene members). Dental hygienists are regulated by the Dental Hygiene Advisory Committee (comprised of three dental hygienists and one public member appointed by the department). Created in the early eighties, its original charge was to develop rules for dental hygiene education and licensure. Now, the committee has authority to originate all dental hygiene rules. Although nominally advisory, it meets and deliberates like a board. The department of health has consistently implemented rules as proposed by the committee.

---

educational program that includes basic science and clinical theory
  (4) Dentists are "preceptors," who provide on-the-job training in the dental office
  (5) Program replaces formal dental hygiene education from an accredited academic program; graduates are not eligible to take the National Board Dental Hygiene Examination; therefore, their practice is limited to Alabama
  (6) Graduates are not eligible for membership in the American Dental Hygienists' Association
9. Updating dental practice acts
  a. Revision or amendments made by state legislatures
  b. Sunset laws—set review of the entire act at a fixed interval (e.g., every 7 years, to keep act updated and relevant to society); if not completed by legislature by designated date or if found to no longer serve its function to society, the act will automatically expire (hence the term *sunset*)
10. Due process requirements for disciplinary action—if a complaint is filed against a professional, with the licensing board, the licensee has a right to:

a. Receive a clear statement of charges
b. Question opposing witnesses
c. Produce witnesses and give testimony (answer charges)
d. The services of an attorney
e. Receive a firm conclusion based on the evidence
f. Contest the board's decision at a court of law
g. If these rights are not provided, the board's decision could be reversed by a court of law
11. Practicing without a license—penalties vary from state to state
  a. Criminal charges—usually result in a fine (~$50 to $500) or imprisonment (usually not to exceed 60 days), or both
  b. Civil suits—may be filed for monetary damages by individuals who have been harmed
  c. Criminal or civil actions, or both, may be brought against the unlicensed person
12. Reporting professional violations—failure to report a violation is grounds for disciplinary action; failure to report is considered unprofessional conduct; reporting a violation requires the following:
  a. Facts must be documented in writing with complete description of violation

b. Report must list other witnesses and clients involved, if applicable

13. National Practitioner Data Bank (NPDB)
   a. Created by the U.S. Department of Health and Human Services in 1990
   b. Purpose—electronic repository that collects information on adverse licensure actions, certain actions restricting clinical privileges and professional society membership actions taken against physicians, dentists, and other practitioners.
   c. Medical and dental regulatory boards are required to report certain actions taken against licensees
   d. Health care entities such as hospitals are required to report certain disciplinary action taken against staff members
   e. Licensees are not required to report incidents
   f. Access to data bank information
      (1) Individuals, who may request their own record
      (2) State licensing boards
      (3) Researchers, health care entities (e.g., hospitals, nursing homes)
      (4) Professional societies
      (5) Attorneys
   g. The law prohibits the release of information in the NPDB to the public

14. Health Care Integrity and Protection Data Bank (HIPDB)
   a. Combats fraud and abuse in health insurance and health care delivery
   b. Flagging system used to alert users
   c. Intended to augment, not replace, traditional forms of review and investigation, serving as an important supplement to a review of a practitioner's, provider's, or supplier's past actions

DENTAL RECORDS AND RECORD KEEPING

A. Purpose of dental records
   1. Provides all privileged parties with information; method of communication with dental and other medical providers
   2. Tool for quality assessment and management
   3. Documents assessment findings, treatment, care provided, and outcomes
   4. Serves as an important document in third-party relationships
   5. Provides evidence of compliance with state record-keeping requirements
   6. Resource in forensic identification

7. Reference in litigation and provides information for the client and provider
8. Useful in research

B. Written record management
   1. Adheres to state dental practice or state medical records guidelines, if required
   2. Legible and written in black ink or ball point, not pencil
   3. Consistent style for all entries; uniformly spaced
   4. Corrections and additions clearly explained
   5. Deletions noted by single line through entry
   6. Signed and initialed by appropriate operator

C. Electronic dental records
   1. Same record keeping principles as those for paper records
   2. System should include protections from tampering
   3. Courts accept as documentation

D. Client records—must be clear, complete, and accurate and include:
   1. Client identification data—client's name, address, employment, home and cell telephone numbers, social security number, birth date, emergency contact, physician's name and phone number, financial information; legal guardian information, if appropriate
   2. Consent forms—informed consent and informed refusal
   3. Health, pharmacologic, and dental histories—before treatment, updated at each visit, signed and dated by the client and oral health care professional
   4. Referrals—referrals made to other professionals, reports of tests, or reports from other providers
   5. Clinical observations—intraoral and extraoral examination results, findings of pathology, periodontal evaluation, radiographs, study models, diagnostic photographs
   6. Progress or treatment notes—chronologic notation of treatment, pretreatment procedures, unusual incidents or circumstances, diagnosis and care plans, oral hygiene recommendations, client noncompliance, postoperative instructions, telephone conversations with the client or other health care providers, medications taken or prescribed with dosage, client's missed or canceled appointments
   7. Failure to maintain or store dental records for a specified period may violate state dental practice acts; considered medical malpractice in some jurisdictions in a court of law
   8. Records also include radiographs, photographs, and models
   9. States regulations may delineate specific costs for duplication of records

E. Confidentiality—client confidentiality is protected by federal and state laws; state laws often regulate the disclosure of substance abuse, mental health history, HIV/AIDS (human immunodeficiency virus/acquired immune deficiency syndrome) status; improper disclosure can result in liability for breach of fiduciary duty, breach of implied contract, or invasion of privacy

1. Health Insurance Portability and Accountability Act (HIPAA)
   a. Purpose—this federal act allows employees to move their health insurance when changing jobs and is in place to develop standards for health information, provide greater safeguards regarding privacy of protected health information (PHI), and reduce health care fraud and abuse
   b. Protects health information by establishing transaction standards for the exchange of health information, security standards, and privacy standards for the use and disclosure of individually identifiable health information (IIHI)
   c. Protected Health Information (PHI) includes all individually identifiable health information that is:
      (1) Sent or stored in any form
      (2) Identifies the client or can be used to identify the client
      (3) Created or received by a covered entity
      (4) About the client's past, present, or future treatment and payment for services
   d. Three major areas addressed relating to requirements for privacy and confidentiality of health information (effective April 14, 2003)
      (1) Privacy standards
         (a) Client notification of privacy policies of office or institution
         (b) Written acknowledgment of receipt of notice of privacy policies
         (c) Written and signed authorization and consent
      (2) Client's rights
         (a) Right to inspect and copy confidential health care information
         (b) Right to amend confidential information in the client record
         (c) Right to obtain a list of disclosures of their protected health information
         (d) Right to confidential communication
         (e) Right to complain to the practice, to the Secretary of Health and Human Services, or to both
      (3) Administrative requirements
         (a) Develop policies, procedures, and documentation

         (b) Provide notice of privacy policy to clients
         (c) Designate a privacy officer and a contact person to receive complaints
         (d) Implement complaint systems
         (e) Provide training for employees
         (f) Execute business associate contracts
         (g) Mitigate any breach of confidentiality
2. Exceptions to nondisclosure of client information—original client records should never be released
   a. Client consent—with written authorization only, specifying name of the client, name of the person authorized to disclose the information, amount and type of information to be released, name of the person or entity to receive the information, the date information is to be released, the date authorization expires, and the client's signature
   b. Relevant copies of a client's medical records may be released to the court where the client's medical condition is put in issue by filing a lawsuit[4]
   c. Duty to disclose—state reporting statutes may require release of client information (e.g., in cases of child or elder abuse); state statutes identify health care providers who are obligated by law to report suspected cases of abuse; statutes also provide immunity from civil liability for health care providers involved in reporting suspected abuse, unless it can be proved that a false report had been made, and the person knew that the report was false; access statutes allow for release of client information with no client authorization required (e.g., worker's compensation statutes)
3. PHI in electronic form is sometimes referred to as ePHI; ePHI can include client information in an email, in an electronic file, or on a CD or a memory stick
4. Health Information and Technology Clinical Health Technology Act (HITECH); effective September 23, 2009; enforced February 2010
   a. Expands HIPAA's privacy and security provisions
   b. Requires covered entities to provide notice of any breaches or unauthorized disclosures of PHI

EMPLOYER AND EMPLOYEE RIGHTS AND RESPONSIBILITIES

A. Employment
1. Employer—person, business, or organization that hires and compensates one or more workers; engages the services of an individual

2. Employee—person who is hired to provide services to a company on a regular basis in exchange for compensation
3. Status
   a. At will; individual can be hired or terminated without notice
      (1) Employees without a contract
      (2) Should a dispute arise relating to termination of employment, courts often examine the office policy and procedure manual in determining an implied contract
   b. Contract—a legally binding agreement between two or more parties
      (1) Elements (to be enforced by a court)
         (a) Offer—one party proposes a bargain
         (b) Acceptance—the other party agrees to the proposed bargain
         (c) Consideration—one party gives up something of value, and the other party makes a promise in exchange for that something of value
         (d) Mutuality—parties must reach an agreement or understanding
         (e) Legal capacity—all parties must have legal capacity (i.e., be the age of majority and mentally competent)
      (2) Contract must be for a lawful purpose
      (3) Breach of contract—failure of performance of a contractual agreement by one or more parties
         (a) Remedies for breach of contract
            [1] Specific performance (the court requires performance of the contract)
            [2] Monetary damage
            [3] Injunctions (the court orders a party to refrain from specific behavior)
      (4) Employment contracts (Box 22-2)
         (a) Define duties and responsibilities of the position; location and hours
         (b) Define salary and benefits
         (c) Describe notice and termination requirements
         (d) Provide written description of understanding between the parties
4. Independent practitioner—one who provides services directly to the public; dental hygienists who perform as independent practitioners may do so only in a state where it is allowed by the dental practice act; a dental hygienist as an independent practitioner must follow the state's (province's) dental practice act and regulations (Box 22-3)

BOX 22-2 Employment Contract Terms

An employment contract spells out the conditions of employment, including wages, hours, and type of work. Depending on the level of employment, the responsibility of the new employee, and the nature of the business, the conditions of employment should be detailed regarding the following elements:
Parties including the name of the employer and the entity and the name of the employee
Time and place: Hours of employment and location
Duties: General and specific, scope of practice, if appropriate
Term and conditions of employment
Compensation, including salary, bonus pay, vacation, sick leave, continuing education policies and reimbursement, and professional memberships
Benefits, including disability, medical, life insurance, and retirement plan
Termination provisions

---

5. Independent contractor—contracted by another person, company, or agency to produce a certain result, but not subject to the control of the employer and may do the work in a manner he or she selects; a dental hygienist as an independent contractor must follow both Internal Revenue Service (IRS) rules and the state's dental practice act and regulations
6. Vicarious liability—one party is responsible for another's action; respondeat superior (Latin, meaning "let the master answer"), an employer is legally responsible for the wrongs committed by an employee acting within the scope of his or her employment; dentist employer may be held responsible for negligent acts of a dental hygienist
   a. Vicarious liability or negligent retention may shield a dental hygienist from liability in tort cases
   b. Dental hygienists are liable for their actions
7. Negligent hiring and retention—employer can be held liable for acts or omissions of employees if the client can show that the employee was incompetent and the employer knew or should have known
B. Employment laws—offer protections for employer and employee
   1. Equal Employment Opportunity Commission (EEOC)—enforces federal laws passed to prevent discrimination in the workplace; investigates complaints and assists an individual or the Department of Justice in bringing a lawsuit
   2. Title VII of the Civil Rights Act of 1964—forbids discrimination against employees by federal,

BOX 22-3 Independent Practice

There is virtually no legal guidance–even in the laws of states which allow it—about what INDEPENDENT PRACTICE means. If one equates it with other health practices one would expect that the practice is a business entity that can be sold to another, be directly reimbursed for services and has patients of record.

Four states which have specific authorization in the practice act law which allows a hygienist to own a dental hygiene practice–Colorado (any hygienist), Maine (hygienists licensed as independent dental hygiene practitioners), New Mexico (hygienists in collaborative practice) and California (RDHAPs–registered dental hygienists in alternative practice). In several other states like Washington and Oregon where dental hygienists may practice with no or little supervision in various types of settings outside the dental office, dental hygienists do own dental hygiene businesses.

If you are interested in what business ownership options there are in a state other than these, you need to review the practice laws to see whether there is an actual or implied prohibition. Some state practice acts specify or strongly imply that a dental hygienist must be employed or be an independent contractor. Others define owning, operating or managing a dental practice as the practice of dentistry.

Keep in mind that supervision issues are different from worker status (employee vs independent contractor) and business option issues. Supervision concerns the degree of oversight of patient treatment that the practice law requires. Even owners of dental hygiene practices in Colorado and Maine must have an agreement with a dentist to provide supervision for some services; New Mexico practitioners need to practice in an agreed protocol with a collaborating dentist, and patients of California RDHAP's need a prescription from a dentist or physician to obtain dental hygiene services.

---

state, and local governments, employers with 15 or more employees, and labor organizations, if the basis of discrimination is race, color, national origin, religion, or gender

3. Civil Rights Act of 1991—expanded rights under federal anti-discrimination law
4. Sexual harassment—"unwelcome sexual conduct that is a term of employment"[5] is considered sexual discrimination and is prohibited under Title VII
   a. Quid pro quo (Latin, meaning "something for something") sexual harassment[6] criteria
      (1) The employee was in a "protected group" (a subordinate position)
      (2) The employee encountered unwelcome sexual advances or requests for sexual favors
      (3) Conduct was sexually motivated (e.g., hostile acts toward an individual because of his or her gender)
      (4) Harassment must affect a "tangible aspect of the job" such as salary, benefits, promotions, and perks
   b. Hostile work environment sexual harassment criteria—"verbal or physical conduct of a sexual nature that has the purpose or effect of creating an intimidating, hostile, or offensive work environment"[7]
      (1) Created by the words or conduct of an employer, colleague, vendor, or client
      (2) Examples
         (a) Unwanted touching
         (b) Suggestive comments about one's appearance
         (c) Display of sexually suggestive objectives or pictures
         (d) Use of diminutive terms such as "honey" or "cutey"
      (3) Employer has legal duty to take action to stop or prevent sexual harassment
      (4) Sexual harassment may occur between members of the opposite sex or members of the same sex
5. Age Discrimination in Employment Act of 1967—forbids discrimination against persons over age 40 by federal, state, and local governments and by employers with 20 or more employees
6. Equal Pay Act of 1963—illegal to pay lower wage to employees of one gender if the jobs have equal responsibility, working conditions, requirements for mental or physical effort, and requirements in experience, education, or training
7. Uniformed Services Employment and Re-employment Rights Act of 1994 protects civilian job rights and benefits for veterans and members of Reserve components
8. Occupational Safety and Health Act of 1970 (OSHA)—see Chapter 10
   a. The dental profession must comply with all General Industry standards[8] of primary importance to the dental practice (i.e., OSHA's Bloodborne Pathogens Standard [1991])
   b. Requirements for employers—employers must:
      (1) Identify employees at risk
      (2) Provide personal protective equipment to employees (gloves, protective eyewear, masks, etc.)
      (3) Provide hepatitis B vaccinations to employees

(4) Provide safety needles for the workplace

(5) Provide puncture-proof containers for sharps

(6) Ensure that standard precautions are practiced in the work environment

(7) Provide prompt treatment to employees who have needlestick or other exposures (includes immediate medical screening and follow-up treatment)

(8) Provide annual employee education relating to bloodborne diseases

c. OSHA amended the Bloodborne Pathogens Standard[6] (2001)—stricter requirements to prevent needlesticks and other exposures to blood (http://www.osha.gov/SLTC/bloodbornepathogens/); employers covered by the standards must:

(1) Provide safety needles

(2) Maintain a log of needlestick or other injuries to employees

(3) Enlist the assistance of employees who provide direct client care to prevent needlestick and other exposures by seeking input regarding equipment selection and work practices

(4) State OSHA laws—if a state has a health and safety law that meets or exceeds federal OSHA standards, enforcement of the law is assumed by the state rather than by a federal agency

(5) Twenty-five states, Puerto Rico, and the Virgin Islands have OSHA-approved State Plans and have adopted their own standards and enforcement policies; for the most part, these states adopt standards that are identical to Federal OSHA; however, some states have adopted different standards applicable to this topic or may have different enforcement policies; contact state agency for copy of the safety and health standards (state plans see http://www.osha.gov/dcsp/osp/)

9. Family and Medical Leave Act of 1993 (FMLA)—protects job security for women and men by allowing unpaid leave for medical reasons (e.g., care of a child, spouse, or parent; birth; adoption; or serious illness); updated January 19, 2009, to include military family leave entitlements

10. Pregnancy Discrimination Act of 1978 (PDA)—protects rights of pregnant women in the workplace; maternity-related medical conditions must be treated as all other medical conditions

a. The FMLA and the ADA; both require an employer to grant medical leave to an employee in certain circumstances; the FMLA and Title VII both have requirements governing leave for pregnancy and pregnancy-related conditions

b. The FMLA covers private employers with 50 or more employees within a 75-mile radius of the workplace; the ADA and Title VII cover private employers with 15 or more employees; only those private employers with 50 or more employees are covered concurrently by the FMLA, the ADA, and Title VII

c. State and local government employers are covered by the ADA and the FMLA, regardless of the number of employees; state and local government employers are covered by Title VII, however, only if they have 15 or more employees

11. Americans with Disabilities Act (ADA of 1990)—prohibits discrimination against qualified applicants and employees on basis of disability; must be mental or physical impairment that substantially limits one or more of the major life activities (disabilities include visual and hearing impairments, epilepsy, HIV-positive status, and AIDS); employer must make reasonable accommodations for employee; updated by the ADA Amendments Act of 2008 and expanded list of major life activities protected by the Act (http://www.ada.gov/pubs.adastatute08mark.htm#12102)

12. Fair Employment Statutes—many federal employment laws apply to workplaces with as many as 50 employees (e.g., Family and Medical Leave Act); therefore, most do not apply to dentistry; most states have passed statutes that enhance these federal laws; each state's statutes differ; contact specific state's Attorney General for information.

13. Worker's Compensation: insurance program regulated by each state's insurance commission; employer must purchase insurance through an insurance company to protect employees, should they become seriously ill or injured as a result of conditions in the workplace; programs vary from state to state; employees are covered on first date of employment, and benefits include medical expenses and income

RISK MANAGEMENT AND AVOIDING LITIGATION

A. Concepts

1. Risk management—Clinical and administrative activities undertaken to identify, evaluate, and reduce the risk of injury to clients, staff, and visitors

2. Risk assessment
   a. Evaluation of personnel, policies, and protocol to identify and address risk factors
   b. Strategies
      (1) Personnel evaluations; conducted by employer or peer review
      (2) Office audits
         (a) Review and updating of staff handbook
         (b) Assessment of policies related to client care (i.e., record keeping, referral policies, documentation)
         (c) Evaluation of equipment (i.e., condition)
         (d) Protocol reviews (i.e., accident protocol)
         (e) Personnel assessment (i.e., current licenses, communication style)
   c. Identified risks are addressed and remedied

B. Individual risk management
   1. Maintain a current license and certifications, if required (e.g., CPR certification)
      a. Be knowledgeable of state dental practice act and statutes or guidelines impacting health care providers
      b. Comply with state guidelines, federal guidelines, or both for infection control, record keeping, reporting requirements, confidentiality, and other specified mandates
   2. Obtain membership in a professional association such as the American Dental Hygienists' Association or the Canadian Dental Hygienists' Association, which provides legal updates through various publications
   3. Provide evidence-informed care in all aspects of client care activities
   4. Maintain competence by participation in continuing education; continuing education is mandatory in 47 states; from a legal perspective, it is advisable to document current competency with tasks routinely performed and those within the scope of practice
   5. Possess knowledge of legally protected employee rights and responsibilities
      a. Use legal or state or federal resources that provide guidance
      b. Document in detail any incidents occurring in the workplace
      c. Seek legal advice, if necessary
   6. Purchase professional liability insurance; keep the policy current
      a. Policy classifications
         (1) Occurrence-based policy—covers injuries arising out of incidents that occurred during the time the insurance was in effect, even if cancelled at a later date (preferred type)
         (2) Claims-made policy—covers injuries occurring and reported during the period in which the policy premiums are paid and in force
      b. Declaration—states policyholder's personal data (name, address, occupation) and limits of liability coverage (dollar figure for each claim and aggregate for policy period)
      c. Exclusions—liabilities not covered by policy; usually injuries resulting from criminal behavior, those involving alcohol or drug abuse on the part of health care provider, or cases involving practice beyond the scope of one's license
      d. Injuries covered—listed in policy (e.g., bodily injury, defamation, invasion of privacy)
      e. Supplemental coverage—lost earnings
      f. Conditions—subrogation of rights, policyholder's right to hire counsel versus insurance company's right to retain counsel
         (1) Policyholder's interest and insurance company's interest may be in conflict
         (2) A conflict of interest could also arise if a health care provider relies on the employer's insurance for liability coverage; protection is broader with an individual policy; an employer's policy provides coverage only when acting within the scope of employment; if the health care provider (by his or her action or failure to act) was liable for the client's injury, the employer (or his or her insurance company) may bring an indemnity claim and recover a portion of dollar amount awarded by the court to the client

C. Professional risk management
   1. Maintain knowledge of professional and legal responsibilities related to the provision of oral health care services
   2. Be familiar with and adhere to the professional code of ethics (ADHA Code of Ethics and Canadian Dental Hygienists Association Code of Ethics)
   3. Maintain a professional and respectful relationship with employers, colleagues, and clients
   4. Provide accurate and appropriate communication to clients, verbally and in writing; poor record keeping can contribute to a poor outcome in a lawsuit
   5. Maintain confidentiality—obtain proper written authorization from the client before release of any client information; ensure that any disclosure is covered by a reporting or access law and is appropriately followed

6. Document informed consent or informed refusal in client record before treatment

7. Ensure that all progress notes and client records are complete, accurate, factual, legible, unaltered, and promptly recorded; failure to do so is considered malpractice; a client's record may be obtained by an opposing party in a lawsuit

8. Be familiar with professional guidelines, including ADHA Standards for Clinical Dental Hygiene

9. Remain up-to-date on state or provincial dental hygiene practice acts and regulations

@ WEB SITE INFORMATION AND RESOURCES

LEGAL RESOURCES	WEB SITE ADDRESS	DESCRIPTION
Find Law	www.findlaw.com	Legal searches at no cost
9to5 National Office	152 W. Wisconsin Ave., Ste. 408 Milwaukee, WI 53203 T: 414-274-0925 http://www.9to5.org	National organization dedicated to putting working women's issues on the public agenda; 9to5's constituents are low-wage women, women in traditionally female jobs, and those who have experienced any form of discrimination; committed to, among other objectives, eliminating workplace discrimination through educating women about legal rights on the job, monitoring enforcement agencies, and expanding anti-discrimination laws
American Dental Hygienists' Association	444 N. Michigan Avenue, Suite 3400 Chicago, IL 60611 T: 312-440-8900 www.adha.org	Largest professional association representing dental hygienists.
National Practitioner Data Bank and Health Care Integrity and Protection Data Bank	http://www.npdb-hipdb.hrsa.gov/index.htm	The U.S. Department of Health and Human Services (HHS), Health Resources and Services Administration (HRSA), Bureau of Health Professions (BHPr), Division of Practitioner Data Banks (DPDB) is responsible for the management of the National Practitioner Data Bank and the Healthcare Integrity and Protection Data Bank
U. S. Equal Employment Opportunity Commission	131 M Street, NE, Washington, DC 20507 T: 202-663-4900 www.eeoc.gov	Responsible for enforcing federal laws that make it illegal to discriminate against a job applicant or an employee because of the person's race, color, religion, sex (including pregnancy), national origin, age (40 or older), disability or genetic information; it is also illegal to discriminate against a person because the person complained about discrimination, filed a charge of discrimination, or participated in an employment discrimination investigation or lawsuit Work is conducted at the headquarters and at 53 field offices throughout the United States
Occupational Safety and Health Administration Seeking legal advice from a qualified attorney is also recommended; the State Bar Association provides referrals to an attorney for legal services in a particular location	200 Constitution Avenue NW, Washington, DC 20210 T: 1.800.321.OSHA www.osha.gov	Ensures safe and healthful working conditions for working persons by setting and enforcing standards and by providing training, outreach, education, and assistance

Continued

@ WEB SITE INFORMATION AND RESOURCES—cont'd

ETHICS RESOURCES	WEB SITE ADDRESS	DESCRIPTION
Center for Health Policy and Ethics, Creighton University Medical Center	www.chpe.creighton.edu	A multi-disciplinary group of scholars dedicated to the study and teaching of ethical dimensions of health care and health policy; also offer roundtables, lectures, and courses
Center for Law, Ethics and Health, University of Michigan School of Public Health	www.sph.umich.edu/cleh	Examines the influence of law and ethics on the health care and public health system; provides publications and other resources
Berman Bioethics Institute, Johns Hopkins University	www.bioethicsinstitute.org	Provides education, conducts research, and provides leadership for the understanding of ethical issues in health care
Center for Ethics and Leadership in the Health Professions, Regis University	www.ethicsandleadership.org	Provides educational and consulting services and ethics simulations

REFERENCES AND LEGAL CITATIONS

1. Garner BA: *Black's law dictionary*, ed 9, 2009, Westlaw School.
2. Norwood Hospital *v* Munoz, 564 NE 2d 1017, 1991.
3. Thor *v* Superior Court, 855 P2d 375, 21 Cal. Rept. 2d 357, 1993.
4. Harlan *v* Lewis, 141 F.D.R. 107, 109, n5.
5. 729 CRF, § 1604.11(a).
6. 29 CRF 1910.1030, Occupational Exposure to Bloodborne Pathogens, Needlestick and Other Sharps Injuries Final Rule-66: 5317–5325 Federal Register January 18, 2001.
7. Harris *v* Forklift Sys. Inc., 510 US 17, 1993.
8. 29 CRF 1910.

SUGGESTED READINGS

American Dental Hygienists' Association: Standards for Clinical Dental Hygiene Practice, Chicago, 2008: Available at http://www.adha.org/downloads/adha_standards08.pdf: Accessed July 2, 2010

American Dental Hygienists' Association: Bylaws—codes of ethics, Chicago, 2010: Available at www.adha.org/downloads/ADHA-Bylaws-Code-of-Ethics.pdf: Accessed July 2, 2010

Beemsterboer PL: *Ethics and law in dental hygiene*, ed 2, St Louis, 2010, Saunders.

Canadian Dental Hygienists' Association: Codes of ethics, Ontario, 2002: Available at http://www.cdha.ca/pdfs/Profession/Resources/CDHA_Code_of_Ethics_public.pdf: Accessed July 2, 2010

Darby ML, Walsh MM: Dental hygiene theory and practice, ed 3, St Louis, 2010, Saunders.

Pamela Zarkowski and the publisher acknowledge the past contribution of Judith A. Davison to this chapter.

CHAPTER 22 REVIEW QUESTIONS

Answers and Rationales to Review Questions are available on this text's accompanying Evolve site. See inside front cover for details.

*e*volve

1. A dental hygienist observes clinical findings that may indicate child abuse. Her employer refuses to report the abuse and suggests if the dental hygienist does take action, she may lose her job. The dental hygienist decides to report the abuse. Which of the following ethical theories do the dental hygienist's actions BEST follow?.
   a. Act utilitarianism
   b. Rule utilitarianism
   c. Act deontology
   d. Rule deontology

2. Which of the following statements from the ADHA Code of Ethics provides guidance to the dental hygienist about obligations to report cases of suspected abuse or violence against adults, children, or both?
   a. Comply with local, state, and federal statutes that promote public health and safety
   b. Avoid self-deception and continually strive for knowledge and personal growth
   c. Serve as an advocate for the welfare of clients
   d. Respect the confidentiality and privacy of data
   e. Comply with local, state, and federal statutes that promote public health and safety; serve as an advocate for the welfare of clients

3. Following a discussion with a client concerning proposed dental hygiene treatment, including the treatment alternatives, risks and benefits, and outcomes, the client accepts and signs an informed consent form. Which of the ethical principles guiding oral health care did the process of obtaining informed consent satisfy?
   a. Autonomy
   b. Confidentiality
   c. Justice
   d. Trust
   e. Veracity

4. The dental hygiene treatment plan includes root planing and scaling, using a local anesthetic agent. The client repeatedly indicates that the dental hygienist "need not work below the gumline." The dental hygienist is aware that the clients' request will result in poor quality (substandard) care. The dental hygienist continues to educate the client about the appropriate treatment. Which of the following ethical principles is guiding the dental hygienist in the interactions with the client?
   a. Beneficence
   b. Confidentiality
   c. Fidelity
   d. Justice
   e. Veracity

5. A local dental hygiene component society collaborates with the faculty in a dental hygiene program conducting a research project about the impact of a new mouthrinse on burning mouth syndrome in perimenopausal women. Which of the following characteristics of a profession does this research project support?
   a. Identifiable membership with autonomy of practice
   b. Strong service orientation
   c. Intellectual work and promotion of a body of knowledge in the field
   d. Self-regulation
   e. Adherence to a code of ethics

6. A client Bill of Rights provides:
   a. A list of the proposed treatment with the associated fees for the services provided
   b. A legal document that provides guidance to a client during a legal proceeding such as a lawsuit
   c. A comprehensive list of all the procedures and services provided in a dental office or dental clinic
   d. An outline of client expectations and guidelines for provider conduct
   e. Rights created by the dental board or dental hygiene board of examiners in each state for client education

7. The Hippocrates' Code of Ethics is an example of an early ethical code that advocated that health providers should do no harm. Which universal ethical principle best identifies the supports this recommendation?
   a. Autonomy
   b. Fidelity
   c. Justice
   d. Nonmaleficence
   e. Veracity

8. A dental hygienist performs a procedure on a client that is outside the state's defined scope of practice. Following a hearing by the state's dental hygiene committee, the dental hygienist's license is suspended for 6 months. As required by state law, the information about the suspension is posted on a Web site that publishes license status and is available to the public. Which of the following characteristics of a profession do these actions support?
   a. Identifiable membership with autonomy of practice
   b. Strong service orientation
   c. Intellectual work and promotion of a body of knowledge in the field
   d. Self-regulation
   e. Adherence to a code of ethics

9. A state dental board or dental hygiene committee monitors the behavior of licensed oral health care providers and recommends sanctions for individuals who violate a state dental practice act because:
   a. It is an obligation outlined in the ADHA Code of Ethics
   b. A federal statute requires states to create a board or committee
   c. State boards or dental hygiene committees are created for the protection of the public
   d. Accrediting agencies require states to create state boards of dentistry or dental hygiene committees
   e. Dental hygiene and dental schools cannot suspend a dental professional's license

10. A city council votes to allocate health department funds for a dental sealant program. After consultation with appropriate individuals, the council determines that children enrolled in either a hot lunch program or a state-funded program for medical services for children from low-income families should receive the sealants. On which principle of allocation of resources is this determination based?
    a. Contribution
    b. Equity
    c. Effort
    d. Need
    e. Merit

11. A dental hygienist has allegations of professional misconduct reported to the state board. A hearing is conducted, and the dental hygienist has an opportunity to hear the allegations and respond to them. These actions best demonstrate:
    a. Protection of freedom of speech
    b. Protection of the dental hygienist's civil rights
    c. Protection of due process
    d. Protection against discrimination
    e. Protection against defamation

12. A former client brings a lawsuit against a dental hygienist for negligence. The client alleges the incident occurred 10 years ago. The state has designed a specific period of only 2 years in which a lawsuit for negligence can be filed. This defined period of time is known as:
    a. Civil rights protections
    b. Tort reform
    c. Statute of limitations
    d. Stare decisis
    e. Caveat

13. A client is scheduled with the dentist who examines the client, develops a treatment plan, and obtains informed consent. The client nods in agreement and indicates that he or she will be scheduling further appointments. On the basis of the dentist's and client's actions, which of the following may exist?
    a. Express contract
    b. Implied contract
    c. Insurance contract
    d. Lease contract
    e. None of the above

14. A dental hygienist is seeking to apply for a dental hygiene license in the state in which the hygienist recently relocated. The license application asks the applicant to indicate whether he has been convicted of any felonies. A felony is:
    a. A violation of the dental or dental hygiene practice act which resulted in harm and a sanction from the state board or dental hygiene committee
    b. A minor crime that involved a fine of less than $1000 and imprisonment of less than 1 year
    c. A serious crime that involved a fine of more than $1000 and imprisonment of more than 1 year
    d. A violation of someone's civil rights resulting in an allegation of discrimination
    e. A licensing application is not allowed to request information about convictions

15. A(n) _____ offense is a wrongful act against a person for which financial satisfaction is sought whereas a(n) _____ offense is a wrongful act against society.
    a. Administrative; civil
    b. Civil; criminal
    c. Criminal; civil
    d. Criminal; administrative
    e. Administrative; criminal

16. A dental provider and a client discuss a proposed dental hygiene treatment plan. The written plan outlines the treatment, the fees, the client's financial obligations, and the expectations of the provider concerning the client's responsibilities. The provider and client sign the treatment plan. The situation BEST describes:
    a. An express contract
    b. An implied contract
    c. An ethical obligation
    d. A noncontractual agreement
    e. An insurance agreement

17. A dental office employs a dental hygiene student approximately 6 months before graduation. The dentist in the office was scheduled to provide a maintenance visit with a client. However, an emergency client is also waiting to be assessed for care. The dentist asks the dental hygiene student to provide a "quick cleaning." Which of the following contractual responsibilities to the client is the dentist violating?
    a. Using standard drugs, materials, and techniques
    b. Maintaining an appropriate level of knowledge
    c. Allowing a licensed individual to exceed their scope of practice
    d. Delegating responsibilities to an unlicensed individual
    e. Providing care in a timely manner

18. The trial for a dental hygienist alleged to have committed negligence is complete. The judge prepares to give the jury instructions specifically the level of proof that the jury must consider to make their decision about the guilt or innocence of the defendant. Which of the following levels of proof will the judge inform the jury that they should consider in their deliberations?
    a. Beyond a reasonable doubt
    b. Preponderance of the evidence
    c. Burden of proof
    d. Substantial proof
    e. Evidence

19. A client's contractual responsibilities include:
    a. The client must provide truthful answers concerning health status
    b. The client must cooperate in care
    c. The client must pay appropriate fees
    d. The client must provide truthful answers concerning health status and must pay an appropriate fees
    e. The client must provide truthful answers concerning health status, must cooperate in care, and must pay an appropriate fee

20. A new client presents to the dental office for treatment. Client demographic and clinical data are collected and reviewed by the dentist and the dental hygienist who together determine that the case is too complex for the office to handle and suggest the client seek another provider. The client is informed that he or she will not be accepted into the practice. Which statement BEST describes this situation?
    a. The dentist cannot refuse to treat any client once data are collected
    b. The dentist can decline accepting the client
    c. The dentist should not have collected the client data
    d. A dentist must treat a client at least once before the referral
    e. None of the above; the dentist must accept and treat the client

21. A dental hygienist has a number of mannerisms that include purposefully using a loud voice and waving syringes and handpieces in a threatening manner. The dental hygienist is aware of the actions and the potential impact it may have on a client. Which of the following intentional torts may the dental hygienist be accused of?
    a. Assault
    b. Battery
    c. Harm
    d. Misrepresentation
    e. Negligence

22. Adam is scheduled for sealants on his four first molars. The chart indicates that Adam is somewhat uncooperative during dental appointments. As the appointment progresses, the dental hygienist and the dental assistant become more aggravated at Adam's uncooperative actions. During the appointment the assistant holds Adam's hands down. At one point, the dental hygienist firmly takes Adam's chin to position his face. At the end of the appointment, red marks are seen on Adam's hands and cheeks. As he enters the reception area, Adam's mother looks at her son and says to the assistant, "What did you do to my son?" Which of the following might the dental hygienist and the assistant be accused of?
    a. Assault
    b. Battery
    c. Harm
    d. Misrepresentation
    e. Negligence

23. All of the following make up the key elements of obtaining an informed refusal EXCEPT one. Which one is the EXCEPTION?
    a. The form must be printed
    b. The client needs to know the oral and general health implications of the refusal
    c. The explanation must be understood by the client
    d. The reasons a procedure is recommended as well as the alternatives need to be outlined
    e. The refusal form should be signed

24. The dental hygienist is root planing and scaling and removes a portion of a client's amalgam during the procedure. The dental hygienist fails to inform the client who later experiences pain and swallows a portion of the remaining restoration. The intentional tort committed is:
    a. Negligence
    b. Assault
    c. Misrepresentation
    d. Abandonment

25. **A dentist colleague of yours is accused of a serious criminal violation against a client. Following the trial, the jury will be asked to judge the facts and make a decision based on the standard:**
    a. Beyond a reasonable doubt
    b. Preponderance of the evidence
    c. Burden of proof
    d. Substantial proof
    e. Harm

26. **The client fails to pay the balance due on dental treatment charges in spite of repeated notices. Which of the following civil violation occurred?**
    a. Client negligence
    b. Dental negligence
    c. Abandonment
    d. Breach of contract
    e. Dental fraud

27. **A 17-year-old client presents to the practice for an appointment. He indicates that he is employed, is living in an apartment, and does not rely on his parents or family members for financial support. This BEST describes:**
    a. A compromised minor
    b. A disenfranchised minor
    c. An emancipated minor
    d. An independent minor

28. **A dental employer has the dental license suspended by the board of dentistry for inappropriate delegation to a dental staff employee. This adverse action requires:**
    a. A report filed with the American Dental Association
    b. A report filed with the American Dental Hygienists' Association
    c. A report filed with the Health Care Integrity and Protection Data Bank
    d. A report filed with the National Practitioner Data Bank
    e. A report filed with the Health Information Portability and Accountability Act

29. **A dental office receives a request for a copy of dental records to assist in identifying recently discovered human remains. For which of the following purposes are the dental records being used?**
    a. Tool for quality assurance and management
    b. Reference material in litigation proceedings
    c. Resource in forensic identification
    d. Assists in providing data for research projects
    e. Resource for members of the dental team

30. **The importance of confidentiality about client information has been supported by the:**
    a. Health Care Integrity and Protection Data Bank
    b. Health Information Portability and Accountability Act
    c. Health Information Technology for Economic and Clinical Health (HITECH) Act
    d. Health Information Portability and Accountability Act and Health Information Technology for Economic and Clinical Health (HITECH) Act
    e. The state dental practice act

31. **Dr. Miller recently joined a private practice as a partner. The office staff can check email or order supplies using the Internet from a computer in the staff lounge. The staff, mostly female, use the staff lounge to eat their lunch. During lunch, Dr. Miller frequently logs on to read his email. He usually reads his email, laughs out loud, and without anyone asking, proceeds to read some of the jokes, poems, and "stories" out loud. Most of the jokes would be considered crude or inappropriate. Which of the following types of sexual harassment may be occurring in this office?**
    a. Carpe diem
    b. Hostile environment
    c. Quid pro quo
    d. Civil rights laws
    e. Caveat

32. **A dental hygienist is terminated from a full-time position in a dental office with 25 employees. The dental hygienist suspects the reason for the termination is based on age, as the dental hygienist recently turned 65. Which of the following federal regulations provides legal protection for the employee?**
    a. Age Discrimination Act of 1967
    b. Civil Rights Act of 1964
    c. Fair employment statutes
    d. The state dental practice act

33. **The state legislature of a Midwest state recently passed legislation to increase the reimbursement for dental services. The services are provided by dentists in the state and funded by the social services division of the state public health department. This increased support was the result of the identification of increased dental needs for citizens in the state and an inability to identify providers willing to provide care because reimbursement rates were minimal. Which of the following aspects of creating public health policy do the actions of the state legislature support?**
    a. Action
    b. Analysis
    c. Goal
    d. Federal–state partnerships
    e. Social justice

34. A dental provider is informed that he will be facing a hearing concerning an allegation that the provider violated the state dental practice act. The notice provides the date of the hearing and indicates that the provider will have an opportunity to respond to the allegations. This situation BEST describes:
    a. Protections provided by the Civil Rights Act of 1964
    b. Protections provided by Due Process
    c. Protections provided by Equal Protection
    d. Protections provided by the Fair Trade Act
    e. Protections provided by Worker's Compensation

35. The level of care a reasonably prudent practitioner would provide in the same or similar circumstances BEST describes:
    a. Duty
    b. Ethical behavior
    c. Professionalism
    d. Scope of practice
    e. Standard of care

36. An employer indicates that an employee will be eligible for a raise if he or she agrees to some requests of a sexual nature. Which type of sexual harassment does this BEST describe?
    a. Employer harassment
    b. Environmental harassment
    c. Gender-based harassment
    d. Hostile environment
    e. Quid pro quo

37. To assist in maintaining competence and reduce the risks of malpractice allegations, it is advisable for a dental provider to:
    a. Maintain membership in a professional organization.
    b. Participate in continuing education courses
    c. Purchase malpractice liability insurance
    d. Understand legally protected employee rights
    e. Rely on colleagues to provide peer feedback

38. A client requests and is allowed to review her dental record. Which of the following regulations supports this?
    a. Health Insurance Portability and Accountability Act (HIPAA)
    b. Occupational Health and Safety Act (OSHA)
    c. Protected Health Information (PHI)
    d. Health Care Integrity and Protection Data Bank (HIPDB)
    e. None of the above; clients do not have a right to review their dental record

39. A dental hygienist realizes that an entry made 2 days ago in a client's dental record incorrectly recorded the number of carpules that were used for anesthesia. The dental hygienist obtains the record to correct the entry. Which is the appropriate method to make a correction?
    a. Use a liquid paper substance to cover the entry; rewrite the correct entry on the next available line
    b. Use a dark marker to cover over the entry; rewrite the correct entry on the next available line
    c. Indicate a correction to the previous entry, and write the correct information on the next available line
    d. Identify the original entry, and write the correction above the incorrect entry
    e. Verbally inform someone at the office of the incorrect entry

40. All of the following statements accurately explain some aspect of ethics EXCEPT one. Which one is the EXCEPTION?
    a. The focus of virtue ethics is on character of the individual
    b. Principalism uses various ethical principles and applies one or more of them
    c. Society is governed by the rules and regulations developed to protect its citizens from harm
    d. An act or behavior may be unethical and illegal
    e. Professional codes of ethics provide guidelines for decision making in one's professional life

41. A dental provider accepts a client and during the course of treatment decides not to complete the treatment because of an antagonistic relationship with the client. Which of the following has occurred?
    a. Client abandonment
    b. Client dismissal
    c. Client referral
    d. Client termination
    e. Client behavior modification

42. A dental provider seeking to obtain informed consent discusses the diagnosis; proposed treatment, including risks and benefits; and anticipated outcomes of the treatment and allows the client to ask questions and provides answers. Which element of informed consent is lacking?
    a. Use of photographs and diagrams to show the proposed treatment
    b. Presence of a witness to the informed consent process
    c. Offering information about alternative forms or treatment
    d. Request for an insurance form from the client
    e. All the elements of informed consent are detailed as required

43. Legislation is passed in a state to allow dental hygienists to administer local anesthetic agents under the direct supervision of a dentist. Direct supervision requires that a licensed dentist has authorized the procedure and:
    a. Need not be physically present when the procedure is performed
    b. Needs to be available for consultation
    c. Remains in the operatory to directly supervise the procedure
    d. Remains on the premises while the procedure is being performed
    e. Remains on the premises while the procedure is being done and checks the client before dismissal

44. Which of the following expanded HIPAA's privacy and security provisions by requiring notification of breaches or unauthorized disclosures of the PHI?
    a. Health Care Reform Act
    b. Health Information Technology for Economic and Clinical Health (HITECH) Act
    c. Medical Injury Compensation Reform Act
    d. Occupational Safety and Health Act
    e. Client Protection and Affordable Care Act

45. What type of professional liability insurance should a dental hygienist purchase?
    a. Claims-made policy
    b. Group policy
    c. Indemnity policy
    d. Occurrence-based policy
    e. None of the above

46. A trial for negligence results in a dental provider being found guilty. The judge awards damages for pain and suffering to the defendant. Which of the following types of damages were awarded?
    a. Contract damages
    b. General damages
    c. Nominal damages
    d. Punitive damages
    e. Special damages

47. All of the following are recommended personal risk management strategies EXCEPT one. Which one is the EXCEPTION?
    a. Maintaining current licensure and certifications
    b. Providing evidence-informed, competent care
    c. Participating in continuing education courses to maintain competency
    d. Relying on employers for information about scope of practice and legal responsibilities
    e. Purchasing professional liability insurance

48. An insurance program that is regulated by the state's insurance commission to protect employees if they become seriously ill or injured as a result of conditions in the workplace BEST describes:
    a. Health Insurance
    b. Malpractice Insurance
    c. Professional Liability Insurance
    d. Employee Benefit Insurance
    e. Worker's Compensation Insurance

49. A dental hygienist is informed that the employment situation is "at will." The employment situation is BEST described as:
    a. The employee is willing to work for the employer
    b. The employee can be terminated without notice
    c. The employee can only be terminated with notice
    d. The employee can work at the hours and compensation he or she chooses
    e. The employee is not subject to any type of employment evaluation

50. A dental hygienist relocates to another state and applies for a dental hygiene license. To obtain a license, the dental hygienist must take and pass the dental hygiene licensing examination. Which of the following regulatory board duties does this situation BEST describe? The board's duty to:
    a. Draft laws pertaining to dental professionals for the legislature
    b. Implement mechanisms to measure applicant competence
    c. Include dental hygienists as members of the regulating board
    d. Monitor educational standards
    e. Monitor continuing education requirements

Simulated National Board Dental Hygiene Examination

Meg Horst Zayan

The Simulated National Board Dental Hygiene Examination parallels the National Board Dental Hygiene Examination (NBDHE) in content and question format. This test allows you the opportunity to mimic the reality of the board examination that you will soon be taking.

Read the test items and record your answers. Each item has one best response. After you have completed the entire test, check your answers on the companion Evolve site. Remember, it is better to guess than to leave an answer blank.

The exam is provided in written format within this textbook and on the companion Evolve website with a timer function for a more realistic testing experience, given that the NBDHE is administered only in computer-based testing format. To provide ample practice and build confidence in test taking, other simulated examinations can be found on the Evovle website.

EXAM FORMAT

Although results are provided in one overall score, the examination is divided into the following two distinct parts:

1. *Component A* consists of 200 randomly ordered multiple-choice questions and testlets (i.e., not grouped by subject area). Major content areas covered include the following:
   - The scientific basis for dental hygiene practice
   - The provision of clinical dental hygiene services
   - Community health research and principles
2. *Component B* (beginning on p. 921) is made up of 150 case-based questions designed to test your knowledge of all content areas. Patient history forms, dental charts, radiographs/digital images, and clinical photographs necessary to answer these questions are provided at the outset of each set of case.

Answers and rationales for all Simulated NBDHE questions are provided on this text's companion Evolve website. (See the inside front cover of the book for details.) Rationales are provided for both correct and incorrect answers to facilitate a more comprehensive understanding of the content.

For additional information on the NBDHE, please visit the official site of the Joint Commission on National Dental Examinations: www.ada.org/2662.aspx. Changes in the NBDHE are ongoing; candidates are advised to access the latest information on the official website, and thoroughly read the most current Candidate's Guide.

COMPONENT A

Answers and rationales for the Component A review questions are located on this text's companion Evolve website. See inside front cover for details. **e**volve

Component A Review Questions and Testlets of the Simulated National Board Dental Hygiene Examination (sometimes referred to as the AM portion, taken in the morning on examination day) are not based solely on information provided in the chapters of this book.

SIMULATED NATIONAL BOARD DENTAL HYGIENE EXAMINATION—COMPONENT A REVIEW QUESTIONS

1. The type of epithelial tissue that is found in the oral cavity is called:
   a. Stratified squamous epithelium
   b. Simple columnar epithelium
   c. Simple cuboidal epithelium
   d. Pseudo-stratified columnar epithelium

2. The cellular part of the blood that caries oxygen but does not contain a nucleus comprises the:
   a. Neutrophils
   b. Basophils
   c. Monocytes
   d. Red blood cells

3. The nasal septum is composed of:
   a. Vomer and perpendicular plate of the ethmoid bone
   b. Greater wing of the sphenoid bone
   c. Mandible and temporal bones
   d. Occipital and parietal bones

4. What bones form the temporomandibular joint (TMJ)?
   a. Vomer and perpendicular plate of the ethmoid bone
   b. Greater wing of the sphenoid and frontal bones
   c. Mandible and temporal bones
   d. Occipital and parietal bones

5. The articulating surface of the condyle rotates within the:
   a. External acoustic meatus
   b. Styloid process
   c. Coronoid notch
   d. Mandibular fossa

6. A circular structure in the cell that contains powerful digestive enzymes and acts as a scavenger is the:
   a. Mitochondrium
   b. Lysosome
   c. Endoplasmic reticulum
   d. Golgi apparatus

7. The localized entrapment of pathogens from a dental infection in a closed tissue space is called:
   a. Paresthesia
   b. Osteomyelitis
   c. Abscess
   d. Pustule

8. Which tooth is known for its bifurcated root?
   a. Mandibular second premolar
   b. Maxillary second premolar
   c. Maxillary first premolar
   d. Mandibular first premolar

9. Which of the following permanent teeth occlude with only one tooth in the opposite arch, assuming ideal relations exist?
   a. Maxillary canine
   b. Maxillary first molar
   c. Mandibular central incisor
   d. Mandibular first premolar

10. The junction of three surfaces on the crown of a tooth is referred to as:
    a. Line angle
    b. Point angle
    c. Occlusal surface
    d. Incisal edge

11. In which one of the following processes does Meckel's cartilage form?
    a. Maxillary
    b. Frontal
    c. Temporal
    d. Mandibular

12. Which cusp on permanent molars generally is the one that gets progressively smaller as you go posterior in the arch?
    a. Mesiobuccal
    b. Distobuccal
    c. Mesiolingual
    d. Distolingual

13. During which stage of tooth development can macrodontia and microdontia occur?
    a. Bud
    b. Cap
    c. Bell
    d. Postdevelopment

14. The muscles of facial expression and taste are controlled by cranial nerve:
    a. V
    b. VII
    c. X
    d. XII

15. **To which salivary gland does the external carotid artery supply blood?**
    a. Minor
    b. Sublingual
    c. Submandibular
    d. Parotid

16. **An individual with type AB blood can give a transfusion to an individual with:**
    a. Type O blood
    b. Type A blood
    c. Type B blood
    d. Type AB blood

17. **Cardiac output is the product of:**
    a. Heart rate and peripheral resistance
    b. Heart rate and stroke volume
    c. Heart rate and strength of contraction
    d. Heart rate and vascular dilation

18. **All of the following are a function of the pancreas EXCEPT one. Which one is the EXCEPTION?**
    a. Secretion of digestive enzymes
    b. Secretion of insulin
    c. Secretion of bile
    d. Secretion of glucagon

19. **Functions of the adult liver include all of the following EXCEPT one. Which one is the EXCEPTION?**
    a. Bile formation
    b. Reticuloendothelial activity
    c. Glycogenesis, glycogenolysis, and gluconeogenesis
    d. Erythropoiesis
    e. Detoxication

20. **What is the difference between renal physiology and nephrology?**
    a. Renal physiology is the study of kidney disease, and nephrology is the study of kidney function
    b. Renal physiology is the treatment of kidney disease, and nephrology is the treatment of kidney function
    c. Renal physiology is the study of kidney function, and nephrology is the study of kidney disease
    d. Renal physiology is the treatment of kidney function, and nephrology is the treatment of kidney disease

21. **Two thirds of the body's water is found in:**
    a. Intracellular fluid
    b. Extracellular fluid
    c. Muscles
    d. Blood

22. **How many 8-ounce glasses of water per day should the average adult drink?**
    a. 5 to 7
    b. 8 to 10
    c. 11 to 12
    d. 13 to 14

23. **What is the amount of extra calories a woman needs during the first trimester of pregnancy?**
    a. 0
    b. 300
    c. 900
    d. 1200

24. **A chemical, biologic, or physical agent that causes birth defects is known as a:**
    a. Gestation
    b. Carcinogen
    c. Teratogen
    d. Free radical

25. **Common allergic foods include all of the following EXCEPT one. Which one is the EXCEPTION?**
    a. Peanuts
    b. Dairy
    c. Vegetables
    d. Wheat
    e. Fish

26. **Protein, fat, and starch digestion takes place primarily in the:**
    a. Stomach
    b. Small intestine
    c. Large intestine
    d. Mouth

27. **Anorexics are commonly deficient in:**
    a. Iron
    b. Zinc
    c. Chromium
    d. Magnesium

28. **Periodontal pathogens are communicable. Research shows that destructive periodontal microorganisms can be passed between parent and child and between spouses through saliva.**
    a. Both statements are TRUE
    b. Both statements are FALSE
    c. The first statement is TRUE, and the second statement is FALSE
    d. The first statement is FALSE, and the second statement is TRUE

29. **All of the following are necessary criteria for bacteria to infect the periodontium EXCEPT one. Which one is the EXCEPTION?**
    a. The host must be susceptible to periodontal pathogens
    b. Bacteria must be present in a virulent form
    c. Bacteria must be organized into complex communities to initiate disease
    d. Bacteria must be aerobic and not viable in the oral cavity

30. The type of bacterium that plays an important role in tissue destruction seen in periodontitis, has a double cell wall, and whose outer membrane contains endotoxins is:
    a. Aerobic
    b. Anaerobic
    c. Gram-positive
    d. Gram-negative

31. The attraction of new bacteria to previously attached bacteria is referred to as:
    a. Bacterial blooms
    b. Colonization
    c. Cell division
    d. Coaggregation

32. Factors that enable bacteria to colonize, invade, and damage tissues are referred to as _____ factors:
    a. Bacterial
    b. Virulence
    c. Facultative
    d. Enzymatic

33. The two main inorganic minerals found in supra-gingival calculus are:
    a. Magnesium and sodium chloride
    b. Sodium and potassium phosphate
    c. Calcium carbonate and zinc oxide
    d. Calcium phosphate and calcium carbonate

34. Bacterial organisms stain differently on the basis of:
    a. The thickness of the slime layer
    b. The thickness of the glycocalyx
    c. Permeability of their cell walls
    d. The thickness of the plaque biofilm

35. Which type of immunity may be immediately provided to a dental hygienist following an accidental curet laceration of the finger accident during hand-activated instrumentation (scaling)?
    a. Natural passive immunity
    b. Artificial passive immunity
    c. Natural active immunity
    d. Artificial active immunity

36. A combination of antibody and antigen is:
    a. Immune complex
    b. Humoral immunity
    c. Rheumatoid factor
    d. Autoimmune disease

37. In which type of immunopathologic disease are the cells of the body no longer tolerated and the immune system treats them as antigens?
    a. Hypersensitivity
    b. Immunodeficiency
    c. Opportunistic infection
    d. Autoimmune diseases

38. What type of lymphocyte matures in the thymus, produces lymphokines, and can affect the humoral immune response?
    a. B lymphocyte
    b. T lymphocyte
    c. Plasma cell
    d. Macrophage

39. All of the following is an example of retrograde cellular change EXCEPT one. Which one is the EXCEPTION?
    a. Atrophy
    b. Degeneration
    c. Necrosis
    d. Hyperplasia

40. A malignant tumor of bone forming tissue is called:
    a. Chondrosarcoma
    b. Angiosarcoma
    c. Osteosarcoma
    d. Hemangiosarcoma

41. The main difference between a verucca vulgaris and a papilloma is that:
    a. One is viral and the other is a true benign neoplasm
    b. Pain is associated with papilloma
    c. Common local recurrence of papilloma
    d. The presence of virus particles in a verucca vulgaris

42. All wounds are subject to certain complications. Which of the following dangers should be given first consideration?
    a. Infection
    b. Edema
    c. Inflammation
    d. Erythema

43. Which of the following cells would be the predominant cell seen in an acute inflammatory reaction?
    a. Monocyte
    b. Neutrophil
    c. Plasma cell
    d. Foreign body giant cell

44. Deposition of calcium salts in a tooth that is either a response to age or is caused by a stimulus is called *pulp calcification*. When this occurs in the pulp cavities, this is a:
    a. Cementoma
    b. Pulp stone
    c. Linear calcification
    d. Dentoma

45. A carious lesion of the first lower permanent molar is observed and a mass of tissue is protruding from the large cavity opening. The client is 10 years old and has no symptoms. What is the mass of tissue called?
   a. Cementoma
   b. Periapical abscess pulpitis
   c. Chronic hyperplastic pulpitis
   d. Periapical granuloma

46. Shingles is caused by the same virus that causes:
   a. Cold sores
   b. Mononucleosis
   c. Mumps
   d. Chickenpox
   e. Measles

47. On x-ray examination, a radiolucent, pear-shaped lesion is found distal to a client's maxillary right lateral incisor causing divergence of the lateral and canine roots. The lesion is probably a(an):
   a. Odontogenic keratocyst
   b. Ameloblastoma
   c. Globulomaxillary cyst
   d. Giant cell tumor

48. Odontogenic keratocysts are of particular clinical importance because they:
   a. Often become malignant
   b. Are frequently found in amelobastomas
   c. Commonly recur after surgical removal
   d. Often occur after endodontic treatment of a radicular cyst

49. Infectious mononucleosis is caused by:
   a. Gram-negative bacteria
   b. Epstein-Barr virus
   c. Thermophilic fungus
   d. Slow virus

50. When reviewing a dentigerous cyst on a radiograph, the radiolucent area will:
   a. Be found in a place of a tooth
   b. Surround the crown of an unerupted or impacted tooth
   c. Surround the root apex of a fully erupted tooth
   d. Surround the root apex of an impacted tooth

51. Which one of the following is MOST characteristic of nitrous oxide abuse?
   a. Is found primarily in food service employees
   b. Can lead to physical dependence
   c. Can cause infertility
   d. Can cause myelocytosis

52. Which one of the following when taken with antacids can result in a decrease in intestinal absorption of the medication?
   a. Meperidine (Demerol)
   b. Penicillin V
   c. Tetracycline
   d. Acetaminophen (Tylenol)

53. When epinephrine is added to a local anesthetic agent, all of the following occur EXCEPT one. Which one is the EXCEPTION?
   a. Cardiac output and heart rate are increased
   b. Coronary arteries dilate causing increase in blood flow
   c. Systolic blood pressure decreases
   d. Overall decrease in cardiac efficiency occurs

54. Which one of the following drugs can increase the risk for developing oral candidiasis?
   a. Phenytoin (Dilantin)
   b. Acetaminophen (Tylenol)
   c. Metoprolol (Lopressor, Toprol XL)
   d. Fluticasone (Flovent)

55. All of the following are side effects associated with oral contraceptives EXCEPT one. Which one is the EXCEPTION?
   a. Headache
   b. Weight gain
   c. Anorexia
   d. Nausea

56. The ceiling dose (effect) relates significantly to:
   a. Efficacy
   b. Threshold dose
   c. Placebo
   d. Affinity

57. Side effects of calcium channel blocking agents include all of the following EXCEPT one. Which one is the EXCEPTION?
   a. Stomatitis
   b. Hypotension
   c. Increased bleeding
   d. Heartburn

58. Which one of the following drugs is NOT used for reducing anxiety?
   a. Diazepam (Valium)
   b. Paroxetine (Paxal)
   c. Escitalopram (Lexapro)
   d. Secobarbital (Seconal)

59. When one drug reduces the absorption of another drug, what is a common strategy to minimize the interaction?
   a. Administration of one of the drugs by injection
   b. Administration of doses 2 hours apart
   c. Withholding of all drugs for 24 hours
   d. Withholding of one of the drugs until therapy with other drug is completed

60. Overuse of nasal decongestant sprays can cause _____.
   a. Dry mouth
   b. Constipation
   c. Sedation
   d. Rebound congestion

61. All of the following are lesions palpable during an intraoral exam EXCEPT one. Which one is this EXCEPTION?
   a. Bulla
   b. Nodule
   c. Papule
   d. Macule
   e. Vesicle

62. During treatment of a client with compromised pulmonary function, all of the following must be done EXCEPT one. Which one is the EXCEPTION?
   a. Avoid using motor-driven polishing devices
   b. Ask the client to be pre-medicated
   c. Avoid aerosol producing mechanized scalers
   d. Ask the client if they would like to be in a more upright position

63. Tachycardia is characterized by an increase in:
   a. Pulse rate
   b. Blood pressure
   c. Body temperature
   d. Respirations

64. Dental biofilm that is capable of demineralizing tooth structure is referred to as:
   a. Cariogenic
   b. Calculogenic
   c. Pathogenic
   d. Periogenic

65. Which of the following factors may increase the risk of bradycardia?
   a. Exercise
   b. Fasting
   c. Stimulants
   d. Anxiety

66. The gingival col area is particularly susceptible to destruction because of:
   a. Absence of keratinization and interproximal location
   b. Keratinization and a rough surface
   c. Facial location, where toothbrushing could easily destroy it
   d. Posterior location, where the client cannot reach

67. The MOST common cause of tooth mobility is caused by:
   a. Excessive occlusal biting forces
   b. Destruction of the periodontium
   c. Aggressive periodontal instrumentation
   d. Generalized gingival recession

68. Which of the following BEST describes bruxism?
   a. Chemical wearing of tooth structure
   b. Grinding of teeth
   c. Breakdown of tooth structure because of bacterial attack
   d. Uneven pitting of the facial surface

69. Which fibers of the principal fiber group run from the alveolar crest to cementum just below the cemento-enamel junction (CEJ)?
   a. Oblique
   b. Horizontal
   c. Alveolar crest
   d. Inter-radicular

70. A fluid-filled skin elevation, which is 1cm or less in diameter and contains serum or mucin, is BEST described as a:
   a. Papule
   b. Vesicle
   c. Lobule
   d. Macule

71. Class II occlusion is a molar relationship of the:
   a. Buccal groove of the mandibular molar is mesial to the mesiobuccal (MB) cusp of the maxillary molar
   b. Buccal groove of the mandibular molar is aligned with the MB cusp of the maxillary molar
   c. Buccal groove of the mandibular molar is distal to the MB cusp of the maxillary molar
   d. MB cusps of the maxillary and mandibular molars are in an end-to-end relationship

72. During the client's periodontal evaluation, the hygienist detects a furcation on tooth #30 and notes that the Nabers probe enters into the furcation area and penetrate through to the opposite side, however, the furcation is still covered with soft tissue. This type of furcation involvement is classified as:
   a. Class I
   b. Class II
   c. Class III
   d. Class IV

73. Which of the following terms BEST describes the involvement of the attached gingiva, the papilla, and the free gingiva?
   a. Localized
   b. Papillary
   c. Diffuse
   d. Marginal

74. All of the following are characteristics of free gingiva EXCEPT one. Which one is the EXCEPTION?
   a. Closely adapts around each tooth
   b. Connects with the attached gingiva
   c. Contains the free gingival groove
   d. Has a stippled surface

75. The color of the marginal gingiva of a client with chronic inflammation is predominantly:
   a. Red, or pink if it is fibrotic
   b. Coral pink with or without melanin pigmentation
   c. Blue
   d. White

76. **Pellicle formation involves:**
    a. Bacterial colonization
    b. Focal areas of mineralization
    c. Adhesion of salivary proteins to the tooth surface
    d. Organized mass of organisms

77. **During radiographic exposure, if the vertical angulation of the cone is too flat, the image on the film becomes distorted. Which of the following terms BEST describes the appearance of the tooth?**
    a. Foreshortened
    b. Overlapped
    c. Elongated
    d. Normal

78. **Which of the following appears as a radiopaque intersection of the maxillary sinus and the nasal cavity as viewed on a dental radiograph?**
    a. Nutrient canal
    b. Anterior nasal spine
    c. Zygomatic process
    d. Inverted Y

79. **In the dental setting, *interpretation* refers to an explanation of what is viewed on a radiograph, whereas the term *diagnosis* refers to the identification of a problem, deficit, or disease by examination or analysis.**
    a. Both statements are TRUE
    b. Both statements are FALSE
    c. The first statement is TRUE; the second statement is FALSE
    d. The first statement is FALSE; the second statement is TRUE

80. **Extraoral radiographs may be used in conjunction with intraoral films. The images seen on an extraoral film are more defined or sharp than the images on an intraoral radiograph.**
    a. Both statements are TRUE
    b. Both statements are FALSE
    c. The first statement is TRUE; the second statement is FALSE
    d. The first statement is FALSE; the second statement is TRUE

81. **In digital radiography, how do the exposure times differ from those required for conventional radiography?**
    a. 10% to 20% more
    b. 10% to 20% less
    c. 50% to 80% more
    d. 50% to 80% less

82. **Which of the following projections is used to evaluate fractures of the zygomatic arch and the position of the condyles and to demonstrate the base of the skull?**
    a. Lateral cephalometric
    b. Posteroanterior
    c. Waters
    d. Submentovertex

83. **Which of the following bitewing-size film is used to examine permanent posterior teeth of children and, when positioned vertically, can be used to examine anterior teeth in adults?**
    a. Size 0
    b. Size 1
    c. Size 2
    d. Size 3

84. **Using 10 milliamperes (mA) with an exposure time of 3 seconds would result in 30 mAs. If the milliamperage is increased to 15, the time must be decreased to _____ seconds to maintain the same density of the exposed radiograph.**
    a. 0.5
    b. 1.0
    c. 1.5
    d. 2.0

85. **Which form of the x-ray beam is MOST detrimental to the client and the operator?**
    a. Primary radiation
    b. Secondary radiation
    c. Scatter radiation
    d. Useful beam

86. **Which of the following forms of electromagnetic radiation has the shortest wavelength?**
    a. Radio waves
    b. Infrared waves
    c. Ultraviolet waves
    d. X-rays and gamma rays

87. **Which of the following types of cells is MOST radiosensitive?**
    a. Nerve
    b. Bone marrow
    c. Muscle
    d. Salivary glands

88. **When taking a radiograph, how many inches is the recommended size of the beam at the client's face?**
    a. 2.75
    b. 3.25
    c. 3.50
    d. 4.00

89. Which of the following terms MOST accurately describes the dose of radiation that the body can endure with little or no chance of injury?
    a. Cumulative dose
    b. Maximum permissible dose
    c. Threshold dose
    d. Erythema dose

90. What is the name of the zone in which structures are clearly demonstrated on panoramic radiograph?
    a. Focal trough
    b. Rectification
    c. Penumbra
    d. Midsagittal plane

91. Hydrogen peroxide has been used in the oral cavity for a variety of purposes. These include all of the following EXCEPT one. Which one is the EXCEPTION?
    a. With baking soda for toothbrushing, called the Keyes technique
    b. As an irrigation agent to get oxygen to the gingival tissues
    c. As part of tooth whitening products
    d. As an essential oil

92. All of the following are risk factors associated with osteoporosis EXCEPT one. Which one is the EXCEPTION?
    a. Low calcium
    b. Female gender
    c. Cigarette smoking
    d. Halitosis
    e. Sedentary lifestyle

93. All of the following are risk factors of a cardiovascular accident (stroke) EXCEPT one. Which one is the EXCEPTION?
    a. Hypertension
    b. Diabetes mellitus
    c. Hyperlipidemia
    d. Asthma

94. The client indicates on the health history form that she has asthma. It may be recommended that she take any of the following medications EXCEPT one. Which one is the EXCEPTION?
    a. Bronchodilator
    b. Prednisone
    c. Aspirin
    d. Triamicinolone

95. On a health history form, a client indicates that his ankles swell, that he is short of breath after climbing one flight of stairs, and that he sleeps with two pillows. Which one of the following diseases should be suspected?
    a. Angina pectoris
    b. Hypertension
    c. Diabetes mellitus
    d. Congestive heart failure

96. All of the following are included in the "5 A's of smoking cessation" EXCEPT one. Which one is the EXCEPTION?
    a. Ask
    b. Advice
    c. Admit
    d. Arrange
    e. Assess

97. The byproducts from smoking are eliminated from the body by:
    a. Exhaling
    b. Liver metabolism
    c. Lung absorption
    d. Blood dissemination

98. Symptoms of nicotine addiction include all of the following EXCEPT one. Which one is the EXCEPTION?
    a. Depression
    b. Anxiety
    c. Decreased appetite
    d. Irritability

99. The abuse of alcohol by a pregnant woman can cause all of the following to the fetus EXCEPT one. Which one is the EXCEPTION?
    a. Low birth weight
    b. Mental illness
    c. Spontaneous abortion
    d. Fetal alcohol syndrome

100. What is the MOST likely cause of early childhood caries (ECC)?
    a. Frequent intake of milk or juice in baby bottles and or prolonged breast feeding
    b. Too early introduction of solid foods
    c. Early tooth eruption into the child's mouth
    d. Excessive alcohol consumption by the mother during pregnancy

101. Which teeth are MOST affected when a child has ECC?
    a. Primary maxillary anterior
    b. Permanent maxillary anterior
    c. Primary mandibular anterior
    d. Permanent mandibular anterior

102. All of the following can decrease the effectiveness of a topical anesthetic agent EXCEPT one. Which one is the EXCEPTION?
    a. Degree of keratinization
    b. Thickness of epithelium
    c. Client nervousness
    d. Presence of saliva

103. Older adults are at an increased risk for root caries because of all of the following EXCEPT one. Which one is the EXCEPTION?
    a. Exposed root surfaces
    b. Biofilm retention
    c. Xerostomia
    d. High protein diet

104. All of the following are considered common upper respiratory infections EXCEPT one. Which one is the EXCEPTION?
- a. Asthma
- b. Laryngitis
- c. Rhinitis
- d. Tonsillitis

105. The prevalence and severity of periodontal disease increases with type 1 and type 2 diabetes. The presence of uncontrolled diabetes increases dental caries risk as a result of reduced saliva secretion and increased glucose in saliva.
- a. Both statements are TRUE
- b. Both statements are FALSE
- c. The first statement is TRUE, and the second statement is FALSE
- d. The first statement is FALSE, and the second statement is TRUE

106. Handwashing is the MOST effective strategy in the prevention of:
- a. Environmental surface infection
- b. Instrument contamination
- c. Infection and disease transmission
- d. Occupational hazards

107. Xerostomia is a common oral manifestation accompanying:
- a. Rheumatic heart disease
- b. Asthmatic attack
- c. Chronic alcoholism
- d. Controlled diabetic mellitus

108. The knowledge, skills and ability to provide oral health care effectively to people who are culturally different from oneself is known as:
- a. Ethnicity
- b. Cognitive learning
- c. Nonverbal communication
- d. Cultural competence

109. The administration of oxygen is indicated in most medical emergencies. In which of the following is oxygen NOT indicated?
- a. Hyperglycemia
- b. Hyperventilation
- c. Syncope
- d. Asthma

110. A face shield does not replace the need for other forms of protective eyewear. Face shields do not provide the same respiratory protection as provided by face masks.
- a. Both statements are TRUE
- b. Both statements are FALSE
- c. The first statement is TRUE, and the second statement is FALSE
- d. The first statement is FALSE, and the second statement is TRUE

111. All of the following are steps indicated when a curet tip breaks during periodontal débridement EXCEPT one. Which one is this EXCEPTION?
- a. Placing the client in a supine position
- b. Examining the mucobuccal fold and floor of mouth
- c. Taking a radiograph to locate the tip
- d. Gently instrumenting the pocket to locate the tip

112. Which one of the following is MOST characteristic of a dull instrument?
- a. Decreased tactile sensitivity
- b. Less working time involved
- c. Light grasp required
- d. Decreased pressure on tooth

113. Pain associated with dentinal hypersensitivity can BEST be described as:
- a. Constant pain
- b. Transient pain
- c. Intermittent pain
- d. Severe pain

114. All of the following are contraindicated for polishing/selective polishing EXCEPT one. Which one is the EXCEPTION?
- a. Implants
- b. Decay
- c. Amalgam
- d. Porcelain

115. To comply with Environmental Protection Agency (EPA) statutes regarding the disposal of infectious waste, health care workers need to:
- a. Discard blood disposables in a biohazard container
- b. Separate regular waste from biohazard waste
- c. Discard blood disposables in regular waste containers
- d. Place all waste in a biohazard container

116. Nitroglycerin is the medication that is usually used to relieve the symptoms of:
- a. Asthma
- b. Congestive heart failure
- c. Chronic hypertension
- d. Angina pectoris

117. Emergency care of a client who is experiencing an epileptic seizure includes all of the following EXCEPT one. Which one is the EXCEPTION?
- a. Placing a bite-block in the mouth to avoid fracturing of teeth
- b. Lowering the dental chair to the horizontal position
- c. Monitoring vital signs
- d. Summoning help from other staff

118. All of the following are appropriate treatment modifications for an individual with chronic obstructive pulmonary disease (COPD) EXCEPT one. Which one is the EXCEPTION?
    a. Placing chair in upright position
    b. Avoiding the use of rubber dam
    c. Administering high-flow oxygen
    d. Avoiding the use of nitrous oxide–oxygen conscious sedation

119. Which of the following treatment considerations is acceptable for myasthenia gravis?
    a. Using air polishing
    b. Avoiding fluoride therapy
    c. Scheduling short morning appointments
    d. Using ultrasonic scalers

120. The following vital signs are taken and recorded: pulse: 86 beats per minute (beats/min); respiration: 16 respirations per minute; blood pressure: 138/88 mm Hg. From these readings, which of the following conclusions is MOST accurate?
    a. Pulse is elevated
    b. Vitals are within normal limits
    c. Blood pressure should be classified as prehypertensive
    d. Systolic pressure is borderline low

121. During an oral assessment, both the appearance and the ability of Stensen's ducts to function adequately are examined while palpating the:
    a. Buccal mucosa
    b. Floor of the mouth
    c. Mucobuccal fold
    d. Palate

122. A tooth desensitizing agent is applied continually:
    a. For 5 minutes
    b. For 20 minutes
    c. According to manufacturer's instruction
    d. Until the dispenser is emptied

123. By what percentage is the blade of a "mini" five instrument shorter than a traditional instrument?
    a. 30%
    b. 40%
    c. 50%
    d. The blades are the same size

124. Through which of the following routes is tuberculosis usually transmitted?
    a. Fecal–oral
    b. Contaminated water
    c. Congenital
    d. Inhalation

125. All of the following are true regarding the progression of inflammation by way of the periodontal ligament space EXCEPT one. Which one is the EXCEPTION?
    a. Uneven bone loss
    b. Vertical bone loss
    c. Progression caused by weakened fiber bundles
    d. Cancellous bone being destroyed first

126. Periodontal pathogens are transmissible within families, and research suggests that certain individuals have a genetic susceptibility to the disease. However, there is evidence that periodontal infections are contagious.
    a. Both statements are TRUE
    b. Both statements are FALSE
    c. The first statement is TRUE, and the second is FALSE
    d. The first statement is FALSE, and the second is TRUE

127. All of the following are types of subgingival plaque EXCEPT one. Which one is the EXCEPTION?
    a. Unattached plaque
    b. Tooth-attached plaque
    c. Connective tissue–attached plaque
    d. Epithelial tissue–attached plaque

128. The purpose of extracellular slime layer found on biofilms is to:
    a. Protect microcolonies from antibiotics and antimicrobials
    b. Protect microcolonies from sessile, mushroom-shaped bacteria
    c. Allow chemical signals to communicate with other bacteria
    d. Allow host defenses to initiate immunity

129. A 25-year-old man with a history of gingivitis is assessed at his 6-month recare appointment. Which of the following clinical signs will MOST likely confirm that his condition has progressed to periodontitis?
    a. Loss of clinical attachment
    b. Bleeding on probing
    c. Change in gingival color
    d. Inflamed gingival tissues

130. A client's probing depths are 4, 4, 4 on tooth #6 facial. The gingival margin is 2 mm apical to the CEJ, and the mucogingival line is 3 mm apical to the gingival margin. What is the MOST likely periodontal diagnosis?
    a. Gingival hyperplasia
    b. Gingival pocket
    c. Long, junctional epithelium
    d. Mucogingival involvement

131. Reduction in probing depth following periodontal debridement is generally caused by:
a. Bone growth
b. Formation of a long junctional epithelium
c. New cementum formation
d. Reattachment of periodontal ligament fibers

132. Full thickness periodontal flaps are commonly used in surgical procedures because they:
a. Allow harvesting of connective tissue from the palatal donor site
b. Expose gingival connective tissue
c. Provide access to tooth roots and alveolar bone
d. Remove excess gingival tissue

133. An osseo-integrated implant is expected to have the following relationship to bone:
a. Hemidesmosomes and basal lamina attachment
b. Functional ankylosis
c. Periodontal ligament attachment
d. Connective tissue fiber insertion into the implant surface

134. Which of the following types of periodontal therapies heals by repair or "scar"?
a. Root debridement
b. Osseous surgery
c. Guided tissue regeneration
d. Connective tissue graft

135. What is the IDEAL situation for guided tissue regeneration surgery?
a. Formation of a long junctional epithelium
b. Regeneration of cementum, periodontal ligament, and alveolar bone
c. Epithelial tissue covering the wound area
d. Keratinization of the gingiva

136. One indication for performing a gingivectomy is a(an):
a. Infrabony pocket
b. Muco-gingival defect
c. Gingival overgrowth
d. Root sensitivity

137. Which of the following phrases regarding healing after periodontal surgery defines the reunion of the connective tissue and root that have been separated by incision or injury but not by disease?
a. Healing by repair
b. Healing by reattachment
c. Healing by new attachment
d. Healing by regeneration

138. Locally applied antimicrobials (LAA) used in conjunction with periodontal debridement for pocket reduction is preferred over antibiotics administered by mouth because LAA's:
a. Deliver antibiotics systemically
b. Reduce dentinal hypersensitivity
c. Suppress the host response
d. Provide a steady release of the drug in the pocket

139. Incisional periodontal surgery is also referred to as:
a. Gingivectomy
b. Periodontal flap surgery
c. Gingivoplasty
d. Muco-gingival surgery

140. One of the objectives of periodontal maintenance is to minimize the recurrence and progression of periodontal disease. The frequency of periodontal maintenance care visits decrease when the self-care practices of clients are less than optimal.
a. Both statements are TRUE
b. Both statements are FALSE
c. The first statement is TRUE, and the second statement is FALSE
d. The first statement is FALSE, and the second statement is TRUE

141. Which of the following findings would indicate failed dental implantation?
a. Implant mobility
b. Absence of bleeding
c. Periodontal implant support
d. Stable bone level height

142. When treating a client who is on an implant maintenance regimen, it is crucial that the dental hygienist use:
a. Stainless steel or carbon-tipped curets
b. Nonplastic or non–Teflon-coated probes
c. Sonic and ultrasonic scalers
d. Plastic instrument curets

143. Which one of the following client factors is an indication for a dental implant?
a. Poor quality and density of bone
b. Osteoporosis
c. Severe malocclusion
d. Single missing tooth

144. Dental sealants are indicated for placement in pit and fissures with incipient carious lesions. They are also indicated for placement in caries-free pits and fissures.
a. Both statements are TRUE
b. Both statements are FALSE
c. First statement is TRUE, and second statement is FALSE
d. First statement is FALSE, and the second statement is TRUE

145. All of the following are contraindications to dental sealant application EXCEPT one. Which one is the EXCEPTION?
a. Presence of proximal decay
b. Dry field can be obtained
c. Previously restored tooth
d. Primary tooth near exfoliation

146. When evaluating the results of pit and fissure sealant placement, the dental hygienist should do all of the following EXCEPT one. Which one is the EXCEPTION?
    a. Flossing the client's teeth to ensure contacts are free of sealant material
    b. Drying the client's teeth and using an explorer to look for surface voids
    c. Determine if high spots are present by checking with articulating paper
    d. Inserting the curet under the gingival margin to confirm that the sealant material is not in the sulcus

147. All of the following antimicrobial agents can be delivered via a cannula into the client's periodontal pocket EXCEPT one. Which one is this EXCEPTION?
    a. Metronidazole gel
    b. Minocycline hydrochloride
    c. Doxycycline hyclate
    d. Chlorhexidine chip

148. If a child accidentally ingests a toxic quantity of fluoride, the hygienist should FIRST:
    a. Induce vomiting by physical or chemical means
    b. Force fluids to dilute the fluoride concentration
    c. Have the child eat high-fiber foods to speed the elimination of the fluoride
    d. Have the child drink a sodium bicarbonate solution to neutralize the toxicity of the fluoride

149. The type of fluoride recommended as a 1.1% (5000 parts per million [ppm]) preparation intended to be brushed on daily is:
    a. Sodium fluoride (NaF)
    b. Acidulated phosphate fluoride (APF)
    c. Stannous fluoride (SnF_2)
    d. Monofluorophosphate

150. Approximately what concentration of fluoride do MOST commercially available dentrifices have?
    a. 1000 ppm
    b. 100,000 ppm
    c. 10%
    d. 4%

151. When a product has "substantivity," it has
    a. To be effective over an extended period with the retention of its potency
    b. To stay in the oral cavity after exposure to the agent
    c. To have binders and filters added to give it more substance
    d. To be bound to the pellicle and tooth surface

152. Approximately how many parts per million of fluoride does a recommended low-potency, over-the-counter fluoride mouthrinse contain?
    a. 9000
    b. 500
    c. 1000
    d. 250

153. Which of the following oral tissues provides sensation or proprioception to the individual with regard to the forces placed on the tooth?
    a. Pulp
    b. Dentin
    c. Periodontium
    d. Gingival tissue

154. For better retention and a longer-lasting sealant, it is best to apply the dental sealant material to _____ quadrant(s) at a time.
    a. One
    b. Two
    c. Three
    d. Four

155. The chemical composition of both plaster and dental stone is:
    a. Calcium chlorate dihydrate
    b. Potassium sulfate
    c. Calcium sulfate hemihydrate
    d. Potassium alginate

156. When mixing alginate material, if warm water is used, it will:
    a. Shorten the gelation time
    b. Lengthen the gelation time
    c. Make the mix unusable
    d. Increase the voids in the impression

157. All of the following conditions are contraindications for dental implant placement EXCEPT one. Which one is the EXCEPTION?
    a. Recurrent dental caries
    b. Poor oral hygiene
    c. Uncontrolled diabetes
    d. Substance abuse

158. The final setting time for study model gypsum products is:
    a. 15 to 30 minutes
    b. 30 to 45 minutes
    c. 45 to 90 minutes
    d. 90 to 120 minutes

159. The primary goal of infection control when handling and disinfecting impressions, dentures, and appliances is to:
    a. Protect the client from laboratory personnel
    b. Protect laboratory personnel from the client
    c. Prevent cross-contamination
    d. Prevent contamination of equipment in the dental laboratory

160. The American Dental Hygienists' Association (ADHA) and the Canadian Dental Hygienists' Association (CDHA) have established codes of ethics. These codes encourage all of the following EXCEPT one. Which one is the EXCEPTION?
   a. Ethical expectations of the dental hygienist by the public
   b. Overseeing the responsibilities of the dentist
   c. Professional and ethical consciousness
   d. Professional judgment and conduct

161. Veracity is an ethical principle of dental hygiene. Veracity is BEST reflected in the word:
   a. Pleasant
   b. Truthful
   c. Effective
   d. Nonmalice

162. Law is divided into three categories—labor, civil and criminal. Criminal law is law established for preventing harm against society and describes a criminal act and its appropriate punishment.
   a. Both statements are TRUE
   b. Both statements are FALSE
   c. The first statement is TRUE, and the second statement is FALSE
   d. The first statement is FALSE, and the second statement is TRUE

163. What type of breach occurs if the dental hygienist discusses an adult client's dental condition with her mother and the identity of the client is revealed?
   a. Informed consent
   b. Confidentiality
   c. Defamation
   d. Statute of limitations

164. Jurisprudence is defined as:
   a. Breach of contract
   b. Malpractice
   c. Philosophy or science of law
   d. Jury deliberation

165. The term for written defamation of character is:
   a. Slander
   b. Libel
   c. Breach of contract
   d. Assault

166. The term for verbal defamation of character is:
   a. Slander
   b. Libel
   c. Breach of contract
   d. Battery

167. It is not the dental hygienists legal and ethical responsibility to assess and document client information during the dental hygiene visit. Nor is it the responsibility of the dental hygienist to inform the dentist if he or she is concerned about the quality of the dentist's work in an edifying way.
   a. Both statements are TRUE
   b. Both statements are FALSE
   c. The first statement is TRUE, and the second statement is FALSE
   d. The first statement is FALSE, and the second statement is TRUE

168. If a client decides to sue a dentist for improper placement of an amalgam restoration, this is considered a category of law called:
   a. Torts
   b. Accidentals
   c. Abandonments
   d. Defamation

169. When restorations are not properly placed in a client's mouth, the dentist is not meeting the profession's:
   a. Licensure
   b. Accreditation
   c. Supervision
   d. Standard of care

170. Dental and dental hygiene practice acts are enacted to protect the:
   a. Profession
   b. Public
   c. Dental hygienist
   d. Dentist

171. Agreement between states for recognition of dental hygiene licensure to practice in those respective states is referred to as:
   a. Reciprocity
   b. Endorsement
   c. Licensure by examination
   d. Licensure by waiver

172. If a dental hygienist's license to practice dental hygiene is in jeopardy, the dental hygienist must first be given notice of the violation, a hearing, and an opportunity to respond before license revocation or suspension. This is an example of:
   a. Equal protection
   b. Tort law
   c. Due process
   d. Statute of limitations

173. A health care providers' code of ethical conduct that focuses on client needs, encourages informed choice, and provides for quality care is a referred to as the:
a. Code of ethics
b. Oath of Hippocrates
c. Principles of medical ethics
d. Patient's bill of rights

174. It is the dental hygienist's responsibility not to use treatment to injure or wrong the client, i.e., inflicting no harm. This provider's duty is referred to as:
a. Nonmaleficence
b. Beneficence
c. Fidelity
d. Veracity

175. What type of supervision occurs when a licensed dentist authorizes dental hygiene procedures and remains in the dental facility while those procedures are being performed?
a. General
b. Direct
c. Indirect
d. Personal

176. Most law suits are caused by poor communication; therefore, it is paramount to treat patients with concern, honesty, and respect, reducing the likelihood of lawsuits.
a. Both statements and the reason are correct and related
b. Both the statements and the reason are correct but not related
c. The statement is correct, but the reason is not correct
d. Neither the statement nor the reason is correct

Test items #177 to 186 refer to the following testlet:

A state-hired full-time public health dentist and dental hygienist are responsible for collecting data on the dental plaque rates of elementary school–aged children. Correlational studies are planned to determine strength of data between genders and among geographical locations of the elementary schools. It was decided to screen children in grades K, 2, 4, and 6 within 25 schools throughout the state. The 25 schools were chosen on the basis of geographic locations and number of students enrolled. All students within each of the chosen grades would be part of the study. Three other public health dental hygienists were hired part time to help in the data collection process. When data collection was completed, analyzed, and interpreted, the public health dentist and the dental hygienist would decide on an oral health program to best meet the needs of the elementary school–aged children of the state.

177. What type of epidemiologic study is exemplified by this research?
a. Retrospective cohort
b. Cross-sectional
c. Case-control
d. Prospective cohort
e. Experimental

178. Which of the following is characteristic of the type of sampling used to collect these data?
a. Simple random
b. Stratified
c. Systematic
d. Convenience

179. The MOST appropriate index to use to measure the plaque rate of these children is:
a. DMTF/DEFT
b. CPITN
c. OHI-S
d. PHP

180. To gain the support of the principals of all these elementary schools, the dentist and dental hygienist decided to meet with each of the 25 school boards. Who should be invited to attend this board meeting?
a. Board of education members only
b. Board of education members and the school principals
c. Board of education members, the school principals, and the parents
d. Board of education members, the school principals, the parents, and the elementary school children

181. If it is decided that future services will be provided in the state that are directed toward the initial stages of disease pathogenesis, what stage of disease pathogenesis do these services exemplify?
a. Primary
b. Secondary
c. Tertiary
d. Quaternary

182. The evaluation of a dental health program that will be implemented in these elementary schools should be PRIMARILY concerned with:
 a. Program effectiveness in reducing plaque scores
 b. Number of children participating in the program
 c. Public support of the program
 d. Cost analysis of program costs

183. Calculation of the plaque score index resulted in an overall mean score of 2.75 on a scale of 0 to 3. The MOST effective approach to improve the plaque scores of elementary students in this state is to:
 a. Reinforce brushing techniques already practiced by the children
 b. Educate the parents on proper oral hygiene habits at home
 c. Initiate a 2-year plaque control program in elementary schools
 d. Provide information on dental disease progression to teachers

184. After calculating the results of the correlation test between geographic location and plaque scores, the correlation coefficient was +0.26. This relationship between these two variables is:
 a. Weak
 b. Moderate
 c. Strong
 d. Not correlated

185. The mean of the correlation between geographic location and plaque scores was compared with the mean of the correlation between gender and plaque scores. What type of research analysis does this exemplify?
 a. Standard deviation
 b. Chi-square
 c. Students t-test
 d. Analysis of variance (ANOVA)

186. Which of the following *P* levels associated with a test of significance would BEST indicate that the researcher's results were MOST likely caused by an independent variable rather than by chance occurrence?
 a. $P \geq 0.01$
 b. $P \geq 0.001$
 c. $P \leq 0.01$
 d. $P \leq 0.001$

Test items #187 to 193 refer to the following testlet:
A Mission of Mercy (M.O.M.) event was planned for an urban city in a southern state of the United States. This 2-day event was designed to meet the critical needs of underserved people of all ages by providing free dental care to as many adults and children as time, volunteers, and supplies would allow. Local dentists, dental hygienists, dental assistants, dental students, dental hygiene students, and dental assisting students volunteered for the event. Local politicians and two state representatives were also in attendance. Before receiving dental treatment, informed consent was required of all patients. A 10-question client survey was distributed, and volunteers reviewed each question with clients while the clients were completing the questionnaire. Confidential questions included information on age, gender, education, family income, address, and past dental experiences. At the end of each client's treatment and before each volunteer completed his or her shift, the client was asked to complete an evaluation survey. There was an 88% response rate, and 79% answered that their experience was positive.

187. Which of the following information is provided to the participant before signing the informed consent?
 a. Guarantee of confidentiality to each client
 b. A review of the cost of each procedure
 c. The dental hygienists credentials
 d. M.O.M. statistics from other states

188. The PRIMARY goal of this dental event was to:
 a. Provide free services to children and adults
 b. Educate the public on the prevention of dental disease
 c. Promote the need to seek future dental care
 d. Reduce the prevalence of dental disease

189. All of the following are reasons for the success of the questionnaire data collection process EXCEPT one. Which one is the EXCEPTION?
 a. The questionnaire was limited to 10 questions
 b. Volunteers helped ensure clients' understanding of each question
 c. Responses to questions were indicated as confidential
 d. Participants were given a deadline to complete the questionnaire

190. What type of data is information such as age, gender, education, family income, and address?
 a. Need
 b. Access
 c. Demographic
 d. Knowledge

191. **What type of evaluation is the feedback provided during this event?**
    a. Process
    b. Formative
    c. Summative
    d. Ongoing

192. **On the basis of the testlet's scenario, the M.O.M. event was designed to prevent future dental problems because the demand for dental care in this southern state is higher than the need for dental care.**
    a. Both the statement and the reason are correct
    b. Both the statement and the reason are not correct
    c. The statement is correct, but the reason is not
    d. The statement is not correct, but the reason is correct

193. **Dental health in populations such as the one treated by the M.O.M. Project is often neglected because of all of the following reasons EXCEPT one. Which one is this EXCEPTION?**
    a. Self-perception of need
    b. Expense of provider services
    c. Undramatic nature of dental disease
    d. Lack of availability of preventive care

Test items #194 to 200 refer to the following testlet:
A university dental hygiene school received a state-funded grant to improve the oral health status of senior citizens in a rural area of the United States. The funding was for $50,000 over a 1-year period and covered expenses for salaries, equipment, supplies, and education. It was determined that high rates of root caries, root sensitivity, and gum disease were present in this population. The dental hygiene school decided to address these needs by implementing an oral health program in its clinic and to determine the effectiveness of two different types of desensitizing agents on treating root sensitivity.

194. **What is (are) the independent variable(s) in the study on the effectiveness of two different types of desensitizing agents on root sensitivity?**
    a. Senior citizen population
    b. Root sensitivity
    c. Desensitizing agents
    d. Plaque scores

195. **The hypothesis for this study states, "There is no statistically significant difference between desensitizing agent A and desensitizing agent B in the treatment of root sensitivity." What type of hypothesis does this exemplify?**
    a. Null
    b. Positive
    c. Research
    d. Standard

196. **During which of the following public health process stages is the final development of program goals and objectives done?**
    a. Assessment
    b. Planning
    c. Implementation
    d. Evaluation

197. **Four dental hygiene clinical instructors will document the client's response to each desensitizing agent. To ensure consistency of documentation among the four instructors, a calibration session is scheduled. This is an example of:**
    a. Research consistency
    b. Data consistency
    c. Rater reliability
    d. Interpreter reliability

198. **The data collection instrument chosen to measure the effect of the desensitizing agent on root sensitivity has been used successfully before and published in the *Journal of Dental Hygiene*. This indicates that the instrument is:**
    a. Reliable
    b. Valid
    c. Systematic
    d. Correctional

199. **The local dental hygienists' association offered its services to provide educational sessions to the senior citizens. During these educational sessions, toothbrushes, dental floss, floss threaders, and denture brushes were made available for distribution. The distribution of dental products as part of a dental health program for senior citizens is indicative of:**
    a. Health promotion
    b. Health prevention
    c. Disease promotion
    d. Disease prevention

200. **The local dental hygienists' association is planning to educate the senior citizens about the presentation and treatment of root caries. Which of the following would be MOST effective for the seniors to retain the information?**
    a. Review of topics presented in pamphlet
    b. Description of oral conditions and therapeutic strategies
    c. Presentation of PowerPoint slides and incorporation of the use of hand mirrors
    d. Having the seniors look at one another's mouth and describe what they see.

COMPONENT B—REVIEW QUESTIONS

Answers and Rationales to Component B Review Questions are located on this text's accompanying Evolve site.

Component B of the Simulated National Board Dental Hygiene Exam (also referred to as the PM portion taken in the afternoon on examination day) is based on Cases A to J. Relevant illustration for each case are followed by test questions relating to the case. Many of the radiographs and clinical photographs used in these pages have been cropped, reduced, or enlarged to enhance the clarity of the structures or lesions they represent.

CASE A

1. Which of the following medications is prescribed for this client's treatment of high blood pressure?
   a. Fosamax
   b. Crestor
   c. Metoprolol
   d. Aspirin

2. The radiopaque line observed on the panoramic radiograph that runs horizontally across the maxilla from molar to molar is caused by the:
   a. Nose
   b. Pterygoid plates
   c. Floor of the maxillary sinus
   d. Tongue
   e. Palate

3. The gingival recession noted on tooth #3 is MOST likely caused by:
   a. Erosion
   b. Abrasion
   c. Attrition
   d. Abfraction

4. Using G. V. Black's classification of dental caries and restorations, which of the following describes the restoration on tooth #3?
   a. Class I
   b. Class II
   c. Class III
   d. Class IV
   e. Class V
   f. Class VI

5. The alignment of teeth #24 and 25 in relation to the client's occlusion are referred to as:
   a. Linguoversion/torsoversion
   b. Torsoversion/labioversion
   c. Labioversion/linguoversion
   d. Infraversion/labioversion

6. Which of the following is the radiolucent area viewed on the apical area of tooth #20?
   a. Periapical abscess
   b. Mandibular fossa
   c. Mental foramen
   d. Apical granuloma

7. Which of the following home care aids would be MOST useful for this client to clean underneath her bridges?
   a. Regular dental tape
   b. Gum stimulator
   c. Tufted dental floss
   d. Soft toothbrush

8. During client preparation for the panoramic radiograph, a lead apron without a thyroid collar should be placed around the client's neck because the thyroid collar:
   a. Blocks part of the beam and obscures important diagnostic information
   b. Affects the complete rotation of the machine during radiographic exposure
   c. Creates a ghost image on anterior teeth on the panoramic radiograph
   d. Causes the client's chin to tip upward during the rotating cycle

9. The redness on the marginal gingiva of tooth #11 is MOST likely caused by:
   a. A reactive lesion caused by local irritant
   b. Denture flange
   c. Age and hormonal changes
   d. Unknown etiology

10. Which of the following BEST describes the contour of the interdental papilla around teeth #23, #24, #25, and #26?
    a. Bulbous
    b. Rolled
    c. Cratered
    d. Blunted

11. The endodontic material used to obturate the roots of teeth #4, #13, and #19 during endodontic therapy is MOST likely:
    a. Zinc oxide and eugenol
    b. Polycarboxylate dental cement
    c. Gutta percha
    d. Calcium hydroxide

SYNOPSIS OF PATIENT HISTORY

Age 72
Sex F
Height 5'5"

CASE A
Medically complex -geriatric

Weight 135 lbs
60 kgs

VITAL SIGNS
Blood pressure 130/85 mmHg
Pulse rate 72 bpm
Respiration rate 18 rpm

1. Under Care of Physician
Yes ☒ No ☐   Condition: Hypertension

2. Hospitalized within the last 5 years
Yes ☒ No ☐   Reason: Open heart surgery

3. Has or had the following conditions
Osteoprosis, high cholestrol

4. Current medications
Metoprolol, Crestor, Fosamax,
Aspirin

5. Smokes or uses tobacco products
Yes ☐ No ☒

6. Is pregnant
Yes ☐ No ☒ N/A ☐

MEDICAL HISTORY:
Had open heart surgery 2 years ago (Aorta valve replaced, mitral valve repaired)

DENTAL HISTORY:
Has history of perio flap surgery. Patient was smoking for 50 years and she quit last 2 years.
Brushes 3x/day
Flosses 2-3 x/week

SOCIAL HISTORY:
Retired and widowed. Has 2 children and one grandchild.

CHIEF COMPLAINT:
I am concerned about my bones because of the osteoprosis and my dental health

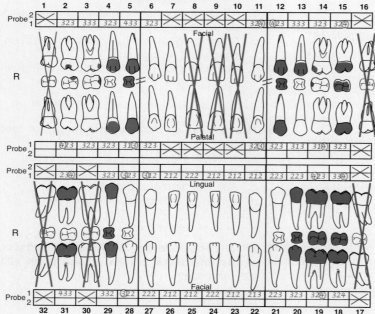

Case A
Medically complex -geriatric

CURRENT ORAL HYGIENE STATUS:
1. Minimal plaque biofilm
2. Limited bleeding on probing
3. Patient brushes two times a day

SUPPLEMENTAL ORAL EXAMINATION FINDINGS:
1. Recession
2. Sensitivity
3. Periodontal surgery
4. Maxillary anterior bridge and mandibular posterior bridge

Restoration

Cavity

Sealant

Clinically missing tooth

Furcation

"Through and through" furcation

Probe 1 : initial probing depth

Probe 2 : probing depth 1 month after scaling and root planing

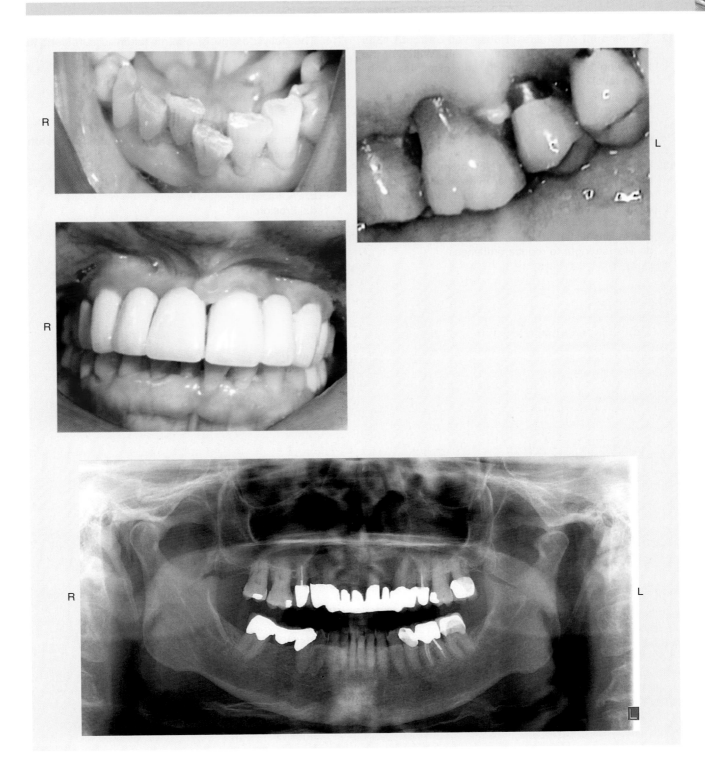

12. The amount of recession observed on tooth #3 is 6 mm, and the pocket depth is 3 mm. Which of the following accurately reflects the clinical attachment level?
    a. 3 mm
    b. 5 mm
    c. 6 mm
    d. 9 mm

13. Which of the following is an advantage of the porcelain-fused-to-metal crowns observed in this client compared with a porcelain-only crown?
    a. Is aesthetically pleasing
    b. Is susceptible to staining
    c. Retains luster
    d. Has strength to reduce brittleness

14. The daily dosage of aspirin taken is sufficient to cause:
    a. Analgesia
    b. Coagulation of blood
    c. Integumental pain relief
    d. Visceral pain relief

15. The incisal edges of the anterior mandibular teeth are characteristic of:
    a. Abrasion
    b. Attrition
    c. Abfraction
    d. Erosion

CASE B

SYNOPSIS OF PATIENT HISTORY	Age	12	VITAL SIGNS	
	Sex	M	Blood pressure	120/80 mmHg
	Height	5'1"	Pulse rate	85 bpm
			Respiration rate	18 rpm

CASE __B__
__Pedodontic__   Weight   98   lbs
                          45   kgs

1. Under Care of Physician
   Yes No
   ☒   ☐   Condition: __Seasonal allergy__
2. Hospitalized within the last 5 years
   Yes No
   ☐   ☒   Reason: _____
3. Has or had the following conditions
   _____
   _____

4. Current medications
   __Loratadine (Claritin),__
   __Iansoprazole (Prevacid) 15 mg__

5. Smokes or uses tobacco products
   Yes No
   ☐   ☒

6. Is pregnant
   Yes No   N/A
   ☐   ☒   ☐

MEDICAL HISTORY:
This client has seasonal allergies and currently he is taking Claritin and Prevacid.

DENTAL HISTORY:
Does not visit the dentist on a regular basis. It is recorded in his chart that he has excessive salivation during dental treatment

SOCIAL HISTORY:
He lives with his parents and has 3 siblings. He enjoys sports baseball and football

CHIEF COMPLAINT:
"Not happy with the white colors on my teeth"

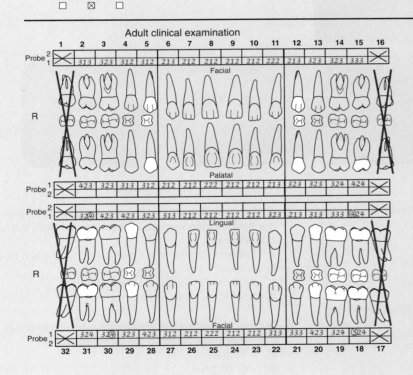

Adult clinical examination

Case B
Pedodontic

CURRENT ORAL HYGIENE STATUS:
1. Good oral hygiene
2. Patient brush twice a day
3. Mouthbreather

SUPPLEMENTAL ORAL EXAMINATION FINDINGS:
1. Permanent dentition.
2. High intake of snacks
3. No carious lesions and no fillings

Restoration
Cavity
Sealant
Clinically missing tooth
Furcation
"Through and through" furcation

Probe 1 : initial probing depth
Probe 2 : probing depth 1 month after scaling and root planing

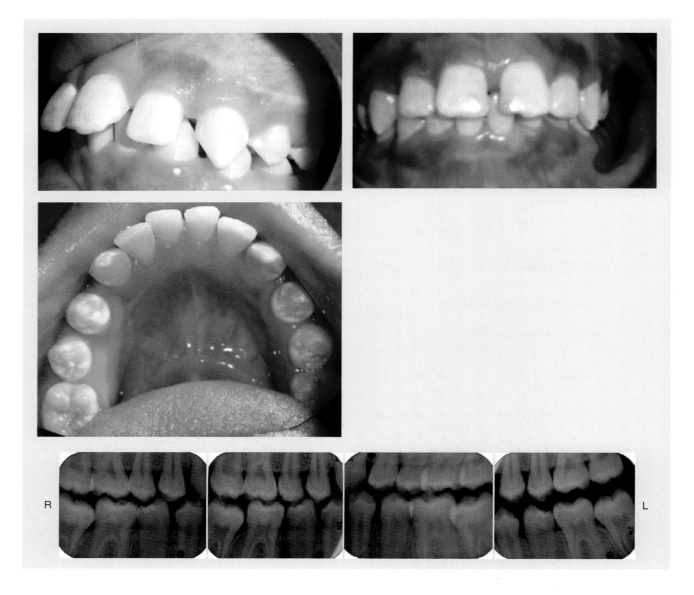

1. **Which of the following BEST describes this client's vital signs?**
   a. Blood pressure is considered low
   b. Respiration is considered low
   c. Pulse rate is considered high
   d. Vital signs are within normal limits

2. **The 15 mg of lansoprazole (Prevacid) taken by this client is indicated for:**
   a. Heartburn
   b. Asthma
   c. Attention deficit disorder
   d. Anxiety

3. **The dark brownish area on the gingival and alveolar mucosa on the area of tooth #10 is caused by:**
   a. Injury
   b. Hereditary factors
   c. Inflammation
   d. Abscess

4. **At the end of oral prophylaxis, the dental hygienist applied fluoride varnish to the client's teeth. Varnish consists of:**
   a. Sodium fluoride in a noncolophony or rosin base
   b. Acidulated phosphate fluoride at 2%
   c. Acidulated phosphate fluoride at 5%
   d. Sodium fluoride at 5%

5. **During the bitewing technique, the central ray of the x-ray beam should be directed at:**
   a. 0 degree
   b. +10 degrees
   c. −10 degrees
   d. −20 degrees

6. During treatment, the dental hygienist noticed excessive salivation in the client. Which of the following salivary glands produce the largest amount of saliva in the mouth?
   a. Parotid
   b. Submandibular
   c. Sublingual
   d. Ebner's

7. Which of the following BEST describes the relationship of the incisal occlusion of anterior teeth?
   a. Edge-to-edge bite
   b. Open bite
   c. Overjet
   d. Cross-bite

8. The cause of the generalized white areas observed on most of the teeth is MOST likely caused by:
   a. Calculus
   b. Decalcification or demineralization
   c. Trauma
   d. Fluorosis

9. The BEST rationale for the 5-mm probe reading on the mesiobuccal of tooth #18 is:
   a. Partially erupted tooth
   b. Plaque biofilm
   c. Open contact spaces
   d. Malocclusion

10. Which of the following is a motivator to help this client improve his home plaque removal routine?
    a. Improvement of appearance
    b. Rewards
    c. Saving money
    d. Reducing pain

11. The dentist has recommended that this client's parents consult with an orthodontist. If the client has orthodontic appliances placed on his teeth, which of the following would you NOT recommend as an adjunct to his home care after his braces are placed?
    a. Interdental brush
    b. Floss threader
    c. Wooden wedges
    d. Floss holder

12. The spacing observed between the anterior maxillary teeth is:
    a. Normal for this client's age and eruption pattern
    b. Excessive and indicates diastemas between the permanent teeth
    c. Minimal and indicates that crowding will occur in the future
    d. No spacing is evident between the anterior maxillary teeth

13. As indicated in the client's dental history, this client is a mouthbreather. All of the following are significant oral conditions common in mouth-breathers EXCEPT one. Which one is the EXCEPTION?
    a. Increase in plaque formation
    b. Fordyce granules
    c. Gingival enlargement
    d. Erythematous incisive papilla

14. During football season, this client would benefit from a mouth protector because of all the following reasons EXCEPT one. Which one is the EXCEPTION?
    a. Promoting mouth protectors to the other players on the team
    b. Preventing the dislocation or fracture of the anterior maxillary teeth
    c. Minimizing lacerations by holding soft tissues away from teeth
    d. Decreasing shock to the temporomandibular joint (TMJ) and the mandibular condyle, which would prevent concussions

15. The type of material used for athletic mouth protectors is referred to as:
    a. Thermoset
    b. Thermoplastic
    c. Reversible hydrocolloid
    d. Irreversible hydrocolloid

CASE C

SYNOPSIS
OF PATIENT
HISTORY

Age _42_
Sex _M_
Height _5'10"_

VITAL SIGNS
Blood pressure _140/90 mmHg_
Pulse rate _60 bpm_
Respiration rate _20 rpm_

CASE _C_
_Medically complex
- special need_

Weight _165_ lbs
_75_ kgs

1. Under Care of Physician
   Yes   No
   ☒   ☐   Condition: _Kidney disease_
2. Hospitalized within the last 5 years
   Yes   No
   ☒   ☐   Reason: _Alcoholism_
3. Has or had the following conditions
   Stage 2 Kidney disease

4. Current medications
   none

5. Smokes or uses tobacco products
   Yes   No
   ☐   ☒

6. Is pregnant
   Yes   No   N/A
   ☐   ☒   ☐

MEDICAL HISTORY:
_This client was diagnosed with kidney disease
one year ago and is an alcoholic who has been
unsuccessful with rehabilitation. Allergic to
penicillin. Family history of kidney disease_

DENTAL HISTORY:
_He has carious lesions, generalized pigmentation
and malalignment. Brushes one time per day and
flosses infrequently_

SOCIAL HISTORY:
Single and has a part-time job in a post office.

CHIEF COMPLAINT:
"I have a decayed tooth"

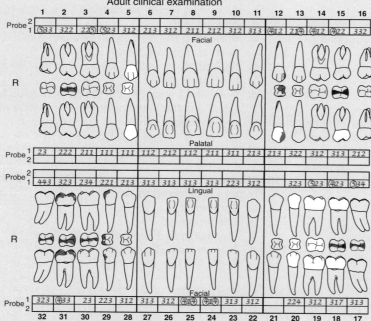

Adult clinical examination

	1	2	3	4	5	6	7	8	9	10	11	12	13	14	15	16
Probe 2/1	⑤33	322	22⑤	⑤23	312	213	312	211	212	312	313	④12	21④	④12	④22	332

Facial

R

Palatal

| Probe 1/2 | 23 | 222 | 211 | 111 | 111 | | 112 | 212 | 112 | 211 | 311 | 213 | 213 | 322 | 312 | 313 | 212 |
| Probe 2/1 | 443 | 323 | 234 | 221 | 213 | | 313 | 313 | 313 | 313 | 223 | 312 | | 323 | ⑤23 | ④23 | ⑤34 |

Lingual

R

Facial

| Probe 1/2 | 323 | ④33 | 23 | 223 | 312 | | 313 | 312 | ④1④ | ④1④ | 313 | 312 | | 224 | 312 | 317 | 313 |

| | 32 | 31 | 30 | 29 | 28 | 27 | 26 | 25 | 24 | 23 | 22 | 21 | 20 | 19 | 18 | 17 |

Case C
Medically complex - special need

CURRENT ORAL HYGIENE STATUS:
1. _Does not use any interdent aids_
2. _Bleeding on probing_

SUPPLEMENTAL ORAL EXAMINATION FINDINGS:
1. _Remaining root_
2. _Dental caries_
3. _Stains_
4. _Malalignment upper anterior_
5. _Fluorosis_

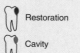

Restoration

Cavity

Sealant

Clinically missing tooth

△ Furcation

▲ "Through and through" furcation

Probe 1 : initial probing depth
Probe 2 : probing depth 1 month after
scaling and root planing

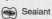
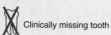

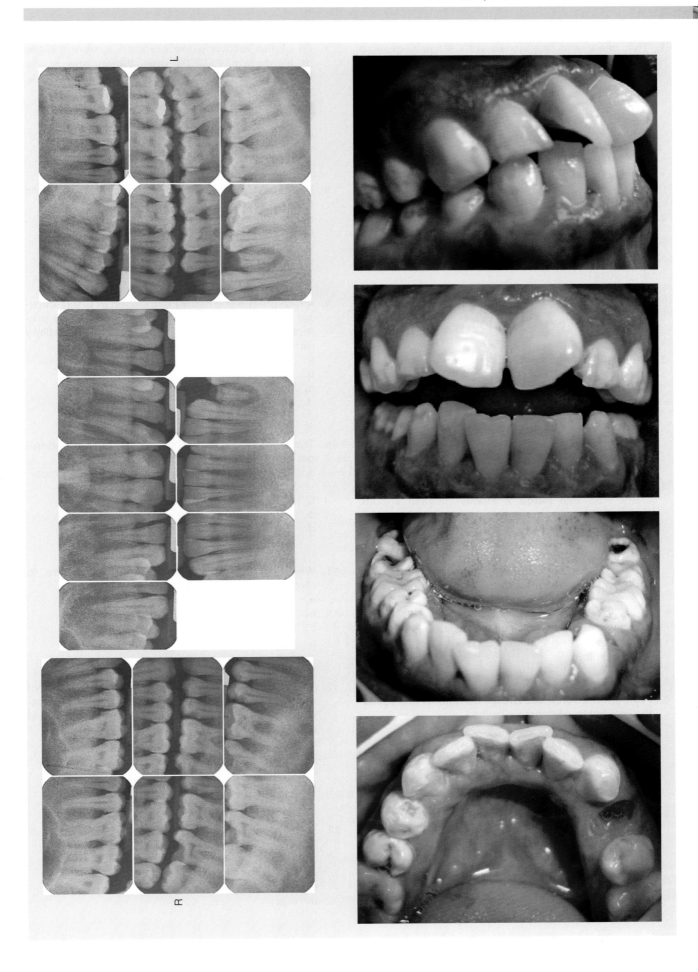

1. This client was diagnosed with stage 2 chronic kidney disease. What does stage 2 imply?
   a. Kidney damage with normal kidney function
   b. Kidney damage with a mild decrease in kidney function
   c. Kidney damage with a moderate decrease in kidney function
   d. Kidney damage with a severe decrease in kidney function
   e. Kidney failure

2. All of the following drugs use the kidneys as a major pathway of elimination and must be used with caution for this client EXCEPT one. Which one is the EXCEPTION?
   a. Xylocaine
   b. Aspirin
   c. Penicillin
   d. Amantadine

3. The impaired kidney function can lead to the following effects EXCEPT one. Which one is the EXCEPTION?
   a. Hypertension
   b. Peripheral edema
   c. Diabetes
   d. Bone changes

4. Recommended dental hygiene care for this client who has stage 2 kidney disease should include:
   a. Maintaining the highest level of oral health to prevent the need for extensive treatment
   b. Addressing and communicating with the client directly and not just through the caregiver
   c. Providing the client with the opportunity to expectorate often because of the increase in salivary flow
   d. Allowing frequent changes in the client's body position during treatment to avoid client discomfort

5. Prolonged alcohol use MOST commonly increases the incidence of damage to the:
   a. Kidney
   b. Heart
   c. Liver
   d. Brain

6. Which of the following oral conditions is this client MOST susceptible to because of his alcoholism?
   a. Dental caries
   b. Benign migratory glossitis
   c. Keratosis
   d. Oral cancer

7. All of the following are common extraoral signs of alcoholism EXCEPT one. Which one is the EXCEPTION?
   a. Tremor of hands, tongue, eyelids
   b. Breath odors of alcohol and tobacco
   c. Redness of forehead, cheeks, and nose
   d. Red, baggy, or puffy eyes
   e. Melanin pigmentation of the face

8. The type of cyst found on the apical area of tooth #21 can be BEST described as a:
   a. Residual cyst
   b. Radicular cyst
   c. Dermoid cyst
   d. Lateral periodontal cyst

9. A radiopaque line mainly composed of dense cortical bone found above the apices of maxillary premolars and molars in this client's posterior maxillary radiographs is known as the:
   a. Maxillary sinus
   b. Nutrient canal
   c. Zygomatic process
   d. Floor of maxillary sinus

10. The technique error in the upper left molar periapical radiograph can be corrected by:
    a. Moving the position-indicating device (PID) more distally
    b. Adjusting the vertical angulation
    c. Instructing the patient not to move
    d. Moving the film more posteriorly

11. Which of the following is the BEST choice to remove subgingival calculus in this client?
    a. Air-powder, air-abrasive, or air polisher
    b. Sickle scaler
    c. Ultrasonic scaler
    d. Oral irrigation device

12. The mandibular occlusal intraoral photograph of this client confirms that one of the following treatment needs was performed first. Which treatment need is it?
    a. Periodontal debridement
    b. Treatment of dental caries
    c. Orthodontic consultation
    d. Extraction of root tip

13. The MOST probable cause for the alignment of teeth #8 and #9 is:
    a. Thumb sucking
    b. Developmental
    c. Inflammation
    d. Injury

14. The classification of dental caries in teeth #29 and #31 can be BEST identified as_____ and _____ respectively:
    a. Class II , Class II
    b. Class II, Class I
    c. Class I, Class II
    d. Class I, Class I

15. This client wants to use a mouthrinse because he believes it will make his mouth feel fresher. You have instructed him to use a fluoridated, essential oils–containing mouthrinse without alcohol with the American Dental Association (ADA) Seal of Acceptance. Other than his alcoholism, the following represent other good reasons for recommending an ADA-accepted mouthrinse with essential oils EXCEPT one. Which one is the EXCEPTION?
    a. Prevention of oral fungal infection
    b. Hydration of oral tissues
    c. An antimicrobial effect
    d. Fresh feeling in the mouth

CASE D

<table>
<tr><td>SYNOPSIS
OF PATIENT
HISTORY</td><td>Age ___65___
Sex ___F___
Height ___5'4"___</td><td>VITAL SIGNS
Blood pressure ___150/90 mmHg___
Pulse rate ___74 bpm___
Respiration rate ___14 rpm___</td></tr>
<tr><td>CASE ___D___
___Geriatric___</td><td>Weight ___110___ lbs
___50___ kgs</td><td></td></tr>
</table>

1. Under Care of Physician
   Yes ☒ No ☐   Condition: ___high cholesterol___
2. Hospitalized within the last 5 years
   Yes ☐ No ☒   Reason: _____
3. Has or had the following conditions
   _____
   _____

4. Current medications
   ___atorvastatin calcium (Lipitor)___

   ___10 mg day___
   _____

5. Smokes or uses tobacco products
   Yes ☐ No ☒

6. Is pregnant
   Yes ☐ No ☒ N/A ☐

MEDICAL HISTORY:
This client has high cholesterol (hyperlipidemia)

DENTAL HISTORY:
She brushes twice a day. Her last dental visit was 2 years ago. Had gingival grafting done by a periodontist.

SOCIAL HISTORY:
Housewife and she seems happy and loves gardening

CHIEF COMPLAINT:
"Time to get my teeth cleaned"

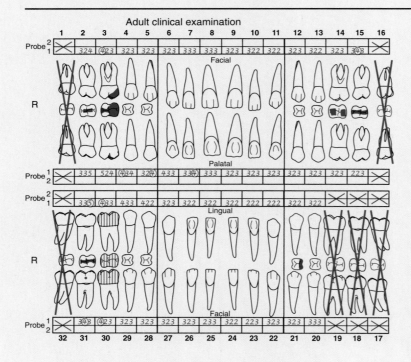

Adult clinical examination

Case D
Geriatric

CURRENT ORAL HYGIENE STATUS:
1. Use hard tooth brush twice a day
2. Localized area of bleeding

SUPPLEMENTAL ORAL EXAMINATION FINDINGS:
1. Decay
2. Deep groove staining
3. Wear facets in teeth 6, 11, 22, 27
4. Attrition and malignment

 Restoration

Cavity

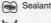 Sealant

 Clinically missing tooth

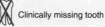 Furcation

 "Through and through" furcation

Probe 1 : initial probing depth

Probe 2 : probing depth 1 month after scaling and root planing

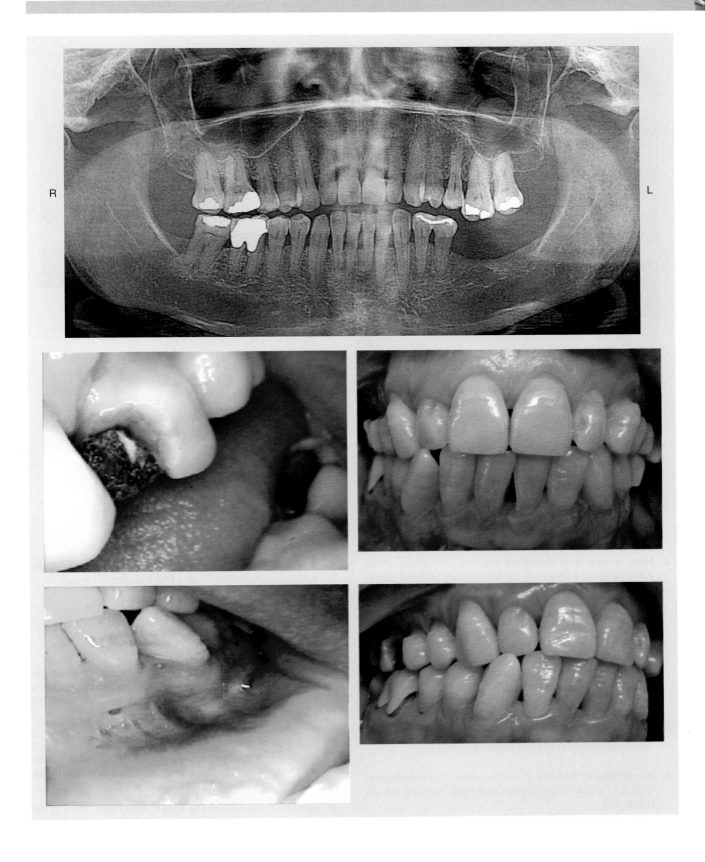

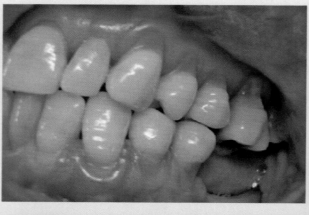
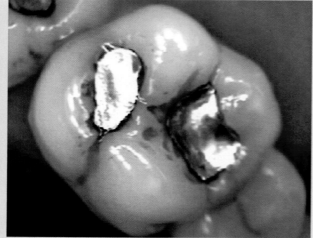
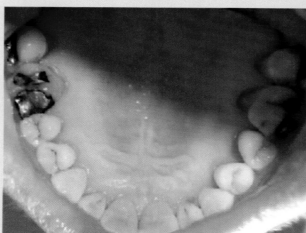

1. **How would you describe the classification of an ASA (American Society of Anesthesiologists) physical status II client?**
   a. A client with severe systemic disease that is a constant threat to life; does require dental treatment modifications
   b. For a healthy client, it is not necessary to modify the dental treatment
   c. A client with moderate to severe systemic disease requires special care, and dental treatment modifications are generally necessary
   d. A client with mild systemic disease that does not interfere with day-to-day activity may require dental treatment modifications

2. **According to Black's classification of restorations, which of the following describes the restoration on tooth #3?**
   a. Class I
   b. Class II
   c. Class III
   d. Class IV
   e. Class V
   f. Class VI

3. **Which of the following terms BEST describes the radiopaque lesion in the left maxillary sinus?**
   a. Osteoma
   b. Ossifying fibroma
   c. Compound odontoma
   d. Periapical granuloma

4. **During the panoramic radiography procedure, what will be the result if the patient's head is positioned too high or is tipped upward and the Frankfort plane is angled upward?**
   a. Loss of details in maxillary incisor region
   b. Lack of visibility of the mandibular condyle
   c. An "exaggerated smile line" that is curved upward
   d. Radiolucent shadow that obscures anterior teeth

5. **Which of the following BEST describes the conditions in the cervical areas of maxillary left and right molars?**
   a. Abrasion
   b. Erosion
   c. Attrition
   d. Abfraction

6. Which of the following is the BEST term for the sign of the disease or disorder on tooth #14?
   a. Recurrent caries
   b. Overeruption
   c. Fractured amalgam
   d. Bruxism

7. An amalgam polishing setup consists of cups and points that are abrasives and impregnated with polishing ingredients to provide fast results without pumice or tin oxide. In which order should the dental hygienist use these cups and points to achieve a good result?
   a. Greenies, brownies, and super-greenies
   b. Brownies, greenies, and super-greenies
   c. Greenies, brownies, and super-brownies
   d. Brownies, greenies, and super-brownies

8. A total cholesterol level of less than 200 mg/dL is a desirable level that places this client at lower risk for coronary artery disease. Low-density lipoprotein (LDL) levels decrease the risk of heart disease, and high-density lipoprotein (HDL) levels increase the risk.
   a. The first statement is TRUE, and second statement is FALSE
   b. The first statement is FALSE, and second statement is TRUE
   c. Both statements are TRUE
   d. Both statements are FALSE

9. On the basis of the client's oral condition, the dental hygienist may instruct the client to use all of the following aids EXCEPT one. Which one is the EXCEPTION?
   a. End-tufted toothbrush
   b. Soft manual toothbrush
   c. Tufted dental floss with threader
   d. Interdental wooden cleaner

10. All of the following statements are true about atorvastatin calcium (Lipitor) medication EXCEPT one. Which one is the EXCEPTION?
    a. Cholesterol-lowering drugs can interact with grapefruit juice and increase the risk of the drugs' potential adverse effects
    b. Common adverse effects include headaches, muscle pain, and diarrhea
    c. This medication can cause birth defects and is therefore contraindicated during pregnancy.
    d. Atorvastatin calcium is a medication used to treat arthritis

11. Which of the client's vital signs needs further assessment?
    a. Blood pressure
    b. Height
    c. Pulse rate
    d. Weight

12. The client's pulp chambers of maxillary molars are slightly obliterated. What is the MOST likely cause for this occurrence?
    a. Abscesses
    b. Traumatic occlusion
    c. Tongue thrusting
    d. Aging process

13. This client has class I mobility on tooth #2. The BEST description for this classification of mobility is:
    a. No more than 1 mm of discernible movement
    b. Combined facial–lingual movement totaling 2 mm, and the tooth is depressible in the socket
    c. Combined facial–lingual movement is between 2 and 3 mm
    d. Combined facial–lingual movement totaling 3 mm or more, and the tooth is depressible in the socket

14. What is the MOST likely cause of midline shift in this client?
    a. Periodontal movement of teeth
    b. Missing mandibular molars
    c. History of gingival grafting
    d. Supernumerary mandibular incisor

15. The bilateral radiolucent area in the molar region inferior to the mylohyoid ridge is known as the:
    a. Mandibular canal
    b. External oblique ridge
    c. Submandibular fossa
    d. Mental foramen

CASE E

SYNOPSIS OF PATIENT HISTORY

Age __57__
Sex __F__
Height __5'8"__

VITAL SIGNS
Blood pressure __138/88 mmHg__
Pulse rate __64 bpm__
Respiration rate __16 rpm__

CASE __E__
Chronic periodontitis

Weight __140__ lbs
__64__ kgs

1. Under Care of Physician
   Yes ☒   No ☐   Condition: ___Psoriasis___
2. Hospitalized within the last 5 years
   Yes ☐   No ☒   Reason: _____
3. Has or had the following conditions
   hyperparathyroidism
   _____

4. Current medications
   Methotrexate (Trexall) 2.5 mg
   _____
   _____

5. Smokes or uses tobacco products
   Yes ☐   No ☒

6. Is pregnant
   Yes ☐   No ☒   N/A ☐

MEDICAL HISTORY:
Patient undergoing dermatological treatment for psoriasis. Had successful parathyroid surgery 3 years ago.

DENTAL HISTORY:
Visits the dental office infrequently. Has no history of cavities.

SOCIAL HISTORY:
Mother of 3 children ages 15, 16, and 21. Works full time work in a bank.

CHIEF COMPLAINT:
"My gums bleed when I brush my teeth and my breath smells"

Adult clinical examination

	1	2	3	4	5	6	7	8	9	10	11	12	13	14	15	16
Probe 2/1	⊠	334	446	534	523	332	324	434	433	(425)	(424)	(435)	(535)	(645)	744)	532)

Facial

R

Palatal

| Probe 1/2 | ⊠ | 334 | 435 | 544 | 534 | 33 | 334 | 323 | 323 | 334 | 323 | 323 | 325 | 535 | 534 | 422 |

| Probe 2/1 | (435) | 544) | ⊠ | 233 | 334) | 333 | 222 | 222 | 222 | 223 | 322 | 334) | 434 | (435) | (535) | (535) |

Lingual

R

Facial

| Probe 1/2 | 323 | 333 | ⊠ | 222 | 234 | 333 | 322 | 434 | 434 | 433 | 323 | 434 | 333 | 433 | 535 | 435 |

| | 32 | 31 | 30 | 29 | 28 | 27 | 26 | 25 | 24 | 23 | 22 | 21 | 20 | 19 | 18 | 17 |

Case E
Chronic periodontitis

CURRENT ORAL HYGIENE STATUS:
1. _Moderate plaque biofilm and calculus_
2. _Bleeding on probing_
3. _Localized area of deep pockets > 84mm_

SUPPLEMENTAL ORAL EXAMINATION FINDINGS:
1. _Wear facets (multiple areas)_
2. _Craized lines_
3. _Missing teeth_

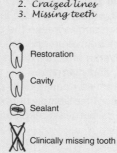

▮ Restoration

▯ Cavity

⊜ Sealant

⊠ Clinically missing tooth

△ Furcation

▲ "Through and through" furcation

Probe 1 : initial probing depth

Probe 2 : probing depth 1 month after scaling and root planing

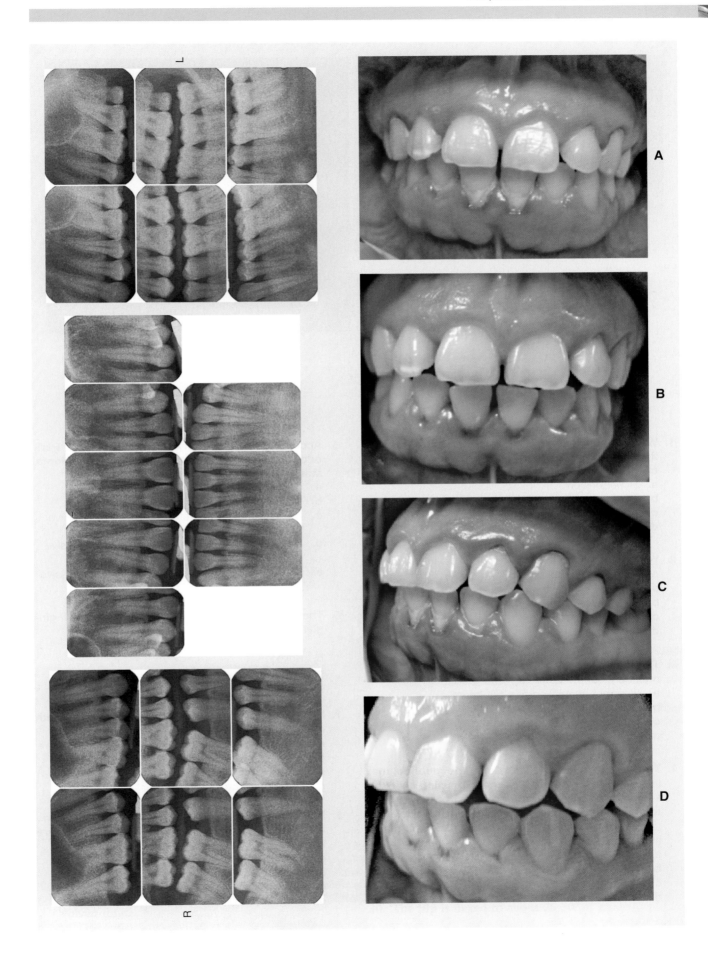

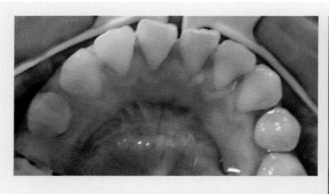

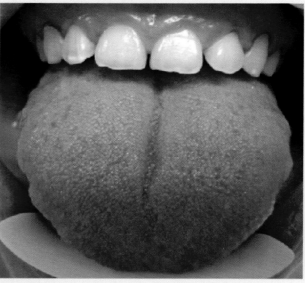

1. **When treating psoriasis with methotrexate (Trexall), it is important NOT to prescribe this medication to clients who exhibit:**
   a. Hypertension
   b. Hyperthyroidism
   c. Anemia
   d. Pregnancy

2. **Which one of the following conditions in the client needs further assessment?**
   a. Weight
   b. Pulse rate
   c. Height
   d. Blood pressure

3. **The major cause for the error on the distal of the maxillary canine films is:**
   a. Incorrect angulation of x-ray beam
   b. Crowding of anterior teeth
   c. Improper placement of film
   d. Aged fixer solution

4. **The dental hygienist has started to debride the lingual aspect of teeth #24 and #25, using a sickle scaler to remove the supragingival calculus. The total number of cutting edges on a sickle scaler is _____ . The face and the terminal shank will meet in an angle of _____.**
   a. 1, 45 degrees
   b. 1, 70 degrees to 80 degrees
   c. 2, 70 degrees to 80 degrees
   d. 2, 45 degrees

5. **According to the American Association of Periodontology, this client's posterior periodontal status is classified as:**
   a. Case Type I: Gingivitis
   b. Case Type II: Slight Chronic Periodontitis
   c. Case Type III: Moderate Chronic or Aggressive Periodontitis
   d. Case Type IV: Advanced Chronic or Aggressive Periodontitis
   e. Case Type V: Refractory, Chronic, or Aggressive Periodontitis

6. **The BEST way to describe the client's overall gingival margin is:**
   a. Blunted
   b. Rolled
   c. Cratered
   d. Fibrotic

7. **The radiopaque area on the mesial surface of tooth #2 in the right premolar bitewing is a (an):**
   a. Overhang amalgam restoration
   b. Interproximal subgingival calculus
   c. Crest of the alveolar bone
   d. Overlapped radiographic error

8. **Mushroom-shaped elevations scattered over the anterior third of the dorsum of the tongue are known as:**
   a. Foliate papillae
   b. Circumvallate papillae
   c. Filiform papillae
   d. Fungiform papillae

9. **After this client undergoes periodontal therapy, the primary purpose of the maintenance phase of care is to:**
   a. Complete all remaining aspects of the treatment plan
   b. Prevent recurrence of the disease
   c. Re-evaluate the results of the initial therapy
   d. Keep the client on a recare system

10. **Which of the following is MOST likely the cause of this client's halitosis?**
    a. Microorganisms that produce foul-smelling compounds
    b. Decaying food particles in the mouth
    c. Frequent consumption of spicy foods
    d. Gastric diseases

11. **The BEST term to describe the client's anterior occlusal relationship is:**
    a. Overbite
    b. Edge-to-edge
    c. Overjet
    d. Normal

12. **Which one of the following instruments is BEST to remove the subgingival calculus on the mesial surface of tooth #2?**
    a. SH 6/7 sickle scaler
    b. SH 5/33 sickle scaler
    c. Gracy 11/12 curet
    d. Gracy 13/14 curet

13. **The client returns 4 weeks after the initial periodontal debridement. Which of the following is the single BEST criterion for evaluating the success of this treatment?**
    a. Removal of all of the calculus
    b. Smooth and glass-like root surfaces
    c. No evidence of bleeding on probing
    d. Reduction in pocket depth

14. **Horizontal bone loss is evident between teeth #20 and #21. The type of pocket formed is referred to as an infrabony pocket.**
    a. The first statement is TRUE, and the second statement is FALSE
    b. The first statement is FALSE , and the second statement is TRUE
    c. Both statements are TRUE
    d. Both statements are FALSE

15. **When comparing photo A with photo B, and photo C with photo D, what should the dental hygienist conclude about the client's gingival healing?**
    a. Calculus remains, and the gingiva cannot begin the healing process
    b. Calculus is removed, and the redness of the gingiva implies infection
    c. Calculus is removed, and the gingiva can begin the healing process
    d. Calculus remains, and the gingiva can begin the healing process

CASE F

SYNOPSIS
OF PATIENT
HISTORY

Age _24_
Sex _M_
Height _6'2"_

CASE _F_
Special needs

Weight _188_ lbs
_85_ kgs

VITAL SIGNS
Blood pressure _122/82 mmHg_
Pulse rate _68 bpm_
Respiration rate _16 rpm_

1. Under Care of Physician
   Yes ☐ No ☒ Condition: _____
2. Hospitalized within the last 5 years
   Yes ☒ No ☐ Reason: _Car accident - Spinal_ _Cord Injury_
3. Has or had the following conditions
   Physical disability - paraplegic - lower limbs
   Recovered from Tonsilitis 2 weeks ago.
4. Current medications
   None
   _____

5. Smokes or uses tobacco products
   Yes ☐ No ☒
6. Is pregnant
   Yes ☐ No ☒ N/A ☐

MEDICAL HISTORY:
Has physical disability due to car accident 4 years ago. Overall he is in good health

DENTAL HISTORY:
Had oral piercing (tongue and lip) for last 2 years. Does not routinely visit dental office

SOCIAL HISTORY:
College student. His hobby is photography. He overcomes all barriers to live as independent as possible. He uses a wheelchair.

CHIEF COMPLAINT:
"concerned about chipped tooth due to oral piercing"

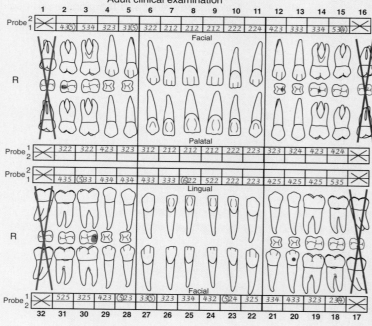

Case F
Special needs

CURRENT ORAL HYGIENE STATUS:
1. _Brushes twice a day_
2. _Minimal plaque biofilm_
3. _Uses a medium bristle tooth brush_

SUPPLEMENTAL ORAL EXAMINATION FINDINGS:
1. _Cross bite 3.4_
2. _Overjet 2 mm_
3. _Recession on mandibular facial aspect_
4. _#25 chipped incisal edge_

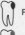 Restoration

 Cavity

 Sealant

 Clinically missing tooth

 Furcation

 "Through and through" furcation

Probe 1 : initial probing depth
Probe 2 : probing depth 1 month after scaling and root planing

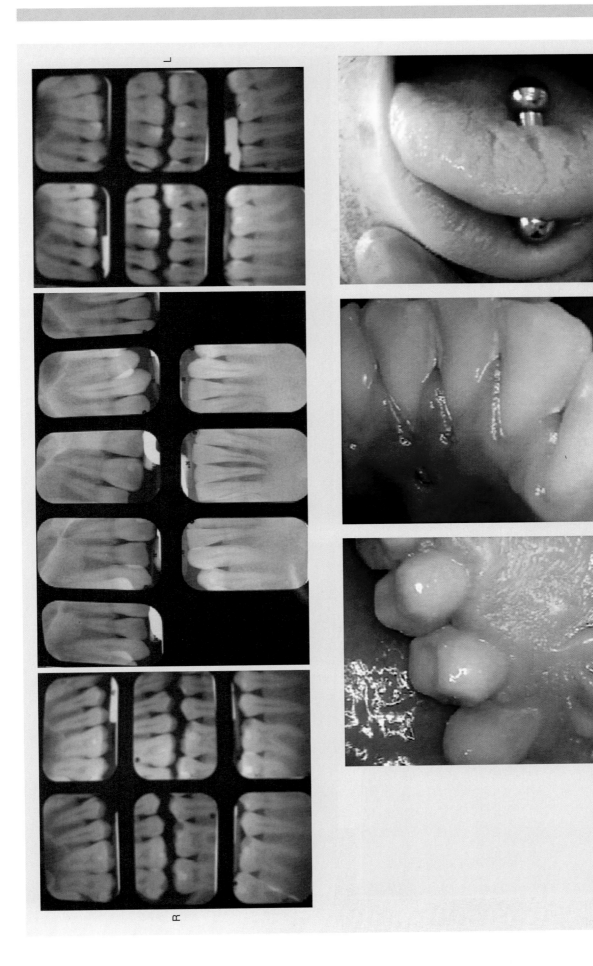

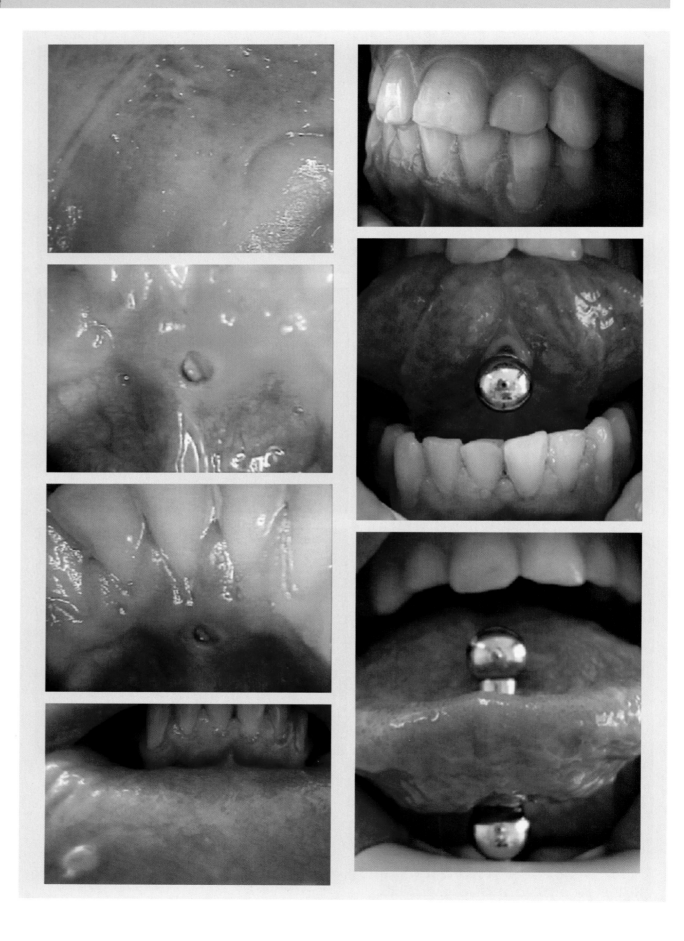

1. It is required by law that health care facilities contain a barrier-free design to accommodate clients who have a physical disability. By which of the following laws that ensure the rights of people with disabilities is this client who is wheelchair bound protected?
   a. 1996 Telecommunications Act
   b. 1973 Rehabilitation Act
   c. 1999 Olmstead Decision
   d. 1990 Americans with Disabilities Act

2. To provide the most optimal treatment to this client, it is the responsibility of the dental hygienist to do all of the following EXCEPT one. Which one is the EXCEPTION?
   a. To take the responsibility of transferring the client from the wheelchair to the dental chair
   b. To assess the client's cognitive awareness
   c. To determine his ability to ambulate with or without assistance
   d. To determine his ability to communicate and interpret information

3. Which of the following vertebrae is affected by the spinal cord injury of this client with paraplegia?
   a. C—cervical
   b. T—thoracic
   c. L—lumbar
   d. S—sacral

4. The inverted Y in the maxillary left canine periapical film represents the intersection of:
   a. Orbital cavity and nasal cavity
   b. Orbital cavity and maxillary sinus
   c. Maxillary sinus and nasal fossa
   d. Nasal fossa and maxillary tuberosity

5. The radiographic error in the maxillary central incisor can be corrected by:
   a. Adjusting the horizontal angulations
   b. Moving the film more distally to the left
   c. Replacing depleted developer and fixer solutions
   d. Removing the bite block from the client's mouth

6. Common signs or symptoms that may occur after tongue piercing include all of the following EXCEPT one. Which one is the EXCEPTION?
   a. Decreased salivary flow
   b. Pain
   c. Swelling
   d. Infection

7. In addition to the chipped tooth, which of the following adverse outcomes secondary to tongue piercing is present in this client?
   a. Increased salivary flow
   b. Damage to restorations
   c. Pulpal sensitivity
   d. Soft tissue injury

8. The full mouth series of radiographs indicate that this client is experiencing all of the following EXCEPT one. Which one is the EXCEPTION?
   a. Dental caries
   b. Recession
   c. Periapical pathosis
   d. Bone loss

9. The client's labial mucosa presents with a fibroma. Which of the following statements regarding fibromas is TRUE?
   a. It is the least common of oral fibrous benign neoplasms
   b. It is a reactive fibrous hyperplasia caused by trauma or local irritation
   c. It is a round-to-ovoid, symptomatic, smooth-surfaced, and firm—sessile, or pedunculated mass
   d. Its diameter ranges from 1 mm to 2 cm

10. On the lingual roots of tooth #23 and tooth #24, a gingival cleft is present, and the marginal alveolar bone is denuded, forming a defect extending apical to the normal level and exposing an abnormal amount of root surface. This is characteristic of:
    a. Fenestration
    b. Dehiscence
    c. Aggressive periodontitis
    d. Necrotizing ulcerative gingivitis (NUG)

11. While performing periodontal debridement of tooth #5, the instrument breaks. All of the following are appropriate actions EXCEPT one. Which one is this EXCEPTION?
    a. Isolating the area with gauze or cotton roll
    b. Drying the area using the air–water syringe
    c. Taking a periapical radiograph of the area
    d. Using another instrument to examine the sulcus

12. The client's mucogingival junction is located 3 mm from the gingival margin on the facial surface of tooth #22. On the basis of the pocket measurement on this surface, what is the amount of attached gingiva at the facial surface of tooth #22?
    a. 0 mm
    b. 1 mm
    c. 2 mm
    d. 3 mm

13. The carious lesion needing the MOST immediate attention is seen on:
    a. Tooth #2
    b. Tooth #14
    c. Tooth #20
    d. Tooth #30

14. To reduce the amount of radiation exposure for this client when taking the full mouth series of radiographs, it is BEST that the dental hygienist use:
    a. A radiation monitoring device
    b. Rectangular collimation
    c. Film holders
    d. Slow-speed film

15. When the client returns for evaluation following his periodontal debridement, gingival bleeding and edema on the mesial and distal of tooth #13 are noticed. Which of the following is the treatment of choice?
    a. Probing the periodontal sulcus
    b. No treatment
    c. Removing residual calculus
    d. Taking a periapical radiograph

CASE G

SYNOPSIS
OF PATIENT
HISTORY

Age _____9_____
Sex _____M_____
Height ___4' 5"___

VITAL SIGNS
Blood pressure ___100/60 mmHg___
Pulse rate _____80 bpm_____
Respiration rate _____20 rpm_____

CASE ___G___
pediatric

Weight ___77___ lbs
       ___35___ kgs

1. Under Care of Physician
   Yes   No
   ☐   ☒   Condition: _____

2. Hospitalized within the last 5 years
   Yes   No
   ☐   ☒   Reason: _____

3. Has or had the following conditions
   None _____
   _____

4. Current medications
   None _____
   _____

5. Smokes or uses tobacco products
   Yes   No
   ☒   ☒

6. Is pregnant
   Yes   No   N/A
   ☐   ☐   ☒

MEDICAL HISTORY:
Healthy child. Came with his mother to see the condition of the metal crown.

DENTAL HISTORY:
He fell when he was 10 months old. It affected his permanant teeth buds.
Sealants
Localized area of gingivitis

SOCIAL HISTORY:
He lives with his parents in southern Texas. He is in grade 6 and he likes to play the piano and video games.

CHIEF COMPLAINT:
" uncomfortable in the lower left side of my mouth"

Adult clinical examination

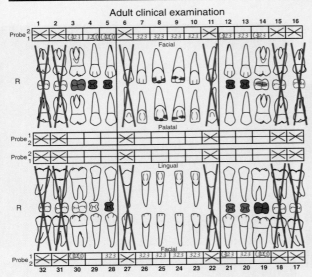

Case G
Pediatric

CURRENT ORAL HYGIENE STATUS:

1. *Pt brushes once every morning and sometime at night*
2. *Plaque index reading was 2*

SUPPLEMENTAL ORAL EXAMINATION FINDINGS:

1. *Fissure sealant placed in teeth # 3, 14, 19, 30*
2. *Stainless steel crown on tooth # T area of tooth 29*
3. *8 and 9 were chipped and replaced with composite*

 Restoration

 Cavity

Sealant

Clinically missing tooth

Furcation

"Through and through" furcation

Probe 1 : initial probing depth

Probe 2 : probing depth 1 month after
          scaling and root planing

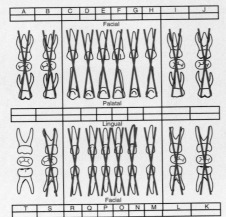

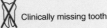

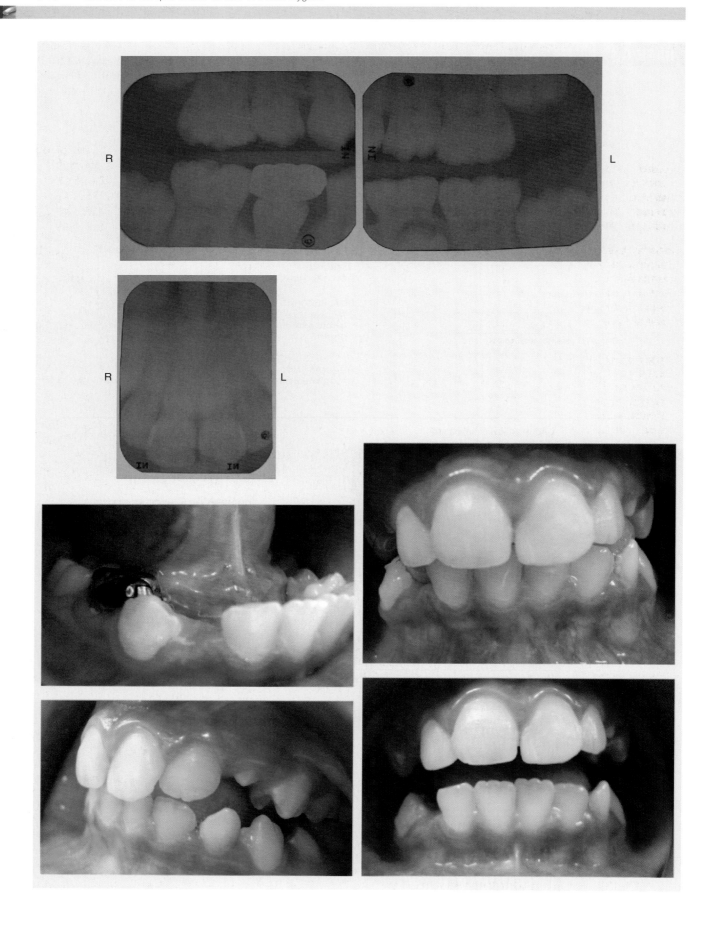

1. **Which of the following BEST describes this client's vital signs?**
   a. Blood pressure rate is considered high
   b. Blood pressure rate is considered low
   c. Respiration rate is considered high
   d. Pulse rate is considered high
   e. Vital sign are within normal limits

2. **Which of the following BEST describes the gingival margin on the facial area of tooth #28?**
   a. Stippled
   b. Blunted
   c. Inflamed
   d. Edematous

3. **The total number of tooth buds that fuse together to form anterior permanent teeth are:**
   a. 2
   b. 3
   c. 4
   d. 5

4. **During the assessment phase of care, the dental hygienist determined that some of the client's premolar teeth are indicated for pit-and-fissure sealants. What percentage of phosphoric acid is contained in the acid-conditioning agent used during the sealant placement?**
   a. 5% to 10%
   b. 15% to 50%
   c. 60% to 80%
   d. 90% to 120%

5. **Which of the following is NOT an indicator for pit-and-fissure sealant application?**
   a. Occlusal contour of tooth
   b. Eruption status of tooth
   c. Frequency of recare or recall appointments or continued care appointments
   d. Presence of a carious lesion on the proximal surface

6. **When examining this client's teeth, the dental hygienist notices that the dental sealant on tooth #14 is partially missing. Which of the following should be undertaken?**
   a. No treatment at this time
   b. Re-etching tooth surface and reapplying the dental sealant
   c. Removing the remainder of the dental sealant and replacing it
   d. Replacing the dental sealant with a restorative material

7. **As the dental hygienist replaces the dental sealant on tooth #14, the sealant dislodges from the tooth when the client is rinsing. Which of the following factors is MOST likely the cause of the failure of sealant placement?**
   a. Moisture contamination
   b. Dated etching solution
   c. Insufficient rinsing time
   d. Omission of a post-application fluoride treatment

8. **The light appearance of this client's dental radiograph is caused by:**
   a. Accidental exposure to white light
   b. Concentrated developer solution
   c. Developer solution being too hot
   d. Inadequate development time

9. **Which primary tooth is in the process of root resorption?**
   a. K
   b. L
   c. S
   d. T

10. **According to the radiographs, which teeth are expected to exfoliate soon?**
    a. Mandibular primary first molars
    b. Maxillary lateral incisors
    c. Mandibular primary second molars
    d. Mandibular second premolars

11. **The client's mother reports that they live in the city and that the community water supply is fluoridated. What is the optimal amount of fluoride appropriate for the city water supply?**
    a. 0.7 parts per million (ppm)
    b. 1.0 ppm
    c. 1.6 ppm
    d. 2.0 ppm

12. **The root of tooth #O appears blunted. Which of the following BEST describes the cause of this blunted root?**
    a. Improper film placement
    b. Pathologic bone lesion
    c. Root fracture
    d. Physiologic root resorption

13. **Which of the following is the MOST appropriate dental caries index to use with this client?**
    a. DMFT/deft
    b. OHI-S
    c. GI
    d. PDI

14. The dental hygienist has been asked to take alginate impressions on the client and the client says
that he is concerned about gagging. Which of the
following will help reduce the client's gagging
sensation?
   a. Asking the client to rinse with an antimicrobial
      rinse
   b. Asking the client to concentrate on breathing
      through his nose
   c. Spraying the client's throat with a topical
      anesthetic
   d. Placing the client in the Trendelenburg position

15. The father of this client asks what the dental office
personnel do to ensure that his son does not contract a disease from other clients. Which of the
following explains the concept of "standard
precautions"?
   a. Precautions are taken when treating a specific
      client
   b. Precautions are taken on the assumption that all
      blood and other bodily fluids of clients are
      infectious
   c. Precautions are taken when treating clients who
      are infected by human immunodeficiency virus
      (HIV)
   d. Precautions that are used in all parts of the
      country are taken

CASE H

SYNOPSIS
OF PATIENT
HISTORY

Age _37_
Sex _M_
Height _5' 5"_

VITAL SIGNS
Blood pressure _140/90 mmHg_
Pulse rate _74 bpm_
Respiration rate _14 rpm_

CASE _H_
Periodontitis

Weight _168_ lbs
_76_ kgs

1. Under Care of Physician
   Yes   No
   ☒   ☐   Condition: _____
2. Hospitalized within the last 5 years
   Yes   No
   ☐   ☒   Reason: _____
3. Has or had the following conditions

   Hypertension

   Back pain
4. Current medications

   Diovin HCT (Valsartan

   Hydrochlorothiazide) 12.5 mg

   Propranolol (Inderal) 10 mg
5. Smokes or uses tobacco products
   Yes   No
   ☒   ☐
6. Is pregnant
   Yes   No   N/A
   ☐   ☐   ☒

MEDICAL HISTORY:
Client has a history of back pain and hypertension. Taking medication.

DENTAL HISTORY:
Client's oral hygiene is poor. He brushes his teeth once per day. Localized areas of suppuration and bone loss.

SOCIAL HISTORY:
Client is married and has 2 children. He does not have any health or dental insurance. He thinks his deteriorating oral condition is due to stress.

CHIEF COMPLAINT:
"It is time to have my teeth cleaned and take care of them"

Adult clinical examination

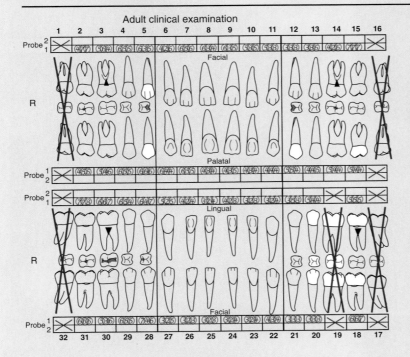

Case H
Periodontitis

CURRENT ORAL HYGIENE STATUS:
1. _Patient brushes one time a day and sometime he forget to brush._
2. _Never use dental floss_
3. _Bleeds easily when brush._

SUPPLEMENTAL ORAL EXAMINATION FINDINGS:
1. _Tooth decay_
2. _Localized areas of wear facets_
3. _Attrition_
4. _Unerupted teeth 17 and 32_
5. _Crowding in # 7 and 8_
6. _1 and 16 are congenitally missing_

 Restoration

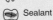 Cavity

Sealant

Clinically missing tooth

△ Furcation

▲ "Through and through" furcation

Probe 1 : initial probing depth
Probe 2 : probing depth 1 month after scaling and root planing

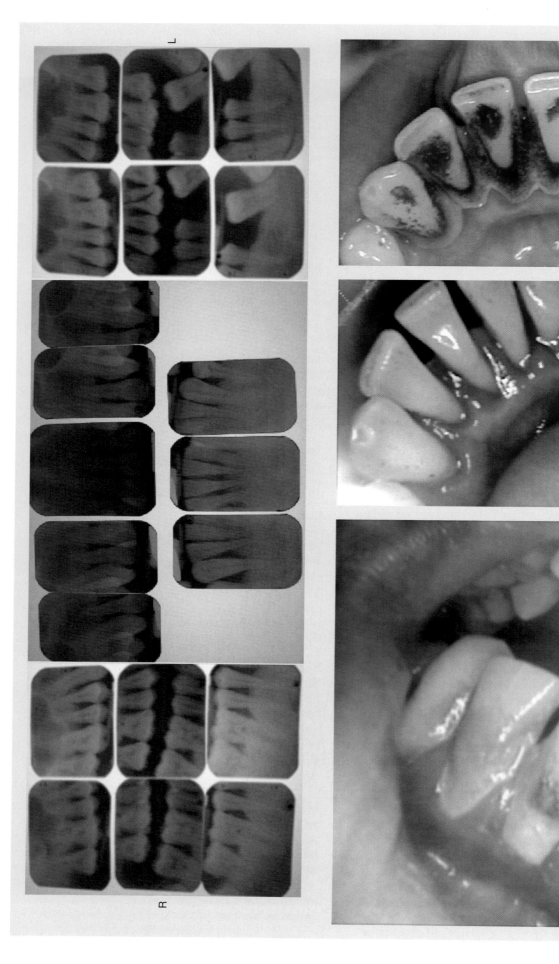

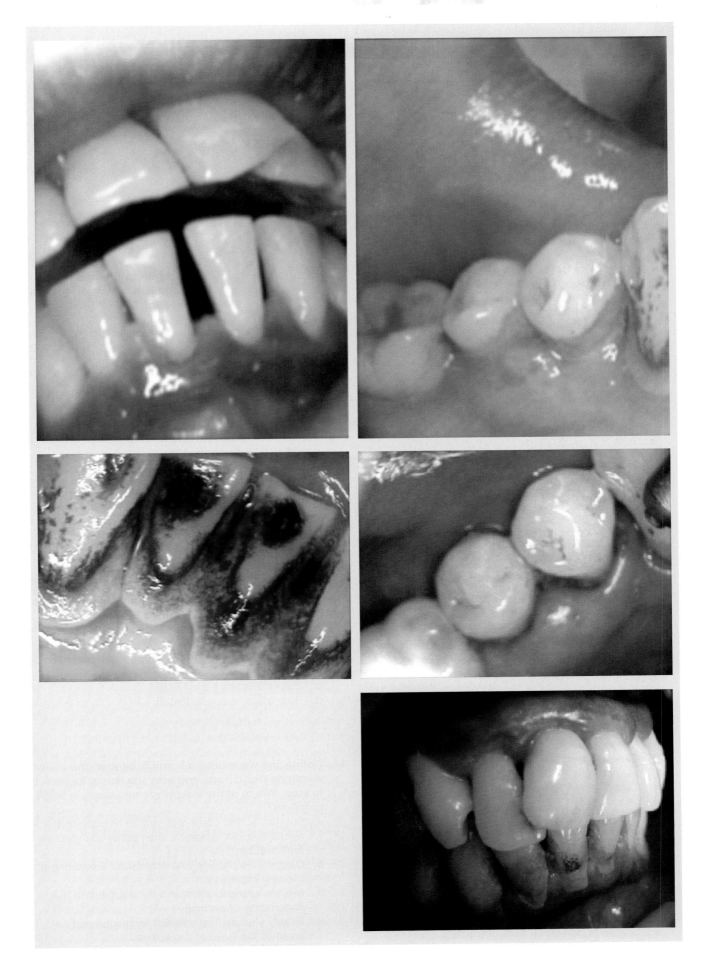

1. All of the following are risk factors for this client's high blood pressure EXCEPT for one. Which one is the EXCEPTION?
   a. Smoking
   b. Stress
   c. Age
   d. Poor oral home care

2. All of the following are true in regards to this client's antihypertensive medication EXCEPT one. Which one is the EXCEPTION?
   a. The majority of hypertensive patients take two types of medications
   b. Beta-blockers are not effective in treating hypertension
   c. Diovin HCT acts as a diuretic and allows blood to flow more easily through the vessels.
   d. In addition to hypertension, propolonol is also used to treat migraines and anxiety

3. According to the American Society of Anesthesiologists classification, this client's physical status can be classified as:
   a. ASA I
   b. ASA II
   c. ASA III
   d. ASA IV
   e. ASA V

4. Which of the following probes is BEST for assessing furcation involvement?
   a. Williams probe
   b. Nabers probe
   c. Marquis probe
   d. Michigan-O probe

5. According to the American Association of Periodontology, this client's periodontal classification is:
   a. Case Type I: Gingivitis
   b. Case Type II: Slight chronic periodontitis
   c. Case Type III: Moderate chronic or aggressive periodontitis
   d. Case Type IV: Advanced chronic or aggressive periodontitis
   e. Case Type V: Refractory, chronic, or aggressive periodontitis

6. The mandibular right first molar exhibits a furcation involvement MOST appropriately classified as?
   a. Class I
   b. Class II
   c. Class III
   d. Class IV
   e. Unable to determine from client data

7. This client has Class II mobility on teeth #6 and #7. Which of the following BEST describes this classification of tooth mobility?
   a. Barely discernible movement
   b. Tooth can be moved up to 1 mm in any direction
   c. Tooth can be moved >1 mm in any direction but is not depressible in socket
   d. Tooth can be moved in a buccolingual direction and is depressible in socket

8. Each of the following factors contributes to difficulty in debriding the mandibular anterior sextant EXCEPT one. Which one is the EXCEPTION?
   a. Sensitivity of the client
   b. Large deposits of supra and subgingival calculus
   c. Mobility of teeth
   d. Rolled gingival margin

9. The dark lines evident on the left premolar bitewing are MOST likely caused by
   a. Bent or creased film
   b. Static electricity
   c. Film overlap during developing
   d. Fingernail use

10. Tobacco use is not considered a strong environmental risk factor for chronic periodontitis. However, it has been found that smoking does impair revascularization during healing.
    a. First statement is TRUE, and second statement is FALSE
    b. First statement is FALSE, and second statement is TRUE.
    c. Both statements are TRUE
    d. Both statements are FALSE

11. During the measuring of probe depths, the client mentions that it hurts and asks the dental hygienist to stop. Which of the following procedures is BEST to follow?
    a. Suggest to the client that you administer local anesthesia per quadrant, then probe and debride that quadrant
    b. Discontinue probing and reconsider measuring at the next recare visit
    c. Ask the client to withstand the pain due to the importance of probing
    d. Modify your instrumentation technique and not insert to the base of the sulcus

12. Anesthetic agents that contain vasopressors are **CONTRAINDICATED** in clients with a history of hypertension because vasopressors increase the risk of cerebrovascular accident, myocardial infarction, and congestive heart failure.
    a. Both the statement and the reason are correct and related
    b. Both the statement and the reason are correct and not related
    c. The statement is correct but the reason is not correct
    d. Neither the statement nor the reason is correct

13. The amide type of local anesthetic agent includes all of the following **EXCEPT** one. Which one is the **EXCEPTION?**
    a. Lidocaine
    b. Prilocaine
    c. Procaine
    d. Mepivacaine

14. Bone loss evident on the radiographs on the mesial of tooth #30 is indicative of what type of pocket?
    a. Suprabony pocket
    b. Subbony pocket
    c. Infrabony pocket
    d. Interbony pocket

15. All of the following are true regarding the stain present on the lingual surfaces of the mandibular anterior teeth **EXCEPT** one. Which one is the **EXCEPTION?**
    a. Brown stain is extrinsic to the tooth
    b. Coloration is due to blood pigments from the diseased pocket tissues
    c. Smoking is a contributing factor
    d. Extrinsic stain removal can occur with debridement of supragingival calculus

CASE I

SYNOPSIS	Age	43	VITAL SIGNS	
OF PATIENT	Sex	M	Blood pressure	116/78 mmHg
HISTORY	Height	5'10"	Pulse rate	64 bpm
			Respiration rate	14 rpm

CASE _I_ / _Medically complex_   Weight   220 lbs   100 kgs

1. Under Care of Physician
   Yes No
   ☒ ☐   Condition: _Heart disease_
2. Hospitalized within the last 5 years
   Yes No
   ☒ ☐   Reason: _Stent implants_
3. Has or had the following conditions
   Fainting spells, dizziness;

   heart attack, high blood pressure
4. Current medications
   Lopresor (metoprolol) 50 mg

   Plavix (clopidogrel bisulfate) 75 mg

   asprin - 2 tablets per day

   Troprol XL (simvastatin) 40 mg
5. Smokes or uses tobacco products
   Yes No
   ☐ ☒

6. Is pregnant
   Yes No N/A
   ☐ ☐ ☒

MEDICAL HISTORY:
Patient has a history of heart attack 2 years ago.

DENTAL HISTORY:
Patient brushes daily 2 times a day. He is a regular patient in the dental clinic and take good care of his oral hygiene.

SOCIAL HISTORY:
He is married with 2 kids. Own his own business.

CHIEF COMPLAINT:
"Time to check my teeth"

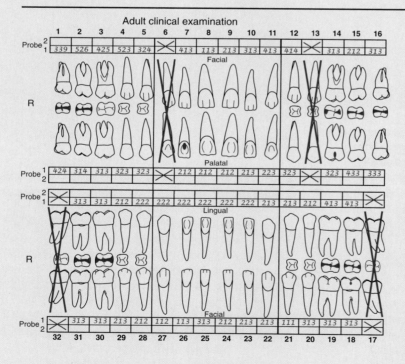

Adult clinical examination

Case I
Medically complex

CURRENT ORAL HYGIENE STATUS:
1. Minimal plaque biofilm
2. Brushes twice a day

SUPPLEMENTAL ORAL EXAMINATION FINDINGS:
1. Multiple amalgam fillings
2. Anterior composite filling
3. Missing tooth #6, 13, 17, and 32
4. Multiple areas of wear facet
5. Multiple areas of attrition
6. Deep groove, staining.

 Restoration

Cavity

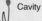 Sealant

Clinically missing tooth

 Furcation

"Through and through" furcation

Probe 1 : initial probing depth

Probe 2 : probing depth 1 month after scaling and root planing

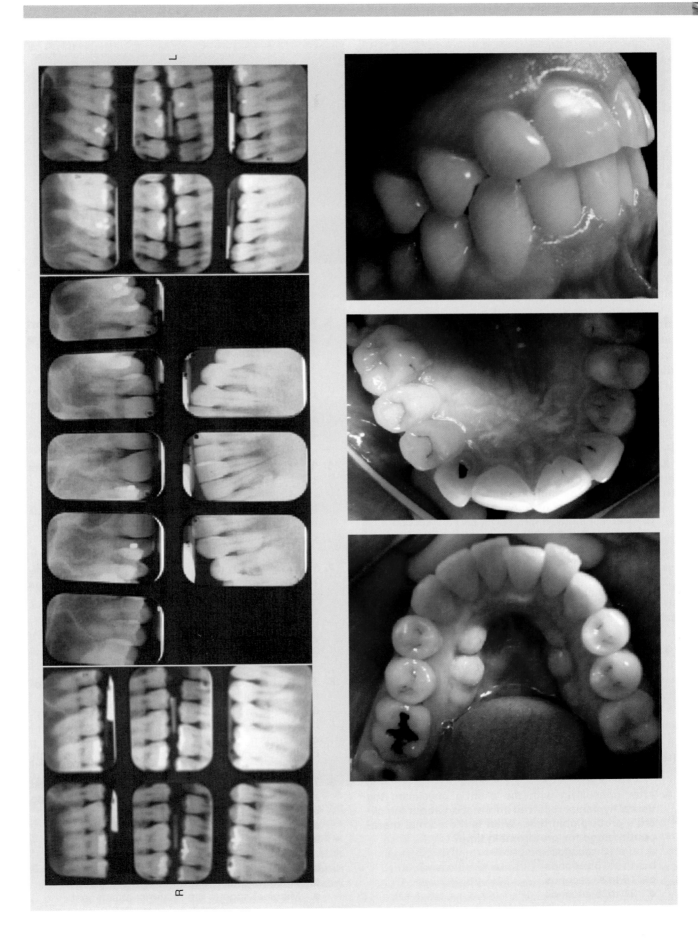

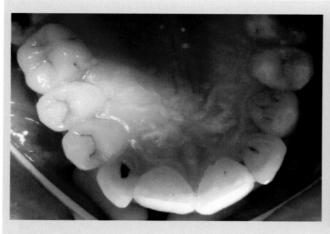 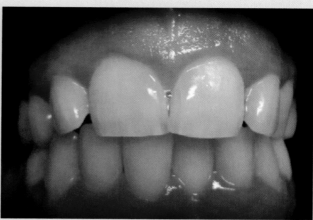

1. **Which of the following medications prescribed to this client is BEST used to reduce the rate of atherothrombosis?**
   a. Metoprolol
   b. Plavix
   c. Aspirin
   d. Simvastatin

2. **Simvastatin, a lipid lowering drug, belongs to the class of pharmaceuticals called statins. The client should avoid grapefruit when taking simvastatitin due to the risk of toxicity.**
   a. The first statement is TRUE, and the second statement is FALSE
   b. The first statement is FALSE, and the second statement is TRUE
   c. Both statements are TRUE
   d. Both statements are FALSE

3. **What is the first action the dental hygienist should take if this client describes that he has chest pain and labored breathing?**
   a. Reassure the client
   b. Administer oxygen
   c. Call for urgent medical assistance
   d. Place client in upright position

4. **After consulting with the client's physician; the dental hygienist received information about the client's prothrombin time. What is the normal therapeutic range for prothrombin time?**
   a. 5 to10 seconds
   b. 11 to15 seconds
   c. 16 to20 seconds
   d. 21 to25 seconds

5. **All of the following are true regarding heart stent implants EXCEPT one. Which one is the EXCEPTION?**
   a. Stents are removed approximately 4 weeks after surgery
   b. Stents are referred to as balloon angioplasty
   c. Stents are indicated for narrow or blocked arteries
   d. Stents cause impaired arteries

6. **The pathological lesion evident between the roots of tooth #8 and tooth #9 is referred to as a**
   a. Globulomaxillary cyst
   b. Median palatine cyst
   c. Nasopalatine cyst
   d. Nasolabial cyst

7. **Which of the following BEST describes the radiopaque areas superimposed on the root surfaces of teeth #20, #21, #22, #27, #28, and #29?**
   a. Supernumerary tooth
   b. Compound odontoma
   c. Radicular cyst
   d. Mandibular tori

8. **The technique error in the mandibular right premolar periapical radiograph can be corrected by**
   a. Decreasing milliamperage setting
   b. Decreasing exposure time
   c. Increasing the KVP setting
   d. Increasing the distance between the PID and tooth

9. **The client has 5 mm pockets on teeth #2, #3, and #4. Which of the following BEST describes how the measurement is determined?**
   a. Alveolar crest to the gingival margin
   b. Cementoenamel junction to the epithelial attachment
   c. Cementoenamel junction to the gingival margin
   d. Epithelial attachment to the gingival margin
   e. Marginal ridge to the epithelial attachment

10. According to G.V Black's classification of caries and restorations, which of the following describes the restoration on tooth #7?
    a. Class I
    b. Class II
    c. Class III
    d. Class IV
    e. Class V
    f. Class VI

11. The fold of tissue that attaches the lip to the oral mucosa below the mandibular central incisors is the:
    a. Lingual frenum
    b. Labial frenum
    c. Incisive papilla
    d. Mucobuccal fold

12. The gingival tissue around the facial of tooth #7 is erythematous and bleeds easily on probing. The client reports that the area has been very tender the past couple of days. Which of the following BEST describes what is happening in this area?
    a. Acute gingivitis
    b. Chronic gingivitis
    c. Acute periodontitis
    d. Chronic periodontitis

13. During the dental charting of this client, you notice a generalized characteristic on the majority of the teeth. What is this generalized observation?
    a. Reddened incisive papilla
    b. Carious lesions on posterior teeth
    c. Staining on the pits and fissures
    d. Dental fluorosis

14. This client has slight gingivitis on the maxillary posterior sextant. How is this condition demonstrated in the radiographic findings?
    a. Change in bone trabeculation
    b. Increase in bone density
    c. Horizontal bone loss
    d. Normal bone pattern

15. During the intraoral assessment, the dental hygienist observes that this client does not have a midline shift although he is missing tooth #6. What is the rationale for the normal alignment of the anterior teeth?
    a. It is documented that he received orthodontic treatment
    b. Bonding of the maxillary central incisors corrected the alignment
    c. Balance of the arch was possible due to missing tooth #13
    d. The midline shift is misaligned

CASE J

SYNOPSIS
OF PATIENT
HISTORY

Age _47_
Sex _F_
Height _5'11"_

VITAL SIGNS
Blood pressure _128/74 mmHg_
Pulse rate _82 bpm_
Respiration rate _16 rpm_

CASE _J_
Medically complex

Weight _260_ lbs
_118_ kgs

1. Under Care of Physician
   Yes   No   _Chronic bronchitis_
   ☒   ☐   Condition: _Diabetes type 1_
2. Hospitalized within the last 5 years
   Yes   No
   ☒   ☐   Reason: _Copious sputum_
3. Has or had the following conditions

   coughing slightly with

   expectoration
4. Current medications

   Inhaled corticosteroid Vanceril,

   Fluticasone and Salmeterol

5. Smokes or uses tobacco products
   Yes   No
   ☐   ☒
6. Is pregnant
   Yes   No   N/A
   ☐   ☐   ☒

MEDICAL HISTORY:
Patient was hospitalized 5 years ago for having
Copious Sputum. She showed a lot of improvement
after quitting smoking for the last 6 years. Has
diabetes mellitus type 1

DENTAL HISTORY:
Has a root canal filling in tooth #8 and
multiple amalgam filling. Localized area
of teeth sensitivity.

SOCIAL HISTORY:
She is a single mother of one son. She own
a store and works full time.

CHIEF COMPLAINT:
"Need oral health improvement"

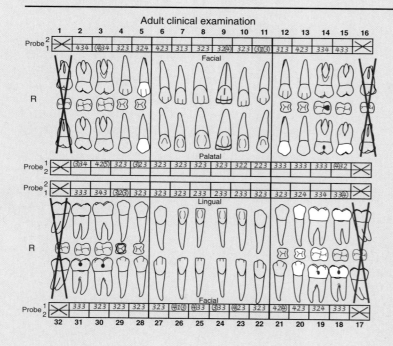

Adult clinical examination

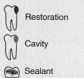

Case J
Medically complex

CURRENT ORAL HYGIENE STATUS:
1. _Minimal plaque control_
2. _Localized area of bleeding_
   while brushing

SUPPLEMENTAL ORAL EXAMINATION FINDINGS:
1. _Composite filling in teeth 9 and 29_
2. _Multiple amalgam filling in teeth_
   14, 18, 19, 30 and 31
3. _Root canal in tooth #9_
4. _Missing teeth 1, 16, 17 and 32_

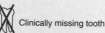

Restoration

Cavity

Sealant

Clinically missing tooth

Furcation

"Through and through" furcation

Probe 1 : initial probing depth

Probe 2 : probing depth 1 month after
         scaling and root planing

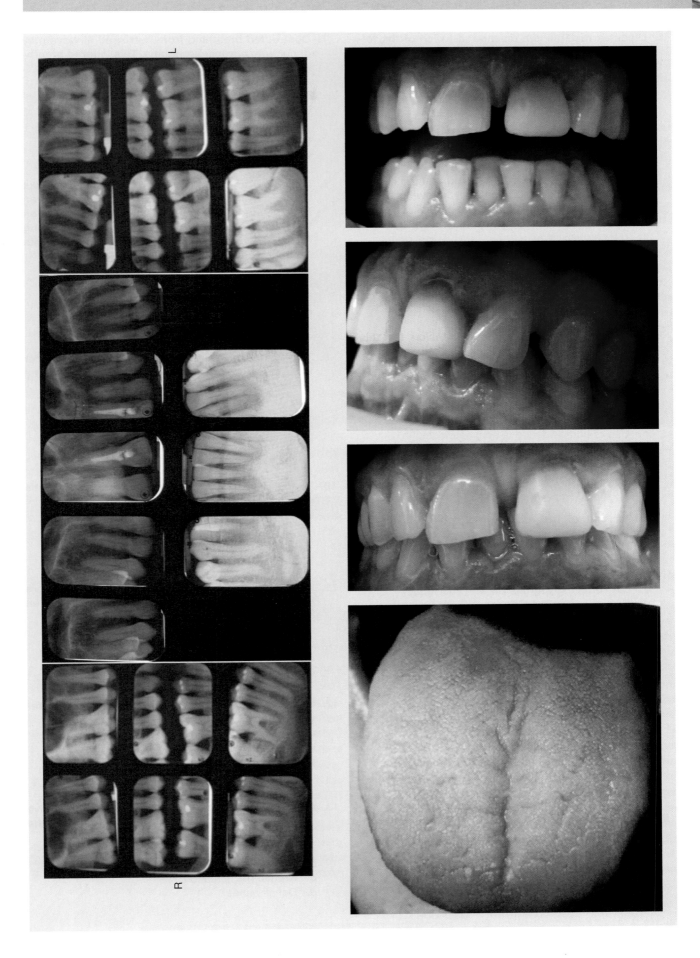

1. Diabetes mellitus is a disease of which of the following organs?
   a. Intestines
   b. Kidneys
   c. Liver
   d. Pancreas

2. In the assessment phase of the process of care, the client reports that she had a fasting plasma glucose test two weeks earlier, and that the results were 120 mg/dl. Which of the following BEST describes the interpretation of this test?
   a. Blood glucose level is below normal and dangerously low
   b. Blood glucose level is normal and well controlled
   c. Blood glucose level is moderately controlled
   d. Blood glucose level is uncontrolled

3. When planning an educational session for this client, which of the following concepts should be included?
   a. Insulin requirements may decrease in the presence of infection
   b. Individuals with type 1 diabetes have a higher risk for coronal caries
   c. Use of home fluoride is contraindicated in individuals who have type 1 diabetes
   d. The presence of infection may make diabetes more difficult to regulate

4. Which one of the following questions is MOST important to ask a client with type 1 diabetes?
   a. Did you take your medications and eat today?
   b. Which of your relatives have had diabetes and what type?
   c. Did you bring your insulin with you today?
   d. Do you have a burning sensation in your mouth or a dry mouth?

5. Which one of the following statements succinctly describes the reason diabetes mellitus is important in the pathogenesis of periodontal disease?
   a. Diabetes has a direct effect on pocket depth
   b. Diabetes can be the direct cause of periodontal disease
   c. Diabetes determines the pattern of bone loss
   d. Diabetes can increase the host's proinflamatory cytokines

6. Gas exchange during respiration takes place in the:
   a. Pleura
   b. Inferior lobe of the lung
   c. Bronchus
   d. Alveoli

7. Obstructed breathing from narrowed airways may occur with chronic bronchitis. This labored breathing is referred to as tachypnea.
   a. The first statement is TRUE, and the second statement is FALSE
   b. The first statement is FALSE, and the second statement is TRUE
   c. Both statements are TRUE
   d. Both statements are FALSE

8. It is important to teach this client about the risks involved with smoking and chronic bronchitis, even if it is second hand or third hand smoking. Although this client does not smoke, all of the following EXCEPT one may develop in chronic smokers with COPD. Which one is the EXCEPTION?
   a. Halitosis
   b. Nicotine stomatitis
   c. Intrinsic tooth stains
   d. Oral cancer
   e. Periodontal disease

9. The fluticasone/salmeterol inhaler is prescribed for this client to enhance which one of the following effects?
   a. Anti-inflammatory
   b. Anti-pyretic
   c. Bronchodilation
   d. Anti-inflammatory and anti-pyretic
   e. Anti-inflammatory and bronchodilation

10. The BEST reason for the presence of this client's maxillary diastema is
    a. periodontal pockets
    b. labial frenum
    c. endodontic treatment
    d. occlusal overbite

11. Some of the radiographic films on this client are light in density. How could this have been prevented?
    a. Increase the temperature of the developer
    b. Increase the exposure time
    c. Decrease milliamperage
    d. Decrease the temperature of the fixer

12. Which of the following developer components prevents rapid oxidation of the developing agents?
    a. Accelerator
    b. Preservative
    c. Developing agent
    d. Restrainer

13. A dark discoloration on the facial marginal gingiva of #9 is MOST likely due to which of the following?
    a. Non vital tooth
    b. Subgingival calculus
    c. Normal pigmentation
    d. Dental caries

14. The radiopaque areas on the mesial surface of tooth #18, and the distal surface of tooth #19 are the result of which of the following?
    a. Dental caries
    b. Amalgam particles
    c. Calculus
    d. Enamel pearls

15. During the intraoral inspection of the tongue, the dental hygienist noted which of the following conditions?
    a. Atrophic glossitis
    b. Fissured tongue
    c. Candidiasis
    d. Elongated papillae
    e. Benign migratory glossitis

APPENDIX
A Medical Terminology

PREFIXES

a-, ab-, abs- From; away; departing from normal
ad- Addition to; toward; nearness
amb-, ambi- Both; ambidextrous, having the ability to work effectively with either hand
amphi- On both sides
ampho- Both
an- Negative; without or not
ana- Upper, away from
andro- Signifying man
ant-, anti- Against
ante-, antero- Front; before
bili- Pertaining to bile
brady- Slow
brom-, bromo- A stench
broncho- Pertaining to the bronchi
cac- Bad
cardi-, cardio- Pertaining to the heart
cata- Down or downward
cervico- Pertaining to the neck
circa- About
circum- Around
co- With or together
con- Together with
contra- Opposite; against
demi- Half
di- Twice
dia- Through
dialy- To separate
en- In
end-, endo-, ento- Inward; within
ep-, epi- On; in addition to
ex- Out; away from
exo- Without, outside of
extra- Outside of; in addition to
fibro- Pertaining to fibers
gaster-, gastr-, gastro- Pertaining to the stomach
hemi- Half

hemo- Pertaining to the blood
hepat-, hepatico-, hepato- Pertaining to the liver
heter-, hetero- Denoting other; relationship to another
homeo- Denoting likeness or resemblance
homo- Denoting sameness
hyal-, hyalo- Transparent
hyper- Above; excessive; beyond
hypo- Below; less than
ideo- Pertaining to mental images
idio- Denoting relationship to one's self or to something separate and distinct
in- Not; in; inside; within; also intensive action
infra- Below
inter- In the midst; between
intra- Within
intro- In or into
iso- Equal or alike
juxta- Of close proximity
karyo- Pertaining to a cell's nucleus
kypho- Humped
laryngo- Pertaining to the larynx
medi- Middle
myelo- Pertaining to the spinal cord or bone marrow
omni- All
ovari-, ovario- Pertaining to the ovary
per- Through; by means of
peri- Around; about
post- Behind or after
postero- Pertaining to the posterior
pre- Before
pro- Before, in front of
pseudo- False
re- Back; again (contrary)
retro- Backward
semi- Half
steato- Fatty
sub- Under; near

syn- Joined together
trans- Across; over
un- Not; reversal

SUFFIXES

-able, -ible, -ble The power to be
-ad Toward; in the direction of
-aemia, -emia Pertaining to blood
-age Put in motion; to do
-agra Denoting a seizure; severe pain
-algia Denoting pain
-ase Forms the name of an enzyme
-blast Designates a cell or a structure
-cele Denoting a swelling
-centesis Denoting a puncture
-ectomy A cutting out
-esthesia Denoting sensation
-facient That which makes or causes
-gene, -genesis, -genetic, -genic Denoting production; origin
-gog, -gogue To make flow
-gram A tracing; a mark
-graph A writing; a record
-iasis Denoting a condition or pathologic state
-id Denoting shape or resemblance
-ite Of the nature of
-itis Denoting inflammation
-logia Denoting discourse, science, or study of
-oid Denoting form or resemblance
-oma Denoting a tumor
-osis Denoting a morbid process
-ostomosis, -ostomy, -stomy Denoting an outlet; to furnish with an opening or mouth
-plasty Denoting molding or shaping
-rrhagia Denoting a discharge; usually bleeding
-rhaphy Denoting suturing or stitching
-rhea Denoting a flow or discharge
-scope, -scopy Generally an instrument for viewing
-tomy Denoting a cutting operation
-trophy Denoting a relationship to nourishment

COMBINING FORMS

aer-, aero- Denoting air or gas
alge-, algesi-, algo- Pertaining to pain
allo- Other; differing from the normal
anomalo- Denoting irregularity
arthro- Pertaining to a joint or joints
brevi- Short
celio- Denoting the abdomen
centro- Center
cheil-, cheilo- Denoting the lip

chol-, chole-, cholo- Pertaining to bile
chondr-, chondri- Pertaining to cartilage
chrom, chromo Pertaining to color
cole-, coleo- Denoting a sheath
colp-, colpo- Pertaining to the vagina
cranio- Pertaining to the cranium of the skull
crymo-, cryo- Denoting cold
crypt- To hide; a pit
cyano- Dark blue
cyclo- Pertaining to a cycle
cysto- Pertaining to a sac or cyst
cyto- Denoting a cell
dacryo- Pertaining to the lacrimal glands
dactylo- Pertaining to digits
dent-, dento- Pertaining to teeth
derma-, dermat- Pertaining to skin
desmo- Pertaining to a bond or ligament
dextro- Right
diplo- Double; twofold
dorsi-, dorso- Pertaining to the back
duodeno- Pertaining to the duodenum
electro- Pertaining to electricity
encephalo- Denoting the brain
entero- Pertaining to the intestines
episio- Pertaining to the vulva
eso- Inward
esthesio- Pertaining to feeling or sensation
facio- Pertaining to the face
gangli-, ganglio- Pertaining to a ganglion
geno- Pertaining to reproduction
gero-, geronto- Denoting old age
giganto- Huge
gingivo- Pertaining to the gingiva or gum
gloss-, glosso- Pertaining to the tongue
gluco- Denoting sweetness
glyco- Pertaining to sugar
gnath-, gnatho- Denoting the jaw
gon- Denoting a seed
grapho- Denoting writing
hapt-, hapte-, hapto- Pertaining to touch or a seizure
helo- Pertaining to a nail or callus
hist-, histio-, histo- Pertaining to tissue
holo- Pertaining to the whole
hydr-, hydro- Denoting water
hygro- Denoting moisture
hyl-, hyle-, hylo- Denoting matter or material
ileo-, ilio- Pertaining to the ileum
ipsi- Denoting self
irido- Pertaining to a colored circle
iso- Equal
jejuno- Pertaining to the jejunum
kerato- Pertaining to the cornea
kino- Denoting movement
labio- Pertaining to the lips
lacto- Pertaining to milk

laparo- Pertaining to the loin or flank
latero- Pertaining to the side
leido-, leio- Smooth
leuk-, leuko- Denoting deficiency of color
lip-, lipo- Pertaining to fat
litho- Denoting a calculus
macr-, macro- Large; long
mast-, masto- Pertaining to the breast
meg-, mega- Great; large
meli- Sweet
meningo- Denoting membranes; covering the brain and the spinal cord
micr-, micro- Small in size or extent
mono- One
morpho- Pertaining to form
multi- Many
my-, myo- Pertaining to muscle
myc-, mycet- Denoting a fungus
myringo- Denoting tympani or the eardrum
myx-, myxo- Pertaining to mucus
narco- Denoting stupor
naso- Pertaining to the nose
necro- Denoting death
neo- New
nephr-, nephro- Denoting the kidney
normo- Normal or usual
oculo- Denoting the eye
odyno- Denoting pain
oleo- Denoting oil
onco- Denoting a swelling or mass
onycho- Pertaining to the nails
oo- Denoting an egg
opisth-, opistho- Backward
ophthal-, ophthalmo- Pertaining to the eye
optico- Pertaining to the eye or vision
orchi-, orcho- Pertaining to the testes
oro- Pertaining to the mouth
ortho- Straight; right
oscillo- Denoting oscillation
osteo- Pertaining to the bones
ot-, oto- Denoting an egg
palato- Denoting the palate
patho- Denoting disease
pedia-, pedo- Denoting a child
perineo- Combining form for the region between the anus and the scrotum or vulva
phago- Denoting a relationship to eating
pharyngo- Pertaining to the pharynx
phleb-, phlebo- Denoting the veins
phon-, phono- Denoting sound
phot-, photo- Pertaining to light
phren- Pertaining to the mind
picr-, picro- Bitter
pilo- Denoting hair
plasmo- Pertaining to plasma or the substance of a cell

pneuma-, pneumono-, pneumoto- Denoting air or gas
pod-, podo- Denoting the foot
poly- Many
proct-, procto- Denoting the anus and rectum
psych-, psycho- Pertaining to the mind
ptyalo- Denoting saliva
pubio-, pubo- Denoting the pubic region
pulmo- Denoting the lung
pupillo- Denoting the pupil
pyel-, pyelo- Denoting the pelvis
pyloro- Pertaining to the pylorus
py-, pyo- Denoting pus
recto- Denoting the rectum
rhin-, rhino- Denoting the nose
salpingo- Denoting a tube, specifically the fallopian tube
schizo- Split
sclero- Denoting hardness
scoto- Pertaining to darkness
sero- Pertaining to serum
sialo- Pertaining to saliva or the salivary glands
sidero- Denoting iron
sinistro- Left
somato- Denoting the body
somni- Denoting sleep
spasmo- Denoting a spasm
spermato-, spermo- Denoting sperm
sphero- Denoting a sphere; round
sphygmo- Denoting a pulse
splen-, spleno- Denoting the spleen
staphyl-, staphylo- Resembling a bunch of grapes
steno- Narrow; short
sterco- Denoting feces
steth-, stetho- Pertaining to the chest
stomato- Denoting the mouth
sym-, syn- With; along
tacho-, tachy- Swift
tarso- Pertaining to the flat of the foot
terato- Denoting a marvel, prodigy, or monster
thoraco- Pertaining to the chest
thrombo- Denoting a clot of blood
toxico-, toxo- Denoting poison
tracheo- Denoting the trachea
trichi-, tricho- Denoting hair
ur-, uro-, urono- Pertaining to urine
varico- Denoting a twisting or swelling
vaso- Denoting a vessel
veno- Denoting a vein
ventri-, ventro- Denoting the abdomen
vertebro- Pertaining to the vertebra
vesico- Denoting the bladder
viscero- Denoting the organs of the body
vivi- Denoting alive
xantho- Denoting yellow
xero- Denoting dryness

TERMINOLOGY FREQUENTLY USED TO DESIGNATE BODY PARTS OR ORGANS

anus Anal, ano-
arm Brachial, brachio-
blood Hem-, hemat-
chest Thoracic, thorax
ear Auricle, oto-
eye Ocular, oculo-, ophthalmo-
foot Pedal, ped-, -pod
gallbladder Chole-, chol-
head Cephalic, cephalo-
heart Cardium, cardiac, cardio-
intestines Cecum, colon, duodenum, ileum, jejunum

kidney Renal, nephric, nephro-
lip Cheil-
liver Hepatic, hepato-
lungs Pulmonary, pulmonic, pneumo-
mouth Oral, os, stoma, stomat-
muscle Myo-
neck Cervix, cervical, cervico-
penis Penile
rectum Rectal
skin Derma, integumentum
stomach Gastric, gastro-
testicle Orchio-, orchi-, orchido-
urinary bladder Cysti-, cysto-
uterus Hystero-, metra
vagina Vulvo, vaginal

APPENDIX B Professional Organizations of Interest to Dental Hygienists

Academy of General Dentistry
211 E. Chicago Avenue, Suite 900
Chicago, IL 60611
Phone: (888) 243-3368
Fax: (312) 440-0559
http://www.agd.org

American Academy of Pediatric Dentistry
211 E. Chicago Avenue, Suite 1700
Chicago, IL 60611-2637
Phone: (312) 337-2169
Fax: (312) 337-6329
http://www.aapd.org
aapdweb@aapd.org

American Association for Dental Research
1619 Duke Street
Alexandria, VA 22314-3406
Phone: (703) 548-0066
Fax: (703) 548-1883
http://www.dentalresearch.org
research@iadr.com

American Association of Public Health Dentistry
3085 Stevenson Dr., Suite 200
Springfield, IL 62703
Phone: (217) 529-6941
Fax: (217) 529-9120
http://www.aaphd.org
natoff@aol.com

American Dental Association
211 E. Chicago Avenue
Chicago, IL 60611
Phone: (312) 440-2500
Fax: (312) 440-2800
http://www.ada.org

American Dental Education Association
1400 K Street NW, Suite 1100
Washington, DC 20005
Phone: (202) 289-7201

Fax: (202) 289-7204
http://www.adea.org

American Dental Hygienists' Association
444 N. Michigan Avenue, Suite 3400
Chicago, IL 60611
Phone: (312) 440-8900
http://www.adha.org

American Public Health Association
800 I Street NW
Washington, DC 20001-3710
Phone: (202) 777-APHA
Fax: (202) 777-2534
http://www.apha.org
comments@apha.org

Association of Schools of Allied Health
   Professions
4400 Jenifer St, NW, Suite 333
Washington, DC 20015
Phone: (202) 237-6481
Fax: (202) 237-6485
http://www.asahp.org

Canadian Dental Association
1815 Alta Vista Dr.
Ottawa, Ontario
Canada K1G 3Y6
Phone: (613) 523-1770
Fax: (613) 523-7736
http://www.cda-adc.ca/
reception@cda-adc.ca

Canadian Dental Hygienists' Association
96 Centrepointe Drive
Nepean, Ontario
Canada K2G 6B1
Phone: (613) 224-5515 or (800) 267-5235
Fax: (613) 224-7283
http://www.cdha.ca
info@cdha.ca

Canadian Public Health Association
300-1565 Carling Avenue
Ottawa, Ontario
Canada K1Z 8R1
Phone: (613) 725-3769
Fax: (613) 725-9826
http://www.cpha.ca
info@cpha.ca

Centers for Disease Control and Prevention
1600 Clifton Road NE
Atlanta, GA 30333
Phone: (800) 232-4636 or (888) 232-6348
http://www.cdc.gov
cdcinfo@cdc.gov

Dental Hygiene Research Center
Gene W. Hirschfeld School of Dental Hygiene
Old Dominion University, Health Sciences Bldg
4608 Hampton Blvd
Norfolk, VA 23529-0499
Phone: (757) 683-3338
http://hs.odu.edu/dental/research/welcome.shtml

FDI World Dental Federation
Tour de Cointrin, Avenve Louis Casni 84,
Case Postale 3,
1216 Geneve-Cointrin,
Switzerland
Phone: 41 22 560 81 50
Fax: 41 22 560 81 40
http://www.fdiworldental.org/home/home.html
info@fdiworlddental.org

Hispanic Dental Association
3085 Stevenson Drive, Suite 200
Springfield, IL 62703
Phone: (800) 852-7921 or (217) 529-6517
Fax: (217) 529-9120
http://www.hdassoc.org
hdassoc@aol.com

International Association for Dental Research
1619 Duke Street
Alexandria, VA 22314-3406
Phone: (703) 548-0066
Fax: (703) 548-1883
http://www.iadr.com
research@iadr.com

International Association for Disability and Oral Health
http://www.iadh.org

International Federation of Dental Hygienists
P.O. Box 957
Merlynston
Victoria, Australia 3058
http://www.ifdh.org
admin@ifdh.org

National Center for Dental Hygiene Research
USC School of Dentistry
925 W. 34th Street, Room 4330
Los Angeles, CA 90089-0641
Phone: (213) 740-8669
Fax: (213) 740-1072
http://www.usc.edu/hsc/dental/dhnet/

National Dental Hygienists' Association/National Dental Association
3517 16th Street NW
Washington, DC 20010
Phone: (202) 588-1697
Fax: (202) 588-1244
http://www.ndaonline.org
admin@ndaonline.org

Special Care Dentistry
401 N. Michigan Avenue, Suite 2200
Chicago, IL 60611
Phone: (312) 527-6764
Fax: (312) 673-6663
http://www.scdonline.org
SCD@online.org

World Health Organization
Avenue Appia 20
1211 Geneva 27
Switzerland
Phone: (+41 22) 791 21 11
Fax: (+41 22) 791 31 11
http://www.who.int
info@who.int

APPENDIX C American Dental Hygienists' Association and Canadian Dental Hygienists Association Codes of Ethics

THE AMERICAN DENTAL HYGIENISTS' CODE OF ETHICS*

1. Preamble

As dental hygienists, we are a community of professionals devoted to the prevention of disease and the promotion and improvement of the public's health. We are preventive oral health professionals who provide educational, clinical, and therapeutic services to the public. We strive to live meaningful, productive, satisfying lives that simultaneously serve us, our profession, our society, and the world. Our actions, behaviors, and attitudes are consistent with our commitment to public service. We endorse and incorporate the Code into our daily lives.

2. Purpose

The purpose of a professional code of ethics is to achieve high levels of ethical consciousness, decision making, and practice by the members of the profession. Specific objectives of the Dental Hygiene Code of Ethics are:

- To increase our professional and ethical consciousness and sense of ethical responsibility.
- To lead us to recognize ethical issues and choices and to guide us in making more informed ethical decisions.
- To establish a standard for professional judgment and conduct
- To provide a statement of the ethical behavior the public can expect from us
  The Dental Hygiene Code of Ethics is meant to influence us throughout our careers. It stimulates our

*Reprinted with permission from the American Dental Hygienists' Association homepage (www.adha.com).

continuing study of ethical issues and challenges us to explore our ethical responsibilities. The Code establishes concise standards of behavior to guide the public's expectations of our profession and supports existing dental hygiene practice, laws, and regulations. By holding ourselves accountable to meeting the standards stated in the Code, we enhance the public's trust on which our professional privilege and status are founded.

3. Key Concepts

Our beliefs, principles, values, and ethics are concepts reflected in the Code. They are the essential elements of our comprehensive and definitive code of ethics, and are interrelated and mutually dependent.

4. Basic Beliefs

We recognize the importance of the following beliefs that guide our practice and provide context for our ethics:

- The services we provide contribute to the health and well-being of society.
- Our education and licensure qualify us to serve the public by preventing and treating oral disease and helping individuals achieve and maintain optimal health.
- Individuals have intrinsic worth, are responsible for their own health, and are entitled to make choices regarding their health.
- Dental hygiene care is an essential component of overall healthcare and we function interdependently with other healthcare providers.
- All people should have access to healthcare, including oral healthcare.
- We are individually responsible for our actions and the quality of care we provide.

5. Fundamental Principles

These fundamental principles, universal concepts, and general laws of conduct provide the foundation for our ethics.

Universality

The principle of universality assumes that if one individual judges an action to be right or wrong in a given situation, other people considering the same action in the same situation would make the same judgment.

Complementarity

The principle of complementarity assumes the existence of an obligation to justice and basic human rights. It requires us to act toward others in the same way they would act toward us if roles were reversed. In all relationships, it means considering the values and perspective of others before making decisions or taking actions affecting them.

Ethics

Ethics are the general standards of right and wrong that guide behavior within society. As generally accepted actions, they can be judged by determining the extent to which they promote good and minimize harm. Ethics compel us to engage in health promotion/disease prevention activities.

Community

This principle expresses our concern for the bond between individuals, the community, and society in general. It leads us to preserve natural resources and inspires us to show concern for the global environment.

Responsibility

Responsibility is central to our ethics. We recognize that there are guidelines for making ethical choices and accept responsibility for knowing and applying them. We accept the consequences of our actions or the failure to act and are willing to make ethical choices and publicly affirm them.

6. Core Values

We acknowledge these values as general guides for our choices and actions.

Individual Autonomy and Respect for Human Beings

People have the right to be treated with respect. People have the right to informed consent prior to treatment, and they have the right to full disclosure of all relevant information so that they can make informed choices about their care.

Confidentiality

We respect the confidentiality of client information and relationships as a demonstration of the value we place on individual autonomy. We acknowledge our obligation to justify any violation of a confidence.

Societal Trust

We value client trust and understand that public trust in our profession is based on our actions and behavior.

Nonmaleficence

We accept our fundamental obligation to provide services in a manner that protects all clients and minimizes harm to them and others involved in their treatment.

Beneficence

We have a primary role in promoting the well-being of individuals and the public by engaging in health promotion/disease prevention activities.

Justice and Fairness

We value justice and support the fair and equitable distribution of healthcare resources. We believe all people should have access to high-quality, affordable oral healthcare.

Veracity

We accept our obligation to tell the truth and assume that others will do the same. We value self-knowledge and seek truth and honesty in all relationships.

7. Standards of Professional Responsibility

We are obligated to practice our profession in a manner that supports our purpose, beliefs, and values in accordance with the fundamental principles that support our ethics. We acknowledge the following responsibilities:

To Ourselves as Individuals ...

- Avoid self-deception, and continually strive for knowledge and personal growth.
- Establish and maintain a lifestyle that supports optimal health.
- Create a safe work environment.
- Assert our own interests in ways that are fair and equitable.
- Seek the advice and counsel of others when challenged with ethical dilemmas.
- Have realistic expectations of ourselves and recognize our limitations.

To Ourselves as Professionals ...

- Enhance professional competencies through continuous learning in order to practice according to high standards of care.
- Support dental hygiene peer-review systems and quality-assurance measures.
- Develop collaborative professional relationships and exchange knowledge to enhance our own life-long professional development.

To Family and Friends ...

- Support the efforts of others to establish and maintain healthy lifestyles and respect the rights of friends and family.

To Clients ...

- Provide oral healthcare utilizing high levels of professional knowledge, judgment, and skill.
- Maintain a work environment that minimizes the risk of harm.
- Serve all clients without discrimination and avoid action toward any individual or group that may be interpreted as discriminatory.
- Hold professional client relationships confidential.
- Communicate with clients in a respectful manner.
- Promote ethical behavior and standards of care by all dental hygienists.
- Serve as an advocate for the welfare of clients.
- Provide clients with the information necessary to make informed decisions about their oral health and encourage their full participation in treatment decisions and goals.
- Refer clients to other healthcare providers when their needs are beyond our ability or scope of practice.
- Educate clients about high-quality oral healthcare.

To Colleagues ...

- Conduct professional activities and programs, and develop relationships in ways that are honest, responsible, and appropriately open and candid.
- Encourage a work environment that promotes individual professional growth and development.
- Collaborate with others to create a work environment that minimizes risk to the personal health and safety of our colleagues.
- Manage conflicts constructively.
- Support the efforts of other dental hygienists to communicate the dental hygiene philosophy of preventive oral care.
- Inform other healthcare professionals about the relationship between general and oral health.
- Promote human relationships that are mutually beneficial, including those with other healthcare professionals.

To Employees and Employers ...

- Conduct professional activities and programs, and develop relationships in ways that are honest, responsible, open, and candid.
- Manage conflicts constructively.
- Support the right of our employees and employers to work in an environment that promotes wellness.
- Respect the employment rights of our employers and employees.

To the Dental Hygiene Profession ...

- Participate in the development and advancement of our profession.
- Avoid conflicts of interest and declare them when they occur.
- Seek opportunities to increase public awareness and understanding of oral health practices.
- Act in ways that bring credit to our profession while demonstrating appropriate respect for colleagues in other professions.
- Contribute time, talent, and financial resources to support and promote our profession.
- Promote a positive image for our profession.
- Promote a framework for professional education that develops dental hygiene competencies to meet the oral and overall health needs of the public.

To the Community and Society ...

- Recognize and uphold the laws and regulations governing our profession.
- Document and report inappropriate, inadequate, or substandard care and/or illegal activities by any healthcare provider to the responsible authorities.
- Use peer review as a mechanism for identifying inappropriate, inadequate, or substandard care and for modifying and improving the care provided by dental hygienists.
- Comply with local, state, and federal statutes that promote public health and safety.
- Develop support systems and quality-assurance programs in the workplace to assist dental hygienists in providing the appropriate standard of care.
- Promote access to dental hygiene services for all, supporting justice and fairness in the distribution of healthcare resources.
- Act consistently with the ethics of the global scientific community of which our profession is a part.
- Create a healthful workplace ecosystem to support a healthy environment.
- Recognize and uphold our obligation to provide pro bono service.

To Scientific Investigation ...

- We accept responsibility for conducting research according to the fundamental principles underlying our ethical beliefs in compliance with universal codes, governmental standards, and professional guidelines for the care and management of experimental subjects. We acknowledge our ethical obligations to the scientific community:

- Conduct research that contributes knowledge that is valid and useful to our clients and society.
- Use research methods that meet accepted scientific standards.
- Use research resources appropriately.
- Systematically review and justify research in progress to ensure the most favorable benefit-to-risk ratio to research subjects.
- Submit all proposals involving human subjects to an appropriate human subject review committee.
- Secure appropriate institutional committee approval for the conduct of research involving animals.
- Obtain informed consent from human subjects participating in research that is based on specifications published in title 21 code of federal regulations part 46.
- Respect the confidentiality and privacy of data.
- Seek opportunities to advance dental hygiene knowledge through research by providing financial, human, and technical resources whenever possible.
- Report research results in a timely manner.
- Report research findings completely and honestly, drawing only those conclusions that are supported by the data presented.
- Report the names of investigators fairly and accurately.
- Interpret the research and the research of others accurately and objectively, drawing conclusions that are supported by the data presented and seeking clarity when uncertain.
- Critically evaluate research methods and results before applying new theory and technology in practice.
- Be knowledgeable concerning currently accepted preventive and therapeutic methods, products, and technology and their application to our practice.

THE CANADIAN DENTAL HYGIENISTS ASSOCIATION CODE OF ETHICS

"Dental hygienists believe that oral health is an integral part of a person's overall health, well-being, and quality of life."

Table of Contents

Dental hygienists believe that oral health is an integral part of a person's overall health, well-being, and quality of life. The profession of dental hygiene is devoted to promoting optimal oral health for all. Dental hygiene has an identified body of knowledge and a distinctive expertise which dental hygienists use to serve the needs of their clients and promote the public good.

The Code of Ethics sets down the ethical principles and ethical practice standards of the dental hygiene profession. The principles express the broad ideals to which dental hygienists aspire and which guide them in their practice. The standards provide more specific direction for conduct. They are more precise and prescriptive as to what a given principle requires under par-ticular circumstances. Clients, colleagues, and the public in general can reasonably expect dental hygienists to be guided by, and to be accountable under, the principles and standards articulated in this Code.

The purpose of the Code of Ethics is to
- Elaborate the ethical principles and standards by which dental hygienists are guided and under which they are accountable;
- Serve as a resource for education, reflection, self-evaluation, and peer review;
- Educate the public about the ethical principles and standards of the profession; and,
- Promote accountability.

The Code of Ethics is a public document that augments and complements the relevant laws and regulations under which dental hygienists practise. By elaborating on the profession's ethical principles and standards, the Code promotes accountability and worthiness of the public's trust.

The Code of Ethics applies to dental hygienists and dental hygiene students in all practice settings including, but not limited to, private practice, institutions, research, education, administration, community health, and industry.

Interpretation and application of the Code in specific circumstances requires individual judgment. Several aids are appended to the Code to assist in this.

Summary of the Main Principles in the Code

The fundamental principle underlying this Code is that the dental hygienist's primary responsibility is to the client, whether the client is an individual or a community.

Principle I: Beneficence

Beneficence involves caring about and acting to promote the good of another. Dental hygienists use their knowledge and skills to assist clients to achieve and maintain optimal oral health and to promote fair and reasonable access to quality oral health services.

Principle II: Autonomy

Autonomy pertains to the right to make one's own choices. By communicating relevant information openly and truthfully, dental hygienists assist clients to make informed choices and to participate actively in achieving and maintaining their optimal oral health.

Principle III: Privacy and Confidentiality

Privacy pertains to the individual's right to decide the conditions under which others will be permitted access to his or her personal life or information. Confidentiality is the duty to hold secret any information acquired in the professional relationship. Dental hygienists respect the privacy of clients and hold in confidence information disclosed to them, subject to certain narrowly defined exceptions.

Principle IV: Accountability

Accountability pertains to the acceptance of responsibility for one's actions and omissions in light of relevant principles, standards, laws, and regulations and the potential to self-evaluate and to be evaluated accordingly. Dental hygienists practise competently in conformity with relevant principles, standards, laws and regulations, and accept responsibility for their behaviour and decisions in the professional context.

Principle V: Professionalism

Professionalism is the commitment to use and advance professional knowledge and skills to serve the client and the public good. Dental hygienists express their professional commitment individually in their practice and communally through their professional associations and regulatory bodies.

Principle I: Beneficence

Beneficence involves caring about and acting to promote the good of another. Dental hygienists use their knowledge and skills to assist clients to achieve and maintain optimal oral health and to promote fair and reasonable access to quality oral health services.

Standards for Principle I
Dental hygienists:
1a. provide services to their clients in a caring and respectful manner, in recognition of the inherent dignity of human beings;
1b. provide services to their clients with respect for their individual needs and values and life circumstances;
1c. provide services fairly and without discrimination, in recognition of fundamental human rights;
1d. put the needs, values, and interests of their clients first and avoid exploiting their clients for personal gain;
1e. seek to improve the quality of care and advance knowledge in the field of oral health through such activities as quality assurance, research, education, and advocacy in the public arena.

Principle II: Autonomy

Autonomy pertains to the right to make one's own choices. By communicating relevant information openly and truthfully, dental hygienists assist clients to make informed choices and to participate actively in achieving and maintaining their optimal oral health.

Standards for Principle II
Dental hygienists:
2a. actively involve clients in their oral health care and promote informed choice by communicating relevant information openly, truthfully, and sensitively in recognition of the client's needs, values, and capacity to understand;
2b. in the case of clients who lack the capacity for informed choice, actively involve and promote informed choice on the part of the client's substitute decision-makers, involving the client to the extent of the client's capacity;
2c. honour the client's informed choices, including refusal of treatment, and regard informed choice as a precondition of treatment;
2d. do not rely upon coercion or manipulative tactics in assisting the client to make informed choices;
2e. recommend or provide only those services they believe are necessary for the client's oral health or as consistent with the client's informed choice.
   Note: Critical elements of informed choice include disclosure (i.e., revealing pertinent information, including risks and benefits); willingness (i.e., the choice is not coerced or manipulated); and capacity (i.e., the cognitive capacity to understand and process the relevant information).

"Informed choice" encompasses what is sometimes referred to as "informed consent."

Principle III: Privacy and Confidentiality

Privacy pertains to the individual's right to decide the conditions under which others will be permitted access to his or her personal life or information. Confidentiality is the duty to hold secret any information acquired in the professional relationship. Dental hygienists respect the privacy of clients and hold in confidence information disclosed to them, subject to certain narrowly defined exceptions.

Standards for Principle III
Dental hygienists:
3a. demonstrate regard for the privacy of their clients;
3b. hold confidential any information acquired in the professional relationship and do not use or disclose it to others without the client's express consent, except:
   3b.i as required by law
   3b.ii as required by the policy of the practice environment (e.g., quality assurance)
   3b.iii in an emergency situation
   3b.iv in cases where disclosure is necessary to prevent serious harm to others
   3b.v to the guardian or substitute decision-maker of a client in these cases, disclose to others only as much information as is necessary to accomplish the purpose for the disclosure;
3c. may infer the client's consent for disclosure to others directly involved in delivering and administering services to the client, provided there is no reason to believe the client would not give express consent if asked;
3d. obtain the client's express consent to use or share information about the client for the purpose of teaching or research;
3e. inform their clients in advance of treatment about how they will use or share their information, in particular about any uses or sharing that may occur without the client's express consent;
3f. promote practices, policies, and information systems that are designed to respect client privacy and confidentiality.

Principle IV: Accountability

Accountability pertains to the acceptance of responsibility for one's actions and omissions in light of relevant principles, standards, laws, and regulations and the potential to self-evaluate and to be evaluated accordingly. Dental hygienists practise competently in conformity with relevant principles, standards, laws and regulations, and accept responsibility for their behaviour and decisions in the professional context.

Standards for Principle IV
Dental hygienists:
4a. accept responsibility for knowing and acting consistently with the principles, standards, laws and regulations under which they are accountable;
4b. accept responsibility for providing safe, quality, competent care including, but not limited to, addressing issues in the practice environment within their capacity that may hinder or impede the provision of such care;
4c. take appropriate action to ensure first and foremost the client's safety and quality of care when they suspect unethical or incompetent care;
4d. practise within the bounds of their competence, scope of practice, personal and/or professional limitations, and refer clients requiring care outside these bounds;
4e. inform the dental hygiene regulatory body when an injury, dependency, infection, condition, or any other serious incapacity has immediately affected, or may affect over time, their continuing ability to practise safely and competently;
4f. promote workplace practices and policies that facilitate professional practice in accordance with the principles, standards, laws and regulations under which they are accountable.

Principle V: Professionalism

Professionalism is the commitment to use and advance professional knowledge and skills to serve the client and the public good. Dental hygienists express their professional commitment individually in their practice and communally through their professional associations and regulatory bodies.

Standards for Principle V
Dental hygienists:
5a. uphold the principles and standards of the profession before clients, colleagues, and others;
5b. maintain and advance their knowledge and skills in dental hygiene through continuing education and the quality of the care they provide through ongoing self-evaluation and quality assurance;
5c. advance general knowledge and skills in the field of oral health by supporting, participating in, or conducting ethically approved research;
5d. participate in professional activities such as meetings, committee work, peer review, and participation in public forums to promote oral health;

5e. participate in mentoring, education, and dissemination of knowledge and skills in oral health care;

5f. support the work of their professional associations and regulatory bodies to promote oral health and professional practice;

5g. inform potential employers about the principles, standards, laws and regulations to which they are accountable and determine whether employment conditions facilitate professional practice accordingly;

5h. collaborate with colleagues in a cooperative, constructive, and respectful manner toward the primary end of providing safe, competent, fair, quality care to clients;

5i. communicate the nature and costs of professional services fairly and accurately.

Appendix A: Ethical Challenges/Problems

No code of ethics can be expected to resolve definitively all ethical challenges or problems that may arise in practice. The analysis below is intended to help dental hygienists understand the nature of ethical challenges or problems and thereby better resolve them.

Ethical challenges or problems faced by practising dental hygienists tend to fall into the categories of ethical violations, ethical dilemmas, and ethical distress.

Ethical violations: when dental hygienists fail to meet or neglect their specific ethical responsibilities as expressed in the Code's standards. An example would be a dental hygienist who recommends unnecessary treatment in order to achieve personal gain at the expense of the client.

Ethical dilemmas: when one or more ethical principles conflict either with other ethical principle(s) or with self-interest(s) and no apparent course of action will satisfy both sides of the dilemma. An example would be a client with a hip prosthesis who may refuse to be pre-medicated prior to receiving invasive dental treatment. In this case, the principle of autonomy conflicts with the principle of beneficence.

Ethical distress: when dental hygienists experience constraints or limitations in relation to which they are or feel powerless and which compromise their ability to practise in full accordance with their professional principles or standards. An example would be a dental hygienist who is expected by the employer to complete dental hygiene treatment in a length of time insufficient to render quality care or to provide an acceptable level of infection control.

This Code is a useful guide in helping dental hygienists to identify, work through, and put into words ethical issues in light of their responsibilities as articulated in the Code's principles and standards, and to decide on an ethically responsible course of action. It is important to realize that some challenges or problems are perceived to be primarily ethical in nature when, in fact, they arise less from conflicting principles than from poor communication or lack of information. Reflecting on a perceived challenge or problem in light of the Code can help determine to what extent the problem or challenge is truly rooted in conflicting ethical principles, and to what extent it can be resolved by improved communication or by new information.

The Code provides clear direction for avoiding ethical violations. When a course of action is mandated by a standard in the Code or by a principle where there exists no opposing principle, ethical conduct requires that course of action.

In the case of ethical dilemmas and ethical distress, the Code cannot always provide a clear direction. The resolution of dilemmas often depends on the specific circumstances of the case in question. Total satisfaction by all parties involved may not be achieved. Resolution may also depend on which opposing ethical principle is considered to be more important, a matter on which reasonable people may disagree. Ethical distress often arises in situations where the dental hygienist is significantly limited by factors beyond his or her immediate control that may not be resolvable in the specific context.

In all cases, dental hygienists are accountable for how they conduct themselves in professional practice. Even in situations of ethical dilemma or distress where the Code does not prescribe a specific course of action, the hygienist can be expected to give account of his or her chosen action in light of the principles and standards expressed in the Code. Ultimately, dental hygienists must reconcile their actions with their consciences in caring for clients.

Appendix B: Reporting Suspected Incompetence or Unethical Conduct

The first consideration of the dental hygienist who suspects incompetence or unethical conduct in colleagues or associates is the welfare of present clients and/or potential harm to future clients. Adherence to the following guidelines could be helpful:

1. First, confirm the facts of the situation.
2. Ensure you are familiar with existing protocols in the practice setting for reporting incidents, incompetence, or unethical care and follow those protocols.
3. Document and report issues that cannot be resolved within the practice setting and report to the appropriate authority or regulatory body.

The dental hygienist who attempts to protect clients threatened by incompetent or unethical conduct should not be placed in jeopardy (e.g., loss of employment). Colleagues and professional organizations are morally obligated to support dental hygienists who fulfil their ethical obligations under the Code.

Appendix C: Decision—Procedure

Guidance Regarding the Process for Resolving Ethical Challenges

Ethical problems or challenges arise in a variety of contexts and require thoughtful analysis and careful judgment. The following guide may be useful to assist dental hygienists faced with an ethical challenge, recognizing that other stakeholders may need to be involved in resolving the matter. Talking with or getting advice from others at any step on the way to a decision can be very helpful.

1. Identify in a preliminary way the nature of the challenge or problem. What is the issue? What kind of issue is it? What ethical principles are at stake?
2. Become suitably informed and gather information (e.g., talk to others to find out the facts; research relevant policy statements) relevant to the challenge or problem, including:
   a. Factual information about the situation. What has happened? What is the sequence of events?
   b. Applicable policies, laws or regulations. Does a workplace policy address the issue? What does the Code say? What does law or regulation say?
   c. Who are the relevant stakeholders? How do they view the situation?
3. Clarify and elaborate the challenge or problem after getting this information. Now that you are better informed, What is the issue? What ethical principles are at stake? What stakeholders need to be consulted or involved in resolving the challenge or problem?
4. Identify various options for actions, recognizing that the best option may not be obvious at first and realizing it may require creativity or imagination.
5. Assess the various options in light of applicable policy, law or regulation, being as clear as possible in your mind of the pluses and minuses of each option as assessed in this light.
6. Decide on a course of action, mindful of how you would justify or defend your decision in light of the applicable policy, law or regulation, if you are called to account.
7. Implement your decision as thoughtfully and sensitively as possible, communicating a willingness to explain or justify the reasons for taking it.
8. Assess the consequences of your decision. Evaluate the process you used to arrive at the decision and the decision itself in light of those consequences. Did things turn out as you thought they would? Would you do the same thing again? What went wrong? Or, what went right?

In all of this, bear in mind that reasonable people can disagree about what is the right thing to do when faced with an ethical challenge or problem. If you cannot be certain whether you have made the right decision, you can at least have some assurance that you came to your decision in a responsible way. The test for this is whether you are able to defend your decision in light of relevant laws, principles, and regulations, and to defend the process by which you came to your decision. Reference to the above guidelines will help in this.

In addition, there is a very rich literature on ethics that can be very helpful for thinking through ethical challenges and problems in dental hygiene or for ongoing professional education and development.

Dental hygienists may also find it useful to familiarize themselves with various ethical theories, which tend to guide or orient ethical thinking along different lines. The main ethical theories current today are briefly described below:

- Deontology guides ethical thinking in terms of duties and rights, which the philosopher immanuel kant grounds in the fundamental imperative to act in relation to others according to principles that apply universally to all people, and that one would also wish for others to apply in their actions in relation to oneself.
- Utilitarianism guides ethical thinking in terms of harms and benefits, which the philosopher j.S. Mill grounds in the fundamental imperative to promote the greatest good for the greatest number.
- The ethic of care guides ethical thinking in terms of preserving and enhancing relationships and service to others. This theory derives from the work of carol gilligan, who found in her research that this style of ethical thinking tends to be more associated with females than with males.
- Virtue ethics guides ethical thinking in terms of habits of acting and assesses actions in terms of virtues and vices of character. This theory derives from the work of the philosopher aristotle, who emphasized that ethics cannot be reduced to rules or formulas and held that the person of good character (the "good man") is the ultimate standard of right and wrong and should be emulated by others as a role model.
- Feminist ethics guides ethical thinking in terms of sensitivity to the power or political dimension of human interaction. The philosopher susan sherwin grounds feminist ethics in the allegiance to those who are oppressed, vulnerable, or

disadvantaged and the imperative to improve their situation.

This is by no means a complete listing of ethical theories, nor is the richness of these theories captured in the condensed descriptions given. Moreover, considerable controversy exists not only among these theories but also among adherents of each theory.

REFERENCES

Canadian Dental Hygienists Association: *Dental Hygiene: Client's Bill of Rights*, Ottawa, October 2001, CDHA.

—: *Code of Ethics*, Ottawa, July 1997, CDHA.

College of Dental Hygienists of Ontario: *Code of Ethics*, Toronto, 1996, CDHO.

College of Dental Hygienists of British Columbia: *Code of Ethics*, Victoria, March 1, 1995, CDHBC.

Canadian Dental Association: *Code of Ethics*, Ottawa, August 1991, CDA.

American Dental Hygienists' Association: *Code of Ethics for Dental Hygienists*, Chicago, 1995, ADHA.

Canadian Dental Assistants Association: *CDAA Code of Ethics*, Ottawa, 2000, CDAA.

Canadian Medical Association: *Code of Ethics of the Canadian Medical Association*, Ottawa, 1997, CMA.

Canadian Nurses Association: *Code of Ethics for Registered Nurses*, Ottawa, March 1997, CNA.

Canadian Dental Hygienists Association
96 Centrepointe Drive
Ottawa, ON K2G 6B1
Telephone (613) 224-5515
1 800 267-5235
Fax (613) 224-7283
www.cdha.ca

INDEX

Note: Pages numbers followed by "b" indicate boxes; "f" figures; "t" tables.

root planing

1-2- All Ant   60-70°   Begin at JE

3-4- Ant premolers   Bal of Post

7-8 - Fal Post

9-10 Bal of molars

11-12 mFL

13-14 D

15-16 M

17-18 D